With more than 4 million of their bestselling *Counter* books in print, Annette Natow and Jo-Ann Heslin have provided their readers with the answers to all their questions about healthy eating, food shopping, and eating out.

Now the nutrition experts present this completely updated and revised second edition of their ultimate encyclopedia of food values, nutrition basics, healthy eating advice, and a comprehensive nutrition dictionary.

THE MOST COMPLETE FOOD COUNTER

- The MOST nutrient values—calories + 12 key nutrients
- The MOST food categories
- The MOST restaurant chains
- The MOST take-out items
- The MOST low carb, low fat, vegetarian, ethnic, and organic foods
- The MOST nutrition information at your fingertips, ready to use to help you make sense of the latest health information

Books by Annette B. Natow and Jo-Ann Heslin

The Calorie Counter (Third Edition)
The Carbohydrate, Sugar and Fiber Counter
The Cholesterol Counter (Sixth Edition)
The Complete Food Counter (Second Edition)
Eating Out Food Counter
The Fat Counter (Sixth Edition)
The Food Shopping Counter (Second Edition)
The Healthy Heart Food Counter
The Most Complete Food Counter
The Pocket Fat Counter (Second Edition)
The Pocket Protein Counter
The Protein Counter (Second Edition)
The Ultimate Carbohydrate Counter
The Vitamin and Mineral Food Counter

THE MOST COMPLETE FOOD COUNTER, 2ND EDITION

ANNETTE B. NATOW, PH.D.
JO-ANN HESLIN, M.A., R.D.
WITH THE ASSISTANCE OF
KAREN J. NOLAN, PH.D.

POCKET BOOKS
New York   London   Toronto   Sydney

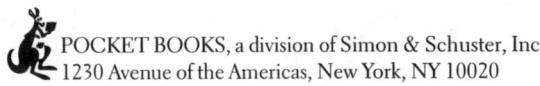 POCKET BOOKS, a division of Simon & Schuster, Inc.
1230 Avenue of the Americas, New York, NY 10020

Library of Congress Cataloging-in-Publication Data
Natow, Annette B.
   The most complete food counter / Annette B. Natow, Jo-Ann Heslin,
with the assistance of Karen J. Nolan. — 2nd ed.
      p.   cm.
   1. Food—Composition—Tables.   I. Heslin, Jo-Ann.   II. Nolan, Karen J.
III. Title.
TX551.N3964   2006
613.2'8—dc22   2005054619

ISBN-13: 978-0-7434-6441-3
ISBN-10:   0-7434-6441-9

First Pocket Books trade paperback printing of this revised edition January 2006

10 9 8 7 6 5 4 3 2 1

For information regarding special discounts for bulk purchases,
please contact Simon & Schuster Special Sales at
1-800-456-6798 or business@simonandschuster.com

To our families,
who support us through every project:
Harry, Allen, Irene, Sarah, Meryl, Laura,
Marty, George, Emily, Steven, Rebecca, Joseph,
Kristen, Brian, Karen, and John.

ACKNOWLEDGMENTS

For graciously sharing her knowledge, Karen J. Nolan, Ph.D.

For all her continuous support and help, our agent, Nancy Trichter.

For her suggestions and editing skills, Sara Clemence.

For his creative computer programming and technical support, Brian Robinson.

Without the tireless cooperation of Stephen Llano and the production department at Pocket Books, *The Most Complete Food Counter, 2nd Edition*, would never have been completed.

A special thank you to our editor, Micki Nuding.

CONTENTS

Introduction   1

Nutrition Basics   2
   Calories   2
   Fat   3
   Saturated Fat   4
   Cholesterol   4
   Protein   5
   Carbohydrates   6
   Sugar   7
   Fiber   8
   Calcium   8
   Sodium   9
   Potassium   10
   Folic Acid   11
   Vitamin C   11

Using *The Most Complete Food Counter*   13

Understanding the Dietary Guidelines   15

Just the Facts—A to Z   20

Definitions   44

Abbreviations   45

Notes   46

Part 1: Brand Name, Nonbranded (Generic), and Take-out Foods   47

Part 2: Restaurant Chains   691

"... foods, though so numerous and so varied in form, can be reduced to rather simple terms."

Mary Swartz Rose, Ph.D.
Feeding the Family
The Macmillan Company, 1919

INTRODUCTION

Listen to any group of people talking and the conversation almost always turns to food—what's the best choice for lunch, the current popular diet, or the latest health report. Everyone loves to talk about food. And everyone has questions about their health.

We wrote *The Most Complete Food Counter* to give you answers. It is the *most complete* food and nutrition resource available, listing nutrient values for more than 21,000 foods, along with information on how to get enough of, or how to limit, each nutrient. You'll find information on how to use the latest Dietary Guidelines for Americans. And if that isn't comprehensive enough, we've also sprinkled the book with **Smart Stuff** information boxes and included a dictionary that explains nutrition terms in simple language. Last night, the TV news mentioned something about trans fats. Not quite sure what that is? Go to page 40 and you'll learn everything you need to know about this type of fat and what it means to your health.

Let's talk about food—it's fun.
Let's talk about nutrition—it's important to your health.

NUTRITION BASICS

Calories, fat, saturated fat, cholesterol, protein, carbohydrate, sugar, fiber, calcium, sodium, potassium, folic acid and vitamin C—the list is long. Because your body is working all the time, even when you are sleeping, you need a source of calories and nutrients to keep you going. It's reassuring to know that you can get all of them from the foods you enjoy. Different foods have different assortments of nutrients. Some foods, like meat and cheese, are high in protein. Milk and yogurt have lots of calcium. Fruits and vegetables are good sources of vitamins and fiber. Eating a variety of foods ensures that you get all the calories and nutrients you need.

For some nutrients—protein, carbohydrate, fiber, calcium, potassium, folic acid, and vitamin C—the goal is to get enough each day for optimum health. For other nutrients—fat, saturated fat, cholesterol, sugar, and sodium—the goal is to limit the amount each day for optimum health. What about calories? Here the goal is simple: eat enough to keep your body running smoothly, but not so many that you gain weight. *The Most Complete Food Counter, 2nd Edition* will show you how to track all these important nutrients and help you determine your individual need for each one. We'll help you make the best choices.

Calories (cals)

Calories are calories, whether they come from apples or chocolate fudge. All foods except water have some. Every time you eat, you take in calories. Your body is a machine that uses food calories as fuel. When the amount of fuel you take in equals the amount of fuel you need for your body to run, your weight remains constant. Eat too many calories, and your body uses what it needs and stores the remainder for future use. You see the storage on your thighs, hips, and waist. Eat too few calories, and your body draws on its fuel reserves. Your thighs, hips, and waist get slimmer as the surplus is depleted.

Calories come from the fat, protein, and carbohydrate in foods. Fat has the most calories of the three—more than twice as many as protein and carbohydrate. One teaspoon of fat has 40 calories, while a teaspoon of either carbohydrates or protein has only 16 calories.

Over and over, studies have shown that if you cut calories, you lose weight. If you eat too many calories—even from healthy foods—you gain weight. It doesn't matter if those calories come from bread, meat, or salad dressing. The key to long-term weight control is to burn as many calories as you eat.

CALCULATING CALORIES

You need to know two things to figure out how many calories you need. First, how much do you want to weigh? Not your current weight, but your target weight. Second, you need to select an activity factor that fits your current activity level.

1. Your target weight is: _____
2. Your activity factor is: _____
   20 = Very active men
   15 = Moderately active men or very active women
   13 = Inactive men, moderately active women, and people over 55
   10 = Inactive women, repeat dieters, and seriously overweight people
3. Target weight × activity factor = calories needed each day

For example, if your target weight is 130 pounds and you are a moderately active woman (factor 13) you need between 1,600 and 1,700 calories a day:

$$130 \text{ pounds} \times 13 \text{ (activity factor)} = 1690 \text{ calories a day}$$

Fat (fat)

Fat has a bad reputation that is undeserved. It's important in the body: providing energy, supplying essential fatty acids that the body cannot make, insulating the body and protecting vital organs, carrying fat soluble vitamins, and becoming part of cell membranes. Just as important, fat makes food taste good.

Fats (or *lipids*, as scientists refer to them) is actually an umbrella term for several similar substances. You get fat from the foods you eat, and your body can also make some fats. Food fats are made up of strands of *fatty acids*. You can think of these fatty acids as strands of beads that vary in combination and number of beads, depending on their chemical composition.

There are three main types of fatty acids—saturated, monounsaturated, and polyunsaturated. Foods contain combinations of all three, but we label foods as sources of saturated (butter), monounsaturated (olive oil), or polyunsaturated (corn oil), based on the predominant fat in the food. Recent research suggests that the *type* of fat you eat may be more important than the *amount* of fat you eat.

HOW MUCH FAT SHOULD YOU EAT?

Experts recommend that your daily fat intake should make up 20 to 35% of your total calories. This means that if you regularly eat 1,800 calories a day, somewhere between 360 (20%) and 630 (35%) calories should come from fat:

$$20\% \times 1{,}800 \text{ calories} = 360 \text{ fat calories a day}$$
$$35\% \times 1{,}800 \text{ calories} = 630 \text{ fat calories a day}$$

To convert fat calories into grams of fat, all you need to know is that 1 gram of fat equals 9 calories. Using the example of 1,800 calories, the grams of fat each day would range from 40 to 70:

$$360 \text{ fat calories } (20\%) \div 9 = 40 \text{ grams of fat}$$
$$630 \text{ fat calories } (35\%) \div 9 = 70 \text{ grams of fat}$$

But we need to set the record straight. Even though the current research suggests that a moderate fat intake may be healthy, no one is suggesting a *high* fat intake is good for you.

Smart Stuff

A recent study found that dieters who were given 35% of their daily calories as fat found it easier to stick with their weight-loss plan and kept their weight off longer.

Saturated Fat (sat fat)

Many experts feel saturated fats are dietary villains because they contribute to raising your blood cholesterol levels. They are found mainly in animal foods—meats, whole milk, and cheese—and also in tropical oils, such as palm and coconut. You can't eliminate all saturated fats from your diet, and you really don't have to, but it is important to limit them. That's easy when it comes to milk, cream, sour cream, and cheese—simply choose the nonfat or lower fat versions. When it comes to meat, choose leaner cuts and smaller portions.

HOW MUCH SATURATED FAT SHOULD YOU EAT?

No specific recommendation has been made for saturated fat; you are simply advised to keep your intake as low as possible. You're probably asking, "How low is low?" The National Cholesterol Education Program has recommended that 7% of daily calories come from saturated fat. Other groups have suggested 10% or less. Using common sense, and knowing that we currently eat between 12 and 14% of our daily calories as saturated fat, anything less than 10% would be a significant reduction and provide you with health benefits.

Using the example above, if you eat 1,800 calories a day:

$$7\% \text{ saturated fat} \times 1{,}800 \text{ calories} = 126 \text{ calories of saturated fat a day}$$

$$126 \div 9 = 14 \text{ grams saturated fat daily}$$

$$10\% \text{ saturated fat} \times 1{,}800 \text{ calories} = 180 \text{ calories of saturated fat daily}$$

$$180 \div 9 = 20 \text{ grams of saturated fat daily}$$

Smart Stuff

When you eat less total fat, you automatically eat less saturated fat.

Cholesterol (chol)

Cholesterol is a white, waxy, fat-like substance found in every cell in your body. It insulates nerve cells and helps skin cells retain moisture. Cholesterol makes up a major part of your brain. It's the main building block from which vitamin D and essential hormones such as cortisone, estrogen, and testosterone are made. But having too much cholesterol in your blood is unhealthy. The extra can be deposited on your artery walls, narrowing them and interfering with normal blood flow.

You get cholesterol every time you eat animal foods—meat, poultry, fish, eggs, milk, yogurt, cheese, or butter. There is no cholesterol in foods that grow in the ground—vegetables, fruits, nuts, seeds, cereals, and grains have none. Cholesterol can also be made in the body. In fact, most people make 3 times more cholesterol than they eat in food.

Smart Stuff

It's simple. If a food grows in the ground, it has no cholesterol. If a food has a face, it has cholesterol.

HOW MUCH CHOLESTEROL SHOULD YOU EAT EACH DAY?

On average, American men eat about 330 milligrams of cholesterol a day; women eat about 240 milligrams. The federal government's National Cholesterol Education Program recommends no more than 200 milligrams of cholesterol a day. The American Heart Association (AHA) recommends that you limit cholesterol to less than 300 milligrams a day, 200 milligrams if you already have heart disease.

Your daily cholesterol intake should be based on the results of your latest blood test. If your total cholesterol and LDL levels are within the desirable range, limit your cholesterol to less than 300 milligrams a day. If your numbers are up, reduce your daily intake to 200 milligrams a day.

Protein (prot)

Your body loses millions of cells each day. They are used up, worn out, rubbed off, and even cut off, like your beard or fingernails. You need a source of protein to replace these lost cells.

Protein is found in every cell, tissue, and substance in your body, except for urine and bile. Bones, teeth, muscles, enzymes, skin, and blood all contain protein. Active tissues such as muscles and glands are high in protein, while less active tissues, such as fat, have less.

Protein is made up of small building blocks called *amino acids*. There are 20 amino acids that the body uses to build different proteins, just like the letters in the alphabet are used to make different words. Of the 20 different amino acids found in food, 9 are *essential. These 9 must be obtained directly from the food you eat.* The remaining 11 can be made in the body. When you eat different foods, you get varying amounts of protein and varying amounts of the different amino acids. That is one of the reasons it's important to eat a variety of foods. Almost all foods you eat contain protein—some more, some less. Fruits have very little protein compared to meat, milk, cheese, beans, grains, and vegetables, all of which have more.

When your body is stressed physically or mentally, protein is lost. When it's too hot or too cold, you need extra protein. Protein is needed to replace nitrogen lost during heavy sweating. Exercise, fever, surgery, injury, infection, and broken bones all increase your need for protein. Even emotional stress, such as losing your job or taking an exam, causes protein loss.

CALCULATING YOUR DAILY PROTEIN NEED

A quick way to estimate your daily protein need is to divide your weight by 2.2. For example, if you weigh 150 pounds, you should be eating 68 grams of protein a day:

150 pounds ÷ 2.2 = 68 grams of protein

Most people eat more than their recommended level of protein daily.

Smart Stuff

The top 10 sources of protein eaten in the U.S. are beef, poultry, milk, yeast bread, cheese, fish, eggs, fresh pork, ham, and pasta.

Carbohydrates (carb)

Carbohydrates include sugars, starches, and fibers found in foods. All plant foods—fruits, vegetables, beans, and grains—are rich in carbohydrates. Fruits have more sugar. Vegetables, beans, and grains have more starch. Both have some fiber.

Sugars and starches are your body's main source of energy, or calories. When the food you eat is digested, sugar molecules move easily into the bloodstream and travel to cells. There they are burned for needed energy to keep your body working. Starch molecules are more complex. They are made up of many sugar molecules bound together. During digestion, these larger starch molecules are slowly broken apart to yield smaller sugar fragments, which are sent to the cells to be converted into energy. If you eat more carbohydrate calories than your body needs for energy, the leftover is stored as fat.

Smart Stuff

Simple carbohydrates are foods that contain a lot of sugar: syrups, jelly, honey, soda, and molasses. Complex carbohydrates are foods that contain a lot of starch: whole grains, cereals, beans, vegetables. These foods are also rich in vitamins, minerals, and fiber.

COUNTING CARBS

Not too long ago, you were told to eat all the carbohydrates you wanted. In fact, most Americans get 50% or more of their daily calories as carb. Today, however, carbs are being blamed for many of our health concerns, especially obesity. So how much carb should you be eating?

The National Academy of Sciences' Recommended Dietary Allowance (RDA) for carbohydrate is 130 grams a day. The Food and Drug Administration (FDA) has set 300 grams of carb as the Daily Value (DV), or the amount needed by the "typical" American consumer.

You can estimate your individual carb intake by first deciding what amount of carbs you want to eat each day. Most food professionals consider a diet where 40% or less of your daily calories come from carbohydrates to be a low carb diet.

Let's use 40% carbohydrate as an example. If you eat 1,800 calories a day:

40% × 1,800 calories = 720 carb calories

To figure out how many grams of carbs to eat each day, you need to know that 1 gram of carb equals 4 calories. Continuing to use the example above:

720 carb calories per day ÷ 4 = 180 grams of carb

These values more than meet the RDA recommendation of at least 130 grams of carbohydrate a day. To make good carb choices, choose more foods that are higher in starch and fiber, and choose fewer foods that are higher in sugar.

Sugar (sugar)

Most of us enjoy sweets. Anthropologists believe that our ability to taste the difference between sweet plants and bitter plants may have helped humans to evolve, since sweet plants are more often edible and bitter ones poisonous.

Today, however, our passion for sweets is creating an epidemic of obesity. Clearly, we are letting sugary foods crowd out more nutritious choices. We drink more soda than milk in this country, and buy far more sugared drinks than fruit juice.

Cereals, grains, fruits, vegetables, milk, and plain yogurt all contain sugars. These are *natural* sugar choices, and the sweet foods come packaged with vitamins, minerals, and fiber. Soda, candy, fruit drinks, cakes, cookies, ice cream, jelly, and syrup, in contrast, offer little more than sweetness and calories, and are loaded with *added sugar*.

HOW MUCH SUGAR IS TOO MUCH?

Americans currently eat 15 to 21% of their daily calories as sugar, with teenagers eating the most. Studies have shown over and over that as sugar intake goes up, vitamin and mineral intake goes down. We should all be eating less sugar, but there is no specific recommendation on how much to eat every day. The U.S. Dietary Reference Intakes (DRIs) suggests 25% of daily calories from added sugar as the maximum. Obviously, people should eat less. The World Health Organization (WHO) has suggested limiting added sugars to no more than 10% of total calories, although some experts feel this amount is unrealistically low.

Without clear-cut recommendations, you need to decide for yourself how much sugar to eat. We suggest attempting to eat closer to the WHO recommendation of 10% total calories as sugar, keeping in mind the 25% recommendation as the healthy upper limit.

If you eat 1,800 calories a day:

10% of 1,800 calories = 180 sugar calories per day

—OR—

25% of 1,800 calories = 450 sugar calories per day

To figure out how many grams of sugar to eat each day, you need to know that 1 gram of sugar equals 4 calories. Continuing to use the example above:

180 (10%) sugar calories per day ÷ 4 =
45 grams of sugar per day

—OR—

450 (25%) sugar calories per day ÷ 4 =
113 grams of sugar per day

To make good sugar choices, choose foods with naturally containing sugars more often, and choose foods with added sugars less often.

Fiber (fiber)

Fiber is a type of carbohydrate that your body doesn't digest and that provides no calories. But it is important. Fiber found in the foods you eat aids in losing weight, helps to manage diabetes, relieves constipation, and protects against colon cancer. It may even lower your risk for heart disease.

Add foods rich in fiber to your diet slowly — beans, berries, bran, fruits, oatmeal, vegetables, popcorn, and whole grains. Don't go overboard, because it takes your body a little time to adjust to the extra bulk passing through your digestive tract. And, drink plenty of fluids. Fiber soaks up fluids like a sponge. The swollen carbs not only help you feel fuller longer but also help form soft, easily passed stools.

HOW MUCH FIBER SHOULD YOU EAT?

Most of us eat too little. We average about 15 grams of fiber a day, far less than we should be eating. Experts recommend the following amounts of fiber daily:

Men

| 19–50 years old | 38 grams of fiber |
| 50 and older | 30 grams of fiber |

Women

19–50 years old	25 grams of fiber
50 and older	21 grams of fiber
Pregnant	28 grams of fiber

Calcium (calci)

We've all heard that calcium builds strong teeth and bones, and protects us against *osteoporosis* (adult bone thinning), but it does much more than that.

Calcium:
- helps blood clot
- helps nerves work normally
- helps muscles work and the heart beat
- helps lower high blood pressure
- aids in weight loss
- helps prevent mid-life weight gain in women

- relieves PMS (premenstrual syndrome)
- protects against complications in pregnancy
- lowers the risk for some cancers
- may help increase HDL (good) cholesterol in postmenopausal women
- lowers the risk for periodontal disease, a leading cause of tooth loss
- protects against infertility
- reduces the risk for kidney stones

Calcium may even influence behavior. A study with rats showed that they became frantic on a low-calcium diet but calmed down when they were fed adequate amounts.

Smart Stuff

Depending on your size and weight, your body may contain up to 3 pounds of calcium, more than any other mineral.

Over half of the calcium in the American diet comes from dairy products: milk, cheese, yogurt, and ice cream. A glass of nonfat milk provides more than one third of your calcium for the day. Calcium-fortified soy milk is the best nondairy source. Other good sources are canned sardines and salmon with bones, oysters, clams, tofu, molasses, almonds, calcium-fortified foods, beans, and dark green leafy vegetables such as Chinese cabbage, kale, and mustard and turnip greens. And as much as 25% of your daily calcium can come from mineral-rich bottled waters!

HOW MUCH CALCIUM DO YOU NEED EACH DAY?

The Dietary Reference Intakes (DRIs) for calcium for adults are:

1,000 milligrams	19 to 50 years old
1,200 milligrams	51 and older

There is no need for additional calcium during pregnancy and breastfeeding. Growing children between the ages of 9 and 18 should be getting slightly more—1,300 milligrams—to help them form strong bones.

Sodium (sod)

Sodium regulates your body's fluid level both outside and inside cells. This monitors your blood volume, blood pressure, and the acidity of your body. The movement of sodium into and out of cells allows other important substances to make this journey, too, helping to transmit nerve impulses and electrical messages that are vital to your body's minute-by-minute functioning.

Most people associate an excess of sodium with high blood pressure. This assumption has been proven by studies done throughout the world. In places where little salt is used, blood pressure docs not go up with age as it does in the United States. Reducing sodium can lower blood pressure in people with high blood pressure, and to a lesser extent in people who have normal blood pressure. About 10 to 15% of all people with high blood pressure are very sensitive to salt. If they reduce the amount of salt they eat, their blood pressure goes down. People who are not salt-sensitive will not get the same dramatic results, but their blood pressure does go down. It's wise to eat less salt, because keeping your blood pressure values within normal range reduces your risk for heart attacks, strokes, and kidney disease.

When people are told to eat less sodium, their first reaction is to stop salting their food. This may not be the the most effective approach, because most of your total daily salt and sodium intake actually comes from:

Salt added and **sodium**-containing
   additives used in food processing   77%
Sodium naturally occurring in food   12%
Salt added in cooking or at the table   11%

HOW MUCH SODIUM SHOULD YOU EAT EACH DAY?

Most of us eat 2,300 to 4,700 milligrams of sodium a day. Experts recommend 1,500 milligrams for adults, with less for older adults, and many believe that healthy adults could do nicely on as few as 500 milligrams of sodium a day.

Experts recommend the following sodium intakes for adults:

1,500 milligrams	19 to 50 year olds
1,300 milligrams	50 to 70 year olds
1,200 milligrams	those over age 70

Smart Stuff

Salt or Sodium?

Table salt is actually a mixture of two minerals: sodium and chloride. In a teaspoon of salt (which equals 5,000 milligrams), 2,000 milligrams are sodium and 3,000 are chloride.

Sodium without chloride is found in MSG (monosodium glutamate), food additives (sodium benzoate, sodium propionate), artificial sweeteners (sodium saccharin), medications (sodium citrate), and naturally in water as the mineral (sodium).

Potassium (potas)

The third most abundant mineral in your body, potassium is found inside every cell. It's important to the firing of nerves and working of muscles. Potassium allows the heart muscle to relax—the opposite action of calcium, which makes it contract. Potassium also helps to regulate high blood pressure. People with high blood pressure who increase their intake of potassium-rich fruits and vegetables usually see their blood pressure come down.

Smart Stuff

More Fruits and Vegetables = Strong Bones

If you want stronger bones, eat potassium-rich fruits and vegetables. As fruit and vegetable intake goes up, bones get stronger. Experts believe that high potassium levels encourage your body to hang on to calcium instead of excreting it—the net result, stronger bones.

HOW MUCH POTASSIUM DO YOU NEED EACH DAY?

Potassium is so abundant in food that no Dietary Reference Intake (DRI) has been set. Experts have set an adult daily minimum requirement of 1,600 to 2,000 milligrams a day. A healthy diet supplies 2,000 to 4,000 milligrams daily. Most people get enough of this mineral every day.

Folic Acid (folic)

Everyone needs the vitamin folic acid to insure that new cells reproduce and develop correctly. Folic acid is involved in making the cell's genetic material and in the production of protein and red blood cells. When you don't have enough folic acid available, red blood cells develop abnormally and have a very short life span.

Because folic acid helps to make the genetic material of every cell, it's essential to support the healthy growth of an unborn child. Pregnant women who take in too little folic acid have a higher risk for miscarriage and birth defects involving the spinal cord and brain. These organs begin to develop very soon after conception, even before you are aware that you are pregnant. Research has also shown that men who have low intakes of folic acid have lower sperm counts and more fragile sperm. So when it comes to a healthy pregnancy, adequate folic acid levels are important for both parents.

In addition to aiding fertility and preventing birth defects, folic acid protects you against heart disease by reducing blood levels of a protein, homocysteine, which is believed to be a risk factor.

Food sources of folic acid are green leafy vegetables, orange juice, dried beans, liver, asparagus, broccoli, strawberries, wheat germ, and peanuts. Fortified sources are enriched bread, pasta, flour, breakfast cereal, and rice.

Smart Stuff

Cooking can destroy 50 to 90% of the folic acid in food. Experts recommend eating folate-rich foods uncooked or cooking them quickly by steaming, stir-frying, or microwaving in small amounts of water.

HOW MUCH FOLIC ACID DO YOU NEED EACH DAY?

The Dietary Reference Intakes (DRIs) for folic acid are:

400 micrograms	Men 14 and older
400 micrograms	Women 14 and older
600 micrograms	Pregnant women
500 micrograms	Breastfeeding women

Scientists estimate that 10% of Americans are folate deficient. Others are not deficient but their normal intake is below the desirable level. Based on this evidence, fortification of bread, cereal, pasta, flour, and rice was begun in 1998. Since the fortification program started, it's estimated that the average American is getting 200 micrograms more folic acid each day, but most still fall short of the daily recommendation.

Vitamin C (vit C)

Lack of vitamin C was the major downfall of early ocean explorers. At sea for months at a time, with no source of fresh fruits or vegetables, many sailors developed and died from scurvy. Vitamin C plays a critical role in the formation of collagen, the connective tissue that holds together the structures of the body. Collagen is found in most of the tissues throughout your body, especially in the heart, brain, pancreas, adrenal glands, thymus, lungs, pituitary gland, and lens of the eyes. The sailors suffered from bleeding gums and aching joints because they were unable to make collagen.

Vitamin C is also an antioxidant. Antioxidants are substances that protect healthy cells against harmful substances called *free radicals*. Antioxidants scoop up free radicals and prevent them from causing damage to cells that could lead to heart disease and cancer. Free radicals result from smoking, air pollution, and sun exposure, and are by-products of normal body functions.

Vitamin C also protects other nutrients such as vitamin E, folic acid, and iron, so they can work effectively in the body.

Excellent food sources of vitamin C are citrus fruits, potatoes, broccoli, strawberries, kiwi, cabbage, spinach and other leafy greens, cantaloupe, green peppers, and vitamin-fortified juices.

Smokers need more vitamin C because smoking depletes the body's stores by promoting more free radicals. Smokers are encouraged to get an extra 35 milligrams each day.

Smart Stuff

An estimated one quarter of the world's adults eat chile peppers every day. By weight, chile peppers are one of the richest sources of vitamin C.

HOW MUCH VITAMIN C DO YOU NEED EACH DAY?

The Dietary Reference Intakes (DRIs) for vitamin C are:

90 milligrams	Men 19 and older
125 milligrams	Men who smoke
75 milligrams	Women 19 and older
110 milligrams	Women who smoke
85 milligrams	Pregnant women
120 milligrams	Breastfeeding women

USING *THE MOST COMPLETE FOOD COUNTER*

The Most Complete Food Counter, 2nd Edition lists the calories, fat, saturated fat, cholesterol, protein, carbohydrate, sugar, fiber, calcium, sodium, potassium, vitamin C, and folic acid in more than 21,000 foods. These are key nutrients for you to consider when you are choosing foods. Fat, saturated fat, cholesterol, sugar, and sodium are nutrients you may want to limit. You can be more liberal with the others, aiming for moderate amounts of calories, protein, and carbohydrates, and higher amounts of the rest. Recommended intakes for all nutrients listed have been described in the chapter called Nutrition Basics. There are still other nutrients needed for good health, but when you eat a variety of foods containing the nutrients listed in this counter, you will get the other necessary nutrients along with them.

Now you can compare the values in your favorite foods and, when necessary, choose substitutes before you go out to shop or eat. This will save you time and help you decide what to buy.

The counter section of the book is divided into two parts: Part 1: Brand-Name, Non-branded (Generic), and Take-out Foods; and Part 2: Restaurant Chains. Each part lists foods or restaurant chains alphabetically.

In Part 1, for each category, you will find non-branded (generic) foods listed first, in alphabetical order, followed by an alphabetical listing of brand name foods. The nonbranded listings will help you estimate calorie values when you don't see your favorite. They can also help you to evaluate store brands. Large categories are divided into subcategories, such as canned, fresh, frozen, and ready-to-eat, to make it easier to find what you're looking for. Some categories have "see" and "see also" notes, to help you find related items.

Because people eat out so often, we listed more than 500 take-out foods in Part 1. These are found in the take-out subcategory in many categories throughout this section. Look there for foods you take out or order in, because these foods are not nutrition labeled.

Most foods are listed alphabetically, but in some cases foods are grouped by category. For example, a tuna sandwich is found in the Sandwich category. Other group categories include:

ASIAN FOOD   Page 55
     includes all types of Asian foods
     except egg rolls and sushi, which
     are found in separate categories

DELI MEATS/COLD CUTS   Page 290
     includes all sandwich meats
     except chicken, ham, and turkey,
     which are found in separate
     categories

DINNER   Page 294

    includes all by brand name, except
    pasta dinners, which are found in
    a separate category

LIQUOR/LIQUEUR   Page 424

    includes all alcoholic beverages
    and mixed drinks except beer,
    champagne, and wine, which
    are found in separate categories

NUTRITION SUPPLEMENTS   Page 454

    includes all dieting aids, meal
    replacements, and drinks, except
    energy bars and energy drinks,
    which are found in separate
    categories

SANDWICHES   Page 565

    includes popular sandwich
    choices

SNACKS   Page 581

    includes a variety of miscellaneous
    snack items such as trail mix, pork
    rinds, and cheese puffs

SPANISH FOOD   Page 622

    includes all types of Spanish and
    Mexican foods except salsa and
    tortillas, which are found in
    separate categories

In Part 2: Restaurant Chains, 107 national and regional restaurants are listed, including candy, coffee, doughnut, ice cream, pizza, burger, seafood, sandwich, and ethnic food chains. Brand-name foods are required by federal law to have nutrition information on labels. Restaurants, however, provide this information voluntarily.

With *The Most Complete Food Counter, 2nd Edition* as your guide, you have at your fingertips the most comprehensive guide to the calories and important nutrients in the foods you eat.

UNDERSTANDING THE DIETARY GUIDELINES

In a nutshell, the Dietary Guidelines for Americans *encourage you to eat fewer calories, be more active, and make wiser food choices.*

Initiated in 1980 by the U.S. Department of Agriculture (USDA) and the Department of Health and Human Services (DHHS), the guidelines are intended primarily for policymakers. They are designed to promote an optimal eating plan, to prevent diseases, and to set standards for federal programs like the National School Lunch Program. The guidelines allow all government agencies and policymakers to share a common approach when it comes to health and nutrition messages given to Americans.

By law, every 5 years, the USDA and DHHS must appoint a committee of experts to review all new scientific information and revise the guidelines. The experts also translate this science-based information into recommendations for average people. Following these recommendations will help reduce your risk for obesity and chronic diseases such as heart disease, diabetes, hypertension, osteoporosis, and cancer.

The 2005 Dietary Guidelines are the sixth and most complex revision, and include the following health messages.

- **Balance your need for important nutrients with your daily calorie need.**

If you limit foods high in sugars, fats, and alcohol, this will free up calories for wiser food choices. Calorie intake remains the same, but food choices improve.

Meeting your daily nutrient needs has to go hand in hand with keeping your total calorie intake under control, so that your weight remains stable.

Smart Stuff

Discretionary what?

Discretionary calories is a new concept with the current guidelines. Once you've eaten enough nutrient-rich foods to meet your daily needs, you can use leftover calories to splurge on foods that add to the pleasure of eating but have few, if any, nutrients, such as sugar, soda, chips, salad dressing, candy, cake, and butter. For most people, 200 to 300 discretionary calories are the most you can count on.

- **Balance food intake and physical activity to manage body weight.**

The energy you use each day should equal the energy (calories) you eat, so that you stay at the same weight.

An important key to weight loss is to eat fewer calories each day while increasing your physical activity.

- **Be physically active every day**

  Regular exercise improves your health and sense of well-being, and helps to maintain your weight.

  The rates of all causes of death are lower in physically active people.

  Exercise lowers your risk for obesity, heart disease, hypertension, type 2 diabetes, osteoporosis, and some cancers.

  Exercise helps to manage depression and anxiety.

  You should try to be physically active at least 30 minutes most days of the week.

  To control your weight and get additional health benefits, aim for 60 to 90 minutes of physical activity daily.

  Children and teens should be physically active 60 minutes or more every day.

  Varying your type of exercise—aerobic, stretching, strength training—will help you achieve maximum physical fitness.

  Short periods of exercise add up. Try to do several 10-minute exercise sessions during the day—taking a short walk, weeding the garden, washing a floor—to reach your daily goal of 30 to 90 minutes.

Smart Stuff

According to the Advisory Committee for the Dietary Guidelines, most Americans don't eat enough of the following important nutrients. Here are some expected and unexpected sources.

__Vitamin A__—liver, carrots, sweet potatoes, spinach, mango, cantaloupe, collards, romaine lettuce, broccoli, tomato juice, watermelon, prunes, and turnips

__Vitamin C__—orange juice, strawberries, brussels sprouts, cantaloupe, mango, cauliflower, watermelon, spinach, pineapple, blueberries, cabbage, and potatoes

__Vitamin E__—wheat germ oil, sunflower seeds, almonds, wheat bran cereal, cottonseed oil, safflower oil, hazelnuts, strawberries, peanuts, and margarine

__Calcium__—milk, calcium-processed tofu, yogurt, cheese, sesame seeds, sardines, soybeans, spinach, canned salmon with bones, and blackeyed peas

__Potassium__—orange juice, tomato juice, banana, sweet potatoes, beans, strawberries, clams, lima beans, halibut, soybeans, potatoes, and baked beans

__Magnesium__—sesame seeds, halibut, almonds, oysters, pumpkin seeds, spinach, cashews, black beans, brown rice, peanut butter, and yogurt

__Fiber__—whole-wheat bread, bran cereal, brown rice, fruit with skin, dried fruit, carrots, beans, lentils, split peas, strawberries, green beans, and popcorn

- **Eat a variety of nutrient-rich foods each day.**

  Eat more whole fruits rather than drinking fruit juices.

  Eat more dark green vegetables, such as broccoli, and orange vegetables, such as carrots and sweet potatoes.

  Eat more peas and beans.

  Have at least 3 servings of fat free milk, yogurt, and low fat cheese each day.

  Scientific evidence shows that the calcium in dairy products protects you from osteoporosis and colon cancer.

Make whole grains half of your cereal, bread, cracker, and pasta choices.

Eat lean protein choices.

Scientific evidence suggests that eating 2 servings of fish a week may reduce your risk of heart disease.

Use some nonmeat protein sources such as tofu, beans, and nuts.

Smart Stuff

It won't be easy, but do your best.

The Dietary Guidelines recommend 5 to 13 servings (2½ to 6½ cups) of fruits and vegetables a day, depending on your daily calorie need (1,200 to 3,200). The average American currently eats only 3 servings, which equal 1½ cups. But studies have shown that you get positive health benefits when you add 1 to 2 servings (½ to 1 cup) a day. Small changes do count.

- **Choose fats wisely.**

  Select a daily total fat intake that equals 20 to 35% of your total calories.

  Keep your intake of saturated fat and cholesterol low by limiting the amount of animal fats—cheese, butter, ice cream, fatty meat, bacon, sausage, and poultry skin—you eat.

  Limit your saturated fat intake to 10% or less of your total daily calories.

  Use more polyunsaturated fats (soybean oil, corn oil, and safflower oil) instead of saturated fats.

  Use more monounsaturated fats (canola oil, olive oil, and sunflower oil) instead of saturated fats.

  Limit your cholesterol intake to 300 milligrams or less each day.

Keep your intake of trans fats low by limiting the amount of food you eat containing hydrogenated vegetables oils.

REDUCING SATURATED FAT

Eat This	Instead of This	Grams of Sat Fat Saved
Low-fat Cheddar cheese	Regular Cheddar cheese	4
Skim milk	Whole milk	4.5
Low-fat frozen yogurt	Regular ice cream	6
Bran bagel	Croissant	6.5
Safflower oil	Lard	4
Soft margarine	Butter	5
Extra-lean ground beef	Regular ground beef	4.6
Roasted chicken breast	Fried chicken leg	2.5
Baked fish	Fried fish	2
Sliced roast beef	Bologna	7.5

Smart Stuff

Less Is Best

The major sources of trans fat are cookies, crackers, cakes, pastries, shortening, stick margarine, deep-fried foods (french fries, doughnuts), partially hydrogenated oil, and hydrogenated vegetable oils. Trans fat raises cholesterol, lowers HDL (good) cholesterol, raises LDL (bad) cholesterol, and increases your risk for heart disease.

- **Choose carbohydrates wisely.**

  Carbohydrates—sugars, starches, and fiber—are important in a healthy diet.

  Fruits, vegetables, beans, grains, and milk are the major sources of carbohydrates in your diet.

  Carbohydrates are the major source of calories in most diets.

  One strategy to control weight and to eat more nutrient-rich foods is to limit your intake of foods and beverages high in added sugar.

  Eat fiber-rich fruits, vegetables, and whole grains daily.

  Eat fiber-rich peas and beans several times a week.

  Make more whole grain choices—whole wheat, oatmeal, popcorn, bulgur, and brown rice.

  Try to eat at least 3 whole grain servings a day.

  Research continues to show that whole grains reduce your risk for heart disease and diabetes.

Smart Stuff

Oh, So Sweet

The major sources of added sugar in your diet are soda, candy, cakes, cookies, pies, sweetened fruit drinks, ice cream, sweetened yogurt, flavored milk, and sweetened cereal and breads. Choose them less often and eat smaller portions.

- **Eat less salt and more potassium.**

  Reducing the amount of salt you eat reduces your risk for high blood pressure.

  Eating potassium-rich fruits and vegetables helps control high blood pressure and supports healthy bones.

  People with normal blood pressure readings have a lower risk for heart disease, stroke, congestive heart failure, and kidney disease.

  Processed foods (canned, frozen, and mixes) and restaurant choices are higher in salt than those prepared at home.

  Bananas, tomato juice, orange juice, lima beans, spinach, cantaloupe, potatoes, and apricots are rich sources of potassium.

- **If you drink alcohol, do it in moderation.**

  Moderate intake is defined as 1 drink a day for women and 2 for men.

  Studies suggest that 1 to 2 drinks a day lowers the risk for heart disease for middle-aged and older adults. Younger adults get little, if any, health benefit from alcohol.

  Alcohol should be avoided by women who are trying to get pregnant, are pregnant, or are breastfeeding.

  Heavy drinking increases the risk of liver disease, hypertension, cancers of the GI tract, injury, and death.

  Alcohol contains calories but few, if any, nutrients.

  If you take medications, check with your doctor since many interact with alcohol.

  If you drink moderately, you may receive some small health benefits. However, the hope of preventing disease is not a good reason to start drinking.

CALORIES IN ALCOHOLIC BEVERAGES

Drink	Amount	Calories
Beer	12 ounces	150
Light Beer	12 ounces	100
White Wine	5 ounces	115
Red Wine	5 ounces	110
Liquor	1.25 ounces	80

A six-pack of beer has 900 calories; a six-pack of light beer has 600.

- **Keep foods safe to eat.**
  Keep hands, counter tops, and food clean.
  Keep raw, cooked, and ready-to-eat foods separate while shopping for, preparing, and storing food.
  Keep cold foods cold.
  Keep hot foods hot.
  Don't keep any foods at room temperature longer than 2 hours.
  Put leftovers in the refrigerator promptly.
  Use up leftovers in 3 to 4 days.
  Thaw foods in the refrigerator or microwave, not on the kitchen counter.
  Use a thermometer and cook meat, fish, and poultry to safe temperatures to prevent foodborne illness.
  To prevent foodborne illness, don't eat unpasteurized milk, raw eggs, raw or rare-cooked meat or poultry, unpasteurized juice, or raw sprouts.
  Don't taste or smell food you think may be spoiled. *When in doubt, throw it out.*

Bottom line: Few people will be able to apply all of these recommendations to their daily lives, but every positive change will make a positive impact on your health. Think about the Dietary Guidelines as just that—guidelines for living a healthier life, not an all-or-nothing rulebook.

Smart Stuff

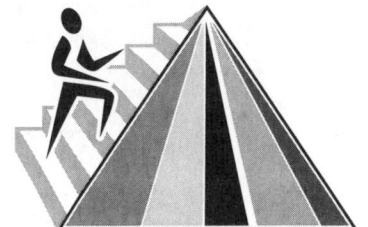

www.MyPyramid.gov
STEPS TO A HEALTHIER YOU

Pyramid Remodeled

Eighty percent of Americans recognize the food pyramid, so the USDA decided the healthy-eating graphic was worth keeping, with a little renovation. The latest edition turns the 1992 version on its side and adds a person climbing a set of stairs. The slogan, "Steps to a healthier you," encourages everyone to be more active and make healthier food choices every day. A website, www.MyPyramid.gov, offers 12 versions of the pyramid personalized by age, sex, and activity level.

Vertical bands of different colors and widths represent the proportions that various food groups should form in our diet. Fruits, vegetables, grains, and milk take up most of the space; there's a narrower band for meats and beans, and a very skinny band for oils and fats. The pyramid visually displays four basic messages: variety, moderation, proportion—eat more of some foods, less of others—and activity.

JUST THE FACTS—A TO Z

*"Science has fulfilled her function when she has
ascertained and enunciated truth."*

Thomas Henry Huxley (1825–95)
British biologist and educator

AFLATOXINS—These are poisons produced by molds in foods. They can cause cancer and birth defects. Grains and peanuts are foods most likely to be contaminated but the USDA tests foods for aflatoxin to prevent potential health problems.

ALCOHOL—Ethyl alcohol (ethanol) is the type found in the alcoholic beverages you drink. Vodka, gin, rye, and scotch average 40 to 50% alcohol, wines 10 to 14%, and beer 2 to 4%. Some over-the-counter drugs and herbal extracts also contain alcohol, which must be noted on the label. Excessive use of alcohol contributes to 3 leading causes of death: cirrhosis of the liver, accidents, and suicide. Moderate drinking (1 drink a day for women and 2 drinks a day for men) may have health benefits. One drink is defined as 12 ounces of beer, 5 ounces of wine, or 1½ ounces of liquor. See also PROOF.

AMERICAN DIETETIC ASSOCIATION (ADA)—The world's largest professional organization of food and nutrition professionals, with over 70,000 members. The ADA serves the public by promoting nutrition and health.

Members must meet minimum education requirements; if they are registered dietitians (R.D.s) they are required to pass a national qualifying exam and to pursue continuing education to maintain R.D. status. The ADA Consumer Hotline (1-800-366-1655) offers food and nutrition information and professional referrals. See also DIETITIAN.

AMINO ACIDS—These are protein fragments that make up larger protein structures. Twenty amino acids are needed in your body. Some are essential and can only be supplied by the protein foods you eat, such as eggs, steak, and fish. Others are nonessential because they can be made in the body. See also PROTEINS.

ANABOLISM—The process by which simple substances and structures in your body are made into more complex substances and structures. It is also called constructive metabolism and is the opposite of catabolism. Catabolism plus anabolism equals metabolism, which is the process by which your body uses energy. See also CATABOLISM and METABOLISM.

ANOREXIA—A lack of appetite which can be temporary or may last a long time. It may occur as the side effect of a disease, disease treatment, medication, pain, or a mental disorder. Anorexia nervosa is an eating disorder in which a person refuses to maintain a minimal normal weight. See also EATING DISORDERS.

ANTIOXIDANTS—Substances that help protect the body against harmful substances called free radicals that damage healthy cells. Free radicals are caused by smoking, air pollution, and sun exposure, and are the by-products of normal body functions. Fruits, vegetables, nuts, and tea are rich sources of antioxidants.

APHRODISIACS—The list of foods that is thought to increase sex drive is long, including oysters (Casanova is reported to have eaten 50 a day), asparagus, ginseng, yohimbe, pomegranates, wild yams, carrots, cucumbers, fertilized duck eggs, cacao beans, caviar, blueberries, and "prairie oysters" (the testicles of bulls and rams). In studies that measured blood flow to the penis and vagina, men appeared to be turned on by smelling lavender and pumpkin pie. Women were aroused by the scents of Good & Plenty candy and cucumber.

APPETITE—Your desire to eat at a given time. It can be affected by hunger, the taste of food, and your social setting, environment, culture, and habits. Appetite affects when you eat, what you eat, and how much you eat. See also HUNGER, SATIATION, and SATIETY.

ARTIFICIAL SWEETENERS—See SUGAR SUBSTITUTES.

ATHEROSCLEROSIS—See CARDIOVASCULAR DISEASE.

B VITAMINS—See VITAMINS.

BARIATRICS—The field of medicine that treats obesity and the diseases associated with obesity.

BETA-CAROTENE—See CAROTENOIDS.

BINGE EATING—Previously called "compulsive eating," this condition is characterized by frequent episodes of eating very large amounts of foods, where the person feels a lack of control over his or her eating behavior. See also EATING DISORDERS.

BLOOD PRESSURE (BP)—This is the force that the blood creates against the wall of the blood vessels every time your heart beats. It is measured with a sphygmomanometer (blood pressure machine). The blood pressure during the contraction of the heart is called systolic pressure. The pressure when the heart relaxes between beats is the diastolic pressure. Blood pressure is reported as systolic over diastolic. A good blood pressure reading for an adult is 120/80 or lower. See also DASH DIET (DIETARY APPROACHES TO STOP HYPERTENSION), HIGH BLOOD PRESSURE, and SODIUM.

BLOOD SUGAR LEVEL (BSL)—The normal level of blood sugar (glucose) is 70 to 110 for adults; 80 to 115 for those over 60; and 60 to 90 for pregnant women. A fasting blood sugar is measured after a person has not eaten for 8 to 12 hours. A normal fasting blood sugar level is 100 or below.

BODY MASS INDEX (BMI)—BMI is used to estimate health risk. As BMI goes up, so does your risk for early death and serious illness. To determine BMI, your weight and height are used to estimate your body fat:

1. Multiply your weight in pounds by 700.
2. Divide the result by your height in inches.

3. Divide the result by your height in inches again.

The National Institutes of Health (NIH) recommends that adults aim for a BMI below 25. A BMI of 18.5 to 24.9 is considered normal. A BMI of less than 18.5 is considered underweight. People with BMIs between 25 to 30 are considered overweight. A BMI over 30 is considered obese. According to these guidelines, over 97 million Americans weigh too much.

BULIMIA—See EATING DISORDERS.

CACHEXIA—Weakness, extreme weight loss, and severe loss of body tissues as the result of long-standing illness, chronic disease, malnutrition, or terminal illness.

CAFFEINE—This stimulant is found in coffee, tea, soda, cocoa, chocolate, and many over-the-counter medications. It is not addictive, but it is habit-forming. Many people can't get going without their morning coffee or cola. Caffeine is absorbed quickly into the body and its effects can be felt within 30 minutes. It stimulates your brain and heart, increasing work capacity, urination, and stomach acid secretion. For some people caffeine disrupts sleep and causes heartburn and stomach upset.

Food	Portion Size	Milligrams of Caffeine
Coffee	1 (5-ounce) cup	110 to 150
Tea	1 (5-ounce) cup	25 to 110
Iced tea	1 (12-ounce) glass	70
Cola drinks	1 (12-ounce) can	30 to 60
Hot chocolate	1 (5-ounce) cup	2 to 20
Chocolate milk	1 (8-ounce) glass	2 to 7
Chocolate candy	1 ounce	1 to 35

CALORIES—The energy stored in food. Every time you eat, you take in calories. Proteins and carbohydrates have 4 calories per gram, fats have 9, and alcohol has 7. Your body is a machine that uses food calories as fuel. When the amount of fuel you use equals the amount of fuel you burn, your weight remains constant. Eat too many calories, and your body uses what it needs and stores the rest. Cut calories and you lose weight. The average woman eats 1,850 calories a day; men eat 2,550 calories a day. Discretionary calories are those calories left over each day, after a person has met his or her daily nutrient need. These calories can be used for any additional foods that a person wishes to eat. Discretionary calories are often used on foods that add to the pleasure of eating but usually have few, if any, nutrients, such as sugar, soda, salad dressing, candy, cake, and butter. See also EMPTY CALORIES and NUTRITION BASICS, pages 2 to 3.

CANCER—A disease that occurs when a cell loses its normal control mechanisms and has unregulated growth. As cancer cells grow and multiply, they form a mass of cancerous tissue that can invade surrounding tissues and spread (metastasize) around the body. See also CARCINOGEN.

CARBOHYDRATES—One of the major sources of energy (calories) found in food, carbohydrates are classified by the amount of sugar units in their structure. Simple carbohydrates are made up of one or two sugar units. Examples are glucose and fructose, found in honey and fruits. Complex carbohydrates are made up of many sugar units and are found in foods such as starches and fibers. Starches can be broken down in your body to provide energy (calories). Fiber cannot be broken down in the body for energy, but it does help to promote regularity and offers protection against some diseases. Carbohydrates are the primary source of energy for your brain and central nervous system. Good sources of carbohydrates are bread, pasta, cereal, rice, vegetables, beans, potatoes, milk, and yogurt. See also FIBER, SUGARS, and NUTRITION BASICS, pages 6 to 7.

CARCINOGEN—A cancer-causing substance that changes a cell's genetic material. It can be a chemical, a virus, radiation, or sunlight. Food can carry carcinogens into the body. See also CANCER.

CARDIOVASCULAR DISEASE (HEART DISEASE)—This refers to diseases of the heart and the blood vessel system in the body. More than 61 million Americans have some form of the condition. In the most common form, atherosclerosis, arteries leading to the heart become progressively blocked, impairing blood flow and depriving the heart of oxygen and nutrients. High levels of cholesterol and fats in the blood contribute to this problem. Eating fewer foods high in cholesterol and saturated fat, and more foods high in fiber, can help reduce your risk for heart disease.

CARNITINE—See VITAMIN-LIKE COMPOUNDS.

CAROB—Candy and other sweet foods made of carob are often found in health food stores. It is used in place of chocolate. Carob comes from the seed pods of a tree and is also called St. John's bread. Some think that carob is healthier than chocolate, but there is no evidence to back up this claim.

CAROTENOIDS—A group of pigments that give the deep yellow, orange, and red colors to fruits and vegetables. The major carotenoids are alpha-carotene, beta-carotene, lutein, zeazanthin, cryptoxanthin, and lycopene. Beta-carotene, found in cantaloupe, carrots, and squash, is the most common. Your body can convert alpha-carotene and beta-carotene into vitamin A. Researchers think that people who regularly eat carotene-rich fruits and vegetables may be at lower risk for some eye diseases and cancer. See also LUTEIN.

CATABOLISM—The process by which complex substances and structures in your body are broken down into simpler compounds. The breakdown results in the release of energy. It is the opposite of anabolism. Catabolism plus anabolism equals metabolism, the process by which your body uses energy. See also ANABOLISM and METABOLISM.

CENTERS FOR DISEASE CONTROL AND PREVENTION (CDC)—An agency of USDHHS that develops techniques for nutritional assessment and whose mission is to promote health and the QUALITY OF LIFE by preventing and controlling disease, injury, and disability. See also FOODBORNE ILLNESS and USDHHS.

CELIAC DISEASE—This disease damages the small intestine and interferes with the absorption of nutrients. People with celiac disease cannot tolerate gluten, a protein found in wheat, rye, barley, and oats. They need to eat a gluten-free diet. Instead of wheat they eat flour, bread, pasta, and crackers made of potato, rice, soy, or bean flour.

CHOLESTEROL—A white, waxy, fat-like substance that is part of every cell in your body. Cholesterol insulates nerve cells and helps skin cells retain moisture. It makes up a major part of your brain, and is the main building block for vitamin D and essential hormones, such as cortisone, estrogen, progesterone, and testosterone. Having too much cholesterol in your blood is unhealthy. The extra cholesterol can be deposited in your artery walls, narrowing them and interfering with normal blood flow. You get cholesterol every time you eat animal foods—meat, poultry, fish, eggs, milk, yogurt, cheese, and butter. This type of cholesterol is called dietary cholesterol. There is no cholesterol in any food that grows in the ground—vegetables, fruits, nuts, seeds, cereals, and grains. Serum cholesterol is the type that travels in your bloodstream. It is a combination of dietary cholesterol and cholesterol that is made in your liver. In fact, most people make 3 times more cholesterol than they eat in food. See also CHOLESTEROL VALUES, HDL (HIGH DENSITY LIPOPROTEINS), LDL (LOW DENSITY LIPOPROTEINS), and NUTRITION BASICS, pages 4 to 5.

CHOLESTEROL VALUES—Blood cholesterol values are measured in milligrams (mg). The number of milligrams (mg) of cholesterol in 1 deciliter (dl), or slightly less than ½ cup, is the value used to describe how much cholesterol is in your blood. For example, 180 mg/dl. Your doctor may just give you the number instead of the complete measurement. The National Cholesterol Education Program (NCEP) recommends that adults over age 20 be screened for cholesterol at least once every 5 years. Those with higher than normal readings should be checked more often. At a screening you'll find out your total cholesterol, LDL cholesterol, HDL cholesterol, and a ratio. Total cholesterol is just that, the total amount of cholesterol in a given volume of blood. You want your levels to be below 200 to have a lower risk of heart disease. LDL cholesterol is often referred to as "bad" cholesterol, so the lower your level, the better. Desirable levels are under 100. HDL cholesterol is referred to as "good" cholesterol. Levels under 40 are considered too low. Having low LDL and high HDL cholesterol re-

duces your risk of developing plaques and lowers your risk of heart disease. Your ratio is determined by dividing HDL cholesterol into total cholesterol. For example, if your total cholesterol is 200 and your HDL cholesterol is 50, your ratio is 4:1. A ratio below 5:1 is good. The optimum is 3.5:1. See also CHOLESTEROL, HDL (HIGH DENSITY CHOLESTEROL), and LDL (LOW DENSITY CHOLESTEROL).

CHOLINE—See VITAMIN-LIKE COMPOUNDS.

CLA (CONJUGATED LINOLEIC ACID)—This is an unsaturated fatty acid (a building block of fat) found in beef and dairy foods. Research is showing that CLA may have anticancer properties and may help to lower blood cholesterol and triglyceride levels. See also FATS.

CONSTIPATION—This condition results in difficult or infrequent passage of stools. Poor nutrition, lack of exercise, and a low fluid intake can all contribute to the problem. Eating well, including more fiber in your meals, and getting adequate fluids will make stool bulkier and easier to pass. People mistakenly believe that they need to have a bowel movement every day. Three bowel movements or more a week is considered normal.

COOL—This abbreviation stand for the mandatory USDA Country-Of-Origin food Labeling program, which tells consumers where their food comes from.

DASH DIET (DIETARY APPROACHES TO STOP HYPERTENSION)—The DASH eating plan helps to lower high blood pressure by focusing on plant foods instead of animal foods. It is an eating plan low in total fat, saturated fat, and cholesterol, but rich in fruits, vegetables, and low fat dairy products. Combining the DASH diet with low sodium eating can lower blood pressure even more. See also HIGH BLOOD PRESSURE and SODIUM.

DEHYDRATION—This word has two meanings: the removal of water from food, such as drying fruit, or the loss of water from the body. When you are mildly dehydrated (3% weight loss) you will experience impaired physical performance and decreased blood volume. At 5% weight loss you will have nausea and difficulty concentrating. At 8% weight loss you will experience dizziness, increased weakness, and have trouble maintaining your body temperature. Ten percent weight loss or greater can be life threatening. It is easy to become mildly or moderately dehydrated after vigorous physical exercise, especially in hot weather. That is one reason why competitive athletes are weighed before and after a competition.

DIABETES MELLITUS—A chronic disease of insulin deficiency or resistance which upsets the body's ability to use the energy (calories) found in foods. Over 16 million Americans have diabetes, but only half of them have been diagnosed. There are 3 types of diabetes: type 1, type 2, and gestational diabetes (diabetes during pregnancy). Type 1, which accounts for 5 to 10% of all cases, can occur at any age but most often is diagnosed in people under the age of 30. Lifestyle changes, insulin replacement, and diet are the usual ways to handle this condition. Type 2 is the most common form of diabetes. Your risk for this condition goes up if there is a family history, you are overweight, and you do little or no exercise. In the past, it occurred more frequently in older adults. Today, as more and more people are overweight, type 2 diabetes is occurring in all age groups, even children. Lifestyle changes, including weight loss and diet, are the usual ways to handle this condition. Gestational diabetes develops in 2 to 5% of all

pregnancies. Although the condition usually disappears at the end of the pregnancy, 20 to 50% of women with gestational diabetes are at risk for type 2 diabetes 5 to 10 years in the future. The condition is usually managed during pregnancy by diet and, when necessary, insulin therapy. See also INSULIN.

DIARRHEA—The passage of frequent, loose, watery stools. Diarrhea can be caused by infections, drugs, stress, and serious medical conditions. High doses of vitamin C, drinking too much apple juice, or eating large amounts of "sugar-free" candy, cookies, or gum sweetened with sorbitol or mannitol can cause diarrhea. It was once believed that eating nothing was the way to stop diarrhea, but the current thinking is to eat anything you desire except fatty foods. Apples, bananas, rice, cottage cheese, dry toast, crackers, pretzels, and tea, in addition to plain water, are all good choices. Most cases of diarrhea last only a day or two. If diarrhea lasts for more than 2 days, see your doctor.

DIET—The usual foods and drinks a person eats. An adequate diet meets all the nutrition requirements for an individual. A therapeutic diet is a selection of foods and drinks that will help prevent or treat a condition. Many think of a diet as a way to control calories and weight, but in actuality that is a weight control diet, and it can be used to either gain or lose weight.

DIETARY GUIDELINES FOR AMERICANS—The federal government's health and nutrition messages for Americans. By law, the guidelines must be reviewed and revised every 5 years. The sixth edition was released in 2005. Following the guidelines will help reduce your risk for obesity and chronic disease. See also UNDERSTANDING THE DIETARY GUIDELINES, pages 15 to 19.

DIETARY SUPPLEMENTS—Any substance that is taken to enhance a person's regular diet in hopes of improving health. A supplement may be in the form of a pill (such as a vitamin pill), powder (such as added fiber), a drink (such as energy drinks), or an herbal supplement that is not part of a whole food. Many dietary supplements are beneficial; others have no scientifically proven value.

DIETITIAN—Someone who specializes in the study of food and nutrition as it relates to health. The credential R.D. stands for registered dietitian, which means that the person has passed a national qualifying exam assuring proficiency in the field. In order to maintain this credential, the person must participate in continuing education so that his or her knowledge remains current. See also AMERICAN DIETETIC ASSOCIATION.

DIGESTION—The process of breaking down the foods you eat into nutrients. Food enters your body through the mouth. The stomach churns it like a blender so that it can be further broken down and absorbed in the small intestines. The absorbed nutrients provide the energy needed to run your body and to build and repair your tissues. The large intestine recycles minerals and water and excretes wastes.

DNA (DEOXYRIBONUCLEIC ACID)—The main carrier of genetic information in your body.

DOUBLE BLIND EXPERIMENT—In this type of study, neither the subjects nor the researchers know which subjects are being given the real treatment and which are receiving a placebo. This keeps researchers from reaching biased conclusions before all the information is collected. See also PLACEBO.

DYSPEPSIA—Also called indigestion, this is an uncomfortable feeling of fullness and bloating after eating.

DYSPHAGIA—Also known as difficulty swallowing. It can occur for a number of reasons, such as inflammation, surgery of the throat, or a stroke. Without the ability to swallow, it is difficult for a person to get adequate nutrition.

EATING DISORDERS—Can be grouped into 3 categories: anorexia nervosa, refusing to maintain a minimal normal weight; bulimia nervosa, eating in binges and then purging; and bulimia, bingeing without purging. Bingeing is the rapid consumption of food in a short period of time, where the person feels out of control. Purging is the use of vomiting, laxatives, diuretics, or enemas to rid the body of food. People with anorexia have distorted body images and restrict their food intake to the point that they suffer severe weight loss. They may also exercise compulsively and use laxatives. They are desparately afraid of gaining weight. Untreated, the condition can result in malnutrition, sterility, damage to vital organs, and even death. People with bulimia nervosa repeatedly and compulsively eat large amounts of food and then they may use laxatives, diet pills, or excessive exercise to control their weight. Often their weight is normal or even above normal, making it harder to detect the problem. Binge eating disorder, or bulimia without purging, is simply the excessive intake of large amounts of food. It usually occurs in people who are overweight or obese and contributes to the problem becoming progressively worse. The more they eat, the heavier they become; the heavier they become, the more they binge.

EDAMAME—The Japanese name for fresh soybeans. Smaller than a lima bean, edamame are jade green and plump, with a creamy texture and pleasant crunch. They can be bought fresh or frozen and can be simmered, steamed, microwaved, or sautéed. Edamame are an excellent source of fiber, protein, and calcium. See also SOY PRODUCTS.

EDEMA—Also called "fluid retention," this is the presence of a large amount of fluid in the body, caused by a disruption to the body's normal ability to control fluid. Pregnant women may experience edema of the ankles and feet late in pregnancy.

EDIBLE FLOWERS—Flowers that can be safely eaten include squash blossoms, roses, pansies, nasturtium, day lilies, sesbania, marigolds, hibiscus, violets, and jasmine. Many flowers are *not* edible, such as lilies of the valley, sweet peas, and delphinium.

EMPTY CALORIES—Foods that contain mainly calories and few if any nutrients, including soda, sugars, syrups, jelly, lard, and short-ening.

ENERGY—Through the process of digestion and absorption, energy is released from the food you eat and can be used or stored by the body. The amount of energy in food is measured in calories. See also CALORIES.

ENZYMES—Substances made in the body that speed up chemical reactions. They help to break down, build up, or change one substance to another. Many enzymes are just proteins, while others have a vitamin or mineral attached to the protein part. The names of many enzymes begin with the name of the substance they act on and end in *ase*. An example is lactase, which breaks down the milk sugar, lactose.

EPIDEMIOLOGICAL STUDIES—This type of study investigates the occurrence of disease in human populations and tries to determine what factors caused the disease.

FASTING BLOOD SUGAR—See BLOOD SUGAR LEVELS.

FAT REPLACERS OR SUBSTITUTES—Substances that are used to replace some of the fat found in food. They can be made of carbohydrate, protein, or even a type of fat that your body cannot use. Olestra and Simplesse are fat replacers found in foods you eat.

FATS (LIPIDS)—One of the major sources of energy (calories) for your body. Fats provide double the amount of calories as the same amounts of protein or carbohydrate. Fats are made up of chains of fatty acids. There are 3 types of fatty acids: saturated, polyunsaturated, and monounsaturated. All food fats are a combination of the different types of fatty acids, but we classify the foods by the predominant fatty acids. Meat, whole milk, cheese, and butter are high in saturated fats. Nuts, vegetables oils, and fish are high in polyunsaturated fats. Olives, olive oil, canola oil, and peanut oil are high in monounsaturated fats. Too much saturated fat puts you at greater risk for heart disease. Too much of any fat may contribute to weight gain. But some fat is necessary for your body to function. Fat provides energy, carries fat-soluble vitamins into your body, protects and cushions your vital organs, helps to keep your body temperature regulated, and lubricates your tissues. See also CLA (CONJUGATED LINOLEIC ACID), OMEGA-3 FATS, OMEGA-6 FATS, STEARIC ACID, TRANS FATS, and NUTRITION BASICS, pages 3 to 4.

FDA (FOOD AND DRUG ADMINISTRATION)—A federal agency within the U.S. Department of Health and Human Services, the FDA is responsible for nutrition labeling, and the approval and use of food additives and drugs.

This agency protects Americans from unsafe or unsanitary foods by watching for fraud, conducting inspections, analyzing food samples, and testing for toxicity, chemical contamination, and pesticide residues. The FDA also prevents the transmission of contagious disease by regulating the movement of foods across state lines. See also USDHHS and NUTRITION LABELING.

FIBER—A type of carbohydrate that cannot be broken down in your body for energy (calories). Fiber provides you with many benefits: it prevents and relieves constipation, protects against certain cancers, reduces cholesterol, aids in weight control, and helps to control diabetes. When you check nutrition labels, look for foods that have 2 or more grams of fiber per serving. See also CARBOHYDRATES and NUTRITION BASICS, pages 6 to 7.

FOOD—Anything taken into the body that nourishes, builds or repairs tissues, supplies energy, or helps regulate body processes. Emotional, cultural, social, and religious factors affect what different groups define as acceptable foods to eat.

FOOD ADDITIVE—Any substance added to food during production, processing, storage, or packaging. Additives are regulated to ensure they are safe to eat.

FOOD FAD—An idea associated with food or a way of eating that becomes popular for a short time, though it may or may not stand up to scrutiny. A fad is often an exaggerated truth that promises a special result. Many weight loss diets are based on fads.

FOOD IRRADIATION—The treatment of food with a carefully controlled amount of gamma rays, X-rays, or ionizing radiation. This process enhances food quality and safety by reducing spoilage and slowing down ripening. The FDA requires that irradiated foods be specially labeled. These foods are safe to eat and their nutritional value is the same as those that have not been irradiated. See also FDA.

FOOD POISONING—See FOODBORNE ILLNESS.

FOODBORNE ILLNESS—Many things can contaminate food—including bacteria, mold, viruses, and chemicals—resulting in illness for anyone who eats the food. Examples of common foodborne organisms are *salmonella*, *E. coli*, and *campylobacter*.

FREE RADICALS—See ANTIOXIDANTS.

FUNCTIONAL FOODS—This term refers to any food or food ingredient that has been modified to provide health benefits. Other terms for this category of foods are designer foods, nutraceuticals, and pharmafoods. Some examples of functional foods are calcium-fortified orange juices, energy drinks, and cholesterol-lowering margarines.

GAS (FLATULENCE)—We all produce gas; some more, some less. If you are lucky and expel it as soon as it is produced, you will not experience bloating and discomfort as gas builds up in your intestine. Everyone swallows some air as they eat or drink. Mouth breathers swallow more. Eating slowly with a closed mouth and drinking through a straw can reduce the amount of air swallowed. Chewing gum and drinking carbonated soda or water increases it. You expel some swallowed air by burping. Bacteria in the intestines also ferment undigested food, producing gas. This gas is expelled through the rectum. Some foods, like beans, have well-deserved reputations as gas producers. Other foods—such as onions, celery, applesauce, bagels, broccoli, cabbage, bananas, pretzels, cucumbers, or prune juice—cause gas in some people and none in others. If you suffer from uncomfortable gas or belching, keep a record of the foods you ate before a gassy episode and you'll be able to figure out which foods cause you discomfort.

GASTRIC BYPASS OR STAPLING—A procedure designed to divert the normal food intake through the intestines as a way to control weight. The surgery literally "bypasses" part of the digestive tract that would normally absorb nutrients and calories.

GI TRACT (GASTROINTESTINAL TRACT)—The passageway that food takes through your body. It is like an enormous beginning at the mouth and ending at your rectum. With all the twists and turns, the average GI tract is 7 times a person's height. It is made up of your mouth, esophagus, stomach, small intestine, large intestine, and rectum. Food must be broken down and absorbed out of the GI tract before it can be used by the body.

GLUTEN-FREE DIET—See CELIAC DISEASE.

GLYCEMIC INDEX—This index ranks a food by how quickly it can be converted into glucose and enter your bloodstream. Foods with a high glycemic index—rice, white bread, potatoes—raise blood sugar levels quickly. Foods with a low glycemic index—beans, whole grains, meat, fat—raise blood sugar levels more slowly, either because they are high in fiber that can't be broken down, or because they don't have any carbohydrates in them. The theory be-

hind the glycemic index is correct: some foods do raise blood sugar quickly; others do not. But in practice, it's not that simple. The glycemic index was devised based on eating one food at a time. Straight glucose was given a rating of 100 and individual foods were measured against it. White bread has a very high glycemic index. But if you add peanut butter, the glycemic response is lowered because peanut butter, a high-fat food, has a low glycemic index. It gets even more complicated. Ripe fruits have a lower glycemic index than unripe fruits. Cooking pasta al dente is fine; overcook it, and its glycemic value goes up. Even sugars vary. Glucose is high on the index, but fructose (fruit sugar) is low. Bottom line: Research into the health effects of the glycemic index is in its infancy. Eating more foods with a low glycemic index may lower the risk for heart disease and help to control diabetes. But if you are trying to lose weight, the best approach is still to reduce calories and increase activity.

GRAM—This is a standard unit of weight in the metric system. Protein, fat, carbohydrate, fiber, and sugar are measured in grams on food labels. Vitamins and minerals may be measured in milligrams (mg), one one-thousandth of a gram, or in micrograms (mcg), one one-millionth of a gram. A kilogram equals 1,000 grams and is the unit used to measure body weight. One pound equals 2.2 kilograms.

HEALTH—This is a state of physical, mental and emotional well-being. Keys to good health are: eating a balanced and adequate diet, exercising regularly, having a positive outlook on life, drinking moderate amounts of alcohol, drinking adequate water, getting enough sleep, avoiding stress, using minimal medication, and not smoking or using illicit drugs.

HDL (HIGH DENSITY LIPOPRO-TEINS)—About ⅓ of the blood's cholesterol is carried by HDL (high density lipoproteins). Experts believe that HDL cholesterol carries cholesterol away from arteries and back to the liver, where it is broken down and removed from the body. Because this may slow down the growth of plaque (blockage), HDL is referred to as "good" cholesterol. Levels under 40 are considered too low. See also CHOLESTEROL, LDL (LOW DENSITY LIPOPROTEINS), and LIPOPROTEINS.

HEALTHY EATING INDEX (HEI)—The Healthy Eating Index is a 100-point tool designed to measure how well a person's diet measures up to recommendations such as the Dietary Guidelines for Americans. The Healthy Eating Index allows researchers to use a standard tool for gathering and analyzing diet patterns and their effects on health outcomes.

HEART DISEASE—See CARDIOVASCULAR DISEASE.

HEARTBURN—Also known as acid indigestion or gastroesophageal reflux disease (GERD), this is a burning sensation felt in the throat or chest near the heart. It has nothing to do with your heart, but the burning sensation can be so strong that it can be mistaken for a heart attack. Heartburn is caused by the back splashing of food and acid from the stomach onto the delicate tissues of the esophagus (the connection between the stomach and throat). Overeating, drinking alcohol, smoking, eating fatty and spicy foods, and lying down after eating all increase your risk for heartburn.

HIGH BLOOD PRESSURE (HYPERTENSION)—The main symptom of this condition is the continued elevation of blood pressure above normal. This means that systolic blood pressure (the top number) is 140 or higher and the diastolic blood pressure (the bottom number) is 90 or higher. High blood pressure affects one in every four Americans. Doctors are on the lookout for adults with prehypertension, a condition in which blood pressure is mildly elevated, between 120/80 and 139/89. These people are at greater risk for developing high blood pressure in the future. Blood pressure increases with higher intakes of salt, alcohol, and protein. Smoking, stress, being overweight, and lack of exercise also increase risk. Blood pressure goes down with adequate intakes of potassium, calcium, and magnesium. Losing weight, exercising, and eating well also help to control blood pressure. See also BLOOD PRESSURE, DASH DIET (DIETARY APPROACHES TO STOP HYPERTENSION), and SODIUM.

HIGH FRUCTOSE CORN SYRUP (HFCS)—A sweetener made by converting cornstarch to syrup. It is widely used in foods and beverages.

HOMOCYSTEINE—Elevated levels of this amino acid increase your risk for heart attacks and strokes. Blood levels between 6 and 12 are considered normal. Moderate risk is 12 to 30; high risk over 30. Levels below 7 are associated with the lowest risk for heart disease. Homocysteine levels can be reduced by getting adequate amounts of folic acid (a B vitamin), B_6, and B_{12}. Fruits and vegetables, especially green leafy vegetables, are rich in folic acid, as are bread, cereal, and pasta that has been enriched with the vitamin. See also AMINO ACIDS and CARDIOVASCULAR DISEASE.

HUMAN GENOME PROJECT—This is an international project to create a map or guide of each human gene. This guide will aid scientists in pinpointing **polymorphism**, common variations in genes seen in less than 1% of the population. Identifying these polymorphic variations will help to more effectively treat people who carry a risk for certain diseases. For most diseases, if you practice prevention, your genes have little effect on your health risk. Information from the Human Genome Project can target prevention for at-risk individuals. These people will be able to alter their diets or environmental factors (like exercise or smoking) early in life, before the disease causes symptoms, reducing their risk and potentially increasing their life span by a dozen years. See also NUTRITIONAL GENOMICS.

HUNGER—This reflects your body's drive to fulfill its need for energy and nutrients. Hunger affects when you eat and how much you eat. See also APPETITE, SATIATION, and SATIETY.

HYDROGENATION—A process by which hydrogen atoms are added to a liquid fat to make it solid at room temperature. You often see this on a food label as hydrogenated vegetable oil or partially hydrogenated vegetable oil. Hydrogenated fats are more stable for deep-frying and work very well in baked goods. But hydrogenation creates a type of fat called trans fat. Eating too many trans fats puts you at risk for heart disease. See also TRANS FATS.

HYPER—A prefix meaning above normal or an excess.

- Hypercholesterolemia—higher than normal levels of cholesterol in the blood
- Hyperglycemia—higher than normal levels of blood sugar
- Hyperkalemia—higher than normal levels of potassium
- Hyperlipidemia—higher than normal levels of one or more fats in the blood, such as cholesterol or triglycerides

- Hypertension—refers to repeated blood pressure readings above 140/90
- Hypetriglyceridemia—higher than normal levels of triglycerides in the blood
- Hypervitaminosis—excessive intake of one or more vitamins at levels that may cause health problems

See also BLOOD PRESSURE, BLOOD SUGAR LEVEL, CHOLESTEROL, CHOLESTEROL VALUES, DASH DIET, HIGH BLOOD PRESSURE, HYPERVITAMINOSIS, POTASSIUM, and TRIGLYCERIDES.

HYPERTENSION—See HIGH BLOOD PRESSURE.

HYPERVITAMINOSIS—Also called vitamin toxicity, this is a condition where the level of a vitamin in the blood or tissues is so high that it causes undesirable symptoms. Hypervitaminosis has been associated with high intakes of vitamins A and D.

HYPO—A prefix meaning below normal, a deficiency, or lack of a substance.

- Hypoglycemia—lower than normal levels of blood sugar
- Hypokalemia—lower than normal levels of potassium

See also BLOOD SUGAR LEVEL and POTASSIUM.

IATROGENIC—This term means "caused by a medical treatment or a diagnostic procedure." Iatrogenic malnutrition is an induced nutrition deficiency caused by drug therapy or medical procedures.

IMMUNE SYSTEM—The role of the immune system is to protect the body against foreign invaders such as microbes, cancer cells, and even transplanted organs. The immune system's main job is to recognize enemies of the body, mobilize forces against them, and finally to attack and conquer the enemy. The organs of the immune system include the bone marrow, thymus, lymph nodes, lymphatic vessels, tonsils, adenoids, and spleen.

INDIGESTION—See DYSPEPSIA.

INOSITOL—See VITAMIN-LIKE COMPOUNDS.

INSULIN—A hormone secreted by the pancreas that helps glucose enter cells to be used for energy. Lower levels of insulin or the complete lack of it causes diabetes. About 25% of all people with diabetes are given insulin. The rest control the condition through diet or with diet and medication that stimulates the pancreas to produce more insulin. Because insulin is a protein, it would be digested in the GI tract if it were taken by mouth. That is why is must be injected.

IU (INTERNATIONAL UNIT)—A system to measure vitamin activity, used less frequently today.

JOULE—The international unit of energy. One joule equals 4.184 calories. See also CALORIES.

KILOGRAM—See GRAM.

LACTOSE INTOLERANCE—This occurs when a person cannot digest lactose, the main sugar in milk. They lack the enzyme lactase, which breaks down this sugar. Common symptoms of lactose intolerance include bloating, gas, cramps, diarrhea, and nausea. To avoid symptoms, it is wise to use smaller portions of regular milk, yogurt, processed cheese, and ice cream, or to eat foods made with a dairy substitute such as soy. Lactose-free foods are also available, as well as drops and tablets that can be taken to help a person better tolerate foods containing lactose.

LDL (LOW DENSITY LIPOPROTEINS)—This is the main carrier of cholesterol in your body. If too much LDL cholesterol circulates in the blood, it can stick to the walls of the arteries that lead to the heart and brain. Optimum values for LDL cholesterol are under 100. See also CHOLESTEROL, HDL, and LIPOPROTEIN.

LEARN—This abbreviation stands for: **L**isten, **E**xplain, **A**cknowledge, **R**ecommend, and **N**egotiate. It serves as a guideline to be used in an intervention process. The LEARN technique might be used to counsel a person to lose weight.

LIPIDS—See FATS.

LIPOIC ACID—See VITAMIN-LIKE COMPOUNDS.

LIPOPROTEIN—A combination of fat and protein. An example is cholesterol, a fatlike substance that is coated with a protein so it can travel in your blood, which is mainly water. The combination is called a lipoprotein. See also HDL and LDL.

LITER—A liter equals 33.8 fluid ounces—1.8 ounces more than a quart, which has 32 ounces. Soda and other beverages are sold in liters.

LUTEIN—This is a substance found in dark green leafy vegetables, bright yellow vegetables, and egg yolks. It is part of the carotenoid family. Several studies have suggested that people who eat more lutein are less likely to have serious eye problems as they age. See also CAROTENOIDS.

MACRONUTRIENTS—Nutrients needed by your body in large amounts, including proteins, fats, and carbohydrates. This group of nutrients provides calories. See also MICRONUTRIENTS.

MAD COW DISEASE (BOVINE SPONGI-FORM ENCEPHALOPATHY OR BSE)—BSE is a contagious, degenerative, and fatal disease that affects the central nervous system of adult cattle. It was first diagnosed in 1986. Researchers believe that people who eat BSE-infected meat are at greater risk of developing a human brain-wasting illness, variant Creutzfeldt-Jakob disease (vCJD). Almost 100 people have died of vCJD in Great Britain, France, Portugal, Germany, Spain, and Ireland. According to the FDA, there have been no re-ported cases of vCJD in the U.S. caused by BSE-infected beef. The FDA, USDA, other federal and state agencies, and industry groups have taken steps over the last 10 years to prevent the introduction of BSE into our food supply. Your chances of eating BSE-contaminated beef in Europe are estimated at 1 in 10 billion. For U.S. travelers in Europe, the CDC suggests avoiding beef and beef products or eating only solid pieces of muscle meat, not ground beef such as burgers and sausages.

MALNUTRITION—This can also be called undernutrition or poor nutrition. It results when too few or too many nutrients and calories are consumed, both of which can jeopardize your health. Too few nutrients may result in starvation or deficiency diseases, such as scurvy (too little vitamin C). Too many nutrients, like calories, can result in obesity. We rarely think of someone who is overweight at malnourished, but their condition truly is the result of poor nutrition.

MEDICAL NUTRITION THERAPY (MNT)—The use of nutrition to treat an illness, injury, or condition.

METABOLIC SYNDROME—Previously re-ferred to as Syndrome X and also called insulin resistant syndrome, this condition identifies a cluster of health problems. When these prob-lems occur together, a person is at greater risk for heart disease. The problems associated with metabolic syndrome are: higher than normal fasting blood glucose, high triglycerides, low HDL cholesterol, high blood pressure, and overweight. Weight loss and exercise are the pri-mary treatment to reduce risks.

METABOLISM—The process by which the body extracts energy (calories) from the food you eat and makes use of it. Metabolism has 2 parts: catabolism and anabolism. Catabolism is the breakdown of complex substances such as food into simpler substances. It results in the re-lease of energy. Anabolism occurs when simple substances are used to build more complex sub-stances. For example, muscles in your body are made from smaller protein fragments. See also ANABOLISM and CATABOLISM.

MICROGRAM (mcg)—See GRAM.

MICRONUTRIENTS—Nutrients needed by the body in small amounts, including vitamins and minerals. This group of nutrients does not provide calories. See also MACRONUTRIENTS.

MILLIGRAM (mg)—See GRAM.

MG/DL The abbreviation for milligrams per deciliter. Blood cholesterol is measured as the amount of cholesterol in a given amount of blood.

MINERALS—Unlike vitamins, minerals can-not be destroyed or have their shape changed by your body. Calcium, for example, is the same whether it is found in seashells, milk, or your bones. Minerals are divided into 2 groups: major minerals and trace minerals. Each day, your body needs 100 milligrams or more of major minerals. Your body needs less than 100 milligrams of trace minerals per day.

Major Minerals	Trace Minerals
Calcium	Chromium
Chloride	Cobalt
Magnesium	Copper
Phosphorous	Fluorine
Potassium	Iodine
Sodium	Iron
Sulfur	Manganese
	Molybdenum
	Selenium
	Zinc

See also NUTRITION BASICS, pages 8 to 10.

MONOUNSATURATED FATS—See FATS.

NATIONAL INSTITUTES OF HEALTH (NIH)—The U.S. Department of Health and Human Services oversees the National Institutes of Health, which is made up of 27 institutes and centers. These individual institutes and centers conduct or support research, training, and education to promote the health of Americans. They include: National Cancer Institute (NCI), National Eye Institute (NEI), National Heart, Lung, and Blood Institute (NHLBI), National Human Genome Research Institute (NHGRI), National Institute on Aging (NIA), National Institute on Alcohol Abuse and Alcoholism (NIAAA), National Institute of Allergy and Infectious Diseases (NIAID), National Institute of Arthritis and Musculoskeletal and Skin Diseases (NIAMS), National Institute of Biomedical Imaging and Bioengineering (NIBIB), National Institutes of Child Health and Human Development (NICHD), National Institute on Deafness and Other Communica-tion Disorders (NIDCD), National Institute of Dental and Craniofacial Research (NIDCR), National Institute of Diabetes and Digestive and Kidney Diseases (NIDDK), National Institute on Drug Abuse (NIDA), National Institute of Environmental Health Sciences (NIEHS), National Institute of General Medical Sciences (NIGMS), National Institute of Mental Health (NIMH), National Institute of Neurological Disorders and Stroke (NINDS), National Institute of Nursing Research (NINR), National Library of Medicine (NLM), Center for Information Technology (CIT), Center for Scientific Review (CSR), John F. Fogarty International Center (FIC), National Center for Complementary and Alternative Medicine (NCCAM), National Center for Research Resources (NCRR), and NIH Clinical Center (CC).

NAUSEA—This general feeling of physical uneasiness often leads to an urge to vomit. It may be caused by early pregnancy, gallbladder disease, food poisoning, a virus, or as the side effect of chemotherapy or medications. See also VOMITING.

NUTRIENT-DENSE FOOD—Foods that are rich in one of more important nutrients. Citrus fruits are rich in vitamin C; milk is rich in calcium.

NUTRIENTS—For nutrition to be complete and adequate, a person must get the right amount of nutrients—carbohydrates, fats, proteins, vitamins, minerals, and water. These nutrients are used by the body to support growth, repairs, and normal functioning. Some nutrients are essential; they must be supplied through the food you eat. Others are nonessential because the body can make as much of the nutrients as it needs.

NUTRITION—The study of how food and the nutrients found in food affect your body and your health. You truly are what you eat.

NUTRITION LABELING—The Nutrition Labeling and Education Act (NLEA) was signed into law in 1994. It requires nutrition information on most packaged foods and allows the use of FDA-approved health claims on labels. The main features of the Nutrition Facts Panel, which appears on food labels, include:

- Serving size
- Servings per container
- Calories
- Total fat, trans fat, saturated fat
- Cholesterol
- Sodium
- Total carbohydrate, dietary fiber, sugars
- Protein

- Daily Values (DVs), which are standards set by the government based on a diet of 2,000 or 2,500 calories a day. Some values are recommended maximums, such as less than 65 grams of fat, less than 20 grams of saturated fat, less than 300 milligrams of cholesterol, and less than 2,400 milligrams of sodium. Others are recommended minimums, such as 300 grams of carbohydrates, and 25 grams of fiber. The Daily Values for a 2,500 calorie diet are slightly higher.
- % Daily Value (%DV) shows how a food fits into your daily eating plan. The %DVs are set for a 2,000 calorie diet. The percentage listed on the label reflects the amount of the daily value found in one serving of food. For example: if the %DV for carbohydrate is 10%, this means 1 serving of that food provides 30 grams of carbohydrate, because the DV for carbohydrates is 300 grams ($10\% \times 300 = 30$).

- Vitamins A and C and the minerals calcium and iron are required to be listed. Food companies may voluntarily include additional VITAMINS and minerals on nutritional labels.
- Health claims that have been approved by the FDA. See also FDA.

NUTRITION SCREENING—A way of examining health variables to see if you are at risk for a specific problem. A nutrition screening could target pregnant women, older adults, or those at risk for certain conditions, like heart disease. Once the screening is complete, a level of risk is assigned. Someone at high risk for a condition, such as heart disease, would be taught how to implement positive health behaviors to lower their risk. Someone at moderate or low risk would be re-evaluated periodically.

NUTRITIONAL GENOMICS—The study of how food, nutrients, and other lifestyle choices influence a person's genes or hereditary makeup. The food you eat and the nutrients found in food communicate with your genes. Carrying certain genetic variations affects your health and your risk for disease. When immigrant groups move to the U.S. and stop eating their native cuisines, their risk for diseases like heart disease and cancer goes up. Geneticists believe that their original gene packages may have evolved to accommodate their native foods, and they are unable to adapt fully to their adopted lifestyle. We also know that obesity increases your genetic risk for certain disease, like type 2 diabetes. By never gaining weight, your genetic risk for type 2 diabetes can be almost totally eliminated. Based on your genetic profile, in the future, you may be able to alter your diet or lifestyle to protect yourself from inborn risks. See also HUMAN GENOME PROJECT.

OBESITY—Also called adiposity, this is a state of malnutrition in which the accumulation of body fat is so excessive that it negatively impacts a person's health. Mild obesity is defined as 20 to 40% over desirable weight or a BMI of 30 to 34.9. Moderate obesity is 60 to 80% over desirable weight or a BMI of 35 to 39.9. Extreme obesity is more than 100% over desirable weight or a BMI over 40. It is estimated that 97 million Americans are overweight or obese, putting them at greater risk for heart disease, diabetes, respiratory problems, stroke, joint problems, and some types of cancer. See also BODY MASS INDEX.

OMEGA-3 FATS—A type of polyunsaturated fat found mainly in fish, shellfish, olive oil, canola oil, and walnuts. We eat less of these than we should. See also FATS and OMEGA-6 FATS.

OMEGA-6 FATS—A type of polyunsaturated fat found mainly in vegetable oils such as soybean, corn, and safflower oil. See also FATS and OMEGA-3 FATS.

ORGANIC FOODS—Foods grown and processed without synthetic chemicals such as pesticides, herbicides, fertilizers, and preservatives, and without the use of irradiation or genetic engineering. Organic animals are raised without hormones and antibiotics, except for vaccines that prevent animal diseases. Organic labeling requirements were established in the United States in 2000. The words "100% organic" or "organic" can be used only on foods that contain at least 95% organic ingredients.

OSTEOPOROSIS—This condition is commonly referred to as adult bone-thinning. It occurs when bone breakdown exceeds bone formation, resulting in porous bones that are prone to fracture. It usually occurs in people over age 50, especially post-menopausal wo-

men. Men and younger adults can also be affected but often to a lesser degree. The primary means of prevention is to have adequate nutrition and calcium early in life to form strong bones. Experts recommend that adults under age 50 take in 1,000 milligrams of calcium a day, 1,200 milligrams for adults 51 and over, and 1,300 milligrams for preteens and teenagers. Exercising, not smoking, limiting caffeine intake, and moderate use of alcohol all decrease your risk for osteoporosis.

OVERWEIGHT—Defined as a body mass index of 25 to 25.9, which is 10 to 20% over a person's ideal weight. More than half of all adults in the U.S. are considered overweight. See also BODY MASS INDEX and OBESITY.

PATHOGEN—An organism that can cause illness.

pH—A numerical scale that measures the acidity or alkalinity of a substance. A pH of 7.0 to 14.0 is alkaline. A pH below 7.0 is acid. Every food has a pH: limes are 2.0, bananas are 4.6, milk is 6.6, and egg whites are 8.0.

PHYSICAL ACTIVITY—This includes all movement that burns calories and increases your heart rate, such as walking, bicycling, weeding, dancing, swimming, or cleaning the house. Physical activity helps to prevent weight gain and reduces your risk for many diseases. See also SEDENTARY LIFESTYLE.

PHYTOCHEMICALS—Naturally occurring plant substances that help protect your body or lower your risk for disease. Fruits, vegetables, grains, beans, seeds, soy, and tea are all rich in phytochemicals. More than 900 different phytochemicals have been found in foods.

PLACEBO—An inactive substance that appears the same as an active substance that is being studied. A placebo is sometimes called a sugar pill. The placebo effect is a physical or emotional change that is the result of the person's expectations and not directly a result of the substance they were given. See also DOUBLE BLIND EXPERIMENT.

POLYUNSATURATED FATS — See FATS.

PORTION SIZE — The amount of food consumed at one time. Restaurant portion sizes are often bigger than amounts you would typically eat at home. Portions sizes vary widely, whereas serving sizes are standardized. See also SERVING SIZE.

POTASSIUM — This mineral helps to maintain balance in the body and is part of many enzyme reactions. Some medications taken to control high blood pressure increase the need for potassium. Eating potassium-rich foods helps to lower blood pressure.

Food High in Potassium:

Apricots	*Milk*
Avocados	*Molasses*
Bananas	*Nuts*
Broccoli	*Potatoes*
Carrots	*Raisins*
Citrus fruits and juices	*Spinach*
Corn	*Tomatoes and*
Dried fruits	*tomato products*
Dried peas and beans	*Whole grains*
Green leafy vegetables	*Yogurt*
Meat	*Yams*
Melons	

See also ENZYMES and MINERALS.

PROBIOTICS — These are cultures of bacteria that are healthful for normal intestinal function.

Yogurt is one of the best examples of a food that contains probiotics.

PROOF — This refers to the concentration of ethanol (alcohol) in a liquid. In the U.S., proof is twice the alcohol content. Gin or vodka may be 80 proof, which means they contain 40% alcohol. Wine is usually 10% to 14% alcohol, which is 20 to 28 proof. Vanilla flavoring is usually alcohol based, as are many other flavor extracts and medications. All will list the percent alcohol on the label; double that number to get the proof. See also ALCOHOL.

PROTEINS — Complex structures that consist of the building blocks known as amino acids. Proteins are strung together to make up body parts, such as muscle, blood, skin, and cartilage. Proteins can also provide energy (calories) to your body. Good sources of protein include: meat, fish, poultry, dry beans, eggs, nuts, nut butters, milk, yogurt, cheese, tofu, bread, cereal, rice, pasta, and some vegetables. See also AMINO ACIDS and NUTRITION BASICS, pages 5 to 6.

QUACKERY — In the field of foods and nutrition, quackery refers to false claims about the power of a food or nutrient to cure or prevent a health problem. The 10 red flags to detect a food fad or food quackery are:

1. Recommendations that promise a quick fix
2. Claims that sound too good to be true
3. Simplistic conclusions drawn from a complex study
4. Recommendations that are based on a single study
5. The use of vague terms such as "cure-all"
6. Advertisements that promote something as "new" or a "scientific breakthrough"

7. Recomendations that ignore the differences between individuals or groups of people
8. Advertisements that do not state any disadvantages to following the advice
9. Lists of "good" and "bad" foods
10. Use of questionable publications to promote claims

QUALITY OF LIFE—Defined by the World Health Organization as "a complete state of physical, mental, and social well-being and not merely the absence of disease or infirmity."

RECOMMENDED DIETARY ALLOWANCES (RDAs)—Daily requirements of individual nutrients for healthy people. The RDA is set for each nutrient for different sexes and age groups. These recommendations are published periodically by the National Academy of Sciences. Beginning in 1989, the RDAs underwent a comprehensive review and revision, the results of which were published in a series of reports called Dietary Reference Intakes (DRIs). Instead of a single reference RDA table, the newer DRIs are made up of several reference recommendations.

RISK—This is the possibility that an event may occur. There are numerous risk factors that can affect your health.

SALT—Table salt is made up of two minerals, 40% sodium and 60% chloride. One teaspoon of table salt has slightly more than 2,000 milligrams of sodium. Kosher salt and sea salt are slightly less salty than table salt because they are less dense and coarser in shape. Most of these coarser salts average between 1,100 and 1,900 milligrams of sodium in a teaspoon. Many cooks prefer coarser salt because they feel it offers more texture and flavor. See also SODIUM.

SATIATION—The sensation that tells you a meal is over and you have eaten enough. It affects how much you eat at a given meal. See also APPETITE, HUNGER, and SATIETY.

SATIETY—The sensation that you experience once a meal is finished. It influences the time between meals and the number of times you eat in a day. It is simply the satisfaction you feel after you have been fed, and how long that satisfaction lasts. See also APPETITE, HUNGER, and SATIATION.

SATURATED FATS—See FATS.

SCOVILLE SCALE—The standard test for measuring the heat of peppers. The scale goes from 0 for bell peppers to 2,500 to 10,000 for jalapeños and chipotles, to a four-alarm 100,000 to 350,000 for habanero and Scotch bonnet peppers. Hot food can be nutritious because peppers are rich in vitamins A and C. The ingredient in peppers that stimulates the sensors in the mouth and creates the burning sensation is capsaicin. The "burn" you feel actually activates pain receptors in your mouth, which causes the brain to release endorphins, a "feel-good" chemical that produces a pleasurable sensation. The result: Your mouth is on fire, but you keep eating. Hot dishes may temporarily speed up your metabolism and help to stimulate the breakdown of fats. These dishes also activate the body's natural cooling system, making you sweat.

SEDENTARY LIFESTYLE—Behaviors that include little or no physical activity. Sedentary behavior increases your risk for gaining weight and for contracting many serious diseases, including heart disease and diabetes. See also PHYSICAL ACTIVITY.

SERVING SIZE—Most foods have standard serving sizes, such as ½ cup of cooked vegetables, 1 slice of bread, 8 ounces of milk, etc. These standard serving sizes are used to calculate diets, give weight control advice, and compare foods. See also PORTION SIZE.

SODIUM—This mineral regulates the fluid level both outside and inside the cells of your body, which in turn affects blood volume, blood pressure, and your body's acidity. The movement of sodium into and out of cells allows other important substances to make this journey, too, helping to transmit nerve impulses and electrical messages vital to your body's minute-by-minute functioning. Most of us eat 3,000 to 6,000 milligrams of sodium a day, but experts recommend 1,500 milligrams or less. Healthy adults can do nicely on as little as 500 milligrams a day. See also HIGH BLOOD PRESSURE, SALT, and NUTRITION BASICS, pages 9 to 10.

SOY PRODUCTS—A number of foods can be prepared from soybeans, including soy milk, soy cheese, soy flour, tempeh, miso, tofu, soy protein, meat substitutes, and soybean oil. Fresh soybeans are called edamame. See also EDAMAME.

STEARIC ACID—This saturated fatty acid (a building block of fat) doesn't act like a typical saturated fat; it doesn't raise cholesterol levels. It's found in meats, milk, and some plant foods. This finding suggests that not all saturated fats are bad for you. See also FATS.

SUGAR SUBSTITUTES—Different types of sugar substitutes have been in use for decades. Sugar alcohols—sorbitol, mannitol, xylitol, isomalt, lactitol, maltitol, and trehalose—contain some calories but are absorbed very slowly by the body, so they have very little effect on blood sugar. High intakes can cause diarrhea. Artificial sweeteners—saccharin, aspartame, acesulfame-K, sucralose, and neotame—don't raise blood sugar and have no calories. Some lose their sweetness when heated, so they cannot be used in cooking.

Artificial Sweetener	Brand Name
Saccharin	Sweet and Low
	Sweet Twin
	Necta Sweet
Aspartame	Nutrasweet
	Equal
	Sugar Twin
Acesulfame-K	Sunette
	Sweet&Safe
	Sweet One
Sucralose	Splenda

SUGARS—Cereals, grains, fruits, vegetables, milk, and plain yogurt all contain sugars. These are natural sugar choices that contain vitamins, minerals, and fiber, too. Soda, candy, fruit drinks, cakes, cookies, ice cream, jelly, and syrup, in contrast, offer little more than sweetness and calories, and are loaded with added sugar. Americans eat 15 to 21% of their daily calories as sugar, with teenagers eating the most. Studies have shown that as sugar intake goes up, vitamin and mineral intake goes down. The U.S. Dietary Reference Intakes suggest that at most 25% of daily calories come from added sugar. Obviously, people should eat less. The World Health Organization (WHO) has suggested limiting added sugars to no more than 10% of total calories, though some experts feel this amount is unrealistically low. Try eating closer to the WHO recommendation of 10% total calories as sugar, keeping in mind that the U.S. Dietary Reference Intake of 25% of daily calories is the healthy upper limit. See also NU-TRITION BASICS, pages 7 to 8.

SYMPTOM—An indication of a disease as the person experiences it, in contrast to a sign, which is an indication of a disease that a doctor can evaluate. For example, a headache is a symptom, but high blood pressure is a sign—a headache can be described but not measured; blood pressure can be measured.

SYNDROME X—The name previously used for the condition now referred to as Metabolic Syndrome. See also METABOLIC SYNDROME.

TASTE—Humans have the ability to taste sweet, sour, salty, and bitter flavors through receptors found on the tongue and in the mouth. Scientists have found a fifth taste sensation called umami, often described as full-bodied, savory, or rich. There are receptors on the tongue specific to umami taste. The umami taste results from the addition of MSG (monosodium glutamate) to foods, and is caused by the amino acid glutamine (also called glutamate). See also AMINO ACIDS.

TAURINE—See VITAMIN-LIKE COMPOUNDS.

THIRST—A sensation that signals your body's need for water. Thirst is normally a good guide for water need, except in infants, the sick, and older adults, who may have a diminished sense of thirst. In extreme heat and during excessive sweating, thirst cannot always keep up with your body's need for water.

TOLERABLE UPPER INTAKE LEVEL (UL)—The highest average amount of a nutrient one can take without causing a problem. The UL for each nutrient is set for different sexes and age groups. As amounts increase over the UL, the potential for problems increases.

TRANS FATS (TRANS FATTY ACIDS)—Almost all the trans fat found in food is created by passing hydrogen gas through vegetable oil, a process called hydrogenation, which makes oils harder and more stable. Most of us eat 1.5 to 2% of our daily calories as trans fats. Even this small amount raises total cholesterol and lowers HDL, or "good" cholesterol. Cutting back or cutting out foods with trans fats is a good idea. Look for the amount of trans fat on the nutrition facts panel, or the words hydrogenated vegetable oil or partially hydrogenated vegetable oil on the ingredient lists for baked goods, snack foods, fried foods, and margarine. See also HYDROGENATION.

TRIGLYCERIDES—The main type of fat found in food, and the major storage form of fat in your body. Triglycerides are transported through the bloodstream to cells where they are burned for energy (calories), or to fat tissues where they are stored for future use. High levels of triglycerides in your bloodstream can be a risk factor for heart disease. Levels above 150 mg/dl are considered high. Your risk for high triglyceride levels goes up if you are overweight, do little exercise, drink too much alcohol, eat a high carbohydrate diet, smoke, or have diabetes.

UNDERWEIGHT—This describes a person with a BMI below 18.5 or who is 10% or more below the normal weight for a person of that age, sex, and height. A weight 30% below normal or a BMI of 15 or less can be life threatening. See also BODY MASS INDEX.

URINE—The fluid excreted by your kidneys. Most people make 1,000 to 1,500 milliliters in 24 hours. You make half the amount of urine at night that you make during the day. The color of your urine is a simple way to tell if you are drinking enough fluids. The deeper the yellow, the more likely it is that you are mildly dehydrated. Pale yellow to clear means good hydration. Urinalysis, a physical, chemical, and microscopic evaluation of a urine sample, is used to evaluate your health and nutritional status. See also DEHYDRATION and WATER.

USDA (UNITED STATES DEPARTMENT OF AGRICULTURE) — This agency is responsible for monitoring the wholesomeness and quality of meat, poultry, and eggs. The USDA has a consumer hotline number at 1-800-535-4555.

USDHHS (UNITED STATES DEPARTMENT OF HEALTH AND HUMAN SERVICES) — This agency is responsible for setting all policies related to human development, general health, and the welfare of all Americans. See also FDA.

VEGETARIAN DIET — A way of eating that excludes some or all animal foods. Vegans, or total vegetarians, eat only plant foods. They do not eat any animal foods. Lacto-ovo vegetarians eat plant foods plus dairy products and eggs. Lacto vegetarians eat plant foods and dairy products. Partial vegetarians or semi-vegetarians eat plant foods but no red meat, and may or may not eat chicken, fish, dairy products, and eggs.

VISCERAL FAT — This type of fat, stored in the trunk or belly region, is also called "intra-abdominal fat." Visceral fat increases a person's risk for heart disease, diabetes, hypertension, and stroke because it can easily be released into the bloodstream. Fat in other areas of the body, called subcutaneous fat, is not so easily released.

VITAMIN-LIKE COMPOUNDS — Your body can make a number of the vitamin-like compounds it needs. These include:

- *Choline*, which helps maintain cell structure and transmits nerve messages. It can be made from an amino acid, methionine. If you eat enough protein, you will be able to make enough choline.
- *Carnitine* helps to deliver needed substances into cells and to remove waste from cells. The liver is able to make carnitine from 2 amino acids. Carnitine is also found in dairy foods and meat.
- *Inositol* is found mainly in brain tissue and is part of cell structures. Your body can make inositol from glucose. Animal foods also are a good source of inositol.
- *Taurine* is found mainly in muscle, blood, and nerve tissues and helps them function properly. It is made in the body from amino acids.
- *Lipoic acid* helps your body to use energy and acts as an antioxidant. It can easily be made in the body. Red meat, liver, and brewer's yeast are good food sources.

See also AMINO ACIDS and VITAMINS.

VITAMINS — The word comes from the Latin *vita*, meaning "life." All vitamins are vital to life, even though they are needed by your body in very small amounts. They help you digest, absorb, and use the fats, carbohydrates, and proteins found in food. Vitamins do not provide energy (calories), and they can be destroyed or have their shape changed. Cooking at high temperatures can destroy vitamins. Your body can also change a vitamin's shape to make it easier to use in certain situations. Vitamins are divided into two groups: fat soluble and water soluble. Fat soluble vitamins are carried into the body by foods containing fat and are stored in your fat tissues, waiting to be used. Water soluble vitamins are absorbed directly into the blood and travel freely around the body in the bloodstream.

Water Soluble	Fat Soluble
Thiamin (B_1)	*Vitamin A*
Riboflavin (B_2)	*Vitamin D*
Niacin (B_3)	*Vitamin E*
Vitamin B_6	*Vitamin K*
Vitamin B_{12}	
Vitamin C	
Biotin	
Folic acid	
Pantothenic acid	

See also VITAMIN-LIKE COMPOUNDS and NUTRITION BASICS, pages 11 to 12.

VOMITING—The process of "throwing up" material from the stomach through the esophagus and out the mouth. It is the body's response to something irritating and can be caused by too much alcohol or caffeine, an infection, or foodborne illness. Vomiting results in weakness, mild dehydration, and the loss of some important minerals, including sodium, magnesium, and chloride. Prolonged vomiting can lead to nutritional deficiencies and severe dehydration. Do not eat anything immediately after vomiting; just relax and give your digestive tract a chance to rest. After an hour with no further vomiting, try a little water. If this stays down, slowly add other drinks, such as tea or ginger ale. Then try crackers, dry toast, pretzels, bananas, applesauce, plain rice, or plain pasta. Most cases of vomiting last for a very short time. If you vomit profusely or if vomiting continues for more than 24 hours, see your doctor.

WATER—A continuous supply of water is one of your most basic nutrition needs. Without water, you can survive for less than a week. It makes up 50 to 80% of your body weight. The fluids in your body are found in 2 places—inside your cells and outside your cells. Fluid inside your cells is called intracellular fluid and the fluid outside your cells is called extracellular fluid. Both types of fluid help your body to function by:

- Giving structure and shape to your cells
- Helping to form structures like protein
- Lubricating your eyes and joints
- Helping to regulate your body's temperature
- Aiding in digestion and absorption of nutrients
- Transporting nutrients to cells
- Carrying waste products away from cells in urine, stools, and perspiration
- Aiding in your body's chemical reactions

Drinking water and other liquids are your major sources of water, but many foods, like fruits and vegetables, are good sources, too.

WEIGHT LOSS—The loss of body weight can only happen if a person decreases food intake, increases physical activity, or does both.

WELLNESS—This defines a lifestyle with appropriate levels of nutrition, exercise, work, and rest to ensure that a person gets the best experience from life.

WHO (WORLD HEALTH ORGANIZATION)—This United Nations organization aims to eliminate disease on a global scale.

WHOLE GRAIN FOODS—Foods made from the entire grain seed. They include brown rice, oatmeal, cracked wheat, popcorn, and whole wheat pasta, cereal, bread, and crackers. You should try to eat at least 3 servings of whole grain foods a day.

XEROSTOMIA—This condition occurs when salivary glands in the mouth do not work properly and the mouth and becomes very dry because there is not enough saliva. Over 70% of older adults have this condition. It affects taste and puts the person at greater risk for tooth decay and mouth infections.

YEAST—Several strains of yeast are used to make foods and beverages. Baker's yeast is used to make dough rise. Brewer's yeast is a bitter-tasting byproduct of the production of beer. It's rich in protein, minerals, and some B vitamins, and it can be bought as a nutritional supplement in flake, powder, or tablet form. Nutritional yeast is grown especially to be used as a dietary supplement and has a pleasant nutty-cheese flavor. Brewer's yeast and nutritional yeast cannot be substituted for baker's yeast in cooking.

YO-YO DIETING—This term refers to repeated dieting where a person loses weight, only to regain all the weight that was lost. They may diet again and again throughout their lifetime, but rarely retain the weight loss for any extended period of time. This up and down weight loss/weight gain syndrome is also called weight cycling, or the "feast and famine diet."

ZEN MACROBIOTIC DIET—This diet is based on the idea that one's health and happiness depends on a proper balance between "yin" and "yang" foods. Macrobiotic diets are vegan and stress whole grains, vegetables, beans, sea vegetables, and soups. Extreme forms of this diet are very limiting, relying mostly on brown rice. See also VEGETARIAN DIET.

DEFINITIONS

as prep (as prepared): refers to food that has been prepared according to package directions

lean and fat: describes meat with some fat on its edges that is not cut away before cooking, or poultry prepared with skin and fat as purchased

lean only: refers to lean meat that is trimmed of all visible fat, or poultry without skin

shelf stable: refers to prepared products found on the supermarket shelf that are ready-to-eat or are ready to be heated and do not require refrigeration

take-out: describes prepared dishes that you purchase ready-to-eat; those included in this book serve as a guide to the calories, fat, saturated fat, cholesterol, protein, carbohydrate, sugar, fiber, calcium, sodium, potassium, folic acid, and vitamin C values of similar products you may purchase

ABBREVIATIONS

avg	=	average
diam	=	diameter
fl	=	fluid
frzn	=	frozen
g	=	gram
in	=	inch
lb	=	pound
lg	=	large
med	=	medium
mg	=	milligram
oz	=	ounce
pkg	=	package
pt	=	pint
prep	=	prepared
qt	=	quart
reg	=	regular
sec	=	second
serv	=	serving
sm	=	small
sq	=	square
tbsp	=	tablespoon
tr	=	trace
tsp	=	teaspoon
w/	=	with
w/o	=	without
<	=	less than

NOTES

CALS = Calories

FAT = Fat
   All fat values are given in grams (g).

SAT FAT = Saturated Fat
   All saturated fat values are given in grams (g).

CHOL = Cholesterol
   All cholesterol values are given in
   milligrams (mg).

PROT = Protein
   All protein values are given in grams (g).

CARB = Carbohydrate
   All carbohydrate values are given in
   grams (g).

SUGAR = Sugar
   All sugar values are given in grams (g).

FIBER = Fiber
   All fiber values are given in grams (g).

CALCI = Calcium
   All calcium values are given in
   milligrams (mg).

SOD = Sodium
   All sodium values are given in
   milligrams (mg).

POTAS = Potassium
   All potassium values are given in
   milligrams (mg).

FOLIC = Folic Acid
   All folic acid values are given in
   micrograms (mcg).

VIT C = Vitamin C
   All vitamin C values are given in
   milligrams (mg).

tr (trace) = less than 1 gram of fat, saturated fat,
   protein, carbohydrate, sugar, or fiber; less
   than 1 milligram of cholesterol, calcium,
   sodium, potassium, and vitamin C; and less
   than 1 microgram of folic acid.
— (dash) indicates data was not available.
0 (zero) indicates that there is none of the nutrient in that food.

Discrepancies in figures are due to rounding,
product reformulation, and reevaluation. Labeling law allows rounding of values. Because
much of our data is analysis data, obtained directly from manufacturers rather than from labels, in some cases our values may not be
exactly the same as label information because
they have not been rounded.

PART ONE

BRAND-NAME, NONBRANDED (GENERIC), AND TAKE-OUT FOODS

> **Smart Stuff**
>
> *If you want to stay healthy—overeating and avoiding exercise is doomed to make you fail!*

FOOD	PORTION	CALS	FAT	SAT FAT	CHOL	PROT	CARB	SUGAR	FIBER	CALCI	SOD	POTAS	FOLIC	VIT C
ABALONE														
fresh fried	3 oz	161	6	1	80	17	9	—	—	32	502	—	5	—
raw	3 oz	89	1	tr	72	15	5	—	—	27	255	—	4	—
ACEROLA														
fresh	1	2	tr	—	0	tr	tr	—	—	1	0	7	—	81
ACEROLA JUICE														
juice	1 cup	51	1	—	0	1	12	—	1	24	7	235	—	3872
ADZUKI BEANS														
canned sweetened	1 cup	702	tr	—	0	11	163	—	—	65	645	352	317	0
dried cooked	1 cup	294	tr	—	0	17	57	—	17	64	18	1224	278	0
AKEE														
fresh	3.5 oz	223	20	—	0	5	5	—	—	40	—	—	—	26
ALCOHOL														
(*see* BEER AND ALE, CHAMPAGNE, LIQUOR/LIQUEUR, MALT, WINE)														
ALE														
(*see* BEER AND ALE)														
ALFALFA														
sprouts	1 cup	40	tr	tr	0	1	1	—	1	10	2	26	12	3
sprouts	1 tbsp	1	tr	tr	0	tr	tr	—	tr	1	0	2	1	tr
ALLIGATOR														
cooked	3 oz	126	2	—	57	28	0	0	0	—	66	—	—	—
ALLSPICE														
ground	1 tsp	5	tr	tr	0	tr	1	—	—	13	1	20	—	1
ALMONDS														
almond butter honey & cinnamon	1 tbsp	96	8	1	0	3	4	—	—	43	2	120	10	tr
almond butter w/ salt	1 tbsp	101	9	1	0	2	3	—	—	43	75	121	10	tr
almond butter w/o salt	1 tbsp	101	10	1	0	2	3	—	—	43	2	121	10	tr
almond meal	1 oz	116	5	tr	0	11	8	—	—	120	2	390	—	—
almond paste	1 oz	127	8	1	0	3	12	—	—	65	3	184	16	tr
dried unblanched	1 oz	167	15	1	0	6	6	—	—	75	3	208	16	tr
dry roasted unblanched	1 oz	167	15	1	0	5	7	—	—	80	3	219	18	tr
dry roasted unblanched salted	1 oz	167	15	1	0	5	7	—	—	80	260	219	18	tr
dry roasted w/ salt	24 nuts (1 oz)	170	15	1	0	6	6	1	3	80	100	210	8	—
jordan almonds	10 (1.4 oz)	190	7	1	0	4	28	24	1	40	0	—	—	0

FOOD	PORTION	CALS	FAT	SAT FAT	CHOL	PROT	CARB	SUGAR	FIBER	CALCI	SOD	POTAS	FOLIC	VIT C
oil roasted blanched	1 oz	174	16	2	0	16	5	—	3	55	3	197	18	tr
oil roasted blanched salted	1 oz	174	16	2	0	5	5	—	—	55	3	197	18	tr
oil roasted unblanched	1 oz	176	16	2	0	6	5	—	—	66	3	194	18	tr
praline	17 pieces (1.4 oz)	210	12	1	0	5	21	17	3	60	45	—	—	0
toasted unblanched	1 oz	167	14	1	0	6	7	—	3	80	3	220	18	tr
AMERICAN ALMOND														
Almond Paste	2 tbsp	140	9	1	0	4	13	11	2	40	0	—	—	0
Marzipan	2 tbsp	130	5	0	0	2	19	17	1	20	0	—	—	0
Roasted Butter	2 tbsp	180	16	2	0	6	6	1	3	100	55	—	—	0
JUDY'S														
Sugar Free Coconut Almond Brittle	¼ piece (1 oz)	90	5	2	0	1	2	0	1	—	0	—	—	—
KETO														
Chocolatey Covered	1 oz	169	13	6	—	6	7	0	5	170	—	—	—	0
LANCE														
Smoked	1 pkg (0.8 oz)	130	10	1	0	6	4	0	3	60	125	135	—	0
LOW CARB CREATIONS														
Soft Almond Brittle	2 pieces (1 oz)	170	12	2	0	6	17	2	2	—	170	—	—	—
MAMA MELLACE'S														
Butter Rum	1 oz	150	10	1	0	4	13	11	2	40	0	—	—	0
Cinnamon Roasted	1 oz	140	9	1	0	4	14	11	2	40	0	—	—	0
MARANATHA														
Almond Butter	2 tbsp	220	18	1	0	8	6	2	3	100	0	—	—	0
Raw Almond Butter	2 tbsp	190	17	2	0	7	7	2	4	80	0	—	—	0
Tamari Almonds	¼ cup	160	14	2	0	6	6	2	3	80	140	—	—	0
SWEET DELIGHTS														
Almond Roasters	⅓ pkg (1 oz)	190	14	—	0	6	6	3	3	—	200	300	—	—
AMARANTH														
leaves cooked	1 cup	28	tr	tr	0	3	5	—	—	276	28	846	75	54
uncooked	1 cup (6.8 oz)	729	13	3	0	28	129	—	30	298	41	714	96	8
ANCHOVY														
canned in oil	5	42	2	tr	—	6	0	—	—	46	734	109	—	—
canned in oil	1 can (1.6 oz)	95	4	1	—	13	0	—	—	104	1651	245	—	—
fresh fillets	3 (0.4 oz)	21	1	—	—	2	tr	—	—	20	—	—	—	0
fresh raw	3 oz	62	4	1	—	17	0	—	—	125	88	325	—	—

FOOD	PORTION	CALS	FAT	SAT FAT	CHOL	PROT	CARB	SUGAR	FIBER	CALCI	SOD	POTAS	FOLIC	VIT C
ANGLERFISH														
raw	3.5 oz	72	1	—	—	15	0	—	—	—	109	235	—	—
ANISE														
seed	1 tsp	7	tr	—	0	tr	1	—	—	14	tr	30	—	—
ANTELOPE														
roasted	3 oz	127	2	1	107	25	0	—	—	4	46	316	—	—
APPLE														
CANNED														
sliced sweetened	1 cup	137	1	tr	0	tr	34	—	4	4	7	138	1	1
DEL MONTE														
Fruit Pleasures Pie Spiced Apples	½ cup (4.1 oz)	70	0	0	0	0	18	17	1	20	10	—	—	0
LUCK'S														
Fried Apples	½ cup (4.7 oz)	130	0	0	0	0	33	20	2	—	0	—	—	—
DRIED														
cooked w/ sugar	1 cup	232	tr	tr	0	1	58	—	5	8	53	274	0	3
cooked w/o sugar	1 cup	145	tr	tr	0	1	39	—	5	8	51	268	0	2
rings	10	155	tr	tr	0	1	42	—	6	9	56	288	0	3
DEL MONTE														
Dried Apples	¼ cup	110	0	0	0	1	26	18	3	100	250	180	—	0
FRESH														
apple	1 med	81	tr	tr	0	tr	21	—	4	10	1	159	4	8
apple	1 sm	63	tr	tr	0	tr	16	—	3	7	0	122	3	6
apple	1 lg	125	1	tr	0	tr	32	—	6	15	0	244	6	12
w/o skin sliced	1 cup	63	tr	tr	0	tr	16	—	2	4	0	124	tr	4
w/o skin sliced & cooked	1 cup	91	tr	tr	0	tr	23	—	4	8	1	150	1	tr
w/o skin sliced & microwaved	1 cup	95	tr	tr	0	tr	25	—	5	8	1	159	1	tr
CHIQUITA														
Apple	1 med (5.4 oz)	80	0	0	0	0	22	16	5	0	0	—	—	5
COOL CUT														
Apples & Caramel Dip	1 pkg (4.25 oz)	180	5	2	5	1	32	26	3	20	80	—	—	42
FROZEN														
sliced w/o sugar	1 cup	83	1	tr	0	tr	21	—	3	7	5	133	2	tr
STOUFFER'S														
Escalloped	1 cup (6 oz)	180	3	0	0	0	37	30	3	0	70	130	—	48
TAKE-OUT														
baked	1 (5.3 oz)	126	tr	tr	0	tr	33	29	3	10	1	159	4	8
baked no sugar	1 (5.9 oz)	82	1	tr	0	tr	21	18	3	14	6	161	4	8

FOOD	PORTION	CALS	FAT	SAT FAT	CHOL	PROT	CARB	SUGAR	FIBER	CALCI	SOD	POTAS	FOLIC	VIT C
APPLE JUICE														
frzn as prep	1 cup	111	tr	tr	0	tr	28	—	—	14	17	301	1	1
frzn not prep	1 can (6 oz)	350	1	tr	0	1	87	—	—	43	54	945	2	188
juice + vitamin C	1 cup	117	tr	tr	0	tr	29	—	tr	16	7	296	0	103
mulled cider	1 serv	265	1	tr	0	1	42	—	6	129	12	409	18	37
APPLE & EVE														
100% Juice	8 fl oz	110	0	0	0	1	26	22	—	—	5	—	—	60
Cider	8 fl oz	110	0	0	0	1	27	24	—	—	10	260	—	—
EDEN														
Organic Juice	8 oz	80	0	0	0	0	23	12	0	0	0	310	—	0
EVERFRESH														
Apple Juice	1 can (8 oz)	110	0	0	0	0	29	29	0	—	10	—	—	—
HANSEN'S														
Junior Juice 100%	1 box (4.23 oz)	60	0	0	0	0	15	14	1	100	0	—	—	60
LANGERS														
100% Cider	8 oz	120	0	0	0	0	28	26	—	—	0	—	—	60
100% Juice	8 oz	120	0	0	0	0	28	26	—	—	0	—	—	60
Diet Cocktail	8 oz	60	0	0	0	0	14	13	—	150	10	95	—	60
LOW CARB CREATIONS														
Apple Cider as prep	1 serv	10	0	0	0	0	2	tr	0	0	5	—	—	0
MOTT'S														
100% Juice	1 box (8 oz)	120	0	0	0	0	29	—	—	—	15	—	—	—
100% Juice	8 fl oz	120	0	0	0	0	29	23	0	0	20	250	—	2
100% Natural	8 fl oz	120	0	0	0	0	29	28	0	—	20	—	—	—
NAKED JUICE														
Just Apple	8 oz	120	0	0	0	0	29	28	0	20	5	—	—	2
NANTUCKET NECTARS														
100% Pressed	8 oz	100	0	0	0	0	25	22	—	0	10	—	—	0
NUTRABALANCE														
Plus Fibre	1 pkg (8 oz)	120	0	0	0	0	29	24	10	10	8	295	—	60
OCEAN SPRAY														
100% Juice	8 oz	110	0	0	0	0	28	28	0	—	35	240	—	0
ODWALLA														
Spiced Harvest Cider	8 fl oz	130	0	0	0	0	30	28	0	20	20	—	—	2
ROBERT & JAMES														
100% Juice	8 oz	110	0	0	0	0	28	28	—	—	35	—	—	78
SNAPPLE														
Diet	8 oz	15	0	0	0	0	4	3	—	—	10	—	—	—
Snapple Apple	8 fl oz	120	0	0	0	0	30	28	—	—	10	—	—	—
SQUEEZIT														
Green Apple	1 bottle (7 oz)	110	0	0	0	0	27	25	0	0	0	—	—	0

FOOD	PORTION	CALS	FAT	SAT FAT	CHOL	PROT	CARB	SUGAR	FIBER	CALCI	SOD	POTAS	FOLIC	VIT C
SWISS MISS														
Hot Apple Cider Mix	1 serv	84	tr	0	0	tr	20	19	1	3	58	—	—	65
Hot Apple Cider Mix Low Calorie	1 serv	14	0	0	0	0	3	tr	0	5	78	—	—	81
TROPICANA														
Season's Best	8 oz	110	0	0	0	tr	28	—	—	20	25	200	—	—
TURKEY HILL														
Herbal Cider w/ Chamomile & Lemongrass	1 cup	100	0	0	0	—	24	24	—	—	—	—	—	—
VERYFINE														
100% Juice	1 bottle (10 oz)	150	0	0	0	0	38	38	0	0	20	—	—	2
Juice-Ups	8 fl oz	120	0	0	0	0	30	30	0	0	35	—	—	60
WHITE HOUSE														
Juice	8 oz	120	0	0	0	0	30	26	—	—	25	—	—	—
ZEIGLER'S														
Old Fashioned Cider	8 oz	120	0	0	0	0	30	26	0	—	25	170	—	1

APPLESAUCE

FOOD	PORTION	CALS	FAT	SAT FAT	CHOL	PROT	CARB	SUGAR	FIBER	CALCI	SOD	POTAS	FOLIC	VIT C
sweetened	½ cup	97	tr	tr	0	tr	25	—	2	5	4	78	1	2
unsweetened	½ cup	52	tr	tr	0	tr	14	—	2	4	2	91	1	2
EDEN														
Organic	½ cup	50	0	0	0	0	15	11	2	0	15	107	0	0
Organic Sweet Cinnamon	½ cup	50	0	0	0	0	19	15	4	0	0	150	0	2
JOK'N'AL														
Low Carb	1 tbsp	10	0	0	0	0	2	1	—	—	0	—	—	—
MOTT'S														
Single-Serve Cinnamon	1 pkg (4 oz)	100	0	0	0	0	26	—	—	—	0	—	—	—
Single-Serve Natural	1 pkg (4 oz)	50	0	0	0	0	12	—	—	—	0	—	—	—
Single-Serve Original	1 pkg (4 oz)	100	0	0	0	0	24	—	—	—	0	—	—	—
MUSSELMAN'S														
Apple Sauce	1 pkg (4 oz)	80	0	0	0	0	20	19	2	0	10	—	—	0
VERMONT VILLAGE														
Organic Unsweetened	½ cup	80	0	0	0	tr	19	13	2	—	1	—	—	60
WHITE HOUSE														
Applesauce	½ cup (4.4 oz)	90	0	0	0	0	23	18	2	—	15	—	—	—
Chunky	½ cup (4.4 oz)	90	0	0	0	0	23	18	2	—	15	—	—	—

FOOD	PORTION	CALS	FAT	SAT FAT	CHOL	PROT	CARB	SUGAR	FIBER	CALCI	SOD	POTAS	FOLIC	VIT C
WHITE HOUSE (CONT.)														
Cinnamon	½ cup (4.5 oz)	100	0	0	0	0	25	21	2	—	15	—	—	—
Natural Plus	½ cup (4.4 oz)	70	0	0	0	0	15	13	2	—	15	—	—	—

APRICOT JUICE

FOOD	PORTION	CALS	FAT	SAT FAT	CHOL	PROT	CARB	SUGAR	FIBER	CALCI	SOD	POTAS	FOLIC	VIT C
nectar	1 cup	141	tr	tr	0	1	36	—	2	17	9	286	3	1
CERES														
Apricot	8 oz	120	0	0	0	0	30	29	0	20	10	190	—	30

APRICOTS

FOOD	PORTION	CALS	FAT	SAT FAT	CHOL	PROT	CARB	SUGAR	FIBER	CALCI	SOD	POTAS	FOLIC	VIT C
CANNED														
halves heavy syrup pack w/ skin	1 cup (9.1 oz)	214	tr	tr	0	1	55	—	—	22	10	361	4	8
halves water pack w/ skin	1 cup (8.5 oz)	65	tr	tr	0	2	16	—	—	19	7	465	4	8
halves water pack w/o skin	1 cup (8 oz)	51	tr	tr	0	2	12	—	—	19	25	350	4	4
heavy syrup	3 halves	99	tr	tr	0	1	26	—	2	12	6	168	3	4
juice pack	3 halves	51	tr	tr	0	1	13	—	2	12	3	177	3	5
puree from heavy syrup pack w/ skin	¾ cup (9.1 oz)	214	tr	tr	0	1	55	—	—	22	10	361	4	8
puree from light pack w/ skin	¾ cup (8.9 oz)	160	tr	tr	0	1	42	—	—	28	10	349	4	7
puree from water pack w/ skin	¾ cup (8.5 oz)	65	tr	tr	0	2	16	—	—	19	7	465	4	8
puree juice pack w/ skin	1 cup (8.7 oz)	119	tr	tr	0	2	31	—	—	30	9	409	—	12
water pack	3 halves	30	tr	tr	0	1	7	—	2	9	3	207	3	4
DEL MONTE														
Halves Unpeeled Lite	½ cup (4.3 oz)	60	0	0	0	0	16	15	1	0	10	—	—	5
Orchard Select Halves Unpeeled	½ cup (4.4 oz)	80	0	0	0	0	21	20	1	0	10	—	—	48
DRIED														
halves	4	32	tr	tr	0	tr	9	—	1	8	0	164	0	0
halves cooked w/o sugar	½ cup	153	tr	tr	0	2	40	—	6	21	4	598	0	2
FRESH														
apricots	1	17	tr	tr	0	tr	4	—	1	5	0	104	3	4

FOOD	PORTION	CALS	FAT	SAT FAT	CHOL	PROT	CARB	SUGAR	FIBER	CALCI	SOD	POTAS	FOLIC	VIT C
CHIQUITA														
Apricots	3 med (4 oz)	60	1	0	0	0	11	11	1	20	0	—	—	12
FROZEN														
sweetened	½ cup	119	tr	tr	0	1	30	—	3	12	5	277	3	11
ARROWHEAD														
corm boiled	1 med	9	tr	—	0	1	2	—	—	1	2	106	1	0
flour	1 cup	457	tr	tr	0	tr	113	—	4	51	3	14	9	0
ARTICHOKE														
CANNED														
PROGRESSO														
Hearts	2 pieces (2.9 oz)	30	0	0	0	2	6	1	1	0	240	—	—	4
Hearts Marinated	2 pieces (1.1 oz)	170	5	1	0	0	2	0	0	0	110	—	—	4
S&W														
Marinated Hearts	2 pieces (1 oz)	20	2	0	0	0	2	0	1	0	80	55	—	6
FRESH														
cooked	1 med	60	tr	tr	0	4	13	—	7	54	114	425	61	12
hearts cooked	½ cup	42	tr	tr	0	3	9	—	5	38	80	297	42	8
FROZEN														
cooked	1 pkg (9 oz)	108	1	tr	0	7	22	—	11	50	127	634	285	12
BIRDS EYE														
Hearts	½ cup	40	0	0	0	—	—	—	6	0	45	—	—	6
ARUGULA														
fresh	½ cup	3	tr	tr	0	tr	tr	—	tr	16	3	37	10	2
ASIAN FOOD														
(*see also* DINNER, EGG ROLLS, SUSHI)														
CANNED														
chow mein chicken	1 cup	95	tr	tr	8	7	18	—	—	45	725	418	—	tr
CHUN KING														
Beef Pepper Oriental BiPack	1 cup (8.8 oz)	98	2	1	14	10	13	0	3	26	865	—	—	20
Chow Mein Beef BiPack	1 cup (8.6 oz)	78	1	tr	6	8	11	3	3	32	718	—	—	14
Chow Mein Chicken BiPack	1 cup (8.8 oz)	98	3	1	6	8	11	2	3	24	1123	—	—	13
Chow Mein Pork BiPack	1 cup (8.6 oz)	78	2	1	10	7	9	0	2	32	1183	—	—	3
Hot & Spicy Chicken BiPack	1 cup (8.6 oz)	98	3	1	19	8	11	0	1	32	857	—	—	4
Sweet & Sour Chicken BiPack	1 cup (8.9 oz)	161	2	1	25	7	29	26	3	32	687	—	—	12

FOOD	PORTION	CALS	FAT	SAT FAT	CHOL	PROT	CARB	SUGAR	FIBER	CALCI	SOD	POTAS	FOLIC	VIT C
LA CHOY														
Beef Pepper Oriental BiPack	1 cup (8.8 oz)	98	2	1	14	10	13	0	3	26	865	—	—	20
Chow Mein Beef BiPack	1 cup (8.6 oz)	78	1	tr	6	8	11	3	3	32	718	—	—	14
Chow Mein Chicken BiPack	1 cup (8.9 oz)	98	3	1	6	8	11	2	3	24	1123	—	—	13
Chow Mein Shrimp BiPack	1 cup (8.6 oz)	52	1	tr	4	4	9	0	3	30	965	—	—	19
Main Entree Chow Mein Chicken	1 cup (9.3 oz)	80	4	1	9	8	6	2	3	87	1325	—	—	1
Oriental Beef w/ Noodles BiPack	1 cup (8.8 oz)	156	3	1	17	18	18	2	4	29	896	—	—	25
Oriental Chicken w/ Noodles BiPack	1 cup (8.7 oz)	154	4	1	23	14	18	3	2	20	1100	—	—	21
Sweet & Sour Chicken BiPack	1 cup (8.9 oz)	161	2	1	25	7	29	26	3	32	687	—	—	12
Teriyaki Chicken BiPack	1 cup (8.6 oz)	109	3	1	20	8	15	5	3	27	1230	—	—	15
FRESH														
wonton wrappers	1	23	tr	tr	1	1	5	—	—	4	46	7	1	0
AZUMAYA														
Round Wraps	10	160	1	0	10	6	31	1	1	20	370	—	—	0
Square Wraps	6	160	1	0	10	6	31	1	1	20	370	—	—	0
Wrappers Large Square	3	170	1	0	10	7	35	1	1	20	410	—	—	0
NASOYA														
Egg Roll Wrapper	3	170	1	0	10	7	35	1	1	20	410	—	—	0
Won Ton Wrappers	8	160	1	0	10	6	31	1	1	20	370	—	—	0
FROZEN														
AMY'S														
Bowls Teriyaki	1 pkg (10 oz)	300	2	0	0	10	59	12	3	—	780	—	—	—
Skillet Meals Teriyaki Stir Fry	1 cup	320	3	0	0	9	64	9	4	—	590	—	—	—
Stir Fry Asian Noodle	1 pkg (10 oz)	240	5	1	0	12	41	6	6	—	680	—	—	—
Stir Fry Thai	1 pkg (9.5 oz)	270	11	7	0	7	36	4	2	—	420	—	—	—
BANQUET														
Fried Rice w/ Chicken & Egg Rolls	1 meal (8.5 oz)	330	9	3	60	12	51	3	5	40	1270	—	—	0

FOOD	PORTION	CALS	FAT	SAT FAT	CHOL	PROT	CARB	SUGAR	FIBER	CALCI	SOD	POTAS	FOLIC	VIT C
BIRDS EYE														
Easy Recipe Creations Oriental Lo Mein	2¼ cups	230	4	1	5	8	40	11	2	60	1200	—	—	9
Easy Recipe Creations Sesame Ginger Teriyaki	2¼ cups	140	2	0	0	6	24	15	4	60	1230	—	—	42
Easy Recipe Creations Spicy Szechuan Cashews	2¼ cups	180	5	1	0	6	29	18	4	40	1410	—	—	27
GREEN GIANT														
Create A Meal LoMein Stir Fry as prep	1¼ cups (10 oz)	320	70	2	60	30	35	9	4	60	980	—	—	18
Create A Meal Sweet & Sour Stir Fry as prep	1¼ cups (10 oz)	290	7	1	60	27	29	16	5	80	460	—	—	18
Create A Meal Szechuan Stir Fry as prep	1¼ cups (10 oz)	340	15	4	60	28	22	10	5	60	1280	—	—	36
Create A Meal Teriyaki Stir Fry as prep	1¼ cups (10 oz)	240	6	1	55	27	18	10	4	60	940	—	—	42
LA CHOY														
Beef Pepper Oriental	1 cup (7.1 oz)	151	1	tr	10	8	30	7	2	26	714	—	—	3
Chow Mein Vegetable	1 cup (8.9 oz)	108	2	tr	0	2	20	3	5	39	1135	—	—	6
LEAN CUISINE														
Everyday Favorites Oriental Style Dumplings	1 pkg (9 oz)	300	6	2	20	10	51	14	2	40	520	500	—	15
Everyday Favorites Teriyaki Stir Fry	1 pkg (10 oz)	290	4	1	20	18	45	9	4	40	590	610	—	0
STOUFFER'S														
Chicken Chow Mein w/ Rice	1 pkg (10.6 oz)	260	5	1	25	13	40	3	3	40	1090	280	—	6
TYSON														
Chicken Fried Rice Kit w/ Sauce	1 pkg (14 oz)	440	6	2	30	27	69	15	5	40	1810	—	—	0
WEIGHT WATCHERS														
Smart Ones Chicken Chow Mein	1 pkg (9 oz)	200	2	1	25	12	34	5	3	20	570	—	—	5

FOOD	PORTION	CALS	FAT	SAT FAT	CHOL	PROT	CARB	SUGAR	FIBER	CALCI	SOD	POTAS	FOLIC	VIT C
WEIGHT WATCHERS (CONT.)														
Smart Ones Hunan Style Rice & Vegetables	1 pkg (10.34 oz)	280	0	2	0	7	45	4	5	40	630	—	—	9
Smart Ones Kung Pao Noodles & Vegetables	1 pkg (10 oz)	250	8	1	5	8	37	12	5	60	650	—	—	1
Smart Ones Spicy Szechuan Style Vegetables & Chicken	1 pkg (9 oz)	220	2	1	10	11	39	1	3	150	730	—	—	2
MIX														
ANNIE CHUN'S														
Meal Kit Black Bean	1 serv	230	3	0	0	8	42	8	2	0	670	—	—	5
Meal Kit Garlic Scallion	1 serv	230	5	1	0	7	39	6	2	20	780	—	—	9
Meal Kit Soy Ginger	1 serv	220	2	0	0	8	42	9	3	20	850	—	—	2
TAKE-OUT														
buddha's delight w/ cellophane noodles fat choi jai	1 serv (7.6 oz)	211	4	1	tr	7	44	3	2	77	772	986	36	59
cashew chicken	1 serv	406	29	5	61	—	—	—	—	—	988	—	—	—
cha siu bao steamed buns w/ chicken filling	1 (2.3 oz)	160	3	1	15	5	26	4	tr	0	300	—	—	0
chop suey cantonese chicken	1 serv	570	17	3	70	—	—	—	—	—	1070	—	—	—
chop suey w/ beef & pork	1 cup	300	17	4	68	26	13	—	—	81	1053	425	—	33
chop suey w/ pork	1 cup	375	29	8	62	19	29	—	2	36	1378	584	24	58
chow mein chicken	1 cup	255	10	4	75	31	10	—	—	58	718	473	—	10
chow mein pork	1 cup	425	24	8	89	32	21	—	3	75	1673	1050	27	15
chow mein shrimp	1 cup	221	10	1	55	13	21	—	3	105	1658	701	28	15
chow mein vegetable	1 serv (8 oz)	90	3	0	0	3	15	2	4	40	1010	—	—	9
filipino chicken adobo	1 serv (15 oz)	555	26	7	116	33	45	tr	1	56	468	366	15	3
fried rice chicken	1 serv	314	89	1	5	—	—	—	—	—	972	—	—	—
fried rice vegetable	1 cup	210	9	1	0	3	30	3	1	10	520	—	—	6

FOOD	PORTION	CALS	FAT	SAT FAT	CHOL	PROT	CARB	SUGAR	FIBER	CALCI	SOD	POTAS	FOLIC	VIT C
TAKE-OUT (CONT.)														
fried rice w/ egg	6.7 oz	395	20	—	—	8	49	—	2	25	—	—	—	tr
general tsao's chicken	1 serv	723	35	5	143	—	—	—	—	—	1775	—	—	—
kung pao chicken	1 cup	409	29	5	60	—	—	—	—	—	988	—	—	—
kung pao chicken w/ rice	1 serv (1.75 cups)	240	3	1	25	12	42	3	4	40	800	—	—	18
lo mein pork	1 serv	323	40	1	7	—	—	—	—	—	1337	—	—	—
moo goo gai pan chicken	1 cup	272	35	4	31	—	—	—	—	—	305	—	—	—
phad thai	1 serv (9.2 oz)	232	9	1	0	11	30	2	1	111	426	282	27	21
sesame seed paste bun	1 (2.5 oz)	220	6	1	0	5	39	12	2	125	53	—	—	0
shrimp & snow peas	1 cup	220	148	2	12	—	—	—	—	—	1067	—	—	—
shrimp chips	1¼ cups (1 oz)	140	6	3	0	2	19	1	0	40	240	—	—	0
shu mai chicken & vegetable dumplings	6 (3.6 oz)	160	5	1	35	10	18	6	1	20	910	—	—	5
soba noodles w/ vegetables	1 serv	276	39	2	8	—	—	—	—	—	1092	—	—	—
spring roll	1 (3.5 oz)	112	2	—	—	12	37	—	5	54	670	244	—	—
stir fry beef & broccoli	2 cups	512	202	10	39	—	—	—	—	—	1473	—	—	—
stir fry garlic green beans	1 serv	68	0	0	1	—	—	—	—	—	357	—	—	—
stir fry vegetable	1 serv	235	70	2	11	—	—	—	—	—	1900	—	—	—
sweet & sour chicken w/o rice	1 serv	416	95	1	6	—	—	—	—	—	442	—	—	—
sweet & sour pork	1 serv (8 oz)	250	8	3	30	6	37	30	2	20	1500	—	—	9
sweet red bean bun	1 (2.5 oz)	130	1	0	0	4	38	17	2	40	95	—	—	0
szechuan chicken w/ lo mein	1 cup (5.3 oz)	190	1	0	5	10	35	3	0	20	560	—	—	1
szechuan cold noodles	1 serv	334	0	1	7	—	—	—	—	—	1531	—	—	—
tempura seafood & vegetable	1 serv	590	185	6	32	—	—	—	—	—	1660	—	—	—
tempura vegetables	5 pieces (4 oz)	270	15	3	0	2	31	3	2	40	210	—	—	1
teriyaki beef w/ sticky rice	1 serv	664	105	—	14	—	—	—	—	—	898	—	—	—
teriyaki chicken plain	¾ cup	399	27	6	92	30	7	—	—	39	2190	511	14	tr

FOOD	PORTION	CALS	FAT	SAT FAT	CHOL	PROT	CARB	SUGAR	FIBER	CALCI	SOD	POTAS	FOLIC	VIT C
TAKE-OUT (CONT.)														
teriyaki chicken w/ rice	1 serv (11 oz)	430	6	1	25	19	77	10	1	60	1210	—	—	12
wonton fried	½ cup (1 oz)	111	8	1	31	2	8	—	1	10	147	33	5	1

ASPARAGUS

FOOD	PORTION	CALS	FAT	SAT FAT	CHOL	PROT	CARB	SUGAR	FIBER	CALCI	SOD	POTAS	FOLIC	VIT C
CANNED														
spears	½ cup	23	1	tr	0	3	3	—	2	19	347	208	116	22
DEL MONTE														
Cuts & Tips	½ cup (4.4 oz)	20	0	0	0	2	3	0	1	0	420	—	—	15
Spears Extra Long	½ cup (4.4 oz)	20	0	0	0	2	3	0	1	0	420	—	—	15
Spears Tender Young	½ cup (4.4 oz)	20	0	0	0	2	3	0	1	0	420	—	—	15
Tips Hand Selected	½ cup (4.4 oz)	20	0	0	0	2	3	0	1	0	420	—	—	15
GREEN GIANT														
Cut Spears	½ cup (4.2 oz)	20	0	0	0	2	3	tr	1	0	420	—	—	9
Cut Spears 50% Less Sodium	½ cup (4.2 oz)	20	0	0	0	2	3	tr	1	0	210	—	—	9
Extra Long Spears	4.5 oz	20	0	0	0	2	3	tr	1	0	400	—	—	12
Spears	4.5 oz	20	0	0	0	2	3	tr	1	0	450	—	—	12
LESUEUR														
Spears Extra Large	4.5 oz	20	0	0	0	2	3	tr	1	0	440	—	—	12
S&W														
Green	6 pieces (4.5 oz)	15	0	0	0	2	4	1	1	0	260	130	—	21
FRESH														
cooked	4 spears	14	tr	tr	0	2	3	—	1	12	7	96	88	7
cooked	½ cup	22	tr	tr	0	2	4	—	1	18	10	144	132	18
raw	½ cup	16	tr	tr	0	2	3	—	1	14	2	183	86	9
raw	4 spears	15	tr	tr	0	tr	1	—	tr	3	0	44	20	2
FROZEN														
cooked	1 pkg (10 oz)	82	1	tr	0	9	14	—	5	68	12	640	395	72
cooked	4 spears	17	tr	tr	0	2	3	—	1	14	2	131	81	15
BIRDS EYE														
Cuts	½ cup	25	0	0	0	—	—	—	2	20	5	—	—	24
Jumbo Spears	3 oz	20	0	0	0	—	—	—	1	0	5	—	—	21
GREEN GIANT														
Harvest Fresh Cuts	⅔ cup (3 oz)	25	0	0	0	2	4	tr	1	0	85	—	—	12

ATEMOYA

FOOD	PORTION	CALS	FAT	SAT FAT	CHOL	PROT	CARB	SUGAR	FIBER	CALCI	SOD	POTAS	FOLIC	VIT C
fresh	½ cup	94	1	—	—	1	24	—	—	—	2	314	—	9

AVOCADO

FOOD	PORTION	CALS	FAT	SAT FAT	CHOL	PROT	CARB	SUGAR	FIBER	CALCI	SOD	POTAS	FOLIC	VIT C
fresh mashed	1 cup	407	40	6	0	5	16	—	11	25	28	1458	152	18
fresh peeled california	1	306	30	4	0	4	12	—	9	19	21	1097	114	14
fresh peeled florida	1	340	27	5	0	5	27	—	16	33	15	1484	161	24

FOOD	PORTION	CALS	FAT	SAT FAT	CHOL	PROT	CARB	SUGAR	FIBER	CALCI	SOD	POTAS	FOLIC	VIT C
BROOKS TROPICAL														
Lite SlimCado	1 tbsp	35	3	1	0	0	3	0	tr	0	—	—	—	2
CHIQUITA														
Fresh	⅓ med (1 oz)	55	5	1	0	1	3	0	3	0	0	—	—	2
TAKE-OUT														
guacamole	1 serv (2.2 oz)	105	10	1	0	1	5	1	2	9	187	378	38	7
BACON														
breakfast strips cooked	3 strips	156	12	4	36	10	tr	—	0	5	714	—	1	0
gammon lean & fat grilled	4.2 oz	274	15	—	—	35	0	—	0	11	—	—	—	0
pan fried	3 strips	109	9	3	16	6	tr	—	0	2	303	—	1	0
ARMOUR														
Star cooked	1 strip	38	3	—	6	—	—	—	—	—	185	—	—	—
BLACK LABEL														
Center Cut cooked	3 slices (0.5 oz)	70	6	2	15	5	0	0	0	0	260	—	—	0
Cooked	2 slices (0.5 oz)	80	7	3	15	5	0	0	0	0	330	—	—	0
Low Salt cooked	2 slices (0.5 oz)	80	7	3	15	5	0	0	0	0	230	—	—	0
HEALTH IS WEALTH														
Uncured Sliced	2 slices (0.5 oz)	70	7	3	10	3	0	—	—	—	380	—	—	—
HORMEL														
Bacon Bits	1 tbsp (7 g)	30	2	1	5	3	0	0	0	0	250	—	—	0
Bacon Pieces	1 tbsp (7 g)	25	2	1	10	3	0	0	0	0	180	—	—	0
Microwave cooked	2 slices (0.5 oz)	70	5	2	15	5	0	0	0	0	230	—	—	0
OLD SMOKEHOUSE														
Cooked	2 slices (0.5 oz)	80	7	3	15	5	0	0	0	0	280	—	—	0
OSCAR MAYER														
Bacon Bits	1 tbsp (0.2 oz)	25	2	1	5	3	0	0	0	0	220	—		0
Bacon Pieces	1 tbsp (0.2 oz)	25	2	1	5	2	0	0	0	0	170	—	—	0
Center Cut cooked	2 slices (0.4 oz)	70	5	2	15	4	0	0	0	0	270	—	—	0
Cooked	2 slices (0.5 oz)	70	6	2	15	4	0	0	0	0	290	—	—	0
Lower Sodium cooked	2 slices (0.5 oz)	70	5	2	15	5	1	0	0	0	200	—	—	0
Thick Cut cooked	1 slice (0.4 oz)	60	5	2	10	4	0	0	0	0	250	—	—	0
RANGE BRAND														
Cooked	2 slices (0.7 oz)	100	9	4	20	7	0	0	0	0	460	—	—	0
READY CRISP														
Fully Cooked	3 slices (0.5 oz)	70	6	3	15	4	0	—	—	—	270	—	—	—
RED LABEL														
Cooked	2 slices (0.5 oz)	80	7	3	15	5	0	0	0	0	330	—	—	0
BACON SUBSTITUTES														
meatless	1 strip	16	1	tr	0	1	tr	—	tr	1	73	9	2	0

FOOD	PORTION	CALS	FAT	SAT FAT	CHOL	PROT	CARB	SUGAR	FIBER	CALCI	SOD	POTAS	FOLIC	VIT C
BAC-OS														
Chips or Bits	1½ tbsp (7 g)	30	2	0	0	3	2	0	0	0	120	120	—	0
LIGHTLIFE														
Fakin' Bacon Bits	1 tsp	45	1	0	0	1	1	0	0	—	25	—	—	—
Smart Bacon	2 strips (0.8 oz)	45	2	0	0	6	2	0	0	—	360	—	—	—
LOUIS RICH														
Turkey Bacon	1 slice (0.5 oz)	35	3	1	15	2	0	0	0	0	180	—	—	0
MORNINGSTAR FARMS														
Breakfast Strips	2 (0.5 oz)	60	5	1	0	2	2	0	tr	0	220	15	—	0
WORTHINGTON														
Stripples	2 strips (0.5 oz)	60	5	1	0	2	2	0	tr	0	220	15	—	0

BAGEL

FOOD	PORTION	CALS	FAT	SAT FAT	CHOL	PROT	CARB	SUGAR	FIBER	CALCI	SOD	POTAS	FOLIC	VIT C
cinnamon raisin	1 lg	359	2	tr	0	13	72	—	3	25	422	194	118	1
cinnamon raisin toasted	1 lg	363	2	tr	0	13	73	—	3	25	426	200	95	1
egg	1 mini	72	1	tr	6	3	14	—	1	3	131	18	23	tr
egg	1 lg	364	3	1	31	14	69	—	3	17	662	89	115	1
mini onion	1 (1.4 oz)	100	0	0	0	4	20	1	1	20	90	—	—	0
oat bran	1 lg	334	2	tr	0	14	70	—	5	16	664	151	106	tr
onion	1 lg	363	2	tr	0	13	71	—	3	98	706	134	92	0
plain	1 mini	72	tr	tr	0	3	14	—	1	19	139	26	23	0
plain	1 lg	360	2	tr	0	13	70	—	3	57	700	132	115	0
poppy seed	1 lg	360	2	tr	0	14	70	—	3	97	700	132	115	0
ATKINS														
Cinnamon Raisin	1	200	4	1	0	20	20	1	11	60	290	—	0	4
Onion	1	190	5	1	0	19	19	3	11	60	290	—	0	1
Plain	1	190	5	1	0	20	18	0	11	40	310	—	0	0
NATURAL OVENS														
Blueberry	1 (3 oz)	190	2	0	0	9	40	10	4	200	220	—	160	0
Brainy	1 (3 oz)	170	2	0	0	8	35	6	6	200	270	—	160	0
Cinnamon Raisin	1 (3 oz)	180	1	0	0	9	40	9	5	200	240	—	160	0
Golden Crunch	1 (3 oz)	190	11	0	0	15	15	5	8	200	200	—	120	0
Hearty Grains & Onion	1 (3 oz)	190	4	1	0	10	37	6	7	200	250	—	160	0
Whole Grain	1 (3 oz)	170	3	0	0	9	35	6	6	200	200	—	160	0
OTIS SPUNKMEYER														
Barnstormin' Blueberry	1 (3.6 oz)	250	3	0	0	10	50	6	3	60	390	—	—	0
Barnstormin' Cinnamon Raisin	1 (3.6 oz)	230	2	0	0	9	47	6	3	60	370	—	—	0
Barnstormin' Onion	1 (3.6 oz)	230	2	0	0	9	47	6	3	60	370	—	—	0
Barnstormin' Plain	1 (3.6 oz)	240	3	0	0	10	49	5	3	60	390	—	—	0

FOOD	PORTION	CALS	FAT	SAT FAT	CHOL	PROT	CARB	SUGAR	FIBER	CALCI	SOD	POTAS	FOLIC	VIT C
PEPPERIDGE FARM														
Mini	1 (1.4 oz)	110	1	0	0	4	22	4	1	20	200	—	—	0
Plain	1 (3.5 oz)	290	1	0	0	11	60	6	2	150	480	—	—	0
SARA LEE														
Blueberry	1 (2.8 oz)	210	1	0	0	8	41	5	2	20	570	—	—	0
Cinnamon Raisin	1 (2.8 oz)	220	1	0	0	8	45	12	3	20	320	—	—	0
Egg	1 (2.8 oz)	210	1	1	0	7	44	7	2	—	460	—	—	0
Oat Bran	1 (2.8 oz)	210	1	0	0	8	42	7	3	—	570	—	—	—
Onion	1 (2.8 oz)	210	0	0	0	7	44	6	2	—	540	—	—	—
Plain	1 (2.8 oz)	210	1	1	0	8	43	3	2	—	500	—	—	0
Poppy Seed	1 (2.8 oz)	210	1	0	0	8	41	5	2	20	570	—	—	0
Sesame Seed	1 (2.8 oz)	210	2	1	0	8	42	5	2	—	530	—	—	0
THOMAS'														
Carb Counting Whole Wheat	1 (2.2 oz)	140	2	1	0	11	22	tr	6	60	330	—	—	0
Everything	1 (3.6 oz)	300	4	1	0	10	56	7	3	100	510	—	—	0
Multi-Grain	1 (3.6 oz)	280	2	1	0	11	55	7	4	80	460	—	—	0
Plain	1 (3.6 oz)	280	2	1	0	10	56	7	2	80	530	—	—	0
UNCLE B'S														
Plain	1 (2.8 oz)	210	1	0	0	8	41	4	2	60	310	—	—	1
WEIGHT WATCHERS														
Original	1 (2.8 oz)	190	2	1	0	10	44	3	10	80	520	—	60	0
WONDER														
Blueberry	1 (3 oz)	210	1	1	0	7	43	9	1	40	450	—	—	0
Cinnamon Raisin	1 (3 oz)	210	1	0	0	8	42	9	2	40	360	—	—	0
Onion	1 (3 oz)	210	1	0	0	8	43	5	1	20	340	—	—	0
Plain	1 (3 oz)	210	1	0	0	8	43	5	2	20	350	—	—	0
Rye	1 (3 oz)	220	1	0	0	9	42	1	2	60	520	—	—	0
Wheat	1 (3 oz)	210	1	0	0	8	43	5	2	20	350	—	—	0
BAKING POWDER														
baking powder	1 tsp	2	0	0	0	0	1	—	—	270	488	1	0	0
low sodium	1 tsp	5	0	0	0	0	2	—	—	217	4	505	0	0
CALUMET														
Baking Powder	¼ tsp (1 g)	0	0	0	0	0	0	0	0	60	100	0	—	0
CLABBER GIRL														
Baking Powder	1 tsp	0	0	0	0	tr	1	—	—	84	435	tr	—	—
DAVIS														
Baking Powder	1 tsp	0	0	0	0	0	0	0	—	80	380	—	—	—
RUMFORD														
Aluminum Free	⅛ tsp	0	0	0	0	0	tr	—	—	80	110	—	—	—
BAKING SODA														
baking soda	1 tsp	0	0	0	0	0	0	—	—	0	1259	0	0	0

FOOD	PORTION	CALS	FAT	SAT FAT	CHOL	PROT	CARB	SUGAR	FIBER	CALCI	SOD	POTAS	FOLIC	VIT C
BALSAM PEAR (BITTER GOURD)														
leafy tips cooked	½ cup	10	tr	—	0	1	2	—	1	12	4	174	26	16
leafy tips raw	½ cup	7	tr	—	0	1	1	—	—	20	3	145	31	21
pods cooked	½ cup	12	tr	—	0	1	3	—	1	6	4	198	32	21
BAMBOO SHOOTS														
canned sliced	1 cup	25	1	tr	0	2	4	—	2	10	9	104	4	1
fresh	½ cup	21	tr	tr	0	2	1	—	2	10	3	405	6	3
fresh cooked	½ cup	12	tr	tr	0	1	2	—	—	5	5	52	2	1
CHUN KING														
Bamboo Shoots	2 tbsp (0.8 oz)	3	tr	0	0	tr	1	tr	tr	tr	0	—	—	0
LA CHOY														
Bamboo Shoots	2 tbsp (0.8 oz)	3	tr	0	0	tr	1	tr	tr	tr	0	—	—	0
BANANA														
banana chips	1 oz	147	10	8	0	1	17	—	2	5	2	152	4	2
fresh	1 med	109	tr	tr	0	1	28	—	3	7	1	467	22	11
fresh mashed	1 cup	207	1	tr	0	2	53	—	5	13	2	890	43	20
fresh sliced	1 cup	138	1	tr	0	2	35	—	4	9	2	594	29	14
powder	1 tbsp	21	tr	tr	0	tr	5	—	1	1	0	92	1	tr
whole dried	1 piece (1.2 oz)	130	1	0	0	1	33	22	2	0	0	—	—	0
CHIQUITA														
Fresh	1 med (4.4 oz)	110	0	0	0	1	29	21	4	—	0	400	—	9
RAINFOREST FARMS														
Slices Dried	5 slices (1.3 oz)	60	0	0	0	1	12	10	—	—	10	—	—	15
BARBECUE SAUCE														
barbecue	1 cup	188	5	1	0	5	32	—	—	48	2038	436	—	18
ATKINS														
Barbecue Sauce	1 tbsp	15	1	0	0	0	tr	0	0	—	180	—	—	—
BULL'S EYE														
Original	2 tbsp	50	0	—	0	—	—	—	—	tr	—	—	—	—
CARB OPTIONS														
Original	2 tbsp	10	0	0	0	0	3	0	0	—	340	—	—	—
HOUSE OF TSANG														
Hong Kong	1 tbsp (0.6 oz)	10	0	0	0	0	2	1	0	0	150	—	—	0
HUNT'S														
Hickory	2 tbsp	45	0	0	0	0	11	9	tr	0	290	75	—	0
Hickory & Brown Sugar	2 tbsp	70	0	0	0	0	16	15	1	20	360	100	—	0
Honey Hickory	2 tbsp (1.2 oz)	50	0	0	0	0	12	11	tr	0	380	100	—	0
Honey Mustard	2 tbsp	50	0	0	0	0	12	10	1	0	310	85	—	0
Hot & Spicy	2 tbsp	45	0	0	0	0	11	8	tr	0	440	90	—	0
Mesquite	2 tbsp	40	0	0	0	0	9	6	tr	0	360	75	—	0
Original	2 tbsp	45	0	0	0	1	11	9	tr	0	290	75	—	0

FOOD	PORTION	CALS	FAT	SAT FAT	CHOL	PROT	CARB	SUGAR	FIBER	CALCI	SOD	POTAS	FOLIC	VIT C
KRAFT														
Char-Grill	2 tbsp (1.3 oz)	60	0	0	0	0	13	11	0	0	460	45	—	0
Extra Rich Original	2 tbsp (1.2 oz)	50	0	0	0	0	12	10	0	0	440	45	—	0
Hickory Smoke	2 tbsp (1.2 oz)	40	0	0	0	0	9	7	0	0	420	30	—	0
Hickory Smoke Onion Bits	2 tbsp (1.2 oz)	45	0	0	0	0	11	9	0	0	360	25	—	0
Honey	2 tbsp (1.3 oz)	50	0	0	0	0	13	11	0	0	360	25	—	0
Honey Hickory	2 tbsp (1.3 oz)	60	0	0	0	0	14	12	0	0	370	30	—	0
Honey Mustard	2 tbsp (1.3 oz)	60	0	0	0	0	13	12	0	0	300	30	—	0
Hot	2 tbsp (1.2 oz)	40	0	0	0	0	9	7	0	0	520	25	—	0
Hot Hickory Smoke	2 tbsp (1.2 oz)	40	0	0	0	0	9	7	0	0	380	35	—	0
Kansas City Style	2 tbsp (1.2 oz)	50	0	0	0	0	11	9	0	0	310	100	—	0
Mesquite Smoke	2 tbsp (1.2 oz)	40	0	0	0	0	9	7	0	0	420	30	—	0
Molasses	2 tbsp (1.3 oz)	70	0	0	0	0	16	14	0	20	390	105	—	0
Onion Bits	2 tbsp (1.2 oz)	45	0	0	0	0	11	9	0	0	360	30	—	0
Original	2 tbsp (1.2 oz)	40	0	0	0	0	9	7	0	0	420	30	—	0
Roasted Garlic	2 tbsp (1.2 oz)	50	0	0	0	0	12	10	0	0	360	40	—	0
Spicy Honey	2 tbsp (1.3 oz)	60	0	0	0	0	14	13	0	0	360	25	—	0
Teriyaki	2 tbsp (1.3 oz)	60	1	0	0	tr	12	10	0	0	440	80	—	0
Thick'N Spicy Brown Sugar	2 tbsp (1.2 oz)	60	0	0	0	0	15	13	0	0	350	60	—	0
Thick'N Spicy Hickory Bacon	2 tbsp (1.2 oz)	60	1	0	0	0	13	11	0	0	570	45	—	0
Thick'N Spicy Hickory Smoke	2 tbsp (1.2 oz)	50	0	0	0	0	12	10	0	0	450	40	—	0
Thick'N Spicy Honey	2 tbsp (1.3 oz)	60	0	0	0	0	13	11	0	0	360	80	—	0
Thick'N Spicy Honey Mustard	2 tbsp (1.3 oz)	60	0	0	0	0	14	12	0	0	310	50	—	0
Thick'N Spicy Kansas City Style	2 tbsp (1.3 oz)	60	0	0	0	0	14	12	0	0	310	110	—	0
Thick'N Spicy Mesquite Smoke	2 tbsp (1.2 oz)	50	0	0	0	0	12	10	0	0	440	40	—	0
MCILHENNY														
Sauce	2 tbsp (1.1 oz)	70	5	1	0	tr	6	3	tr	0	290	—	—	0
MUIR GLEN														
Garlic Mesquite	2 tbsp (1.3 oz)	40	0	0	0	0	6	6	tr	20	265	—	—	5
Hot & Smoky	2 tbsp (1.2 oz)	40	0	0	0	0	6	6	tr	20	265	—	—	5
Original	2 tbsp (1.2 oz)	40	0	0	0	0	6	6	tr	20	265	—	—	5
STEEL'S														
Sugar Free	2 tbsp	15	0	0	0	0	2	0	0	—	200	—	—	—
BARLEY														
flour	1 cup	511	2	tr	0	15	110	—	15	47	6	457	12	0
malt flour	1 cup	585	3	1	0	17	127	—	12	60	18	363	62	1

FOOD	PORTION	CALS	FAT	SAT FAT	CHOL	PROT	CARB	SUGAR	FIBER	CALCI	SOD	POTAS	FOLIC	VIT C
pearled cooked	1 cup (5.5 oz)	193	1	tr	0	4	44	—	6	17	5	146	25	0
pearled uncooked	1 cup	704	2	tr	0	20	155	—	31	58	18	560	46	0
MOTHER'S														
Quick Cooking	⅓ cup	170	1	0	0	5	37	—	5	—	0	—	—	—

BARRACUDA
fresh	3 oz	122	8	—	66	14	0	0	0	11	57	234	—	0

BASIL
fresh chopped	2 tbsp	1	tr	tr	0	tr	tr	—	tr	8	0	24	3	1
ground	1 tsp	4	tr	—	0	tr	1	—	—	30	tr	48	—	1
leaves fresh	5	1	tr	tr	0	tr	tr	—	tr	4	0	12	2	1

BASS
freshwater raw	3 oz	97	3	1	58	16	0	—	—	68	59	303	—	—
sea cooked	3 oz	105	2	1	45	20	0	—	—	11	74	279	—	—
sea raw	3 oz	82	2	tr	35	16	0	—	—	9	58	218	—	—
striped baked	3 oz	105	3	1	87	19	0	—	—	—	75	—	—	—
striped bass farm raised	4 oz	110	3	1	90	20	0	0	0	20	80	—	—	0

BAY LEAF
crumbled	1 tsp	2	tr	tr	0	tr	tr	—	—	5	tr	3	—	tr

BEAN SPROUTS
(*see* ALFALFA, SPROUTS)

BEANS
(*see also individual names*)

CANNED
baked beans plain	½ cup	118	1	tr	0	6	26	—	6	64	504	376	30	4
baked beans vegetarian	½ cup	118	1	tr	0	6	26	—	6	64	504	376	30	4
baked beans w/ beef	½ cup	161	5	2	29	8	22	—	—	60	632	426	57	2
baked beans w/ franks	½ cup	184	9	3	8	9	20	—	9	61	551	301	39	3
baked beans w/ pork	½ cup	134	2	1	9	7	25	—	7	66	522	389	46	3
baked beans w/ pork & sweet sauce	½ cup	140	2	1	9	7	26	—	7	77	423	335	47	4
baked beans w/ pork & tomato sauce	½ cup	124	1	tr	9	7	24	—	7	70	554	378	28	4
refried beans	½ cup	134	1	1	—	8	23	—	—	59	534	495	—	8
AMY'S														
Vegetarian Baked	½ cup	120	5	1	0	5	24	9	6	—	480	—	—	—
B&M														
Barbeque Baked Beans	½ cup (4.6 oz)	210	1	0	0	8	42	19	9	60	570	—	—	4
Maple Baked	½ cup	150	1	0	0	6	28	12	6	40	340	—	—	0

FOOD	PORTION	CALS	FAT	SAT FAT	CHOL	PROT	CARB	SUGAR	FIBER	CALCI	SOD	POTAS	FOLIC	VIT C
B&M (CONT.)														
Vegetarian 99% Fat Free	½ cup	150	1	0	0	6	28	12	6	40	340	—	—	0
BUSH'S														
Barbecue	½ cup (4.6 oz)	160	1	0	0	6	32	13	6	60	510	—	—	0
Country Style	½ cup	170	1	0	0	7	33	16	7	60	680	—	—	1
Homestyle	½ cup	150	2	0	5	6	28	8	8	40	480	—	—	0
Maple Cured Bacon	½ cup	150	1	1	0	7	28	11	7	60	620	—	—	1
Original	½ cup	150	1	0	0	7	29	5	7	60	550	—	—	0
Vegetarian	½ cup (4.6 oz)	130	0	0	0	6	24	4	6	40	550	—	—	1
CAMPBELL'S														
Pork & Beans	½ cup	140	1	1	<5	6	27	9	7	40	460	—	—	0
CHI-CHI'S														
Refried	½ cup (4.2 oz)	100	1	0	0	5	18	1	4	20	580	—	—	0
Refried Beans Fat Free	½ cup (4.2 oz)	120	0	0	0	5	17	1	4	20	570			0
Refried Beans Vegetarian	½ cup (4.2 oz)	100	1	0	0	5	18	1	4	20	580	—	—	0
EDEN														
Organic Baked w/ Sorghum & Mustard	½ cup (4.6 oz)	150	0	0	0	8	27	6	7	100	130	460	0	0
GEBHARDT														
Chili	½ cup (4.6 oz)	134	1	tr	0	7	31	1	7	64	630	—	—	2
Refried Jalapeño	½ cup (4.5 oz)	105	3	1	1	7	19	3	6	4	380	—	—	0
Refried No Fat	½ cup (4.5 oz)	92	tr	0	0	7	20	2	6	43	480	—	—	0
Refried Traditional	½ cup (4.5 oz)	109	3	1	1	6	20	2	6	43	497	—	—	0
Refried Vegetarian	½ cup (4.5 oz)	118	2	tr	tr	8	21	3	7	41	550	—	—	0
GREEN GIANT														
Pork And Beans w/ Tomato Sauce	½ cup (4.5 oz)	120	1	0	0	5	23	4	4	60	490	—	—	0
Spicy Chili	½ cup (4.5 oz)	110	1	0	0	6	20	1	5	40	490	—	—	0
Three Bean Salad	½ cup (4.2 oz)	90	0	0	0	3	20	10	4	60	490	—	—	0
HEALTH VALLEY														
Honey Baked	½ cup	110	0	0	0	7	25	11	7	40	135	—	—	12
Honey Baked No Salt	½ cup	110	0	0	0	7	25	11	7	40	25	—	—	12
HEINZ														
Vegetarian	1 cup	250	1	0	0	11	48	24	9	100	840	—	—	0
HORMEL														
Beans & Wieners	1 can (7.5 oz)	290	12	4	50	11	34	12	6	60	1310	—	—	0
HUNT'S														
Big John's Beans & Fixin's	½ cup (4.7 oz)	127	4	1	3	7	23	11	6	72	590	—	—	3

FOOD	PORTION	CALS	FAT	SAT FAT	CHOL	PROT	CARB	SUGAR	FIBER	CALCI	SOD	POTAS	FOLIC	VIT C
HUNTS (CONT.)														
Homestyle Country Kettle	½ cup (4.6 oz)	152	2	1	1	7	31	11	7	85	425	—	—	4
Homestyle Special Recipe	½ cup (4.7 oz)	185	3	1	1	7	36	22	8	91	687	—	—	11
Mix & Serve	½ cup (4.7 oz)	125	3	1	1	2	30	16	8	74	575	—	—	2
Pork & Beans	½ cup (4.5 oz)	130	1	tr	tr	6	28	16	4	45	516	—	—	2
Pork & Beans	½ cup (4.6 oz)	157	5	2	2	6	27	11	7	73	621	—	—	4
KID'S KITCHEN														
Microwave Meals Beans & Weiners	1 cup (7.5 oz)	310	13	5	45	13	37	13	8	80	760	—	—	6
OLD EL PASO														
Refried Fat Free	½ cup	100	0	0	0	6	18	1	6	40	580	—	—	0
OPEN RANGE														
Ranch	½ cup (4.4 oz)	124	3	1	1	6	23	5	8	55	628	—	—	2
PRINGLES														
Vegetarian	1 cup (7.9 oz)	250	1	0	0	11	48	24	9	100	840	—	—	0
ROSARITA														
3 Bean Recipe Bacon & Jalapeño	½ cup (4.6 oz)	117	2	0	1	8	22	1	5	49	543	—	—	4
3 Bean Recipe Chiles & Chicken	½ cup (4.6 oz)	115	1	0	1	7	22	3	4	44	517	—	—	4
3 Bean Recipe Chilies & Chorizo	½ cup (4.6 oz)	111	2	0	1	8	19	3	4	47	591	—	—	7
3 Bean Recipe Onions & Peppers	½ cup (4.6 oz)	104	1	0	1	7	20	2	5	48	539	—	—	3
Fiesta Beans Bacon & Jalapeños	½ cup (4.6 oz)	117	2	0	1	8	22	1	5	49	543	—	—	4
Fiesta Beans Chicken & Chilies	½ cup (4.6 oz)	115	1	0	1	7	22	3	4	44	517	—	—	4
Fiesta Beans Chilies & Chorizo	½ cup (4.6 oz)	110	2	0	1	8	19	3	4	47	591	—	—	7
Fiesta Beans Onions & Peppers	½ cup (4.6 oz)	104	1	0	1	8	20	2	5	48	539	—	—	3
Refried Bacon	½ cup (4.5 oz)	116	3	1	1	6	19	2	8	42	489	—	—	1
Refried Green Chile	½ cup (4.5 oz)	110	3	2	1	6	20	2	7	41	495	—	—	1
Refried Low Fat Black	½ cup (4.5 oz)	107	1	0	0	8	23	tr	7	65	569	—	—	0

FOOD	PORTION	CALS	FAT	SAT FAT	CHOL	PROT	CARB	SUGAR	FIBER	CALCI	SOD	POTAS	FOLIC	VIT C
ROSARITA (CONT.)														
Refried Nacho Cheese	½ cup (4.5 oz)	108	2	1	2	8	19	1	6	46	574	—	—	0
Refried No Fat	½ cup	90	0	0	0	7	17	tr	5	40	590	—	—	—
Refried No Fat Green Chiles & Lime	½ cup (4.5 oz)	101	tr	0	0	8	22	1	8	58	565	—	—	3
Refried No Fat w/ Zesty Salsa	½ cup (4.5 oz)	105	tr	0	0	6	24	1	6	62	599	—	—	2
Refried Onion	½ cup (4.5 oz)	114	3	1	1	6	21	2	6	46	508	—	—	1
Refried Spicy	½ cup (4.5 oz)	118	3	1	0	7	22	2	6	46	574	—	—	0
Refried Traditional	½ cup (4.5 oz)	108	1	1	0	5	19	1	5	32	510	—	—	0
Refried Vegetarian	½ cup (4.5 oz)	237	5	1	tr	15	42	6	13	80	1101	—	—	0
S&W														
Barbecue Beans Ranch Recipe	½ cup (4.5 oz)	100	2	1	0	6	25	9	8	40	640	500	—	5
TACO BELL														
Home Originals Fat Free Refried Beans	½ cup (4.6 oz)	110	0	0	0	7	21	1	6	40	460	—	—	0
Home Originals Fat Free Refried Beans w/ Mild Chilies	½ cup (4.5 oz)	110	0	0	0	7	20	tr	5	40	480	—	—	0
Home Originals Refried Beans	½ cup (4.7 oz)	140	3	1	0	5	23	1	7	40	530	—	—	0
VAN CAMP														
Baked Fat Free	½ cup (4.6 oz)	132	tr	tr	0	6	29	11	5	4	505	—	—	tr
Baked Original	½ cup	140	1	0	0	7	30	12	6	60	540	—	—	0
Baked Southern Style Sauteed Onion	½ cup (4.8 oz)	145	1	tr	1	6	35	18	8	67	555	—	—	0
Baked Sweet Hickory & Bacon	1 can (4.8 oz)	143	1	tr	tr	6	32	14	6	66	471	—	—	0
Beanee Weenee Baked	1 cup (9.1 oz)	410	14	4	40	18	58	25	10	80	1210	—	—	0
Beanee Weenee BBQ	1 cup (7.7 oz)	290	12	3	35	14	36	12	7	60	970	—	—	5
Beanee Weenee Microwave	1 cup (7.5 oz)	260	11	3	35	14	29	8	6	40	1020	—	—	4
Beanee Weenee Original	1 cup (9.1 oz)	320	14	4	40	16	35	10	8	60	1240	—	—	5
Beanee Weenee Zestful	1 cup (7.7 oz)	300	12	3	35	14	40	16	7	60	1030	—	—	4
Brown Sugar	½ cup (4.6 oz)	170	3	1	5	7	31	13	6	40	410	—	—	0
Pork And Beans	½ cup (4.6 oz)	110	2	1	0	6	23	7	6	40	490	—	—	1
Vegetarian	½ cup (4.6 oz)	110	1	0	0	6	23	7	5	40	400	—	—	0

FOOD	PORTION	CALS	FAT	SAT FAT	CHOL	PROT	CARB	SUGAR	FIBER	CALCI	SOD	POTAS	FOLIC	VIT C
FROZEN														
NATURAL TOUCH														
Nine Bean Loaf	1 in slice (3 oz)	160	8	2	<5	8	13	tr	5	40	350	190	—	1
MIX														
MELTING POT														
Terrazza Napoli Mixed Beans	1 cup	200	2	0	<5	9	41	7	2	20	460	—	—	6
TAKE-OUT														
baked beans	½ cup	161	5	2	29	8	22	—	—	60	632	426	57	2
barbecue beans	3.5 oz	120	tr	tr	0	4	26	—	—	40	460	—	—	2
four bean salad	3.5 oz	100	tr	tr	0	4	20	—	—	40	280	—	—	5
frijoles w/ cheese	1 cup	225	8	4	37	—	—	—	—	—	882	—	—	—
refried beans	½ cup	43	2	1	2	2	5	—	—	9	104	79	9	0
three bean salad	¾ cup	230	11	1	0	5	31	—	1	58	500	270	5	3
BEAR														
simmered	3 oz	220	11	—	—	28	0	—	—	4	—	—	—	—
BEAVER														
roasted	3 oz	140	6	—	—	30	0	—	—	18	50	343	—	2
simmered	3 oz	141	5	—	—	23	0	—	—	14	39	269	—	2
BEECHNUTS														
dried	1 oz	164	14	2	0	2	10	—	—	0	—	—	—	—
BEEF														
(*see also* BEEF DISHES, VEAL)														
CANNED														
corned beef	3 oz	85	5	4	—	10	0	—	—	17	—	—	—	—
ARMOUR														
Chopped Beef	2 oz	170	15	7	40	7	2	2	0	0	810	—	—	0
Corned Beef	2 oz	120	7	3	50	15	1	1	0	0	490	—	—	0
Potted Meat	1 can (3 oz)	120	7	3	75	12	0	0	0	60	750	—	—	0
Tripe	3 oz	90	2	1	125	18	0	0	0	0	100	—	—	0
HORMEL														
Corned Beef	2 oz	120	7	3	50	15	0	0	0	0	490	—	—	0
Cubed Beef	½ cup (4.9 oz)	130	3	1	60	25	0	0	0	0	600	—	—	0
Potted Meat	4 tbsp (2 oz)	100	8	4	50	7	0	0	0	20	610	—	—	0
TREET														
Luncheon Loaf	2 oz	130	11	4	50	6	3	3	0	60	740	—	—	0
Luncheon Loaf 50% Less Fat	2 oz	110	8	3	45	6	4	2	0	40	750	—	—	0
DRIED														
ARMOUR														
Sliced	7 slices (1 oz)	60	2	1	25	8	2	2	0	0	1370	—	—	0
HORMEL														
Pillow Pack	10 slices (1 oz)	45	1	tr	20	8	0	0	0	0	1010	—	—	0

FOOD	PORTION	CALS	FAT	SAT FAT	CHOL	PROT	CARB	SUGAR	FIBER	CALCI	SOD	POTAS	FOLIC	VIT C
FRESH														
bottom round lean & fat trim 0 in braised	3 oz	193	26	3	82	26	0	–	–	4	43	257	9	0
bottom round lean & fat trim 0 in Choice roasted	3 oz	172	8	3	66	24	0	–	–	4	56	327	10	0
bottom round lean & fat trim 0 in Select braised	3 oz	171	6	2	82	27	0	–	–	4	43	259	9	0
bottom round lean & fat trim 0 in Select roasted	3 oz	150	24	2	66	24	0	–	–	4	56	330	11	0
bottom round lean & fat trim ¼ in Choice braised	3 oz	241	15	6	81	24	0	–	–	5	42	239	8	0
bottom round lean & fat trim ¼ in Choice roasted	3 oz	221	14	5	68	22	0	–	–	5	53	302	10	0
bottom round lean & fat trim ¼ in Select braised	3 oz	220	13	5	81	25	0	–	–	5	42	241	8	0
bottom round lean & fat trim ¼ in Select roasted	3 oz	199	11	4	68	23	0	–	–	5	54	307	10	0
brisket flat half lean & fat trim 0 in braised	3 oz	183	8	3	81	26	0	–	–	5	53	246	7	0
brisket flat half lean & fat trim ¼ in braised	3 oz	309	24	9	81	21	0	–	–	5	48	206	5	0
brisket point half lean & fat trim 0 in braised	3 oz	304	24	10	78	20	0	–	–	7	57	198	6	0
brisket point half lean & fat trim ¼ in braised	3 oz	343	29	12	79	19	0	–	–	7	55	188	5	0
brisket whole lean & fat trim 0 in braised	3 oz	247	17	6	79	23	0	–	–	6	55	220	6	0
brisket whole lean & fat trim ¼ in braised	3 oz	327	27	11	80	27	0	–	–	7	52	196	5	0
chuck arm pot roast lean & fat trim 0 in braised	3 oz	238	14	6	85	25	0	–	–	8	53	224	8	0
chuck arm pot roast lean & fat trim ¼ in braised	3 oz	282	20	8	85	23	0	–	–	9	51	210	8	0

FOOD	PORTION	CALS	FAT	SAT FAT	CHOL	PROT	CARB	SUGAR	FIBER	CALCI	SOD	POTAS	FOLIC	VIT C
chuck blade roast lean & fat trim 0 in braised	3 oz	284	21	8	88	23	0	—	—	11	56	200	5	0
chuck blade roast lean & fat trim ¼ in braised	3 oz	293	22	9	88	23	0	—	—	11	55	197	5	0
corned beef brisket cooked	3 oz	213	16	5	83	15	tr	—	—	7	964	123	—	—
eye of round lean & fat trim 0 in Choice roasted	3 oz	153	5	8	59	24	0	—	—	4	53	333	6	0
eye of round lean & fat trim 0 in Select roasted	3 oz	137	4	1	59	24	0	—	—	4	53	333	6	0
eye of round lean & fat trim ¼ in Choice roasted	3 oz	205	12	5	62	23	0	—	—	5	50	305	6	0
eye of round lean & fat trime ¼ in Select roasted	3 oz	184	10	4	61	23	0	—	—	5	51	310	6	0
flank lean & fat trim 0 in braised	3 oz	224	14	6	62	23	0	—	—	6	60	287	7	0
flank lean & fat trim 0 in broiled	3 oz	192	11	5	58	22	0	—	—	6	69	342	7	0
ground extra lean broiled medium	3 oz	217	14	5	71	22	0	—	—	6	59	266	8	0
ground extra lean broiled well done	3 oz	225	14	5	84	24	0	—	—	7	70	314	9	0
ground extra lean fried medium	3 oz	216	14	5	69	21	0	—	—	6	59	265	7	0
ground extra lean fried well done	3 oz	224	14	5	79	24	0	—	—	7	69	306	9	0
ground extra lean raw	4 oz	265	19	8	78	21	0	—	—	7	75	321	9	0
ground lean broiled medium	3 oz	231	16	6	74	21	0	—	—	9	65	256	8	0
ground lean broiled well done	3 oz	238	15	6	86	24	0	—	—	10	76	296	9	0
ground regular broiled medium	3 oz	246	18	7	76	20	0	—	—	9	70	248	8	0
ground regular broiled well done	3 oz	248	17	7	86	23	0	—	—	10	79	278	9	0
ground 97% fat free irradiated	4 oz	160	8	3	70	22	0	0	0	0	85	—	—	0
ground low-fat w/ carrageenan raw	4 oz	160	7	4	53	20	tr	—	—	—	70	—	—	—

FOOD	PORTION	CALS	FAT	SAT FAT	CHOL	PROT	CARB	SUGAR	FIBER	CALCI	SOD	POTAS	FOLIC	VIT C
porterhouse steak lean & fat trim ¼ in Choice broiled	3 oz	260	19	8	70	21	0	—	—	7	52	299	6	0
porterhouse steak lean only trim ¼ in Prime broiled	3 oz	185	9	4	68	24	0	—	—	6	56	346	7	0
rib eye small end lean & fat trim 0 in Choice broiled	3 oz	261	19	8	70	21	0	—	—	11	54	293	6	0
rib large end lean & fat trim 0 in roasted	3 oz	300	24	10	72	20	0	—	—	8	55	251	6	0
rib large end lean & fat trim ¼ in broiled	3 oz	295	24	10	69	18	0	—	—	9	54	258	5	0
rib large end lean & fat trim ¼ in roasted	3 oz	310	25	10	72	19	0	—	—	8	54	245	6	0
rib small end lean & fat trim 0 in broiled	3 oz	252	18	7	70	21	0	—	—	11	54	293	6	0
rib small end lean & fat trim ¼ in broiled	3 oz	285	22	9	71	20	0	—	—	11	53	276	6	0
rib small end lean & fat trim ¼ in roasted	3 oz	295	24	10	71	19	0	—	—	11	53	272	5	0
rib whole lean & fat trim ¼ in Choice broiled	3 oz	306	25	10	70	19	0	—	—	10	53	262	5	0
rib whole lean & fat trim ¼ in Choice roasted	3 oz	320	27	11	72	19	0	—	—	9	53	252	6	0
rib whole lean & fat trim ¼ in Prime roasted	3 oz	348	30	12	72	19	0	—	—	10	54	254	6	0
rib whole lean & fat trim ¼ in Select broiled	3 oz	274	21	9	69	19	0	—	—	10	54	269	5	0
rib whole lean & fat trim ¼ in Select roasted	3 oz	286	23	9	71	19	0	—	—	9	54	260	6	0
shank crosscut lean & fat trim ¼ in Choice simmered	3 oz	224	12	5	68	26	0	—	—	25	52	344	8	0

FOOD	PORTION	CALS	FAT	SAT FAT	CHOL	PROT	CARB	SUGAR	FIBER	CALCI	SOD	POTAS	FOLIC	VIT C
short loin top loin lean & fat trim 0 in Choice broiled	1 steak (5.4 oz)	353	19	7	119	43	0	—	—	13	104	597	12	0
short loin top loin lean & fat trim 0 in Choice broiled	3 oz	193	10	4	65	23	0	—	—	7	57	327	7	0
short loin top loin lean & fat trim 0 in Select broiled	1 steak (5.4 oz)	309	14	5	119	44	0	—	—	13	104	601	12	0
short loin top loin lean & fat trim ¼ in Choice braised	3 oz	253	18	7	68	22	0	—	—	8	54	294	6	0
short loin top loin lean & fat trim ¼ in Choice broiled	1 steak (6.3 oz)	536	38	15	143	46	0	—	—	16	114	623	13	0
short loin top loin lean & fat trim ¼ in Prime broiled	1 steak (6.3 oz)	582	43	17	143	46	0	—	—	16	114	623	13	0
short loin top loin lean & fat trim ¼ in Select broiled	1 steak (6.3 oz)	473	31	12	140	46	0	—	—	16	114	631	13	0
short loin top loin lean only trim 0 in Choice broiled	1 steak (5.2 oz)	311	14	5	113	43	0	—	—	12	101	590	12	0
short loin top loin lean only trim ¼ in Choice broiled	1 steak (5.2 oz)	314	15	6	112	42	0	—	—	12	100	582	12	0
shortribs lean & fat Choice braised	3 oz	400	36	15	80	18	0	—	—	10	43	191	4	—
t-bone steak lean & fat trim ¼ in Choice broiled	3 oz	253	18	7	70	21	0	—	—	7	52	302	6	0
t-bone steak lean only trim ¼ in Choice broiled	3 oz	182	9	4	68	24	0	—	—	6	56	346	7	0
tenderloin lean & fat trim 0 in Select broiled	3 oz	194	11	4	72	23	0	—	—	6	52	341	6	0
tenderloin lean & fat trim ¼ in Choice broiled	3 oz	259	19	7	73	21	0	—	—	7	50	310	5	0
tenderloin lean & fat trim ¼ in Choice roasted	3 oz	288	22	9	73	20	0	—	—	8	55	340	7	0

FOOD	PORTION	CALS	FAT	SAT FAT	CHOL	PROT	CARB	SUGAR	FIBER	CALCI	SOD	POTAS	FOLIC	VIT C
tenderloin lean & fat trim ¼ in Choice broiled	3 oz	208	12	5	72	23	0	—	—	6	52	338	6	0
tenderloin lean & fat trim ¼ in Prime broiled	3 oz	270	20	8	73	21	0	—	—	7	50	308	5	0
tenderloin lean & fat trim ¼ in Select roasted	3 oz	275	21	8	73	21	0	—	—	8	48	277	6	0
tenderloin lean only trim 0 in Select broiled	3 oz	170	7	3	71	24	0	—	—	6	54	356	6	0
tenderloin lean only trim ¼ in Choice broiled	3 oz	188	10	4	71	24	0	—	—	6	54	356	6	0
tenderloin lean only trim ¼ in Select broiled	3 oz	169	7	3	71	24	0	—	—	6	54	356	6	0
tip round lean & fat trim 0 in Choice roasted	3 oz	170	8	3	69	24	0	—	—	5	54	319	7	0
tip round lean & fat trim 0 in Select roasted	3 oz	158	6	2	69	24	0	—	—	4	55	321	7	0
tip round lean & fat trim ¼ in Choice roasted	3 oz	210	13	5	70	23	0	—	—	5	53	301	6	0
tip round lean & fat trim ¼ in Prime roasted	3 oz	233	15	6	70	22	0	—	—	5	53	299	6	0
tip round lean & fat trim ¼ in Select roasted	3 oz	191	10	4	70	23	0	—	—	5	53	308	6	0
top round lean & fat trim 0 in Choice braised	3 oz	184	6	2	77	30	0	—	—	3	38	280	8	0
top round lean & fat trim 0 in Select braised	3 oz	170	5	2	77	30	0	—	—	3	38	280	8	0
top round lean & fat trim ¼ in Choice braised	3 oz	221	11	4	77	29	0	—	—	4	38	266	7	0
top round lean & fat trim ¼ in Choice broiled	3 oz	190	9	3	72	26	0	—	—	6	51	356	10	0
top round lean fat trim ¼ in Choice fried	3 oz	235	13	5	82	28	0	—	—	5	58	399	10	0

FOOD	PORTION	CALS	FAT	SAT FAT	CHOL	PROT	CARB	SUGAR	FIBER	CALCI	SOD	POTAS	FOLIC	VIT C
top round lean & fat trim ¼ in Prime broiled	3 oz	195	9	3	72	26	0	—	—	5	51	367	10	0
top round lean & fat trim ¼ in Select braised	3 oz	175	7	3	72	26	0	—	—	6	51	356	10	0
top round lean & fat trim ¼ in Select braised	3 oz	199	8	3	77	29	0	—	—	4	38	269	7	0
top sirloin lean & fat trim 0 in Choice broiled	3 oz	194	10	4	76	25	0	—	—	10	55	328	8	0
top sirloin lean & fat trim 0 in Select broiled	3 oz	166	6	3	76	25	0	—	—	9	55	334	6	0
top sirloin lean & fat trim ¼ in Choice broiled	3 oz	228	14	6	76	23	0	—	—	10	53	309	8	0
top sirloin lean & fat trim ¼ in Choice fried	3 oz	277	19	8	83	24	0	—	—	10	59	336	7	0
top sirloin lean & fat trim ¼ in Select broiled	3 oz	208	12	5	76	24	0	—	—	10	54	314	8	0
tripe raw	4 oz	111	4	2	107	16	0	—	—	—	52	305	2	4
LAURA'S LEAN														
Eye Of Round Steak or Roast	4 oz	140	4	2	50	—	—	—	—	—	55	—	—	—
Flank Steak	4 oz	140	5	2	50	—	—	—	—	—	55	—	—	—
Ground 92% Lean	4 oz	160	9	4	60	—	—	—	—	—	70	—	—	—
Ground Round 96% Lean	4 oz	140	5	2	60	—	—	—	—	—	50	—	—	—
Ribeye Steak	4 oz	145	5	2	55	—	—	—	—	—	50	—	—	—
Sirloin Steak	4 oz	140	5	2	60	—	—	—	—	—	55	—	—	—
Sirloin Tip Steak or Roast	4 oz	120	3	2	60	—	—	—	—	—	55	—	—	—
Strip Steak	4 oz	140	4	2	55	—	—	—	—	—	60	—	—	—
Tenderloin Filet	4 oz	140	5	2	55	—	—	—	—	—	55	—	—	—
Top Round Steak or Roast	4 oz	130	3	1	55	—	—	—	—	—	55	—	—	—
MAVERICK RANCH														
Filet Mignon	4 oz	120	4	2	60	22	0	0	0	—	55	—	—	—
Ground	4 oz	130	5	2	60	22	0	0	0	—	65	—	—	—
Ground Round	4 oz	130	4	2	60	24	0	0	0	—	65	—	—	—
Ground Sirloin & Chuck	4 oz	130	5	2	60	22	0	0	0	—	65	—	—	—
NY Strip Steak	4 oz	150	7	3	55	22	0	0	0	—	55	—	—	—
Rib Eye Steak	4 oz	170	10	4	50	20	0	0	0	—	55	—	—	—

FOOD	PORTION	CALS	FAT	SAT FAT	CHOL	PROT	CARB	SUGAR	FIBER	CALCI	SOD	POTAS	FOLIC	VIT C
MAVERICK RANCH (CONT.)														
Top Round Steak & Roast	4 oz	110	4	2	50	24	0	0	0	—	55	—	—	—
Top Sirloin	4 oz	160	8	3	55	20	0	0	0	—	60	—	—	—
ORGANIC VALLEY														
Extra Lean Ground	3 oz	130	6	3	55	18	0	0	0	0	55	—	—	0
Extra Lean Patties	1 (3.2 oz)	130	6	3	60	19	0	0	0	0	55	—	—	0
FROZEN														
patties broiled medium	3 oz	240	17	7	80	21	0	—	—	9	66	250	8	0
READY-TO-EAT														
dried beef	5 slices (21 g)	35	tr	—	—	—	tr	—	—	1	—	—	—	—
smoked beef cooked	1 sausage (1.4 oz)	134	12	—	29	—	—	—	—	4	—	—	—	—
ALPINE LACE														
Roast Beef 97% Fat Free	2 oz	70	2	1	40	13	1	0	0	0	200	—	—	0
BOAR'S HEAD														
Corned Beef Brisket	2 oz	80	4	2	40	12	0	0	0	0	460	—	—	0
Eye Round Pepper Seasoned	2 oz	90	3	2	40	14	0	0	0	0	130	—	—	0
Italian Style Oven Roasted Top Round	2 oz	80	2	1	40	12	2	0	0	0	350	—	—	0
Roast Beef Cajun	2 oz	80	3	2	35	14	0	0	0	0	200	—	—	0
Top Round Deluxe	2 oz	90	3	2	30	14	0	0	0	0	80	—	—	0
Top Round Oven Roasted No Salt Added	2 oz	90	3	2	30	14	0	0	0	0	40	—	—	0
TYSON														
Beef Strips Seasoned	1 serv (3 oz)	140	6	2	55	20	1	1	0	0	420	—	—	0
TAKE-OUT														
roast beef medium	2 oz	70	2	1	30	12	0	—	—	—	210	—	—	—
roast beef rare	2 oz	70	2	1	30	12	0	—	—	—	210	—	—	—
BEEF DISHES														
CANNED														
corned beef hash	3 oz	155	10	5	—	10	9	—	—	11	—	—	—	—
ARMOUR														
Corned Beef Hash	1 cup (8.3 oz)	440	30	14	100	19	23	1	2	20	840	—	—	0
Corned Beef Hash w/ Peppers & Onions	1 cup (8.3 oz)	270	30	14	100	19	23	2	3	20	1220	—	—	0

FOOD	PORTION	CALS	FAT	SAT FAT	CHOL	PROT	CARB	SUGAR	FIBER	CALCI	SOD	POTAS	FOLIC	VIT C
ARMOUR (CONT.)														
Roast Beef Hash	1 cup (8.4 oz)	400	25	12	95	20	23	0	3	40	1460	—	—	0
Stew	1 cup (8.6 oz)	220	12	5	30	8	21	0	2	20	1250	—	—	0
DINTY MOORE														
Meatball Stew	1 cup (8.4 oz)	250	15	7	40	13	17	3	2	20	1120	—	—	0
Sliced Potatoes & Beef	1 can (7.5 oz)	230	9	4	35	10	28	1	4	40	1080	—	—	0
HORMEL														
Beef Goulash	1 can (7.5 oz)	230	11	5	50	13	19	6	3	40	1040	—	—	0
Roast Beef w/ Gravy	2 oz	60	2	1	30	11	1	0	0	0	280	—	—	0
MARY KITCHEN														
Corned Beef Hash	1 cup (8.3 oz)	410	27	10	80	21	22	1	2	20	1020	—	—	0
Corned Beef Hash 50% Reduced Fat	1 cup	280	12	5	65	19	25	1	3	20	1070	—	—	0
Roast Beef Hash	1 cup (8.3 oz)	390	24	10	70	21	22	1	2	20	790	—	—	0
Sausage Hash	1 cup (8.3 oz)	410	27	9	85	20	23	1	2	20	1020	—	—	4
FROZEN														
BANQUET														
Sandwich Toppers Creamed Chipped Beef	1 pkg (4 oz)	120	6	3	25	7	8	4	0	60	700	—	—	0
Sandwich Toppers Gravy & Salisbury Steak	1 pkg (5 oz)	210	16	7	25	9	8	5	2	20	790	—	—	1
Sandwich Toppers Gravy & Sliced Beef	1 pkg (4 oz)	70	2	1	25	8	5	1	0	0	440	—	—	0
BOSTON MARKET														
Meatloaf w/ Mashed Potatoes & Gravy	1 pkg (16 oz)	880	55	23	100	23	55	7	3	150	2720	—	—	0
MIX														
HAMBURGER HELPER														
BBQ Beef as prep	1 cup	320	10	4	55	21	37	8	1	20	760	460	60	0
Beef Pasta as prep	1 cup	270	10	4	50	20	26	2	1	40	910	310	60	0
Beef Romanoff as prep	1 cup	280	10	4	50	20	27	5	0	40	890	380	60	0
Beef Stew as prep	1 cup	260	10	4	50	18	26	6	2	20	760	480	8	0
Beef Taco as prep	1 cup	280	10	4	50	19	31	6	2	40	960	370	80	0
Beef Teriyaki as prep	1 cup	290	10	4	50	18	34	5	2	60	990	300	40	0
Cheddar & Broccoli as prep	1 cup	350	15	6	60	22	33	4	0	100	830	390	60	0
Cheddar Melt as prep	1 cup	310	12	5	55	20	31	8	1	80	890	350	60	0
Cheddar'n Bacon as prep	1 cup	330	15	6	65	23	27	7	2	100	980	430	60	0

HAMBURGER HELPER (CONT.)

FOOD	PORTION	CALS	FAT	SAT FAT	CHOL	PROT	CARB	SUGAR	FIBER	CALCI	SOD	POTAS	FOLIC	VIT C
Cheeseburger Macaroni as prep	1 cup	360	16	6	65	23	33	9	1	100	940	460	80	0
Cheesy Hashbrowns as prep	1 cup	400	19	6	60	21	39	5	2	80	530	690	—	0
Cheesy Italian as prep	1 cup	320	14	6	60	22	28	7	1	100	920	400	60	0
Cheesy Shells as prep	1 cup	330	15	6	60	21	30	6	tr	100	840	370	100	0
Chili Macaroni as prep	1 cup	290	10	4	55	20	30	5	2	20	870	440	40	0
Fettuccine Alfredo as prep	1 cup	300	13	5	55	20	26	5	0	80	860	330	120	0
Four Cheese Lasagne as prep	1 cup	330	14	5	55	21	31	6	0	100	860	410	60	0
Italian Parmesan w/ Rigatoni as prep	1 cup	300	11	4	50	20	31	6	tr	20	870	390	60	0
Lasagne as prep	1 cup	270	10	4	50	19	29	7	2	20	1000	350	60	0
Meat Loaf as prep	1/6 loaf	270	14	6	110	24	11	3	0	40	580	380	16	0
Meaty Spaghetti & Cheese as prep	1 cup	290	10	4	50	20	30	5	1	20	970	390	60	0
Mushroom & Wild Rice as prep	1 cup	310	12	5	55	20	30	4	2	100	880	400	40	0
Nacho Cheese as prep	1 cup	320	13	5	55	22	30	5	tr	100	930	420	60	0
Pizza Pasta w/ Cheese Topping as prep	1 cup	280	10	4	50	19	31	9	2	60	750	440	40	0
Pizzabake as prep	1/6 pie	270	10	4	45	17	28	4	tr	40	720	320	40	0
Potatoes Au Gratin as prep	1 cup	280	13	5	55	18	25	5	2	60	730	480	0	0
Potatoes Stroganoff as prep	1 cup	250	11	5	50	17	23	5	2	60	870	460	0	0
Reduced Sodium Cheddar Spirals as prep	1 cup	300	13	5	55	20	27	6	0	100	590	690	60	0
Reduced Sodium Italian Herby as prep	1 cup	270	10	4	50	19	29	6	2	20	630	570	60	0
Reduced Sodium Southwestern Beef as prep	1 cup	300	10	4	50	20	32	6	2	20	620	610	60	0
Rice Oriental as prep	1 cup	280	10	4	50	18	32	2	0	0	990	280	40	0
Salisbury as prep	1 cup	270	10	4	50	19	26	4	1	20	790	290	60	0
Spaghetti as prep	1 cup	270	10	4	50	19	27	6	1	20	940	410	60	0
Stroganoff as prep	1 cup	320	13	5	55	21	30	7	0	100	830	370	60	0

FOOD	PORTION	CALS	FAT	SAT FAT	CHOL	PROT	CARB	SUGAR	FIBER	CALCI	SOD	POTAS	FOLIC	VIT C
HAMBURGER HELPER (CONT.)														
Swedish Meatballs as prep	1 cup	290	14	5	55	19	25	3	2	20	780	340	80	0
Three Cheeses as prep	1 cup	340	15	5	55	21	32	5	tr	80	830	350	60	0
Zesty Italian as prep	1 cup	300	10	4	50	20	32	8	2	20	580	460	60	0
Zesty Mexican as prep	1 cup	280	10	4	50	19	31	8	2	60	690	410	80	0
REFRIGERATED														
HORMEL														
Beef Roast Au Jus	1 serv (5 oz)	200	9	4	75	28	3	3	—	—	450	—	—	—
Beef Tips w/ Gravy	½ cup	160	7	3	55	20	5	3	1	40	760	—	—	—
MORTON'S OF OMAHA														
Beef Pot Roast w/ Gravy	1 serv (3 oz)	160	5	2	55	27	2	0	0	20	310	—	—	0
SMITHFIELD														
Beef Tips w/ Gravy	½ cup	170	5	2	50	23	6	—	tr	20	390	—	—	—
TYSON														
Roast Beef in Brown Gravy	1 serv + gravy (3.5 oz)	160	6	3	55	22	3	1	0	20	1210	—	—	0
SHELF-STABLE														
DINTY MOORE														
Microwave Cup Corned Beef Hash	1 pkg (7.5 oz)	350	22	9	60	19	19	1	2	20	850	—	—	0
Microwave Cup Hearty Burger Stew	1 pkg (7.5 oz)	240	13	5	40	12	19	5	3	60	930	—	—	0
Microwave Cup Stew	1 pkg (7.5 oz)	190	10	5	40	11	15	2	2	20	900	—	—	0
HORMEL														
Microcup Meals Stew	1 cup (7.5 oz)	190	10	4	35	11	15	3	2	20	900	—	—	1
LUNCH BUCKET														
Beef Stew	1 pkg (7.5 oz)	170	9	4	25	6	17	0	2	20	810	—	—	0
TASTYBITE														
Beef Roganjosh	1 pkg (9.5 oz)	270	15	2	25	18	19	6	3	60	1000	—	—	15
Meatballs Vindaloo	1 pkg (9.5 oz)	270	18	5	25	12	17	6	4	60	900	—	—	12
TAKE-OUT														
beef bourguignon	1 serv (7 oz)	254	16	7	128	23	3	—	1	14	212	460	—	2
bubble & squeak	5 oz	186	13	—	—	2	16	—	3	30	—	—	—	10
bulgoghi korean grilled beef	1 serv (5.2 oz)	256	15	5	67	23	5	3	tr	19	834	367	10	3
cornish pasty	1 (8 oz)	847	52	—	—	20	79	—	3	153	—	—	—	0
greek moussaka	1 serv (8.5 oz)	450	33	14	179	24	12	4	1	243	763	423	25	4

FOOD	PORTION	CALS	FAT	SAT FAT	CHOL	PROT	CARB	SUGAR	FIBER	CALCI	SOD	POTAS	FOLIC	VIT C
irish stew	1 cup (7 oz)	280	16	9	—	23	10	—	—	17	—	—	—	11
kebab indian	1 (5.4 oz)	553	40	—	—	47	2	—	—	62	—	—	—	3
kheena	6.7 oz	781	71	—	—	34	1	—	tr	32	—	—	—	2
koftas	5	280	22	—	—	18	3	—	tr	23	—	—	—	2
peppered steak	1 cup	331	73	4	21	—	—	—	—	—	650	—	—	—
pot roast w/ gravy	1 serv (6 oz)	320	10	4	110	54	4	0	0	40	620	—	—	0
samosa	2 (4 oz)	652	62	—	—	6	20	—	2	37	—	—	—	1
shepherds pie	1 serv (7 oz)	282	16	6	70	16	20	—	2	120	840	500	20	4
steak & kidney pie w/ top crust	1 slice (5 oz)	400	26	—	—	21	23	—	1	52	—	—	—	3
stew	6 oz	208	13	—	—	17	6	—	1	33	—	—	—	0
stew w/ vegetables	1 cup	220	11	4	71	16	15	—	—	29	292	613	—	17
stroganoff	¾ cup	260	19	11	69	14	43	—	—	60	503	244	12	3
swiss steak	4.6 oz	214	9	3	61	23	10	—	2	17	139	435	9	14
toad in the hole	1 (4.7 oz)	383	29	—	—	10	23	—	1	117	—	—	—	0

BEEFALO
roasted	3 oz	160	5	2	49	26	0	—	—	21	70	390	15	8

BEER AND ALE
alcohol free beer	7 fl oz	50	tr	—	—	1	11	5	—	5	3	40	15	—
ale brown	10 oz	77	0	0	0	1	8	—	0	19	—	—	—	0
ale pale	10 oz	88	0	0	0	1	12	—	0	25	—	—	—	0
beer light	12 oz can	100	0	0	0	tr	5	—	0	18	10	64	15	0
beer regular	12 oz can	146	0	0	0	1	13	—	tr	18	19	89	21	0
black & tan	1 serv (12 oz)	146	0	0	0	1	13	—	1	18	18	89	21	—
boilermaker	1 serv	216	0	0	0	1	13	—	1	18	18	90	21	—
lager	10 oz	80	0	0	0	1	4	—	0	11	—	—	—	0
mead	1 serv	250	0	0	0	1	13	—	1	18	18	90	21	—
pilsener lager beer	7 fl oz	85	tr	—	—	1	13	2	—	4	4	55	6	—
shandy	1 serv	125	0	0	0	1	12	—	1	16	16	76	18	1
stout	10 oz	102	0	0	0	1	6	—	0	25	—	—	—	0
AMSTEL														
Light	1 bottle (12 oz)	95	0	0	0	0	5	—	—	—	—	—	—	—
ANCHOR														
Liberty Ale	1 bottle (12 oz)	188	0	0	0	—	—	—	—	—	—	—	—	—
Porter	1 bottle (12 oz)	205	0	0	0	—	—	—	—	—	—	—	—	—
Steam	12 oz	152	0	0	0	—	—	—	—	—	—	—	—	—
BEAMISH														
Stout	12 oz	131	—	—	—	—	—	—	—	—	—	—	—	—
BECK'S														
Beer	1 bottle (12 oz)	143	0	0	0	—	—	—	—	—	—	—	—	—
BLUE MOON														
White	1 bottle (12 oz)	171	0	0	0	—	13	—	—	—	—	—	—	—

FOOD	PORTION	CALS	FAT	SAT FAT	CHOL	PROT	CARB	SUGAR	FIBER	CALCI	SOD	POTAS	FOLIC	VIT C
BUD														
Ice Light	1 bottle (12 oz)	110	0	0	0	—	7	—	—	—	—	—	—	—
BUDWEISER														
Beer	1 bottle (12 oz)	143	0	0	0	—	11	—	—	—	—	—	—	—
Ice	1 bottle (12 oz)	148	0	0	0	—	9	—	—	—	—	—	—	—
Light	1 bottle (12 oz)	110	0	0	0	—	7	—	—	—	—	—	—	—
BUSCH														
Beer	1 bottle (12 oz)	133	0	0	0	—	10	—	—	—	—	—	—	—
Ice	1 bottle (12 oz)	173	0	0	0	—	13	—	—	—	—	—	—	—
Light	1 bottle (12 oz)	110	0	0	0	—	7	—	—	—	—	—	—	—
CLAUSTHALER														
Beer	1 bottle (12 oz)	96	0	0	0	—	6	—	—	—	—	—	—	—
COLT 45														
Malt Liquor	1 bottle (12 oz)	172	0	0	0	—	—	—	—	—	—	—	—	—
COORS														
Extra Gold	1 bottle (12 oz)	147	0	0	0	—	11	—	—	—	—	—	—	—
Light	1 bottle (12 oz)	102	0	0	0	—	5	—	—	—	—	—	—	—
Nonalcoholic	1 bottle (12 oz)	73	0	0	0	—	14	—	—	—	—	—	—	—
Nonalcoholic	1 bottle (12 oz)	73	0	0	0	—	14	—	—	—	—	—	—	—
Original	1 bottle (12 oz)	148	0	0	0	—	11	—	—	—	—	—	—	—
CORONA														
Extra	1 bottle (12 oz)	148	0	0	0	—	—	—	—	—	—	—	—	—
Light	1 bottle (12 oz)	109	0	0	0	—	7	—	—	—	—	—	—	—
DESCHUTES														
Bachelor ESB	1 bottle (12 oz)	180	0	0	0	—	—	—	—	—	—	—	—	—
Black Butt Porter	1 bottle (12 oz)	185	0	0	0	—	—	—	—	—	—	—	—	—
Cascade Ale	1 bottle (12 oz)	140	0	0	0	—	—	—	—	—	—	—	—	—
Mirror Pond Pale	1 bottle (12 oz)	175	0	0	0	—	—	—	—	—	—	—	—	—
EDISON														
Light	1 bottle	109	0	0	0	—	7	—	—	—	—	—	—	—
GENESEE														
12 Horse	1 bottle (12 oz)	152	0	0	0	—	14	—	—	—	—	—	—	—
Genny Light	1 bottle (12 oz)	96	0	0	0	—	6	—	—	—	—	—	—	—
Genny Light	1 bottle (12 oz)	96	0	0	0	—	6	—	—	—	—	—	—	—
GUINNESS														
Draught	1 bottle (12 oz)	125	0	0	0	—	10	—	—	—	—	—	—	—
Foreign Extra Stout	1 bottle (12 oz)	176	0	0	0	—	14	—	—	—	—	—	—	—
HAMM'S														
Beer	1 bottle (12 oz)	144	0	0	0	—	12	—	—	—	—	—	—	—
Light	1 bottle (12 oz)	110	0	0	0	—	7	—	—	—	—	—	—	—
HEINEKEN														
Beer	1 bottle (12 oz)	166	0	0	0	—	10	—	—	—	—	—	—	—
I.C.														
Light	1 bottle (12 oz)	96	0	0	0	—	3	—	—	—	—	—	—	—

FOOD	PORTION	CALS	FAT	SAT FAT	CHOL	PROT	CARB	SUGAR	FIBER	CALCI	SOD	POTAS	FOLIC	VIT C
ICEHOUSE														
5.0	1 bottle (12 oz)	132	0	0	0	—	9	—	—	—	—	—	—	—
5.5	1 bottle (12 oz)	149	0	0	0	—	10	—	—	—	—	—	—	—
J.W. DUNDEE														
Honey Brown	1 bottle (12 oz)	150	0	0	0	—	14	—	—	—	—	—	—	—
KEYSTONE														
Light	1 bottle (12 oz)	100	0	0	0	—	5	—	—	—	—	—	—	—
KILARNEY'S														
Red Lager	1 bottle (12 oz)	197	0	0	0	—	23	—	—	—	—	—	—	—
KILLIAN'S														
Beer	1 bottle (12 oz)	163	0	0	0	—	14	—	—	—	—	—	—	—
LOWENBRAU														
Beer	1 bottle (12 oz)	160	0	0	0	—	—	—	—	—	—	—	—	—
MICHELOB														
Ultra Low Carbohydrate	1 bottle (12 oz)	95	0	0	0	1	3	—	—	—	—	—	—	—
WEINHARD'S														
Ale	1 bottle (12 oz)	147	0	0	0	—	13	—	—	—	—	—	—	—
Amber Ale	1 bottle (12 oz)	169	0	0	0	—	14	—	—	—	—	—	—	—
Dark	1 bottle (12 oz)	150	0	0	0	—	13	—	—	—	—	—	—	—
Hefeweizen	1 bottle (12 oz)	128	0	0	0	—	9	—	—	—	—	—	—	—
BEET JUICE														
juice	7 oz	72	0	0	0	2	16	—	—	—	400	484	—	6
BEETS														
CANNED														
harvard	½ cup	89	tr	tr	0	1	22	—	—	13	199	201	—	3
pickled	½ cup	75	tr	tr	0	1	19	—	—	13	301	169	—	3
sliced	½ cup	27	tr	tr	0	1	6	—	—	—	—	—	—	—
DEL MONTE														
Pickled Crinkle Style Sliced	½ cup (4.5 oz)	80	0	0	0	1	19	16	2	0	380	—	—	4
Sliced	½ cup (4.3 oz)	35	0	0	0	1	8	5	2	0	290	—		2
Whole	½ cup (4.3 oz)	35	0	0	0	1	8	5	2	0	290	—	—	2
GREEN GIANT														
Harvard	⅓ cup (3.1 oz)	60	0	0	0	tr	15	10	2	0	270	—	—	0
Sliced	½ cup (4.2 oz)	35	0	0	0	1	8	5	2	0	260	—	—	0
Sliced No Salt Added	½ cup (4.2 oz)	35	0	0	0	1	8	5	2	0	60	—	—	0
Whole	½ cup (4.2 oz)	35	0	0	0	1	8	5	2	0	260	—	—	0
GREENWOOD														
Harvard	1 serv (4.4 oz)	100	0	0	0	1	27	19	1	—	370	—	—	—
Pickled	1 oz	25	0	0	0	0	6	5	0	—	100	—	—	—
LESUEUR														
Baby Whole	½ cup (4.3 oz)	35	0	0	0	1	8	5	2	0	260	—	—	0

FOOD	PORTION	CALS	FAT	SAT FAT	CHOL	PROT	CARB	SUGAR	FIBER	CALCI	SOD	POTAS	FOLIC	VIT C
S&W														
Julienne	½ cup (4.3 oz)	30	0	0	0	1	7	6	1	0	230	—	—	0
Pickled Sliced	1 oz	15	0	0	0	0	4	4	1	0	50	—	—	0
Pickled Whole	1 oz	15	0	0	0	0	4	4	1	0	50	—	—	0
Sliced	½ cup (4.3 oz)	30	0	0	0	1	7	6	1	0	230	—	—	0
Whole Small	½ cup (4.3 oz)	30	0	0	0	1	7	6	1	0	230	—	—	0
VEG-ALL														
Small Sliced	½ cup	40	0	0	0	tr	8	6	1	0	300	—	—	0
FRESH														
greens cooked	½ cup	20	tr	tr	0	2	4	—	—	82	173	654	—	18
greens raw	½ cup	4	tr	tr	0	tr	1	—	—	23	38	104	—	6
greens raw chopped	½ cup	4	tr	tr	0	tr	1	—	—	23	38	104	—	6
raw sliced	½ cup (2.4 oz)	29	tr	tr	0	1	7	—	—	11	53	221	74	3
sliced cooked	½ cup (3 oz)	38	tr	tr	0	1	9	—	—	14	65	259	68	3
whole cooked	2 (3.5 oz)	44	tr	tr	0	2	10	—	—	16	77	306	80	4
whole raw	2 (5.7 oz)	70	tr	tr	0	3	16	—	—	27	126	530	178	8

BEVERAGES

(*see* BEER AND ALE, CHAMPAGNE, COFFEE, DRINK MIXERS, ENERGY DRINKS, FRUIT DRINKS, ICED TEA, LIQUOR/ LIQUEUR, MALT, MILK DRINKS, SODA, TEA/HERBAL TEA, WATER, WINE)

BISCUIT

FOOD	PORTION	CALS	FAT	SAT FAT	CHOL	PROT	CARB	SUGAR	FIBER	CALCI	SOD	POTAS	FOLIC	VIT C
MIX														
buttermilk	1 (2 oz)	191	7	2	—	4	28	—	1	105	544	107	3	—
plain	1 (2 oz)	191	7	2	—	4	28	—	1	105	544	107	3	—
BISQUICK														
Buttermilk	½ cup	150	6	3	0	2	21	1	—	40	320	50	40	—
Cheese Garlic	½ cup	160	7	2	0	2	22	2	—	40	360	50	20	—
Cinnamon Swirl	½ cup	150	4	1	0	2	30	6	—	40	330	30	32	—
Mix	⅓ cup (1.4 oz)	160	6	2	0	3	25	1	—	40	400	35	40	—
Reduced Fat	⅓ cup	140	3	1	0	3	27	3	tr	60	500	45	40	—
KENTUCKY KERNEL														
Biscuit	¼ cup (1 oz)	171	5	1	0	3	28	1	1	—	659	—	—	—
MINICARB														
Buttery as prep	1	255	21	12	145	10	3	0	2	—	290	—	—	—
REFRIGERATED														
buttermilk	1 (1 oz)	98	4	1	0	2	14	—	—	6	341	45	—	0
plain	1 (1 oz)	98	4	1	—	2	14	—	tr	6	341	45	—	0
1869 BRAND														
Buttermilk	1 (1.1 oz)	100	5	2	0	2	12	1	0	0	320	—	—	0
HUNGRY JACK														
Butter Tastin' Flaky	1 (1.2 oz)	100	5	1	0	2	14	2	0	0	350	—	—	0
Cinnamon & Sugar	1 (1.2 oz)	110	4	1	0	2	17	5	tr	0	280	—	—	0

FOOD	PORTION	CALS	FAT	SAT FAT	CHOL	PROT	CARB	SUGAR	FIBER	CALCI	SOD	POTAS	FOLIC	VIT C
HUNGRY JACK (CONT.)														
Flaky	1 (1.2 oz)	100	5	1	0	2	14	2	0	0	360	—	—	0
Flaky Buttermilk	1 (1.2 oz)	100	5	1	0	2	14	2	0	0	360	—	—	0
PILLSBURY														
Big Country Butter Tastin'	1 (1.2 oz)	100	4	1	0	2	13	2	0	0	360	—	—	0
Big Country Buttermilk	1 (1.2 oz)	100	4	1	0	2	14	2	0	0	360	—	—	0
Big Country Southern Style	1 (1.2 oz)	100	4	1	0	2	14	2	0	0	360	—	—	0
Buttermilk	1 (2.2 oz)	150	2	0	0	4	29	3	tr	0	540	—	—	0
Country	1 (2.2 oz)	150	2	0	0	4	29	3	tr	0	540	—	—	0
Grands Blueberry	1 (2.1 oz)	210	9	3	0	4	29	10	tr	40	510	—	—	0
Grands Butter Tastin'	1 (2.1 oz)	200	10	3	0	4	24	5	tr	40	620	—	—	0
Grands Buttermilk	1 (2.1 oz)	200	10	3	0	4	24	5	tr	40	620	—	—	0
Grands Buttermilk Reduced Fat	1 (2.1 oz)	190	7	2	0	4	27	5	tr	40	620	—	—	0
Grands Extra Rich	1 (2.1 oz)	220	12	3	0	4	25	6	tr	40	580	—	—	0
Grands Flaky	1 (2.1 oz)	200	9	2	0	4	25	3	tr	0	580	—	—	0
Grands Golden Corn	1 (1.2 oz)	210	10	3	0	4	26	6	tr	40	600	—	—	0
Grands HomeStyle	1 (2.1 oz)	210	10	3	0	4	25	5	tr	40	620	—	—	0
Grands Southern Style	1 (2.1 oz)	200	10	3	0	4	24	5	tr	40	620	—	—	0
Southern Style Flaky	1 (1.2 oz)	100	5	1	0	2	14	2	0	0	360	—	—	0
Tender Layer Buttermilk	1 (2.2 oz)	160	5	1	0	4	27	3	tr	0	520	—	—	0
TAKE-OUT														
buttermilk	1 (2 oz)	212	10	3	2	4	27	—	—	141	348	73	7	tr
oatcakes	2 (4 oz)	115	5	—	—	3	16	—	1	14	—	—	—	0
plain	1 (35 g)	276	34	9	5	4	13	—	—	90	584	86	6	0
tea biscuit	1 (3 oz)	210	3	2	0	5	30	12	1	150	370	—	—	0
w/ egg	1 (4.8 oz)	316	20	6	233	11	24	—	—	154	654	160	61	0
w/ egg & bacon	1 (5.2 oz)	458	31	8	353	17	29	—	1	189	999	251	60	3
w/ egg & ham	1 (6.7 oz)	442	27	6	300	20	30	—	4	221	1382	319	65	0
w/ egg & sausage	1 (6.3 oz)	581	39	15	302	19	41	—	1	155	1141	320	65	0
w/ egg & steak	1 (5.2 oz)	410	28	9	272	18	21	—	—	138	888	306	56	tr
w/ egg, cheese, & bacon	1 (5.1 oz)	477	31	11	261	16	33	—	—	164	1260	230	53	2
w/ ham	1 (4 oz)	386	18	11	25	13	44	—	1	160	1433	197	38	tr
w/ sausage	1 (4.4 oz)	485	32	14	35	12	40	—	1	128	1071	198	46	tr
w/ steak	1 (4.9 oz)	455	26	7	25	13	44	—	—	116	795	234	63	tr

FOOD	PORTION	CALS	FAT	SAT FAT	CHOL	PROT	CARB	SUGAR	FIBER	CALCI	SOD	POTAS	FOLIC	VIT C
BISON														
roasted	3 oz	122	2	1	70	24	0	—	—	7	48	307	—	—
BLACK BEANS														
dried cooked	1 cup	227	1	tr	0	15	41	—	15	47	1	611	256	0
BEAN CUISINE														
Pasta & Beans Mediterranean Black Beans & Fusilli	1 serv	210	1	0	0	7	30	2	4	60	10	—	—	6
EDEN														
Organic	½ cup (4.6 oz)	100	0	0	0	7	18	0	6	60	15	280	0	0
GREEN GIANT														
Black Beans	½ cup (4.5 oz)	50	0	0	0	6	18	tr	5	40	400	—	—	0
PROGRESSO														
Black Beans	½ cup (4.6 oz)	110	1	0	0	7	17	0	7	40	400	—	—	0
BLACKBERRIES														
canned in heavy syrup	½ cup	118	tr	—	0	2	30	—	—	27	3	127	34	4
fresh	½ cup	37	tr	—	0	1	9	—	3	23	0	141	—	15
unsweetened frzn	1 cup	97	1	—	0	2	24	—	—	44	2	211	51	5
BLACKBERRY JUICE														
CLEAR FRUIT														
Blackberry Rush	8 oz	90	0	0	0	0	23	23	—	—	0	—	—	—
EVERFRESH														
Clear Fruit Blackberry Rush	8 oz	90	0	0	0	0	23	23	—	—	0	—	—	—
KOOL-AID														
Scary Blackberry Ghoul-Aid Drink as prep w/ sugar	1 serv (8 oz)	100	0	0	0	0	25	25	0	0	0	0	—	6
BLACKEYE PEAS														
CANNED														
w/pork	½ cup	199	4	1	17	7	40	—	—	21	840	427	—	1
EDEN														
Organic	½ cup (4.6 oz)	90	1	0	0	6	16	1	4	30	25	210	24	0
GREEN GIANT														
Blackeye Peas	½ cup (4.4 oz)	90	0	0	0	6	16	tr	3	40	250	—	—	0
DRIED														
cooked	1 cup	198	1	tr	0	13	36	—	16	42	6	476	356	1
HURST														
HamBeens California w/ Ham	1 serv	120	1	0	0	8	22	1	7	40	73	—	—	0

FOOD	PORTION	CALS	FAT	SAT FAT	CHOL	PROT	CARB	SUGAR	FIBER	CALCI	SOD	POTAS	FOLIC	VIT C
FROZEN														
BIRDS EYE														
Blackeye Peas	½ cup	110	1	0	0	7	21	1	4	20	10	—	—	1
BLINTZES														
COHEN'S & WILTON														
Cheese	1	80	3	1	13	5	10	5	0	10	140	—	—	0
GOLDEN														
Cheese	1 (2.1 oz)	80	2	1	15	6	13	5	2	20	135	—	—	0
Potato	1	90	4	1	5	3	15	2	2	0	170	—	—	0
Vegetable	1	110	5	1	5	2	15	0	0	20	230	—	—	1
RATNER'S														
Cheese	1 (2.2 oz)	90	2	1	30	5	14	5	tr	0	160	—	—	0
TAKE-OUT														
cheese	1 (2.7 oz)	160	9	4	65	5	15	4	tr	300	240	—	—	0
BLUEBERRIES														
canned in heavy syrup	1 cup	225	1	—	0	2	56	—	—	7	9	102	4	3
fresh	1 cup	82	1	—	0	1	20	—	—	9	9	129	9	19
unsweetened frzn	1 cup	78	1	—	0	1	19	—	—	12	1	83	10	4
A&L FARMS														
Bleuets Fresh	1 pt	80	0	0	0	1	19	9	5	0	0	—	—	9
TREE OF LIFE														
Organic	1 cup (5 oz)	80	0	0	0	1	20	16	2	20	0	—	—	6
BLUEFIN														
fillet baked	4.1 oz	186	6	1	88	30	0	—	—	10	90	558	2	tr
BLUEFISH														
fresh baked	3 oz	135	5	1	64	22	0	—	—	8	65	405	2	tr
BOAR														
wild roasted	3 oz	136	4	1	—	24	0	—	—	13	—	—	—	—
BOK CHOY														
(*see* CABBAGE)														
BONITO														
fresh	3 oz	117	4	—	—	20	0	0	0	24	—	—	—	0
BORAGE														
fresh chopped	½ cup	9	tr	—	0	1	1	—	—	41	35	207	—	15
fresh chopped cooked	3.5 oz	25	1	—	0	2	4	—	—	102	88	491	—	33
BOTTLED WATER														
(*see* WATER)														
BOYSENBERRIES														
in heavy syrup	1 cup	226	tr	—	0	3	57	—	—	23	9	230	88	16
unsweetened frzn	1 cup	66	tr	—	0	1	16	—	—	36	2	183	84	4

FOOD	PORTION	CALS	FAT	SAT FAT	CHOL	PROT	CARB	SUGAR	FIBER	CALCI	SOD	POTAS	FOLIC	VIT C
BRAINS														
beef pan-fried	3 oz	167	13	3	1696	11	0	—	—	8	134	301	5	3
beef simmered	3 oz	136	11	2	1746	9	0	—	—	8	102	204	6	1
lamb braised	3 oz	124	9	2	1737	11	0	—	—	10	114	175	4	10
lamb fried	3 oz	232	19	5	2128	14	0	—	—	18	133	304	6	20
pork braised	3 oz	117	8	2	2169	10	0	—	0	8	77	—	3	12
veal braised	3 oz	115	8	—	2635	10	0	—	—	13	133	181	3	11
veal fried	3 oz	181	14	—	1802	12	0	—	—	9	150	401	5	12
ARMOUR														
Pork Brains In Milk Gravy	⅔ cup (5.5 oz)	150	5	3	3500	16	10	0	0	0	550	—	—	6
BRAN														
corn	1 cup (2.7 oz)	170	1	tr	0	6	65	—	65	32	5	33	3	0
oat	½ cup (1.6 oz)	116	3	1	0	8	31	—	7	27	2	266	25	0
oat cooked	½ cup (3.8 oz)	44	1	tr	0	4	13	—	3	11	1	101	7	0
rice	½ cup (2.1 oz)	187	12	2	0	8	29	—	12	34	3	786	37	0
wheat	½ cup (2 oz)	63	1	tr	0	5	19	—	12	21	1	343	23	0
HODGSON MILL														
Oat	¼ cup	120	3	1	0	6	23	0	6	20	3	40	20	—
Wheat Unprocessed	¼ cup	30	0	0	0	2	10	0	7	0	0	50	12	—
QUAKER														
Oat Bran	½ cup (1.4 oz)	150	3	1	0	7	25	1	6	20	0	230	8	—
BRAZIL NUTS														
dried unblanched	1 oz	186	19	5	0	4	4	—	—	50	0	170	1	tr
BREAD														
CANNED														
boston brown	1 slice (1.6 oz)	88	1	tr	—	2	20	—	2	31	284	143	3	0
FROZEN														
MARIE CALLENDER'S														
Cornbread & Honey Butter	1 piece + butter	210	11	5	15	2	28	2	1	20	370	—	—	0
Original Garlic	1 piece	190	8	6	<5	4	23	5	2	20	330	—	—	0
Parmesan & Romano Garlic	1 piece	200	10	3	5	5	23	2	2	200	430	—	—	0
NEW YORK														
Garlic	1 slice (2 oz)	190	8	2	0	3	27	1	1	0	390	—	—	0
Garlic Reduced Fat	1 slice (2 oz)	160	4	1	0	4	29	1	1	0	340	—	—	0
Texas Garlic Toast	1 in slice (1.4 oz)	160	9	2	0	3	17	1	1	0	260	—	—	0
MIX														
cornbread	1 piece (2 oz)	189	6	2	37	4	29	—	1	44	467	77	7	tr

FOOD	PORTION	CALS	FAT	SAT FAT	CHOL	PROT	CARB	SUGAR	FIBER	CALCI	SOD	POTAS	FOLIC	VIT C
ATKINS														
Caraway Rye as prep	1 slice	150	0	0	0	12	8	0	5	0	150	—	—	0
Country White as prep	1 slice	70	0	0	0	12	8	0	5	0	135	—	—	0
Sourdough as prep	1 slice	70	0	0	0	12	8	0	5	0	170	—	—	0
BUITONI														
Focaccia Rosemary & Garlic	1 piece (1 oz)	110	1	0	0	4	22	2	1	20	250	0	—	2
Foccacia Italian Herb & Cheese	1 slice	110	2	1	0	3	21	3	0	20	390	—	—	0
CARBOLITE														
Bread Mix as prep	1 slice	45	5	1	0	6	4	—	—	—	130	—	—	—
HODGSON MILL														
European Cheese & Herb	¼ cup (1.2 oz)	130	1	0	0	5	21	3	tr	20	250	—	—	0
Honey Whole Wheat	¼ cup (1.2 oz)	120	1	0	0	5	22	2	2	—	160	—	—	4
KETO														
Quick Bread All Flavors as prep	1 slice	55	0	0	0	5	3	—	—	—	95	100	—	—
MINICARB														
Country White as prep	1 slice	80	3	0	0	9	7	0	4	—	115	—	—	—
SASSAFRAS														
12 Grain & Sunflower	1 slice (1.4 oz)	150	2	0	0	5	28	4	1	20	160	—	—	0
READY-TO-EAT														
baguette parisian	2 oz	120	0	0	0	5	26	0	tr	0	270	—	—	0
baguette whole wheat	2 oz	140	0	0	0	6	29	tr	1	0	360	—	—	0
challah	1 slice (2 oz)	160	3	1	0	3	29	5	1	0	250	—	—	0
cracked wheat	1 slice	65	1	tr	—	2	12	—	1	11	135	44	10	—
egg	1 slice (1.4 oz)	115	2	1	20	4	19	—	—	37	197	46	28	0
french	1 slice (1 oz)	78	1	tr	0	3	15	—	1	21	172	32	9	0
french	1 loaf (1 lb)	1270	18	4	0	43	230	—	—	499	2633	409	—	tr
gluten	1 slice	47	tr	tr	0	2	8	—	—	24	104	—	7	0
italian	1 loaf (1 lb)	1255	4	1	0	41	256	—	—	77	2656	336	—	0
italian	1 slice (1 oz)	81	1	tr	0	3	15	—	1	23	175	33	9	0
navajo fry	1 (5 in diam)	296	9	2	0	6	48	—	—	210	625	67	11	0
navajo fry	1 (10.5 in diam)	527	15	3	0	11	85	—	—	373	1112	118	20	0
oat bran	1 slice	71	1	tr	0	3	12	—	1	19	122	—	—	—
oat bran reduced calorie	1 slice	46	1	tr	0	2	10	—	—	13	81	24	—	0
oatmeal	1 slice	73	1	tr	—	2	13	—	1	18	162	38	7	—

FOOD	PORTION	CALS	FAT	SAT FAT	CHOL	PROT	CARB	SUGAR	FIBER	CALCI	SOD	POTAS	FOLIC	VIT C
oatmeal reduced calorie	1 slice	48	1	tr	0	2	10	—	—	26	89	—	—	—
pita	1 sm (1 oz)	78	tr	tr	0	3	16	—	1	24	152	34	7	0
pita	1 reg (2 oz)	165	1	tr	0	5	33	—	1	52	322	72	14	0
pita whole wheat	1 sm (1 oz)	76	1	tr	0	3	16	—	2	4	151	48	—	0
pita whole wheat	1 reg (2 oz)	170	2	tr	0	6	35	—	5	10	340	108	—	0
potato scallion	1 slice (2 oz)	120	1	0	0	4	24	1	0	20	340	—	—	4
protein	1 slice	47	tr	tr	0	2	8	—	—	24	104	—	7	0
pumpernickel	1 slice	80	1	tr	0	3	15	—	2	22	215	661	11	0
raisin	1 slice	71	1	tr	0	2	14	—	—	17	101	59	9	—
rice bran	1 slice	66	1	tr	0	1	12	—	—	19	119	—	—	—
rye	1 slice	83	1	tr	0	3	16	—	2	23	211	53	16	—
rye reduced calorie	1 slice	47	1	tr	0	2	9	—	—	18	93	23	—	—
seven grain	1 slice	65	1	tr	0	3	12	—	2	24	127	53	12	tr
sourdough	1 slice (1 oz)	78	1	tr	0	3	15	—	1	21	172	32	9	0
vienna	1 slice (1 oz)	78	1	tr	0	3	15	—	1	21	172	32	9	0
wheat reduced calorie	1 slice	46	1	tr	—	2	10	—	3	18	117	—	—	—
wheat berry	1 slice	65	1	tr	0	2	12	—	1	26	132	50	—	0
wheat bran	1 slice	89	1	tr	0	3	17	—	3	27	175	82	—	—
wheat germ	1 slice	74	1	tr	—	3	14	—	—	25	157	72	16	—
white	1 slice	67	1	tr	0	2	12	—	1	27	135	30	8	0
white reduced calorie	1 slice	48	1	tr	0	2	10	—	2	22	104	18	—	—
white toasted	1 slice	67	1	tr	0	2	13	—	—	27	136	30	6	0
white cubed	1 cup	80	1	tr	0	2	15	—	—	38	154	34	—	tr
whole wheat	1 slice	70	1	tr	—	3	13	—	2	20	149	71	14	—
ARNOLD														
Bran'nola Country Oat	1 slice (1.3 oz)	110	2	0	0	4	20	3	3	40	160	—	—	0
Carb Counting Multigrain	1 slice	60	—	—	—	5	9	—	3	—	—	—	—	—
Country White	1 slice (1.3 oz)	110	2	0	0	3	21	4	tr	40	250	—	60	0
Country Classics Buttermilk	1 slice	110	2	0	0	4	19	4	tr	60	180	—	—	0
Country Classics Wheat	1 slice (1.3 oz)	110	2	0	0	4	19	4	2	20	190	—	—	0
Natural 100% Whole Wheat	1 slice (1.3 oz)	90	1	0	0	4	16	2	3	0	170	—	—	0
Raisin Cinnamon	1 slice (1 oz)	80	2	0	0	2	15	6	1	0	95	—	40	0
ATKINS														
Rye	1 slice	60	1	1	5	7	8	0	5	40	110	—	—	0
White	1 slice	60	1	1	5	7	8	0	5	40	115	—	—	0
BEEFSTEAK														
Rye Soft	1 slice	70	1	0	0	2	14	1	0	0	200	—	16	0

FOOD	PORTION	CALS	FAT	SAT FAT	CHOL	PROT	CARB	SUGAR	FIBER	CALCI	SOD	POTAS	FOLIC	VIT C
BREAD DU JOUR														
French	3 in slice (2 oz)	140	1	0	0	5	26	3	1	80	310	—	40	0
DAMASCUS														
Pita	1 (2 oz)	130	0	0	0	6	29	0	2	40	150	—	—	0
Pita Whole Wheat	1 (2 oz)	160	0	0	0	6	32	0	3	40	230	—	—	1
Wraps Honey Wheat	½ wrap (2 oz)	130	0	0	0	5	28	0	1	0	150	—	60	0
Wraps Plain	½ wrap (2 oz)	130	0	0	0	5	29	tr	1	0	150	—	60	0
Wraps Spinach	1 (4 oz)	280	0	0	0	10	52	tr	2	80	460	—	160	0
Wraps Tomato	1 12-inch (4 oz)	240	0	0	0	10	58	1	2	40	440	—	120	0
ECCE PANIS														
Country Wheat	1 slice (2 oz)	150	0	0	0	4	32	tr	2	0	320	—	—	0
European Baguette	2 oz	150	0	0	0	5	34	tr	1	0	370	—	—	0
FREIHOFER'S														
100% Whole Wheat	1 slice	90	2	0	0	45	17	3	3	40	160	—	32	0
Whole Wheat Light	2 slices	80	1	0	0	5	19	3	5	20	160	—	16	0
GOLD MEDAL														
100% Whole Wheat	1 slice	70	2	0	0	2	13	1	2	20	180	—	—	0
HOME PRIDE														
Carb Action Multigrain	1 slice	60	—	—	—	6	8	—	1	—	—	—	—	—
Carb Action White Fiber	1 slice	60	—	—	—	4	10	—	4	—	—	—	—	—
Wheat	1 slice (1 oz)	80	1	0	0	2	14	2	1	20	190	—	16	0
LA MEXICANA														
Wraps Chocolate	1 (1.3 oz)	120	3	1	0	4	18	1	1	60	360	—	—	0
Wraps Southwestern Mild Chili	1 (1.3 oz)	120	4	1	0	4	18	1	1	100	360	—	—	0
Wraps Spinach	1 (1.3 oz)	120	4	1	0	4	18	1	1	60	360	—	—	0
Wraps Tomato Basil	1 (1.3 oz)	120	4	1	0	4	18	1	1	100	360	—	—	0
MILTON'S														
Healthy Multi-Grain	1 slice (1.4 oz)	110	1	0	0	3	24	6	3	20	150	—	—	6
NATURAL OVENS														
100% Whole Grain	1 slice	60	1	0	0	4	14	1	5	100	80	—	40	0
7 Grain Herb	1 slice	70	1	0	0	4	16	1	4	100	70	—	60	0
Better White	1 slice	80	1	0	0	4	19	1	2	100	75		40	0
Cracked Wheat	1 slice	80	1	0	0	4	16	1	3	100	70	—	60	0

FOOD	PORTION	CALS	FAT	SAT FAT	CHOL	PROT	CARB	SUGAR	FIBER	CALCI	SOD	POTAS	FOLIC	VIT C
NATURAL OVENS (CONT.)														
English Muffin Bread	1 slice	80	1	0	0	4	16	1	2	100	70	—	40	0
Glorious Cinnamon Raisin	1 slice	70	1	0	0	3	15	3	2	100	70	—	40	0
Happiness Raisin Pecan	1 slice	70	1	0	0	3	15	3	3	100	70	—	80	0
Health Max	1 slice	80	1	0	0	3	16	2	3	100	80	—	60	0
Hunger Filler	1 slice	60	1	0	0	4	13	1	4	60	90	—	40	0
Lo Carb Golden Crunch	1 slice	70	4	0	0	8	7	2	4	100	80	—	60	0
Lo Carb Original	1 slice	60	2	0	0	7	8	2	5	100	70	0	60	0
Mild Rye	1 slice	70	1	0	0	3	13	0	4	100	70	—	80	0
Multi-Grain Stay Slim	1 slice	60	1	0	0	3	14	1	5	60	90	—	40	0
Nutty Natural	1 slice	70	1	0	0	3	16	1	5	100	70	—	60	0
Right Wheat	1 slice	60	1	0	0	2	13	1	5	60	90	—	40	0
Soft Wheat	1 slice	70	1	0	0	3	15	1	3	100	70	—	40	0
Sunny Millet	1 slice	60	1	0	0	3	14	1	4	100	80	—	40	0
PEPPERIDGE FARM														
Apple Cinammon	1 slice (1 oz)	80	2	0	0	4	15	4	1	0	120	—	—	0
Deli Rye Seedless	1 slice	80	1	1	0	3	15	tr	1	20	210	—	24	0
Deli Swirl Rye & Pump	1 slice	80	1	0	0	3	15	tr	1	20	220	—	—	0
Farmhouse Butter Topped Wheat	1 slice	110	2	1	0	4	21	3	2	40	210	—	32	0
Farmhouse Country Wheat	1 slice	110	2	0	0	4	21	3	2	40	190	—	40	0
Farmhouse Hearty White	1 slice (1.5 oz)	110	2	0	<5	5	20	5	tr	40	260	—	24	0
Farmhouse Sesame Wheat	1 slice	110	2	0	0	4	19	2	2	40	190	—	32	0
Farmhouse Soft Oatmeal	1 slice	110	1	0	0	4	21	3	1	40	200	—	32	0
Farmhouse Sourdough	1 slice (1.5 oz)	110	2	1	0	4	20	2	1	40	220	—	60	0
Jewish Rye	1 slice	80	1	0	0	3	15	tr	2	20	210	—	24	0
Natural Whole Grain Whole Wheat	1 slice (1.2 oz)	90	1	0	0	4	16	2	2	40	135	—	8	0
Natural Whole Grain Honey Oat	1 slice (1.2 oz)	90	2	0	0	4	15	2	2	20	135	—	16	0
Sandwich Pocket Wheat	1 (2 oz)	160	1	1	0	6	30	2	3	60	260	—	—	0
Sandwich Pocket White	1 (2 oz)	150	1	0	0	6	30	2	2	40	290	—	—	0

FOOD	PORTION	CALS	FAT	SAT FAT	CHOL	PROT	CARB	SUGAR	FIBER	CALCI	SOD	POTAS	FOLIC	VIT C
PEPPERIDGE FARM (CONT.)														
Swirl Cinnamon	1 slice (1 oz)	90	3	1	0	2	15	tr	1	0	110	—	—	0
Swirl French Vanilla	1 slice	140	4	1	0	4	23	7	tr	0	190	—	40	0
Swirl Raisin Cinnamon	1 slice (1 oz)	80	2	0	0	3	14	6	1	0	105	—	—	0
STROEHMANN														
100% Whole Wheat	1 slice (1.3 oz)	90	1	0	0	5	17	3	2	40	180	—	8	0
D'Italiano Italian No Seeds	1 slice (1 oz)	80	1	0	0	2	15	tr	tr	40	170	—	32	0
D'Italiano Italian Seeded	1 slice (1 oz)	80	1	0	0	2	15	tr	tr	40	170	—	32	0
Family White	1 slice (0.8 oz)	65	1	0	0	2	13	1	0	20	135	—	24	0
Homestyle Split Top Wheat	1 slice (0.8 oz)	60	0	0	0	2	13	2	tr	20	110	—	24	0
Homestyle Split Top White	1 slice (0.8 oz)	65	1	0	0	2	12	1	1	20	110	—	24	0
Honey Cracked Wheat	1 slice	90	1	0	0	3	16	2	1	20	140	—	24	0
King White	1 slice (0.8 oz)	65	1	0	0	2	13	1	0	20	135	—	24	0
New York Rye	1 slice (1 oz)	80	1	0	0	3	15	1	1	20	150	—	24	0
Potato	1 slice (1.2 oz)	100	2	0	0	3	19	3	tr	40	170	—	32	0
Ranch White	1 slice (0.8 oz)	65	1	0	0	2	13	1	0	20	135	—	24	0
Rye	1 slice (1.1 oz)	80	1	0	0	3	15	tr	tr	20	180	—	24	0
Twelve Grain	1 slice (1.2 oz)	90	1	0	0	3	17	3	1	20	140	—	32	0
TASTYBITE														
Nan Kontos Massala	½ loaf (1.4 oz)	120	3	1	0	7	15	1	1	40	160	76	—	0
Nan Kontos Onion	½ loaf (1.4 oz)	120	4	1	0	7	15	1	1	40	160	—	—	0
Nan Kontos Roghani	½ loaf (1.4 oz)	125	3	2	0	4	19	3	1	20	240	—	—	0
Nan Kontos Tandoori	½ loaf (1.4 oz)	120	3	2	0	4	19	3	1	20	240		—	0
Roti Kontos Missy	½ loaf (1.4 oz)	125	4	2	0	5	18	2	2	20	185	—	—	0
THOMAS'														
Toasting Cinnamon	1 slice	130	5	2	0	3	20	6	1	40	170	—	—	0
Toasting Cinnamon Raisin	1 slice	120	3	1	0	3	22	10	1	40	170	—	—	0
TOUFAYAN														
Wraps Sundried Tomato Basil	1 (2 oz)	183	5	1	0	6	30	1	2	50	537	—	—	0
Wraps Wheat	1 (2 oz)	183	5	1	0	6	29	1	3	50	354	—	—	0
VALLEY LAIIVOSH														
Valley Wraps	1 (1 oz)	100	1	0	0	4	19	3	1	20	125	—	—	0

FOOD	PORTION	CALS	FAT	SAT FAT	CHOL	PROT	CARB	SUGAR	FIBER	CALCI	SOD	POTAS	FOLIC	VIT C
REFRIGERATED														
PILLSBURY														
Crusty French Loaf	⅕ loaf (2.2 oz)	150	2	1	0	5	27	3	tr	0	390	—	—	0
Grands Wheat	1 (2.1 oz)	200	8	2	0	4	27	6	2	40	600	—	—	0
TAKE-OUT														
chapatis as prep w/ fat	1 bread (1.6 oz)	95	2	1	3	3	18	1	3	10	180	101	11	0
chapatis as prep w/o fat	1 (2½ oz)	141	1	—	—	5	31	—	5	42	—	—	—	0
cornbread	2 in x 2 in (1.4 oz)	107	2	1	28	4	18	—	—	44	276	75	—	tr
cornstick	1 (1.3 oz)	101	4	1	30	2	13	—	tr	37	195	36	4	tr
focaccia	1 piece (2 oz)	130	3	0	0	4	23	3	1	0	310	—	—	0
focaccia onion	1 piece (4.6 oz)	282	10	1	0	6	43	2	2	20	536	114	43	2
focaccia rosemary	1 piece (3.5 oz)	251	7	1	0	6	40	1	2	13	535	68	38	tr
focaccia tomato olive	1 piece (4.7 oz)	270	8	1	0	6	42	1	2	31	683	122	39	3
garlic bread	2 slices (2 oz)	190	8	2	0	3	27	1	1	0	290	—	—	0
irish soda bread	1 slice (2 oz)	174	3	1	11	4	34	—	—	49	239	160	6	1
naan	1 bread (3.5 oz)	286	9	5	46	7	43	3	2	54	546	107	53	tr
papadums fried	2 (1.5 oz)	81	4	—	—	4	9	—	2	15	—	—	—	0
paratha	1 bread (2.1 oz)	201	10	7	27	4	23	1	2	10	268	78	11	0
BREAD COATING														
DON'S CHUCK WAGON														
Chicken Baking Mix	¼ cup (1 oz)	95	0	0	0	3	21	0	1	0	850	—	—	0
Fish & Chips Mix	¼ cup (1 oz)	100	0	0	0	3	21	0	1	0	740	—	—	0
Fish Mix	¼ cup (1 oz)	95	0	0	0	4	21	0	1	0	940	—	—	0
Mushroom Batter Mix	¼ cup (1 oz)	95	0	0	0	3	21	0	1	0	990	—	—	0
Onion Ring Mix	¼ cup (1 oz)	100	0	0	0	3	21	0	1	0	690	—	—	0
Seafood Bake & Fry Mix	¼ cup (1 oz)	95	0	0	0	2	21	0	1	0	990	—	—	0
LUZIANNE														
Cajun Chicken Coating Mix	2 tbsp (1 oz)	100	1	0	0	3	20	2	1	0	1260	—	—	0
OVEN FRY														
Extra Crispy For Chicken	⅛ pkg (0.5 oz)	60	1	0	0	2	10	2	0	0	420	30	—	0
Extra Crispy For Pork	⅛ pkg (0.5 oz)	60	2	0	0	2	11	1	0	0	340	20	—	0

FOOD	PORTION	CALS	FAT	SAT FAT	CHOL	PROT	CARB	SUGAR	FIBER	CALCI	SOD	POTAS	FOLIC	VIT C
SHAKE 'N BAKE														
Buffalo Wings	1/10 pkg (0.4 oz)	40	1	0	0	0	8	3	0	0	300	15	—	0
Classic Italian Chicken or Pork	1/8 pkg (0.4 oz)	40	1	0	0	1	7	tr	0	0	270	30	—	0
Country Mild Recipe	1/8 pkg (0.3 oz)	35	2	1	0	0	5	0	0	0	240	10	—	0
Glazes Barbecue Chicken Or Pork	1/8 pkg (0.4 oz)	45	1	0	0	0	9	5	0	0	410	35	—	0
Glazes Honey Mustard Chicken Or Pork	1/8 pkg (0.4 oz)	45	1	0	0	0	9	6	0	0	300	20	—	0
Glazes Tangy Honey Chicken Or Pork	1/8 pkg (0.4 oz)	45	1	0	0	0	9	6	0	0	300	45	—	0
Home Style Flour Recipe For Chicken	1/8 pkg (0.4 oz)	40	1	0	0	tr	7	0	0	0	470	15	—	0
Hot & Spicy Chicken Or Pork	1/8 pkg (0.4 oz)	40	1	0	0	1	7	tr	0	0	170	20	—	0
Original For Chicken	1/8 pkg (0.4 oz)	40	1	0	0	1	7	tr	0	0	220	20	—	0
Original For Fish	1/4 pkg (0.7 oz)	80	2	0	0	2	14	tr	tr	0	350	25	—	0
Original For Pork	1/8 pkg (0.4 oz)	45	1	0	0	1	8	tr	0	0	230	20	—	0
BREAD MACHINE MIX														
BETTY CROCKER														
Harvest Wheat	1/11 loaf	140	3	1	0	4	25	3	2	—	220	75	24	—
Home-Style White	1/11 loaf	130	2	0	0	4	25	2	0	—	220	45	40	—
CARBSENSE														
Harvest Wheat as prep	1 slice	60	0	0	0	11	4	0	1	—	120	—	—	—
FLEISCHMANN'S														
Apple Cinnamon	1/8 loaf	160	1	0	0	5	32	12	2	0	160	—	—	1
Cinnamon Raisin	1/8 loaf	160	1	0	0	5	33	4	2	0	170	—	—	1
Country White	1/8 loaf (1.6 oz)	170	3	1	0	6	31	4	2	20	170	—	—	1
Cranberry Orange	1/10 loaf	150	2	0	0	2	33	4	2	20	150	—	—	1
Honey Oatmeal	1/8 loaf	160	1	0	0	5	33	5	3	0	270	—	—	1
Italian Herb	1/8 loaf	160	2	1	0	5	29	2	2	0	310	—	—	1
Sourdough	1/8 loaf	150	2	1	0	5	29	3	2	20	160	—	—	0
Stoneground Wheat	1/8 loaf	160	1	0	0	5	32	4	3	0	180	—	—	1
KETO														
Cinnamon Raisin as prep	1 slice	79	0	0	0	13	6	tr	3	—	95	—	—	—
French Loaf as prep	1 slice	79	0	0	0	13	5	tr	3	—	95	—	—	—
Sourdough Rye as prep	1 slice	79	1	—	—	13	5	tr	3	—	95	—	—	—

FOOD	PORTION	CALS	FAT	SAT FAT	CHOL	PROT	CARB	SUGAR	FIBER	CALCI	SOD	POTAS	FOLIC	VIT C
KETOGENICS														
Low Carb Honey Wheat as prep	1 slice	80	1	1	0	0	7	1	5	—	60	—	—	—
Low Carb Original White as prep	1 slice	62	0	0	0	13	2	—	—	—	277	—	—	—
Low Carb Pumpernickel Rye as prep	1 slice	80	2	1	0	11	7	1	5	—	—	—	—	—
BREADCRUMBS														
dry	1 cup	426	6	1	—	14	78	—	5	245	930	239	—	—
dry seasonsed	1 cup (4 oz)	441	3	1	—	17	85	—	5	119	3180	324	—	—
fresh	⅔ cup	76	1	tr	0	4	14	—	1	31	153	34	10	0
ARNOLD														
Italian	¼ cup	110	2	0	0	4	19	1	1	40	560	—	—	0
KETO														
Low Carb Cajun	½ cup	185	1	—	—	13	13	—	9	—	595	—	—	—
Low Carb Italian	½ cup	185	1	—	—	13	13	—	9	—	480	—	—	—
Low Carb Original	½ cup	185	1	—	—	13	13	—	9	—	480	—	—	—
PROGRESSO														
Garlic & Herb	¼ cup (1 oz)	100	2	0	0	4	18	1	1	40	530	—	—	0
Italian Style	¼ cup (1 oz)	110	2	0	0	4	20	1	1	40	430	—	—	0
Parmesan	¼ cup (1 oz)	100	2	0	0	4	17	1	1	40	870	—	—	0
Plain	¼ cup (1 oz)	110	2	0	0	4	19	1	1	40	210	—	—	0
RONZONI														
Italian Flavored	¼ cup	120	2	1	0	4	21	2	2	40	330	—	—	1
BREADFRUIT														
fresh	¼ small	99	tr	—	0	1	26	—	—	17	2	470	—	28
seeds cooked	1 oz	48	1	tr	0	2	9	—	—	12	—	—	—	—
seeds raw	1 oz	54	2	tr	0	2	8	—	—	10	—	—	—	2
seeds roasted	1 oz	59	tr	tr	0	2	11	—	—	24	—	—	—	—
BREADNUTTREE SEEDS														
dried	1 oz	104	tr	tr	0	2	23	—	—	27	—	—	13	—
BREADSTICKS														
onion poppyseed	1	64	1	—	10	2	11	—	—	19	69	—	—	—
plain	1 sm	25	1	tr	0	1	4	—	—	2	66	12	—	0
plain	1	41	1	tr	0	1	7	—	—	2	66	12	—	0
ANGONOA														
Deli Style Sesame	3 (0.5 oz)	730	3	0	0	2	10	tr	tr	20	110	—	—	0
BREAD DU JOUR														
Original	1 (1.9 oz)	130	1	0	0	5	25	3	1	80	290	—	40	0
Sourdough	1 (1.9 oz)	130	1	0	0	5	25	1	1	150	280	—	40	0
JOHN WM MACY'S														
CheeseSticks Original Cheddar	3 (1 oz)	130	6	3	11	6	14	0	1	60	190	—	—	0

FOOD	PORTION	CALS	FAT	SAT FAT	CHOL	PROT	CARB	SUGAR	FIBER	CALCI	SOD	POTAS	FOLIC	VIT C
NEW YORK														
Garlic Soft	1 (1.5 oz)	140	4	1	0	3	23	1	1	0	220	—	—	0
PEPPERIDGE FARM														
Snack Sticks Wheat	9 (1 oz)	130	4	1	0	3	22	4	1	0	370	—	—	0
PILLSBURY														
Soft	1 (1.4 oz)	110	2	0	0	3	19	2	tr	0	290	—	—	0
Soft Garlic & Herb	1 (2.1 oz)	180	7	2	0	4	25	3	tr	0	580	—	—	0
STELLA D'ORO														
Grissini Style Fat Free	3 (0.5 oz)	60	0	0	0	2	12	1	0	0	130	—	—	0
Original	1 (0.4 oz)	45	1	0	0	1	7	0	0	0	40	—	—	0
Potato 'N Onion	1 (0.4 oz)	45	1	0	0	1	8	tr	0	0	210	—	—	0
Roasted Garlic	1	45	1	0	0	1	8	tr	0	0	230	—	—	0
Sesame	1 (0.4 oz)	50	3	0	0	1	7	tr	tr	20	45	—	—	0
Snack Stix Cracked Pepper	4 (0.5 oz)	70	2	0	0	2	11	tr	0	0	290	—	—	0
Snack Stix Salted	4 (0.5 oz)	70	2	0	0	2	11	tr	0	0	290	—	—	0
Sodium Free	1 (0.4 oz)	45	1	0	0	1	7	tr	0	0	0	—	—	0
Wheat	1 (0.3 oz)	40	1	0	0	1	6	tr	0	0	20	—	—	0

BREAKFAST BARS

(*see* CEREAL BARS, ENERGY BARS)

BREAKFAST DRINKS

FOOD	PORTION	CALS	FAT	SAT FAT	CHOL	PROT	CARB	SUGAR	FIBER	CALCI	SOD	POTAS	FOLIC	VIT C
orange drink powder	3 rounded tsp	93	0	0	0	0	24	—	—	46	4	40	116	98
orange drink powder as prep w/water	6 oz	86	0	0	0	0	22	—	—	46	9	37	107	91
CARNATION														
Instant Breakfast French Vanilla as prep w/ 2% milk	1 serv	250	5	—	—	13	40	—	—	500	220	620	100	30
Instant Breakfast French Vanilla as prep w/ fat free milk	1 serv	220	1	—	—	13	40	—	—	500	230	650	100	30
Instant Breakfast French Vanilla as prep w/ whole milk	1 serv	280	8	—	—	13	39	—	—	500	220	610	100	30

BROAD BEANS

FOOD	PORTION	CALS	FAT	SAT FAT	CHOL	PROT	CARB	SUGAR	FIBER	CALCI	SOD	POTAS	FOLIC	VIT C
canned	1 cup	183	1	tr	0	14	32	—	—	67	1161	620	84	5
dried cooked	1 cup	186	1	tr	0	13	33	—	—	62	8	456	177	1
fresh cooked	3½ oz	56	tr	tr	0	5	10	—	—	18	41	193	—	20

FOOD	PORTION	CALS	FAT	SAT FAT	CHOL	PROT	CARB	SUGAR	FIBER	CALCI	SOD	POTAS	FOLIC	VIT C
BROCCOFLOWER														
fresh raw	½ cup (1.8 oz)	16	tr	tr	0	1	3	—	—	16	12	150	29	44
BROCCOLI														
FRESH														
chinese broccoli (gai lan) cooked	1 cup (3.1 oz)	19	1	tr	0	1	3	—	2	88	6	230	87	0
chopped cooked	½ cup	22	tr	tr	0	2	4	—	2	36	20	228	39	58
raw chopped	½ cup	12	tr	tr	0	1	2	—	1	21	12	143	31	41
FROZEN														
chopped cooked	½ cup	25	tr	tr	0	3	5	—	—	47	22	166	52	37
spears cooked	10 oz pkg	69	tr	tr	0	8	13	—	4	127	60	451	76	100
spears cooked	½ cup	25	tr	tr	0	3	5	—	3	127	22	166	28	37
BIRDS EYE														
Chopped	⅓ cup	25	0	0	0	—	—	—	2	20	15	—	—	42
Cuts	½ cup	25	0	0	0	—	—	—	3	20	30	—	—	60
Florets	1 cup	25	0	0	0	2	4	1	2	40	35	—	—	54
In Cheese Sauce	½ cup	70	4	2	5	3	7	3	2	—	500	—	—	—
FRESH LIKE														
Spear	3.5 oz	26	tr	—	—	3	5	—	1	55	32	224	—	57
GREEN GIANT														
Butter Sauce	4 oz	50	2	1	<5	2	7	2	2	40	330	—	—	42
Cheese Sauce	⅔ cup (3.9 oz)	70	3	1	<5	3	9	5	2	60	520	—	—	42
Chopped	¾ cup (2.8 oz)	25	0	0	0	2	4	1	2	20	25	—	—	30
Cuts	1 cup (2.9 oz)	25	0	0	0	2	4	1	2	20	25	—	—	36
Harvest Fresh Cut	⅔ cup (3.2 oz)	25	0	0	0	2	4	tr	2	20	150	—	—	42
Harvest Fresh Spears	3.5 oz	25	0	0	0	2	4	1	2	40	125	—	—	36
Select Florets	1⅓ cups (2.9 oz)	25	0	0	0	2	4	1	2	20	25	—	—	36
Select Spears	3 oz	25	0	0	0	2	4	2	2	20	25	—	—	30
HEALTH IS WEALTH														
Broccoli Munchees	2 (1 oz)	60	2	0	0	2	10	0	1	20	170	—	—	2
STOUFFER'S														
Au Gratin	1 serv (4 oz)	100	4	2	10	5	10	3	2	100	450	230	—	18
TREE OF LIFE														
Cuts	1 cup (3.1 oz)	25	0	0	0	2	4	1	2	20	20	—	—	36
BROWNIE														
FROZEN														
GREENFIELD														
Fat Free Homestyle	1 (1.3 oz)	110	0	0	0	2	27	19	0	0	60	—	—	0
OTIS SPUNKMEYER														
Blue Yonder w/ Walnuts	1 (2 oz)	230	10	3	20	3	34	22	2	0	170	—	—	0

FOOD	PORTION	CALS	FAT	SAT FAT	CHOL	PROT	CARB	SUGAR	FIBER	CALCI	SOD	POTAS	FOLIC	VIT C
WEIGHT WATCHERS														
Brownie A La Mode	1 (3.14 oz)	190	4	2	30	5	33	15	2	100	190	—	—	0
Double Fudge Brownie Parfait	1 (5.3 oz)	190	3	2	5	6	39	20	2	200	170	—	—	0
MIX														
plain	1 (1.2 oz)	139	7	1	9	1	20	—	1	6	83	61	—	—
plain low calorie	1 (0.8 oz)	84	2	1	0	1	16	—	1	3	21	69	1	0
ATKINS														
Kitchen Fudge as prep	1 (2 inch)	60	0	0	0	3	17	0	4	—	80	—	—	—
AUNT PAULA'S														
Low Carb Chef Fudge Brownie as prep	1 (2.5 inch)	89	5	2	3	7	9	0	2	—	—	—	—	—
BETTY CROCKER														
Chocolate Chunk as prep	1	180	9	2	21	1	25	18	—	20	90	—	8	—
Dark Chocolate Fudge as prep	1	170	7	1	21	1	24	17	—	20	120	—	8	—
Dark Chocolate w/ Syrup as prep	1	170	7	1	21	2	25	16	—	20	105	—	8	—
Fudge as prep	1	170	7	1	21	1	23	17	—	20	100	90	8	—
German Chocolate Coconut Pecan Filling as prep	1	200	8	2	21	1	29	21	1	20	115	—	8	—
Hot Fudge as prep	1	170	8	2	21	2	23	16	—	20	105	—	8	—
Original as prep	1	180	6	1	21	1	27	19	—	20	135	—	8	—
Peanut Butter as prep	1	180	8	3	21	3	23	17	—	20	105	—	8	—
Stir'n Bake w/ Mini Kisses as prep	1 scrv	220	7	3	0	2	38	27	1	—	160	—	8	—
Turtle w/ Caramel & Pecans as prep	1	170	8	1	21	1	25	16	—	20	95	—	8	—
Walnut as prep	1	180	9	1	21	2	23	15	—	20	90	—	8	—
BIG TRAIN														
Low Carb Chocolate Chip as prep	1 (2 inch)	140	9	5	42	2	15	4	4	20	45	—	—	0
ESTEE														
Brownie Mix as prep	2	100	4	2	0	tr	23	10	1	—	0	140	—	—
KETO														
Chocolate Fudge as prep	1	59	3	—	—	6	2	0	1	—	50	—	—	—

FOOD	PORTION	CALS	FAT	SAT FAT	CHOL	PROT	CARB	SUGAR	FIBER	CALCI	SOD	POTAS	FOLIC	VIT C
MINICARB														
Chocolate Brownie as prep	1	220	17	4	50	5	10	1	8	—	75	—	—	—
NO PUDGE!														
All Flavors	1	100	0	0	0	2	21	13	tr	40	90	—	—	0
SWEET REWARDS														
Low Fat Fudge as prep	1	130	3	1	0	2	27	18	1	60	115	—	8	0
Reduced Fat Supreme as prep	1	140	3	1	21	2	27	19	—	60	110	90	8	—
READY-TO-EAT														
plain	1 lg (2 oz)	227	9	2	10	3	36	—	1	16	175	84	—	—
plain	1 sm (1 oz)	115	5	1	5	1	18	—	1	8	88	42	—	—
w/ nuts	1 (1 oz)	100	4	2	14	1	16	—	—	13	59	50	—	tr
DOLLY MADISON														
Fudge	1 (3 oz)	330	11	4	45	3	54	11	1	40	190	—	—	0
ENTENMANN'S														
Little Bites	3 (2.2 oz)	290	16	3	45	3	37	26	1	20	200	—	—	0
Ultimate Fudge	1 (1.6 oz)	220	13	4	50	3	27	18	2	0	60	—	—	0
GREENFIELD														
Blondie Fat Free Apple Spice	1 (1.3 oz)	110	0	0	0	2	26	19	0	0	60	—	—	0
HEALTH VALLEY														
Bar w/ Fudge Filling	1 bar	110	0	0	0	3	26	17	4	20	30	—	—	1
HOSTESS														
Brownie Bites	3 (1.3 oz)	170	9	2	30	2	21	17	1	0	80	—	—	0
Fudge	1 (3 oz)	330	11	4	45	3	54	11	1	40	190	—	—	0
Light	1 (1.4 oz)	140	3	1	1	1	28	19	1	0	80	—	—	0
LANCE														
Fudge Nut	1 (2.25 oz)	340	13	3	20	3	56	26	2	20	180	15	—	0
LITTLE DEBBIE														
Brownie Lights	1 (2 oz)	190	3	0	0	3	39	27	1	23	200	130	—	tr
Brownie Loaves	1 (2.1 oz)	260	15	3	40	3	31	21	1	14	160	169	—	tr
Fudge	1 pkg (2.1 oz)	270	13	3	15	2	39	24	tr	21	170	88	—	tr
TASTYKAKE														
Fudge Walnut	1 (3 oz)	370	17	4	80	5	52	37	1	20	150	—	—	0
TOM'S														
Fudge Nut	1 pkg (2.5 oz)	300	13	3	5	3	45	19	0	20	95	—	—	0
REFRIGERATED														
TOLL HOUSE														
Brownie Dough	¹⁄₁₂ pkg (1.5 oz)	180	7	3	15	2	26	18	2	0	160	—	—	0
TAKE-OUT														
plain	1 2 in sq (2.1 oz)	243	10	3	10	3	39	—	—	25	153	83	17	3

FOOD	PORTION	CALS	FAT	SAT FAT	CHOL	PROT	CARB	SUGAR	FIBER	CALCI	SOD	POTAS	FOLIC	VIT C
BRUSSELS SPROUTS														
FRESH														
cooked	½ cup	30	tr	tr	0	2	7	—	3	28	17	247	47	48
cooked	1 sprout	8	tr	tr	0	1	2	—	—	7	4	67	13	13
raw	1 sprout	8	tr	tr	0	1	2	—	1	8	5	74	12	16
raw	½ cup	19	tr	tr	0	1	4	—	—	18	11	171	27	37
FROZEN														
cooked	½ cup	33	tr	tr	0	3	6	—	—	19	18	254	79	36
BIRDS EYE														
Brussels Sprouts	11 sprouts	35	0	0	0	3	7	2	3	20	15	—	—	54
GREEN GIANT														
Butter Sauce	⅔ cup (3.6 oz)	60	2	2	<5	3	9	3	4	20	270	—	—	42
BUCKWHEAT														
groats roasted cooked	1 cup (5.9 oz)	647	1	tr	0	6	34	—	5	12	7	148	24	0
groats roasted uncooked	1 cup (5.7 oz)	567	4	1	0	19	123	—	17	28	18	525	69	0
BUFFALO														
burger	4 oz	150	5	3	50	24	1	0	0	0	80	—	—	0
water buffalo roasted	3 oz	111	2	1	52	23	0	—	—	13	48	266	8	—
BULGUR														
cooked	1 cup (6.3 oz)	151	tr	tr	0	7	34	—	8	18	9	124	33	0
uncooked	1 cup (4.9 oz)	479	2	tr	0	17	106	—	26	49	24	574	38	0
TAKE-OUT														
tabbouleh	½ cup	120	4	0	0	—	—	—	—	—	252	—	—	—
BURBOT (FISH)														
fresh baked	3 oz	98	1	tr	65	65	0	—	—	54	106	440	—	—
BURDOCK ROOT														
cooked	1 cup	110	tr	—	0	3	26	—	—	62	5	450	—	—
fresh	1 cup	85	tr	—	0	2	20	—	—	48	6	363	—	4
BUTTER														
clarified butter	3½ oz	876	99	62	256	tr	0	—	—	tr	—	—	—	0
ghee cow's milk	1 tbsp	126	14	—	39	—	—	—	0	—	0	0	0	0
ghee vegetable oil	1 tbsp	126	14	—	0	—	—	—	0	—	0	0	0	—
stick	1 stick (4 oz)	813	92	57	248	1	tr	—	—	27	937	29	3	0
stick	1 pat (5 g)	36	4	3	11	tr	tr	—	—	1	41	1	tr	0
whipped	1 pat (4 g)	27	3	2	8	tr	tr	—	—	1	31	1	tr	—
whipped	4 oz	542	61	38	165	1	tr	—	—	18	625	20	2	0
whipped	1 tbsp	70	7	5	20	0	0	0	0	—	0	—	—	—
BREAKSTONE'S														
Salted	1 tbsp (0.5 oz)	100	11	7	30	0	0	—	—	—	85	—	—	—

FOOD	PORTION	CALS	FAT	SAT FAT	CHOL	PROT	CARB	SUGAR	FIBER	CALCI	SOD	POTAS	FOLIC	VIT C
CABOT														
Butter	1 tbsp	100	11	7	30	0	0	0	0	0	90	—	—	0
Unsalted	1 tbsp	100	11	7	30	0	0	0	0	—	0	—	—	—
CORMAN														
Light	1 tbsp	55	6	3	5	tr	0	0	0	0	60	—	—	0
HOTEL BAR														
Stick	1 tbsp (0.5 oz)	100	11	7	30	0	0	—	—	—	90	—	—	—
KELLER'S														
European	1 tbsp (0.5 oz)	100	11	7	30	0	0	0	0	0	0	—	—	0
LAND O LAKES														
Salted	1 tbsp (0.5 oz)	100	11	8	30	0	0	—	—	—	85	—	—	—
Ultra Creamy Salted	1 tbsp (0.5 oz)	110	12	8	30	0	0	—	—	—	85	—	—	—
ORGANIC VALLEY														
Butter	1 tbsp (0.5 oz)	100	11	8	30	0	0	0	0	0	75	—	—	0
Unsalted	1 tbsp (0.5 oz)	110	12	8	30	0	0	0	0	0	0	—	—	0
BUTTER BEANS														
CANNED														
GREEN GIANT														
Butter Beans	½ cup (4.5 oz)	90	0	0	0	6	16	1	4	40	450	—	—	0
VAN CAMP														
Butter Beans	½ cup (4.6 oz)	110	1	0	0	8	22	0	7	40	430	—	—	0
FROZEN														
BIRDS EYE														
Speckled	½ cup	100	0	0	0	6	20	1	4	20	130	—	—	2
BUTTER SUBSTITUTES														
stick	1 stick	811	91	32	99	1	1	—	—	31	1013	40	2	tr
KETO														
Butta	1 tsp	43	5	5	0	0	0	0	0	—	0	—	—	—
MOLLY MCBUTTER														
Natural Butter	1 tsp	5	0	0	0	0	1	—	—	—	180	0	—	—
Natural Cheese	1 tsp	5	0	0	0	0	1	—	—	—	125	0	—	—
Roasted Garlic	1 tsp	5	0	0	0	0	1	—	—	—	125	0	—	—
OLIVIO														
Spread	1 tbsp	80	8	1	0	0	0	0	0	0	95	—	—	0
BUTTERBUR														
canned fuki chopped	1 cup	3	tr	—	0	tr	tr	—	—	42	5	15	—	15
fresh fuki	1 cup	13	tr	—	0	tr	3	—	—	97	7	616	—	30
BUTTERFISH														
baked	3 oz	159	9	—	71	19	0	—	—	—	97	409	—	—
fillet baked	1 oz	47	3	—	21	6	0	—	—	—	29	120	—	—
BUTTERNUTS														
dried	1 oz	174	16	tr	0	7	3	—	—	15	0	119	—	—

FOOD	PORTION	CALS	FAT	SAT FAT	CHOL	PROT	CARB	SUGAR	FIBER	CALCI	SOD	POTAS	FOLIC	VIT C
BUTTERSCOTCH														
(see also CANDY)														
HERSHEY'S														
Chips	1 tbsp	80	4	4	0	tr	10	—	—	—	10	—	—	—
NESTLE														
Morsels	1 tbsp	80	4	4	0	0	9	9	0	0	15	—	—	0
CABBAGE														
(see also COLESLAW)														
chinese bok choy shredded cooked	½ cup	10	tr	tr	0	1	2	—	—	79	29	315	—	22
chinese pak-choi raw shredded	½ cup	5	tr	tr	0	1	1	—	—	37	23	88	—	16
chinese pe-tsai raw shredded	1 cup	12	tr	tr	0	1	2	—	—	58	7	181	60	21
chinese pe-tsai shredded cooked	1 cup	16	tr	tr	0	2	3	—	—	38	11	268	64	19
danish raw	1 head (2 lbs)	228	2	tr	0	13	49	—	18	431	164	2231	392	292
danish raw shredded	½ cup (1.2 oz)	9	tr	tr	0	1	2	—	tr	17	6	86	15	11
danish shredded cooked	½ cup (2.6 oz)	17	tr	tr	0	1	3	—	1	23	6	73	15	15
green raw	1 head (2 lbs)	228	2	tr	0	12	49	—	18	431	164	2231	392	292
green raw shredded	½ cup (1.2 oz)	9	tr	tr	0	1	2	—	tr	17	6	86	15	11
green shredded cooked	½ cup (2.6 oz)	17	tr	tr	0	1	3	—	1	23	6	73	15	15
napa cooked	1 cup (3.8 oz)	13	tr	0	0	1	2	—	0	32	12	95	47	0
red raw shredded	½ cup	10	tr	tr	0	tr	2	—	1	18	4	72	7	20
red shredded cooked	½ cup	16	tr	tr	0	1	3	—	—	28	6	105	9	26
savoy raw shredded	½ cup	10	tr	tr	0	1	2	—	—	12	10	81	—	11
savoy shredded cooked	½ cup	18	tr	tr	0	1	4	—	—	22	17	134	—	12
GREENWOOD														
Sweet & Sour Red	½ cup	100	0	0	0	1	24	14	0	40	380	—	—	5
LOHMANN														
Red Cabbage Sweet & Sour	¼ cup	40	0	0	0	0	10	8	0	0	110	—	—	2
TAKE-OUT														
korean kimchee	½ cup	22	tr	—	0	2	4	—	4	34	—	—	—	16
northern white kimchi	½ cup	79	1	—	0	3	18	—	7	—	—	—	—	—
stuffed cabbage	1 (6 oz)	373	22	12	95	25	18	—	—	339	1007	335	22	7
sweet & sour red cabbage	4 oz	61	3	—	—	1	8	—	3	43	—	—	—	14

FOOD	PORTION	CALS	FAT	SAT FAT	CHOL	PROT	CARB	SUGAR	FIBER	CALCI	SOD	POTAS	FOLIC	VIT C
CACTUS														
napoles fresh sliced	½ cup (1.5 oz)	7	tr	—	0	1	1	—	—	70	9	137	1	6
pricklypear fresh	1 cup (5.3 oz)	56	1	—	0	2	13	—	4	—	—	—	—	29
CAKE														
(*see also* CAKE MIX)														
angelfood	1 cake (11.9 oz)	876	3	tr	0	20	197	—	5	477	2548	318	—	0
battenburg cake	1 slice (2 oz)	204	10	—	—	3	28	—	1	48	—	—	—	0
boston cream pie frzn	⅙ cake (3.2 oz)	232	8	2	34	2	40	—	1	21	132	36	7	—
carrot w/ cream cheese icing	1 cake 10 in diam	6175	328	66	1183	63	775	—	—	707	4470	1720	—	23
cheesecake	⅙ cake (2.8 oz)	256	18	9	44	4	20	—	2	50	165	72	12	—
cheesecake	1 cake 9 in diam	3350	213	120	2053	60	317	—	—	622	2464	1088	—	56
cherry fudge w/ chocolate frosting	⅛ cake (2.5 oz)	187	9	3	—	2	27	—	—	34	160	118	—	10
coffeecake fruit	⅛ cake (1.8 oz)	156	5	1	—	3	26	—	—	23	192	45	9	tr
cream puff shell	1 (2.3 oz)	239	17	4	129	6	15	—	—	24	368	64	14	0
crumpet	1 (2.3 oz)	131	1	—	0	4	31	—	2	79	535	61	6	0
devil's food cupcake w/ chocolate frosting	1	120	4	4	19	2	20	—	—	21	92	46	—	tr
devil's food w/ creme filling	1 (1 oz)	105	4	2	15	1	17	—	—	21	105	34	—	0
eccles cake	1 slice (2 oz)	285	16	—	—	2	36	—	1	47	—	—	—	0
eclair	1 (1.4 oz)	149	10	—	—	2	15	—	tr	19	—	—	—	tr
fruitcake	1 piece (1.5 oz)	139	4	tr	2	1	27	—	—	14	116	66	—	—
fruitcake dark	1 cake 7½ in x 2¼ in	5185	228	48	640	74	738	—	—	1293	2123	6138	—	504
jelly roll lemon filled	1 slice (3 oz)	210	2	1	35	3	48	29	tr	20	300	—	0	1
madeira cake	1 slice (1 oz)	98	4	—	—	1	15	—	1	11	—	—	—	0
pound	⅒ cake (1 oz)	117	6	3	66	2	15	—	—	11	119	36	—	—
pound	1 cake (8½ x 3½ x 3 in)	1935	94	52	1100	26	257	—	—	146	1857	443	—	0
pound fat free	1 cake (12 oz)	961	4	1	0	18	208	—	—	146	1158	373	14	1
sheet cake w/ white frosting	1 cake 9 in sq	4020	129	42	636	37	694	—	—	548	2488	669	—	2
sheet cake w/o frosting	1 cake 9 in sq	2830	108	30	552	35	434	—	—	497	2331	614	—	2

FOOD	PORTION	CALS	FAT	SAT FAT	CHOL	PROT	CARB	SUGAR	FIBER	CALCI	SOD	POTAS	FOLIC	VIT C
sheet cake w/o frosting	1/9 cake	315	12	3	61	4	48	—	—	55	258	68	—	tr
sour cream pound	1/10 cake (1 oz)	117	5	1	17	1	16	—	tr	19	120	32	—	—
sponge	1/12 cake (1.3 oz)	110	1	tr	39	2	23	—	—	26	93	38	5	0
sponge cake dessert shell	1 (0.8 oz)	70	2	1	20	1	12	7	0	30	150	—	—	0
sponge w/ creme filling	1 (1.5 oz)	155	5	1	7	1	27	—	—	19	155	—	—	—
tiramisù	1 cake (4.4 lbs)	5732	421	217	2395	101	439	234	3	1602	1107	2953	221	8.3
toaster pastry apple	1 (1¾ oz)	204	5	1	—	2	37	—	—	14	218	58	42	—
toaster pastry blueberry	1 (1¾ oz)	204	5	1	—	2	37	—	—	14	218	58	42	—
toaster pastry brown sugar cinnamon	1 (1¾ oz)	206	7	2	—	3	34	—	—	17	212	57	40	—
toaster pastry cherry	1 (1¾ oz)	204	5	1	—	2	37	—	—	14	218	58	42	—
toaster pastry strawberry	1 (1¾ oz)	204	5	1	—	2	37	—	—	14	218	58	42	—
treacle tart	1 slice (2.5 oz)	258	10	—	—	3	42	—	1	43	—	—	—	0
vanilla slice	1 slice (2½ oz)	248	13	—	—	3	30	—	1	59	—	—	—	1
white w/ white frosting	1 cake 9 in diam	4170	148	33	46	43	670	—	—	536	2827	832	—	0
white w/ white frosting	1/16 cake	260	9	2	3	3	42	—	—	33	176	52	—	0
yellow w/ chocolate frosting	1/8 cake (2.2 oz)	242	11	3	35	2	36	—	1	24	216	114	—	—
yellow w/ chocolate frosting	1 cake 9 diam	3895	175	92	609	40	620	—	—	366	3080	1972	—	0
AMY'S														
Toaster Pops Apple	1	140	3	0	0	5	26	6	tr	—	130	—	—	—
Toaster Pops Strawberry	1	140	3	0	0	5	26	6	tr	—	130	—	—	—
BABY WATSON														
Cheesecake	1 slice (3 oz)	260	18	11	65	4	19	15	tr	0	150	—	—	0
CAROUSEL														
New York Cheese Cake	1 cake (3 oz)	250	19	11	95	4	16	15	1	80	180	—	—	0
DOLLY MADISON														
Angel Food	1 slice (2.1 oz)	160	2	0	0	3	34	30	1	80	190	—	—	0
Apple Crumb	1 (1.6 oz)	160	5	2	15	2	28	19	0	0	160	—	—	0
Banana Dream Flip	1 (3.5 oz)	390	16	3	30	3	59	26	1	40	240	—	—	0
Bear Claw	1 (2.75 oz)	270	10	4	25	5	40	16	1	60	330	—	—	0

FOOD	PORTION	CALS	FAT	SAT FAT	CHOL	PROT	CARB	SUGAR	FIBER	CALCI	SOD	POTAS	FOLIC	VIT C
DOLLY MADISON (CONT.)														
Carrot	1 (4 oz)	360	8	3	0	4	67	46	1	40	500	—	—	0
Chocolate Snack Squares	1 (1.6 oz)	210	10	6	10	2	28	22	0	40	150	—	—	0
Cinnamon Buttercrumb	1 (1.6 oz)	170	6	2	15	2	28	20	0	20	170	—	—	0
Cinnamon Buttercrumb Low Fat	1 (1.5 oz)	140	2	0	0	1	29	24	0	20	150	—	—	0
Cinnamon Stix	1 (1.3 oz)	170	9	4	15	1	21	14	0	60	140	—	—	0
Creme Cakes	2 (1.9 oz)	210	8	4	25	1	32	21	0	20	230	—	—	0
Cupcakes Chocolate	1 (2 oz)	210	7	3	5	2	35	20	1	100	330	—	—	0
Cupcakes Spice	1 (2 oz)	230	10	4	20	2	33	25	0	20	160	—	—	0
Dunkin' Stix	1 (1.3 oz)	170	9	4	15	1	20	14	0	60	130	—	—	0
Frosty Angel	1 (3.5 oz)	330	6	4	0	4	65	50	1	80	270	—	—	0
Holiday Cupcakes	1 (1.9 oz)	180	3	1	5	1	35	22	0	100	190	—	—	0
Honey Bun	1 (3.7 oz)	440	25	11	15	6	49	22	1	60	260	—	—	0
Koo Koos	1 (1.8 oz)	200	9	6	5	1	29	23	0	20	90	—	—	0
Mini Coconut Loaf	1 (3.5 oz)	350	10	2	5	3	62	35	1	20	350	—	—	0
Mini Pound Cake	1 (3.2 oz)	310	11	5	15	5	48	28	1	20	390	—	—	0
Raspberry Square	1 (1.8 oz)	190	8	4	5	1	28	23	0	0	110	—	—	0
Sweet Roll Apple	1 (2.2 oz)	200	6	2	5	3	33	16	0	40	240	—	—	0
Sweet Roll Cherry	1 (2.2 oz)	210	6	3	10	3	34	19	1	20	180	—	—	0
Sweet Roll Cinnamon	1 (2.2 oz)	230	7	3	10	3	36	15	1	60	200	—	—	0
Texas Cinnamon Bun	1 (4.2 oz)	440	15	6	25	7	69	33	1	20	410	—	—	0
Zingers Devil's Food	2 (2.6 oz)	270	8	4	5	2	46	26	1	40	230	—	—	0
Zingers Lemon	1 (1.4 oz)	150	6	3	5	1	22	18	0	20	90	—	—	0
Zingers Raspberry	1 (1.4 oz)	150	6	3	5	1	22	18	0	20	90	—	—	0
Zingers Yellow	2 (2.5 oz)	280	8	3	5	2	50	29	1	20	160	—	—	0
DRAKE'S														
Coffee Cake Low Fat	1 (1.1 oz)	110	2	1	10	1	21	12	0	0	110	—	—	0
Coffee Cakes	1 (1.2 oz)	140	6	2	5	1	20	11	0	0	100	—	—	0
Yodel's	1 (1 oz)	150	9	—	5	2	16	—	—	tr	65	—	—	tr
DUTCH MILL														
Dessert Shells Chocolate Covered	1 (0.5 oz)	80	5	2	0	1	8	6	0	0	—	—	—	0
ENTENMANN'S														
Apple Puffs	1 (3 oz)	270	13	4	0	2	37	20	1	0	230	—	—	0

FOOD	PORTION	CALS	FAT	SAT FAT	CHOL	PROT	CARB	SUGAR	FIBER	CALCI	SOD	POTAS	FOLIC	VIT C
ENTENMANN'S (CONT.)														
Coffee Cake Cheese Filled Crumb	1 serv (1.9 oz)	200	10	3	35	4	25	11	tr	40	190	—	—	0
Coffee Cake Crumb	1 serv (2 oz)	250	12	3	10	3	33	13	1	20	210	—	—	0
Hot Cross Buns	1 (2.3 oz)	230	7	2	20	4	37	20	2	60	160	—	—	2
Light Loaf Cake Fat Free	⅛ cake (1.7 oz)	120	0	0	0	2	27	16	0	0	190	—	—	0
Loaf All Butter	⅙ cake (2.4 oz)	220	9	6	0	3	31	19	0	20	290	—	—	0
Louisiana Crunch	⅑ cake (2.9 oz)	330	14	4	45	3	49	35	tr	150	35	—	—	0
Stollen Fruit	⅛ cake (2 oz)	210	7	2	15	3	34	17	1	20	125	—	—	2
Ultimate Crumb Cake	⅒ cake	250	13	3	15	2	32	15	tr	20	280	—	—	0
FILLO FACTORY														
Apple Turnovers Vegan	5 (5 oz)	270	5	0	0	5	53	4	2	—	125	—	—	—
GOODY MAN														
Happy Birthday Cupcake Chocolate	1 (1.75 oz)	200	6	3	20	2	34	24	tr	40	190	—	16	0
Happy Birthday Cupcake White	1 (1.75 oz)	190	5	2	20	2	36	26	0	60	230	—	16	0
GREENFIELD														
Blondie Fat Free Chocolate Chip	1 (1.3 oz)	110	0	0	0	2	27	19	0	0	60	—	—	0
HOSTESS														
Angel Food	⅛ cake (2 oz)	160	2	0	0	3	33	29	1	80	180	—	—	0
Chocodiles	1 (1.6 oz)	240	11	8	20	2	33	22	1	0	180	—	—	0
Chocolicious	1 (1.6 oz)	190	7	3	10	1	30	19	1	0	210	—	—	0
Coffee Crumb	1 (1.1 oz)	130	5	2	10	1	19	10	0	0	110	—	—	0
Crumb Cake Light	1 (1 oz)	100	2	0	0	1	18	11	0	20	130	—	—	0
Cupcakes Chocolate	1 (1.8 oz)	180	6	3	5	2	30	17	1	100	290	—	—	0
Cupcakes Orange	1 (1.5 oz)	160	5	2	10	1	27	20	0	60	160	—	—	0
Cupcakes Light Chocolate	1 (1.6 oz)	140	2	1	0	2	29	19	1	0	190	—	—	0
Ding Dongs	2 (2.7 oz)	360	19	12	15	3	44	32	2	20	240	—	—	0
Ho Ho's	2 (2 oz)	250	12	8	20	2	34	23	1	20	150	—	—	0
Honey Bun Glazed	1 (2.7 oz)	320	19	9	15	4	34	25	1	40	210	—	—	0
Honey Bun Iced	1 (3.4 oz)	410	24	11	10	5	42	31	1	40	270	—	—	0
Shortcake Dessert Cups	1 (1 oz)	100	2	1	15	1	17	10	0	0	120	—	—	0
Sno Balls	1 (1.8 oz)	180	5	3	5	1	31	19	1	0	190	—	—	0
Suzy Q's	1 (2 oz)	230	9	4	10	2	35	22	1	20	270	—	—	0
Sweet Roll Cherry	1 (2.2 oz)	210	6	3	10	3	34	19	1	20	180	—	—	0

FOOD	PORTION	CALS	FAT	SAT FAT	CHOL	PROT	CARB	SUGAR	FIBER	CALCI	SOD	POTAS	FOLIC	VIT C
HOSTESS (CONT.)														
Sweet Roll Cinnamon	1 (2.2 oz)	230	7	3	10	3	36	15	1	60	200	—	—	0
Twinkies	1 (1.5 oz)	150	5	2	20	1	25	14	0	0	200	—	—	0
Twinkies Light	1 (1.5 oz)	130	2	1	10	1	27	16	0	0	190	—	—	0
JELL-O														
Dessert Delights Cheesecake	1 bar (1.4 oz)	160	7	3	5	2	20	13	tr	20	100	—	—	0
Dessert Delights Chocolate Fudge Pudding	1 bar (1.4 oz)	150	6	3	0	2	23	15	1	20	80	—	—	0
KELLOGG'S														
Pop-Tarts Apple Cinnamon	1 (1.8 oz)	210	6	1	0	2	37	16	1	0	180	15	40	0
Pop-Tarts Blueberry	1 (1.8 oz)	210	5	1	0	2	36	16	1	0	190	50	40	0
Pop-Tarts Brown Sugar Cinnamon	1 (1.8 oz)	210	6	1	0	3	35	14	1	0	190	70	40	0
Pop-Tarts Cherry	1 (1.8 oz)	200	5	1	0	2	37	15	1	0	180	60	40	0
Pop-Tarts Chocolate Graham	1 (1.8 oz)	210	6	2	0	3	35	17	1	0	230	80	40	0
Pop-Tarts Frosted Apple Cinnamon	1 (1.8 oz)	190	3	1	0	2	39	19	1	0	230	30	40	0
Pop-Tarts Frosted Blueberry	1 (1.8 oz)	200	5	1	0	2	37	18	1	0	170	50	40	0
Pop-Tarts Frosted Brown Sugar Cinnamon	1 (1.8 oz)	210	7	2	0	3	34	17	1	0	180	55	40	0
Pop-Tarts Frosted Cherry	1 (1.8 oz)	200	5	1	0	2	38	19	1	0	170	50	40	0
Pop-Tarts Frosted Chocolate Vanilla Creme	1 (1.8 oz)	200	5	1	0	3	37	19	1	0	220	60	40	0
Pop-Tarts Frosted Chocolate Fudge	1 (1.8 oz)	200	5	1	0	3	37	19	1	0	220	80	40	0
Pop-Tarts Frosted Grape	1 (1.8 oz)	200	5	1	0	2	38	18	1	0	170	60	40	0
Pop-Tarts Frosted Raspberry	1 (1.8 oz)	210	5	1	0	2	37	18	1	0	170	45	40	0
Pop-Tarts Frosted S'mores	1 (1.8 oz)	200	6	1	0	3	36	18	1	0	200	65	40	0
Pop-Tarts Frosted Strawberry	1 (1.8 oz)	200	5	1	0	2	38	19	1	0	170	45	40	0
Pop-Tarts Frosted Wild Berry	1 (2 oz)	210	5	1	0	2	39	20	1	0	170	45	40	0
Pop-Tarts Frosted Wild Watermelon	1 (2 oz)	210	5	1	0	2	39	20	1	0	170	35	40	0

FOOD	PORTION	CALS	FAT	SAT FAT	CHOL	PROT	CARB	SUGAR	FIBER	CALCI	SOD	POTAS	FOLIC	VIT C
KELLOGG'S (CONT.)														
Pop-Tarts Low Fat Blueberry	1 (1.8 oz)	190	3	1	0	2	39	17	1	0	230	30	40	0
Pop-Tarts Low Fat Cherry	1 (1.8 oz)	190	3	1	0	2	39	17	1	0	230	30	40	0
Pop-Tarts Low Fat Frosted Brown Sugar Cinnamon	1 (1.8 oz)	190	3	1	0	2	39	20	1	0	230	30	40	0
Pop-Tarts Low Fat Frosted Chocolate Fudge	1 (1.8 oz)	190	3	1	0	3	39	18	2	0	270	60	40	0
Pop-Tarts Low Fat Frosted Strawberry	1 (1.8 oz)	190	3	1	0	2	39	20	1	0	210	25	40	0
Pop-Tarts Low Fat Strawberry	1 (1.8 oz)	190	3	1	0	2	39	17	1	0	230	30	40	0
Pop-Tarts Strawberry	1 (1.8 oz)	200	5	1	0	2	37	15	1	0	190	50	40	0
LANCE														
Dunking Sticks	1 (2.75 oz)	180	10	3	<5	2	22	15	tr	0	130	—	—	0
Fig Cake	½ piece (2.1 oz)	110	2	5	0	1	21	14	1	20	70	80	—	0
Fig Cake Fat Free	½ piece (2.1 oz)	100	0	0	0	1	22	13	1	20	85	70	—	0
Honey Bun	1 (3 oz)	330	13	5	0	4	47	13	4	40	200	70	—	0
Pecan Twirls	1 pkg (2 oz)	220	9	4	5	3	32	17	1	20	140	50	—	0
Swiss Rolls	1 (2.5 oz)	170	9	5	10	1	23	13	tr	0	130	60	—	0
LITTLE DEBBIE														
Angel Cakes Lemon	1 (1.6 oz)	130	1	0	0	2	29	22	0	—	135	—	—	—
Angel Cakes Raspberry	1 (1.6 oz)	130	1	0	0	2	29	23	0	—	125	—	—	—
Banana Nut Loaves	1 (1.9 oz)	220	10	2	10	2	31	19	tr	18	220	110	—	2
Banana Twins	1 (2.2 oz)	250	10	3	10	2	39	29	0	11	170	35	—	0
Be My Valentine Chocolate	1 (2.2 oz)	280	13	3	0	2	38	25	1	16	140	62	—	0
Be My Valentine Vanilla	1 (2.2 oz)	290	14	3	0	2	38	26	0	6	125	20	—	0
Blueberry Loaves	1 (2 oz)	220	10	2	0	3	29	16	tr	18	200	42	—	tr
Chocolate Chip	1 (2.4 oz)	310	15	4	0	2	41	32	tr	11	210	81	—	0
Christmas Tree Cake	1 pkg (1.5 oz)	190	10	2	0	1	26	19	0	4	100	14	—	0
Coconut Creme	1 (1.7 oz)	210	10	3	0	1	30	24	0	7	140	28	—	0
Coffee Cake Apple	1 (2.1 oz)	230	7	2	10	2	39	23	0	17	190	59	—	tr
Cupcake Creme Filled Chocolate	1 (1.6 oz)	180	9	2	5	2	26	18	tr	12	135	92	—	0

FOOD	PORTION	CALS	FAT	SAT FAT	CHOL	PROT	CARB	SUGAR	FIBER	CALCI	SOD	POTAS	FOLIC	VIT C
LITTLE DEBBIE (CONT.)														
Cupcake Creme Filled Orange	1 (1.7 oz)	210	10	3	0	1	29	22	0	6	110	18	—	0
Cupcake Creme Filled Strawberry	1 (1.7 oz)	210	10	3	0	1	29	22	tr	6	100	19	—	0
Devil Cremes	1 (1.6 oz)	190	8	2	0	1	29	20	0	9	170	63	—	0
Devil Squares	1 (2.2 oz)	270	13	3	0	2	39	31	1	16	180	57	—	0
Easter Basket Cake Chocolate	1 (2.4 oz)	300	14	4	0	3	40	29	tr	17	160	59	—	0
Easter Basket Cake Vanilla	1 (2.5 oz)	320	10	4	0	2	43	32	0	8	150	26	—	0
Fall Party Cake Chocolate	1 (2.4 oz)	290	14	3	0	2	42	29	tr	11	170	57	—	0
Fall Party Cake Vanilla	1 (2.5 oz)	310	15	4	0	2	44	31	0	8	170	26	—	0
Fancy Cakes	1 (2.4 oz)	300	15	4	0	1	42	33	0	8	190	25	—	0
Frosted Fudge	1 (1.5 oz)	200	10	3	<5	2	25	18	tr	9	105	69	—	0
Golden Cremes	1 (1.5 oz)	150	5	2	10	1	26	18	0	—	120	—	—	—
Holiday Cake Roll Cherry Creme	1 (2.1 oz)	260	12	3	13	2	37	24	tr	27	170	64	—	0
Holiday Snack Cake Chocolate	1 (2.4 oz)	300	14	3	0	3	41	29	1	11	150	57	—	0
Holiday Snack Cake Vanilla	1 (2.5 oz)	320	15	4	0	2	41	29	0	9	180	31	—	0
Honey Bun	1 (1.8 oz)	220	13	4	<5	3	24	13	tr	53	170	1	—	2
Pecan Spinwheels	1 (1 oz)	110	4	1	0	1	16	7	0	—	80	—	—	—
Snack Cake Chocolate	1 (2.5 oz)	310	15	4	0	2	44	30	1	12	180	70	—	0
Strawberry Shortcake Roll	1 (2.1 oz)	230	8	2	15	1	41	29	0	9	230	22	—	0
Swiss Rolls	1 (2.1 oz)	270	12	3	15	2	38	25	1	21	140	43	—	0
Zebra Cakes	1 (2.6 oz)	330	16	4	0	2	45	33	0	9	160	34	—	0
LOW CARB CREATIONS														
Cheesecake Blueberry Swirl	1 slice (3 oz)	220	16	10	95	5	21	2	0	40	150	—	—	1
Cheesecake Chocolate	1 slice (3 oz)	250	20	12	115	6	19	2	0	60	180	—	—	0
Cheesecake Key Lime	1 slice (3 oz)	250	20	12	115	6	19	2	0	40	180	—	—	0
Cheesecake New York	1 slice (3 oz)	250	15	9	85	6	19	1	0	60	140	—	—	0
Cheesecake Pumpkin Swirl	1 slice (3 oz)	220	16	10	90	5	22	2	0	40	140	—	—	0
MARIE CALLENDER'S														
Cobbler Apple	1 serv (4.25 oz)	370	20	9	0	2	45	31	2	0	170	—	—	30
Cobbler Berry	1 serv (4.25 oz)	370	21	5	<5	3	41	29	1	20	220	—	—	4

FOOD	PORTION	CALS	FAT	SAT FAT	CHOL	PROT	CARB	SUGAR	FIBER	CALCI	SOD	POTAS	FOLIC	VIT C
MARIE CALLENDER'S (CONT.)														
Cobbler Cherry	1 serv (4.25 oz)	380	19	8	5	3	50	32	0	0	240	—	—	1
Cobbler Peach	1 serv (4.25 oz)	380	18	6	0	3	47	24	0	0	240	—	—	4
NATURAL TOUCH														
Toaster Square Blueberry	1 (2.8 oz)	180	2	1	0	6	33	12	6	0	65	140	—	0
Toaster Square Date Walnut	1 (2.8 oz)	200	3	1	0	6	36	9	8	0	50	200	—	0
PEPPERIDGE FARM														
Apple Turnover	1 (3.1 oz)	330	14	3	0	4	48	5	6	40	180	—	—	0
Blueberry Turnover	1 (3.1 oz)	340	16	3	0	4	45	5	6	20	200	—	—	6
Cherry Turnover	1 (3.1 oz)	320	13	3	0	4	46	6	6	0	190	—	—	5
Large Layer Chocolate Fudge	⅛ cake (2.4 oz)	260	11	3	30	3	31	20	1	0	160	—	—	0
Large Layer Coconut	⅛ cake (2.4 oz)	260	11	3	35	2	35	24	0	0	115	—	—	0
Large Layer Vanilla	⅛ cake (2.4 oz)	250	11	3	25	2	35	25	0	0	120	—	—	0
Mini Turnover Apple	1 (1.4 oz)	140	8	2	0	2	15	10	1	0	80	—	—	0
Mini Turnover Cherry	1 (1.4 oz)	140	8	2	0	2	16	7	1	0	70	—	—	1
Mini Turnover Strawberry	1 (1.4 oz)	140	7	2	0	2	18	10	0	0	100	—	—	2
Peach Turnover	1 (3.1 oz)	340	15	3	0	4	47	5	6	0	180	—	—	36
Raspberry Turnover	1 (3.1 oz)	330	14	3	0	4	47	6	6	0	190	—	—	36
PHILADELPHIA														
Snack Bars Classic Cheesecake	1 (1.5 oz)	200	13	6	35	2	17	12	0	20	85	—	—	0
PILLSBURY														
Apple Turnovers	1 (2 oz)	170	8	2	0	2	23	11	tr	0	310	—	—	0
Cherry Turnovers	1 (2 oz)	180	8	2	0	2	24	12	0	0	310	—	—	1
SARA LEE														
Cheesecake 25% Reduced Fat	¼ cake (4.2 oz)	310	13	8	70	9	40	28	2	100	310	—	—	0
Cheesecake Cherry Cream	¼ cake (4.7 oz)	350	12	5	35	6	55	35	2	40	310	—	—	15
Cheesecake Chocolate Chip	¼ cake (4.2 oz)	410	21	14	65	8	47	43	2	60	300	—	—	1
Cheesecake French	⅙ cake (3.9 oz)	350	21	13	20	5	24	22	1	40	280	—	—	1
Cheesecake French Strawberry	⅙ cake (4.3 oz)	320	14	9	20	4	43	26	1	40	230	—	—	12

FOOD	PORTION	CALS	FAT	SAT FAT	CHOL	PROT	CARB	SUGAR	FIBER	CALCI	SOD	POTAS	FOLIC	VIT C
SARA LEE (CONT.)														
Cheesecake Strawberry Cream	¼ cake (4.7 oz)	330	12	5	40	6	49	36	2	40	330	—	—	18
Coffee Cake Butter Streusel	⅙ cake (1.9 oz)	220	12	6	35	4	25	11	1	20	240	—	—	0
Coffee Cake Crumb	⅛ cake (2 oz)	220	9	2	15	3	32	17	1	20	210	—	—	0
Coffee Cake Pecan	⅙ cake (1.9 oz)	230	12	5	25	4	24	9	1	20	170	—	—	0
Coffee Cake Raspberry	⅙ cake (1.9 oz)	220	8	3	15	3	27	13	1	—	220	—	—	0
Coffee Cake Reduced Fat Cheese	⅙ cake (1.9 oz)	180	6	2	20	3	28	11	0	40	230	—	—	0
Layer Cake Coconut	⅛ cake (2.8 oz)	260	14	10	15	2	33	25	1	20	210	—	—	0
Layer Cake Double Chocolate	⅛ cake (2.8 oz)	260	13	9	10	3	33	24	2	20	230	—	—	0
Layer Cake Fudge Golden	⅛ cake (2.8 oz)	260	13	10	15	2	34	23	1	0	200	—	—	0
Layer Cake German Chocolate	⅛ cake (2.9 oz)	280	14	9	15	3	35	26	1	20	250	—	—	0
Layer Cake Vanilla	⅛ cake (2.8 oz)	260	14	10	15	2	32	22	0	20	210	—	—	0
Original Cheesecake	¼ cake (4.2 oz)	350	18	9	50	7	39	30	1	80	320	—	—	0
Pound Cake All Butter	¼ cake (2.7 oz)	320	16	9	85	4	38	21	1	20	280	—	—	—
Pound Cake Chocolate Swirl	¼ cake (2.9 oz)	330	16	8	75	5	42	31	tr	60	350	—	—	—
Pound Cake Family Size	⅙ cake (2.7 oz)	310	17	9	75	4	36	15	1	20	360	—	—	—
Pound Cake Reduced Fat	¼ cake (2.7 oz)	280	11	3	65	4	42	26	tr	20	350	—	—	—
Pound Cake Strawberry Swirl	¼ cake (2.9 oz)	290	11	3	60	4	44	25	tr	40	140	—	—	—
Strawberry Shortcake	⅛ cake (2.5 oz)	180	7	5	15	2	27	15	1	20	140	—	—	9
SNACK & SMILE														
Mini Loaf Apple Cinnamon	1 loaf (2 oz)	190	8	2	10	2	29	16	0	0	260	—	24	0
Mini Loaf Banana	1 loaf (2 oz)	200	8	2	10	2	30	17	0	0	260	—	24	0
Mini Loaf Blueberry	1 loaf (2 oz)	190	8	2	10	2	29	16	tr	0	260	—	24	0
Mini Loaf Carrot	1 loaf (2 oz)	200	8	2	10	2	30	16	0	0	260	—	24	0

FOOD	PORTION	CALS	FAT	SAT FAT	CHOL	PROT	CARB	SUGAR	FIBER	CALCI	SOD	POTAS	FOLIC	VIT C
SNACKWELL'S														
Streusel Squares Apple Cinnamon	1 (1.5 oz)	150	3	0	0	1	31	17	tr	40	90	—	—	0
Streusel Squares Cherry	1 (1.5 oz)	150	3	0	0	1	31	16	tr	40	110	—	—	0
SUPER														
Bun	1 (2.5 oz)	270	16	4	10	5	24	9	tr	200	230	—	—	21
TASTYKAKE														
Banana Creamie	1 (1.5 oz)	170	7	1	5	1	25	18	0	0	105	—	—	0
Bear Claw Apple	1 (3 oz)	280	7	2	0	4	50	24	0	40	320	—	—	4
Bear Claw Cinnamon	1 (3 oz)	300	8	2	0	5	53	27	tr	60	310	—	—	4
Big Texas	1 (3 oz)	300	9	2	0	5	51	21	tr	60	360	—	—	4
Breakfast Bun Chocolate Raisin	1 (3.2 oz)	330	8	2	0	5	59	32	1	60	320	—	—	4
Bunny Trail Treats	1 (1.3 oz)	150	6	1	30	1	25	16	0	0	105	—	—	0
Chocolate Creamie	1 (1.5 oz)	180	8	1	15	1	25	17	0	20	120	—	—	0
Chocolate Krimpies	2 (2.2 oz)	240	10	2	45	3	38	24	1	20	250	—	—	0
Coffee Roll Glazed	1 (3 oz)	300	9	2	0	5	51	22	tr	60	360	—	—	4
Coffee Roll Vanilla	1 (3.2 oz)	320	9	2	0	5	56	27	tr	60	360	—	—	4
Cupcakes	2 (2.1 oz)	200	5	1	10	2	37	22	1	20	240	—	—	0
Cupcakes Butter Cream Filled Iced	2 (2.2 oz)	240	8	2	10	2	40	26	1	20	250	—	—	0
Cupcakes Chocolate Cream Filled Iced	2 (2.2 oz)	230	8	1	10	2	39	25	1	20	240	—	—	0
Cupcakes Low Fat Vanilla Cream Filled	2 (2.2 oz)	190	2	0	0	2	42	28	0	20	210	—	—	0
Cupid Kake	1 (1.3 oz)	150	6	1	30	1	25	16	0	0	105	—	—	0
Honey Bun Glazed	1 (3.2 oz)	350	17	4	10	5	47	22	0	100	210	—	—	0
Honey Bun Iced	1 (3.2 oz)	350	17	4	10	5	47	22	0	100	210	—	—	0
Junior Chocolate	1 (3.3 oz)	330	12	2	80	4	54	34	1	20	180	—	—	0
Junior Coconut	1 (3.3 oz)	310	8	4	75	3	54	35	0	40	180	—	—	0
Junior Koffee Kake	1 (2.5 oz)	270	9	2	45	3	42	22	1	20	200	—	—	0
Junior Pound Kake	1 (3 oz)	320	13	5	100	5	45	28	1	40	320	—	—	0
Kandy Kakes Chocolate	3 (2 oz)	250	13	8	0	2	35	24	2	20	90	—	—	0
Kandy Kakes Coconut	2 (2.7 oz)	330	18	13	5	3	43	30	2	—	105	—	—	—
Kandy Kakes Peanut Butter	2 (1.3 oz)	190	9	5	10	3	21	14	1	20	85	—	—	0

FOOD	PORTION	CALS	FAT	SAT FAT	CHOL	PROT	CARB	SUGAR	FIBER	CALCI	SOD	POTAS	FOLIC	VIT C
TASTYKAKE (CONT.)														
Koffee Kakes Cream Filled	2 (2 oz)	240	10	2	30	2	35	20	0	20	130	—	—	0
Koffee Kakes Low Fat Apple	2 (2 oz)	170	2	0	0	2	34	20	1	20	170	—	—	1
Koffee Kakes Low Fat Lemon	2 (2 oz)	180	3	0	10	2	36	21	0	20	180	—	—	0
Koffee Kakes Low Fat Raspberry	2 (2 oz)	170	2	0	0	2	36	16	1	20	180	—	—	0
Koffee Kakes	1 (2 oz)	210	7	1	30	2	34	18	tr	20	160	—	—	0
Kreepy Kakes	2 (2.2 oz)	240	8	2	20	2	38	27	0	20	230	—	—	0
Kreme Krimpies	2 (2 oz)	230	9	1	55	2	34	21	0	20	200	—	—	0
Krimpets Butterscotch Iced	2 (2 oz)	210	5	1	60	2	38	24	0	20	250	—	—	0
Krimpets Jelly Fillled	2 (2 oz)	190	3	1	45	2	38	23	1	20	170	—	—	0
Krimpets Strawberry	2 (2 oz)	210	5	1	65	2	37	22	0	20	220	—	—	0
Kringle Kake	1 (1.3 oz)	150	6	1	30	1	25	16	0	0	105	—	—	0
Santa Snacks	2 (2.2 oz)	240	8	2	20	2	38	27	0	20	230	—	—	0
Sparkle Kake	1 (1.3 oz)	150	6	1	30	1	25	16	0	0	105	—	—	0
Tasty Tweets	2 (2.2 oz)	240	8	2	20	2	38	27	0	20	230	—	—	0
Tropical Delight Coconut	2 (2 oz)	190	9	5	30	3	26	16	0	20	230	—	—	0
Tropical Delight Guava	2 (2 oz)	190	7	4	15	2	30	20	0	20	200	—	—	0
Tropical Delight Papaya	2 (2 oz)	200	7	4	20	2	32	22	0	20	220	—	—	0
Tropical Delight Pineapple	2 (2 oz)	200	7	4	20	2	32	22	0	20	220	—	—	0
Vanilla Creamie	1 (1.5 oz)	190	9	1	35	1	25	18	0	20	115	—	—	0
Witchy Treat	1 (1.3 oz)	150	6	1	30	1	24	15	0	0	90	—	—	0
TOM'S														
Honey Bun	1 pkg (3 oz)	360	20	—	10	4	41	15	2	100	200	—	—	0
Honey Bun Jelly Filled	1 pkg (4 oz)	490	29	10	0	6	52	20	2	100	490	—	—	0
Marble Pound	1 pkg (2.5 oz)	300	16	4	50	4	35	24	1	0	380	—	—	0
Texas Cinnamon Roll	1 pkg (4 oz)	360	6	2	0	7	71	56	0	200	470	—	—	0
TORTUGA														
Cayman Island Rum Cake	1 piece (2 oz)	194	9	2	0	2	27	8	0	0	198	—	—	0
WEIGHT WATCHERS														
Chocolate Raspberry Royale	1 (3.5 oz)	190	3	1	20	4	38	22	2	100	220	—	—	0
Chocolate Eclair	1 (2.1 oz)	150	4	1	30	2	25	13	1	40	170	—	—	0

FOOD	PORTION	CALS	FAT	SAT FAT	CHOL	PROT	CARB	SUGAR	FIBER	CALCI	SOD	POTAS	FOLIC	VIT C
WEIGHT WATCHERS (CONT.)														
Danish Coffee Cake Apple Cinnamon	1 piece (1.9 oz)	160	3	1	0	3	30	13	1	0	170	—	—	0
Danish Coffee Cake Cheese	1 piece (1.9 oz)	160	3	1	5	4	29	11	1	20	200	—	—	0
Danish Coffee Cake Raspberry	1 piece (1.9 oz)	160	3	1	0	4	30	13	1	0	170	—	—	0
Double Fudge	1 piece (2.75 oz)	190	4	2	25	4	36	19	2	80	200	—	—	0
French Style Cheesecake	1 piece (3.9 oz)	170	4	2	15	7	28	19	2	100	230	—	—	2
New York Style Cheesecake	1 piece (2.5 oz)	150	5	3	15	6	21	18	1	80	140	—	—	0
Strawberry Parfait Royale	1 (5.24 oz)	180	2	1	10	5	35	22	0	250	100	—	—	0
Triple Chocolate Eclair	1 (2.14 oz)	160	5	1	30	3	25	13	1	40	190	—	—	0
TAKE-OUT														
angelfood	1/12 cake (1 oz)	73	tr	tr	0	2	16	—	1	40	212	26	—	0
apple crisp	1/2 cup (5 oz)	230	5	1	0	37	46	—	—	40	257	137	7	3
baklava	1 oz	126	9	4	23	2	10	—	1	23	78	62	8	1
basbousa namoura	1 piece (1 oz)	60	3	0	0	2	—	10	2	30	144	—	—	—
boston cream pie	1/6 cake (3.3 oz)	293	12	4	43	4	43	—	1	93	309	95	8	tr
cannoli w/ cannoli cream	1	369	21	—	—	6	42	28	—	52	—	—	—	0
carrot w/ cream cheese icing	1/12 cake (3.9 oz)	484	29	5	60	5	52	—		27	273	124	14	1
cheesecake w/ cherry topping	1/12 cake (5 oz)	359	23	13	106	6	33	—		54	254	116	12	1
chocolate w/ chocolate frosting	1/8 cake (2.2 oz)	235	11	3	—	3	35	—	2	28	213	128		—
coffeecake cheese	1/6 cake (2.7 oz)	258	12	4	—	5	38	—	1	45	257	—	—	—
coffeecake crumb topped cheese	1/6 cake (2.7 oz)	258	12	4	—	5	38	—	1	45	257	—	—	—
coffeecake crumb topped cinnamon	1/9 cake (2.2 oz)	263	15	4	20	4	29	—	2	34	221	77	20	—
cream puff w/ custard filling	1 (4.6 oz)	336	20	5	174	9	30	—	—	86	444	149	20	tr
dutch honey cake	1 slice (0.8 oz)	70	0	0	0	1	17	8	0	0	25	—	—	0
eclair w/ chocolate icing & custard filling	1	205	10	—	35	—	—	—	—	10	—	—	—	—
french apple tart	1 (3.5 oz)	302	15	9	60	4	37	15	2	14	326	93	2	3
fruitcake	1/36 cake (2.9 oz)	302	10	1	24	3	54	—	3	55	121	259	8	4
gingerbread	1/9 cake (2.6 oz)	264	12	3	24	3	36	—	2	52	242	325	6	tr

FOOD	PORTION	CALS	FAT	SAT FAT	CHOL	PROT	CARB	SUGAR	FIBER	CALCI	SOD	POTAS	FOLIC	VIT C
panettone	1/12 cake (2.9 oz)	300	12	9	90	6	43	21	2	40	120	—	—	0
petit fours	2 (0.9 oz)	120	7	3	0	1	15	12	0	20	15	—	—	0
pineapple upside down	1/9 cake (4 oz)	367	14	3	25	4	58	—	—	137	367	129	8	1
pound	1 slice (1 oz)	120	5	1	32	2	15	—	—	20	96	28	—	tr
pound fat free	1 oz	80	tr	tr	0	2	17	—	—	12	96	31	1	0
sacher torte	1 slice (2.2 oz)	240	11	5	50	4	30	11	4	—	120	—	—	—
sheet cake w/ white frosting	1/9 cake	445	14	5	70	4	77	—	—	61	275	74	—	tr
strudel apple	1 piece (2½ oz)	195	8	2	—	2	29	—	2	11	191	—	—	1
tiramisù	1 piece (5.1 oz)	409	30	15	171	7	31	17	tr	114	79	211	16	1
torte chocolate ganache	1 slice (3.5 oz)	400	26	10	90	7	40	24	6	40	120	—	—	0
trifle w/ cream	6 oz	291	16	—	—	4	34	—	1	119	—	—	—	7
yellow w/ vanilla frosting	1/8 cake (2.2 oz)	239	9	2	—	2	38	—	—	39	220	34	—	—

CAKE ICING

FOOD	PORTION	CALS	FAT	SAT FAT	CHOL	PROT	CARB	SUGAR	FIBER	CALCI	SOD	POTAS	FOLIC	VIT C
chocolate ready-to-use	1/12 pkg (1.3 oz)	151	7	2	0	tr	24	21	—	3	70	74	0	—
glaze home recipe	1/12 recipe (1 oz)	97	2	tr	1	tr	20	—	—	6	25	8	0	0
vanilla ready-to-use	1/12 pkg (1.3 oz)	159	6	2	0	tr	26	26	—	1	34	14	0	0
BETTY CROCKER														
HomeStyle Mix Coconut Pecan as prep	2 tbsp	160	2	3	0	tr	21	17	tr	—	5	—	—	—
HomeStyle Mix White Fluffy as prep	6 tbsp	100	0	0	0	tr	24	23	—	—	60	—	—	—
Party Frosting Chocolate w/ Stars	2 tbsp (1.2 oz)	140	5	2	0	0	22	20	—	—	90	75	—	—
Rich & Creamy Butter Cream	2 tbsp (1.3 oz)	140	5	2	0	0	23	20	—	—	75	15	—	—
Rich & Creamy Cherry	2 tbsp (1.2 oz)	140	5	2	0	0	23	20	—	—	75	10	—	—
Rich & Creamy Chocolate	2 tbsp (1.2 oz)	130	5	2	0	0	21	17	—	—	90	75	—	—
Rich & Creamy Cream Cheese	2 tbsp (1.2 oz)	140	5	2	0	0	23	20	—	—	80	10	—	—
Rich & Creamy Dark Chocolate	2 tbsp (1.3 oz)	130	6	2	0	1	23	16	1	—	90	115	—	—
Rich & Creamy French Vanilla	2 tbsp (1.2 oz)	140	5	2	0	0	23	20	—	—	70	10	—	—

FOOD	PORTION	CALS	FAT	SAT FAT	CHOL	PROT	CARB	SUGAR	FIBER	CALCI	SOD	POTAS	FOLIC	VIT C
BETTY CROCKER (CONT.)														
Rich & Creamy Milk Chocolate	2 tbsp (1.3 oz)	130	5	2	0	0	21	18	—	—	90	60	—	—
Rich & Creamy Rainbow Chip	2 tbsp (1.2 oz)	140	5	2	0	0	23	20	—	—	65	20	—	—
Rich & Creamy Vanilla	2 tbsp (1.2 oz)	140	5	2	0	0	23	20	—	—	70	10	—	—
Toppers Milk Chocolate	2 tbsp (1.2 oz)	130	5	2	0	0	22	18	—	—	85	60	—	—
Toppers Vanilla	2 tbsp (1.2 oz)	140	5	2	0	0	24	20	—	—	70	10	—	—
DUNCAN HINES														
Chocolate Creamy Homestyle	2 tbsp	130	5	2	0	0	20	19	2	—	95	—	—	—
Milk Chocolate Creamy Homestyle	2 tbsp	130	5	2	0	0	20	19	1	—	95	—	—	—
Vanilla Creamy Homestyle	2 tbsp	140	5	2	0	0	22	21	1	—	60	—	—	—
ESTEE														
Frosting as prep	⅓ pkg	100	0	0	0	0	20	0	0	—	0	0	—	—
SWEET REWARDS														
Ready-To-Spread Reduced Fat Chocolate	2 tbsp (1.2 oz)	120	2	1	0	tr	24	22	—	—	55	—	—	—
Ready-To-Spread Reduced Fat Vanilla	2 tbsp (1.2 oz)	130	2	1	0	0	27	25	—	—	60	—	—	—
CAKE MIX														
angelfood	¹⁄₁₂ cake (1.8 oz)	129	tr	tr	0	3	29	—	1	42	255	68	—	0
angelfood	10 in cake (20.9 oz)	1535	2	tr	0	36	350		9	503	3036	808	—	0
carrot w/o frosting	2 layers (29.6 oz)	2886	133	22	—	43	395	—	—	927	3001	1011	—	—
carrot w/o frosting	¹⁄₁₂ cake (2.5 oz)	239	11	2	—	4	33	—	—	77	249	64	—	—
chocolate pudding type w/o frosting	2 layers (32.4 oz)	3234	172	35	—	43	409	—	—	765	4815	1926	—	—
chocolate pudding type w/o frosting	¹⁄₁₂ cake (2.7 oz)	270	14	3	—	4	34	—	—	64	402	161	—	—
chocolate w/o frosting	¹⁄₁₂ cake (2.3 oz)	198	8	2	35	4	32	—	—	70	370	153	—	0
chocolate w/o frosting	2 layers (26.8 oz)	2393	92	21	425	44	384	—	—	843	4464	1851	—	0

FOOD	PORTION	CALS	FAT	SAT FAT	CHOL	PROT	CARB	SUGAR	FIBER	CALCI	SOD	POTAS	FOLIC	VIT C
coffeecake crumb topped cinnamon	⅛ cake (2 oz)	178	5	1	28	3	30	—	2	76	236	63	—	—
devil's food w/o frosting	1/12 cake (2.3 oz)	198	8	2	35	4	32	—	—	70	370	153	—	0
devil's food w/ chocolate frosting	1/16 cake	235	8	4	37	3	40	—	—	41	181	90	—	tr
devil's food w/ chocolate frosting	1 cake 9 in diam	3755	136	56	598	49	645	—	—	653	2900	1439	—	1
fudge w/o frosting	1/12 cake (2.3 oz)	198	8	2	35	4	32	—	—	70	370	153	—	0
gingerbread	⅑ cake (2.4 oz)	207	7	2	24	3	34	—	2	46	307	162	—	—
gingerbread	1 cake 8 in sq	1575	39	10	6	18	291	—	—	513	1733	1562	—	1
white w/o frosting	2 layer cake (26 oz)	2265	57	9	—	30	410	—	—	1016	3593	700	—	—
white w/o frosting	1/12 cake (2.2 oz)	190	5	1	—	3	34	—	—	85	301	59	—	—
yellow w/ chocolate frosting	1/16 cake	235	8	3	36	3	40	—	—	63	157	75	—	tr
yellow w/o frosting	2 layers (26.5 oz)	2415	71	12	437	35	411	—	—	761	3580	552	—	—
yellow w/o frosting	1/12 cake (2.2 oz)	202	6	1	37	3	34	—	—	64	299	46	—	—
yellow w/ chocolate frosting	1 cake 9 in diam	3895	175	92	609	40	620	—	—	366	3080	1972	—	0
BETTY CROCKER														
Angel Food Fat Free	1/12 cake	140	0	0	0	3	32	24	—	60	320	—	—	—
Angel Food Fat Free Confetti as prep	1/12 cake	150	0	0	0	3	34	24	—	60	320	—	—	—
Cheesecake Chocolate Chip as prep	⅛ cake	410	28	13	99	3	32	23	1	80	230	125	—	—
Cheesecake Original as prep	⅛ cake	400	27	12	102	2	30	20	—	80	240	100	16	—
Cheesecake Strawberry Swirl as prep	⅛ cake	380	25	11	96	2	32	21	—	60	220	90	16	—
Pineapple Upside Down as prep	⅙ cake	420	14	3	36	2	64	43	—	80	280	—	40	—
Quick Bread Banana	1/12 cake	170	7	1	36	2	25	13	—	—	190	35	64	—

FOOD	PORTION	CALS	FAT	SAT FAT	CHOL	PROT	CARB	SUGAR	FIBER	CALCI	SOD	POTAS	FOLIC	VIT C
BETTY CROCKER (CONT.)														
Quick Bread Cinnamon Streusel as prep	1/14 cake	180	7	2	30	3	26	15	—	40	150	20	16	—
Quick Bread Cranberry Orange as prep	1/12 cake	170	6	2	36	2	29	16	—	—	170	15	24	—
Quick Bread Lemon Poppy as prep	1/12 cake	170	7	1	36	2	25	12	—	20	150	20	16	—
Stir'n Bake Carrot Cake w/ Cream Cheese Frosting as prep	1/6 cake	260	7	2	—	2	46	32	—	40	290	—	16	—
Stir'n Bake Coffee Cake w/ Cinnamon Streusel as prep	1/6 cake	230	2	1	12	2	36	20	—	60	120	—	24	—
Stir'n Bake Devils Food w/ Chocolate Frosting as prep	1/6 cake	240	7	2	0	2	42	27	1	40	270	—	16	—
Stir'n Bake Yellow w/ Chocolate Frosting as prep	1/8 cake	240	7	2	9	2	43	26	1	80	240	—	24	—
SuperMoist Butter Pecan as prep	1/12 cake	240	10	2	54	1	35	20	—	80	260	—	64	—
SuperMoist Butter Yellow as prep	1/12 cake	260	11	6	75	2	36	20	—	80	270	—	64	—
SuperMoist Carrot as prep	1/10 cake	320	15	3	63	2	42	24	—	100	340	55	64	—
SuperMoist Cherry Chip	1/10 cake	300	13	3	63	2	41	23	—	60	330	25	24	—
SuperMoist Chocolate Fudge as prep	1/12 cake	270	12	3	54	2	35	21	1	40	320	—	24	—
SuperMoist Golden Vanilla as prep	1/12 cake	240	10	2	54	1	35	20	—	80	270	—	64	—
SuperMoist Lemon as prep	1/12 cake	240	10	2	54	1	35	20	—	80	270	—	64	—
SuperMoist Milk Chocolate as prep	1/12 cake	240	10	2	54	2	34	20	1	100	290	—	24	—
SuperMoist Pineapple as prep	1/12 cake	250	7	2	54	1	25	20	—	80	270	—	64	—
SuperMoist Spice as prep	1/12 cake	240	10	2	54	1	36	20	—	80	270	—	24	—
SuperMoist Strawberry as prep	1/12 cake	250	10	2	39	1	35	21	—	80	260	—	—	64

FOOD	PORTION	CALS	FAT	SAT FAT	CHOL	PROT	CARB	SUGAR	FIBER	CALCI	SOD	POTAS	FOLIC	VIT C
BETTY CROCKER (CONT.)														
SuperMoist White as prep	½₂ cake	230	14	2	0	2	34	18	—	40	290	25	24	—
SuperMoist White Light as prep	⅒ cake	210	3	1	0	2	43	24	—	100	380	—	—	—
BISQUICK														
Mix	⅓ cup (1.4 oz)	160	6	2	0	3	25	1	—	40	400	35	40	—
Reduced Fat	⅓ cup (1.4 oz)	140	3	1	0	3	27	3	tr	60	500	45	40	—
CARBOLITE														
Cheesecake Chocolate as prep	⅛ cake	260	25	—	280	6	2	—	—	—	80	—	—	—
CARBSENSE														
Zero Carb Baking Mix	1 oz	110	1	1	0	22	4	0	4	—	380	—	—	—
DROMEDARY														
Date Bread	⅟₁₁ cake (2 oz)	190	7	2	0	2	29	16	1	20	288	—	—	0
Date Nut Roll	½ in slice	80	2	—	—	1	13	—	—	20	160	60	—	—
Gingerbread	1 piece (2 in x 2 in)	100	2	—	—	1	19	—	—	20	190	90	—	—
Pound	½ in slice	150	6	—	—	2	21	—	—	20	160	65	—	—
DUNCAN HINES														
Angel Food as prep	½₂ pkg (1.3 oz)	140	0	0	0	4	31	23	1	15	310	—	—	0
Butter Recipe Golden as prep	½₂ cake	320	16	7	80	3	42	29	—	60	190	—	—	—
Cupcake Yellow as prep	1	180	0	2	6	1	29	—	—	20	140	—	—	—
Dark Chocolate Fudge as prep	½₂ cake	290	15	3	55	4	34	20	—	60	360	—	—	—
Devil's Food Moist Deluxe as prep	½₂ cake (1.5 oz)	290	15	3	55	4	34	20	1	60	360	—	—	0
French Vanilla as prep	½₂ cake (1.5 oz)	250	11	2	55	3	—	—	—	80	290	—	—	—
Fudge Marble Moist Deluxe as prep	½₂ cake (1.5 oz)	250	17	2	45	3	36	22	0	80	290	—	—	0
Lemon Supreme Moist Deluxe as prep	½₂ cake (1.5 oz)	250	17	2	55	3	36	22	0	80	290	—	—	0
White Moist Deluxe as prep	½₂ cake	190	6	1	0	3	34	20	—	60	300	—	—	—
Yellow Moist Deluxe as prep	½₂ cake (1.5 oz)	250	17	11	55	3	36	—	—	—	270	—	—	—
Yellow Moist Deluxe as prep	½₂ cake	250	11	2	55	3	36	22	—	80	290	—	—	—

FOOD	PORTION	CALS	FAT	SAT FAT	CHOL	PROT	CARB	SUGAR	FIBER	CALCI	SOD	POTAS	FOLIC	VIT C
ESTEE														
Chocolate as prep	⅕ cake	190	4	2	0	2	36	25	1	—	240	240	—	—
White as prep	⅕ cake	200	4	2	0	2	38	24	tr	—	170	70	—	—
HODGSON MILL														
Gingerbread Whole Wheat	¼ cup (1 oz)	110	0	0	0	2	24	10	2	300	260	—	—	0
JELL-O														
No Bake Cherry Cheesecake as prep	⅛ cake (4.8 oz)	340	12	5	5	5	52	33	tr	150	400	280	—	0
No Bake Double Layer Chocolate as prep	⅛ cake (4.4 oz)	260	12	5	<5	4	34	21	1	100	410	220	—	0
No Bake Double Layer Cookies And Creme as prep	⅛ cake (4.5 oz)	390	19	7	<5	5	51	32	1	80	480	150	—	0
No Bake Double Layer Lemon as prep	⅛ cake (4.4 oz)	260	12	4	<5	4	36	25	tr	80	370	125	—	0
No Bake Homestyle Cheesecake as prep	⅙ cake (4.6 oz)	360	15	4	10	7	50	35	tr	200	550	280	—	0
No Bake Peanut Butter Cup as prep	⅛ cake (3.8 oz)	380	23	10	<5	5	41	28	1	100	380	180	—	0
No Bake Reduced Fat Strawberry Swirl Cheesecake as prep	⅛ cake (4 oz)	250	6	2	5	7	44	33	0	200	430	310	—	1
Real Cheesecake as prep	⅛ cake (4.6 oz)	360	16	6	5	7	47	33	1	200	510	320	—	0
MINICARB														
Carrot as prep	1 slice	280	20	3	45	16	10	0	6	—	190	—	—	—
Chocolate as prep	1 slice	230	18	4	60	8	16	0	12	—	110	—	—	—
Zero Carb Baking Mix not prep	½ cup	55	1	0	0	10	2	2	2	—	160	—	—	—
SWEET REWARDS														
Reduced Fat White as prep	¹⁄₁₂ cake	180	3	1	0	2	36	20	—	60	300	—	24	—
Reduced Fat Yellow as prep	¹⁄₁₂ cake	200	5	1	30	2	37	21	—	80	280	—	32	—
CALABAZA														
fresh	½ cup	32	tr	—	—	1	8	—	—	—	3	246	—	18

FOOD	PORTION	CALS	FAT	SAT FAT	CHOL	PROT	CARB	SUGAR	FIBER	CALCI	SOD	POTAS	FOLIC	VIT C
CALZONE														
TAKE-OUT														
beef and cheese	1	330	35	5	11	—	—	—	—	—	1120	—	—	—
cheese	1 (12 oz)	1020	54	24	100	48	86	26	8	700	1760	—	—	1
pepperoni	1	450	19	9	10	—	—	—	—	—	930	—	—	—
CANADIAN BACON														
grilled	1 pkg (6 oz)	257	12	4	81	34	2	—	0	14	2149	—	6	0
BOAR'S HEAD														
Canadian Bacon	2 oz	70	3	1	30	12	1	1	0	0	560	—	—	0
HORMEL														
Sandwich Style	3 slices (2 oz)	70	3	2	30	10	0	0	0	0	640	—	—	0
JONES														
Slices	3	70	3	1	30	11	0	0	0	—	590	—	—	9
OSCAR MAYER														
Canadian Bacon	2 slices (1.6 oz)	50	2	1	25	8	0	0	0	0	620	—	—	0
REAL CANADIAN BACON														
Peameal	4 oz	130	5	2	40	16	4	—	—	—	1120	—	—	—
YORKSHIRE FARMS														
Uncured	3 oz	100	4	2	44	17	9	—	—	—	350	—	—	—
CANADIAN BACON SUBSTITUTES														
YVES														
Canadian Veggie Bacon	1 serv (2 oz)	80	1	0	0	17	1	1	1	20	480	170	—	0
CANDY														
boiled sweets	¼ lb	327	0	—	—	0	87	—	0	5	—	—	—	0
butterscotch	1 piece (6 g)	24	tr	tr	1	0	6	—	—	0	3	0	0	0
candied cherries	1 (4 g)	12	tr	tr	0	0	3	—	—	tr	—	—	—	0
candied citron	1 oz	89	tr	—	0	tr	23	—	—	24	82	34	—	—
candied lemon peel	1 oz	90	tr	—	0	tr	23	—	—	—	14	3	—	—
candied orange peel	1 oz	90	tr	—	0	tr	23	—	—	—	14	3	—	—
candied pineapple slice	1 slice (2 oz)	179	tr	tr	0	tr	45	—	—	17	—	—	—	13
candy corn	1 oz	105	0	0	0	tr	27	—	—	2	57	1	—	0
caramels	1 piece (8 g)	31	1	1	1	tr	6	—	—	11	20	17	0	—
caramels chocolate	1 bar (2.3 oz)	231	2	tr	0	1	56	—	—	—	—	—	—	—
caramels chocolate	1 piece (6 g)	22	tr	tr	0	tr	6	—	—	—	—	—	—	—
carob bar	1 (3.1 oz)	453	28	7	—	11	42	—	—	391	—	785	27	—
crisped rice bar almond	1 bar (1 oz)	130	6	1	0	2	18	—	1	21	66	65	0	—
crisped rice bar chocolate chip	1 bar (1 oz)	115	4	1	0	4	21	9	1	6	79	48	40	—

FOOD	PORTION	CALS	FAT	SAT FAT	CHOL	PROT	CARB	SUGAR	FIBER	CALCI	SOD	POTAS	FOLIC	VIT C
dark chocolate	1 oz	150	10	6	0	1	16	—	—	7	5	86	—	tr
fondant	1 piece (0.6 oz)	57	0	—	0	0	15	—	—	0	6	3	0	0
fondant chocolate coated	1 piece (0.4 oz)	40	1	1	0	tr	9	—	—	2	3	18	—	—
fondant mint	1 oz	105	0	0	0	tr	27	—	—	2	57	1	—	0
fruit pastilles	1 tube (1.4 oz)	101	0	—	—	2	25	—	—	16	—	—	—	0
fudge brown sugar w/ nuts	1 piece (0.5 oz)	56	1	tr	1	tr	11	—	—	16	14	52	1	tr
fudge chocolate marshmallow	1 piece (0.7 oz)	84	3	2	5	1	14	—	—	9	21	28	0	0
fudge chocolate marshmallow w/ nuts	1 piece (0.8 oz)	96	4	2	5	1	15	—	—	11	21	37	1	tr
fudge chocolate w/ nuts	1 piece (0.7 oz)	81	3	1	3	1	14	—	—	9	11	30	2	tr
fudge peanut butter	1 piece (0.6 oz)	59	1	tr	1	1	13	—	—	7	12	21	2	0
fudge vanilla w/ nuts	1 piece (0.5 oz)	62	2	1	2	tr	11	—	—	7	9	17	2	tr
gumdrops	10 lg (3.8 oz)	420	0	0	0	0	108	—	—	3	48	5	—	—
gumdrops	10 sm (0.4 oz)	135	0	0	0	0	35	—	—	1	15	2	—	—
hard candy	1 oz	106	0	0	0	0	28	—	—	1	11	1	—	—
jelly beans	10 lg (1 oz)	104	tr	—	0	0	26	—	—	1	7	11	—	0
jelly beans	10 sm (0.4 oz)	40	tr	—	0	0	10	—	—	0	3	4	—	0
lollipop	1 (6 g)	22	0	0	0	0	6	—	—	0	2	0	—	—
marzipan	1 oz	128	7	1	0	3	15	—	2	24	5	82	16	tr
milk chocolate	1 bar (1.55 oz)	226	14	8	10	3	26	—	—	84	36	169	4	tr
milk chocolate crisp	1 bar (1.45 oz)	203	11	7	8	3	28	—	—	70	59	141	3	tr
milk chocolate w/ almonds	1 bar (1.45 oz)	215	14	7	8	4	22	20	—	92	30	182	—	tr
nougat nut cream	0.5 oz	49	4	—	—	1	8			2	—	—	—	—
peanut bar	1 (1.4 oz)	209	14	2	—	6	19	—	—	31	91	163	—	—
peanut brittle	1 oz	128	5	1	4	2	20	—	—	8	128	59	20	0
peanuts chocolate covered	10 (1.4 oz)	208	13	6	4	5	20	—	—	42	16	201	3	0
peanuts chocolate covered	1 cup (5.2 oz)	773	50	22	13	19	74	—	—	155	61	748	12	0
praline	1 piece (1.4 oz)	177	10	1	0	1	24	—	—	12	24	82	6	tr
pretzels chocolate covered	1 (0.4 oz)	50	2	1	—	1	8	—	—	8	10	—	—	tr
pretzels chocolate covered	1 oz	130	5	2	—	2	20	—	—	21	—	—	—	tr

FOOD	PORTION	CALS	FAT	SAT FAT	CHOL	PROT	CARB	SUGAR	FIBER	CALCI	SOD	POTAS	FOLIC	VIT C
sesame crunch	20 pieces (1.2 oz)	181	12	2	0	4	18	—	—	—	—	—	—	—
sweet chocolate	1 oz	143	10	6	0	1	17	—	—	7	5	82	—	—
sweet chocolate	1 bar (1.45 oz)	201	14	8	0	2	25	—	—	10	7	119	—	—
taffy	1 piece (0.5 oz)	56	1	tr	1	0	14	—	—	0	13	1	0	0
toffee	1 piece (0.4 oz)	65	4	2	13	tr	8	—	—	4	22	6	0	0
truffles	1 piece (0.4 oz)	59	4	3	6	1	5	—	—	19	8	37	0	tr
100 GRAND														
Bar	1 bar (1.5 oz)	200	8	5	10	2	30	27	tr	40	75	—	—	0
5TH AVENUE														
Bar	1 (0.56 oz)	80	4	2	0	1	10	—	—	—	25	—	—	—
ALMOND JOY														
Bar	1 (0.68 oz)	90	5	4	0	1	11	9	—	—	30	—	—	—
ALTOIDS														
All Flavors	3 pieces	10	0	0	0	0	2	2	—	—	0	—	—	—
ANDES														
Chocolate Covered Mint Patties	1 (0.5 oz)	60	1	1	0	0	13	12	0	0	2	—	—	0
AT LAST!														
Chocolate Almond	1 bar	120	10	6	0	2	13	0	6	—	20	—	—	—
Chocolate Crisp	1 bar	110	9	6	0	3	14	0	6	—	40	—	—	—
Chocolate Mint	1 bar	110	10	6	0	2	15	0	7	—	25	—	—	—
Chocolate Peanut Butter	1 bar	120	11	7	0	2	14	0	5	—	20	—	—	—
Chocolate Peanut Butter	1 bar	100	8	5	0	2	15	0	5	—	50	—	—	—
ATKINS														
Endulge Caramel Nut Chew	1 bar (1.23 oz)	140	9	4	5	6	17	1	tr	20	70	—	—	0
Endulge Chocolate Bar	1 bar (1.1 oz)	150	12	7	5	1	2	0	3	20	5	—	—	0
Endulge Chocolate Crunch	1 bar (1 oz)	150	12	7	<5	3	15	0	3	—	7	—	—	—
Endulge Peanut Butter Cups	3 pieces	160	13	6	0	3	17	0	0	0	70	—	—	0
BABY RUTH														
Bar	1 bar (2.1 oz)	270	13	7	0	4	36	27	2	20	130	—	—	0
Fun Size	1 bar (1 oz)	130	6	4	0	3	17	13	tr	0	60	—	—	0

FOOD	PORTION	CALS	FAT	SAT FAT	CHOL	PROT	CARB	SUGAR	FIBER	CALCI	SOD	POTAS	FOLIC	VIT C
BARRICINI														
Dark Chocolate Raspberry Creme Shells	1 piece (0.3 oz)	47	3	1	0	0	5	4	0	0	4	—	—	0
BITTYFINGER														
Bars	2	170	7	4	0	2	27	18	tr	0	85	—	—	0
BODY SMARTS														
Chocolate Peanut Crunch	2 bars (1.8 oz)	210	6	4	<5	5	34	20	2	200	70	—	—	6
BUTTERFINGER														
Bar	1 (2.1 oz)	270	11	5	0	3	42	29	1	0	130	—	—	0
BB's	1 pkg (1.7 oz)	230	9	6	0	2	33	25	1	0	95	—	—	0
Fun Size	1 bar	100	4	2	0	1	15	10	0	0	45	—	—	0
CADBURY														
Milk Chocolate Roast Almond	10 blocks (1.4 oz)	220	13	7	10	4	21	18	1	100	80	—	—	0
CAPE COD PROVISIONS														
Cranberry Bog Frogs	3 pieces (1.9 oz)	250	12	10	7	3	34	27	tr	60	65	—	—	0
CARBOLITE														
Caramel	1 bar	100	5	3	5	1	18	0	0	—	10	—	—	—
CarbAway	1 bar	100	5	3	5	1	17	0	0	—	15	—	—	—
CarboSnack	1 bar	110	6	3	5	1	20	0	1	—	15	—	—	—
Chocolate Truffle	1 bar (1 oz)	122	8	5	<5	2	17	0	1	—	54	—	—	—
Chocolate Almond	1 bar (1.75 oz)	298	21	11	7	9	3	tr	2	—	57	—	—	—
Chocolate Crisp	1 bar (1.75 oz)	256	14	11	14	7	3	0	1	—	0	—	—	—
Chocolate Peanut Butter	1 bar (1.75 oz)	256	21	7	7	—	3	0	0	—	50	—	—	—
Crisy Caramel	1 bar (1 oz)	130	9	5	5	3	17	0	0	—	50	—	—	—
Milk Chocolate	1 bar (1.75 oz)	263	18	11	7	7	1	0	1	—	6	—	—	—
Peanut Butter Cup	1	170	14	7	5	3	17	0	1	—	35	—	—	—
Pecan Cluster	1 bar	120	8	3	5	1	15	0	1	—	10	—	—	—
CARBSLIM														
Crunch Bites Chocolate Caramel	1 pkg	122	14	12	3	6	21	0	9	—	78	—	—	—
Crunch Bites Peanut Butter	1 pkg	171	14	12	2	8	21	0	9	—	123	—	—	—
CARMELLO														
Snack Size	1 (0.66 oz)	90	4	3	<5	1	12	—	—	—	20	—	—	—
CARY'S OF OREGON														
English Toffee Milk Chocolate Almond	1 piece (0.75 oz)	110	8	4	10	1	12	10	tr	—	65	—	—	—

FOOD	PORTION	CALS	FAT	SAT FAT	CHOL	PROT	CARB	SUGAR	FIBER	CALCI	SOD	POTAS	FOLIC	VIT C
CHARLESTON CHEW														
Chocolate	½ bar	120	3	—	—	—	—	—	—	—	—	—	—	—
Strawberry	½ bar	120	3	—	—	—	—	—	—	—	—	—	—	—
Vanilla	½ bar	120	3	—	—	—	—	—	—	—	—	—	—	—
CHARMS														
Blow Pop	1 (0.6 oz)	70	0	0	0	0	17	14	—	—	0	—	—	—
Lollipop Sour	1 (0.6 oz)	70	0	0	0	0	18	17	—	—	0	—	—	—
Lollipop Sweet	1 (0.6 oz)	70	0	0	0	0	18	17	—	—	0	—	—	—
CHUNKY														
Bar	1 (1.4 oz)	210	11	6	5	3	24	21	1	40	20	—	—	0
CLASSIC CARAMELS														
Chocolate Creme Filled	3 pieces	80	3	2	<5	tr	13	—	—	—	30	—	—	—
Soft & Chewy	3 pieces	80	2	2	<5	tr	13	—	—	—	45	—	—	—
CLOUD NINE														
Australian Orange Peel	½ bar (1.5 oz)	220	13	7	0	2	25	19	2	20	5	—	—	1
Butter Nut Toffee	½ bar (1.5 oz)	230	14	8	5	3	25	21	1	60	30	—	—	1
Cool Mint Crisp	½ bar (⅕ oz)	220	13	7	5	2	26	22	2	20	5	—	—	1
Espresso Bean Crunch	½ bar (1.5 oz)	220	14	8	0	2	23	19	2	20	5	—	—	1
Malted Milk Crunch	½ bar (1.5 oz)	230	14	8	5	3	26	23	1	60	40	—	—	1
Milk Chocolate	½ bar (1.5 oz)	230	15	8	5	3	25	23	1	60	25	—	—	1
Oregon Red Raspberry	½ bar (1.5 oz)	230	15	8	0	2	25	20	2	20	5	—	—	2
Peanut Butter Brittle	½ bar (1.5 oz)	230	15	8	5	3	24	21	1	60	40	—	—	1
Sundried Cherry	½ bar (1.5 oz)	230	13	8	5	3	26	22	1	60	25	—	—	1
Toasted Coconut Crisp	½ bar (1.5 oz)	230	14	9	5	2	25	22	2	60	45	—	—	1
Vanilla Dark	½ bar (1.5 oz)	230	15	8	0	3	25	20	2	20	10	—	—	1
CRUNCH														
Fun Size	4 bars	210	11	7	10	2	26	22	tr	60	60	—	—	0
DABOGA														
Organic Milk Chocolate	1 bar (2 oz)	318	20	14	10	4	30	28	6	40	60	—	—	0
DEL MONTE														
Radical Raizins Cinnamon	1 pkg (0.7 oz)	70	0	0	0	0	18	16	0	0	0	—	—	15
Radical Raizins Rainbow	1 pkg (0.7 oz)	70	0	0	0	0	18	16	0	0	0	—	—	15
DOCTOR'S CARBRITE														
Sugar Free Dark Chocolate	1 oz	124	8	—	—	2	2	0	2	—	0	—	—	—

FOOD	PORTION	CALS	FAT	SAT FAT	CHOL	PROT	CARB	SUGAR	FIBER	CALCI	SOD	POTAS	FOLIC	VIT C
DOCTOR'S CARBRITE (CONT.)														
Sugar Free Dark Chocolate w/ Almonds	4 sq (1 oz)	132	10	4	0	8	16	0	4	—	20	—	—	—
Sugar Free Milk Chocolate	1 oz	128	9	—	—	0	0	0	0	—	0	—	—	—
Sugar Free Milk Chocolate w/ Peanuts	4 sq (1 oz)	132	10	4	4	8	12	0	0	—	20	—	—	—
Sugar Free Milk Chocolate w/ Soy Crisps	4 sq (1 oz)	120	8	4	4	4	12	0	2	—	40	—	—	—
Sugar Free Mint Chocolate	1 oz	128	9	—	—	0	0	0	0	—	0	—	—	—
ESTEE														
Caramels Vanilla & Chocolate	5	115	5	1	0	1	26	3	0	—	65	155	—	—
Dark Chocolate	½ bar (1.4 oz)	200	14	8	10	2	23	15	0	—	10	140	—	—
Milk Chocolate	½ bar (1.4 oz)	230	17	10	20	4	17	15	0	—	65	210	—	—
Milk Chocolate w/ Almonds	½ bar (1.4 oz)	230	17	9	20	4	16	14	0	—	65	220	—	—
Milk Chocolate w/ Crisp Rice	½ bar (1.2 oz)	370	26	15	30	7	29	24	0	—	110	340	—	—
Milk Chocolate w/ Fruit & Nuts	½ bar (1.4 oz)	220	16	9	20	4	18	15	0	—	65	220	—	—
Mint Chocolate	½ bar (1.4 oz)	200	14	8	10	2	23	15	0	—	10	140	—	—
Peanut Brittle	⅓ box (1.3 oz)	160	9	2	10	3	28	1	1	—	115	90	—	—
Peanut Butter Cups	5	200	12	7	<5	5	19	13	1	—	70	240	—	—
Sugar Free Assorted Fruit	5	30	0	0	0	0	16	0	0	—	0	0	—	—
Sugar Free Assorted Mint	5	30	0	0	0	0	16	0	0	—	0	0	—	—
Sugar Free Butterscotch	2	25	0	0	0	0	17	0	0	—	50	0	—	—
Sugar Free Fruit Gum Drops	23	80	0	0	0	0	36	0	0	—	0	0	—	—
Sugar Free Gourmet Jelly Beans	26	70	0	0	0	0	24	0	0	—	30	0	—	—
Sugar Free Gummy Apple Rings	5	70	0	0	0	0	28	0	0	—	5	0	—	—
Sugar Free Gummy Bears Assorted Fruit	17	100	0	0	0	3	30	0	0	—	5	0	—	—

FOOD	PORTION	CALS	FAT	SAT FAT	CHOL	PROT	CARB	SUGAR	FIBER	CALCI	SOD	POTAS	FOLIC	VIT C
ESTEE (CONT.)														
Sugar Free Licorice Gum Drops	11	90	0	0	0	1	36	0	0	—	65	0	—	—
Sugar Free Peppermint Swirl	3	30	0	0	0	0	14	0	0	—	0	0	—	—
Sugar Free Sour Citrus Slices	9	60	0	0	0	0	30	0	0	—	50	0	—	—
Sugar Free Toffee	5	30	0	0	0	0	16	0	0	—	0	0	—	—
Sugar Free Tropical Fruit	5	30	0	0	0	0	16	0	0	—	0	0	—	—
FAUCHON														
Chocolate Assortment	3 pieces (1.1 oz)	170	11	5	<5	3	19	15	2	40	15	—	—	0
FAVORITE BRANDS														
Candy Corn	24 pieces (1.4 oz)	150	0	0	—	0	37	34	—	—	110	—	—	—
Cinnamon Imperials	52 (0.5 oz)	80	0	0	—	0	14	12	—	—	5	—	—	—
Circus Peanuts	5 pieces (1.6 oz)	160	0	0	—	1	39	33	—	—	10	—	—	—
Gummallo Apple Ring	5 pieces (1.4 oz)	120	0	0	—	2	27	20	—	—	0	—	—	—
Gummallo Peach Ring	5 pieces (1.4 oz)	120	0	0	—	2	27	20	—	—	5	—	—	—
Gummi Bears	18 pieces (1.4 oz)	130	0	0	—	2	30	19	—	—	15	—	—	—
Gummi Dinos	7 pieces (1.3 oz)	120	0	0	—	2	28	18	—	—	15	—	—	—
Gummi Worms	4 pieces (1.4 oz)	130	0	0	—	2	29	18	—	—	15	—	—	—
Jelly Beans	13 (1.4 oz)	150	0	0	—	0	37	28	—	—	20	—	—	—
Marshmallow Eggs	3 (1.3 oz)	140	0	0	—	0	34	32	—	—	10	—	—	—
Neon Worms	4 pieces (1.4 oz)	120	0	0	—	2	28	22	—	—	0	—	—	—
Sour Gummi Bears	16 pieces (1.4 oz)	110	0	0	—	2	26	20	—	—	0	—	—	—
Sour Gummi Worms	4 pieces (1.6 oz)	130	0	0	—	2	29	23	—	—	0	—	—	—
FERRERO ROCHER														
Candy	3 pieces (1.3 oz)	140	15	5	0	4	17	16	1	60	35	—	—	1

FOOD	PORTION	CALS	FAT	SAT FAT	CHOL	PROT	CARB	SUGAR	FIBER	CALCI	SOD	POTAS	FOLIC	VIT C
GODIVA														
Chocolatier Dark Chocolate w/ Raspberry	1 bar (1.5 oz)	220	11	4	3	2	28	22	0	20	10	—	—	2
Chocolatier Milk Chocolate	1 bar (1.5 oz)	230	13	5	10	3	26	25	0	100	30	—	—	0
Chocolatier Milk Chocolate w/ Almonds	1 bar (1.5 oz)	230	15	4	5	5	20	18	0	100	20	—	—	0
Mochaccino Mousse	2 pieces (1.25 oz)	210	15	4	4	2	17	14	0	40	10	—	—	0
Truffles Assorted	2 pieces (1.5 oz)	220	13	6	10	2	24	20	0	40	15	—	—	0
GOETZE'S														
Caramel Creams	3 pieces	130	3	1	0	2	23	13	tr	20	50	—	—	0
Cow Tales	1 pkg (1 oz)	110	3	1	tr	1	20	11	tr	20	40	—	—	0
GOLD LITE														
Milk Chocolate Crisp	1 bar	125	9	6	6	1	15	0	0	—	18	—	—	—
Seashell Truffle	1 piece	54	3	0	0	1	6	0	1	—	0	—	—	—
GOLDENBERG'S														
Peanut Chews	3 pieces	180	8	2	0	4	22	14	1	20	40	—	—	0
GOLIGHTLY														
Sugar Free Caramels	5 pieces	150	6	3	10	1	31	0	—	—	30	—	—	—
Sugar Free Doublers Chews Peach & Creme	7 pieces	150	7	3	10	0	31	0	tr	—	0	—	—	—
Sugar Free Fudgie Rolls	6 pieces	130	5	2	5	1	28	0	—	—	25	—	—	—
Sugar Free Hard Candy	4 pieces	45	0	0	0	0	15	0	—	—	0	—	—	—
GOOBERS														
Peanuts	1 pkg (1.38 oz)	210	13	5	5	4	20	17	1	40	15	—	—	0
GOOD & PLENTY														
Snack Size	1 box (0.6 oz)	60	0	0	0	0	14	—	—	—	40	—	—	—
GOOD 'N FRUITY														
Snack Size	1 box (0.6 oz)	60	0	0	0	0	15	—	—	—	10	—	—	—
HAVILAND														
Chocolate Covered Thin Mints	6 (1.5 oz)	170	5	3	0	1	33	32	1	0	5	—	—	0
HEATH														
Snack Size	1 bar (0.3 oz)	50	3	1	<5	0	6	—	—	—	35	—	—	—

FOOD	PORTION	CALS	FAT	SAT FAT	CHOL	PROT	CARB	SUGAR	FIBER	CALCI	SOD	POTAS	FOLIC	VIT C
HERSHEY'S														
Bites Almond Joy	8 pieces	100	6	4	<5	tr	10	—	—	—	5	—	—	—
Bites Cookies 'N' Creme	8 pieces	90	5	3	0	2	10	—	—	—	35	—	—	—
Bites Milk Chocolate w/ Almond	7 pieces	90	6	3	<5	2	8	—	—	—	10	—	—	—
Bites Reese's	7 pieces	90	5	3	0	2	10	—	—	—	30	—	—	—
Bites York	9 pieces	90	2	1	0	0	19	—	—	—	10	—	—	—
Candy Coated Milk Chocolate Eggs	4 pieces	90	5	3	<5	1	12	—	—	—	10	—	—	—
Hugs	1 piece	25	2	1	0	0	3	—	—	—	0	—	—	—
Kisses	1 piece	25	2	1	0	0	3	—	—	—	0	—	—	—
Kisses w/ Almonds	1 piece	25	2	1	0	0	3	—	—	—	0	—	—	—
Milk Chocolate	1 bar (0.6 oz)	90	5	4	<5	1	10	9	0	20	15	—	—	0
Milk Chocolate w/ Almonds	1 bar (0.6 oz)	100	6	3	<5	2	9	—	—	—	10	—	—	—
Miniature Special Dark	1 (0.3 oz)	45	3	2	0	0	3	—	—	—	0	—	—	—
Nuggets Cookies 'N' Creme	1	50	3	2	0	tr	5	—	—	—	20	—	—	—
Nuggets Dark Chocolate w/ Almonds	4	220	14	6	<5	3	20	16	3	20	0	—	—	0
Nuggets Milk Chocolate	4	230	13	8	10	3	24	21	1	80	35	—	—	0
Nuggets Milk Chocolate w/ Almonds	1	60	4	2	0	tr	5	—	—	—	5	—	—	—
Nuggets Milk Chocolate w/ Almonds & Toffee	1	50	4	2	<5	tr	5	—	—	—	10	—	—	—
Nuggets Milk Chocolate w/ Raisins & Almonds	1	50	3	2	0	tr	6	—	—	—	10	—	—	—
Pot Of Gold	3 pieces	130	5	4	<5	1	21	18	tr	20	45	—	—	0
Sweet Escapes Caramel & Peanut Butter Crispy	1 bar	80	3	1	0	1	13	—	—	—	70	—	—	—
Sweet Escapes Crispy Caramel Fudge	1 bar	70	2	1	0	tr	13	—	—	—	50	—	—	—
Sweet Escapes Crunchy Peanut Butter	1 bar (0.7 oz)	90	3	1	0	2	13	—	—	—	40	—	—	—

FOOD	PORTION	CALS	FAT	SAT FAT	CHOL	PROT	CARB	SUGAR	FIBER	CALCI	SOD	POTAS	FOLIC	VIT C
HERSHEY'S (CONT.)														
Sweet Escapes Triple Chocolate Wafer	1 bar	80	3	2	0	tr	13	—	—	—	30	—	—	—
Take 5	2 pkg (1.5 oz)	220	11	5	<5	4	25	18	1	20	180	—	—	0
Tastetations Butterscotch	3 pieces	60	2	1	<5	0	12	—	—	—	85	—	—	—
Tastetations Caramel	3 pieces	60	2	1	<5	0	12	—	—	—	85	—	—	—
Tastetations Chocolate	3 pieces	60	21	1	<5	0	12	—	—	—	30	—	—	—
HINT MINT														
All Flavors	2 pieces	10	0	0	0	0	2	2	—	0	0	—	—	0
JOLLY RANCHER														
All Flavors	3 pieces	70	0	0	0	0	17	—	—	—	10	—	—	—
Lollipops All Flavors	1 (0.6 oz)	60	0	0	0	0	16	12	—	—	10	—	—	—
JOYVA														
Halvah Chocolate Covered	1 serv (2 oz)	380	25	5	0	5	20	19	3	0	95	—	—	0
Halvah Marble	1 serv (2 oz)	390	25	4	0	6	18	10	2	0	120	—	—	0
JUDY'S														
Sugar Free Almond Caramel Cluster	1 piece (1.5 oz)	200	15	4	<5	5	10	0	2	—	0	—	—	—
Sugar Free Cashew Caramel Cluster	1 piece (1.5 oz)	190	14	5	5	2	12	1	1	—	5	—	—	—
Sugar Free English Toffee	1 piece (1.5 oz)	220	17	5	5	4	9	0	3	—	25	—	—	—
Sugar Free Macadamia Caramel Cluster	1 piece (1.5 oz)	220	20	5	<5	2	9	tr	2	—	0	—	—	—
Sugar Free Peanut Brittle	¾ cup	100	6	1	0	3	2	0	tr	—	70	—	—	—
Sugar Free Pecan Almond Cluster	1 piece (1.5 oz)	220	19	4	<5	2	9	0	2	—	0	—	—	—
JUNIOR MINTS														
Snack Size	1 box (0.7 oz)	75	1	1	0	tr	16	16	tr	0	5	—	—	0
JUST BORN														
Hot Tamales	1 pkg (2.1 oz)	220	0	0	0	0	55	34	—	—	25	—	—	—
Mike and Ike Berry Fruits	1 pkg (2.1 oz)	220	0	0	0	0	55	34	—	—	85	—	—	—
Mike and Ike Cherry & Bubble Gum	1 pkg (2.1 oz)	220	0	0	0	0	55	34	—	—	25	—	—	—

FOOD	PORTION	CALS	FAT	SAT FAT	CHOL	PROT	CARB	SUGAR	FIBER	CALCI	SOD	POTAS	FOLIC	VIT C
JUST BORN (CONT.)														
Mike and Ike Chewy Grape	1 pkg (2.1 oz)	220	0	0	0	0	55	34	—	—	25	—	—	—
Mike and Ike Lemon	1 pkg (2.1 oz)	220	0	0	0	0	55	34	—	—	25	—	—	—
Mike and Ike Original	1 pkg (1.2 oz)	220	0	0	0	0	55	34	—	—	25	—	—	—
Mike and Ike Strawberry & Banana	1 pkg (2.1 oz)	220	0	0	0	0	55	34	—	—	25	—	—	—
Mike and Ike Tropical Fruits	1 pkg (2.1 oz)	220	0	0	0	0	55	34	—	—	25	—	—	—
Super Hot Tamales	1 pkg (2.1 oz)	220	0	0	0	0	55	34	—	—	25	—	—	—
Teenee Beanee Assorted Fruits	36 pieces (1.4 oz)	150	0	0	0	0	36	23	—	—	15	—	—	—
Teenee Beanee Berry Berry	36 pieces (1.4 oz)	150	0	0	0	0	36	23	—	—	15	—	—	—
Teenee Beanee Tropical Mix	36 pieces (1.4 oz)	150	0	0	0	0	36	23	—	—	15	—	—	—
KIT KAT														
Bar	1 (0.6 oz)	80	4	3	0	tr	10	—	—	—	10	—	—	—
KLEIN														
Sugar Free Hard Candy All Flavors	3 pieces	12	0	0	0	0	5	0	0	—	0	—	—	—
KRACKEL														
Bar	1 (0.6 oz)	90	4	3	0	tr	12	—	—	—	20	—	—	—
Miniature	1	45	3	2	0	tr	5	—	—	—	5	—	—	—
LAMBERTZ														
Petits Soleils Chocolate Coated Gingerbread	1 piece (0.4 oz)	47	2	1	0	1	7	5	tr	7	8	—	—	0
LANCE														
Chocolaty Peanut Bar	1 (2 oz)	290	15	4	0	9	32	23	2	20	90	270	—	0
Cinnamon Chews	1 pkg (1.06 oz)	120	1	0	0	0	28	22	0	0	0	—	—	0
Fruit Chews	1 pkg (1.06 oz)	120	1	0	0	0	28	22	0	0	0	—	—	0
Gum Ball Pops	1 (0.45 oz)	45	0	0	0	0	12	12	tr	0	0	—	—	0
K-Nuts	4 pieces (1.5 oz)	240	15	5	5	4	23	17	0	0	130	—	—	0
Mint Chews	1 pkg (1.06 oz)	120	1	0	0	0	28	22	0	0	0	—	—	0
Peanut Bar	1 (1.75 oz)	270	15	3	0	10	23	15	2	0	80	250	—	0
Pop-A-Lance	1 piece (0.42 oz)	45	0	0	0	0	11	10	0	0	0	—	—	0
Popcorn'n'Carmel	1 bar (0.75 oz)	90	0	0	0	0	20	14	0	0	120	—	—	0
Starlight Mints	3 pieces (1 oz)	60	0	0	0	0	15	11	0	0	0	—	—	0

FOOD	PORTION	CALS	FAT	SAT FAT	CHOL	PROT	CARB	SUGAR	FIBER	CALCI	SOD	POTAS	FOLIC	VIT C
LANCE (CONT.)														
Strawberry Chews	1 pkg (1.06 oz)	120	1	0	0	0	28	22	0	0	0	—	—	0
Suckers	3 pieces (0.5 oz)	50	0	0	0	0	13	10	0	0	6	—	—	0
Whistle Pop	1 (0.67 oz)	70	0	0	0	0	19	17	tr	0	0	—	—	0
LANDIES CANDIES														
Sugar Free Almond Clusters	2 pieces (1.5 oz)	240	17	7	<5	7	17	tr	2	40	105	—	—	0
Sugar Free Bon Bons Peanut Butter	2 (1.5 oz)	240	17	7	<5	7	17	0	tr	20	150	—	—	0
Sugar Free Coconut Clusters	2 pieces (1.5 oz)	250	18	12	10	5	18	tr	1	20	120	—	—	0
Sugar Free Cookies & Cream	2 pieces (1.5 oz)	240	15	8	5	4	23	0	tr	0	150	—	—	0
Sugar Free Dark Almond Bark	1 piece (1.5 oz)	230	15	7	<5	3	23	0	2	20	85	—	—	0
Sugar Free Dark Miniature Bars	7 pieces (1.5 oz)	230	14	8	<5	2	26	0	2	0	0	—	—	0
Sugar Free Milk Miniature Bars	7 pieces (1.5 oz)	240	15	9	5	6	21	0	tr	20	140	—	—	0
Sugar Free Mint Discs	7 pieces (1.5 oz)	240	15	9	5	6	21	0	tr	20	140	—	—	0
Sugar Free Peanut Clusters	2 (1.5 oz)	240	17	7	<5	7	17	0	2	20	100	—	—	0
Sugar Free White Almond Bark	1 piece (1.5 oz)	230	15	10	<5	2	21	0	tr	100	90	—	—	0
Sugar Free White Caps	6 pieces (1.5 oz)	230	15	8	5	3	24	0	0	0	85	—	—	0
LEAN PROTEIN BITES														
Milk Chocolate	1 pkg (1 oz)	120	6	3	3	14	1	0	0	—	180	—	—	—
Peanut Butter	1 pkg (1 oz)	120	5	4	1	14	1	1	0	—	200	—	—	—
White Chocolate	1 pkg (1 oz)	120	4	2	3	16	2	2	0	—	200	—	—	—
LIFESAVERS														
Gummi Shapes Barnum's Animals	1 pkg (0.8 oz)	70	0	0	0	1	18	13	—	—	0	—	—	—
LINDT														
Dark Chocolate 70% Cocoa	4 blocks (1.4 oz)	220	17	10	0	3	13	11	2	40	20	—	—	0
Lindor Truffles Dark Chocolate	3 pieces	220	18	13	5	2	15	13	0	20	10	—	—	0
Lindor Truffles Milk Chocolate	3 pieces	220	17	12	5	2	16	15	0	60	20	—	—	0

FOOD	PORTION	CALS	FAT	SAT FAT	CHOL	PROT	CARB	SUGAR	FIBER	CALCI	SOD	POTAS	FOLIC	VIT C
LOW CARB CHEF														
Gummi Bears	14 pieces	138	0	0	0	0	30	0	0	—	0	—	—	—
Jelly Beans	37 pieces	120	0	0	0	0	36	0	0	—	10	—	—	—
Sugar Free Caramel Marshmallow Treats	3 pieces	140	7	5	<5	1	28	0	0	—	15	—	—	—
Sugar Free Cherry Cordials	3 pieces	250	8	5	<5	tr	28	0	tr	—	10	—	—	—
Sugar Free Coconut Clusters	4 pieces	210	18	13	<5	2	19	0	3	—	15	—	—	—
Sugar Free Milk Chocolate Covered Vanilla Caramels	3 pieces	160	8	5	10	1	27	0	0	—	10	—	—	—
Sugar Free Peanut Butter Cups	1 piece	200	16	8	<5	3	19	0	1	—	5	—	—	—
Sugar Free Peanut Butter Truffes	2 pieces	200	16	8	<5	3	19	0	1	—	5	—	—	—
Sugar Free Peanut Clusters	4 pieces	210	17	5	<5	5	16	0	2	—	5	—	—	—
Sugar Free Pecan Turtles	1 piece	120	13	6	5	1	20	0	1	—	10	—	—	—
Sugar Free Peppermint Patties	3 pieces	150	9	5	10	tr	28	0	3	—	50	—	—	—
M&M'S														
Plain	1 pkg (1.7 oz)	240	10	6	5	2	34	31	1	40	30	—	—	—
MAPLE GROVE FARMS														
Maple Sugar Candy	5 pieces (1.3 oz)	140	0	0	0	0	36	32	—	—	0	—	—	—
MAUNA LOA														
Kona Coffee Crunch Chocolate	1 bar (1.8 oz)	270	16	9	—	3	29	24	4	—	0	—	—	—
Macadamia Crisp Milk Chocolate	1 bar (1.8 oz)	270	17	9	10	4	29	25	tr	—	55	—	—	—
Macadamia Milk Chocolate	1 bar (1.8 oz)	280	18	9	10	4	27	25	1	—	45	—	—	—
MON CHERI														
Hazelnut	4 pieces	260	18	9	5	4	20	20	1	90	25	—	—	1
MOUNDS														
Bar	1 (0.7 oz)	90	5	4	0	tr	11	9	—	—	30	—	—	—
MR. GOODBAR														
Bar	1 (0.6 oz)	100	6	3	0	2	9	—	—	—	5	—	—	—
Miniatures	1 (0.3 oz)	45	3	2	0	tr	5	—	—	—	5	—	—	—

FOOD	PORTION	CALS	FAT	SAT FAT	CHOL	PROT	CARB	SUGAR	FIBER	CALCI	SOD	POTAS	FOLIC	VIT C
NECCO														
Bridge Mix	¼ cup (1.5 oz)	180	9	5	5	2	27	23	tr	60	35	—	—	0
Chocolate Covered Raisins	30 pieces (1.5 oz)	170	7	5	0	1	30	27	1	40	35	—	—	0
Malted Milk Balls	11 pieces (1.5 oz)	180	6	6	0	1	28	25	tr	40	35	—	—	0
Mint	1 piece	12	tr	—	0	—	—	—	—	—	—	—	—	—
SkyBar	1 bar (1.5 oz)	190	9	5	5	2	28	25	0	40	45	—	—	0
NESTLÉ														
Buncha Crunch	1 pkg (1.4 oz)	90	10	6	10	2	26	20	tr	40	60	—	—	0
Crunch	1 bar (1.55 oz)	230	12	7	10	2	29	24	tr	60	65	—	—	0
Crunch Disk	1 (1.2 oz)	180	9	6	5	2	22	19	tr	40	50	—	—	0
Crunchkins	5 pieces	190	10	6	5	2	24	21	tr	60	45	—	—	0
Jingles Milk Chocolate Butterfinger	5 pieces	180	8	4	<5	2	26	20	tr	20	55	—	—	0
Jingles Milk Chocolate Crunch	7 pieces	220	11	7	10	2	28	23	tr	60	65	—	—	0
Jingles White Crunch	7 pieces	230	14	8	10	3	24	21	0	100	80	—	—	0
Milk Chocolate	1 bar (1.45 oz)	220	13	8	10	2	26	24	tr	60	25	—	—	0
Nesteggs Milk Chocolate Butterfinger	5 pieces	210	10	5	5	3	28	23	tr	40	55	—	—	0
Nesteggs Milk Chocolate Crunch	5 pieces	190	10	6	5	2	24	21	tr	60	45	—	—	0
Nesteggs White Crunch	7 pieces	230	14	8	10	3	24	21	0	100	75	—	—	0
Pearson's Egg Nog	2 pieces	60	2	1	0	0	11	7	0	0	40	—	—	0
Toll House Brownie Bar	2 pieces (2 oz)	250	12	5	5	2	36	23	1	20	240	—	—	0
Toll House Cookie Bar	1 piece (1 oz)	130	6	3	<5	tr	18	11	tr	0	90	—	—	0
Treasures Butterfinger	3 pieces	180	9	5	5	2	24	19	tr	40	40	—	—	0
Treasures Crunch	4 pieces (1.4 oz)	210	11	7	10	2	26	21	tr	60	60	—	—	0
Treasures Peanut Butter	4 pieces	250	17	7	5	4	23	21	1	60	90	—	—	0
Turtles Bite Size	1 piece (0.4 oz)	50	2	1	1	1	6	5	tr	15	11	—	—	0
White Crunch	1 bar (1.4 oz)	220	13	8	10	3	23	20	0	80	70	—	—	0
NEWMAN'S OWN														
Organic Peanut Butter Cups Dark Chocolate	3 pieces (1.2 oz)	180	12	6	0	3	18	14	tr	0	55	—	—	0

FOOD	PORTION	CALS	FAT	SAT FAT	CHOL	PROT	CARB	SUGAR	FIBER	CALCI	SOD	POTAS	FOLIC	VIT C
NEWMAN'S OWN (CONT.)														
Organic Peanut Butter Cups Milk Chocolate	3 pieces (1.2 oz)	180	12	6	0	4	18	14	tr	60	70	—	—	0
Organic Peppermint Cups	3 pieces (1.2 oz)	180	12	6	0	2	20	18	tr	20	15	—	—	0
NIBS														
Licorice	9 pieces	35	0	0	0	0	9	—	—	—	60	—	—	—
NIPS														
Butter Rum	2 pieces	60	2	1	0	0	11	7	0	0	40	—	—	0
Caramel	2 pieces	60	2	1	0	0	11	7	0	0	40	—	—	0
Chocolate	2 pieces	60	2	1	0	0	11	7	0	0	40	—	—	0
Chocolate Parfait	2 pieces	60	2	1	0	0	10	7	0	0	30	—	—	0
Coffee	2 pieces	50	2	2	0	0	10	7	0	0	40	—	—	0
Vanilla Almond Cafe	2 pieces	50	1	1	0	0	10	7	0	0	40	—	—	0
OH HENRY!														
Bar	1 (1.8 oz)	120	5	3	<5	2	16	12	0	20	60	—	—	0
PALMER														
Milk Chocolate Lollipop	1 (0.9 oz)	130	7	4	4	1	16	15	2	100	35	—	—	0
PAYDAY														
Snack Size	1 (0.7 oz)	90	5	1	0	2	10	—	—	—	65	—	—	—
PEARSON'S														
Irish Cream Parfait	2 pieces	60	2	2	0	0	10	6	0	0	30	—	—	0
Mint Patties	1	30	1	tr	0	tr	6	5	tr	0	14	—	—	0
PERLEGE														
Sugar Free Belgium Chocolate All Flavors	1 bar (3.5 oz)	532	42	—	—	14	14	0	3	—	112	—	—	—
Sugar Free Cream Filled Belgian Chocolate All Flavors	1 bar (1.5 oz)	226	16	10	14	2	22	0	0	—	32	—	—	—
PEZ														
Candy	1 roll (0.3 oz)	35	0	0	0	0	9	9	—	—	0	—	—	—
Candy Sugar Free	1 roll (0.3 oz)	30	0	0	0	0	8	0	—	—	0	—	—	21
PLANTERS														
Original Peanut Bar	1 pkg (1.6 oz)	230	14	2	0	6	22	13	2	20	70	210	—	0
PURE DE-LITE														
Caramel	1 bar	120	5	4	3	2	19	0	1	—	110	—	—	—
Caramel Crisp	1 bar	120	6	4	3	3	18	0	1	—	115	—	—	—

FOOD	PORTION	CALS	FAT	SAT FAT	CHOL	PROT	CARB	SUGAR	FIBER	CALCI	SOD	POTAS	FOLIC	VIT C
PURE DE-LITE (CONT.)														
Caramel Nougat	1 bar	110	5	3	3	2	20	0	1	—	146	—	—	—
Caramel Peanut Butter	1 bar	120	6	3	2	2	17	0	1	—	58	—	—	—
Caramel Pecan	1 bar	130	7	4	3	2	17	0	1	—	94	—	—	—
Sugar Free Dark Chocolate	1 bar	173	14	8	1	2	1	0	4	—	37	—	—	—
Sugar Free Milk Choclate w/ Mint	1 bar	187	14	9	8	3	3	0	1	—	32	—	—	—
Sugar Free Milk Chocolate	1 bar	187	14	9	8	3	3	0	1	—	32	—	—	—
Sugar Free Milk Chocolate w/ Almonds	1 bar	190	14	9	8	3	4	0	2	—	30	—	—	—
Sugar Free Milk Chocolate w/ Coconut	1 bar	190	14	9	8	3	4	0	1	—	31	—	—	—
Sugar Free Milk Chocolate w/ Orange	1 bar	187	14	9	8	3	3	0	1	—	32	—	—	—
Sugar Free Milk Chocolate w/ Peanuts	1 bar	190	14	9	9	3	4	0	1	—	30	—	—	—
Sugar Free White Chocolate	1 bar	187	14	9	26	2	3	0	0	—	96	—	—	—
Truffle Bar Caramel	1 bar	140	8	5	5	2	16	0	0	—	25	—	—	—
Truffle Bar Dark Mint	1 bar	160	12	8	5	2	13	0	1	—	20	—	—	—
Truffle Bar Hazelnut	1 bar	160	12	7	10	2	12	0	1	—	20	—	—	—
Truffle Bar Peanut Butter	1 bar	160	11	7	5	2	13	0	1	—	20	—	—	—
RAISINETS														
Candy	1 pkg (1.58 oz)	200	8	5	<5	2	31	28	1	40	15	—	—	0
Fun Size	3 pkg	200	8	5	5	2	43	29	2	40	15	—	—	0
REESE'S														
Nutrageous	1 bar (0.6 oz)	95	6	2	0	2	9	8	1	20	25	—	—	0
Peanut Butter Cups	1 (0.28 oz)	40	3	1	0	tr	4	—	—	—	20	—	—	—
Peanut Butter Eggs	1	90	5	2	0	2	9	—	—	—	60	—	—	—
Pieces	25	90	5	3	0	3	11	—	—	—	40	—	—	—
RITTER SPORT														
Dark Chocolate Whole Hazelnuts	6 pieces (1.3 oz)	210	15	8	<2	2	16	14	7	20	<5	—		0

FOOD	PORTION	CALS	FAT	SAT FAT	CHOL	PROT	CARB	SUGAR	FIBER	CALCI	SOD	POTAS	FOLIC	VIT C
ROBIN EGGS														
Large	2 pieces	70	2	2	0	0	14	—	—	—	40	—	—	—
Medium	4 pieces	90	3	2	0	0	16	—	—	—	45	—	—	—
Mini	10 pieces	70	3	2	0	0	13	—	—	—	40	—	—	—
ROKEACH														
Cotton Candy	2 cups (1 oz)	110	0	0	0	0	28	28	0	0	0	—	—	0
ROLO														
Caramels In Milk Chocolate	3 pieces (0.64 oz)	90	3	2	<5	tr	12	—	—	—	35	—	—	—
RUSSELL STOVER														
Looney Tunes Peanut Butter Nougat w/ Peanuts in Milk Chocolate	1 snack size (0.7 oz)	90	5	2	<5	1	14	7	tr	20	60	—	—	0
Low Carb Pecan Delights	1 pkg (1 oz)	130	9	5	0	2	16	0	tr	0	25	—	—	0
Peanut Butter & Grape Jelly	1 piece (0.8 oz)	100	6	2	<5	2	10	8	tr	20	30	—	—	0
Peanut Butter & Red Raspberry Cups	2 (1.2 oz)	140	9	3	<5	3	14	12	tr	20	40	—	—	0
Pecan Delights	1 pkg (2 oz)	280	18	5	10	3	27	20	tr	60	65	—	—	1
Pecan Roll	1 (1.75 oz)	260	18	2	<5	3	23	19	2	20	80	—	—	1
S'mores	3 (1.4 oz)	210	12	7	<5	2	22	18	tr	40	80	—	—	0
Sugar Free Peanut Butter Cups	4 pieces (1.3 oz)	200	13	6	0	5	17	—	2	0	140	—	—	0
Sugar Free Pecans & Caramel	2 pieces (1.2 oz)	170	12	3	0	2	17	—	0	0	30	—	—	0
SIMPLY LITE														
Sugar Free Li'l Bits Chocolately	36 pieces (1.4 oz)	130	5	5	0	3	28	0	1	0	55	—	—	0
Sugar Free Li'l Bits Peanut Buttery	36 pieces (1.4 oz)	140	5	5	0	4	26	0	1	0	50	—	—	0
Sugar Free Patteez	5 pieces (1.3 oz)	110	3	2	0	1	29	0	1	0	10	—	—	0
SIXLETS														
Sixlets	3 tubes	90	4	3	0	0	14	—	—	—	50	—	—	—
SMUCKER'S														
Fruit Fillers Strawberry	1 pkg (0.9 oz)	80	0	0	0	1	19	13	—	—	25	—	—	15
SNICKERS														
Almond	1 bar (1.76 oz)	240	11	5	5	3	32	27	1	60	80	—	—	0
Bar	1 (2.07 oz)	280	14	5	5	4	35	30	1	40	140	—	—	0
Cruncher	1 bar (1.56 oz)	230	13	5	5	4	25	17	1	40	140	—	—	0

FOOD	PORTION	CALS	FAT	SAT FAT	CHOL	PROT	CARB	SUGAR	FIBER	CALCI	SOD	POTAS	FOLIC	VIT C
SNO CAPS														
Candies	1 pkg (2.3 oz)	300	13	8	0	2	48	38	3	0	0	—	—	0
SPEAKEASY														
Organic Mints All Flavors	4 pieces (2 g)	10	0	0	0	0	2	2	—	—	0	—	—	—
STEEL'S														
Salt Water Taffy Assorted	3 pieces (1 oz)	90	1	0	0	0	22	16	0	0	50	—	—	4
SUGAR BABIES														
Tidbits	1 pkg	180	2	—	—	—	—	—	—	—	20	—	—	—
SWEDISH FISH														
Original	19 pieces (1.4 oz)	160	0	0	0	0	39	24	0	0	25	—	—	0
SWEET'N LOW														
Sugar Free Butter Toffee	4 pieces (0.5 oz)	30	1	1	<5	0	15	—	—	—	80	—	—	—
Sugar Free Butterscotch	1 piece	7	0	0	0	0	4	—	—	—	0	—	—	—
Sugar Free Cinnamon	1 piece	7	0	0	0	0	4	—	—	—	0	—	—	—
Sugar Free Fancy Fruit	1 piece	7	0	0	0	0	4	—	—	—	0	—	—	—
Sugar Free Fruit Flavors	1 piece	7	0	0	0	0	4	—	—	—	0	—	—	—
Sugar Free Hard Candy Coffee	4 pieces (0.5 oz)	30	0	0	0	0	14	—	—	—	20	—	—	—
Sugar Free Peppermint	1 piece	7	0	0	0	0	4	—	—	—	0	—	—	—
Sugar Free Soft Candy Fruitie Flavors	1 piece	11	tr	—	—	tr	4	—	—	—	0	—	—	—
Sugar Free Soft Candy Tropical Flavors	1 piece	11	tr	—	—	tr	4	—	—	—	0	—	—	—
Sugar Free Watermelon	1 piece	7	0	0	0	0	4	—	—	—	0	—	—	—
Sugar Free Wild Cherry	1 piece	7	0	0	0	0	4	—	—	—	0	—	—	—
SYMPHONY														
Bar	1 (0.6 oz)	90	5	3	<5	1	10	—	—	—	15	—	—	—
THE CHOCOLATE TRAVELER														
Carb Controlled Wedges Bittersweet	4 pieces	120	9	6	0	1	12	0	0	0	20	—	—	0
Carb Controlled Wedges Dark Chocolate Coffee	4 pieces	110	8	5	0	1	15	0	2	20	0	—	—	0

FOOD	PORTION	CALS	FAT	SAT FAT	CHOL	PROT	CARB	SUGAR	FIBER	CALCI	SOD	POTAS	FOLIC	VIT C
THE CHOCOLATE TRAVELER (CONT.)														
Carb Controlled Wedges Dark Chocolate Mint	4 pieces	110	8	5	0	1	15	0	2	20	0	—	—	0
Carb Controlled Wedges Milk Chocolate	4 pieces	120	8	5	5	1	15	0	tr	60	0	—	—	0
Wedges Bittersweet	4 pieces	130	10	5	0	3	10	7	4	20	20	—	—	1
Wedges Dark Chocolate Coffee	4 pieces	130	8	5	0	1	15	12	2	0	0	—	—	0
Wedges Dark Chocolate Mint	4 pieces	130	8	5	0	1	15	12	2	0	0	—	—	0
Wedges Milk Chocolate	4 pieces	130	8	5	5	1	15	14	0	20	10	—	—	0
TOBLER														
Orange Dark Chocolate	5 pieces (1.5 oz)	240	13	8	<5	2	28	25	3	0	10	—	—	0
TOBLERONE														
Bittersweet Chocolate w/ Honey & Almond Nougat	⅓ bar (1.2 oz)	170	9	5	<5	1	20	16	2	0	5	—	—	0
Milk Chocolate w/ Honey & Almond Nougat	⅓ bar (1.76 oz)	170	9	5	10	2	21	18	tr	40	15	—	—	0
TOM'S														
Cherry Sours	1 pkg (2.25 oz)	210	0	0	0	0	53	38	0	0	30	—	—	0
Jelly Beans	1 pkg (2.25 oz)	230	0	0	0	0	58	44	0	0	30	—	—	0
TOOTSIE														
Pop	1	60	0	0	0	0	12	11	—	—	10	—	—	—
TORRAS														
Sugar Free Dark Chocolate	1 oz	136	10	6	2	2	15	0	0	—	0	—	—	—
Sugar Free Milk Chocolate	1 oz	140	10	6	8	2	17	0	0	—	0	—	—	—
Sugar Free Milk Chocolate w/ Almonds	1 oz	146	10	5	6	2	15	0	0	—	0	—	—	—
Sugar Free Milk Chocolate w/ Hazelnuts	1 oz	148	11	6	6	2	15	0	0	—	0	—	—	—
Sugar Free White Chocolate	1 oz	138	10	6	6	2	17	0	0	—	0	—	—	—
TROPICAL SOURCE														
Butterscotch Dream	4 pieces (0.5 oz)	60	0	0	0	0	14	11	0	—	30	—	—	—

FOOD	PORTION	CALS	FAT	SAT FAT	CHOL	PROT	CARB	SUGAR	FIBER	CALCI	SOD	POTAS	FOLIC	VIT C
TROPICAL SOURCE (CONT.)														
Chocolate Dairy Free California Raisin & Currant	½ bar (1.5 oz)	230	13	8	0	3	25	25	1	0	15	—	—	0
Chocolate Dairy Free Hazelnut Espresso Crunch	½ bar (1.5 oz)	250	17	8	0	3	21	19	1	0	15	—	—	0
Chocolate Dairy Free Maple Almond Granola	½ bar (1.5 oz)	230	15	9	0	3	24	23	1	0	15	—	—	0
Chocolate Dairy Free Mint Candy Crunch	½ bar (1.5 oz)	220	13	8	0	2	24	24	1	0	15	—	—	0
Chocolate Dairy Free Red Raspberry Crush	½ bar (1.5 oz)	230	15	9	0	2	22	22	1	0	15	—	—	0
Chocolate Dairy Free Sundried Jungle Banana	½ bar (1.5 oz)	230	13	8	0	2	26	22	2	0	15	—	—	0
Chocolate Dairy Free Toasted Almond	½ bar (1.5 oz)	250	17	8	0	3	21	19	1	0	15	—	—	0
Chocolate Dairy Free Wild Rice Crisp	½ bar (1.5 oz)	230	14	8	0	3	26	23	1	0	15	—	—	0
Cool Peppermint	4 pieces (0.5 oz)	60	0	0	0	0	14	11	0	—	0	—	—	—
Lollipops All Flavors	1	24	0	0	0	0	6	4	0	—	0	—	—	—
Mango Papaya	4 pieces (0.5 oz)	60	0	0	0	0	14	11	0	—	1	—	—	—
TWIX														
Caramel	1 fun size (0.5 oz)	80	4	2	0	1	10	8	0	—	30	—	—	—
TWIZZLERS														
Cherry	1 piece	30	0	0	0	0	8	—	—	—	25	—	—	—
Chocolate	1 piece	25	0	0	0	0	6	—	—	—	20	—	—	—
Licorice	1 piece	30	0	0	0	0	7	—	—	—	45	—	—	—
Pull'N'Peel Cherry	1 piece	100	0	0	0	1	25	—	—	—	85	—	—	—
Strawberry Snack Size	3 pkgs	130	1	—	0	1	30	19	—	—	100	—	—	—
UNIQUE ORIGIN														
Guaranda Dark Chocolate	1 piece (0.3 oz)	54	4	3	0	1	4	3	1	9	2	—	—	0
WERTHER'S														
Original	3 pieces (0.5 oz)	60	1	1	<5	0	13	11	0	0	60	—	—	0

FOOD	PORTION	CALS	FAT	SAT FAT	CHOL	PROT	CARB	SUGAR	FIBER	CALCI	SOD	POTAS	FOLIC	VIT C
WHATCHAMACALLIT														
Bar	1 (0.57 oz)	80	4	3	0	1	10	—	—	—	50	—	—	—
WHITMAN'S														
Sampler	3 pieces (1.4 oz)	190	10	5	5	2	24	19	tr	40	55	—	—	0
Snoopy Treats Caramel Peanuts Milk Chocolate	1 snack size (1.4 oz)	80	5	3	5	2	24	18	tr	40	90	—	—	1
WHOPPERS														
Malted Milk Balls	9 pieces	90	4	3	0	tr	15	13	tr	40	65	—	—	0
YAMATE CHOCOLATIER														
No Sugar Almonds & Caramel	1 piece (0.6 oz)	70	6	3	0	1	9	1	1	0	0	—	—	0
YORK														
Peppermint Patty	1 (0.49 oz)	50	1	1	0	0	11	8	—	—	0	—	—	—
ZAGNUT														
Snack Size	1 piece	70	3	2	0	tr	9	—	—	—	25	—	—	—
ZERO														
Bar	1	70	3	2	0	tr	12	—	—	—	35	—	—	—
CANTALOUPE														
dried	3.5 pieces (1.4 oz)	140	0	0	0	0	34	32	1	40	110	—	—	0
fresh cubed	1 cup	57	tr	—	0	1	13	—	1	17	14	494	27	68
fresh half	½	94	1	—	0	2	22	—	2	28	23	825	46	113
CHIQUITA														
Wedge	¼ med (4.7 oz)	50	0	0	0	0	12	11	1	20	25	—	—	48
CARAWAY														
seed	1 tsp	7	tr	tr	0	tr	1	—	—	14	tr	28	—	—
CARDAMOM														
ground	1 tsp	6	tr	tr	0	tr	1	—	—	8	tr	22	—	—
CARDOON														
fresh cooked	3½ oz	22	tr	tr	0	1	5	—	—	72	176	392	—	2
fresh shredded	½ cup	36	tr	tr	0	1	4	—	—	62	151	356	—	2
CARIBOU														
roasted	3 oz	142	4	1	93	25	0	—	—	19	51	264	4	3
CARISSA														
fresh	1	12	tr	—	0	tr	3	—	—	2	1	52	—	8
CAROB														
carob mix	3 tsp	45	0	0	0	tr	11	—	—	—	12	—	—	0
carob mix as prep w/ whole milk	9 oz	195	8	5	33	8	23	—	—	291	132	370	12	2
flour	1 tbsp	14	tr	tr	0	tr	7	—	—	28	3	66	2	0
flour	1 cup	185	1	tr	0	5	92	—	—	359	36	852	30	tr

FOOD	PORTION	CALS	FAT	SAT FAT	CHOL	PROT	CARB	SUGAR	FIBER	CALCI	SOD	POTAS	FOLIC	VIT C
SUNSPIRE														
Carob Chips Unsweetened	13 pieces (0.5 oz)	70	3	3	0	2	8	5	0	100	65	—	—	1
Carob Chips Vegan	13 pieces (0.5 oz)	70	3	3	0	0	11	5	0	0	5	—	—	0
CARP														
fresh	3 oz	108	5	1	56	15	0	—	—	15	42	283	—	1
fresh cooked	3 oz	138	6	1	72	19	0	—	—	44	54	363	—	1
fresh cooked	1 fillet (6 oz)	276	12	2	143	39	0	—	—	89	107	726	—	3
roe raw	1 oz	37	tr	—	103	7	tr	—	—	—	—	—	—	4
roe salted in olive oil	2 tbsp (1 oz)	40	—	—	100	—	6	—	0	0	1400	—	—	—
CARROT JUICE														
canned	6 oz	73	tr	tr	0	2	17	—		44	54	538	7	16
NAKED JUICE														
Just Carrot	8 oz	80	0	0	0	2	13	13	0	20	90	—	—	5
CARROTS														
CANNED														
slices	½ cup	17	tr	tr	0	tr	4	—	1	19	176	131	7	2
slices low sodium	½ cup	17	tr	tr	0	tr	4	—	1	19	31	131	7	2
DEL MONTE														
Sliced	½ cup (4.3 oz)	35	0	0	0	0	8	5	3	20	300	—	—	4
GREEN GIANT														
Sliced	½ cup (4.2 oz)	25	0	0	0	tr	6	3	2	40	380	—	—	12
LESUEUR														
Baby Whole	½ cup (4.2 oz)	35	0	0	0	tr	8	5	3	40	410	—	—	0
S&W														
Julienne	½ cup (4.3 oz)	30	0	0	0	1	5	4	2	0	390	—	—	0
Sliced	½ cup (4.3 oz)	30	0	0	0	1	5	4	2	0	390	—	—	0
Whole Small	½ cup (4.3 oz)	30	0	0	0	1	5	4	2	0	390	—	—	0
FRESH														
baby raw	1 (½ oz)	6	tr	tr	0	tr	1	—	—	3	5	42	5	1
raw	1 (2.5 oz)	31	tr	tr	0	1	7	—	2	19	25	233	10	7
raw shredded	½ cup	24	tr	tr	0	1	6	—	2	15	19	178	8	5
slices cooked	½ cup	35	tr	tr	0	1	8	—	—	24	52	177	11	2
BOLTHOUSE FARMS														
Baby	1 pkg (2.25 oz)	25	0	0	0	1	7	4	2	20	33	230	—	5
DOLE														
Shredded	1 cup (3 oz)	40	0	0	0	1	9	5	2	20	45	—	—	6
EARTHBOUND FARMS														
Organic Mini Peeled	½ cup	30	0	0	0	1	7	4	3	20	30	—	—	6
FROZEN														
slices cooked	½ cup	26	tr	tr	0	1	6	—	—	21	43	115	8	2

FOOD	PORTION	CALS	FAT	SAT FAT	CHOL	PROT	CARB	SUGAR	FIBER	CALCI	SOD	POTAS	FOLIC	VIT C
BIRDS EYE														
Baby Whole	½ cup	40	0	0	0	—	—	—	2	20	45	—	—	5
Sliced	½ cup	35	0	0	0	—	—	—	3	20	45	—	—	4
FRESH LIKE														
Carrots Slice	3.5 oz	42	tr	—	—	1	10	—	—	33	42	194	—	5
GREEN GIANT														
Harvest Fresh Baby	⅔ cup (3 oz)	20	0	0	0	0	5	3	2	20	70	—	—	0
Select Baby Cut	¾ cup (2.8 oz)	30	0	0	0	tr	7	3	3	20	40	—	—	0
CASABA														
cubed	1 cup	45	tr	—	0	2	11	—	—	9	20	357	—	27
fresh	⅒	43	tr	—	0	1	10	—	—	8	20	344	—	26
CASHEWS														
cashew butter w/o salt	1 tbsp	94	8	2	0	3	4	—	—	7	2	87	11	0
dry roasted salted	1 oz	163	13	3	0	4	9	—	—	13	213	160	20	0
dry roasted w/ salt	18 nuts (1 oz)	160	13	3	0	4	9	—	1	13	180	160	16	—
oil roasted	1 oz	163	14	3	0	5	8	—	—	12	5	151	19	0
oil roasted salted	1 oz	163	14	3	0	5	8	—	—	12	209	151	19	0
BOWLBY'S														
Bits Cashew	½ cup	200	19	3	0	4	5	1	1	0	95	—	—	0
FRITO LAY														
Salted	1 oz	180	15	3	0	5	7	2	1	—	190	—	—	—
LANCE														
Cashews	1 pkg (1⅛ oz)	200	16	3	0	6	8	3	3	0	90	200	—	0
MARANATHA														
Cashew Butter	2 tbsp	190	15	3	0	5	11	2	2	20	5	—	—	0
Tamari Cashews	¼ cup	160	13	3	0	5	9	2	1	0	142	—	—	0
SWEET DELIGHTS														
Cashew Roasters	⅓ pkg (1 oz)	170	14	—	0	4	10	1	2	—	220	300	—	—
CASSAVA														
fresh	3½ oz	120	tr	tr	0	3	27	—	—	91	8	764	—	48
CATFISH														
channel breaded & fried	3 oz	194	11	3	69	15	7	—	—	37	238	289	—	0
channel raw	3 oz	99	4	1	49	15	0	—	—	34	54	296	—	—
CAULIFLOWER														
FRESH														
cooked	½ cup (2.2 oz)	14	tr	tr	0	1	3	—	1	10	9	88	27	28
flowerets cooked	3 (2 oz)	12	tr	tr	0	1	2	—	1	9	8	76	24	24
flowerets raw	3 (2 oz)	14	tr	tr	0	1	3	—	1	12	17	170	32	26
green cooked	1½ cups (3.2 oz)	29	tr	tr	0	3	6	—	3	29	21	250	40	0

FOOD	PORTION	CALS	FAT	SAT FAT	CHOL	PROT	CARB	SUGAR	FIBER	CALCI	SOD	POTAS	FOLIC	VIT C
green raw	1 head (18 oz)	158	2	tr	0	15	31	—	16	169	118	1533	291	450
green raw	1 cup (2.2 oz)	20	tr	tr	0	2	4	—	2	21	15	192	36	22
green raw floweret	1 (0.9 oz)	8	tr	tr	0	1	2	—	1	8	6	75	14	22
raw	½ cup (1.8 oz)	13	tr	tr	0	1	3	—	1	11	15	151	28	23
FROZEN														
cooked	½ cup	17	tr	tr	0	1	3	—	—	15	16	125	37	28
BIRDS EYE														
Cauliflower	½ cup	20	0	0	0	—	—	—	2	20	15	—	—	42
FRESH LIKE														
Florets	3.5 oz	26	tr	—	—	2	5	—	1	21	48	195	—	52
GREEN GIANT														
Cheese Sauce	½ cup (3.5 oz)	60	3	1	<5	2	8	4	2	60	510	—	—	18
Florets	1 cup (2.8 oz)	25	0	0	0	2	4	1	2	0	25	—	—	24
CAVIAR														
black	1 tbsp	40	3	—	94	4	1	—	—	—	240	—	—	—
red	1 tbsp	40	3	—	94	4	1	—	—	—	240	—	—	—
CELERIAC														
fresh cooked	3½ oz	25	tr	—	0	1	6	—	—	26	61	173	—	4
raw	½ cup	31	tr	—	0	1	7	—	—	34	78	234	—	6
CELERY														
diced cooked	½ cup	13	tr	tr	0	1	3	—	—	32	68	213	16	5
fresh	1 stalk (1.3 oz)	6	tr	tr	0	tr	1	—	1	16	35	115	11	3
raw diced	½ cup	10	tr	tr	0	tr	2	—	1	24	52	172	17	4
seed	1 tsp	8	tr	tr	0	tr	1	—	—	35	3	28	—	—
DOLE														
Stalks	2 med (3 oz)	15	0	0	0	1	3	0	2	20	100	—	—	6
CELTUCE														
raw	3½ oz	22	tr	—	0	1	4	—	—	39	11	330	—	20
CEREAL														
bran flakes	¾ cup (1 oz)	90	1	tr	0	4	22	—	—	14	264	180	—	0
corn flakes	1¼ cup (1 oz)	110	tr	tr	0	2	24	—	—	1	351	26	—	15
corn flakes low sodium	1 cup (0.9 oz)	100	tr	tr	0	2	22	—	tr	11	3	18	2	0
corn grits white regular & quick as prep w/ water & salt	¾ cup (6.4 oz)	109	tr	tr	0	3	24	—	tr	0	406	40	56	0
corn grits white regular or quick as prep	¾ cup (6.4 oz)	109	tr	tr	0	3	24	—	tr	0	0	40	56	0
corn grits yellow regular & quick as prep w/ water & salt	¾ cup (6.4 oz)	109	tr	tr	0	3	24	—	tr	0	406	40	56	0

FOOD	PORTION	CALS	FAT	SAT FAT	CHOL	PROT	CARB	SUGAR	FIBER	CALCI	SOD	POTAS	FOLIC	VIT C
corn grits yellow regular & quick not prep	1 cup (5.5 oz)	579	2	tr	0	14	124	—	3	3	2	214	292	0
crispy rice	1 cup (1 oz)	111	tr	tr	0	2	25	—	tr	5	206	27	138	15
crispy rice low sodium	1 cup (0.9 oz)	105	tr	tr	0	1	23	—	tr	17	3	20	3	0
farina as prep w/ water	¾ cup (6.1 oz)	88	tr	tr	0	2	19	—	2	4	0	23	40	0
farina not prep	1 tbsp (0.4 oz)	40	tr	0	0	1	9	—	tr	2	0	10	19	0
granola	½ cup (2.1 oz)	285	15	3	0	9	32	—	6	45	15	328	53	1
oatmeal instant as prep w/ water	1 cup (8.2 oz)	138	2	tr	0	6	24	—	4	215	377	131	199	0
oatmeal instant w/ cinnamon & spice as prep w/ water	1 pkg (5.6 oz)	177	2	tr	0	5	35	—	3	172	280	105	153	0
oatmeal instant w/ raisins & spice as prep w/ water	1 cup (5.5 oz)	161	2	tr	0	4	32	—	2	166	226	150	150	0
oatmeal regular & quick as prep w/ water	¾ cup (6.1 oz)	149	2	tr	0	5	19	—	3	14	2	98	7	0
oatmeal regular & quick not prep	⅓ cup (0.9 oz)	104	2	tr	0	4	18	—	3	14	1	95	9	0
oatmeal instant cooked w/o salt	1 cup	145	2	tr	0	6	25	—	—	19	2	131	—	0
oatmeal quick cooked w/o salt	1 cup	145	2	tr	0	6	25	—	—	19	2	131	—	0
oatmeal regular cooked w/o salt	1 cup	145	2	tr	0	6	25	—	—	19	2	131	—	0
puffed rice	1 cup (0.5 oz)	56	tr	tr	0	1	13	—	tr	1	0	16	3	0
puffed wheat	1 cup (0.4 oz)	44	tr	tr	0	2	10	—	1	3	0	42	4	0
shredded mini wheats	1 cup (1.1 oz)	107	1	tr	0	3	24	—	3	11	3	108	14	0
shredded wheat rectangular	1 biscuit (0.8 oz)	85	tr	tr	0	3	19	—	2	10	0	77	12	0
shredded wheat round	2 biscuits (1.3 oz)	136	1	tr	0	4	31	—	4	15	1	124	19	0
sugar-coated corn flakes	¾ cup (1 oz)	110	1	tr	0	1	26	—	—	1	230	18	—	15
whole wheat hot natural as prep w/ water	¾ cup (6.4 oz)	113	1	tr	0	4	25	—	3	13	0	129	20	0
ALBERS														
Hominy Quick Grits uncooked	¼ cup	140	1	0	0	3	31	0	1	0	0	—	—	0

FOOD	PORTION	CALS	FAT	SAT FAT	CHOL	PROT	CARB	SUGAR	FIBER	CALCI	SOD	POTAS	FOLIC	VIT C
ALPEN														
Corn Flakes	1 serv (1 oz)	110	tr	—	—	2	25	0	tr	13	2	22	—	0
No Salt No Sugar	1 serv (2 oz)	200	3	—	—	7	34	10	6	130	35	300	—	3
Regular	1 serv (2 oz)	200	3	—	—	7	37	17	4	122	100	270	—	3
ATKINS														
Banana Nut Harvest	⅔ cup	100	3	0	0	12	11	1	6	—	100	—	—	—
Blueberry Bounty w/ Almonds	⅔ cup	100	2	0	0	13	10	1	6	—	105	—	—	—
Crunchy Almond Crisp	⅔ cup	100	2	0	0	15	8	1	5	—	100	—	—	—
AUNT PAULA'S														
Hot Flax Cereal	1 serv (1½ oz)	100	5	5	0	10	8	0	5	—	140	—	—	—
BACK TO NATURE														
Hi-Protein	⅔ cup	140	1	0	0	12	25	10	3	0	130	—	—	0
Muesli	½ cup	160	3	1	0	3	32	11	4	0	70	—	—	0
Puff Wheat	½ cup	160	3	1	0	3	32	11	4	0	70	—	—	0
Ultra Flax	¾ cup	150	2	1	0	7	28	11	3	0	0	—	—	0
BARBARA'S BAKERY														
Apple Cinnamon O's	¾ cup	110	1	0	0	3	24	11	2	—	90	—	—	—
Bite Size Shredded Oats	1¼ cups (2 oz)	220	3	1	0	6	46	12	6	—	260	—	—	—
Cinnamon Puffins	1¼ cups (2 oz)	100	1	0	0	2	26	6	6	—	150	—	—	—
Cocoa Crunch Stars	1 cup (1 oz)	110	1	0	0	2	26	8	1	—	140	—	—	—
Frosted Corn Flakes	1 cup (1 oz)	110	1	0	0	2	27	8	4	—	100	—	—	—
Fruit Juice Sweetened Breakfast O's	1 cup (1 oz)	120	2	0	0	5	22	2	3	—	115	—	—	—
Fruit Juice Sweetened Brown Rice Crisps	1 cup (1 oz)	120	1	0	0	2	25	2	1	—	125	—	—	—
Fruit Juice Sweetened Corn Flakes	1 cup (1 oz)	110	0	0	0	2	26	3	2	—	130	—	—	—
GrainShop	⅔ cup (1 oz)	90	1	0	0	3	24	5	8	—	110	—	—	—
Honey Crunch Stars	1 cup (1 oz)	110	0	0	0	2	26	8	2	—	50	—	—	—
Honey Nut Toasted O's	¾ cup	120	2	1	0	3	23	11	2	—	90	—	—	—
Organic Fruity Punch	1 cup (1 oz)	110	1	0	0	2	26	8	0	—	120	—	—	—
Organic Soy Essence	¾ cup (1 oz)	100	1	0	0	3	25	5	5	—	110	—	—	—

FOOD	PORTION	CALS	FAT	SAT FAT	CHOL	PROT	CARB	SUGAR	FIBER	CALCI	SOD	POTAS	FOLIC	VIT C
BARBARA'S BAKERY (CONT.)														
Puffins	¾ cup (0.9 oz)	90	1	0	0	2	23	5	5	—	190	—	—	—
Shredded Spoonfuls	¾ cup	120	2	0	0	4	24	5	4	20	200	125	—	5
Shredded Wheat	2 biscuits (1.4 oz)	140	1	0	0	4	31	0	5	—	0	—	—	—
CARBSENSE														
Hot Cereal Country Spice not prep	½ cup	130	6	1	0	14	15	0	12	—	130	—	—	—
Hot Cereal Roasted Hazelnut not prep	½ cup	140	9	1	0	25	15	0	12	—	140	—	—	—
COUNTRY CHOICE														
Instant Oatmeal Apples 'N' Cinnamon	1 pkg	140	2	0	0	4	27	11	3	20	85	—	—	0
Instant Oatmeal Maple Syrup	1 pkg	170	2	0	0	6	32	9	4	20	80	—	—	0
Instant Oatmeal Organic Plus French Vanilla	1 pkg	180	3	0	0	7	32	12	3	350	140	—	—	0
Instant Oatmeal Organic Plus Golden Brown Sugar	1 pkg	180	3	0	0	7	32	12	3	350	140	—	—	0
Instant Oatmeal Regular	1 pkg	110	1	0	0	4	19	tr	3	20	0	—	—	0
Oatmeal Steel Cut not prep	½ cup	150	3	0	0	5	27	0	4	20	0	—	—	0
Oats Old Fashioned not prep	½ cup	150	3	1	0	5	27	1	4	20	0	—	—	0
Oats Quick not prep	½ cup	150	3	1	0	5	27	1	4	20	0	—	—	0
Organic Multi Grain Hot Cereal not prep	½ cup	130	2	0	0	6	29	2	5	0	0	—	—	0
DELICIOUSLY SLIM														
Granola Cranberry Cashew	¾ cup	230	13	1	0	9	29	2	12	20	100	—	—	0
Granola Strawberry Almond	¾ cup	230	13	1	0	9	29	2	12	20	100	—	—	4
EREWHON														
Apple Stroodles	¾ cup	110	1	0	0	3	25	4	1	20	15	—	—	0
Aztec	1 cup	110	0	0	0	2	26	1	1	0	70	—	—	0
Banana O's	¾ cup	110	0	0	0	2	26	7	2	0	15	—	—	0

FOOD	PORTION	CALS	FAT	SAT FAT	CHOL	PROT	CARB	SUGAR	FIBER	CALCI	SOD	POTAS	FOLIC	VIT C
EREWHON (CONT.)														
Brown Rice Cream	¼ cup	170	1	0	0	5	36	0	1	20	30	—	—	0
Corn Flakes	1¼ cups	210	3	0	0	5	45	tr	3	0	100	—	—	1
Crispy Brown Rice	1 cup	110	0	0	0	2	25	1	1	20	180	—	—	1
Crispy Brown Rice No Salt Added	1 cup	110	0	0	0	2	25	1	1	20	10	—	—	1
Fruit'n Wheat	¾ cup	170	2	0	0	51	39	12	5	20	105	—	—	0
Kamut Flakes	⅔ cup	110	0	0	0	5	25	1	4	60	75	—	—	0
Raisin Bran	1 cup	170	1	0	0	5	40	10	6	40	100	—	—	1
Rice Twice	¾ cup	120	0	0	0	2	28	8	0	0	80	—	—	0
Whole Wheat Flakes	1 cup	180	1	0	0	6	42	tr	6	40	135	—	—	1
EXPERT FOODS														
Low Carb Hot Cereal Sub	½ cup	24	0	0	0	4	2	—	—	—	65	—	—	—
GENERAL MILLS														
Basic 4	1 cup (1.9 oz)	200	2	0	0	4	42	14	3	250	320	150	100	0
Boo Berry	1 cup (1 oz)	120	1	0	0	1	27	14	—	20	210	15	100	6
Cheerios	1 cup (1 oz)	110	2	0	0	3	22	1	3	100	280	95	200	6
Cheerios Apple Cinnamon	¾ cup	120	2	0	0	2	25	13	1	100	115	55	200	6
Cheerios Frosted	1 cup (1 oz)	120	1	0	0	2	25	13	1	100	210	55	200	6
Cheerios Honey Nut	1 cup (1 oz)	120	2	0	0	3	24	11	2	100	270	90	200	6
Cheerios Multi Grain	1 cup (1 oz)	110	1	0	0	3	24	8	3	100	200	85	400	15
Cheerios Team	1 cup (1 oz)	120	1	0	0	2	25	11	1	100	210	70	200	6
Chex Corn	1 cup (1 oz)	110	0	0	0	2	26	3	0	100	280	25	200	6
Chex Honey Nut	¾ cup	120	1	0	0	1	26	9	—	100	220	30	100	6
Chex Morning Mix Cinnamon	1 pkg (1.1 oz)	130	4	1	0	2	24	8	1	100	180	75	180	0
Chex Morning Mix Fruit & Nut	1 pkg (1.1 oz)	180	4	1	0	2	24	8	1	100	190	75	180	0
Chex Morning Mix Honey Nut	1 pkg (1.1 oz)	130	4	1	0	2	24	8	1	100	190	80	180	0
Chex Multi-Bran	1 cup (2 oz)	200	2	0	0	4	49	12	8	100	380	220	400	6
Chex Rice	1¼ cups (1.1 oz)	120	0	0	0	2	27	2	0	100	290	35	200	6
Cinnamon Grahams	¾ cup (1 oz)	120	1	0	0	1	26	11	1	100	240	—	100	6
Cinnamon Toast Crunch	¾ cup (1 oz)	130	4	1	1	1	24	10	1	100	210	45	100	6
Cocoa Puffs	1 cup (1 oz)	120	1	0	0	1	26	14	—	100	170	50	100	6
Cookie Crisp	1 cup (1 oz)	120	1	0	0	1	26	13	0	100	180	25	100	6
Count Chocula	1 cup (1 oz)	120	1	0	0	1	26	14	0	20	180	—	100	6
Country Corn Flakes	1 cup (1 oz)	120	0	0	0	2	26	2	—	250	270	30	200	6

GENERAL MILLS (CONT.)

FOOD	PORTION	CALS	FAT	SAT FAT	CHOL	PROT	CARB	SUGAR	FIBER	CALCI	SOD	POTAS	FOLIC	VIT C
Fiber One	½ cup (1 oz)	60	1	0	0	2	24	0	14	100	130	210	100	6
Franken Berry	1 cup (1 oz)	120	1	0	0	1	27	14	—	20	210	15	100	6
French Toast Crunch	¾ cup (1 oz)	120	1	0	0	1	26	12	0	60	180	—	100	6
Gold Medal Raisin Bran	1⅓ cups (1.9 oz)	170	2	0	0	5	41	12	6	700	330	330	400	0
Golden Grahams	¾ cup (1 oz)	120	1	0	0	1	25	10	1	350	270	50	100	6
Harmony	1¼ cups (1.9 oz)	200	4	0	0	5	44	13	2	600	350	90	400	30
Honey Nut Clusters	1 cup (1.9 oz)	210	3	0	0	4	46	17	3	20	270	135	100	6
Kaboom	1¼ cups (1 oz)	120	1	0	0	2	24	8	1	100	290	65	200	6
Kix	1⅓ cups (1 oz)	120	1	0	0	2	26	3	1	150	270	35	200	6
Kix Berry Berry	¾ cup (1 oz)	120	2	0	0	1	26	9	0	40	180	25	100	6
Lucky Charms	1 cup (1 oz)	120	1	0	0	2	25	13	1	100	210	60	200	6
Nature Valley Low Fat Fruit Granola	⅔ cup (1.9 oz)	210	3	0	0	4	44	19	3	20	210	150	—	0
Newquick	¾ cup (1 oz)	120	2	0	0	1	25	12	—	100	190	65	100	6
Oatmeal Crisp Almond	1 cup (1.9 oz)	220	5	1	0	5	42	16	4	20	240	180	100	6
Oatmeal Crisp Apple Cinnamon	1 cup (1.9 oz)	210	2	0	0	5	45	19	4	20	250	170	100	6
Oatmeal Crisp Raisin	1 cup (1.9 oz)	210	2	0	0	5	44	18	4	20	220	200	100	0
Para Su Familia Cinnamon Stars	1 cup (1 oz)	120	1	0	0	1	28	6	—	100	240	25	200	6
Para Su Familia Fruitis	1 cup (1 oz)	120	1	0	0	1	25	6	—	100	210	20	200	6
Para Su Familia Raisin Bran	1¼ cups (2 oz)	170	2	0	0	5	41	12	6	700	320	330	400	0
Raisin Nut Bran	¾ cup (1.9 oz)	200	4	1	0	4	41	18	4	20	250	230	100	0
Reese's Puffs	¾ cup	130	3	1	0	2	23	13	0	100	170	45	100	6
Snack'N Dash Cinnamon Toast Crunch	1 pkg (1.2 oz)	140	4	1	0	2	27	12	1	100	230	—	100	6
Snack'N Dash Honey Nut Cheerios	1 pkg (1 oz)	110	1	0	0	3	23	10	2	80	250	—	180	4
Snack'N Dash Lucky Charms	1 pkg (1 oz)	110	1	0	0	2	24	12	1	80	100	—	180	4
Sunrise Organic	¾ cup (1 oz)	110	1	0	0	1	26	10	1	0	190	50	100	6
Total Brown Sugar & Oat	¾ cup (1 oz)	110	1	0	0	2	23	9	1	1000	200	80	400	60
Total Protein	¾ cup	120	4	0	0	13	11	2	3	100	270	75	400	60
Total Raisin Bran	1 cup	170	1	0	0	4	41	20	5	1000	240	350	400	0

FOOD	PORTION	CALS	FAT	SAT FAT	CHOL	PROT	CARB	SUGAR	FIBER	CALCI	SOD	POTAS	FOLIC	VIT C
GENERAL MILLS (CONT.)														
Total Whole Grain	¾ cup (1 oz)	110	1	0	0	2	23	5	3	1000	190	90	400	60
Trix	1 cup (1 oz)	120	1	0	0	1	27	13	1	100	190	15	100	6
Wheat Hearts	¼ cup (1.3 oz)	130	1	0	0	5	26	1	2	0	0	130	—	0
Wheaties	1 cup (1 oz)	110	1	0	0	3	24	4	3	20	220	105	200	6
Wheaties Energy Crunch	1 cup (1.9 oz)	210	3	0	0	6	42	13	4	350	310	140	400	12
Wheaties Frosted	¾ cup (1 oz)	110	1	0	0	1	27	12	—	100	200	35	400	6
Wheaties Raisin Bran	1 cup (1.9 oz)	180	1	0	0	4	45	18	5	20	250	230	200	0
GRAINFIELD'S														
Brown Rice	1 serv (1 oz)	110	1	—	—	3	24	1	tr	14	4	81	—	0
Crisp Rice	1 serv (1 oz)	112	tr	—	—	3	25	0	tr	6	3	31	—	0
Raisin Bran	1 serv (1 oz)	90	2	—	—	2	20	tr	2	16	4	130	—	3
Wheat Flakes	1 serv (1 oz)	100	1	—	—	3	20	tr	2	28	2	99	—	1
GRAM'S GOURMET														
Cream Of Flax not prep	½ cup	142	5	1	0	18	11	1	8	—	305	—	—	—
Crunch Granolas All Flavors	½ cup	349	30	6	2	10	10	1	6	—	40	—	—	—
HANSEN'S														
Orange & Chocolate	½ cup	230	14	4	0	11	35	6	4	700	200	60	340	36
Strawberry & Yogurt	½ cup	230	9	4	0	6	30	11	6	700	220	80	340	36
Toasted Nut Crunch	½ cup	230	6	1	0	6	39	6	7	700	75	80	340	60
Tropical Cluster	½ cup	210	5	3	0	5	36	15	6	700	140	60	340	36
HEALTH VALLEY														
10 Bran O's Apple Cinnamon	¾ cup	100	0	0	0	3	23	4	3	0	90	—	—	0
Bran w/ Apples & Cinnamon	¾ cup	160	0	0	0	5	41	10	7	0	10	—	—	0
Golden Flax	½ cup	190	3	—	0	6	38	8	6	60	30	—	—	0
Granola 98% Fat Free Date Almond	⅔ cup	180	1	—	0	5	43	10	6	20	90	—	—	2
Healthy Crunches & Flakes Almond	¾ cup	130	0	0	0	3	31	4	4	0	35	—	—	0
Healthy Crunches & Flakes Apple Cinnamon	¾ cup	130	0	0	0	3	31	4	4	0	35	—	—	0
Healthy Crunches & Flakes Honey Crunch	¾ cup	130	0	0	0	3	31	4	4	0	35	—	—	0
Hot Cereal Cups Amazing Apple!	1 pkg	220	2	—	0	9	43	9	4	20	230	—	—	0

FOOD	PORTION	CALS	FAT	SAT FAT	CHOL	PROT	CARB	SUGAR	FIBER	CALCI	SOD	POTAS	FOLIC	VIT C
HEALTH VALLEY (CONT.)														
Hot Cereal Cups Banana Gone Nuts	1 pkg	240	3	—	0	10	45	9	4	20	240	—	—	0
Hot Cereal Cups Maple Madness!	1 pkg	240	2	—	0	9	47	19	4	20	290	—	—	0
Hot Cereal Cups Terrific 10 Grain!	1 pkg	220	3	—	0	12	41	8	5	20	210	—	—	0
98% Fat Free Raisin Cinnamon	⅔ cup	180	1	—	0	5	43	10	6	20	90	—	—	2
98% Fat Free Tropical	⅔ cup	180	1	—	0	5	43	10	6	20	90	—	—	2
Oat Bran O'S	¾ cup	100	0	0	0	3	23	5	3	0	90	—	—	0
Organic Amaranth Flakes	¾ cup	100	0	0	0	3	24	4	4	0	35	—	—	0
Organic Blue Corn Bran Flakes	¾ cup	100	0	0	0	3	24	4	4	0	10	—	—	0
Organic Bran w/ Raisin	¾ cup	160	0	0	0	5	40	10	6	0	10	—	—	0
Organic Fiber 7 Flakes	¾ cup	100	0	0	0	3	24	4	4	0	15	—	—	0
Organic Healthy Fiber Flakes	¾ cup	100	0	0	0	3	23	3	4	0	10	—	—	0
Organic Oat Bran Flakes	¾ cup	100	0	0	0	3	24	4	4	0	15	—	—	0
Organic Oat Bran Flakes w/ Raisins	¾ cup	110	0	0	0	3	26	6	4	0	15	—	—	0
Puffed Honey Sweetened Corn	1 cup	110	0	0	0	2	28	7	2	0	0	—	—	0
Puffed Honey Sweetened Crisp Brown Rice	1 cup	110	0	0	0	1	28	5	2	0	0	—	—	0
Raisin Bran Flakes	1¼ cups	190	0	0	0	5	47	13	5	0	90	—	—	0
Real Oat Bran	½ cup	200	3	—	0	6	34	9	5	0	90	—	—	0
HEALTHY CHOICE														
Almond Crunch With Raisins	1 cup (2 oz)	210	3	0	0	5	46	16	5	20	230	200	100	0
Golden Multi-Grain Flakes	¾ cup (1.1 oz)	110	0	0	0	3	26	6	3	0	180	100	100	0
Toasted Brown Sugar Squares	1 cup (2 oz)	190	1	0	0	5	44	9	5	0	5	210	100	0
HI-LO														
Low Carb Cereal	½ cup	90	2	0	0	12	11	1	6	—	150	—	—	—
HODGSON MILL														
Bulgur Wheat w/ Soy Grits	¼ cup	116	1	0	0	10	22	0	3	20	0	80	28	—

FOOD	PORTION	CALS	FAT	SAT FAT	CHOL	PROT	CARB	SUGAR	FIBER	CALCI	SOD	POTAS	FOLIC	VIT C
HODGSON MILL (CONT.)														
Cracked Wheat	¼ cup	110	1	0	0	4	26	0	8	0	3	—	16	0
Multi Grain w/ Flaxseed & Soy	⅓ cup	160	3	1	0	7	25	1	6	20	0	20	28	—
KASHI														
Breakfast Pilaf as prep	½ cup (4.9 oz)	170	3	—	0	6	30	0	6	20	15	—	—	0
Go Apple Spice	½ cup (4.9 oz)	270	3	—	0	7	56	10	6	20	0	—	8	0
Go Banana Almond	½ cup (4.9 oz)	280	4	—	0	7	57	11	6	20	5	—	8	1
Go Blueberry Bliss	½ cup (4.9 oz)	260	3	—	0	7	55	8	6	20	5	—	8	1
Go Cherry Vanilla	½ cup (4.9 oz)	260	3	—	0	7	54	15	6	20	15	—	8	1
Go Just Peachy	½ cup (4.9 oz)	260	3	—	0	7	54	17	6	20	0	—	8	1
GoLean	1 cup	140	1	0	0	13	30	6	10	60	85	480	—	0
Good Friends	1 cup	170	2	0	0	5	43	9	12	0	130	260	—	0
Heart To Heart	¾ cup	110	2	0	0	4	25	5	5	0	90	120	400	30
Honey Puffed	1 cup (1 oz)	120	1	—	0	3	25	7	2	0	6	—	8	0
Medley	½ cup (1 oz)	100	1	—	0	4	20	5	2	0	50	—	8	0
Organic Promise Cranberry Sunshine	1 cup	110	1	0	0	2	26	9	2	0	100	65	—	0
Pillows Apple	¾ cup (1.9 oz)	200	1	—	0	3	45	19	2	20	30	—	—	1
Pillows Chocolate	¾ cup (1.9 oz)	200	1	—	0	3	45	19	2	20	50	—	8	0
Pillows Strawberry Crisp	¾ cup (1.9 oz)	200	1	—	0	3	46	19	2	20	25	—	—	1
Puffed	1 cup (0.9 oz)	70	tr	—	0	3	13	0	2	0	0	—	—	0
KELLOGG'S														
All-Bran	½ cup (1.1 oz)	80	1	0	0	4	24	6	10	150	65	390	100	15
All-Bran Bran Buds	⅓ cup (1 oz)	80	1	0	0	3	24	8	13	0	210	290	100	15
All-Bran Extra Fiber	½ cup (0.9 oz)	50	1	0	0	3	20	0	13	100	120	270	100	15
Apple Jacks	1 cup (1.2 oz)	120	0	0	0	2	30	16	1	0	150	35	100	15
Cocoa Frosted Flakes	¾ cup (1.1 oz)	120	0	0	0	1	28	13	0	0	210	20	100	15
Cocoa Krispies	¾ cup (1.1 oz)	120	1	1	0	1	27	13	0	0	220	65	100	15
Complete Oat Bran Flakes	¾ cup (1 oz)	110	1	0	0	4	23	6	4	0	270	120	100	0
Complete Wheat Bran Flakes	¾ cup (1 oz)	90	1	0	0	3	23	5	5	0	220	170	100	15
Corn Flakes	1 cup (1 oz)	100	0	0	0	2	24	2	1	0	300	25	100	15
Corn Pops K-Sentials	1 oz	100	0	0	0	1	25	13	0	0	110	20	80	12
Cracklin' Oat Bran	¾ cup (1.7 oz)	190	7	2	0	4	35	15	6	20	170	220	100	15
Crispix	1 cup (1 oz)	110	0	0	0	2	25	3	1	0	210	35	100	15
Froot Loops k-Sentials	1 oz	100	1	0	0	2	24	11	0	80	130	30	80	12

FOOD	PORTION	CALS	FAT	SAT FAT	CHOL	PROT	CARB	SUGAR	FIBER	CALCI	SOD	POTAS	FOLIC	VIT C
KELLOGG'S (CONT.)														
Frosted Flakes	¾ cup (1.1 oz)	120	0	0	0	1	28	13	1	0	200	20	100	15
Granola Low Fat	½ cup (1.7 oz)	190	3	1	0	4	39	14	3	20	120	120	100	2
Honey Crunch Corn Flakes	¾ cup (1.1 oz)	120	1	0	0	2	26	10	1	—	210	30	100	15
Just Right Crunchy Nuggets	1 cup (2 oz)	210	2	0	0	4	46	12	3	0	320	120	100	0
Just Right Fruit & Nut	1 cup (2.1 oz)	220	2	0	0	4	49	15	3	0	280	170	100	0
Just Right Low Fat w/ Raisins	⅔ cup (2.1 oz)	220	3	1	0	5	47	16	3	20	150	170	100	4
Mini-Wheats Frosted	1 cup (1.8 oz)	180	1	0	0	5	41	10	5	0	5	170	100	0
Mini-Wheats Strawberry Squares	¾ cup (1.8 oz)	170	1	0	0	4	40	9	5	20	15	170	100	0
Mini-Wheats Apple Cinnamon Squares	¾ cup (1.9 oz)	180	1	0	0	4	44	12	5	20	20	170	100	0
Mini-Wheats Blueberry Squares	¾ cup (1.9 oz)	180	1	0	0	4	43	11	5	0	20	180	100	0
Mini-Wheats Frosted Bite Size	24 pieces (2.1 oz)	200	1	0	0	6	48	12	6	0	5	200	100	0
Mini-Wheats Raisin Squares	¾ cup (1.9 oz)	180	1	0	0	5	42	12	5	0	5	250	100	0
Mueslix Apple & Almond Crunch	¾ cup (1.9 oz)	200	5	1	0	5	39	12	5	40	260	200	100	0
Mueslix Raisin & Almond	⅔ cup (1.9 oz)	200	3	0	0	5	41	17	4	20	160	240	100	0
Nutri-Grain Almond Raisin	1¼ cups (1.7 oz)	180	3	0	0	4	38	7	4	150	170	190	100	0
Nutri-Grain Golden Wheat	¾ cup (1 oz)	100	1	0	0	3	23	0	4	0	210	110	100	0
Product 19	1 cup (1 oz)	100	0	0	0	2	25	4	1	0	210	50	400	60
Raisin Bran	1 cup (2.1 oz)	200	2	0	0	6	47	18	8	40	370	360	100	0
Rice Krispies	1¼ cups (1.2 oz)	120	0	0	0	2	29	3	0	0	350	40	100	15
Rice Krispies Razzle Dazzle	¾ cup (1 oz)	110	0	0	0	1	25	10	0	0	170	25	100	15
Rice Krispies Treats	¾ cup (1 oz)	120	2	0	0	1	26	9	0	0	190	25	100	15
Smacks	¾ cup (1 oz)	100	1	0	0	2	24	15	1	0	50	40	100	15
Smart Start	1 cup	190	1	0	0	3	43	14	3	0	280	90	400	15
Special K	1 cup (1.1 oz)	110	0	0	0	6	21	4	1	0	220	60	140	15

FOOD	PORTION	CALS	FAT	SAT FAT	CHOL	PROT	CARB	SUGAR	FIBER	CALCI	SOD	POTAS	FOLIC	VIT C
KETO														
Cocoa Crisp	½ cup	110	2	0	0	21	4	0	1	—	370	—	—	—
Frosted Flakes All Flavors	¾ cup	110	1	0	0	17	9	tr	2	—	180	—	—	—
Hot Cereal Apple Cinnamon	2 scoops	150	4	1	0	17	12	tr	9	—	210	—	—	—
Hot Cereal Strawberry & Creme	2 scoops	150	4	1	0	17	12	tr	9	—	210	—	—	—
Low Carb Crispy Soy	¾ cup	110	2	—	—	22	2	0	0	—	370	—	—	—
Oatmeal Old Fashioned	2 scoops	150	4	1	0	17	12	tr	9	—	210	—	—	—
LIQUID CEREAL														
Apple & Cinnamon	1 can (11 oz)	160	1	0	5	7	32	21	1	300	170	300	—	18
Chocolate	1 can (11 oz)	170	1	0	5	7	33	21	1	300	125	540	—	18
Fruit	1 can (11 oz)	150	0	0	5	7	31	31	tr	300	135	380	—	18
Peanut Butter	1 can (11 oz)	170	2	0	5	7	32	21	1	300	110	320	—	18
LUNDBERG														
Purely Organic Hot'n Creamy Rice	⅓ cup	190	2	0	0	4	43	0	3	0	0	—	—	0
MCCANN'S														
Irish Oatmeal Instant Apples & Cinnamon	1 pkg (1 oz)	130	2	0	0	3	26	13	2	100	130	—	100	0
Irish Oatmeal Instant Maple & Brown Sugar	1 pkg (1 oz)	160	2	0	0	4	32	14	3	100	220	—	100	0
Irish Oatmeal Instant Regular	1 pkg (1 oz)	100	2	0	0	4	18	1	3	200	80	—	100	0
MINICARB														
Milk Chocolate Hot Cereal not prep	½ cup	140	6	1	10	12	17	2	13	—	170	—	—	—
MORNING TRADITIONS														
Banana Nut Crunch	1 cup (2 oz)	250	6	1	0	5	43	12	4	0	240	170	100	0
Blueberry Morning	1¼ cups (1.9 oz)	220	3	1	0	4	43	13	2	20	250	95	100	0
Cranberry Almond Crunch	1 cup (1.9 oz)	220	3	0	0	4	44	15	3	0	200	100	100	0
Great Grains Crunchy Pecan	⅔ cup (1.9 oz)	220	6	1	0	5	38	9	4	0	190	150	100	0
Great Grains Raisins Dates & Pecans	⅔ cup (1.9 oz)	210	5	1	0	4	39	14	4	0	160	120	120	0

FOOD	PORTION	CALS	FAT	SAT FAT	CHOL	PROT	CARB	SUGAR	FIBER	CALCI	SOD	POTAS	FOLIC	VIT C
MOTHER'S														
Cinnamon Oat Crunch	1 cup	230	3	1	0	6	48	15	5	40	250	320	—	0
Cocoa Bumpers	1 cup	120	1	0	0	2	29	15	1	40	170	260	—	0
Groovy Grahams	¾ cup	100	1	0	0	2	24	13	1	20	240	210	—	0
Honey Round-Ups	¾ cup	110	1	0	0	2	25	10	1	0	160	65	—	0
Multigrain Hot Cereal	½ cup	130	1	0	0	5	29	0	5	—	0	—	—	—
Oat Bran Hot Cereal	½ cup	150	3	1	0	7	25	1	6	20	0	—	—	—
Oatmeal Instant	½ cup	150	3	1	0	5	27	1	4	—	0	—	—	—
Peanut Butter Bumpers	1 cup	130	3	1	0	3	26	10	1	20	270	210	—	0
Rolled Oats	½ cup	150	3	1	0	5	27	1	4	0	0	—	—	0
Toasted Oat Bran	¾ cup	120	2	0	0	4	24	5	3	20	200	160	—	0
Whole Wheat Hot Cereal	½ cup	130	1	0	0	5	30	0	4	0	0	—	—	0
NABISCO														
100% Bran	⅓ cup (1 oz)	80	1	0	0	4	23	7	8	20	120	270	100	0
Frosted Shredded Wheat Bite Size	1 cup (1.8 oz)	190	1	0	0	4	44	12	5	0	10	170	100	0
Honey Nut Shredded Wheat Bite Size	1 cup (1.8 oz)	200	2	0	0	5	43	12	4	0	40	200	100	0
Original Shredded Wheat	2 biscuits (1.6 oz)	160	1	0	0	5	38	0	5	20	0	200	16	0
Original Shredded Wheat 'N Bran	1¼ cups (2.1 oz)	200	1	0	0	7	47	tr	8	20	0	250	24	0
Original Shredded Wheat Spoon Size	1 cup (1.7 oz)	170	1	0	0	5	41	0	5	20	0	200	16	0
NATURAL OVENS														
Great Granola	¼ cup	110	4	1	0	5	18	3	5	50	10	—	40	0
Paul's Oatmeal not prep	⅓ cup	120	3	0	0	4	22	3	3	30	100	—	40	0
POST														
Alpha-Bits	1 cup (1 oz)	130	2	0	0	3	27	13	1	0	210	60	100	0
Alpha-Bits Marshmallow	1 cup (1 oz)	120	1	0	0	2	25	14	0	0	160	30	100	0
Bran Flakes	¾ cup (1 oz)	100	1	0	0	3	24	6	5	0	220	190	100	0
Cocoa Pebbles	¾ cup (1 oz)	120	1	1	0	1	26	13	0	0	160	40	100	0
Fruit & Fibre Peaches Raisins & Almonds	1 cup (1.9 oz)	210	3	1	0	4	42	14	5	20	260	260	120	0
Fruity Pebbles	¾ cup (1 oz)	110	1	0	0	tr	24	12	0	0	160	30	100	0
Golden Crisp	¾ cup (1 oz)	110	0	0	0	1	25	15	0	0	40	35	100	0
Grape-Nuts	½ cup	200	1	0	0	7	47	5	6	20	310	260	200	0
Grape-Nuts Flakes	¾ cup (1 oz)	100	1	0	0	3	24	5	3	0	140	80	100	0

FOOD	PORTION	CALS	FAT	SAT FAT	CHOL	PROT	CARB	SUGAR	FIBER	CALCI	SOD	POTAS	FOLIC	VIT C
POST (CONT.)														
Great Grains Raisins Dates & Pecans	½ cup	210	5	1	0	4	40	14	4	0	130	210	100	0
Honey Bunches Of Oats	¾ cup (1 oz)	120	2	1	0	2	25	6	1	0	190	50	100	0
Honey Bunches Of Oats w/ Almonds	¾ cup (1.1 oz)	130	3	1	0	3	24	7	1	0	180	65	100	0
Honeycomb	1⅓ cups (1 oz)	110	1	0	0	2	26	11	tr	0	220	35	100	0
Post Toasties	1 cup (1 oz)	100	0	0	0	2	24	2	1	0	270	30	100	0
Raisin Bran	1 cup (2 oz)	190	1	0	0	4	47	20	8	20	300	340	140	0
Selects Blueberry Morning	¾ cup (1.3 oz)	140	2	0	0	2	30	9	2	0	150	60	60	—
Shredded Wheat Spoon Size	1 cup	170	1	0	0	6	40	0	6	20	0	190	—	0
Waffle Crisp	1 cup (1 oz)	130	3	0	0	2	24	11	0	0	120	35	100	0
QUAKER														
Instant Grits Original	1 pkg (1 oz)	100	0	0	0	2	22	—	1	—	300	—	40	—
Multigrain	½ cup (1.4 oz)	130	2	0	0	5	29	1	5	0	10	160	9	—
Oatmeal Instant	1 pkg (1 oz)	100	2	0	0	4	19	0	3	100	80	105	80	—
Oatmeal Instant Apples & Cinnamon	1 pkg (1.2 oz)	130	2	1	0	3	27	12	3	100	170	—	80	—
Oatmeal Instant Bananas & Cream	1 pkg (1.2 oz)	130	3	1	0	3	26	11	2	100	170	105	80	—
Oatmeal Instant Blueberries & Cream	1 pkg (1.2 oz)	130	3	1	0	3	26	11	2	100	160	85	80	—
Oatmeal Instant Cinnamon & Spice	1 pkg (1.6 oz)	170	2	1	0	4	35	16	3	100	250	—	80	0
Oatmeal Instant Kid's Choice Chocolate Chip Cookie	1 pkg (1.5 oz)	160	3	1	0	4	32	12	3	100	200	115	80	—
Oatmeal Instant Kid's Choice Cookie'n Cream	1 pkg (1.5 oz)	160	3	1	0	4	31	12	2	100	200	115	80	—
Oatmeal Instant Kid's Choice Fruity Marshmallow	1 pkg (1.4 oz)	150	2	1	0	4	31	13	3	100	190	110	80	—
Oatmeal Instant Kid's Choice Oatmeal Raisin Cookie	1 pkg (1.5 oz)	160	2	1	0	3	32	14	2	100	220	120	80	—

FOOD	PORTION	CALS	FAT	SAT FAT	CHOL	PROT	CARB	SUGAR	FIBER	CALCI	SOD	POTAS	FOLIC	VIT C
QUAKER (CONT.)														
Oatmeal Instant Kid's Choice Radical Raspberry	1 pkg (1.4 oz)	150	3	1	0	4	29	11	3	100	180	115	80	—
Oatmeal Instant Kid's Choice Strawberries'n Stuff	1 pkg (1.4 oz)	150	2	1	0	3	30	13	3	100	180	115	80	—
Oatmeal Instant Kid's Choice Twisted Strawberry Banana	1 pkg (1.4 oz)	150	2	1	0	3	31	13	3	100	180	110	80	—
Oatmeal Instant Maple & Brown Sugar	1 pkg (1.5 oz)	160	2	0	0	4	32	13	3	100	260	—	80	0
Oatmeal Instant Peaches & Cream	1 pkg (1.2 oz)	140	3	1	0	3	27	12	2	100	170	100	80	—
Oatmeal Instant Raisin & Spice	1 pkg (1.5 oz)	150	2	1	0	3	33	16	3	100	250	160	80	—
Oatmeal Instant Raisin Date & Walnut	1 pkg (1.3 oz)	140	3	1	0	3	27	13	3	100	240	135	80	—
Oatmeal Instant Strawberries & Cream	1 pkg (1.2 oz)	140	3	1	0	3	27	11	2	100	170	100	80	—
Oatmeal Instant Supreme Banana Walnut	1 pkg (1.4 oz)	150	3	1	0	4	28	9	3	100	280	—	80	0
Oatmeal Nutrition for Women Golden Brown Sugar	1 pkg (1.6 oz)	170	2	1	0	5	33	13	3	350	310	135	140	0
Oatmeal Quick'n Hearty Microwave	1 pkg (1 oz)	110	2	1	0	4	19	1	2	100	150	110	80	—
Oatmeal Quick'n Hearty Microwave Apple Spice	1 pkg (1.6 oz)	170	2	1	0	4	35	15	3	100	280	140	80	—
Oatmeal Quick'n Hearty Microwave Brown Sugar Cinnamon	1 pkg (1.5 oz)	150	2	1	0	4	31	12	3	100	260	125	80	—
Oatmeal Quick'n Hearty Microwave Cinnamon Double Raisin	1 pkg (1.6 oz)	170	2	1	0	4	35	16	3	100	280	190	80	—
Oatmeal Quick'n Hearty Microwave Honey Bran	1 pkg (1.4 oz)	150	2	1	0	4	30	12	3	100	250	120	80	—

FOOD	PORTION	CALS	FAT	SAT FAT	CHOL	PROT	CARB	SUGAR	FIBER	CALCI	SOD	POTAS	FOLIC	VIT C
QUAKER (CONT.)														
Oats Quick	½ cup (1.4 oz)	150	3	1	0	5	27	1	4	0	0	140	16	—
Oats Steel Cut	½ cup (1.4 oz)	150	3	1	0	5	27	1	4	0	0	140	16	—
Old Fashion Oats not prep	½ cup	150	3	1	0	5	27	1	4	0	0	140	16	0
Whole Wheat Hot Natural	½ cup (1.4 oz)	130	1	0	0	5	30	0	4	0	0	170	16	—
RALSTON														
Raisin Bran	1 cup	200	2	0	0	6	47	18	8	20	370	340	100	0
SUNBELT														
Berry Basic	½ cup (1.9 oz)	220	6	2	0	6	40	12	5	—	200	—	—	—
Granola Banana Nut	½ cup (1.9 oz)	250	9	4	0	5	37	13	4	—	60	—	—	—
Granola Cinnamon Raisins	½ cup (1.9 oz)	200	3	1	0	5	42	20	4	—	80	—	—	—
Granola Fruit & Nut	½ cup (1.9 oz)	240	7	2	0	4	40	21	3	—	70	—	—	—
Muesli 5 Whole Grains	½ cup (1.9 oz)	210	2	1	0	4	44	17	3	—	70	—	—	—
UNCLE SAM														
Cereal	1 cup (1.9 oz)	190	1	0	0	7	38	tr	10	40	135	—	—	1
WEETABIX														
Cereal	2 biscuits (1.2 oz)	100	1	—	—	3	21	2	3	28	106	106	—	1
WHEATENA														
Cereal	⅓ cup (1.4 oz)	150	1	0	0	5	33	0	5	200	0	150	—	0

CEREAL BARS

(*see also* ENERGY BARS)

FOOD	PORTION	CALS	FAT	SAT FAT	CHOL	PROT	CARB	SUGAR	FIBER	CALCI	SOD	POTAS	FOLIC	VIT C
granola	1 bar (1 oz)	134	7	1	0	3	18	7	2	17	83	95	7	tr
BARBARA'S BAKERY														
Nature's Choice Apple Cinnamon	1 bar (1.3 oz)	120	2	0	0	2	27	11	2	—	75	—	—	—
Nature's Choice Blueberry	1 bar (1.3 oz)	120	2	0	0	2	27	11	2	—	75	—	—	—
Nature's Choice Cherry	1 bar (1.3 oz)	120	2	0	0	2	27	11	2	—	75	—	—	—
Nature's Choice Granola Carob Chip	1 bar (0.7 oz)	80	2	0	0	2	16	8	2	—	5	—	—	—
Nature's Choice Granola Cinnamon & Raisin	1 bar (0.7 oz)	80	2	0	0	2	16	7	3	—	5	—	—	—
Nature's Choice Granola Oats 'N Honey	1 bar (0.7 oz)	80	2	0	0	2	15	7	2	—	5	—	—	—

FOOD	PORTION	CALS	FAT	SAT FAT	CHOL	PROT	CARB	SUGAR	FIBER	CALCI	SOD	POTAS	FOLIC	VIT C
BARBARA'S BAKERY (CONT.)														
Nature's Choice Granola Peanut Butter	1 bar (0.7 oz)	80	3	0	0	2	14	7	2	—	5	—	—	—
Nature's Choice Raspberry	1 bar (1.3 oz)	120	2	0	0	2	27	11	2	—	75	—	—	—
Nature's Choice Strawberry	1 bar (1.3 oz)	120	2	0	0	2	27	11	2	—	75	—	—	—
Nature's Choice Triple Berry	1 bar (1.3 oz)	120	2	0	0	2	27	11	2	—	75	—	—	—
DOLLY MADISON														
Apple	1 (1.3 oz)	120	2	0	0	1	25	14	1	20	90	—	120	0
Blueberry	1 (1.3 oz)	120	2	0	0	1	25	14	1	20	90	—	120	0
Raspberry	1 (1.3 oz)	120	2	0	0	1	24	14	1	20	100	—	120	0
Strawberry	1 (1.3 oz)	120	2	0	0	1	24	14	1	20	100	—	120	0
ENTENMANN'S														
Apple Cinnamon	1 (1.3 oz)	140	3	1	0	1	25	15	tr	0	85	—	120	0
Blueberry	1 (1.3 oz)	140	3	1	0	1	25	15	tr	0	90	—	120	0
Multi-Grain Chocolate Chip	1	140	3	1	0	2	28	16	2	100	100	—	100	0
Multi-Grain Rainbow Chip	1	180	8	3	5	1	26	15	tr	0	100	—	—	0
Multi-Grain Real Raspberry	1	140	3	1	0	1	26	16	1	100	110	—	100	0
Oatmeal Apple Cinnamon	1 (1.3 oz)	140	3	1	0	1	27	15	1	0	110	—	120	0
Oatmeal Apple Raisin	1 (1.3 oz)	140	3	0	0	1	27	15	1	0	110	—	120	0
Raspberry	1 (1.3 oz)	140	3	0	0	1	27	15	1	0	110	—	120	0
Strawberry	1 (1.3 oz)	140	3	1	0	1	25	15	tr	0	90	—	120	0
ESTEE														
Rice Crunchie Chocolate	1 (0.7 oz)	50	0	0	0	1	15	0	tr	—	40	0	—	—
Rice Crunchie Chocolate Chip	1 (0.7 oz)	50	0	0	0	1	15	0	0	—	40	0	—	—
ESTEE (CONT.)														
Rice Crunchie Peanut Butter	1 (0.7 oz)	60	1	0	0	1	15	0	0	—	35	0	—	—
Rice Crunchie Vanilla	1 (0.7 oz)	60	0	0	0	1	14	0	0	—	35	15	—	—
GENERAL MILLS														
Milk 'N Cereal Bars Chex	1 bar (1.6 oz)	160	4	2	0	6	26	13	—	250	150	105	200	9
Milk 'N Cereal Bars Cinnamon Toast Crunch	1 bar (1.6 oz)	180	4	2	0	6	30	19	1	250	160	115	200	9

FOOD	PORTION	CALS	FAT	SAT FAT	CHOL	PROT	CARB	SUGAR	FIBER	CALCI	SOD	POTAS	FOLIC	VIT C
GENERAL MILLS (CONT.)														
Oatmeal Crisp Apple	1 bar (1.4 oz)	150	2	0	0	2	31	15	1	200	110	—	100	15
Oatmeal Crisp Strawberry	1 bar (1.4 oz)	140	2	0	0	3	30	14	1	200	115	—	100	15
GLENNY'S														
Chocolate Crunch Creamy Low Fat	1 bar (1.75 oz)	190	3	1	0	3	36	17	4	0	113	—	—	2
Chocolate Crunch Roasted Peanut	1 bar (1.75 oz)	200	4	1	0	4	36	14	6	0	100	—	—	2
Chocolate Crunch Toasted Almond	1 bar (1.75 oz)	200	4	0	0	4	36	14	6	0	100	—	—	2
HEALTH VALLEY														
Blueberry	1	140	0	0	0	2	35	14	3	20	5	—	—	1
Breakfast Bakes Apple Cinnamon	1 bar	110	0	0	0	2	26	13	3	20	25	—	—	2
Breakfast Bakes California Strawberry	1 bar	110	0	0	0	2	26	13	3	20	25	—	—	2
Breakfast Bakes Mountain Blueberry	1 bar	110	0	0	0	2	26	13	3	40	25	—	—	1
Breakfast Bakes Red Raspberry	1 bar	110	0	0	0	2	26	13	3	40	25	—	—	1
Chocolate Chip	1	140	0	0	0	2	35	14	3	20	5	—	—	1
Crisp Rice Bars Apple Cinnamon	1	110	0	0	0	1	26	15	1	20	5	—	—	6
Crisp Rice Bars Orange Date	1	110	0	0	0	1	26	15	1	20	5	—	—	2
Crisp Rice Bars Tropical Fruit	1	110	0	0	0	1	26	15	1	20	5	—	—	0
Date Almond	1	140	0	0	0	2	35	14	3	20	5	—	—	1
Fiber 7 Flakes w/ Strawberry	1 bar	110	0	0	0	2	26	13	3	20	25	—	—	2
Oat Bran Flakes w/ Blueberry	1 bar	110	0	0	0	2	26	13	3	20	25	—	—	2
O's Almond	¾ cup	120	0	0	0	3	26	3	3	0	90	—	—	0
O's Apple Cinnamon	¾ cup	120	0	0	0	3	26	3	3	0	90	—	—	0
O's Honey Crunch	¾ cup	120	0	0	0	3	26	3	3	0	90	—	—	0
Raisin	1	140	0	0	0	2	35	14	3	20	5	—	—	1
Raisin Bran Flakes w/ Apple Raisin	1 bar	110	0	0	0	2	26	13	3	20	25	—	—	2
Raspberry	1	140	0	0	0	2	35	14	3	20	5	—	—	1
Strawberry	1	140	0	0	0	2	35	14	3	20	5	—	—	1

FOOD	PORTION	CALS	FAT	SAT FAT	CHOL	PROT	CARB	SUGAR	FIBER	CALCI	SOD	POTAS	FOLIC	VIT C
HERSHEY'S														
Crispy Rice Peanut Butter	1 bar (0.5 oz)	60	2	1	0	tr	9	—	—	—	55	—	—	—
Crisy Rice Snacks Peanut Butter	1 bar (0.5 oz)	60	2	tr	0	1	9	5	tr	40	57	—	—	1
HOSTESS														
Apple	1 (1.3 oz)	120	2	0	0	1	25	14	1	20	90	—	120	0
Banana Nut	1 (1.3 oz)	120	2	0	0	2	25	14	2	20	80	—	120	0
Blueberry	1 (1.3 oz)	120	2	0	0	1	25	14	1	20	90	—	120	0
Raspberry	1 (1.3 oz)	120	2	0	0	1	24	14	1	20	100	—	120	0
Strawberry	1 (1.3 oz)	120	2	0	0	1	24	14	1	20	100	—	120	0
KELLOGG'S														
Special K Blueberry	1 bar	90	2	1	0	2	18	8	tr	20	95	—	—	0
Special K Cranberry Apple	1 bar	90	2	1	0	2	17	9	tr	20	90	—	—	0
KUDOS														
Apple Nut Crunch	1	90	3	1	0	1	15	8	1	200	65	—	—	0
Chocolate Chip	1	120	5	3	0	1	20	13	1	200	85	—	—	6
Peanut Butter	1	190	6	2	0	2	18	19	1	200	90	—	—	0
Snickers	1	100	4	2	0	1	16	10	0	200	105	—	—	0
With M&M's	1	100	9	2	0	1	17	10	0	150	115	—	—	0
LITTLE DEBBIE														
Raspberry	1 (1.3 oz)	130	3	0	0	1	28	18	tr	6	75	33	—	1
S'mores Granola Treats	1 (1 oz)	130	5	2	0	2	21	12	1	22	45	64	—	tr
Strawberry	1 (1.3 oz)	130	3	0	0	1	28	18	tr	6	75	43	—	4
NABISCO														
Nutter Butter Granola Bar	1 (1 oz)	120	8	1	0	2	21	9	tr	0	45	—	—	0
Oreo Granola Bar	1 (1 oz)	120	4	1	0	2	21	9	1	0	65	—	—	0
NATURAL OVENS														
Great Granola Chocolate Almond	1 bar	150	6	1	0	4	23	14	3	40	110	0	24	0
NATURAL OVENS (CONT.)														
Great Granola Fruit & Lemon	1 bar	130	3	0	0	4	24	8	3	60	140	0	60	18
Great Granola Mixed Fruit	1 bar	130	3	0	0	4	24	8	3	60	140	0	60	18
NATURE VALLEY														
Chewy Trail Mix Fruit & Nut	1 bar	140	4	1	0	3	25	13	2	—	95	—	—	—

FOOD	PORTION	CALS	FAT	SAT FAT	CHOL	PROT	CARB	SUGAR	FIBER	CALCI	SOD	POTAS	FOLIC	VIT C
NUTRI-GRAIN														
Apple Cinnamon	1 (1.3 oz)	140	3	1	0	2	27	13	1	20	110	75	40	0
Blueberry	1 (1.3 oz)	140	3	1	0	2	27	13	1	20	110	75	40	0
Cherry	1 (1.3 oz)	140	3	1	0	2	27	13	1	20	110	70	40	0
Fruit-full Squares Apple	1 (1.7 oz)	180	4	1	0	3	35	17	1	0	95	—	40	0
Fruit-full Squares Banana	1 (1.7 oz)	190	5	1	0	3	35	17	1	0	95	—	40	0
Fruit-full Squares Cinnamon Raisin	1 (1.7 oz)	180	4	1	0	3	35	17	1	0	95	—	40	0
Minis Strawberry	1 pkg (1.5 oz)	160	3	1	0	2	32	18	1	200	115	—	40	0
Mixed Berry	1 (1.3 oz)	140	3	1	0	2	27	13	1	20	110	80	40	0
Twists Low Fat Apple Cinnamon	1 (1.3 oz)	140	3	1	0	1	27	12	1	200	105	—	—	0
Twists Low Fat Banana Strawberry	1 (1.3 oz)	140	3	1	0	1	26	14	1	200	100	—	—	0
Twists Low Fat Strawberry Blueberry	1 (1.3 oz)	140	3	1	0	1	27	12	1	200	110	—	—	0
QUAKER														
Chewy Chocolate Chip	1 (1 oz)	120	4	2	0	2	21	9	1	—	70	—	—	—
Chewy Cookies 'n Cream	1 (1 oz)	110	3	1	0	2	22	10	1	—	80	—	—	—
Chewy Peanut Butter Chocolate Chunk	1 (1 oz)	120	3	1	0	2	20	9	1	—	105	—	—	—
Chewy Graham Slam Chocolate Chip	1 (1 oz)	110	2	—	0	2	22	10	1	—	75	—	—	—
Chewy Graham Slam Peanut Butter	1 (1 oz)	110	2	—	0	2	22	9	1		80	—	—	—
Chewy Low Fat Chocolate Chunk	1 (1 oz)	110	2	—	0	2	22	10	1	—	80	—	—	—
Chewy Low Fat Oatmeal Raisin	1 (1 oz)	110	2	1	0	1	22	10	1	—	70	—	—	—
Chewy Low Fat S'mores	1 (1 oz)	110	2	1	0	1	22	10	1	—	80	—	—	—
Fruit & Oatmeal Bites Apple Crisp	1 pkg	140	3	0	0	2	27	15	1	200	85	—	100	0
Fruit & Oatmeal Bites Strawberry	1 pkg	140	3	0	0	2	27	14	1	200	120	—	100	0
Fruit & Oatmeal Bites Very Berry	1 pkg	140	3	0	0	2	27	14	1	200	110	—	100	0

FOOD	PORTION	CALS	FAT	SAT FAT	CHOL	PROT	CARB	SUGAR	FIBER	CALCI	SOD	POTAS	FOLIC	VIT C
QUAKER (CONT.)														
Fruit & Oatmeal Cranberry Orange Muffin	1 (1.3 oz)	130	3	0	0	1	27	17	1	200	95	—	100	0
Fruit & Oatmeal Low Fat Cherry Cobbler	1 (1.3 oz)	140	3	—	0	2	26	15	1	200	95	—	100	—
Fruit & Oatmeal Low Fat Strawberry	1 (1.3 oz)	140	3	—	0	2	26	15	1	200	125	—	100	—
Fruit & Oatmeal Low Fat Strawberry Banana	1 (1.3 oz)	130	3	—	0	1	26	15	tr	200	100	—	100	—
Fruit & Oatmeal Low Fat Strawberry Cheesecake	1 (1.3 oz)	130	3	1	0	2	26	14	tr	200	125	—	100	—
RICE KRISPIES														
Treats Peanut Butter Chocolate	1 (0.8 oz)	110	4	1	0	2	16	9	0	0	100	—	32	0
Treats Cocoa	1 (0.8 oz)	100	4	1	0	1	16	7	0	0	105	—	—	0
Treats Original	1 (0.8 oz)	90	2	1	0	1	18	8	0	0	100	—	24	0
SKIPPY														
Peanut Butter	1 bar	180	11	3	0	4	18	11	1	—	95	—	—	—
Peanut Butter & Fudge	1 bar	190	12	3	0	4	18	11	1	—	95	—	—	—
Peanut Butter & Marshmallow	1 bar	140	12	3	0	4	14	11	1	—	170	—	—	—
Peanut Butter & Strawberry	1 bar	170	12	3	0	4	14	11	1	—	170	—	—	—
SNACKWELL'S														
Country Fruit Medley	1 (1.3 oz)	130	3	0	0	1	27	13	tr	20	75	—	—	0
Fat Free Apple Cinnamon	1 (1.3 oz)	120	0	0	0	1	28	15	1	20	115	—	—	0
Fat Free Blueberry	1 (1.3 oz)	120	0	0	0	1	28	15	1	20	85	—	—	0
Fat Free Strawberry	1 (1.3 oz)	120	0	0	0	1	28	16	1	20	115	—	—	0
Hearty Fruit'n Grain Crisp Autumn Apple	1 (1.3 oz)	130	3	0	0	1	25	14	1	20	95	—	—	0
Hearty Fruit'n Grain Mixed Berry	1 (1.3 oz)	120	3	0	0	1	25	14	1	20	95	—	—	0
Hearty Fruit'n Grain Orchard Cherry	1 (1.3 oz)	130	5	1	0	1	26	14	1	20	90	—	—	0

FOOD	PORTION	CALS	FAT	SAT FAT	CHOL	PROT	CARB	SUGAR	FIBER	CALCI	SOD	POTAS	FOLIC	VIT C
SUNBELT														
Apple	1 (1.3 oz)	130	3	0	0	1	28	18	tr	5	75	37	—	tr
Blueberry	1 (1.3 oz)	130	3	0	0	1	28	18	tr	5	75	31	—	tr
Chewy Granola Almond	1 (1 oz)	130	7	2	0	2	17	8	1	25	65	79	—	tr
Chewy Granola Apple Cinnamon	1 (1.2 oz)	140	3	0	0	2	28	14	2	15	105	67	—	tr
Chewy Granola Chocolate Chip	1 (1.2 oz)	160	7	3	0	2	23	12	2	20	70	85	—	tr
Chewy Granola Oatmeal Raisin	1 (1.2 oz)	130	3	0	0	2	27	15	1	16	100	100	—	tr
Chewy Granola Oats & Honey	1 (1 oz)	120	5	2	0	2	19	9	1	16	65	—	—	tr
Granola Fudge Dipped Chocolate Chip	1 (1.5 oz)	200	10	4	0	2	27	16	2	20	70	92	—	tr
Granola Fudge Dipped Macaroon	1 (1.4 oz)	190	10	4	0	2	24	14	1	19	65	96	—	tr
WEIGHT WATCHERS														
Apple Cinnamon	1 (1 oz)	100	2	1	0	1	21	12	2	0	95	—	—	0
Blueberry	1 (1 oz)	100	2	1	0	1	21	10	1	0	90	—	—	0
Raspberry	1 (1 oz)	100	2	1	0	1	21	12	2	0	90	—	—	0

CHAMPAGNE

FOOD	PORTION	CALS	FAT	SAT FAT	CHOL	PROT	CARB	SUGAR	FIBER	CALCI	SOD	POTAS	FOLIC	VIT C
mimosa	1 serv	117	tr	tr	0	1	12	—	tr	10	1	186	28	47
punch	1 serv	113	0	0	0	0	5	—	0	3	tr	tr	—	—
sekt german	3.5 fl oz	84	0	0	0	tr	5	—	—	—	—	—	—	—
ANDRE														
Blush	4 fl oz	88	0	0	0	0	4	—	—	—	4	—	—	—
Brut	4 fl oz	84	0	0	0	0	4	—	—	—	4	—	—	—
Cold Duck	4 fl oz	100	0	0	0	0	8	—	—	—	4	—	—	—
Extra Dry	4 fl oz	92	0	0	0	0	4	—	—	—	4	—	—	—
BALLATORE														
Spumante	4 fl oz	92	0	0	0	0	8	—	—	—	8	—	—	—
EDEN ROC														
Brut	4 fl oz	92	0	0	0	0	4	—	—	—	4	—	—	—
Brut Rosé	4 fl oz	99	0	0	0	0	8	—	—	—	4	—	—	—
Extra Dry	4 fl oz	84	0	0	0	0	4	—	—	—	4	—	—	—
TOTT'S														
Blanc de Noir	4 fl oz	88	0	0	0	0	8	—	—	—	4	—	—	—
Brut	4 fl oz	80	0	0	0	0	tr	—	—	—	4	—	—	—
Extra Dry	4 fl oz	84	0	0	0	0	4	—	—	—	4	—	—	—

FOOD	PORTION	CALS	FAT	SAT FAT	CHOL	PROT	CARB	SUGAR	FIBER	CALCI	SOD	POTAS	FOLIC	VIT C
CHAYOTE														
fresh cooked	1 cup	38	1	—	0	1	8	—	—	21	1	276	—	13
raw	1 (7 oz)	49	1	—	0	2	11	—	—	39	8	305	—	22
raw cut up	1 cup	32	tr	—	0	1	7	—	—	25	198	34	—	15
CHEESE														
american	1 oz	93	7	4	18	6	2	—	—	163	337	79	—	0
american cheese food	1 pkg (8 oz)	745	56	35	145	45	17	—	—	1303	2700	633	—	0
american cheese spread	1 jar (5 oz)	412	30	19	78	23	12	—	—	798	1910	343	10	0
american cheese spread	1 oz	82	6	4	16	5	2	—	—	159	381	69	2	0
american cold pack	1 pkg (8 oz)	752	56	35	144	45	19	—	—	1129	2193	824	12	0
beaufort	1 oz	115	9	6	34	8	tr	tr	0	297	128	33	1	0
bel paese	1 oz	112	9	—	—	7	0	—	—	173	—	—	—	—
blue	1 oz	100	8	6	21	6	1	—	—	150	396	73	10	0
blue crumbled	1 cup (4.7 oz)	477	39	25	102	29	3	—	—	712	1884	346	49	0
brick	1 oz	105	8	5	27	7	1	—	—	191	159	38	6	0
brie	1 oz	95	8	—	28	8	tr	—	—	52	178	43	18	0
cacio di roma sheep's milk cheese	1 oz	130	10	6	30	8	0	—	—	300	170	—	—	—
caerphilly	1.4 oz	150	13	—	—	9	0	—	0	220	—	—	—	tr
camembert	1 oz	85	7	4	20	6	tr	—	—	110	239	53	18	0
camembert	1 wedge (1⅓ oz)	114	9	6	27	8	tr	—	—	147	320	71	24	0
cantal	1 oz	105	9	6	26	7	tr	tr	0	277	269	39	6	0
caraway	1 oz	107	8	—	—	7	1	—	—	191	196	—	—	0
chabichou	1 oz	95	8	5	23	6	tr	tr	0	86	189	69	36	0
chaource	1 oz	83	7	4	20	5	tr	tr	0	111	230	27	27	0
cheddar	1 oz	114	9	6	30	7	tr	—	—	204	176	28	5	0
cheddar low fat	1 oz	49	2	1	6	9	1	—	—	118	174	19	3	0
cheddar low sodium	1 oz	113	9	6	28	7	1	—	—	200	6	32	5	0
cheddar reduced fat	1.4 oz	104	6	—	—	13	0	—	0	336	—	—	—	tr
cheddar shredded	1 cup	455	37	24	119	28	1	—	—	815	701	111	21	0
cheshire	1 oz	110	9	—	29	7	1	—	—	182	198	27	—	0
cheshire reduced fat	1.4 oz	108	6	—	—	13	tr	—	0	260	—	—	—	tr
colby	1 oz	112	9	6	27	7	1	—	—	194	171	36	—	0
colby low fat	1 oz	49	2	1	6	9	1	—	—	118	174	19	3	0
colby low sodium	1 oz	113	9	6	28	7	1	—	—	200	6	32	5	0
comte	1 oz	114	9	5	34	8	tr	tr	0	251	105	34	1	0
coulommiers	1 oz	88	7	5	23	6	tr	tr	0	70	195	46	19	0
crottin	1 oz	105	9	6	23	6	tr	tr	0	33	133	83	—	0

FOOD	PORTION	CALS	FAT	SAT FAT	CHOL	PROT	CARB	SUGAR	FIBER	CALCI	SOD	POTAS	FOLIC	VIT C
derby	1.4 oz	161	14	—	—	10	0	—	0	272	—	—	—	tr
edam	1 oz	101	8	5	25	7	tr	—	—	207	274	53	5	0
edam reduced fat	1.4 oz	92	4	—	—	13	tr	—	0	—	—	—	—	tr
emmentaler	1 oz	115	9	—	26	8	tr	—	—	291	129	31	tr	tr
feta	1 oz	75	6	4	25	4	1	—	—	140	316	18	—	0
fontina	1 oz	110	9	5	33	7	tr	—	—	156	—	—	—	0
frais	1.6 oz	51	3	—	—	3	3	—	0	40	—	—	—	tr
gjetost	1 oz	132	8	5	—	3	12	—	—	113	170	—	1	0
gloucester double	1.4 oz	162	14	—	—	10	0	—	0	264	—	—	—	tr
goat fresh	1 oz	23	2	1	5	1	tr	tr	0	31	18	—	—	—
goat hard	1 oz	128	10	7	30	9	1	—	—	254	98	14	—	—
goat semisoft	1 oz	103	8	6	22	6	1	—	—	84	146	45	—	—
goat soft	1 oz	76	6	4	13	5	tr	—	—	40	104	7	—	—
gorgonzola	1 oz	107	9	—	—	5	tr	—	—	175	—	—	tr	—
gouda	1 oz	101	8	5	32	7	1	—	—	198	232	34	6	0
gruyère	1 oz	117	9	5	31	8	tr	—	—	287	95	23	3	0
lancashire	1.4 oz	149	12	—	—	9	0	—	0	224	—	—	—	tr
leicester	1.4 oz	160	14	—	—	10	0	—	0	264	—	—	—	tr
limburger	1 oz	93	8	5	26	8	tr	—	—	141	227	36	16	0
lymeswold	1.4 oz	170	16	—	—	6	tr	—	0	108	—	—	—	tr
maroilles	1 oz	97	8	5	26	6	tr	tr	0	229	300	37	3	0
monterey	1 oz	106	9	—	—	7	tr	—	—	212	152	23	—	0
morbier	1 oz	99	8	5	23	7	tr	tr	0	217	283	29	6	0
mozzarella	1 lb	1276	98	60	356	88	10	—	—	2345	1692	304	32	0
mozzarella	1 oz	80	6	4	22	6	1	—	—	147	106	19	1	0
mozzarella fresh	1 oz	80	6	4	20	6	tr	0	0	150	160	—	—	0
mozzarella low moisture	1 oz	90	7	4	25	6	1	—	—	163	118	21	2	0
mozzarella part skim	1 oz	72	5	3	16	7	1	—	—	183	132	24	2	0
muenster	1 oz	104	9	5	27	7	tr	—	—	203	178	38	3	0
parmesan grated	1 tbsp (5 g)	23	2	1	4	2	tr	—	—	69	93	5	tr	0
parmesan grated	1 oz	129	9	5	22	12	1	—	—	390	528	30	2	0
parmesan hard	1 oz	111	7	5	19	10	1	—	—	336	454	26	2	0
picodon	1 oz	99	8	5	23	6	tr	tr	0	29	—	—	—	0
pimento	1 oz	106	9	6	27	6	tr	—	—	174	405	46	2	—
pont l'eveque	1 oz	86	7	4	20	6	tr	tr	0	134	191	39	3	0
port du salut	1 oz	100	8	5	35	7	tr	—	—	184	151	—	5	0
provolone	1 oz	100	8	5	20	7	1	—	—	214	248	39	3	0
pyrenees	1 oz	101	8	5	26	6	tr	tr	0	181	235	19	7	0
quark 20% fat	1 oz	33	1	—	5	4	1	—	—	24	10	25	tr	tr
quark 40% fat	1 oz	48	3	—	11	3	1	—	—	27	10	23	—	1
quark made w/ skim milk	1 oz	22	tr	—	tr	4	1	—	—	26	11	27	tr	tr
queso anego	1 oz	106	9	5	30	6	1	—	—	193	321	25	0	0

FOOD	PORTION	CALS	FAT	SAT FAT	CHOL	PROT	CARB	SUGAR	FIBER	CALCI	SOD	POTAS	FOLIC	VIT C
queso asadero	1 oz	101	8	5	30	6	1	—	—	188	186	25	2	0
queso chichuahua	1 oz	106	8	5	30	6	2	—	—	185	175	15	1	0
queso fresco	1 oz	41	2	—	—	4	1	—	0	194	—	—	—	0
queso manchego	1 oz	107	8	—	27	8	tr	—	0	237	341	57	6	—
queso panela	1 oz	74	5	—	—	6	1	—	0	195	—	—	—	0
raclette	1 oz	102	8	5	26	7	tr	tr	0	157	217	32	15	0
reblochon	1 oz	88	7	5	23	6	tr	tr	0	179	240	54	7	0
ricotta part skim	1 cup (8.6 oz)	340	19	12	76	28	13	—	—	669	307	308	—	0
ricotta part skim	½ cup (4.4 oz)	171	10	6	38	14	6	—	—	337	155	155	—	0
ricotta whole milk	½ cup (4.4 oz)	216	16	10	63	14	4	—	—	257	104	130	—	0
ricotta whole milk	1 cup (8.6 oz)	428	32	20	124	28	7	—	—	509	207	257	—	0
romadur 40% fat	1 oz	83	6	—	—	7	tr	—	—	115	—	—	—	—
romano	1 oz	110	8	—	29	9	1	—	—	302	340	—	2	0
roquefort	1 oz	105	9	5	26	6	1	—	—	188	513	26	14	0
rouy	1 oz	95	8	5	23	7	tr	tr	0	143	138	21	—	0
saint marcellin	1 oz	94	8	5	23	5	tr	tr	0	49	171	53	38	0
saint nectaire	1 oz	97	8	5	23	6	tr	tr	0	169	169	36	6	0
saint paulin	1 oz	85	6	4	20	7	tr	tr	0	223	174	23	6	0
sainte maure	1 oz	99	8	5	23	6	tr	tr	0	51	411	—	—	0
selles sur cher	1 oz	93	8	5	20	5	tr	tr	0	28	181	—	—	0
stilton blue	1.4 oz	164	14	—	—	9	0	—	0	128	—	—	—	tr
stilton white	1.4 oz	145	13	—	—	8	0	—	0	100	—	—	—	tr
swiss	1 oz	107	8	5	26	8	1	—	—	272	74	31	2	0
swiss cheese food	1 pkg (8 oz)	734	55	—	186	50	10	—	—	1642	3523	645	—	0
swiss processed	1 oz	95	7	5	24	7	1	—	—	219	388	61	—	0
tilsit	1 oz	96	7	5	29	7	1	—	—	198	213	18	—	0
tomé	1 oz	92	7	5	23	6	tr	tr	0	115	231	22	6	0
triple creme	1 oz	113	11	7	34	3	tr	tr	0	28	86	46	3	tr
vacherin	1 oz	92	8	5	23	5	tr	tr	0	200	129	34	3	0
wensleydale	1.4 oz	151	13	—	—	9	0	—	0	224	—	—	—	tr
whey cheese	1 oz	126	8	5	—	4	9	0	0	97	146	—	—	1
yogurt cheese	1 oz	80	7	3	15	6	0	0	0	350	60	—	—	—
ALOUETTE														
Garlic & Herbs	2 tbsp (0.8 oz)	70	7	5	30	1	1	tr	0	20	135	—	—	0
ALPINE LACE														
American Jalapeño Peppers	1 slice (1 oz)	80	6	4	20	6	2	0	0	250	260	—	—	—
American Less Fat Less Sodium White	1 slice (1 oz)	50	6	4	20	6	2	0	0	250	200	—	—	—
American Less Fat Less Sodium Yellow	1 slice (1 oz)	80	6	4	20	6	2	0	0	250	200	—	—	—

FOOD	PORTION	CALS	FAT	SAT FAT	CHOL	PROT	CARB	SUGAR	FIBER	CALCI	SOD	POTAS	FOLIC	VIT C
ALPINE LACE (CONT.)														
Cheddar Reduced Fat	1 slice (1 oz)	70	5	3	15	8	1	0	0	200	170	—	—	—
Colby Reduced Fat	1 slice (1 oz)	80	5	3	15	9	1	0	0	350	115	—	—	—
Fat Free Parmesan	2 tsp (5 g)	10	0	0	0	1	0	0	0	40	65	—	—	—
Feta Reduced Fat	1 oz	50	3	2	10	5	1	0	0	50	370	—	—	—
Feta Reduced Fat Sun Dried Tomato & Basil	1 oz	50	3	2	10	5	1	0	0	50	370	—	—	0
Goat Reduced Fat	1 oz	40	3	2	5	2	tr	0	0	—	130	—	—	—
Mozzarella Reduced Fat	1 oz	70	3	2	10	8	1	0	0	250	200	—	—	—
Muenster Reduced Sodium	1 slice (1 oz)	100	9	5	25	7	1	0	0	300	85	—	—	—
Provolone Smoked Reduced Fat	1 slice (1 oz)	70	5	3	15	9	1	0	0	350	120	—	—	—
Swiss Reduced Fat	1 slice (1 oz)	90	6	4	20	8	1	0	0	250	35	—	—	—
ATHENOS														
Feta	1 oz	80	6	4	20	5	tr	0	0	60	320	—	—	0
BOAR'S HEAD														
American	1 oz	100	9	6	25	6	1	0	0	150	380	—	—	0
Baby Swiss	1 oz	110	9	6	25	7	tr	0	0	200	135	—	—	0
Canadian Cheddar	1 oz	110	10	6	35	7	0	0	0	200	170	—	—	0
Double Glouster Yellow	1 oz	110	10	6	35	7	0	0	0	200	200	—	—	0
Feta	1 oz	60	4	3	10	5	1	0	0	60	370	—	—	0
Havarti	1 oz	110	10	7	35	6	0	0	0	200	210	—	—	0
Havarti w/ Dill	1 oz	110	10	7	35	6	0	0	0	200	210	—	—	0
Havarti w/ Jalapeño	1 oz	110	10	7	35	6	0	0	0	200	210	—	—	0
Lacey Swiss	1 oz	90	6	4	15	9	0	0	0	250	35	—	—	0
Longhorn Colby	1 oz	110	9	5	30	7	tr	0	0	200	170	—	—	0
Monterey Jack	1 oz	100	9	6	25	6	0	0	0	200	170	—	—	0
Monterey Jack w/ Jalapeño	1 oz	100	9	6	25	6	0	0	0	200	170	—	—	0
Mozzarella	1 oz	90	7	4	25	6	tr	0	0	250	140	—	—	0
Muenster	1 oz	100	8	5	25	6	0	0	0	200	180	—	—	0
Muenster Low Sodium	1 oz	100	8	5	20	6	0	0	0	200	75	—	—	0
Provolone Picante Sharp	1 oz	100	8	5	25	7	1	0	0	200	250	—	—	0
Swiss	1 oz	110	8	5	20	8	tr	0	0	250	65	—	—	0
BOAR'S HEAD (CONT.)														
Swiss No Salt Added	1 oz	110	8	5	25	8	tr	0	0	250	10	—	—	0

FOOD	PORTION	CALS	FAT	SAT FAT	CHOL	PROT	CARB	SUGAR	FIBER	CALCI	SOD	POTAS	FOLIC	VIT C
BONBEL														
Mini Babybel	1 piece (0.7 oz)	70	6	4	20	5	0	0	0	150	170	—	—	0
BORDEN														
Lite Line Sharp Cheddar	1 oz	50	2	—	—	—	—	—	—	200	—	—	—	—
Lite Line Swiss	1 oz	50	2	—	—	—	—	—	—	200	—	—	—	—
BOURSIN														
Garlic & Fine Herbs	2 tbsp	120	13	9	35	2	tr	—	—	20	180	—	—	—
BREAKSTONE'S														
Ricotta	¼ cup (2.2 oz)	110	8	5	25	7	3	3	0	250	90	105	—	0
CABOT														
American	1 slice (0.7 oz)	80	7	4	20	7	1	0	0	100	270	—	—	0
Cheddar	1 oz	110	9	5	30	7	tr	0	0	200	180	25	—	0
Cheddar Smoked	1 oz	110	9	5	30	7	tr	0	0	200	180	—	—	0
Cheddar Light 50% Reduced Fat	1 oz	70	5	3	15	8	1	0	0	200	170	—	—	0
Cheddar Light 50% Reduced Fat Jalapeño	1 oz	70	5	3	15	8	1	0	0	200	170	—	—	0
Cheddar Light 75% Reduced Fat	1 oz	60	3	2	10	9	tr	0	0	200	200	35	—	0
Colby Jack	1 oz	110	9	5	30	1	7	0	0	200	170	—	—	0
Fancy Blend Shredded	¼ cup	100	7	4	20	7	1	0	0	200	180	—	—	0
Monterey Jack	1 oz	110	9	5	30	7	tr	0	0	200	170	20	—	0
Mozzarella Shredded	¼ cup	80	6	4	15	8	1	0	0	200	170	—	—	0
Pepper Jack	1 oz	110	9	5	30	7	tr	0	0	200	170	—	—	0
Swiss Slices	1 slice (1 oz)	110	8	5	30	9	1	0	0	250	60	—	—	0
CEDAR GROVE														
Marble Colby	1 oz	110	9	6	30	7	0	0	0	200	185	—	—	0
Organic Tomato Basil Cheddar	1 oz	110	9	6	30	7	0	0	0	200	185	—	—	0
CHAVRIE														
Goat's Milk	2 tbsp	50	4	3	20	3	1	1	0	20	120	—	—	0
CHEEZ WHIZ														
Light	2 tbsp (1.2 oz)	80	3	2	15	6	6	3	0	150	540	110	—	0
CONNOISSEUR														
Asiago Spread	1 tbsp	90	7	4	20	5	2	2	0	150	240	—	—	0
CRACKER BARREL														
Baby Swiss	1 oz	110	9	6	25	7	0	0	0	200	110	15	—	0
Cheddar Extra Sharp	1 oz	120	10	7	30	6	0	0	0	200	180	30	—	0

FOOD	PORTION	CALS	FAT	SAT FAT	CHOL	PROT	CARB	SUGAR	FIBER	CALCI	SOD	POTAS	FOLIC	VIT C
CRACKER BARREL (CONT.)														
Cheddar Marbled Sharp	1 oz	110	9	6	30	7	tr	0	0	200	180	30	—	0
Cheddar New York Aged	1 oz	120	10	7	30	6	0	0	0	200	180	30	—	0
Cheddar Sharp	1 oz	120	10	7	30	6	0	0	0	200	180	30	—	0
Cheddar Vermont Sharp	1 oz	110	9	6	30	7	tr	0	0	200	180	30	—	0
Reduced Fat Cheddar Sharp	1 oz	90	6	4	20	7	tr	0	0	200	240	45	—	0
Reduced Fat Cheddar Vermont Sharp	1 oz	90	6	4	20	7	tr	0	0	200	240	45	—	0
Sharp Cheddar 2% Milk	1 oz	90	6	4	20	7	tr	0	0	200	240	—	—	0
Whipped Spreadable Cream Cheese & Extra Sharp Cheddar	2 tbsp (0.9 oz)	80	8	5	20	3	tr	0	0	80	180	25	—	0
Whipped Spreadable Cream Cheese & Sharp Cheddar	2 tbsp (0.9 oz)	80	8	5	20	3	tr	0	0	80	180	20	—	0
Whipped Spreadable Cream Cheese & Sharp Cheddar w/ Herbs	2 tbsp (0.9 oz)	80	8	5	20	3	tr	0	0	80	180	25	—	0
DI GIORNO														
Parmesan Grated	2 tsp (5 g)	25	2	1	5	2	0	0	0	60	85	10	0	0
Parmesan Shredded	2 tsp (5 g)	20	2	1	5	2	0	0	0	40	75	0	0	0
Romano Grated	2 tsp (5 g)	25	2	1	5	2	0	0	0	60	90	0	0	0
Romano Shredded	2 tsp (5 g)	20	2	1	5	2	0	0	0	40	70	0	0	0
FINLANDIA														
Muenster	1 slice (1.1 oz)	120	10	7	30	8	tr	0	0	200	200	—	—	0
FLEURS DE FRANCE														
Brie	3.5 oz	311	25	18	—	21	tr	0	tr	50	200	—	—	0
HANDI-SNACKS														
Cheez'n Breadsticks	1 pkg (1.1 oz)	120	6	3	15	4	12	3	0	60	320	55	—	0
Cheez'n Crackers	1 pkg (1.1 oz)	110	7	3	15	3	9	2	0	60	300	45	—	0
Cheez'n Pretzels	1 pkg (1 oz)	100	5	3	15	4	11	2	tr	60	410	50	—	0
Mozzarella String Cheese	1 piece (1 oz)	80	6	4	20	7	0	0	0	150	240	35	—	0
Nacho Stix'n Cheez	1 pkg (1.1 oz)	110	6	3	15	4	11	2	0	60	320	55	—	0

FOOD	PORTION	CALS	FAT	SAT FAT	CHOL	PROT	CARB	SUGAR	FIBER	CALCI	SOD	POTAS	FOLIC	VIT C
HOLLOW ROAD FARMS														
Sheep's Milk	1 oz	45	3	—	15	3	1	—	—	61	65	—	—	—
KRAFT														
Cheddar Extra Sharp	1 oz	120	10	7	30	6	0	0	0	200	180	30	—	0
Cheddar Medium	1 oz	110	9	6	30	7	tr	5	0	200	180	30	—	0
Cheddar Mild	1 oz	110	9	6	30	7	tr	0	0	200	180	30	—	0
Cheddar Sharp	1 oz	120	10	7	30	6	0	0	0	200	180	30	—	0
Cheddary Melts Medium Cheddar	1 oz	110	9	6	30	5	2	1	0	150	390	50	—	0
Cheddary Melts Mild Cheddar	1 oz	110	9	6	30	5	2	1	0	150	390	50	—	0
Cheddary Melts Shreds Medium Cheddar	¼ cup (1.1 oz)	120	9	6	30	6	2	1	0	150	420	55	—	0
Cheddary Melts Shreds Mild Cheddar	¼ cup (1.1 oz)	120	9	6	30	6	2	1	0	150	420	55	—	0
Cheese Food w/ Garlic	1 oz	90	7	5	20	5	2	2	0	150	370	75	—	0
Cheese Food w/ Jalapeño Peppers	1 oz	90	7	5	20	5	2	2	0	150	370	80	—	0
Colby	1 oz	110	9	6	30	7	tr	0	0	200	180	15	—	0
Colby Monterey Jack	1 oz	110	9	6	30	7	0	0	0	200	180	15	—	0
Deluxe American	1 oz	100	9	6	25	6	tr	0	0	150	430	25	—	0
Deluxe American White	1 oz	100	9	6	25	6	tr	0	0	150	430	25	—	0
Deluxe Singles American	1 (1 oz)	110	9	6	30	6	tr	0	0	150	460	25	—	0
Deluxe Singles American	1 (0.7 oz)	70	6	4	15	4	tr	0	0	100	310	15	—	0
Deluxe Singles Pimento	1 (1 oz)	100	8	6	25	6	tr	0	0	150	430	25	—	0
Deluxe Singles Swiss	1 slice (0.7 oz)	70	5	4	20	5	0	0	0	150	310	15	—	0
Deluxe Singles Swiss	1 (1 oz)	90	7	5	25	6	0	0	0	200	410	20	—	0
Free Grated	2 tsp (5 g)	15	0	0	0	tr	3	tr	0	0	75	10	—	0
Free Shredded Cheddar	¼ cup (0.9 oz)	40	0	0	<5	9	1	0	0	250	270	35	—	0
Free Shredded Mozzarella	¼ cup (1 oz)	45	0	0	<5	9	2	0	tr	250	340	30	—	0
Grated Parm Plus! Garlic Herb	2 tsp (5 g)	15	0	0	0	tr	2	0	0	0	110	20	—	0
Grated Parm Plus! Zesty Red Pepper	2 tsp (5 g)	15	0	0	0	tr	2	0	0	20	110	15	—	0

FOOD	PORTION	CALS	FAT	SAT FAT	CHOL	PROT	CARB	SUGAR	FIBER	CALCI	SOD	POTAS	FOLIC	VIT C
KRAFT (CONT.)														
Grated Parmesan	2 tsp (5 g)	20	2	1	5	2	0	0	0	60	85	10	—	0
Grated Romano	2 tsp (5 g)	20	2	1	<5	2	0	0	0	60	70	10	—	0
Marbled Cheddar Mild	1 oz	110	9	6	30	7	tr	0	0	200	180	30	—	0
Marbled Cheddar & Monterey Jack	1 oz	110	9	6	30	7	tr	0	0	200	190	20	—	0
Marbled Cheddar & Whole Milk Mozzarella	1 oz	100	8	5	25	6	tr	0	0	200	190	25	—	0
Marbled Colby Monterey Jack	1 oz	110	9	6	30	7	0	0	0	200	180	15	—	0
Monterey Jack	1 oz	110	9	6	30	6	0	0	0	200	190	15	—	0
Monterey Jack w/ Jalapeño Peppers	1 oz	110	9	6	30	7	tr	0	0	200	190	15	—	0
Mozzarella Part Skim Low Moisture	1 oz	80	5	4	15	8	tr	0	0	200	200	20	—	0
Mozzarella String Cheese Low Moisture Part Skim	1 piece (1 oz)	80	6	4	20	7	0	0	0	150	240	35	—	0
Pizza Shredded Four Cheese	¼ cup (0.9 oz)	90	7	5	20	6	tr	0	0	200	220	20	—	0
Pizza Shredded Mozzarella & Cheddar	⅓ cup (1.1 oz)	120	9	6	30	7	1	0	0	200	220	30	—	0
Pizza Shredded Mozzarella & Provolone w/ Smoke Flavor	¼ cup (0.9 oz)	90	7	5	20	6	tr	0	0	150	200	20	—	0
Reduced Fat Cheddar Mild	1 oz	90	6	4	20	7	tr	0	0	200	240	45	—	0
Reduced Fat Cheddar Sharp	1 oz	90	6	4	20	7	tr	0	0	200	240	45	—	0
Reduced Fat Colby	1 oz	80	6	4	20	7	0	0	0	200	220	50	—	0
Reduced Fat Monterey Jack	1 oz	80	6	4	20	7	tr	0	0	200	240	45	—	0
Shredded Cheddar Medium	¼ cup (0.9 oz)	100	8	6	30	6	tr	0	0	200	170	25	—	0
Shredded Cheddar Mild	¼ cup (0.9 oz)	100	8	6	30	6	tr	0	0	200	170	25	—	0
Shredded Cheddar Sharp	¼ cup (0.9 oz)	110	9	6	25	6	tr	0	0	150	170	25	—	0

FOOD	PORTION	CALS	FAT	SAT FAT	CHOL	PROT	CARB	SUGAR	FIBER	CALCI	SOD	POTAS	FOLIC	VIT C
KRAFT (CONT.)														
Shredded Cheddar & Monterey Jack	¼ cup (0.9 oz)	100	8	6	25	6	tr	0	0	200	170	20	—	0
Shredded Colby & Monterey Jack	¼ cup (0.9 oz)	100	8	6	25	6	tr	0	0	150	170	15	—	0
Shredded Hearty Italian	⅓ cup (1.1 oz)	100	8	5	25	7	2	0	0	200	230	35	—	0
Shredded Italian Style Classic Garlic	⅓ cup (1.1 oz)	100	8	5	25	7	2	0	tr	200	240	45	—	0
Shredded Italian Style Mozzarella & Parmesan	⅓ cup (1.1 oz)	100	8	5	25	7	1	0	0	200	240	25	—	0
Shredded Lower Fat Cheddar Mild	¼ cup (0.9 oz)	80	6	4	20	7	tr	0	0	200	220	40	—	0
Shredded Lower Fat Cheddar Sharp	¼ cup (0.9 oz)	80	6	4	20	7	tr	0	0	200	220	40	—	0
Shredded Lower Fat Colby & Monterey Jack	¼ cup (0.9 oz)	80	5	4	15	7	tr	0	0	200	210	40	—	0
Shredded Lower Fat Mozzarella	⅓ cup (1.1 oz)	80	5	3	15	9	tr	0	0	250	210	25	—	0
Shredded Lower Fat Pizza Cheese	⅓ cup (1.1 oz)	90	6	4	20	9	1	0	0	250	240	40	—	0
Shredded Mexican Style Cheddar & Monterey Jack	⅓ cup (1.1 oz)	120	10	7	30	7	tr	0	0	200	200	25	—	0
Shredded Mexican Style Cheddar & Monterey Jack w/ Jalapeño Peppers	⅓ cup (1.1 oz)	120	10	6	30	7	tr	0	0	200	200	25	—	0
Shredded Mexican Style Four Cheese	⅓ cup (1.1 oz)	120	10	7	30	7	tr	0	0	200	210	25	—	0
Shredded Mexican Style Taco Cheese	⅓ cup (1.1 oz)	120	10	7	30	7	1	0	0	200	240	25	—	0
Shredded Monterey Jack	¼ cup (0.9 oz)	100	8	6	25	6	tr	0	0	150	170	15	—	0
Shredded Parmesan	2 tsp (5 g)	20	2	1	2	2	0	0	0	40	75	0	—	0
Shredded Part Skim Mozzarella	¼ cup (1.1 oz)	90	6	4	20	8	tr	0	0	250	220	20	—	0
Shredded Swiss	¼ cup (0.9 oz)	100	8	5	25	7	tr	0	0	250	25	45	—	0

FOOD	PORTION	CALS	FAT	SAT FAT	CHOL	PROT	CARB	SUGAR	FIBER	CALCI	SOD	POTAS	FOLIC	VIT C
KRAFT (CONT.)														
Shredded Whole Milk Mozzarella	¼ cup (1.1 oz)	100	8	5	25	7	1	0	0	200	220	25	—	0
Shredded Finely Cheddar Mild	¼ cup (1.1 oz)	120	10	6	30	7	tr	0	0	200	190	30	—	0
Shredded Finely Cheddar Sharp	¼ cup (1.1 oz)	120	10	7	30	7	tr	0	0	200	190	30	—	0
Shredded Finely Colby & Monterey Jack	¼ cup (1 oz)	110	9	6	30	7	tr	0	0	200	190	15	—	0
Shredded Finely Lower Fat Cheddar Mild	⅓ cup (1.1 oz)	100	7	5	20	8	1	0	0	200	260	50	—	0
Shredded Finely Lower Fat Cheddar Sharp	⅓ cup (1.1 oz)	100	7	5	20	8	1	0	0	200	260	50	—	0
Shredded Finely Part Skim Mozzarella	¼ cup (1.1 oz)	90	6	4	20	8	tr	0	0	250	220	20	—	0
Shredded Finely Swiss	¼ cup (0.9 oz)	110	8	6	25	7	tr	0	0	250	45	20	—	0
Singles American	1 (0.6 oz)	60	5	3	15	3	2	1	0	150	260	45	—	0
Singles American	1 (1.2 oz)	110	8	6	25	6	3	2	0	200	460	80	—	0
Singles American	1 (0.7 oz)	60	5	3	15	3	2	1	0	100	260	45	—	0
Singles Mild Mexican	1 (0.7 oz)	70	5	4	15	4	2	1	0	100	280	50	—	0
Singles Monterey	1 (0.7 oz)	70	5	4	15	4	2	1	0	100	290	55	—	0
Singles Pimento	1 (0.7 oz)	60	5	3	15	4	1	tr	0	100	260	50	—	0
Singles Reduced Fat American	1 (0.7 oz)	50	3	2	10	5	2	2	0	150	320	60	—	0
Singles Reduced Fat American White	1 (0.7 oz)	50	3	2	10	4	2	2	0	150	320	60	—	0
Singles Sharp	1 (0.7 oz)	70	6	4	20	4	tr	0	0	100	300	25	—	0
Singles Swiss	1 (0.7 oz)	70	5	4	15	4	1	1	0	150	320	55	—	0
Singles Nonfat American	1 (0.7 oz)	30	0	0	<5	4	3	2	0	150	270	60	—	0
Singles Nonfat American White	1 (0.7 oz)	30	0	0	<5	4	3	2	0	150	270	60	—	0
Singles Nonfat Sharp Cheddar	1 (0.7 oz)	35	0	0	<5	5	3	2	0	150	300	65	—	0
Singles Nonfat Swiss	1 (0.7 oz)	30	0	0	<5	5	3	2	0	150	270	55	—	0
Slices Cheddar Mild	1 (1 oz)	110	9	6	30	7	tr	0	0	200	180	30	—	0
Slices Colby	1 (1.6 oz)	180	14	10	45	11	tr	0	0	300	290	25	—	0
Slices Part Skim Mozzarella	1 (1.5 oz)	120	8	5	25	12	tr	0	0	350	310	30	—	0

FOOD	PORTION	CALS	FAT	SAT FAT	CHOL	PROT	CARB	SUGAR	FIBER	CALCI	SOD	POTAS	FOLIC	VIT C
KRAFT (CONT.)														
Slices Part Skim Mozzarella	1 (1.6 oz)	130	8	6	25	12	tr	0	0	350	320	30	—	0
Slices Provolone Smoke Flavor	1 (1.5 oz)	150	11	8	35	11	tr	0	0	300	370	35	—	0
Slices Swiss	1 (1.3 oz)	150	12	8	40	10	tr	0	0	350	65	25	—	0
Slices Swiss	1 (0.8 oz)	90	7	5	25	6	0	0	0	200	40	15	—	0
Slices Swiss	1 (1.5 oz)	170	13	9	45	12	tr	0	0	400	45	75	—	0
Slices Swiss	1 (1.6 oz)	180	14	9	45	12	tr	0	0	400	45	75	—	0
Slices Swiss Aged	1 (1.5 oz)	170	13	9	45	12	tr	0	0	400	75	30	—	0
Slices Deli-Thin Part Skim Mozzarella	1 (1 oz)	80	5	4	15	8	tr	0	0	200	200	20	—	0
Slices Deli-Thin Swiss	1 (0.8 oz)	90	7	5	25	6	0	0	0	200	40	15	—	0
Slices Deli-Thin Swiss Aged	1 (0.8 oz)	90	7	5	25	6	0	0	0	200	40	15	—	0
Slices Reduced Fat Swiss	1 (1.3 oz)	130	9	6	25	11	tr	0	0	400	90	55	—	0
Spread Bacon	2 tbsp (1.1 oz)	90	8	5	25	5	tr	0	0	150	570	20	—	0
Spread Olive & Pimento	2 tbsp (1.1 oz)	70	6	4	20	2	3	2	0	20	220	50	—	0
Spread Pimento	2 tbsp (1.1 oz)	80	6	4	20	2	3	2	0	20	170	60	—	0
Spread Pineapple	2 tbsp (1.1 oz)	70	5	4	15	2	4	4	0	20	115	55	—	0
Spread Roka Brand Blue	2 tbsp (1.1 oz)	90	8	5	25	5	tr	0	0	150	520	15	—	0
Swiss	1 oz	110	9	6	30	8	0	0	0	250	50	20	—	0
LAND O LAKES														
American	1 slice (0.7 oz)	80	6	5	20	4	1	0	0	150	320	—	—	0
American Jalapeño	1 slice (0.6 oz)	70	6	4	15	3	1	tr	0	100	320	—	—	0
American Light	1 oz	70	5	3	20	7	2	0	0	200	400	—	—	0
American Reduced Salt	1 oz	110	9	6	30	6	tr	0	0	200	270	—	—	0
American Sharp	2 slices (1 oz)	100	9	6	30	5	1	tr	0	150	420	—	—	0
American & Swiss	1 slice (0.6 oz)	70	5	4	15	4	1	0	0	100	310	—	—	0
Baby Swiss	1 oz	110	9	6	25	6	0	0	0	200	125	—	—	0
Chedarella	1 oz	100	8	5	25	7	0	0	0	200	200	—	—	0
Cheddar	1 oz	100	9	5	30	6	tr	0	0	200	180	—	—	0
Cheddar Extra Sharp	1 oz	110	8	6	30	6	tr	0	0	150	360	—	—	0
Cheddar Sharp	1 oz	110	9	5	30	7	tr	0	0	200	180	—	—	0
Cheese Spread Golden Velvet	1 oz	80	6	4	20	5	2	2	0	150	370	—	—	0
Colby	1 oz	110	9	6	30	7	tr	0	0	200	180	—	—	0
Jalapeño Light	1 oz	70	4	3	15	7	1	0	0	200	400	—	—	0
Monterey Jack	1 oz	110	8	5	30	6	tr	0	0	200	170	—	—	0

FOOD	PORTION	CALS	FAT	SAT FAT	CHOL	PROT	CARB	SUGAR	FIBER	CALCI	SOD	POTAS	FOLIC	VIT C
LAND O LAKES (CONT.)														
Monterey Jack Hot Pepper	1 oz	110	8	5	30	6	tr	0	0	200	140	—	—	0
Mozzarella	1 oz	80	6	4	15	7	tr	0	0	200	190	—	—	0
Muenster	1 oz	100	8	5	25	6	0	0	0	200	220	—	—	0
Parmesan Grated	1 tbsp	35	4	2	10	3	0	0	0	100	95	—	—	0
Provolone	1 oz	100	8	5	20	7	tr	0	0	200	240	—	—	0
Swiss	1 oz	110	8	6	25	8	tr	0	0	250	75	—	—	0
Swiss Light	1 oz	80	4	3	15	9	tr	0	0	250	60	—	—	0
LIGHT N'LIVELY														
Singles American	1 (0.7 oz)	45	3	2	10	5	2	1	0	150	280	50	—	0
NORTHFIELD														
Naturally Slender	1 oz	90	7	—	10	—	—	—	—	250	—	—	—	—
OLD ENGLISH														
American Sharp	1 slice (1 oz)	100	9	6	30	6	tr	0	0	150	460	20	—	0
ORGANIC VALLEY														
Aged Swiss Unpasteurized	1 oz	100	8	5	25	8	tr	0	0	250	60	—	—	0
Cheddar Reduced Fat Low Sodium	1 oz	90	6	4	15	8	1	0	0	250	135	—	—	0
Cheddar Sharp & Mild	1 oz	110	9	6	25	7	1	0	0	200	190	—	—	1
Cheddar Sharp & Mild Unpasteurized	1 oz	110	9	6	25	7	1	0	0	200	190	—	—	1
Colby	1 oz	110	9	5	28	7	1	0	0	200	175	—	—	0
Colby Unpasteurized	1 oz	110	9	5	28	7	1	0	0	200	175	—	—	0
Farmer Reduced Fat	1 oz	90	6	4	15	7	1	0	0	200	110	—	—	1
Feta	1 oz	90	7	5	20	6	0	0	0	100	180	—	—	1
Monterey Jack	1 oz	100	8	6	20	6	1	0	0	200	170	—	—	0
Monterey Jack Reduced Fat	1 oz	80	5	3	15	8	1	0	0	250	170	—	—	1
Mozzarella Part Skim	1 oz	80	5	3	16	8	1	0	0	200	170	—	—	0
Muenster	1 oz	100	8	5	25	6	1	0	0	200	165	—	—	0
Pepper Jack	1 oz	110	9	6	20	6	1	0	0	200	160	—	—	0
Provolone	1 oz	100	8	4	20	7	1	0	0	210	245	—	—	0
String Part Skim	1 oz	80	5	3	16	8	1	0	0	200	170	—	—	0
Wisconsin Raw Milk Cheese	1 oz	100	8	6	20	6	1	0	0	200	170	—	—	0

FOOD	PORTION	CALS	FAT	SAT FAT	CHOL	PROT	CARB	SUGAR	FIBER	CALCI	SOD	POTAS	FOLIC	VIT C
POLLY-O														
Ricotta Lite	¼ cup	70	3	2	10	8	3	2	0	250	80	90	—	0
String Lite	1 piece (1 oz)	60	3	2	10	7	tr	tr	0	150	230	—	—	0
String-Ums	1 stick (1 oz)	80	6	4	20	7	tr	0	0	150	220	—	—	0
PRESIDENT														
Feta	1 inch cube (1 oz)	90	7	5	15	5	2	0	0	60	410	—	—	0
ROUGE ET NOIR														
Breakfast	1 oz	86	7	4	—	5	1	—	—	30	—	—	—	—
Brie	1 oz	86	7	4	—	5	1	—	—	30	—	—	—	—
Camembert	1 oz	86	7	4	—	5	1	—	—	30	—	—	—	—
Schloss	1 oz	86	7	4	—	5	1	—	—	30	—	—	—	—
SARGENTO														
Blue Crumbled	¼ cup (1 oz)	100	8	5	20	6	1	0	0	150	380	—	—	0
Cheddar Extra Sharp	1 oz	110	9	5	30	7	1	0	0	200	180	—	—	0
Cheddar Shredded	¼ cup (1 oz)	110	9	6	30	6	1	tr	0	200	160	—	—	0
Cheese For Nachos & Tacos Shredded	¼ cup (1 oz)	110	9	5	25	6	1	0	0	200	240	—	—	0
Cheese For Pizza Shredded	¼ cup (1 oz)	90	6	4	20	7	0	0	0	200	210	—	—	0
Cheese For Tacos Shredded	¼ cup (1 oz)	110	9	6	25	6	1	0	0	200	220	—	—	2
Colby	1 slice (1 oz)	110	9	6	30	6	0	0	0	200	190	—	—	0
Colby-Jack Shredded	¼ cup (1 oz)	110	9	6	25	6	tr	0	0	200	190	—	—	0
Jarlsberg	1 slice (1.2 oz)	120	9	5	20	9	1	0	0	300	160	—	—	0
Monterey Jack	1 slice (1 oz)	100	9	5	30	6	0	0	0	200	190	—	—	0
Monterey Jack Shredded	¼ cup (1 oz)	100	9	6	30	6	0	0	0	200	190	—	—	0
MooTown Snackers Cheddar	1 piece (0.8 oz)	100	8	5	25	5	1	0	0	150	130	—	—	0
MooTown Snackers Cheddar Mild Light	1 piece (0.8 oz)	60	4	3	10	7	tr	0	0	200	170	—	—	0
MooTown Snackers Cheese & Pretzels	1 pkg (0.9 oz)	90	3	2	10	3	12	1	0	60	320	—	—	0
MooTown Snackers Colby-Jack	1 piece (0.8 oz)	90	8	5	20	5	tr	0	0	150	160	—	—	0
MooTown Snackers Pizza Cheese & Sticks	1 pkg (1 oz)	100	4	3	10	3	13	3	0	60	260	—	—	0

FOOD	PORTION	CALS	FAT	SAT FAT	CHOL	PROT	CARB	SUGAR	FIBER	CALCI	SOD	POTAS	FOLIC	VIT C
SARGENTO (CONT.)														
MooTown Snackers String Light	1 piece (0.8 oz)	60	3	2	10	7	tr	0	0	200	200	—	—	0
Mozzarella	1 slice (1.5 oz)	130	9	6	25	11	2	0	0	300	230	—	—	0
Mozzarella Shredded	¼ cup (1 oz)	80	6	4	15	7	1	0	0	200	150	—	—	0
Muenster	1 slice (1 oz)	100	9	6	25	6	tr	0	0	200	200	—	—	0
Parmesan Grated	1 tbsp (5 g)	25	2	1	<5	2	0	0	0	60	75	—	—	0
Parmesan Shredded	¼ cup (1 oz)	110	7	5	25	9	1	0	0	250	300	—	—	0
Parmesan & Romano Shredded	¼ cup (1 oz)	110	7	5	25	9	1	0	0	250	340	—	—	0
Parmesan & Romano Grated	1 tbsp (5 g)	25	2	1	<5	2	0	0	0	60	70	—	—	0
Pizza Double Cheese Shredded	¼ cup (1 oz)	90	6	5	20	7	1	0	0	200	150	—	—	0
Preferred Light Cheddar Mild Shredded	¼ cup (1 oz)	70	5	3	10	8	tr	0	0	250	200	—	—	0
Preferred Light Mozzarella	1 slice (1.5 oz)	90	5	3	15	11	0	0	0	350	230	—	—	0
Preferred Light Mozzarella Shredded	¼ cup (1 oz)	70	3	2	10	8	tr	0	0	200	140	—	—	0
Preferred Light Swiss	1 slice (1 oz)	80	4	3	15	9	tr	0	0	300	50	—	—	0
Provolone	1 slice (1 oz)	100	8	5	25	7	0	0	0	200	190	—	—	0
Recipe Blend 4 Cheese Mexican Shredded	¼ cup (1 oz)	110	9	6	25	6	tr	0	0	200	200	—	—	0
Recipe Blend 6 Cheese Italian Shredded	¼ cup (1 oz)	90	7	4	20	7	0	0	0	200	180	—	—	0
Reduced Fat 4 Cheese Mexican Shredded	¼ cup (1 oz)	80	6	3	20	8	tr	0	0	250	200	—	—	0
Ricotta Light	¼ cup (2.2 oz)	60	3	2	15	5	3	3	0	100	55	—	—	0
Ricotta Old Fashioned	¼ cup (2.2 oz)	90	6	4	25	7	3	3	0	150	75	—	—	0
Ricotta Part-Skim	¼ cup (2.2 oz)	80	5	3	20	7	2	3	0	150	75	—	—	0
String	1 piece (0.8 oz)	70	5	3	15	6	tr	0	0	150	200	—	—	0
Swiss	1 slice (0.7 oz)	80	6	4	20	6	0	0	0	200	30	—	—	0
Swiss Shredded	¼ cup (1 oz)	110	8	5	30	8	0	0	0	250	40	—	—	0
Swiss Wafer Thin	2 slices (1 oz)	110	9	5	25	5	0	0	0	250	40	—	—	0

FOOD	PORTION	CALS	FAT	SAT FAT	CHOL	PROT	CARB	SUGAR	FIBER	CALCI	SOD	POTAS	FOLIC	VIT C
SORRENTO														
Mozzarella Part Skim Jalapeño	1 oz	80	5	3	15	8	1	0	0	200	180	—	—	0
Mozzarella w/ Tomato & Basil Shredded	¼ cup	80	5	3	15	8	1	1	0	200	180	—	—	1
Pizza Cheese Shredded	¼ cup	90	7	5	20	7	1	0	0	150	200	—	—	0
Stringsters	1 stick (1 oz)	80	5	3	15	8	1	0	0	200	170	—	—	0
SUISSE DELICAT														
Healthy Swiss	1 oz	90	6	5	25	9	0	0	0	250	82	—	—	—
TREE OF LIFE														
Cheddar 33% Reduced Fat Organic Milk	1 oz	90	6	4	15	8	1	—	—	250	135	—	—	1
Colby	1 oz	110	9	6	30	7	1	—	—	200	170	—	—	—
Colby Organic Milk	1 oz	120	10	6	30	7	1	—	—	200	190	—	—	—
Farmer Part-Skim Organic Milk	1 oz	90	6	4	15	7	1	—	—	200	110	—	—	1
Jalapeño Organic Milk	1 oz	110	9	6	20	6	1	—	—	200	190	—	—	—
Monterey Jack 35% Reduced Fat Organic Milk	1 oz	80	5	3	15	8	1	—	—	250	190	—	—	1
Monterey Jack Organic Milk	1 oz	100	8	6	20	6	1	—	—	200	185	—	—	—
Mozzarella Organic Milk	1 oz	80	5	3	16	8	1	—	—	200	170	—	—	—
Muenster Organic Milk	1 oz	100	8	5	25	6	1	—	—	200	185	—	—	—
Provolone	1 oz	100	8	5	20	7	1	—	—	200	250	—	—	—
VELVEETA														
Light	1 oz	60	3	2	10	5	3	2	0	150	440	90	—	0
Shredded	¼ cup (1.3 oz)	130	9	6	30	8	3	3	0	200	500	100	—	0
Shredded Mild Mexican w/ Jalapeño Pepper	¼ cup (1.3 oz)	120	9	6	30	8	3	2	0	200	520	95	—	0
Spread	1 oz	90	6	4	25	5	3	2	0	150	420	95	—	0
Spread Hot Mexican	1 oz	90	6	4	20	5	3	2	0	150	420	90	—	0
Spread Mild Mexican	1 oz	90	6	4	25	5	3	2	0	150	420	90	—	0
WEIGHT WATCHERS														
Cheddar Mild Yellow	1 oz	80	5	3	15	8	1	0	0	200	180	—	—	0
Cheddar Sharp Yellow	1 oz	80	5	3	15	8	1	0	0	200	180	—	—	0

FOOD	PORTION	CALS	FAT	SAT FAT	CHOL	PROT	CARB	SUGAR	FIBER	CALCI	SOD	POTAS	FOLIC	VIT C
WEIGHT WATCHERS (CONT.)														
Fat Free Grated Italian Topping	1 tbsp	20	0	0	0	2	2	1	0	20	60	—	—	0
Fat Free Reduced Sodium Yellow	2 slices (0.75 oz)	30	0	0	0	5	3	2	0	150	160	—	—	0
Fat Free Sharp Cheddar	2 slices (0.75 oz)	30	0	0	0	5	3	2	0	150	320	—	—	0
Fat Free Swiss	2 slices (0.75 oz)	30	0	0	0	5	2	2	0	150	320	—	—	0
Fat Free White	2 slices (0.75 oz)	30	0	0	0	5	3	2	0	150	320	—	—	0
Fat Free Yellow	2 slices (0.75 oz)	30	0	0	0	5	3	2	0	150	320	—	—	0
WHOLESOME VALLEY														
Organic American Reduced Fat	1 slice (0.7 oz)	50	3	2	10	4	2	2	0	100	290	—	—	0

CHEESE DISHES

FROZEN

BANQUET

FOOD	PORTION	CALS	FAT	SAT FAT	CHOL	PROT	CARB	SUGAR	FIBER	CALCI	SOD	POTAS	FOLIC	VIT C
Mozzarella Nuggets	6	260	18	8	40	9	19	3	1	150	1060	—	—	0
FILLO FACTORY														
Tyropita Cheese Fillo Appetizers	5 (5 oz)	340	12	7	30	14	44	1	2	—	480	—	—	—
HEALTH IS WEALTH														
Mozzarella Sticks	2 (1.3 oz)	120	5	3	15	5	14	0	0	80	250	—	—	0
STOUFFER'S														
Welsh Rarebit	½ cup (2.5 oz)	120	9	4	20	5	5	2	0	150	280	90	—	0
TAKE-OUT														
fondue	½ cup (3.8 oz)	247	15	9	49	15	4	—	—	514	142	113	5	0
fried mozzarella sticks	9	840	—		—	—	—	—	—	—	—	—	—	—
soufflé	1 serv (7 oz)	504	38	17	370	23	18	5	1	446	848	274	38	tr
welsh rarebit	1 slice	228	16	—	—	8	14	—	1	204	—	—	—	tr

CHEESE SUBSTITUTES

FOOD	PORTION	CALS	FAT	SAT FAT	CHOL	PROT	CARB	SUGAR	FIBER	CALCI	SOD	POTAS	FOLIC	VIT C
mozzarella	1 oz	70	3	1	0	3	7	—	—	173	194	129	3	0
SARGENTO														
Cheddar Shredded	¼ cup (1 oz)	90	7	2	0	5	2	0	0	150	420	—	—	0
Mozzarella Shredded	¼ cup (1 oz)	80	6	1	0	6	tr	0	0	150	320	—	40	0
YVES														
Good Slice American	1 slice (0.7 oz)	35	2	0	0	4	0	0	0	100	290	—	—	0
Good Slice Cheddar	1 slice (0.7 oz)	35	2	0	0	4	1	0	1	100	280	—	—	0

FOOD	PORTION	CALS	FAT	SAT FAT	CHOL	PROT	CARB	SUGAR	FIBER	CALCI	SOD	POTAS	FOLIC	VIT C
YVES (CONT.)														
Good Slice Jalapeño Jack	1 slice (0.7 oz)	35	2	0	0	4	0	0	0	100	250	—	—	0
Good Slice Mozzarella	1 slice (0.7 oz)	30	2	0	0	4	0	0	0	100	270	—	—	0
Good Slice Swiss	1 slice (0.7 oz)	35	2	0	0	4	1	0	0	100	260	—	—	0
CHERIMOYA														
fresh	1	515	2	—	0	7	131	—	—	126	—	—	—	49
CHERRIES														
CANNED														
sour in heavy syrup	½ cup	232	tr	tr	0	2	60	—	—	26	18	238	19	5
sour in light syrup	½ cup	189	tr	tr	0	2	49	—	—	26	18	238	19	5
sour water packed	1 cup	87	tr	tr	0	2	22	—	—	26	17	240	20	5
sweet in heavy syrup	½ cup	107	tr	tr	0	1	27	—	—	12	3	187	—	5
sweet in light syrup	½ cup	85	tr	tr	0	1	22	—	—	12	3	186	—	5
sweet juice packed	½ cup	68	tr	tr	0	1	17	—	—	17	3	163	—	3
sweet water packed	½ cup	57	tr	tr	0	1	15	—	—	13	2	162	—	3
DEL MONTE														
Dark Pitted In Heavy Syrup	½ cup (4.2 oz)	100	0	0	0	1	24	24	1	0	10	—	—	4
DRIED														
bing unsulfured	¼ cup	130	0	0	0	0	31	21	2	20	10	—	—	0
montmorency tart pitted	⅓ cup	160	1	0	0	2	36	24	2	20	0	—	—	0
rainier unsulfured	⅓ cup	140	1	0	0	1	32	30	2	20	0	—	—	6
yogurt covered	¼ cup	170	6	6	0	1	29	22	5	40	20	—	—	0
FRESH														
sour	1 cup	51	tr	tr	0	1	13	—	—	16	3	178	8	10
sweet	10	49	1	tr	0	1	11	—	—	10	0	152	3	5
CHIQUITA														
Cherries	21	90	1	0	0	2	22	19	9	20	0	—	—	9
SUPER CHERRY														
Rainier	21	90	0	0	0	1	19	14	3	20	0	—	—	6
FROZEN														
dark sweet unsweetened	1 cup	110	1	0	0	1	25	20	3	0	0	—	—	1
sour unsweetened	1 cup	72	1	tr	0	1	17	—	—	20	1	192	7	3
sweet sweetened	1 cup	232	tr	tr	0	3	58	—	—	31	3	514	—	3
CHERRY JUICE														
CAPRI SUN														
Wild Cherry Drink	1 pkg (7 oz)	100	0	0	0	0	30	30	0	0	20	25	—	0
EDEN														
Montmorency Juice	8 oz	140	1	0	0	1	33	25	0	20	30	370	—	0

FOOD	PORTION	CALS	FAT	SAT FAT	CHOL	PROT	CARB	SUGAR	FIBER	CALCI	SOD	POTAS	FOLIC	VIT C
JUICY JUICE														
Drink	1 box (4.23 oz)	70	0	0	0	0	17	16	0	0	10	90	—	60
Drink	1 box (8.5 oz)	140	0	0	0	0	34	32	0	0	15	190	—	78
KOOL-AID														
Black Cherry Drink as prep w/ sugar	1 serv (8 oz)	100	0	0	0	0	25	25	0	0	15	0	—	6
Bursts Cherry Drink	1 (7 oz)	100	0	0	0	0	25	25	0	0	30	15	—	0
Cherry as prep	1 serv (8 oz)	60	0	0	0	0	16	16	0	0	0	0	—	6
Splash Drink	1 serv (8 oz)	110	0	0	0	0	29	29	0	0	35	15	—	0
Sugar Free Drink Mix as prep	1 serv (8 oz)	5	0	0	0	0	0	0	0	0	5	0	—	6
MOTT'S														
Cherry	1 box (8 oz)	120	0	0	0	0	31	—	—	—	15	—	—	—
OCEAN SPRAY														
Black Cherry	8 oz	140	0	0	0	0	33	33	0	—	35	0	—	60
SQUEEZIT														
Cherry Cola	1 bottle (7 oz)	110	0	0	0	0	27	25	0	0	0	—	—	0
Chucklin' Cherry	1 bottle (7 oz)	110	0	0	0	0	28	26	0	0	0	—	—	0
VERYFINE														
Juice-Ups	8 fl oz	130	0	0	0	0	33	33	0	0	15	—	—	60
CHERVIL														
seed	1 tsp	1	tr	—	0	tr	tr	—	—	8	tr	28	—	—
CHESTNUTS														
chinese cooked	1 oz	44	tr	tr	0	1	10	—	—	3	1	87	—	—
chinese dried	1 oz	103	tr	tr	0	2	23	—	—	8	2	206	—	—
chinese raw	1 oz	64	tr	tr	0	1	14	—	—	5	1	127	—	10
chinese roasted	1 oz	68	tr	tr	0	1	15	—	—	5	1	135	—	—
cooked	1 oz	37	tr	tr	0	1	8	—	—	13	8	203	—	—
creme de marrons	1 oz	73	tr	tr	0	1	18	10	1	4	1	49	9	0
dried peeled	1 oz	105	1	tr	0	1	22	—	—	18	11	281	—	—
japanese cooked	1 oz	16	tr	tr	0	tr	4	—	—	3	1	34	—	—
japanese dried	1 oz	102	tr	tr	0	1	23	—	—	20	10	218	—	17
japanese raw	1 oz	44	tr	tr	0	1	10	—	—	9	4	94	—	8
japanese roasted	1 oz	57	tr	tr	0	1	13	—	—	10	—	—	—	8
raw peeled	1 oz	56	tr	tr	0	tr	13	—	—	5	1	137	—	—
roasted	1 cup	350	3	1	0	5	76	—	—	42	3	846	100	37
roasted	2 to 3 (1 oz)	70	1	tr	0	1	15	—	—	8	1	168	10	7
CHEWING GUM														
bubble gum	1 block (8 g)	27	0	0	0	0	8	—	—	—	0	0	—	0
stick	1 (3 g)	10	0	0	0	0	3	—	—	—	0	0	—	0
AQUAFRESH														
Peppermint	2 pieces	5	0	0	0	0	2	—	—	—	0	—	—	—

FOOD	PORTION	CALS	FAT	SAT FAT	CHOL	PROT	CARB	SUGAR	FIBER	CALCI	SOD	POTAS	FOLIC	VIT C
ARM & HAMMER														
Dental Care Spearmint or Peppermint	2 pieces (2.5 g)	5	0	0	0	0	2	—	—	40	30	—	—	—
CAREFREE														
Koolerz Lemonaide	1 piece	5	0	0	0	0	2	0	0	—	0	—	—	—
DENTYNE														
Ice Peppermint	2 pieces (3 g)	5	0	0	0	0	2	0	—	—	0	—	—	—
DOUBLEMINT														
Chewing Gum	1 piece	10	tr	—	0	tr	2	—	—	—	0	—	—	—
ECLIPSE														
Spearmint	2 pieces	5	0	0	0	0	2	—	—	—	0	—	—	—
EXTRA SUGAR FREE														
Cinnamon	1 piece	8	tr	—	0	tr	tr	—	—	—	0	—	—	—
Winter Fresh	1 piece	8	tr	—	0	tr	tr	—	—	—	0	—	—	—
GLEE GUM														
Peppermint	2 pieces (2.5 g)	5	0	0	0	0	2	2	—	—	0	—	—	—
HUBBA BUBBA														
Bubble Gum Cola	1 piece	23	tr	—	0	tr	6	—	—	—	0	—	—	—
Bubble Gum Sugarfree Grape	1 piece	13	tr	—	0	tr	tr	—	—	—	0	—	—	—
Bubble Gum Sugarfree Original	1 piece	14	tr	—	0	tr	tr	—	—	—	0	—	—	—
Original	1 piece	23	tr	—	0	tr	6	—	—	—	0	—	—	—
Strawberry Grape Raspberry	1 piece	23	tr	—	0	tr	6	—	—	—	0	—	—	—
LANCE														
Big Red Cinnamon	1 piece (3 g)	10	0	0	0	0	2	2	0	0	0	0	—	0
Double Bubble	1 piece (7 g)	25	0	0	0	0	6	5	0	0	0	6	—	0
Double Mint	1 piece (3 g)	10	0	0	0	0	2	2	0	0	0	0	—	0
SPEAKEASY														
Natural Rainforest All Flavors	2 pieces	10	0	0	0	5	2	2	—	—	5	—	—	—
WINTERFRESH														
Stick	1 stick (3 g)	10	0	0	0	0	2	2	—	—	0	—	—	—
WRIGLEY'S														
Orbit	1 piece	5	0	0	0	0	1	—	—	—	0	—	—	—
Spearmint	1 stick	10	tr	—	0	tr	2	—	—	—	0	—	—	—
XYLICHEW														
Licorice	2 pieces	4	0	0	0	0	2	0	0	—	0	—	—	—
CHIA SEEDS														
dried	1 oz	134	7	3	0	5	14	—	—	150	—	—	—	—

CHICKEN

(*see also* CHICKEN DISHES, CHICKEN SUBSTITUTES, DINNER, HOT DOG)

FOOD	PORTION	CALS	FAT	SAT FAT	CHOL	PROT	CARB	SUGAR	FIBER	CALCI	SOD	POTAS	FOLIC	VIT C
CANNED														
chicken spread	1 oz	55	3	—	—	4	2	—	—	35	—	—	—	—
chicken spread	1 tbsp	25	2	—	—	2	1	—	—	16	—	—	—	—
chicken spread barbeque flavored	1 oz	55	3	—	—	4	2	—	—	35	—	—	—	1
w/ broth	1 can (5 oz)	234	11	3	—	31	0	—	—	20	714	196	—	3
w/ broth	½ can (2.5 oz)	117	6	2	—	15	0	—	—	10	357	98	—	1
FRESH														
broiler/fryer breast w/ skin batter dipped & fried	2.9 oz	218	11	3	72	21	8	—	—	17	231	169	5	0
broiler/fryer breast w/ skin batter dipped & fried	½ breast (4.9 oz)	364	18	5	119	35	13	—	—	28	385	282	8	0
broiler/fryer breast w/ skin roasted	2 oz	115	5	1	49	17	0	—	—	8	41	142	2	0
broiler/fryer breast w/ skin roasted	½ breast (3.4 oz)	193	8	2	83	29	0	—	—	14	69	240	3	0
broiler/fryer breast w/ skin stewed	½ breast (3.9 oz)	202	8	2	83	30	0	—	—	14	68	195	3	0
broiler/fryer breast w/o skin fried	½ breast (3 oz)	161	4	1	78	29	tr	—	—	14	68	237	4	0
broiler/fryer breast w/o skin roasted	½ breast (3 oz)	142	3	1	73	27	0	—	—	13	63	220	3	0
broiler/fryer breast w/o skin stewed	2 oz	86	2	tr	44	17	0	—	—	7	36	107	2	0
broiler/fryer drumstick w/ skin batter dipped & fried	1 (2.6 oz)	193	11	3	62	16	6	—	—	12	194	134	6	0
broiler/fryer drumstick w/ skin floured & fried	1 (1.7 oz)	120	7	2	44	13	1	—	—	6	44	112	4	0
broiler/fryer drumstick w/ skin roasted	1 (1.8 oz)	112	6	2	48	14	0	—	—	6	47	119	4	0
broiler/fryer drumstick w/ skin stewed	1 (2 oz)	116	6	2	48	14	0	—	—	7	43	105	4	0
broiler/fryer drumstick w/o skin fried	1 (1.5 oz)	82	3	1	40	12	0	—	—	5	40	105	4	0

FOOD	PORTION	CALS	FAT	SAT FAT	CHOL	PROT	CARB	SUGAR	FIBER	CALCI	SOD	POTAS	FOLIC	VIT C
broiler/fryer drumstick w/o skin roasted	1 (1.5 oz)	76	2	1	41	12	0	—	—	5	42	108	4	0
broiler/fryer drumstick w/o skin stewed	1 (1.6 oz)	78	3	1	40	13	0	—	—	5	37	92	4	0
broiler/fryer leg w/ skin batter dipped & fried	1 (5.5 oz)	431	26	7	142	34	14	—	—	28	442	299	14	0
broiler/fryer leg w/ skin floured & fried	1 (3.9 oz)	285	16	4	105	30	3	—	—	15	99	261	9	0
broiler/fryer leg w/ skin roasted	1 (4 oz)	265	15	4	105	30	0	—	—	14	99	256	8	0
broiler/fryer leg w/ skin stewed	1 (4.4 oz)	275	16	4	105	30	0	—	—	14	92	220	8	0
broiler/fryer leg w/o skin fried	1 (3.3 oz)	195	9	2	93	27	1	—	—	12	90	239	8	0
broiler/fryer leg w/o skin roasted	1 (3.3 oz)	182	8	2	89	26	0	—	—	12	87	230	8	0
broiler/fryer leg w/o skin stewed	1 (3.5 oz)	187	8	2	90	26	0	—	—	11	78	192	8	0
broiler/fryer neck w/ skin stewed	1 (1.3 oz)	94	7	2	27	7	0	—	—	10	20	41	1	0
broiler/fryer neck w/o skin stewed	1 (.6 oz)	32	1	tr	14	4	0	—	—	8	12	25	tr	0
broiler/fryer skin batter dipped & fried	from ½ chicken (6.7 oz)	748	55	14	140	20	44	—	—	49	1105	143	17	0
broiler/fryer skin floured & fried	from ½ chicken (2 oz)	281	24	7	41	24	5	—	—	8	30	70	2	0
broiler/fryer skin roasted	from ½ chicken (2 oz)	254	23	6	46	11	0	—	—	8	36	76	1	0
broiler/fryer skin stewed	from ½ chicken (2.5 oz)	261	24	7	45	11	0	—	—	9	40	84	1	0
broiler/fryer thigh w/ skin batter dipped & fried	1 (3 oz)	238	14	4	80	19	8	—	—	16	248	165	8	0
broiler/fryer thigh w/ skin floured & fried	1 (2.2 oz)	162	9	3	60	17	2	—	—	8	55	147	5	0
broiler/fryer thigh w/ skin roasted	1 (2.2 oz)	153	10	3	58	16	0	—	—	8	52	137	4	0
broiler/fryer thigh w/ skin stewed	1 (2.4 oz)	158	10	3	57	16	0	—	—	8	49	115	4	0

FOOD	PORTION	CALS	FAT	SAT FAT	CHOL	PROT	CARB	SUGAR	FIBER	CALCI	SOD	POTAS	FOLIC	VIT C
broiler/fryer thigh w/o skin fried	1 (1.8 oz)	113	5	1	53	15	1	—	—	7	49	134	4	0
broiler/fryer thigh w/o skin roasted	1 (1.8 oz)	109	6	2	49	13	0	—	—	6	46	124	4	0
broiler/fryer thigh w/o skin stewed	1 (1.9 oz)	107	5	1	49	14	0	—	—	6	41	101	4	0
broiler/fryer w/ skin floured & fried	½ chicken (11 oz)	844	47	13	283	90	10	—	—	52	264	735	20	0
broiler/fryer w/ skin fried	½ chicken (16.4 oz)	1347	81	22	404	81	44	—	—	97	1360	863	35	0
broiler/fryer w/ skin roasted	½ chicken (10.5 oz)	715	41	11	263	82	0	—	—	45	244	667	16	0
broiler/fryer w/ skin stewed	½ chicken (11.7 oz)	730	42	12	262	82	0	—	—	44	224	556	16	0
broiler/fryer w/ skin neck & giblets batter dipped & fried	1 chicken (2.3 lbs)	2987	180	48	1054	235	93	—	—	218	2921	1951	241	4
broiler/fryer w/ skin neck & giblets roasted	1 chicken (1.5 lbs)	1598	90	25	730	183	tr	—	—	105	536	1447	201	4
broiler/fryer w/ skin neck & giblets stewed	1 chicken (1.6 lbs)	1625	93	26	726	184	tr	—	—	104	494	1224	200	4
broiler/fryer w/o skin fried	1 cup	307	13	3	131	43	2	—	—	24	127	360	10	0
broiler/fryer w/o skin roasted	1 cup (5 oz)	266	10	3	125	41	0	—	—	21	120	340	8	0
broiler/fryer w/o skin stewed	1 oz	54	3	1	22	7	0	—	—	6	18	41	2	0
broiler/fryer w/o skin stewed	1 cup (5 oz)	248	9	3	116	38	0	—	—	19	98	252	8	0
broiler/fryer wing w/ skin batter dipped & fried	1 (1.7 oz)	159	11	3	39	10	5	—	—	10	157	68	3	0
broiler/fryer wing w/ skin floured & fried	1 (1.1 oz)	103	7	2	26	8	1	—	—	5	25	57	1	0
broiler/fryer wing w/ skin roasted	1 (1.2 oz)	99	7	2	29	9	0	—	—	5	28	62	1	0
broiler/fryer wing w/ skin stewed	1 (1.4 oz)	100	7	2	28	9	0	—	—	5	27	56	1	0
capon w/ skin neck & giblets roasted	1 chicken (3.1 lbs)	3211	165	46	1458	402	1	—	—	211	704	3439	367	6
cornish hen w/ skin roasted	1 hen (8 oz)	595	42	12	299	51	0	—	—	31	146	562	5	1

FOOD	PORTION	CALS	FAT	SAT FAT	CHOL	PROT	CARB	SUGAR	FIBER	CALCI	SOD	POTAS	FOLIC	VIT C
cornish hen w/o skin & bone roasted	1 hen (3.8 oz)	144	4	1	113	25	0	—	—	14	67	268	2	1
cornish hen w/o skin & bone roasted	½ hen (2 oz)	72	2	1	57	13	0	—	—	7	34	134	1	tr
cornish hen w/skin roasted	½ hen (4 oz)	296	21	6	149	25	0	—	—	15	73	280	3	1
roaster dark meat w/o skin roasted	1 cup (5 oz)	250	12	3	104	33	0	—	—	15	133	313	9	0
roaster light meat w/o skin roasted	1 cup (5 oz)	214	6	2	105	38	0	—	—	18	71	330	5	0
roaster w/ skin neck & giblets roasted	1 chicken (2.4 lbs)	2363	140	39	1003	257	1	—	—	136	760	2183	251	4
roaster w/ skin roasted	½ chicken (1.1 lbs)	1071	64	18	365	115	0	—	—	58	349	1014	22	0
roaster w/o skin roasted	1 cup (5 oz)	469	28	3	160	9	0	—	—	25	105	321	7	0
stewing dark meat w/o skin stewed	1 cup (5 oz)	361	21	6	132	39	0	—	—	17	133	285	12	0
stewing w/ skin neck & giblets stewed	1 chicken (1.3 lbs)	1636	107	29	603	157	tr	—	—	78	419	1052	211	3
stewing w/ skin stewed	½ chicken (9.2 oz)	744	49	13	205	70	0	—	—	33	190	476	13	0
stewing w/ skin stewed	6.2 oz	507	34	9	140	34	0	—	—	22	130	325	9	0
AMISH SELECT														
Boneless Skinless Breast w/ Honey Dijon Mustard	1 serv (4 oz)	130	2	0	60	24	4	3	0	40	390	—	—	0
MURRAY'S														
Breast Boneless & Skinless	4 oz	110	1	0	70	26	0	0	0	0	50	—	—	0
Ground	3 oz	130	7	2	90	17	0	0	0	—	55	—	—	—
Whole Lean	4 oz	170	9	3	90	21	0	0	0	0	75	—	—	0
PERDUE														
Boneless Skinless Breasts Cooked	3 oz	110	2	tr	70	25	0	—	—	—	30	—	—	—
Boneless Breast Roasted Garlic Herb	1 piece (3 oz)	90	1	—	50	18	3	—	—	—	620	—	—	1
Breaded Breast Strips Barbecue	3 oz	120	1	—	30	12	16	4	—	80	720	—	—	—
Breaded Breast Strips Hot & Spicy	3 oz	110	1	—	30	12	13	1	—	80	930	—	—	2

FOOD	PORTION	CALS	FAT	SAT FAT	CHOL	PROT	CARB	SUGAR	FIBER	CALCI	SOD	POTAS	FOLIC	VIT C
PERDUE (CONT.)														
Breaded Breast Strips Original	3 oz	120	1	—	35	14	14	1	—	100	750	—	—	—
Burger Cooked	1 (3 oz)	160	10	3	110	17	0	—	—	—	55	—	—	—
Chicken Breast Seasoned Italian Cooked	1 piece (3 oz)	90	1	tr	50	18	3	1	—	—	610	—	—	1
Chicken Breast Seasoned Teriyaki Cooked	1 piece (3 oz)	90	1	tr	50	18	3	1	—	—	560	—	—	0
Ground Cooked	3 oz	170	11	4	125	18	0	—	—	40	50	—	—	—
Ground Breast Cooked	3 oz	80	1	—	55	19	0	—	—	—	60	—	—	—
Honey Rotisserie Dark Meat	3 oz	200	16	5	80	12	1	1	—	—	300	—	—	2
Honey Rotisserie White Meat	3 oz	140	8	3	70	19	1	1	—	—	290	—	—	0
Oven Stuffer Dark Meat Roasted	3 oz	210	15	5	100	18	0	—	—	—	60	—	—	—
Oven Stuffer Drumstick Roasted	1 (3.6 oz)	190	11	4	120	22	0	—	—	—	100	—	—	—
Oven Stuffer White Meat Roasted	3 oz	170	9	3	80	21	0	—	—	—	50	—	—	—
Oven Stuffer Wingette Roasted	3 (3.4 oz)	220	15	5	120	21	0	—	—	—	80	—	—	—
Ovenables Breast Lemon Pepper Cooked	1 piece (3 oz)	90	1	—	50	18	2	—	—	—	380	—	—	1
Seasoned Roasting Chicken Toasted Garlic Dark Meat	3 oz	190	14	4	100	16	1	—	—	20	330	—	—	—
Seasoned Roasting Chicken Toasted Garlic White Meat	3 oz	160	9	3	75	19	1	—	—	0	320	—	—	—
Seasoned Strips Parmesan Garlic cooked	3 oz	100	2	1	55	20	2	—	—	20	710	—	—	1
Seasoned Strips Savory Classic cooked	3 oz	90	1	tr	55	19	1	0	—	—	500	—	—	0
Seasoned Strips Spicy Fiesta cooked	3 oz	140	7	2	75	16	3	1	—	—	630	—	—	4

FOOD	PORTION	CALS	FAT	SAT FAT	CHOL	PROT	CARB	SUGAR	FIBER	CALCI	SOD	POTAS	FOLIC	VIT C
PERDUE (CONT.)														
Split Breast Cooked	1 piece (6.8 oz)	370	20	6	180	48	0	—	—	20	100	—	—	—
Thin Sliced Breast Rosemary Garlic Thyme	1 piece (3 oz)	90	2	1	60	20	1	—	—	—	820	—	—	—
Thin Sliced Breast Tomato Herb	1 piece (3 oz)	90	2	—	60	20	1	—	—	—	740	—	—	—
Whole Dark Meat cooked	3 oz	150	16	5	110	17	0	—	—	—	55	—	—	—
Whole White Meat Cooked	3 oz	170	10	3	85	21	0	—	0	—	45	—	—	—
Wings Roasted	2 (3.2 oz)	210	15	5	115	19	0	—	—	—	75	—	—	—
TYSON														
Broth Marinated Breast Filet	1 (4.7 oz)	140	4	1	70	26	0	0	0	0	330	—	—	0
Broth Marinated Drums	2 (4 oz)	140	7	2	90	17	0	0	0	0	290	—	—	0
Broth Marinated Thighs	1 (4.9 oz)	380	34	10	110	17	1	1	0	0	350	—	—	0
Broth Marinated Wings	4 pieces (4.2 oz)	240	18	5	95	20	0	0	0	20	340	—	—	0
Chicken Broccoli & Cheese	1 piece (5.9 oz)	320	16	5	50	20	23	3	3	60	670	—	—	0
Chicken Stuffed w/ Wild Rice & Mushroom	1 piece (5.9 oz)	300	12	3	50	23	25	4	1	40	860	—	—	0
Cordon Bleu	1 piece (5.9 oz)	350	17	6	55	25	24	3	3	150	640	—	—	0
Cornish Hen	1 serv (4 oz)	180	12	4	130	18	0	0	0	20	65	—	—	0
Kiev	1 piece (5.9 oz)	460	32	16	115	20	24	3	2	40	570	—	—	0
WAMPLER														
Breast Tenders	4 oz	130	2	1	70	27	0	—	—	20	55	—	—	—
FROZEN														
BANQUET														
Breast Nuggets	7	280	20	5	40	13	11	2	1	0	500	—	—	0
Breast Patties Grilled Honey BBQ	1	110	5	2	40	13	3	2	0	40	440	—	—	0
Breast Patties Grilled Honey Mustard	1	120	5	2	25	13	5	3	0	40	500	—	—	0
Breast Tenders Our Original	3	250	15	4	40	12	15	1	tr	0	480	—	—	1
Breast Tenders Southern	3 pieces	260	16	4	40	12	16	1	1	0	460	—	—	1

FOOD	PORTION	CALS	FAT	SAT FAT	CHOL	PROT	CARB	SUGAR	FIBER	CALCI	SOD	POTAS	FOLIC	VIT C
BANQUET (CONT.)														
Country Fried	1 serv (3 oz)	270	18	5	65	14	13	1	1	80	620	—	—	4
Fat Free Baked Breast Patties	1	100	0	0	20	9	15	3	1	0	400	—	—	0
Fried Our Original	1 serv (3 oz)	280	18	5	65	14	15	1	1	20	830	—	—	4
Honey BBQ Skinless Fried	1 serv (3 oz)	230	13	3	55	18	9	1	1	20	480	—	—	2
Hot 'n Spicy Fried	1 serv (3 oz)	260	18	5	65	14	13	1	1	20	730	—	—	4
Nuggets Our Original	6	270	19	4	35	14	12	2	1	0	540	—	—	0
Nuggets Southern Fried	5	270	18	4	35	12	16	4	2	20	570	—	—	1
Patties Our Orignal	1	190	14	3	30	7	10	2	1	0	440	—	—	0
Patties Southern Fried	1	190	12	3	25	8	10	tr	tr	0	430	—	—	1
Skinless Fried	1 serv (3 oz)	220	13	3	65	18	7	1	2	20	480	—	—	2
Smokehouse Big Wings	2	200	17	4	70	14	4	3	0	0	300	—	—	0
Southern Fried	1 serv (3 oz)	280	18	5	65	14	15	1	1	40	700	—	—	4
Wings Firehouse Big	2	190	14	4	70	14	1	0	0	0	650	—	—	0
Wings Honey BBQ	4	380	24	10	70	31	15	4	1	40	570	—	—	1
Wings Hot & Spicy	4 pieces	280	20	5	90	18	9	0	tr	20	450	—	—	1
BELL & EVANS														
Breaded Breast Nuggets	1 serv (4 oz)	190	6	1	45	20	13	1	1	20	440	—	—	0
Breaded Whole Breast Tenders	1 (4 oz)	190	6	1	45	20	13	1	1	20	440	—	—	0
Burgers	1 (3 oz)	120	6	2	85	16	tr	0	0	0	130	—	—	0
Chicken Sandwich Steaks	1 serv (2 oz)	60	1	tr	40	14	tr	0	0	0	25	—	—	0
COUNTRY SKILLET														
Bites	5	270	16	3	20	12	18	2	1	20	720	—	—	0
Breast Tenders	3	240	14	4	25	11	16	1	1	20	450	—	—	0
Chunks	5	270	18	3	20	12	18	2	1	20	720	—	—	0
Fried	3 oz	270	18	5	65	14	13	1	1	80	620	—	—	4
Nuggets	10	280	17	4	25	14	16	2	1	20	610	—	—	0
Patties	1	190	12	3	20	9	12	3	1	0	490	—	—	0
Southern Fried Chunks	5	270	18	4	20	11	17	4	1	20	550	—	—	0
Southern Fried Patties	1	190	12	3	20	9	12	3	1	0	440	—	—	1

FOOD	PORTION	CALS	FAT	SAT FAT	CHOL	PROT	CARB	SUGAR	FIBER	CALCI	SOD	POTAS	FOLIC	VIT C
HEALTH IS WEALTH														
Nuggets	4 (3 oz)	150	6	2	40	14	9	0	0	20	180	—	—	0
Patties	1 (3 oz)	150	6	2	40	13	9	0	0	20	180	—	—	0
Tenders	3 (3 oz)	130	3	1	35	14	11	0	0	20	230	—	—	0
KID CUISINE														
Dino Mite Nuggets	4 pieces	300	23	6	40	11	10	3	1	0	540	—	—	0
Radical Racin' Nuggets w/ Cheese	4 pieces	300	23	7	35	11	12	3	tr	60	620	—	—	0
WEAVER														
Breast Strips	3 pieces (3.3 oz)	210	11	2	35	14	13	1	2	0	430	—	—	0
Breast Tenders	5 pieces (3 oz)	220	15	3	35	14	8	0	1	0	290	—	—	0
Croquettes	1 serv (3.5 oz)	290	18	5	45	11	22	4	2	80	540	—	—	0
Dutch Frye Nuggets	5 pieces (3.3 oz)	280	20	5	45	14	12	0	2	20	410	—	—	0
Honey Battered Tenders	5 pieces (2.9 oz)	230	15	3	35	12	12	3	1	0	380	—	—	0
Hot Wings Buffalo Style	3 pieces (2.7 oz)	190	13	4	95	18	0	0	0	20	370	—	—	0
Mini Drums Crispy	5 pieces (3.3 oz)	250	16	3	40	14	14	2	1	20	410	—	—	0
Nuggets	4 pieces (2.7 oz)	210	15	4	35	11	9	0	1	0	360	—	—	0
Patties	1 (2.6 oz)	180	11	3	30	10	10	1	1	20	430	—	—	0
Rondelet	1 (2.6 oz)	170	10	3	20	10	10	1	1	20	410	—	—	0
Rondelet Dutch Frye	1 (2.6 oz)	230	16	4	35	11	10	1	1	0	360	—	—	0
Rondelet Italian	1 (2.6 oz)	210	14	3	20	10	12	1	1	60	470	—	—	0
READY-TO-EAT														
chicken roll light meat	2 oz	90	4	1	28	11	1	—	—	24	331	129	—	—
chicken roll light meat	1 pkg (6 oz)	271	13	3	85	33	4	—	—	73	992	388	—	—
poultry salad sandwich spread	1 oz	238	4	1	9	3	2	—	—	3	107	52	1	0
poultry salad sandwich spread	1 tbsp (13 g)	109	2	tr	4	2	1	—	—	1	49	24	1	0
BANQUET														
Fat Free Baked Breast Tenders	3	120	0	0	30	13	16	0	2	0	480	—	—	0
BOAR'S HEAD														
Breast Hickory Smoked	2 oz	60	1	0	30	11	tr	0	0	0	440	—	—	0
Breast Oven Roasted	2 oz	50	1	0	30	11	tr	0	0	0	420	—	—	0

FOOD	PORTION	CALS	FAT	SAT FAT	CHOL	PROT	CARB	SUGAR	FIBER	CALCI	SOD	POTAS	FOLIC	VIT C
BOAR'S HEAD (CONT.)														
Breast Bar B Q Sauce Basted	2 oz	60	1	0	30	11	3	1	0	0	490	—	—	0
BUTTERBALL														
Crispy Baked Breasts Italian Style Herb	1 piece (0.5 oz)	190	6	2	55	17	16	0	1	0	710	—	—	1
Crispy Baked Breasts Lemon Pepper	1 piece (0.5 oz)	200	7	3	50	16	16	2	tr	0	420	—	—	1
Crispy Baked Breasts Original	1 piece (0.5 oz)	180	6	2	45	16	16	2	1	0	500	—	—	0
Crispy Baked Breasts Parmesan	1 piece (0.5 oz)	200	7	3	55	17	16	5	tr	20	650	—	—	1
Crispy Baked Breasts Southwestern	1 piece (0.5 oz)	170	6	2	35	17	13	0	2	0	590	—	—	1
Tenders Baked Breast	3 pieces	170	6	2	35	14	15	2	1	0	410	—	—	0
Tenders Hickory Smoked Grilled	4 pieces + sauce	160	5	2	50	17	12	9	1	20	570	—	—	2
Tenders Oriental Grilled	4 pieces + sauce	160	5	2	45	17	12	10	1	0	560	—	—	1
CARL BUDDIG														
Chicken Sliced	1 pkg (2.5 oz)	110	7	2	40	12	1	1	—	20	680	—	—	—
Lean Slices Honey Smoked Breast	1 pkg (2.5 oz)	70	1	1	30	12	3	3	—	—	630	—	—	—
Lean Slices Roasted Breast	1 pkg (2.5 oz)	60	1	1	30	13	1	1	—	—	630	—	—	—
CHICKEN BY GEORGE														
Cajun	1 breast (4 oz)	130	4	1	60	21	3	0	0	0	700	—	—	1
Caribbean Grill	1 breast (4 oz)	150	4	1	60	22	8	6	0	0	550	—	—	2
Garlic & Herb	1 breast (4 oz)	120	3	1	60	21	3	1	0	0	600	—	—	0
Italian Bleu Cheese	1 breast (4 oz)	130	5	1	60	20	2	0	0	20	790	—	—	1
Lemon Herb	1 breast (4 oz)	120	3	1	60	20	3	2	0	0	800	—	—	1
Lemon Oregano	1 breast (4 oz)	130	4	1	50	20	3	1	0	0	600	—	—	2
Mesquite Barbecue	1 breast (4 oz)	130	3	1	60	21	5	3	0	0	700	—	—	1
Mustard Dill	1 breast (4 oz)	140	5	1	60	20	2	1	0	20	650	—	—	1
Roasted	1 breast (4 oz)	110	3	1	55	20	1	0	0	0	500	—	—	1
Teriyaki	1 breast (4 oz)	130	3	1	55	21	6	4	0	0	530	—	—	1
Tomato Herb With Basil	1 breast (4 oz)	140	5	1	60	20	5	4	0	0	630	—	—	1
HILLSHIRE FARM														
Smoked Breast	6 slices (2 oz)	60	1	0	25	11	2	1	0	0	600	—	—	0

FOOD	PORTION	CALS	FAT	SAT FAT	CHOL	PROT	CARB	SUGAR	FIBER	CALCI	SOD	POTAS	FOLIC	VIT C
LOUIS RICH														
Carving Board Classic Baked	2 slices (1.6 oz)	45	1	0	25	9	2	0	0	0	510	—	—	0
Carving Board Grilled	2 slices (1.6 oz)	45	1	0	25	9	2	0	0	0	510	—	—	0
Deli-Thin Oven Roasted Breast	4 slices (1.8 oz)	50	1	1	25	10	1	tr	0	0	620	—	—	0
Oven Roasted Deluxe Breast	1 slice (1 oz)	30	1	0	15	5	1	0	0	0	330	—	—	0
OSCAR MAYER														
Free Oven Roasted Breast	4 slices (1.8 oz)	45	0	0	25	10	1	tr	0	0	650	—	—	0
PERDUE														
Breast Cutlets Homestyle	1 (2.9 oz)	110	1	—	35	14	12	—	—	—	730	—	—	—
Breast Cutlets Italian Style	1 (2.9 oz)	120	2	1	40	15	11	—	—	—	690	—	—	1
Breast Filets In Barbecue Sauce	1 piece + 3 tbsp sauce (5.9 oz)	200	1	—	70	24	24	23	—	—	1100	—	—	9
Breast Strips In Garlic & Herb Sauce	1 serv (5 oz)	100	1	—	50	18	4	1	2	—	1010	—	—	—
Breast Strips In Marinara Sauce	1 serv (5 oz)	120	3	1	50	18	5	1	—	20	1130	—	—	9
Breast Strips In Teriyaki Sauce	1 serv (5 oz)	190	1	—	50	20	26	22	—	—	1660	—	—	—
Carved Breast Honey Roasted	½ cup (2.5 oz)	100	2	1	45	18	2	1	—	—	450	—	—	—
Carved Breast Original Roasted	½ cup (2.5 oz)	90	2	1	50	19	1	—	—	—	500	—	—	—
Cutlets Cooked	1 (3.5 oz)	220	11	3	55	15	15	—	—	—	600	—	—	—
Nuggets	5 (3.4 oz)	210	11	3	50	15	15	—	—	—	580	—	—	—
Nuggets Chicken & Cheese	5 (3.4 oz)	230	13	5	55	15	15	—	—	60	670	—	—	—
Short Cuts Entrees In Teriyaki Sauce	5 oz	190	1	—	50	20	26	22	—	—	1660	—	—	—
Short Cuts Grilled Italian	½ cup	80	1	—	40	15	4	1	—	—	500	—	—	4
Short Cuts Lemon Pepper	½ cup (2.5 oz)	100	3	1	60	19	1	—	—	—	490	—	—	—
Short Cuts Southwestern	½ cup (2.5 oz)	100	3	1	60	18	1	—	—	—	410	—	—	—
SHADY BROOK														
Slow Roasted Breast	2 oz	60	1	0	30	12	—	—	—	—	400	—	—	—
TYSON														
Breaded Breast Chunks	6 pieces (2.9 oz)	230	16	5	20	9	13	0	1	0	440	—	—	0

FOOD	PORTION	CALS	FAT	SAT FAT	CHOL	PROT	CARB	SUGAR	FIBER	CALCI	SOD	POTAS	FOLIC	VIT C
TYSON (CONT.)														
Breaded Breast Fillet	2 pieces (2.8 oz)	180	8	2	25	12	15	0	1	20	440	—	—	0
Breaded Breast Pattie	1 (2.6 oz)	190	12	3	25	11	9	2	1	0	320	—	—	0
Breaded Breast Tenders	5 pieces (3 oz)	220	15	3	35	14	8	0	1	0	290	—	—	0
Breaded Chicken Chunks	6 pieces (3 oz)	220	14	3	40	13	11	1	0	20	480	—	—	0
Chicken Bits Southern Fried	6 pieces (2.9 oz)	260	19	5	40	11	11	0	1	20	540	—	—	0
Chicken Strips Southwestern	1 serv (3 oz)	110	3	1	40	18	2	1	0	20	400	—	—	0
Chick'n Quick Chick'n Cheddar	1 patty (2.6 oz)	220	14	4	40	11	12	1	0	60	270	—	—	0
Country Fried Chicken Fritters	5 pieces (2.9 oz)	260	18	4	40	11	13	0	1	60	470	—	—	0
Drumsticks Hot BBQ Style	2 (3.5 oz)	160	7	2	100	22	3	2	1	20	620	—	—	2
Glazed Grilled Breast Pattie	1 (2.7 oz)	120	7	2	40	12	1	0	0	0	440	—	—	0
Grilled Breast Strips	1 serv (3 oz)	120	4	1	60	21	1	—	0	0	500	—	—	0
Grilled Chicken Pattie	1 (2.9 oz)	170	12	4	55	13	1	0	0	20	340	—	—	0
Nuggets Breaded White Meat	6 pieces (2.9 oz)	250	18	5	35	11	12	0	1	20	450	—	—	0
Patties Southern Fried	1 (2.9 oz)	260	19	5	40	11	11	0	1	20	540	—	—	0
Roasted Drumsticks	3 (5.6 oz)	320	15	5	230	44	2	2	0	20	1200	—	—	0
Roasted Drumsticks w/o Skin	2 (3.3 oz)	140	5	2	120	22	1	1	0	20	730	—	—	0
Roasted Half Chicken	1 serv (3 oz)	160	11	4	75	16	1	1	0	0	490	—	—	0
Roasted Whole Chicken w/ Skin	1 serv (3 oz)	160	11	4	75	16	1	1	0	0	490	—	—	0
Roasted Breast Boneless w/o Skin	1 (3.7 oz)	130	3	1	70	26	1	1	0	20	580	—	—	0
Roasted Breast Half w/o Skin	1 (4.3 oz)	150	3	1	80	30	1	1	0	0	660	—	—	0
Roasted Half Breast w/ Skin	1 (5.1 oz)	260	13	4	110	34	1	1	0	0	670	—	—	0
Roasted Half Chicken w/o Skin	1 serv (3 oz)	120	6	2	75	17	1	1	0	0	510	—	—	0

FOOD	PORTION	CALS	FAT	SAT FAT	CHOL	PROT	CARB	SUGAR	FIBER	CALCI	SOD	POTAS	FOLIC	VIT C
TYSON (CONT.)														
Roasted Tabasco Wings	3 (3 oz)	190	13	4	100	16	1	1	1	20	520	—	—	0
Roasted Thigh w/ Skin	1 (3.6 oz)	270	21	7	120	19	1	1	0	20	650	—	—	0
Roasted Thigh w/o Skin	1 (2.9 oz)	150	8	3	95	19	1	1	0	20	560	—	—	0
Roll White Meat	2 oz	90	6	2	25	10	0	0	0	20	440	—	—	0
Southern Fried Breaded Breast Pattie	1 (2.6 oz)	180	12	3	30	11	8	0	0	0	360	—	—	0
Southern Fried Breast Fillets	2 pieces (3.4 oz)	210	11	2	30	15	14	0	1	20	480	—	—	0
Southern Fried Chunks	6 pieces (2.9 oz)	260	19	5	40	11	11	0	1	20	540	—	—	0
Tenders Breaded Honey Battered	5 pieces (2.9 oz)	230	15	3	35	12	12	3	1	0	380	—	—	0
Tenders Breaded Pattie	3 pieces (3.2 oz)	100	0	0	0	13	11	1	1	20	540	—	—	0
Thick'n Crispy Pattie	1 (2.6 oz)	200	14	3	40	10	10	1	1	20	320	—	—	0
Wings BBQ	3 pieces (3.2 oz)	200	13	4	110	19	2	2	0	20	330	—	—	1
Wings Hot N'Spicy	4 (3.2 oz)	210	14	4	100	18	1	0	0	20	1020	—	—	1
Wings Teriyaki	4 pieces (3.4 oz)	190	12	3	120	21	2	1	2	20	210	—	—	2
Wings Of Fire	4 pieces (3.4 oz)	220	15	4	110	20	1	0	0	20	560	—	—	0
TAKE-OUT														
oven roasted breast of chicken	2 oz	60	1	0	25	11	0	—	—	—	470	—	—	—

CHICKEN DISHES

CANNED

BUMBLE BEE

FOOD	PORTION	CALS	FAT	SAT FAT	CHOL	PROT	CARB	SUGAR	FIBER	CALCI	SOD	POTAS	FOLIC	VIT C
Chicken Salad	1 pkg (3.5 oz)	230	10	2	25	10	25	8	0	40	540	—	—	0
DINTY MOORE														
Noodles & Chicken	1 can (7.5 oz)	180	8	2	30	7	19	2	1	20	1010	—	—	0
Stew	1 cup (8.5 oz)	220	11	3	40	12	16	3	2	20	980	—	—	1
MIX														
CHICKEN SKILLET HELPER														
Stir-Fried Chicken as prep	1 cup	270	9	2	105	18	30	1	1	60	760	210	60	0

FOOD	PORTION	CALS	FAT	SAT FAT	CHOL	PROT	CARB	SUGAR	FIBER	CALCI	SOD	POTAS	FOLIC	VIT C
HAMBURGER HELPER														
Reduced Sodium Cheddar Spirals Chicken Recipe as prep	1 cup	240	6	2	40	20	27	6	0	100	630	690	60	0
Reduced Sodium Italian Herb Chicken Recipe as prep	1 cup	200	2	1	35	19	29	6	2	20	630	570	60	0
Reduced Sodium Southwestern Beef Chicken Recipe as prep	1 cup	220	3	1	35	20	32	6	2	20	600	610	60	0
TYSON														
Mandarin Wrap Kit	1½ wraps (14.6 oz)	630	15	4	50	30	92	8	5	80	1840	—	—	0
REFRIGERATED														
salad low fat	½ cup	90	2	—	20	8	9	—	—	—	440	—	—	—
LLOYD'S														
Barbecue Shredded Chicken	¼ cup (2 oz)	90	2	1	15	6	11	9	—	—	440	—	—	—
OLD EL PASO														
For Tacos Shredded Chicken	¼ cup	60	2	1	25	5	4	1	1	20	430	—	—	0
OSCAR MAYER														
Lunchables Chicken Wraps	1 pkg	440	13	5	40	17	64	25	3	300	860	—	—	60
SHADY BROOK														
Chicken Breast w/ Rice Pilaf	1 serv (12 oz)	350	13	4	120	46	—	—	—	—	270	—	—	—
Teriyaki Breast	1 serv (12 oz)	490	3	1	15	34	—	—	—	—	1600	—	—	—
TYSON														
Chicken Breast Medallions In Tomato & Herb Sauce	1 serv (5 oz)	120	4	1	40	18	5	2	0	0	640	—	—	0
WAMPLER														
Cacciatore	1 cup	260	9	—	90	30	10	—	—	—	600	—	—	—
Fajitas	1 cup	210	7	—	70	23	13	—	—	—	1360	—	—	—
Salad	⅓ cup	200	14	—	30	9	9	—	—	—	420	—	—	—
Salad Lite	⅓ cup	130	7	—	25	9	9	—	—	—	370	—	—	—
Smokey Barbecue Chicken	1 cup	430	15	—	140	42	31	—	—	—	1020	—	—	—
Sweet-n-Sour	1 cup	250	4	—	55	20	35	—	—	—	510	—	—	—

FOOD	PORTION	CALS	FAT	SAT FAT	CHOL	PROT	CARB	SUGAR	FIBER	CALCI	SOD	POTAS	FOLIC	VIT C
SHELF-STABLE														
DINTY MOORE														
Microwave Cup Chicken & Dumpling	1 pkg (7.5 oz)	200	6	2	35	15	21	1	1	20	890	—	—	0
Microwave Cup Stew	1 pkg (7.5 oz)	180	8	2	30	10	18	2	2	20	920	—	—	5
LUNCH BUCKET														
Chicken Fiesta	1 pkg (7.5 oz)	160	2	1	5	6	30	6	5	20	530	—	—	0
Dumplings'n Chicken	1 pkg (7.5 oz)	140	5	2	10	5	21	2	1	20	780	—	—	0
TASTYBITE														
Chicken Moglai	1 pkg (9.5 oz)	300	16	3	45	21	20	5	3	100	1080	—	—	9
TAKE-OUT														
boneless breaded & fried w/ barbecue sauce	6 pieces (4.6 oz)	330	18	6	61	17	25	—	—	21	830	319	28	tr
boneless breaded & fried w/ honey	6 pieces (4 oz)	339	18	5	61	17	27	—	—	17	537	255	11	tr
boneless breaded & fried w/ mustard sauce	6 pieces (4.6 oz)	323	17	6	62	17	21	—	—	25	791	280	12	tr
boneless breaded & fried w/ sweet & sour sauce	6 pieces (4.6 oz)	346	18	6	61	17	29	—	—	20	791	280	12	tr
boneless breast w/ apple stuffing	1 serv (5 oz)	260	9	2	80	32	10	2	1	30	250	—	—	1
breast & wing breaded & fried	2 pieces (5.7 oz)	494	30	8	149	36	20	—	—	60	975	566	9	0
b'stilla chicken pie	1 serv	926	227	21	64	—	—	—	—	—	1242	—	—	—
chicken & dumplings	¾ cup	256	12	4	109	23	12	—	tr	61	1283	163	10	4
chicken & noodles	1 cup	365	18	5	103	22	26	—	—	26	600	149	—	tr
chicken à la king	1 cup	470	34	13	221	27	12	—	—	127	760	404	—	12
chicken cacciatore	¾ cup	394	24	6	99	33	9	—	2	45	671	149	18	40
chicken paprikash	1½ cups	296	10	—	90	—	—	—	—	99	—	—	—	—
chicken pie w/ top crust	1 slice (5.6 oz)	472	31	—	—	19	32	—	1	122	—	—	—	0
chicken cordon bleu	1 serv (5 oz)	280	13	4	70	29	10	0	0	30	800	—	—	1
drumstick breaded & fried	2 pieces (5.2 oz)	430	27	7	165	30	16	—	—	36	756	446	10	0
grilled breast strips	4 strips (3 oz)	100	2	1	50	20	0	0	0	0	310	—	—	0
groundnut stew hkatenkwan	1 serv (15.7 oz)	576	40	10	116	38	18	3	4	79	1009	973	51	21
jamaican jerk wings	4 wings (9.9 oz)	709	51	14	172	57	3	tr	tr	51	1045	402	10	4

FOOD	PORTION	CALS	FAT	SAT FAT	CHOL	PROT	CARB	SUGAR	FIBER	CALCI	SOD	POTAS	FOLIC	VIT C
TAKE-OUT (CONT.)														
kobete turkish chicken w/ pastry	1 serv	513	13	4	71	—	—	—	—	—	551	—	—	—
sancocho de pollo dominican chicken stew	1 serv	702	30	8	195	71	34	4	1	72	653	1324	52	49
souvlaki	1 serv	392	54	3	17	—	—	—	—	—	337	—	—	—
thigh breaded & fried	2 pieces (5.2 oz)	430	27	7	165	30	16	—	—	36	756	446	10	0

CHICKEN SUBSTITUTES

FOOD	PORTION	CALS	FAT	SAT FAT	CHOL	PROT	CARB	SUGAR	FIBER	CALCI	SOD	POTAS	FOLIC	VIT C
HEALTH IS WEALTH														
Buffalo Wings	3 pieces (2.2 oz)	100	2	0	0	10	11	0	3	40	490	—	—	2
Chicken-Free Nuggets	3 pieces (2.25 oz)	90	1	0	0	10	11	0	2	20	330	—	—	0
Chicken-Free Patties	1 (3 oz)	120	2	0	0	14	15	0	2	60	440	—	—	0
LOMA LINDA														
Chicken Supreme Mix not prep	⅓ cup (0.9 oz)	90	1	0	0	15	6	0	4	20	720	450	—	0
Chik Nuggets	5 pieces (3 oz)	240	16	3	0	12	13	tr	5	40	710	150	—	0
Fried Chik'n w/ Gravy	2 pieces (2.8 oz)	160	10	2	0	12	4	tr	2	0	440	35	—	0
MORNINGSTAR FARMS														
Chik Nuggets	4 pieces (3 oz)	160	4	1	0	13	17	2	5	20	670	330	—	0
Chik Patties	1 (2.5 oz)	150	6	1	0	9	15	1	2	0	570	150	—	0
Meatless Buffalo Wings	5 pieces (3 oz)	200	9	2	0	13	16	1	3	40	730	390	—	0
QUORN														
Cutlets	1 (3.5 oz)	200	8	1	0	10	20	2	4	60	610	—	—	0
Naked Cutlets	1 (2.4 oz)	80	3	1	5	11	5	0	2	50	420	—	—	0
Nuggets	3–4 pieces (3 oz)	180	8	1	0	8	18	2	3	40	650	—	—	0
Patties	1 patty (2.6 oz)	160	7	1	0	8	12	2	3	20	525	—	—	0
Tenders	1 cup (3 oz)	90	2	1	0	12	8	1	3	40	350	—	—	0
WORTHINGTON														
Chicken Sliced or Roll	2 slices (2 oz)	80	5	1	0	9	1	0	tr	0	370	280	—	0
Chicken Sliced	2 slices (2 oz)	80	5	1	0	9	1	0	tr	0	270	280	—	0
Chic-Ketts	2 slices (1.9 oz)	120	7	1	0	13	2	0	2	0	390	30	—	0
ChikStiks	1 (1.6 oz)	110	7	1	0	9	3	tr	2	0	360	60	—	0
CrispyChik Patties	1 (2.5 oz)	150	6	1	0	8	15	1	2	0	600	200	—	0
Cutlets	1 slice (2.1 oz)	70	1	0	0	11	3	0	2	0	340	30	—	0
Diced Chik	¼ cup (1.9 oz)	40	0	0	0	7	1	0	1	0	270	100	—	0
FriChik	2 pieces (3.2 oz)	120	8	1	0	10	1	0	1	0	430	150	—	0

FOOD	PORTION	CALS	FAT	SAT FAT	CHOL	PROT	CARB	SUGAR	FIBER	CALCI	SOD	POTAS	FOLIC	VIT C
WORTHINGTON (CONT.)														
FriChik Low Fat	2 pieces (3 oz)	80	3	0	0	10	2	0	1	0	430	150	—	0
Golden Croquettes	4 pieces (3 oz)	210	10	2	0	14	14	1	6	40	600	190	—	0
YVES														
Veggie Chicken Burgers	1 (3 oz)	120	3	0	0	17	6	1	3	80	390	300	—	5
CHICKPEAS														
CANNED														
chickpeas	1 cup	285	3	tr	0	12	54	—	—	78	718	413	160	9
GREEN GIANT														
Garbanzo	½ cup (4.4 oz)	110	2	0	0	6	18	tr	5	40	380	—	—	0
PROGRESSO														
Chick Peas	½ cup (4.6 oz)	120	3	0	0	5	20	3	5	40	280	—	—	0
Garbanzo	½ cup (4.4 oz)	110	2	0	0	6	18	tr	5	40	380	—	—	0
DRIED														
cooked	1 cup	269	4	tr	0	15	45	—	—	80	11	477	282	2
CHICORY														
greens raw chopped	½ cup	21	tr	tr	0	2	4	—	—	90	41	378	—	22
root raw	1 (2.1 oz)	44	tr	tr	0	1	11	—	—	25	30	174	—	3
roots raw cut up	½ cup (1.6 oz)	33	tr	tr	0	1	8	—	—	18	23	131	—	2
witloof head raw	1 (1.9 oz)	9	tr	tr	0	tr	2	—	—	10	1	112	20	2
witloof raw	½ cup (1.6 oz)	8	tr	tr	0	tr	2	—	—	9	1	95	17	1
CHILI														
chile pepper paste	1 tbsp	6	1	—	—	tr	1	—	1	21	1445	40	—	—
chili w/ beans	1 cup	286	14	6	43	15	30	—	—	119	1330	932	—	4
dried ancho	1 tsp	3	tr	—	0	tr	1	—	tr	1	0	24	1	0
dried casabel	1 tsp	3	tr	—	0	tr	1	—	tr	1	—	—	—	1
dried guajillo	1 tsp	3	tr	—	0	tr	1	—	tr	1	—	—	—	1
dried mulato	1 tsp	3	tr	—	0	tr	1	—	tr	1	—	—	—	1
dried pasilla	1 tsp	3	tr	—	0	tr	1	—	tr	1	1	22	2	0
dried smoked chipotle	1 tsp	3	tr	—	0	tr	1	—	tr	3	—	—	—	0
powder	1 tsp	8	tr	—	0	tr	1	—	—	7	26	50	—	2
AMY'S														
Chili & Cornbread	1 pkg (10.5 oz)	320	6	2	10	11	59	14	8	—	680	—	—	—
Organic Black Bean	1 cup	200	2	0	0	11	31	3	15	—	680	—	—	—
Organic Medium	1 cup	190	6	1	0	8	26	5	7	—	590	—	—	—
Organic Medium w/ Vegetables	1 cup	190	6	1	0	7	29	6	8	—	590	—	—	—

FOOD	PORTION	CALS	FAT	SAT FAT	CHOL	PROT	CARB	SUGAR	FIBER	CALCI	SOD	POTAS	FOLIC	VIT C
ARMOUR														
Chili No Beans	1 cup (8.7 oz)	390	29	13	70	14	18	0	0	40	1200	—	—	0
Chili w/ Beans	1 cup (8.9 oz)	370	21	9	50	13	33	2	10	80	1220	—	—	0
Chili w/ Beans Hot	1 cup (8.9 oz)	370	21	9	50	13	33	2	10	80	1220	—	—	0
Chili w/ Beans Western Style	1 cup (8.8 oz)	370	22	10	60	14	29	4	9	60	1130	—	—	0
Vienna Sausage & Chili	1 cup (8.7 oz)	410	27	11	80	14	27	4	15	100	1270	—	—	2
BUSH'S														
Chili Beans Mild Sauce	½ cup	120	1	1	0	6	20	0	6	20	480	—	—	1
Original No Beans	1 cup	240	14	5	25	13	16	5	3	80	1380	—	—	6
CARROLL SHELBY'S														
Original Texas Chili Kit	2 tbsp	60	1	0	0	2	12	0	0	40	1320	—	—	0
CHEF BOYARDEE														
Chili Mac	½ can (7 oz)	260	11	—	30	10	30	5	3	—	1480	—	—	—
CHILI MAN														
Seasoning Mix	1 tbsp (7 g)	25	1	—	—	1	4	—	2	20	330	—	—	1
DEL MONTE														
Sauce	1 tbsp (0.6 oz)	20	0	0	0	0	5	4	0	0	480	—	—	1
GEBHARDT														
Chili Powder	¼ tsp (0.3 g)	1	tr	0	0	tr	tr	tr	tr	tr	tr	—	—	tr
Chili Quik Seasoning	1 tbsp (0.3 oz)	43	1	0	0	1	8	1	2	29	985	—	—	tr
Plain	1 cup (9.4 oz)	232	19	7	0	7	11	0	3	36	737	—	—	6
With Beans	1 cup (9.4 oz)	322	15	6	29	15	32	tr	15	0	673	—	—	0
GRINGO BILLY'S														
Chili Mix	1 tbsp	24	1	0	0	0	2	0	2	—	319	—	—	—
HEALTH VALLEY														
Burrito	1 cup	160	1	—	0	13	28	7	12	40	360	—	—	12
Enchilada	1 cup	160	1	—	0	13	28	7	12	40	320	—	—	12
Fajita	1 cup	80	0	0	0	7	15	4	7	20	160	—	—	12
In A Cup Black Bean Mild	¾ cup	120	1	—	0	10	21	3	6	60	290	—	—	4
In A Cup Texas Style Spicy	¾ cup	120	1	—	0	10	21	3	6	60	290	—	—	4
Vegetarian Lentil Mild	1 cup	160	1	—	0	13	28	6	12	40	200	—	—	9
Vegetarian Lentil No Salt	1 cup	80	0	0	0	7	14	3	6	20	50	—	—	6
Vegetarian Mild	1 cup	160	1	—	0	13	28	7	12	50	200	—	—	12
Vegetarian Mild No Salt	1 cup	160	1	—	0	13	28	7	12	40	65	—	—	12
Vegetarian Spicy	1 cup	160	1	—	0	13	28	7	12	40	200	—	—	12

FOOD	PORTION	CALS	FAT	SAT FAT	CHOL	PROT	CARB	SUGAR	FIBER	CALCI	SOD	POTAS	FOLIC	VIT C
HEALTH VALLEY (CONT.)														
Vegetarian Spicy No Salt	1 cup	160	1	—	0	13	28	7	12	40	65	—	—	12
Vegetarian w/ 3 Beans Mild	1 cup	160	1	—	0	13	28	7	12	40	320	—	—	12
Vegetarian w/ Black Beans Mild	1 cup	160	1	—	0	13	28	7	12	40	320	—	—	12
Vegetarian w/ Black Beans Spicy	1 cup	160	1	—	0	13	28	7	12	40	320	—	—	12
HEALTHY CHOICE														
Bowls Chili & Cornbread	1 meal (9.5 oz)	350	8	3	35	21	49	18	8	100	600	—	—	4
HORMEL														
Chunky w/ Beans	1 cup (8.7 oz)	270	7	3	35	18	34	5	7	60	1240	—	—	0
Hot No Beans	1 cup (8.3 oz)	210	9	3	35	16	17	3	3	40	910	—	—	0
Hot w/ Beans	1 cup (8.7 oz)	270	7	3	35	18	33	5	7	60	1240	—	—	0
Microcup Meals Chili Mac	1 cup (7.5 oz)	200	9	4	25	11	17	3	2	0	980	—	—	0
Microcup Meals Hot w/ Beans	1 cup (7.3 oz)	220	6	3	30	15	27	4	6	40	1050	—	—	0
Microcup Meals No Beans	1 cup (7.3 oz)	190	8	3	30	14	15	3	2	20	800	—	—	0
Microcup Meals w/ Beans	1 cup (7.3 oz)	220	6	3	30	15	27	4	6	40	1050	—	—	0
No Beans	1 cup (8.3 oz)	210	9	3	35	16	17	3	3	40	910	—	—	0
Turkey No Beans	1 cup (8.3 oz)	190	3	1	75	24	17	4	3	100	1250	—	—	0
Turkey w/ Beans	1 cup (8.7 oz)	210	3	1	35	17	30	6	5	80	1180	—	—	1
Vegetarian	1 cup (8.7 oz)	200	1	0	0	12	38	6	7	60	780	—	—	0
With Beans	1 cup (8.7 oz)	270	7	3	35	18	33	5	7	60	1240	—	—	0
HUNT'S														
Chili Beans	½ cup (4.5 oz)	87	1	0	0	6	17	8	6	41	597	—	—	1
Family Favorites Chili Sauce	¼ cup	25	0	0	0	1	5	3	1	20	400	—	—	4
HURST														
HamBeens Chili Beans	1 serv	130	1	0	0	8	22	1	10	40	170	—	—	0
INSTANT INDIA														
Chili Ginger Paste	2 tbsp (1 oz)	90	7	1	0	1	6	5	0	0	470	—	—	0
JUST RITE														
With Beans	1 cup (9 oz)	379	27	13	35	18	31	0	13	101	51	—	—	4
LEAN CUISINE														
Everyday Favorites Three Bean Chili w/ Rice	1 pkg (10 oz)	250	6	2	10	11	37	7	9	150	590	780	—	18

FOOD	PORTION	CALS	FAT	SAT FAT	CHOL	PROT	CARB	SUGAR	FIBER	CALCI	SOD	POTAS	FOLIC	VIT C
LUNCH BUCKET														
Chili w/ Beans	1 pkg (7.5 oz)	260	12	5	25	12	25	1	8	60	1040	—	—	6
MANWICH														
Homestyle Fixins	½ cup (4.6 oz)	84	1	tr	0	6	19	7	6	36	858	—	—	7
MARIE CALLENDER'S														
Chili & Cornbread	1 meal (16 oz)	560	21	9	60	27	67	25	7	80	2110	—	—	0
MCCORMICK														
Mexican Style Chili Powder	¼ tsp	0	0	0	0	0	0	0	0	—	20	—	—	—
Original Chili Seasoning	1⅓ tbsp (9 g)	30	1	—	0	—	5	tr	2	0	310	—	—	0
NATURAL CHOICE														
Organic Vegan Three Bean	½ cup (4.6 oz)	140	1	0	0	9	24	4	7	60	510	—	—	12
NATURAL TOUCH														
Vegetarian	1 cup (8.1 oz)	170	1	0	0	18	21	2	11	40	870	480	—	0
NATURE'S ENTREE														
Texas Chili	1 pkg (12 oz)	320	7	2	15	26	43	5	11	200	960	—	—	2
OPEN RANGE														
Plain	1 cup (8.8 oz)	353	26	12	48	18	19	6	6	63	1216	—	—	12
With Beans	1 cup (9 oz)	281	16	7	26	17	25	7	10	111	1291	—	—	49
SOY7														
Chili Mix as prep	1 cup	150	2	0	0	16	24	3	7	—	400	—	—	—
STOUFFER'S														
With Beans	1 pkg (8.75 oz)	270	10	4	35	15	29	7	8	100	1130	610	—	4
ULTIMATE														
No Beans Hot	1 cup (8.7 oz)	420	30	13	85	20	18	4	5	60	1420	—	—	0
Turkey w/ Beans	1 cup (8.7 oz)	260	9	3	50	17	28	4	9	100	930	—	—	0
With Beans	1 cup (8.7 oz)	320	16	7	50	18	25	4	9	80	920	—	—	0
With Beans Hot	1 cup (8.7 oz)	320	16	7	50	18	25	4	9	80	920	—	—	0
VAN CAMP														
Beanee Weenee Chilee	1 cup (7.7 oz)	240	12	3	35	14	27	1	9	40	1090	—	—	6
Chili w/ Beans	1 cup (8.9 oz)	350	21	8	45	19	28	1	7	40	1020	—	—	6
Mexican Style Chili Beans	½ cup (4.6 oz)	110	2	1	0	7	21	1	8	20	430	—	—	0
WAMPLER														
Turkey	1 cup	250	7	—	75	23	22	—	—	—	1840	—	—	—
WICK FOWLER'S														
2 Alarm Chili Kit	3 tbsp	60	2	0	0	2	10	0	0	20	980	—	—	0
False Alarm Chili Kit	2 tbsp	50	2	0	0	2	9	0	0	20	980	—	—	0
WORTHINGTON														
Chili	1 cup (8.1 oz)	290	15	3	0	19	21	2	9	40	1130	420	—	0
Low Fat	1 cup (8.1 oz)	170	1	0	0	18	21	2	11	40	870	480	—	0

FOOD	PORTION	CALS	FAT	SAT FAT	CHOL	PROT	CARB	SUGAR	FIBER	CALCI	SOD	POTAS	FOLIC	VIT C
YVES														
Veggie Chili	1 pkg (10.5 oz)	230	1	0	0	21	37	7	14	150	850	1010	—	30
TAKE-OUT														
con carne w/ beans	8.9 oz	254	8	3	133	25	22	—	—	67	1008	691	30	2

CHILI PEPPER
(*see* PEPPERS)

CHINESE FOOD
(*see* ASIAN FOOD)

CHINESE PRESERVING MELON

FOOD	PORTION	CALS	FAT	SAT FAT	CHOL	PROT	CARB	SUGAR	FIBER	CALCI	SOD	POTAS	FOLIC	VIT C
cooked	½ cup	11	tr	tr	0	tr	3	—	—	16	93	5	—	9

CHIPS

FOOD	PORTION	CALS	FAT	SAT FAT	CHOL	PROT	CARB	SUGAR	FIBER	CALCI	SOD	POTAS	FOLIC	VIT C
barbecue	1 bag (7 oz)	971	64	16	0	15	105	—	—	96	1486	2498	164	67
barbecue	1 oz	139	9	2	0	2	15	—	—	14	213	358	24	10
corn	1 bag (7 oz)	1067	66	9	0	13	113	—	9	251	1248	281	40	0
corn	1 oz	153	10	1	0	2	16	—	1	36	179	40	6	0
corn barbecue	1 oz	148	9	1	0	2	16	—	1	37	216	67	—	1
corn barbecue	1 bag (7 oz)	1036	65	9	0	14	111	—	10	259	1511	468	—	3
corn cones	1 oz	145	8	6	0	2	18	—	—	1	290	23	—	—
corn cones nacho	1 oz	152	9	8	—	2	17	—	—	10	270	35	—	—
corn onion	1 oz	142	6	1	0	2	19	—	—	8	278	40	—	—
potato	1 oz	152	10	3	0	2	15	—	—	7	168	361	13	9
potato	1 bag (8 oz)	1217	79	25	0	16	120	—	—	54	1347	2894	103	71
potato cheese	1 oz	140	8	2	—	2	16	—	—	20	225	433	—	15
potato cheese	1 bag (6 oz)	842	46	15	—	14	98	—	—	122	1348	2597	—	92
potato light	1 bag (6 oz)	801	35	7	0	12	114	—	—	35	836	2955	—	44
potato light	1 oz	134	6	1	0	2	19	—	—	6	139	495	—	7
potato sour cream & onion	1 oz	150	10	3	2	2	15	—	—	20	177	377	18	11
potato sour cream & onion	1 bag (7 oz)	1051	67	18	14	16	102	—	—	143	1237	2634	122	74
potato sticks	1 pkg (1 oz)	148	10	3	0	2	15	—	—	5	71	351	11	13
potato sticks	½ cup (0.6 oz)	94	6	2	0	1	10	—	1	3	45	223	7	9
potato sticks	1 oz	148	10	3	0	2	15	—	1	5	71	351	11	13
taco	1 oz	136	7	1	—	2	18	—	—	44	223	61	—	—
taco	1 bag (8 oz)	1089	55	11	—	18	143	—	—	352	1788	492	—	—
taro	10 (0.8 oz)	115	6	1	0	1	16	—	—	14	79	174	—	1
taro	1 oz	141	7	2	0	1	19	—	—	17	97	214	—	1
tortilla	1 oz	142	7	1	0	2	18	—	2	44	150	56	—	0
tortilla	1 bag (7.5 oz)	1067	56	11	0	15	134	—	14	327	1124	419	—	0
tortilla nacho	1 bag (8 oz)	1131	58	11	0	18	142	—	12	354	1606	491	32	4
tortilla nacho	1 oz	141	7	1	0	2	18	—	2	42	201	61	4	1
tortilla nacho light	1 bag (6 oz)	757	26	5	0	15	122	—	—	270	1705	462	—	tr
tortilla nacho light	1 oz	126	4	1	0	3	20	—	—	45	284	77	—	tr

FOOD	PORTION	CALS	FAT	SAT FAT	CHOL	PROT	CARB	SUGAR	FIBER	CALCI	SOD	POTAS	FOLIC	VIT C
tortilla ranch	1 bag (7 oz)	969	47	9	1	15	128	—	—	280	1212	483	—	2
tortilla ranch	1 oz	139	7	1	0	2	18	—	—	40	174	69	—	tr
ATKINS														
Crunchers Barbeque	1 pkg (1 oz)	100	3	0	0	13	8	0	4	80	430	—	—	2
Crunchers Nacho Cheese	1 pkg (1 oz)	100	3	0	0	13	8	1	3	80	400	—	—	2
Crunchers Original	1 pkg (1 oz)	90	3	0	0	13	8	0	4	60	440	500	—	0
Crunchers Sour Cream & Onion	1 pkg (1 oz)	100	4	1	5	12	8	0	3	80	410	—	—	0
BARBARA'S BAKERY														
Potato	1¼ cup (1 oz)	150	10	1	0	2	15	0	1	—	180	—	—	—
Potato No Salt Added	1¼ cups (1 oz)	150	10	1	0	2	15	0	1	—	20	—	—	—
Potato Ripple	1¼ cups (1 oz)	150	10	1	0	2	15	0	1	—	180		—	—
Potato Yogurt & Green Onion	1¼ cups (1 oz)	150	9	1	0	2	15	tr	1	—	240	—	—	—
Tortilla Blue Corn	15 chips (1 oz)	140	7	tr	0	3	16	tr	1	—	40	—	—	—
Tortilla Blue Corn No Salt	15 chips (1 oz)	140	7	tr	0	3	16	tr	1	—	0	—	—	—
Tortilla Pinta Salsa	15 chips (1 oz)	130	6	1	0	2	19	0	2	—	210	—	—	—
BRUNO & LUIGI'S														
Pasta Chips Garlic & Herb	1 oz	117	1	0	0	4	23	0	1	40	25	—	—	0
CAPE COD														
Potato Golden Russet	1 pkg (0.5 oz)	70	4	1	0	1	8	0	tr	0	75	—	—	6
CHESTER'S														
Flamin' Hot	1 oz	140	8	2	0	2	17	6	tr	—	250	—	—	—
Salsa	1 oz	140	7	2	0	2	18	0	tr	—	290	—	—	—
DELICIOUSLY SLIM														
Tortilla Black Bean & Sour Cream	1 oz	140	9	2	0	5	13	1	5	40	125	—	—	0
Tortilla Lightly Salted	1 oz	140	8	2	0	4	13	0	5	20	150	—	—	1
Tortilla Ranch	1 oz	140	9	2	0	5	13	1	5	40	140	—	—	0
DORITOS														
3D's Cooler Ranch	27 (1 oz)	140	6	2	<5	2	18	2	1	—	350	—	—	—
3D's Nacho Cheesier	27 (1 oz)	140	7	2	<5	2	17	2	1	—	360	—	—	—
Cooler Ranch	12 (1 oz)	140	7	2	0	2	18	tr	1	—	170	—	—	—
Flamin' Hot	11 (1 oz)	140	7	2	0	2	17	3	1	—	210	—	—	—
Nacho Cheesier	11 (1 oz)	140	7	1	0	2	17	2	1	—	200	—	—	—
Salsa Verde	12 (1 oz)	150	7	2	0	2	20	1	1	—	210	—	—	—

FOOD	PORTION	CALS	FAT	SAT FAT	CHOL	PROT	CARB	SUGAR	FIBER	CALCI	SOD	POTAS	FOLIC	VIT C
DORITOS (CONT.)														
Smokey Red	12 (1 oz)	150	7	2	0	2	21	1	1	—	210	—	—	—
Spicy Nacho	12 (1 oz)	140	6	2	0	2	18	1	1	—	210	—	—	—
Toasted Corn	13 (1 oz)	140	7	2	0	2	18	0	1	—	120	—	—	—
Wow Nacho Cheesier	1 pkg (0.75 oz)	70	1	0	0	2	13	tr	1	40	180	—	—	0
DURANGOS														
Tortilla	15 (1 oz)	150	7	1	0	2	20	0	2	20	105	—	—	0
EDEN														
Brown Rice Chips	1 oz	150	7	2	0	2	19	0	0	0	100	35	—	0
Sea Vegetable Chips	1 oz	140	5	2	0	1	23	2	0	20	220	35	—	0
FRITOS														
Chili Cheese	31 (1 oz)	160	10	2	0	2	16	tr	1	—	240	—	—	—
Corn Chips BBQ	29 (1 oz)	150	9	1	0	2	16	tr	1	—	290	—	—	—
Corn Chips King Size	12 (1 oz)	150	10	2	0	2	16	0	1	—	150	—	—	—
Corn Chips Sabrositas Flamin' Hot	30 (1 oz)	150	9	2	0	2	16	1	1	—	180	—	—	—
Corn Chips Sabrositas Lime'N Chile	28 (1 oz)	150	9	2	0	2	17	0	1	—	240	—	—	—
Corn Chips Wild N'Mild Ranch	28 (1 oz)	160	10	2	0	2	15	tr	1	—	160	—	—	—
Original	32 (1 oz)	160	10	2	0	2	15	tr	1	20	170	—	—	0
Scoops	11 (1 oz)	160	10	1	0	2	17	0	1	—	105	—	—	—
Texas Grill Honey BBQ	15 (1 oz)	150	9	2	0	2	16	1	1	—	200	—	—	—
GENISOY														
Soy Crisps	1 oz	110	2	0	0	7	14	1	2	80	290	—	—	0
Soy Crisps Apple Cinnamon Crunch	1 oz	120	2	0	0	7	17	4	2	80	160	—	—	1
Soy Crisps Creamy Ranch	1 oz	110	2	0	0	7	15	1	2	100	330	—	—	1
Soy Crisps Deep Sea Salt	1 oz	110	2	0	0	7	14	1	2	80	260	—	—	0
Soy Crisps Rich Cheddar Cheese	1 oz	110	2	0	0	7	14	1	2	80	320	—	—	0
Soy Crisps Roasted Garlic & Onion	1 oz	100	2	0	0	7	14	1	2	80	280	—	—	1
Soy Crisps Zesty Barbeque	1 oz	110	2	0	0	7	17	2	2	80	160	—	—	1

FOOD	PORTION	CALS	FAT	SAT FAT	CHOL	PROT	CARB	SUGAR	FIBER	CALCI	SOD	POTAS	FOLIC	VIT C
GUILTLESS GOURMET														
Guiltless Carbs Salsa Verde	1 oz	110	3	0	0	14	9	0	3	60	460	—	—	4
Guiltless Carbs Southwestern Ranch	1 oz	110	3	0	0	14	9	0	3	60	420	—	—	0
Guiltless Carbs Three Pepper	1 oz	110	3	0	0	14	9	0	3	60	300	—	—	1
Tortilla Blue Corn	18 (1 oz)	110	2	0	0	3	22	0	2	60	140	—	—	0
Tortilla Chili Lime	18 (1 oz)	110	2	0	0	2	22	0	2	60	200	—	—	0
Tortilla Chili Verde	18 (1 oz)	120	2	0	0	2	22	1	2	60	200	—	—	5
Tortilla Chipotle	18 (1 oz)	120	2	0	0	2	22	1	2	60	200	—	—	0
Tortilla Mucho Nacho	18 (1 oz)	110	2	0	0	2	20	1	3	0	200	—	—	0
Tortilla Organic Red Corn	18 (1 oz)	110	2	0	0	3	22	0	2	60	160	—	—	0
Tortilla Spicy Black Bean	18 (1 oz)	110	2	0	0	3	22	0	2	60	200	—	—	0
Tortilla Sweet White Corn	18 (1 oz)	110	2	0	0	3	22	0	2	60	160	—	—	0
Tortilla Yellow Corn	18 (1 oz)	110	2	0	0	3	22	0	2	60	160	—	—	0
Tortilla Yellow Corn Unsalted	18 (1 oz)	110	1	0	0	2	22	0	2	60	26	—	—	0
HERR'S														
Potato	1 oz	140	8	3	0	2	16	0	1	0	180	—	—	6
Tortilla Restaurant Style White Corn	10 (1 oz)	140	6	1	0	3	18	1	2	0	90	—	—	0
HUSMAN'S														
Deli Style Tortilla	11	150	7	1	0	3	19	0	1	20	200	—	—	0
Potato	18 (1 oz)	160	11	3	0	2	14	0	1	0	75	—	—	9
Potato Sour Cream & Onion	18 (1 oz)	150	9	3	0	2	14	1	1	20	200	—	—	5
Potato Sweet N'Sassy	18 (1 oz)	155	10	3	0	1	15	1	1	0	110	—	—	9
KETO														
Low Carb Tortilla All Flavors	1 oz	150	8	1	0	12	8	0	4	—	240	—	—	—
LANCE														
BBQ	22 (1 oz)	160	10	3	0	2	15	1	1	0	170	300	—	4
Cajun	15 (1 oz)	150	10	3	0	2	14	0	1	0	290	300	—	6
Corn Chips	39 (1.25 oz)	200	11	3	0	2	14	0	1	0	140	310	—	4
Corn Chips Hot BBQ	35 (1.25 oz)	210	13	4	0	2	20	0	1	40	210	60	—	0
Hot Fries	1 pkg (0.9 oz)	140	10	3	0	2	11	0	1	0	190	0	—	0
Mesquite BBQ	22 (1 oz)	150	10	3	0	2	15	0	1	0	280	320	—	4
Potato	23 (1 oz)	160	10	3	0	2	15	0	1	0	130	310	—	4

FOOD	PORTION	CALS	FAT	SAT FAT	CHOL	PROT	CARB	SUGAR	FIBER	CALCI	SOD	POTAS	FOLIC	VIT C
LANCE (CONT.)														
Ripple	15 (1 oz)	160	11	3	0	1	14	0	1	0	150	320	—	4
Salt & Vinegar	22 (1 oz)	160	10	3	0	2	14	0	2	0	340	320	—	5
Sour Cream & Onion	22 (1 oz)	160	10	3	0	2	15	1	1	0	170	300	—	4
Tortilla Fiesta Salsa Triangles	16 (1 oz)	140	7	2	0	2	18	0	2	40	200	75	—	0
Tortilla Nacho Mini Round	46 (1.5 oz)	180	9	3	0	3	21	0	2	40	240	95	—	0
Tortilla Nacho Triangles	15 (1 oz)	140	14	4	0	2	18	1	1	20	200	70	—	0
LAY'S														
Adobadas	16 (1 oz)	170	10	3	0	2	18	1	1	—	240	—	—	—
Baked KC Masterpiece BBQ	11 (1 oz)	120	3	0	0	2	22	2	2	—	210	—	—	—
Baked Original	11 (1 oz)	110	2	0	0	2	23	2	2	—	150	—	—	—
Baked Roasted Herb	12 (1 oz)	130	3	1	0	2	25	2	2	—	190	—	—	—
Baked Sour Cream & Onion	12 (1 oz)	120	2	0	0	2	21	3	2	—	210	—	—	—
Classic	20 (1 oz)	150	10	3	0	2	15	0	1	—	180	—	—	—
Deli Style Hot N'Tangy BBQ	18 (1 oz)	150	10	3	0	2	16	1	1	—	220	—	—	—
Deli Style Jalapeño	17 (1 oz)	150	10	3	0	2	16	0	1	—	230	—	—	—
Deli Style Original	17 (1 oz)	140	10	3	0	1	16	0	1	—	180	—	—	—
Deli Style Salt & Vinegar	16 (1 oz)	90	10	3	0	1	16	1	1	—	380	—	—	—
Flamin' Hot	17 pieces (1 oz)	150	10	3	0	2	16	5	1	—	180	—	—	—
KC Masterpiece BBQ	15 (1 oz)	150	10	3	0	2	15	2	1	—	200	—	—	—
Onion & Garlic	19 (1 oz)	150	9	3	0	2	16	1	1	—	200	—	—	—
Original Baked	1 pkg (1⅛ oz)	130	2	0	0	2	26	2	2	40	170	—	—	1
Salt & Vinegar	17 pieces (1 oz)	150	10	3	0	2	15	1	1	—	300	—	—	—
Sour Cream & Onion	17 pieces (1 oz)	160	11	3	<5	2	12	1	1	—	200	—	—	—
Toasted Onion & Cheese	17 pieces (1 oz)	160	10	3	0	2	14	0	1	—	240	—	—	—
Wavy	11 pieces (1 oz)	150	10	3	0	2	15	0	1	0	180	—	—	6
Wavy Au Gratin	13 (1 oz)	150	10	3	<5	2	14	tr	1	—	200	—	—	—
Wavy Ranch	11 (1 oz)	160	11	3	0	2	14	0	1	—	150	—	—	—
Wow Mesquite BBQ	20 (1 oz)	75	0	0	0	2	17	1	1	—	250	—	—	—

FOOD	PORTION	CALS	FAT	SAT FAT	CHOL	PROT	CARB	SUGAR	FIBER	CALCI	SOD	POTAS	FOLIC	VIT C
LAY'S (CONT.)														
Wow Original	1 pkg (0.75 oz)	55	0	0	0	1	13	0	1	0	130	—	—	5
Wow Original	20 (1 oz)	75	0	0	0	2	18	0	1	—	200	—	—	—
Wow Sour Cream & Chive	19 (1 oz)	80	0	0	0	2	17	tr	1	—	230	—	—	—
MET-RX														
Pro Chips Bar-B-Que	1 pkg (2 oz)	260	9	1	0	38	8	4	0	—	440	—	—	—
Pro Chips Nacho	1 pkg (2 oz)	260	10	2	0	38	6	2	0	—	500	—	—	—
OLD DUTCH FOODS														
Potato	12–15 chips (1 oz)	150	8	1	0	2	16	1	1	0	130	370	—	9
Potato BBQ	12–15 chips (1 oz)	150	9	1	0	2	15	1	1	0	300	360	—	5
Potato BBQ Ripple	12–15 chips (1 oz)	150	9	1	0	2	16	1	tr	0	180	320	—	6
Potato Cajun Ripple	12–15 chips (1 oz)	150	10	1	0	2	15	tr	1	0	160	300	—	18
Potato Cheddar & Sour Cream Ripple	12–15 chips (1 oz)	160	9	2	0	2	16	tr	1	20	190	350	—	5
Potato Cheddar & Sour Cream Ripple	12–15 chips (1 oz)	150	9	2	0	2	15	1	1	0	190	310	—	5
Potato Dill	12–15 chips (1 oz)	140	8	1	0	2	16	2	1	0	310	380	—	9
Potato Dutch Crunch	15–20 chips (1 oz)	130	6	1	0	2	18	0	2	0	140	340	0	6
Potato French Onion Ripple	12–15 chips (1 oz)	150	10	1	0	2	15	2	1	0	180	330	—	2
Potato Jalapeño & Cheddar Dutch Crunch	15–20 chips (1 oz)	130	6	2	0	2	17	0	1	0	190	390	16	4
Potato Jalapeño Cheese	12–15 chips (1 oz)	150	9	1	0	2	16	tr	1	0	170	330	—	6
Potato Mesquite BBQ Dutch Crunch	15–20 chips (1 oz)	130	6	1	0	2	19	1	2	0	230	330	—	5
Potato Onion & Garlic	12–15 chips (1 oz)	140	8	1	0	2	16	1	1	0	210	390	—	12
Potato Outback Spicy BBQ	12–15 chips (1 oz)	150	10	1	0	2	15	1	1	0	170	320	—	21
Potato Ripple	12–15 chips (1 oz)	150	9	1	0	2	15	0	1	0	115	340	—	4

FOOD	PORTION	CALS	FAT	SAT FAT	CHOL	PROT	CARB	SUGAR	FIBER	CALCI	SOD	POTAS	FOLIC	VIT C
OLD DUTCH FOODS (CONT.)														
Potato Salt & Vinegar Dutch Crunch	15–20 chips (1 oz)	130	6	1	0	0	18	1	1	0	360	350	0	5
Potato Sour Cream & Onion	12–15 chips (1 oz)	150	9	1	0	2	15	2	1	40	230	380	—	9
Tortilla Bite Size White Corn	20 chips (1 oz)	150	8	1	0	2	18	0	1	0	105	—	—	0
Tortilla Nacho Cheese	15 chips (1 oz)	150	7	1	0	2	19	0	1	40	150	65	—	0
Tortilla Restaurant Style White	9 chips (1 oz)	140	7	1	0	2	20	0	2	0	95	50	—	0
Tostados White Corn	11 chips (1 oz)	140	7	1	0	2	20	0	2	0	115	45	—	0
Tostados Yellow Corn	11 chips (1 oz)	140	6	1	0	2	21	0	1	0	90	55	—	0
PITA-SNAX														
Cheddar Cheese	34 (1 oz)	110	2	0	0	3	21	1	tr	20	240	—	—	0
Chili & Lime	34 (1 oz)	120	2	0	0	3	20	1	tr	0	210	—	—	0
Cinnamon	34 (1 oz)	120	2	0	0	3	22	2	tr	0	60	—	—	0
Dill Ranch	34 (1 oz)	120	2	0	0	3	21	0	tr	20	170	—	—	0
Garlic	34 (1 oz)	120	2	0	0	3	22	0	tr	0	120	—	—	0
Lightly Salted	34 (1 oz)	110	1	0	0	3	22	0	tr	0	170	—	—	0
PRINGLES														
BBQ	14 chips (1 oz)	150	10	3	0	2	15	1	1	—	200	275	—	4
Cheese & Onion	14 chips (1 oz)	160	11	2	0	1	15	1	1	20	220	—	—	4
Cheez-ums	14 chips (1 oz)	150	10	3	0	2	14	1	1	—	190	175	—	4
Original	14 chips (1 oz)	160	11	3	0	2	15	—	1	—	170	275	—	4
Pizzalicious	14 chips (1 oz)	160	11	3	0	1	14	1	1	—	200	—	—	4
Ranch	14 chips (1 oz)	150	10	3	0	2	15	1	1	—	130	275	—	4
Salt & Vinegar	14 chips (1 oz)	160	11	3	0	1	15	1	1	—	200	—	—	4
Sour Cream & Onion	14 chips (1 oz)	160	10	3	0	2	15	1	1	—	135	275	—	4
RACQUET														
Wheat Chips All Flavors	6 chips	30	1	0	0	1	4	0	0	—	30	—	—	—
REVIVAL														
Baked Soy Pasta Chips Lightly Salted Sunshine	1 bag (0.9 oz)	100	2	0	0	7	13	0	0	14	180	<2	—	—
Baked Soy Pasta Chips Naturally Nice	1 bag (0.9 oz)	80	1	0	0	7	12	0	0	13	120	<2	—	—
Baked Soy Pasta Chips Rev It Up Ranch	1 bag (0.9 oz)	105	3	0	0	7	12	1	0	17	190	7	—	—
ROBERT'S AMERICAN GOURMET														
Spirulina Spirals	1 oz	120	2	0	0	2	22	4	3	—	110	—	—	—

FOOD	PORTION	CALS	FAT	SAT FAT	CHOL	PROT	CARB	SUGAR	FIBER	CALCI	SOD	POTAS	FOLIC	VIT C
RUFFLES														
Baked	10 (1 oz)	110	2	0	0	2	23	2	2	—	180	—	—	—
Baked Cheddar & Sour Cream	9 (1 oz)	120	3	0	0	2	21	2	2	—	270	—	—	—
Buffalo Style	11 chips (1 oz)	160	10	3	0	2	16	0	1	—	230	—	—	—
Cheddar & Sour Cream	11 chips (1 oz)	160	10	3	0	2	14	2	1	—	190	—	—	—
French Onion	11 (1 oz)	150	10	3	0	2	15	tr	1	—	190	—	—	—
MC Masterpiece Mesquite BBQ	11 (1 oz)	150	10	3	0	1	15	tr	1	—	190	—	—	—
Original	1 pkg (1.5 oz)	240	16	4	0	3	22	0	2	0	250	—	—	9
Original	12 chips (1 oz)	150	10	3	0	2	14	0	1	—	180	—	—	—
Ranch	13 (1 oz)	150	9	3	0	2	15	1	1	—	280	—	—	—
Reduced Fat	16 (1 oz)	130	7	1	0	2	18	0	1	—	130	—	—	—
The Works	12 (1 oz)	160	11	3	0	2	14	2	1	—	210	—	—	—
Wow Cheddar & Sour Cream	15 (1 oz)	75	0	0	0	3	16	tr	1	—	230	—	—	—
Wow Cheddar & Sour Cream	15 (1 oz)	75	0	0	0	3	16	tr	1	—	230	—	—	—
Wow Original	17 (1 oz)	75	0	0	0	2	17	0	1	—	200	—	—	—
SANTITAS														
100% White Corn	6 (1 oz)	130	6	1	0	2	19	0	1	—	110	—	—	—
Restaurant Style Chips	7 (1 oz)	130	6	1	0	2	19	0	1	—	110	—	—	—
Restaurant Style Strips	10 (1 oz)	130	6	1	0	2	19	0	1	—	110	—	—	—
SKINNY														
BBQ	1½ cups	90	2	1	0	2	17	1	1	0	210	—	—	0
Corn	1½ cups	90	2	1	0	2	17	0	1	0	90	—	—	0
Nacho Cheese	1½ cups	90	3	1	0	2	15	1	1	0	200	—	—	0
Sour Cream & Onion	1½ cups	90	2	1	0	2	17	1	1	0	110	—	—	0
Sticks Garden Veggie	1 oz	140	6	1	0	1	17	2	1	60	280	—	—	4
Sticks Island Lime Chili	1 oz	140	6	1	0	1	17	2	1	60	280	—	—	4
Sticks Maui Wowie	1 oz	140	6	1	0	1	17	2	1	60	280	—	—	4
Sticks Original Spud	1 oz	140	6	1	0	1	17	2	1	60	280	—	—	4
SNYDER'S OF HANOVER														
Barbeque Corn	1.5 oz	230	14	2	0	3	22	0	2	—	350	—	—	0
BBQ Rib	1 oz	140	7	2	0	2	17	tr	tr	0	290	—	—	12
Cheddar Bacon	1 oz	150	6	2	0	2	20	tr	3	0	270	—	—	9
Corn Chips	1.5 oz	230	15	2	0	3	22	0	2	80	220	—	—	0
Grilled Steak & Onion	1 oz	140	6	2	0	2	20	0	4	0	140	—	—	9

FOOD	PORTION	CALS	FAT	SAT FAT	CHOL	PROT	CARB	SUGAR	FIBER	CALCI	SOD	POTAS	FOLIC	VIT C
SNYDER'S OF HANOVER (CONT.)														
Hot Buffalo	1 oz	150	7	2	0	2	20	0	4	0	330	—	—	9
Kosher Dill	1 oz	140	6	2	0	2	20	1	3	0	360	—	—	9
No Salt	1 oz	140	6	2	0	2	19	0	3	0	0	—	—	9
Potato	1 oz	140	6	2	0	2	19	0	3	0	90	—	—	21
Ripple	1 oz	140	6	2	0	2	18	0	4	0	100	—	—	9
Salt & Vinegar	1 oz	140	6	2	0	2	19	tr	4	0	150	—	—	9
Sausage Pizza	1 oz	150	6	2	0	2	20	tr	4	0	250	—	—	9
Sour Cream & Onion	1 oz	150	7	2	0	2	19	tr	4	0	150	—	—	9
Tasty Veggie Potato Chips	1 oz	150	6	2	0	3	20	1	4	0	260	—	—	9
Tortilla Nacho	1 oz	140	7	1	0	2	19	tr	1	20	130	—	—	0
Tortilla No Salt Yellow Corn	1 oz	140	6	1	0	2	19	tr	1	20	0	—	—	0
Tortilla White Corn	1 oz	140	6	1	0	2	20	tr	1	20	130	—	—	0
Tortilla Yellow Corn	1 oz	140	6	1	0	2	19	tr	1	20	130	—	—	0
Tortilla Yellow Corn Mini	1 oz	160	8	1	0	2	20	tr	1	20	130	—	—	0
Veggie Crisps	1 pkg (1.5 oz)	190	9	1	0	1	26	0	2	0	470	—	—	1
SOYA KING														
Soy Mongolian BBQ	23 chips (1 oz)	140	7	1	0	1	19	—	3	—	115	—	—	—
Soy Original	23 chips (1 oz)	140	7	1	0	1	19	—	3	—	115	—	—	—
Soy Sour Cream & Onion	23 chips (1 oz)	140	7	1	0	1	19	—	3	—	115	—	—	—
Soy Taco	23 chips (1 oz)	140	7	1	0	1	19	—	3	—	115	—	—	—
STACY'S														
Pita Chips Cinnamon Sugar	1 oz	130	4	0	0	3	18	—	3	0	130	—	—	0
Pita Chips Parmesan Garlic & Herb	1 oz	130	4	0	0	3	18	—	3	0	200	—	—	0
Pita Chips Simply Naked	1 oz	130	4	0	0	3	18	—	3	0	140	—	—	0
Twisted Pasta Low Fat	1 oz	110	2	0	0	3	21	1	1	40	135	—	—	0
SUNCHIPS														
French Onion	13 (1 oz)	140	7	1	0	2	18	2	2	—	115	—	—	—
Harvest Cheddar	13 (1 oz)	140	6	1	0	2	19	2	2	—	115	—	—	—
Original	14 (1 oz)	140	6	1	0	2	19	2	2	—	115	—	—	—
TERRA CHIPS														
Spiced Sweet Potato	1 pkg (½ oz)	190	13	1	0	1	17	3	3	40	180	—	—	3

FOOD	PORTION	CALS	FAT	SAT FAT	CHOL	PROT	CARB	SUGAR	FIBER	CALCI	SOD	POTAS	FOLIC	VIT C
TORENGOS														
Chips	13 chips (1 oz)	140	9	1	0	2	15	0	1	20	150	—	—	0
TOSTITOS														
Baked Bite Size	20 (1 oz)	110	1	0	0	3	24	0	2	—	200	—	—	—
Baked Bite Size Salsa & Cream Cheese	16 (1 oz)	120	3	1	0	2	21	1	1	—	190	—	—	—
Baked Original	13 (1 oz)	110	1	0	3	3	21	0	1	—	200	—	—	—
Bite Size	15 (1 oz)	140	8	1	0	2	17	0	1	—	110	—	—	—
Crispy Rounds	13 (1 oz)	150	8	1	0	2	17	tr	1	—	85	—	—	—
Nacho Style	6 (1 oz)	140	6	1	0	2	19	tr	1	—	100	—	—	—
Restaurant Style	7 (1 oz)	140	6	1	0	2	19	0	1	—	110	—	—	—
Restaurant Style Hint Of Lime	6 (1 oz)	140	6	1	0	2	19	tr	1	—	160	—	—	—
Santa Fe Gold	7 (1 oz)	140	6	1	0	2	19	0	1	—	80	—	—	—
Wow Original	6 (1 oz)	90	1	0	0	2	20	0	1	—	105	—	—	—
TYSON														
Tortilla Salted	13 (1 oz)	150	7	1	0	2	20	0	2	40	65	—	—	0
Tortilla Yellow Corn Salted	13 (1 oz)	150	7	1	0	2	20	0	2	40	65	—	—	0
UTZ														
Baked Crisps	12 (1 oz)	110	2	0	0	2	23	2	2	60	180	—	—	0
Carolina Barbeque	20 (1 oz)	150	9	2	0	2	14	tr	1	0	270	350	—	6
Cheddar & Sour Cream	20 (1 oz)	160	10	3	0	2	14	tr	1	0	200	360	—	6
Corn Chips	24 (1 oz)	160	10	2	0	2	16	0	1	20	160	—	—	0
Corn Chips Barbecue	24 (1 oz)	160	10	2	0	2	16	tr	1	20	180	—	—	0
Grandma	20 (1 oz)	140	8	3	5	2	14	0	1	0	120	410	—	9
Grandma BBQ	20 (1 oz)	140	8	3	5	2	15	2	1	0	240	390	—	6
Home Style Kettle	20 (1 oz)	140	8	2	0	2	14	0	1	0	120	400	—	9
Home Style Kettle BBQ	20 (1 oz)	140	8	2	0	2	15	2	1	0	240	390	—	6
Kettle Classics Crunchy	20 (1 oz)	150	9	2	0	2	15	0	1	0	95	370	—	9
Kettle Classics Crunchy Mesquite BBQ	20 (1 oz)	150	9	2	0	2	15	2	1	0	200	350	—	9
No Salt Added	20 (1 oz)	150	9	2	0	2	14	0	1	0	5	370	—	9
Onion & Garlic	20 (1 oz)	150	9	2	0	2	14	tr	1	0	180	350	—	6
Potato	20 (1 oz)	150	9	2	0	2	14	0	1	0	95	370	—	9
Reduced Fat BBQ	22 (1 oz)	140	6	2	0	2	19	1	1	0	190	—	—	9
Reduced Fat Ripple	24 (1 oz)	140	7	2	0	2	18	0	1	0	120	—	—	9
Ripple	20 (1 oz)	150	10	3	0	2	14	0	1	0	95	370	—	9

FOOD	PORTION	CALS	FAT	SAT FAT	CHOL	PROT	CARB	SUGAR	FIBER	CALCI	SOD	POTAS	FOLIC	VIT C
UTZ (CONT.)														
Ripple Sour Cream & Onion	20 (1 oz)	160	10	3	0	2	14	tr	1	0	140	350	—	6
Ripple Barbeque	20 (1 oz)	150	10	3	0	2	14	1	1	0	200	350	—	6
Salt'N Vinegar	20 (1 oz)	150	9	2	0	2	14	tr	1	0	270	350	—	6
The Crab Chip	20 (1 oz)	150	9	2	0	2	14	tr	1	0	300	350	—	6
Tortilla Black Bean & Salsa	13 (1 oz)	150	7	1	0	2	19	1	1	20	230	—	—	0
Tortilla Low Fat Baked	10 (1 oz)	120	2	0	0	2	24	0	2	40	200	—	—	0
Tortilla Nacho	13 (1 oz)	150	8	1	0	2	19	tr	1	20	200	—	—	0
Tortilla Restaurant Style	6 (1 oz)	140	7	1	0	2	18	0	1	20	120	—	—	0
Tortilla Spicy Nacho	13 (1 oz)	150	8	1	0	2	19	tr	1	20	220	—	—	0
Tortilla White Corn	12 (1 oz)	140	7	1	0	2	18	0	1	20	120	—	—	0
Wavy	20 chips (1 oz)	150	9	2	0	2	14	0	1	0	95	370	—	9
Yes! Fat Free	20 (1 oz)	75	0	0	0	2	17	0	1	0	180	—	—	9
Yes! Fat Free Barbeque	20 (1 oz)	75	0	0	0	2	16	1	1	0	210	—	—	6
Yes! Fat Free Ripple	20 (1 oz)	75	0	0	0	2	17	0	1	0	180	—	—	9
CHITTERLINGS														
pork cooked	3 oz	258	24	9	122	9	0	—	0	23	33	—	3	0
CHIVES														
freeze-dried	1 tbsp	1	tr	tr	0	tr	tr	—	—	2	—	6	—	1
fresh chopped	1 tbsp	1	tr	tr	0	tr	tr	—	—	3	0	9	3	2
fresh chopped	1 tsp	0	tr	tr	0	tr	tr	—	—	1	0	3	1	1

CHOCOLATE

(*see also* CANDY, CHOCOLATE SPREAD, CHOCOLATE SYRUP, COCOA, HOT CHOCOLATE, ICE CREAM TOPPINGS, MILK DRINKS)

FOOD	PORTION	CALS	FAT	SAT FAT	CHOL	PROT	CARB	SUGAR	FIBER	CALCI	SOD	POTAS	FOLIC	VIT C
BAKING														
baking	1 oz	145	15	9	0	3	8	—	—	22	1	235	—	0
grated unsweetened	1 cup	689	73	43	0	14	37	—	20	98	18	1100	9	0
liquid unsweetened	1 oz	134	14	7	0	3	10	—	5	15	3	331	5	0
squares unsweetened	1 square (1 oz)	146	16	9	0	3	8	—	4	21	4	236	2	0
BAKER'S														
Bittersweet	½ square (0.5 oz)	70	6	3	0	1	7	5	1	0	0	75	—	0
German's Sweet	2 squares (0.5 oz)	60	4	2	0	1	8	8	tr	0	0	50	—	0

FOOD	PORTION	CALS	FAT	SAT FAT	CHOL	PROT	CARB	SUGAR	FIBER	CALCI	SOD	POTAS	FOLIC	VIT C
BAKER'S (CONT.)														
Semi-Sweet	½ square (0.5 oz)	70	5	3	0	1	8	7	1	0	0	70	—	0
Unsweetened	½ square (0.5 oz)	70	7	5	0	2	4	0	2	0	0	140	—	0
White	½ square (0.5 oz)	80	5	3	<5	1	8	8	0	20	15	45	—	0
NESTLÉ														
Choco Bake	½ oz	80	8	5	0	1	5	0	2	0	0	—	—	0
Premier White Bar	½ oz	80	5	3	<5	1	8	8	0	40	15	—	—	0
Premier White Morsels	1 tbsp	80	4	4	0	tr	9	9	0	20	20	—	—	0
Semi-Sweet Bar	½ oz	70	4	3	0	<1	9	8	tr	0	0	—	—	0
Unsweetened Bar	½ oz	80	7	5	0	2	4	0	2	0	0	—	—	0
CHIPS														
milk chocolate	1 cup (6 oz)	862	52	31	38	12	100	—	—	321	138	646	14	1
semisweet	60 pieces (1 oz)	136	9	5	0	1	18	—	—	9	3	104	1	0
semisweet	1 cup (6 oz)	804	50	30	0	7	106	—	—	54	19	614	4	0
BAKER'S														
Real Milk Chocolate	½ oz	70	4	2	0	1	9	8	0	20	10	50	—	0
Real Semi-Sweet	½ oz	60	4	2	0	1	9	8	1	0	0	60	—	0
Semi-Sweet	½ oz	70	4	3	0	0	10	9	0	0	15	55	—	0
CLOUD NINE														
Double Dark Chocolate	13 pieces (0.5 oz)	80	4	3	5	1	9	9	0	0	0	—	—	0
GHIRARDELLI														
Semi-Sweet	33 pieces (0.5 oz)	70	4	3	0	1	9	7	tr	0	0	—	—	0
HERSHEY'S														
Holiday Baking Bits	1 tbsp	70	3	2	0	tr	11	—	—	—	0	—	—	—
Milk Chocolate	1 tbsp	80	5	3	<5	1	9	—	—	—	10	—	—	—
Mini Milk Chocolate	1 tbsp	80	4	3	0	tr	10	—	—	—	0	—	—	—
Mini Kisses For Baking	11 pieces	80	5	3	<5	1	9	—	—	—	15	—	—	—
Premier White Milk Chips	1 tbsp	80	4	3	0	1	9	—	—	—	30	—	—	—
Raspberry Chips	1 tbsp	80	4	3	0	tr	10	—	—	—	0	—	—	—
Semi-Sweet	1 tbsp	80	4	3	0	tr	10	—	—	—	0	—	—	—
Semi-Sweet Mini	1 tbsp	80	4	3	0	tr	10	—	—	—	0	—	—	—
Skor English Toffee Baking Bits	1 tbsp	70	5	3	10	0	7	—	—	—	60	—	—	—

FOOD	PORTION	CALS	FAT	SAT FAT	CHOL	PROT	CARB	SUGAR	FIBER	CALCI	SOD	POTAS	FOLIC	VIT C
NESTLÉ														
Crunch Baking Pieces	1½ tbsp	80	4	2	0	tr	10	8	0	0	25	—	—	0
Milk Chocolate Morsels	1 tbsp	70	4	3	<5	tr	9	8	0	0	0	—	—	0
Mint Chocolate Morsels	1 tbsp	70	4	3	0	tr	9	8	tr	0	0	—	—	0
Morsels Semi-Sweet	1 tbsp	70	4	3	0	tr	9	8	tr	0	0	—	—	0
Semi-Sweet Mega Morsels	1 tbsp	70	4	3	0	tr	9	8	tr	0	0	—	—	0
Semi-Sweet Mini Morsels	1 tbsp	70	4	3	0	tr	9	8	tr	0	0	—	—	0
SUNSPIRE														
Chocolate Sundrops	47 pieces (1.4 oz)	190	5	3	0	2	27	26	1	80	50	—	—	0
Dark Chocolate Grain Sweetened	13 pieces (0.5 oz)	70	4	3	0	0	10	5	1	0	1	—	—	0
Organic	13 pieces (0.5 oz)	70	5	3	0	1	9	7	0	20	0	—	—	0
TOLL HOUSE														
Mint-Chocolate	2 tbsp (1.5 oz)	130	3	2	0	1	25	22	1	0	30	0	—	0
Semi-Sweet	2 tbsp (1.5 oz)	130	4	2	0	1	24	22	1	0	30	0	—	0
TROPICAL SOURCE														
Espresso Roast Dairy Free	13 pieces (1.5 oz)	70	4	4	0	1	9	9	1	0	1	—	—	0
Semi-Sweet Dairy Free	13 pieces (1.5 oz)	80	4	3	5	1	9	9	0	0	0	—	—	0
MIX														
powder	2–3 heaping tsp	75	1	tr	0	1	20	—	—	8	45	128	—	tr
powder as prep w/ whole milk	9 oz	226	9	5	33	9	31	—	—	300	165	498	12	3
QUIK														
Chocolate Powder	2 tbsp (0.8 oz)	90	1	1	0	1	19	18	1	0	30	150	—	0
Chocolate Powder No Sugar	2 tbsp (0.4 oz)	40	1	1	0	1	7	1	2	0	45	170	—	0

CHOCOLATE MILK

(*see* MILK DRINKS)

CHOCOLATE SPREAD

FOOD	PORTION	CALS	FAT	SAT FAT	CHOL	PROT	CARB	SUGAR	FIBER	CALCI	SOD	POTAS	FOLIC	VIT C
TWIST														
Sugar Free Chocolate Spread	2 tbsp	170	12	2	0	2	2	0	0	—	55	—	—	—

FOOD	PORTION	CALS	FAT	SAT FAT	CHOL	PROT	CARB	SUGAR	FIBER	CALCI	SOD	POTAS	FOLIC	VIT C
CHOCOLATE SYRUP														
chocolate fudge	1 cup (11.9 oz)	1176	46	19	—	15	200	—	—	340	442	731	—	—
chocolate fudge	1 tbsp (0.7 oz)	73	3	1	—	1	12	—	—	21	27	45	—	—
syrup	1 cup	653	3	2	0	6	177	—	—	42	287	672	12	1
syrup	2 tbsp	82	tr	tr	0	1	22	—	—	5	36	84	2	tr
syrup as prep w/ whole milk	9 oz	232	9	5	33	9	34	—	—	297	156	455	14	2
AH!LASKA														
Organic	2 tbsp	85	0	0	0	2	20	18	—	—	5	—	—	—
COLAC														
Chocolate Topping	1 tbsp	37	1	tr	0	0	15	0	0	—	5	—	—	—
DAVINCI GOURMET														
Sugar Free	2 tbsp	15	0	0	0	1	5	0	1	—	0	—	—	—
ESTEE														
Chocolate	2 tbsp	15	0	0	0	tr	5	—	0	—	40	—	—	—
HERSHEY'S														
Chocolate Fudge	1 tbsp	70	3	2	<5	tr	10	—	—	—	25	—	—	—
Double Chocolate	1 tbsp	50	0	0	0	0	13	—	—	—	15	—	—	—
Lite	2 tbsp	50	0	0	0	0	12	—	—	—	35	—	—	—
Syrup	2 tbsp	100	0	0	0	1	24	—	—	—	25	—	—	—
QUIK														
Chocolate	2 tbsp (1.3 oz)	100	1	0	0	1	23	17	tr	0	30	75	—	0
SMUCKER'S														
Plate Scapers Chocolate	2 tbsp	100	5	—	—	1	23	11	1	—	20	—	—	—
TOLL HOUSE														
Mint Chocolate	2 tbsp (1.5 oz)	130	3	2	0	1	25	22	1	0	30	0	—	0
Semi-Sweet	2 tbsp (1.5 oz)	130	4	2	0	1	24	22	1	0	30	0	—	0
WALDEN FARMS														
Sugar Free	2 tbsp	0	0	0	0	0	0	0	0	—	35	—	—	—
WHOPPERS														
Chocolate Malt	2 tbsp	100	0	0	0	tr	25	—	—	—	55	—	—	—
CHUTNEY														
apple	1.2 oz	68	0	—	—	tr	18	—	1	9	—	—	—	1
apple cranberry	1 tbsp	16	0	—	0	tr	4	—	—	4	1	—	—	—
coconut	¼ cup	74	7	6	0	1	4	—	2	—	5	—	—	—
mango	1 tbsp	54	2	—	0	tr	10	—	tr	4	207	11	—	0
tomato	1 tbsp	32	tr	—	0	tr	8	—	tr	5	26	62	2	1
WILD THYME FARMS														
Apricot Cranberry Walnut	1 tbsp	15	0	0	0	0	3	3	—	—	0	—	—	5
Pineapple Peach Lime	1 tbsp	14	0	0	0	0	6	5	—	—	0	—	—	5

FOOD	PORTION	CALS	FAT	SAT FAT	CHOL	PROT	CARB	SUGAR	FIBER	CALCI	SOD	POTAS	FOLIC	VIT C
CILANTRO														
fresh	1 cup (1.6 oz)	11	tr	tr	0	1	2	—	1	31	25	235	29	1
fresh	1 tsp (2 g)	tr	tr	0	0	tr	tr	—	tr	1	1	8	1	1
CINNAMON														
ground	1 tsp	6	tr	tr	0	tr	2	—	—	28	1	11	—	1
sticks	0.5 oz	39	tr	tr	—	1	8	0	3	175	4	—	—	4
GRINGO BILLY'S														
Cinnamon Sweetener	½ tsp	0	0	0	0	0	0	0	0	—	57	—	—	—
CISCO														
raw	3 oz	84	2	tr	—	16	0	—	—	—	47	301	—	—
smoked	3 oz	151	10	1	27	14	0	—	—	22	409	249	2	—
smoked	1 oz	50	3	tr	9	5	0	—	—	7	135	82	1	—
CLAMS														
CANNED														
liquid only	1 cup	6	tr	—	—	1	tr	—	—	31	516	—	—	—
liquid only	3 oz	2	tr	—	—	tr	tr	—	—	11	183	—	—	—
meat only	3 oz	126	2	tr	57	22	4	—	—	78	95	534	—	—
meat only	1 cup	236	3	tr	107	41	8	—	—	148	179	1005	158	—
BUMBLE BEE														
Baby	2 oz	50	1	1	40	9	2	0	0	—	270	—	—	—
PROGRESSO														
Creamy Clam Sauce	½ cup (4.2 oz)	110	6	2	10	5	8	0	0	0	440	—	—	0
Minced	¼ cup (2.1 oz)	25	0	0	10	4	2	0	0	0	250	—	—	0
Red Clam Sauce	½ cup (4.4 oz)	60	1	0	10	4	8	4	1	20	350	—	—	0
White Clam Sauce	½ cup (4.4 oz)	150	10	2	20	9	5	tr	0	40	710	—	—	1
FRESH														
cooked	3 oz	126	2	tr	57	22	4	—	—	78	95	534	—	—
cooked	20 sm	133	2	tr	60	23	5	—	—	83	100	565	—	—
raw	3 oz	63	1	tr	29	11	2	—	—	39	47	267	—	—
raw	20 sm (6.3 oz)	133	2	tr	60	23	5	—	—	83	100	565	—	—
raw	9 lg (6.3 oz)	133	2	tr	60	23	5	—	—	83	100	565	—	—
TAKE-OUT														
breaded & fried	20 sm	379	21	5	115	27	19	—	—	119	684	612	—	—
CLEMENTINES														
HADDON HOUSE														
In Light Syrup	½ cup	80	0	0	0	0	19	18	1	20	10	—	—	4
TINA														
Fresh	1	50	1	0	0	1	15	12	3	40	0	—	—	30
CLOVES														
ground	1 tsp	7	tr	tr	0	tr	1	—	—	14	5	23	—	2

FOOD	PORTION	CALS	FAT	SAT FAT	CHOL	PROT	CARB	SUGAR	FIBER	CALCI	SOD	POTAS	FOLIC	VIT C
COCOA														
(*see also* HOT CHOCOLATE)														
powder unsweetened	1 tbsp (5 g)	11	1	tr	0	1	3	—	2	6	1	76	2	0
powder unsweetened	1 cup (3 oz)	197	12	7	0	17	47	—	29	110	18	1310	27	0
AH!LASKA														
Organic	2 tbsp	100	0	0	0	2	23	20	5	80	35	—	—	0
Organic Bakers Cocoa	1 tbsp	20	0	0	0	1	3	—	1	—	0	—	—	—
HERSHEY'S														
Cocoa	1 tbsp	20	1	0	0	1	3	—	—	—	0	—	—	—
European Cocoa	1 tbsp	20	1	0	0	1	3	—	—	—	0	—	—	—
NESTLÉ														
Cocoa	1 tbsp	15	1	0	0	1	3	0	1	0	0	—	—	0
COCONUT														
dried sweetened flaked	1 cup	351	24	21	0	2	35	—	—	10	189	234	—	0
dried sweetened flaked	7 oz pkg	944	64	57	0	7	95	—	—	28	509	629	—	0
dried sweetened flaked canned	1 cup	341	24	22	0	3	32	—	—	11	15	249	—	—
dried sweetened shredded	7 oz pkg	997	71	63	0	6	95	—	—	30	522	670	—	1
dried sweetened shredded	1 cup	466	33	29	0	2	44	—	—	14	244	313	—	1
dried toasted	1 oz	168	13	12	0	2	13	—	—	8	11	157	—	—
dried unsweetened	1 oz	187	18	16	0	2	7	—	—	7	11	154	3	tr
fresh	1 piece (1.5 oz)	159	15	13	0	2	7	—	4	6	9	160	12	2
fresh shredded	1 cup	283	27	24	0	3	12	—	7	12	16	285	21	3
BAKER'S														
Angel Flake	1 tbsp (0.5 oz)	70	5	5	0	1	6	5	1	0	45	55	—	0
Angel Flake (canned)	2 tbsp (0.5 oz)	70	6	5	0	1	6	5	1	0	0	65	—	0
Premium Shred	2 tbsp (0.5 oz)	70	5	5	0	1	6	5	1	0	45	60	—	0
COCONUT JUICE														
coconut water	1 cup	46	tr	tr	0	2	9	—	—	58	252	600	—	6
coconut water	1 tbsp	3	tr	tr	0	tr	1	—	—	4	16	38	—	tr
cream canned	1 cup	568	52	47	0	8	25	—	—	4	149	299	—	—
cream canned	1 tbsp	36	3	3	0	1	2	—	—	0	10	19	—	—
milk canned	1 cup	445	48	43	0	5	6	—	—	40	29	497	—	2
milk canned	1 tbsp	30	3	3	0	tr	tr	—	—	3	2	33	—	tr

FOOD	PORTION	CALS	FAT	SAT FAT	CHOL	PROT	CARB	SUGAR	FIBER	CALCI	SOD	POTAS	FOLIC	VIT C
milk frozen	1 tbsp	30	3	3	0	tr	1	—	—	1	2	35	—	—
milk frozen	1 cup	486	50	44	0	4	13	—	—	11	29	556	—	—
AMY & BRIAN														
Juice	8 oz	76	0	0	0	0	19	10	—	20	42	—	—	—
THAI KITCHEN														
Milk	2 oz	124	12	7	0	1	3	1	0	—	13	—	—	—
VITA COCO														
Coconut Water	1 box	65	0	0	0	0	17	17	—	50	65	530	—	—
ZICO														
Coconut Water Mango	11 oz	60	0	0	0	1	15	14	0	40	60	670	—	—
Coconut Water Natural	11 oz	60	0	0	0	1	15	14	0	40	60	670	—	—

COD

FOOD	PORTION	CALS	FAT	SAT FAT	CHOL	PROT	CARB	SUGAR	FIBER	CALCI	SOD	POTAS	FOLIC	VIT C
atlantic canned	1 can (11 oz)	327	3	1	171	71	0	—	—	66	680	1647	—	1
atlantic canned	3 oz	89	1	tr	47	19	0	—	—	18	185	449	—	1
atlantic dried	3 oz	246	2	tr	129	53	0	—	—	136	5973	1239	—	3
atlantic fresh cooked	1 fillet (6.3 oz)	189	2	tr	99	41	0	—	—	25	141	440	—	2
atlantic fresh cooked	3 oz	89	1	tr	47	19	0	—	—	12	66	208	—	1
atlantic fresh raw	3 oz	70	1	tr	37	15	0	—	—	13	46	351	—	1
pacific fresh baked	3 oz	95	1	tr	43	21	0	—	—	8	82	465	—	—
roe canned	1 oz	34	1	—	—	6	tr	—	—	4	—	—	—	—
roe raw	1 oz	37	tr	—	103	7	tr	—	—	—	—	—	—	4
roe tarama	3.5 oz	547	55	—	—	8	6	tr	—	29	600	111	—	—
TAKE-OUT														
roe baked w/butter & lemon juice	1 oz	36	1	—	—	6	tr	—	—	43	21	38	—	—

COFFEE

(*see also* COFFEE BEVERAGES, COFFEE SUBSTITUTES)

FOOD	PORTION	CALS	FAT	SAT FAT	CHOL	PROT	CARB	SUGAR	FIBER	CALCI	SOD	POTAS	FOLIC	VIT C
INSTANT														
decaffeinated	1 rounded tsp	4	0	0	0	tr	1	—	—	3	0	63	0	0
decaffeinated as prep	6 oz	4	0	0	0	tr	1	—	—	6	6	63	0	0
regular as prep	1 cup (6 oz)	4	0	0	0	tr	1	—	0	5	5	64	0	0
regular w/ chicory	1 rounded tsp	6	0	0	0	tr	1	—	—	2	5	61	—	—
regular w/ chicory as prep	6 oz	6	0	0	0	tr	1	—	—	6	10	61	—	—
NESCAFÉ														
Decafe	1 tsp (2 g)	0	0	0	0	tr	tr	0	0	0	0	—	—	0
Decafe w/ Chicory	1 tsp (2 g)	0	0	0	0	tr	tr	0	0	0	0	—	—	0
French Vanilla	1 tsp (2 g)	5	0	0	0	0	1	0	0	0	0	—	—	0

FOOD	PORTION	CALS	FAT	SAT FAT	CHOL	PROT	CARB	SUGAR	FIBER	CALCI	SOD	POTAS	FOLIC	VIT C
NESCAFÉ (CONT.)														
French Vanilla Decaf	1 tsp (2 g)	5	0	0	0	0	1	0	0	0	0	—	—	0
Hazelnut	1 tsp (2 g)	5	0	0	0	0	1	0	0	0	0	—	—	0
Irish Creme	1 tsp (2 g)	5	0	0	0	0	1	0	0	0	0	—	—	0
Regular	1 tsp (2 g)	0	0	0	0	tr	tr	0	0	0	0	50	—	0
With Chicory	1 tsp (2 g)	5	0	0	0	0	1	0	0	0	0	45	—	0
REGULAR														
brewed	8 oz	2	0	0	0	tr	tr	—	—	1	1	16	0	0
roasted beans	1 oz	64	4	—	—	4	18	—	2	42	—	—	—	—
NESCAFE														
Cafe Mocha	1 can (10 oz)	140	3	3	10	3	27	24	1	80	115	270	—	0
Caffe Latte	1 can (10 oz)	130	3	2	15	3	22	20	1	100	130	330	—	0
Caffe Latte Decaffeinated	1 can (10 oz)	130	3	2	15	3	22	20	0	100	100	300	—	0
Espresso	1 tsp (2 g)	0	0	0	0	tr	tr	0	0	0	0	50	—	0
Espresso Cafe Latte	1 pkg (0.6 oz)	70	2	1	10	3	10	6	0	100	50	340	—	0
Espresso Cafe Mocha	1 pkg (1 oz)	110	3	2	10	3	20	15	1	80	35	450	—	0
Espresso Cappuccino	1 pkg (0.6 oz)	80	3	2	10	3	11	6	0	100	40	390	—	0
Espresso Roast	1 can (10 oz)	90	1	1	<5	1	21	14	0	40	75	280	—	0
French Vanilla	1 can (10 oz)	150	4	3	15	4	25	21	2	100	140	320	—	0
Hazelnut	1 can (10 oz)	130	3	2	15	3	22	20	0	100	100	300	—	0
Roasted Ground as prep	1 cup (6 oz)	0	0	0	0	tr	tr	0	0	0	0	—	—	0
Roasted Ground Decaffeinated as prep	1 cup (6 oz)	0	0	0	0	tr	tr	0	0	0	0	—	—	0
REVIVAL														
Soy Caramel Corn	1 cup (8 oz)	0	0	0	0	0	0	0	0	—	0	—	—	—
Soy Hazelnut	1 cup (8 oz)	0	0	0	0	0	0	0	0	—	0	—	—	—
Soy Original Roast	1 cup (8 oz)	0	0	0	0	0	0	0	0	—	0	—	—	—
COFFEE BEVERAGES														
cappuccino mix as prep	7 oz	62	2	2	—	tr	11	—	—	7	104	119	0	0
french mix as prep	7 oz	57	3	3	—	1	7	—	—	8	—	137	—	—
mocha mix as prep	7 oz	51	2	2	—	1	8	—	—	7	36	119	0	0
ACHIEVONE														
All Flavors	1 bottle (9.5 oz)	120	0	—	20	20	5	4	—	250	200	—	180	15
AMERICA'S BEST BREW														
Iced Coffee All Flavors	8 oz	110	2	0	0	3	25	22	—	80	15	—	—	—

FOOD	PORTION	CALS	FAT	SAT FAT	CHOL	PROT	CARB	SUGAR	FIBER	CALCI	SOD	POTAS	FOLIC	VIT C
ARIZONA														
Iced Latte Supreme	8 oz	110	2	1	6	3	21	16	1	120	95	—	—	0
Iced Mocha Latte	8 oz	110	2	1	5	4	21	19	1	170	98	—	—	0
BIG TRAIN														
Low Carb Blended Ice Mocha as prep	1 serv (16 oz)	90	5	1	0	6	14	2	1	150	190	340	—	1
CHOCK FULL O'NUTS														
New York Cappuccino French Vanilla	1 pkg (0.9 oz)	90	2	2	0	2	19	14	0	40	115	—	—	0
New York Cappuccino Hazelnut	1 pkg. (0.9 oz)	90	2	2	0	2	19	14	0	40	115	—	—	0
COFFEE HOUSE USA														
All Flavors	1 bottle (9.5 oz)	100	4	3	15	4	29	28	tr	150	160	360	—	1
FLAVOUR CREATIONS														
Coffee Flavoring Tablets All Flavors	1 tablet	0	0	0	0	0	tr	tr	0	—	0	—	—	—
GEHL'S														
Iced Cappuccino	1 can (11 oz)	190	2	1	13	11	33	31	0	330	330	—	—	0
GENERAL FOODS														
Cappuccino Coolers French Vanilla as prep w/ 2% milk	1 serv	180	5	3	21	—	27	—	0	300	120	—	—	1
International Coffees Sugar Free Cafe Vienna as prep	1 serv (8 oz)	30	2	1	0	tr	3	0	0	0	75	110	—	0
International Coffees Sugar Free Fat Free Suisse Mocha as prep	1 serv (8 oz)	25	0	0	0	0	5	0	tr	0	35	110	—	0
International Coffees Café Français as prep	1 serv (8 oz)	60	4	1	0	tr	7	4	0	0	95	130	—	0
International Coffees Cafe Vienna as prep	1 serv (8 oz)	70	3	1	0	tr	11	9	tr	0	110	130	—	0
International Coffees Decaffeinated French Vanilla Café as prep	1 serv (8 oz)	60	3	1	0	tr	10	7	0	0	55	75	—	0

FOOD	PORTION	CALS	FAT	SAT FAT	CHOL	PROT	CARB	SUGAR	FIBER	CALCI	SOD	POTAS	FOLIC	VIT C
GENERAL FOODS (CONT.)														
International Coffees Decaffeinated Suisse Mocha as prep	1 serv (8 oz)	60	2	1	0	tr	9	7	0	0	35	110	—	0
International Coffees French Vanilla Cafe as prep	1 serv (8 oz)	60	3	1	0	tr	10	7	0	0	55	80	—	0
International Coffees Hazelnut Belgian Cafe as prep	1 serv (8 oz)	70	2	1	0	tr	12	9	0	0	60	115	—	0
International Coffees Irish Creme Cafe as prep	1 serv (8 oz)	60	2	1	0	tr	10	8	0	0	45	70	—	0
International Coffees Italian Cappuccino as prep	1 serv (8 oz)	60	2	1	0	tr	10	8	0	0	50	85	—	0
International Coffees Kahlúa Cafe as prep	1 serv (8 oz)	60	2	1	0	tr	10	7	0	0	55	80	—	0
International Coffees Orange Cappuccino as prep	1 serv (8 oz)	70	2	1	0	tr	11	9	tr	0	100	140	—	0
International Coffees Suisse Mocha as prep	1 serv (8 oz)	60	2	1	0	tr	8	7	0	0	35	115	—	0
International Coffees Viennese Chocolate Cafe as prep	1 serv (8 oz)	50	2	1	0	tr	10	9	0	0	30	70	—	0
International Coffees Sugar Free Fat Free Decaffeinated French Vanilla as prep	1 serv (8 oz)	25	0	0	0	0	5	0	0	0	65	65	—	0
International Coffees Sugar Free Fat Free Decaffeinated Suisse Mocha as prep	1 serv (8 oz)	25	0	0	0	0	5	0	tr	0	35	105	—	0

FOOD	PORTION	CALS	FAT	SAT FAT	CHOL	PROT	CARB	SUGAR	FIBER	CALCI	SOD	POTAS	FOLIC	VIT C
GENERAL FOODS (CONT.)														
International Coffees Sugar Free Fat Free French Vanilla Cafe as prep	1 serv (8 oz)	25	0	0	0	0	5	0	0	0	65	70	—	0
JAKADA														
Latte Mocha	1 bottle (10.5 oz)	180	3.5	0	10	5	33	32	0	150	70	—	—	0
Latte Vanilla	1 bottle (10.5 oz)	180	4	2	10	4	32	31	0	150	70	—	—	0
LOW CARB CREATIONS														
Cappuccino	1 cup	30	2	0	0	0	3	tr	0	0	39	—	—	0
MAXWELL HOUSE														
Cafe Cappuccino Amaretto as prep	1 serv (8 oz)	90	1	0	0	1	19	18	0	60	65	95	—	0
Cafe Cappuccino Decaffeinated Mocha as prep	1 serv (8 oz)	100	3	1	0	2	17	16	0	80	70	160	—	0
Cafe Cappuccino Decaffeinated Vanilla as prep	1 serv (8 oz)	90	1	0	0	1	19	18	0	60	65	90	—	0
Cafe Cappuccino Irish Cream as prep	1 serv (8 oz)	90	1	0	0	1	19	18	0	60	65	105	—	0
Cafe Cappuccino Mocha as prep	1 serv (8 oz)	100	3	1	0	2	17	16	0	80	65	170	—	0
Cafe Cappuccino Sugar Free Mocha as prep	1 serv (8 oz)	60	3	1	0	1	7	0	tr	0	80	90	—	0
Cafe Cappuccino Sugar Free Vanilla as prep	1 serv (8 oz)	60	3	1	0	tr	7	0	0	0	85	65	—	0
Iced Cappuccino as prep w/ 2% milk	1 serv (8 oz)	180	5	3	20	8	27	27	tr	300	125	460	—	1
SILK														
Coffee Soylatte	1 bottle (11 oz)	220	5	1	0	7	38	31	0	400	70	100	24	0
SIPPER SWEETS														
Sugar Free Low Carb Cappuccino	1 serv	50	3	0	0	1	3	0	0	—	80	—	—	—
STARBUCKS														
Frappuccino	1 bottle (9.5 oz)	190	3	2	12	6	39	30	0	220	110	—	—	0
Frappuccino Mocha	1 bottle (9.5 oz)	190	3	2	12	6	39	30	0	220	110	—	—	0

FOOD	PORTION	CALS	FAT	SAT FAT	CHOL	PROT	CARB	SUGAR	FIBER	CALCI	SOD	POTAS	FOLIC	VIT C
STARBUCKS (CONT.)														
Frappuccino Vanilla	1 bottle (9.5 oz)	190	3	2	12	6	39	30	0	220	110	—	—	0
TAKE-OUT														
café amaretto w/ alcohol	1 serv	192	9	6	33	1	15	—	0	25	14	197	1	tr
café au lait	1 cup (8 fl oz)	77	4	3	17	4	6	7	—	148	62	249	6	1
café brûlot	1 cup	48	0	0	0	tr	3	3	—	2	2	64	tr	0
café brûlot w/ alcohol	1 serv	130	tr	tr	0	1	16	—	3	55	4	162	12	24
cappuccino	1 cup (8 fl oz)	77	4	3	17	4	6	7	—	148	62	249	6	1
cafe con leche	1 cup (8 fl oz)	77	4	3	17	4	6	7	—	148	62	249	6	1
espresso	1 cup (3 fl oz)	2	0	0	0	tr	tr	0	—	2	2	48	tr	0
irish coffee	1 serv	226	11	7	41	1	6	—	0	25	15	121	1	tr
latte w/ skim milk	13 oz	88	tr	tr	4	8	12	11	0	304	128	470	13	2
latte w/ whole milk	13 oz	152	8	5	33	8	12	11	0	293	122	434	12	2
mocha	1 mug (9.6 fl oz)	202	15	9	40	3	17	12	—	67	28	228	2	tr

COFFEE SUBSTITUTES

FOOD	PORTION	CALS	FAT	SAT FAT	CHOL	PROT	CARB	SUGAR	FIBER	CALCI	SOD	POTAS	FOLIC	VIT C
powder	1 tsp	9	tr	tr	0	tr	2	—	—	1	2	42	—	—
powder as prep	6 oz	9	tr	tr	0	tr	2	—	—	5	7	43	—	—
powder as prep w/ milk	6 oz	121	6	4	25	6	10	—	—	219	91	319	9	2
NATURAL TOUCH														
Kaffree Roma	1 tsp (2 g)	10	0	0	0	0	2	0	0	0	0	20	—	0
Roma Cappuccino	3 tbsp (0.4 oz)	50	3	3	0	1	5	4	0	0	15	70	—	0
POSTUM														
Instant as prep	1 serv (8 oz)	10	0	0	0	0	3	0	0	0	0	110	—	0
Instant Coffee Flavor as prep	1 serv (8 oz)	10	0	0	0	0	3	0	0	0	0	110	—	0

COFFEE WHITENERS

FOOD	PORTION	CALS	FAT	SAT FAT	CHOL	PROT	CARB	SUGAR	FIBER	CALCI	SOD	POTAS	FOLIC	VIT C
liquid nondairy frzn	1 tbsp (0.5 oz)	20	2	tr	0	tr	2	—	—	1	12	29	0	0
powder nondairy	1 tsp	11	tr	1	0	tr	1	—	—	tr	4	16	0	0
N-RICH														
Coffee Creamer	1 tsp (2 g)	10	1	tr	0	tr	1	0	0	tr	4	—	—	0
SILK														
Creamer	1 tbsp	15	1	0	0	0	1	0	0	0	5	—	—	0
Creamer French Vanilla	1 tbsp	20	1	0	0	0	3	3	0	0	5	—	—	0
Creamer Hazelnut	1 tbsp	15	1	0	0	0	1	0	0	0	5	—	—	0

FOOD	PORTION	CALS	FAT	SAT FAT	CHOL	PROT	CARB	SUGAR	FIBER	CALCI	SOD	POTAS	FOLIC	VIT C
COLESLAW														
FRESH EXPRESS														
Cole Slaw Kit as prep	2 cups	120	8	1	5	1	12	10	2	40	135	—	—	24
TAKE-OUT														
coleslaw w/ dressing	½ cup	42	2	tr	5	1	7	—	—	27	14	109	16	20
vinegar & oil coleslaw	3.5 oz	150	9	1	0	1	16	—	—	20	480	—	—	30
COLLARDS														
fresh cooked	½ cup	17	tr	—	0	1	4	—	—	15	10	84	4	8
frzn chopped cooked	½ cup	31	tr	—	0	3	6	—	—	179	42	214	65	23
raw chopped	½ cup	6	tr	—	0	tr	1	—	—	5	4	30	2	4
BIRDS EYE														
Chopped Greens frzn	1 cup	30	0	0	0	2	2	1	2	80	20	—	—	15
COOKIES														
MIX														
chocolate chip	1 (0.56 oz)	79	4	1	7	1	10	—	—	7	47	34	—	0
oatmeal	1 (0.6 oz)	74	3	1	7	1	10	—	tr	5	75	30	—	—
oatmeal raisin	1 (0.6 oz)	74	3	1	7	1	10	—	tr	5	75	30	—	—
AUNT PAULA'S														
Low Carb Chef Chocolate Chip as prep	1	66	4	1	2	9	4	0	1	—	—	—	—	—
Low Carb Chef Peanut Butter as prep	1	66	4	1	2	9	4	0	1	—	—	—	—	—
BETTY CROCKER														
Chocolate Peanut Butter as prep	1 bar	180	9	2	18	2	25	18	—	—	150	60	8	—
Date Bar as prep	1 bar	150	6	2	0	1	23	14	1	—	30	—	8	—
Oatmeal as prep	2	150	6	1	12	2	22	12	1	—	100	45	8	—
BIG TRAIN														
Low Carb Chocolate Chip as prep	2	140	9	4	42	2	11	5	4	20	45	—	—	0
Low Carb Peanut Butter as prep	2	140	9	4	24	2	9	2	4	20	120	—	—	0
GOLDNBROWN														
Fat Free	1 (1.1 oz)	120	0	0	0	2	27	15	0	20	135	—	24	0
KETO														
Chocolate Chip as prep	1	47	2	—	—	3	2	1	1	—	25	—	—	—

FOOD	PORTION	CALS	FAT	SAT FAT	CHOL	PROT	CARB	SUGAR	FIBER	CALCI	SOD	POTAS	FOLIC	VIT C
KETO (CONT.)														
Oatmeal Raisin as prep	2	59	3	—	—	6	2	0	1	—	50	—	—	—
MINICARB														
All Flavors as prep	1	110	2	0	5	4	7	1	5	—	45	—	—	—
READY-TO-EAT														
animal crackers	11 crackers (1 oz)	126	4	1	—	2	21	—	—	12	112	28	4	0
animal crackers	1 (2.5 g)	11	tr	tr	—	tr	2	—	—	1	10	2	0	0
animal crackers	1 box (2.4 oz)	299	9	4	11	4	51	—	—	11	274	57	22	tr
australian anzac biscuit	1	98	3	1	0	1	17	—	1	11	59	—	—	—
butter	1 (5 g)	23	1	1	—	tr	3	—	tr	1	18	6	0	0
chocolate chip	1 box (1.9 oz)	233	12	5	12	3	36	—	—	20	188	82	16	tr
chocolate chip	1 (0.4 oz)	48	2	1	—	1	7	—	tr	2	32	14	1	0
chocolate chip low fat	1 (0.25 oz)	45	2	tr	0	1	7	—	—	2	38	12	—	—
chocolate chip low sugar low sodium	1 (0.24 oz)	31	1	1	0	tr	5	—	—	—	1	14	—	0
chocolate chip soft-type	1 (0.5 oz)	69	4	1	0	1	9	—	tr	2	49	14	1	0
chocolate w/ creme filling	1 (0.35 oz)	47	2	tr	—	1	7	—	tr	3	36	18	0	0
chocolate w/ creme filling chocolate coated	1 (0.60 oz)	82	5	1	—	1	11	—	—	6	55	41	—	—
chocolate w/ creme filling sugar free low sodium	1 (0.35 oz)	46	2	1	—	1	7	—	—	—	24	29	—	—
chocolate w/ extra creme filling	1 (0.46 oz)	65	3	1	—	1	9	—	—	3	64	16	—	0
chocolate wafer	1 (0.2 oz)	26	1	tr	0	tr	4	—	—	2	35	13	—	—
cream cheese	1 (1.1 oz)	141	9	6	25	2	14	6	tr	12	53	24	4	0
digestive biscuits plain	2	141	7	—	—	2	21	—	1	28	—	—	—	0
fig bars	1 (0.56 oz)	56	1	tr	—	1	11	—	1	10	56	33	2	—
fortune	1 (0.28 oz)	30	tr	tr	—	tr	7	—	tr	1	22	3	1	0
fudge	1 (0.73 oz)	73	1	tr	—	1	17	—	tr	7	40	29	—	—
gingersnaps	1 (0.24 oz)	29	1	tr	0	tr	5	—	—	5	48	24	—	0
graham	1 square (0.24 oz)	30	1	tr	0	1	5	—	—	2	42	9	1	0
graham chocolate covered	1 (0.49 oz)	68	3	2	0	1	9	—	—	8	41	29	—	0
graham honey	1 (0.24 oz)	30	1	tr	0	1	5	—	tr	2	42	9	1	0
hermits	1 (1 oz)	117	5	2	23	2	18	10	1	16	54	76	5	tr

FOOD	PORTION	CALS	FAT	SAT FAT	CHOL	PROT	CARB	SUGAR	FIBER	CALCI	SOD	POTAS	FOLIC	VIT C
jumbles coconut	1 (1 oz)	121	7	5	26	1	13	7	1	5	19	31	4	tr
ladyfingers	1 (0.38 oz)	40	1	tr	40	1	7	—	—	5	16	12	4	tr
macaroons	1 (0.8 oz)	97	3	3	0	1	17	—	—	12	59	38	1	0
madeleines	1 (0.8 oz)	86	5	3	46	2	10	5	tr	7	34	17	5	tr
marshmallow chocolate coated	1 (0.46 oz)	55	2	1	—	1	9	—	—	6	22	24	—	—
marshmallow pie chocolate coated	1 (1.4 oz)	165	7	2	—	2	26	—	—	18	66	72	—	—
meringue	1 (0.3 oz)	20	0	0	0	tr	5	5	0	0	20	—	—	0
molasses	1 (0.5 oz)	65	2	tr	0	1	11	—	—	11	69	52	—	0
neapolitan tri-color cookie	1 (0.6 oz)	79	5	2	17	1	8	5	tr	12	10	36	4	tr
oatmeal	1 (0.6 oz)	81	3	1	0	1	12	—	1	7	69	26	—	—
oatmeal soft-type	1 (0.5 oz)	61	2	tr	—	1	10	—	tr	13	52	20	—	—
oatmeal raisin	1 (0.6 oz)	81	3	1	0	1	12	—	1	7	69	26	—	—
oatmeal raisin low sugar no sodium	1 (0.24 oz)	31	1	1	0	tr	5	—	—	—	1	12	—	—
oatmeal raisin soft-type	1 (0.5 oz)	61	2	tr	—	1	10	—	tr	13	52	20	—	—
peanut butter sandwich	1 (0.5 oz)	67	3	1	0	1	9	—	—	7	52	27	—	0
peanut butter sandwich sugar free low sodium	1 (0.35 oz)	54	3	1	—	1	5	—	—	—	41	29	—	0
peanut butter soft-type	1 (0.5 oz)	69	4	1	0	1	9	—	tr	2	50	16	1	0
pinenut cookies	1 (1.1 oz)	134	9	1	0	4	11	8	1	29	11	130	7	tr
raisin soft-type	1 (0.5 oz)	60	2	1	0	1	10	—	—	7	51	21	—	—
reginette queen'a biscuit	1 (0.8 oz)	86	3	1	tr	2	13	4	tr	27	83	32	8	tr
shortbread	1 (0.28 oz)	40	2	tr	2	1	5	—	—	3	36	8	—	0
shortbread pecan	1 (0.49 oz)	79	5	1	5	1	8	—	tr	4	39	10	—	—
spritz	1 (0.4 oz)	42	2	1	6	1	6	3	tr	4	9	11	2	tr
sugar	1 (0.52 oz)	72	3	1	8	1	10	—	—	3	53	9	—	—
sugar low sugar sodium free	1 (0.24 oz)	30	1	tr	0	1	5	—	—	—	0	7	—	0
sugar wafers w/ creme filling	1 (0.12 oz)	18	1	tr	0	tr	3	—	—	1	5	2	—	0
sugar wafers w/ creme filling sugar free sodium free	1 (0.14 oz)	20	1	tr	0	tr	3	—	—	2	0	2	0	0
toll house original	1 (0.8 oz)	105	6	2	15	2	13	9	tr	15	57	57	4	tr
vanilla sandwich	1 (0.35 oz)	48	2	tr	0	tr	7	—	tr	3	35	9	0	0
vanilla wafers	1 (0.21 oz)	28	1	tr	—	tr	4	—	—	2	18	6	—	—
zeppole	1 (0.8 oz)	78	6	2	24	1	6	4	tr	3	14	9	3	0

FOOD	PORTION	CALS	FAT	SAT FAT	CHOL	PROT	CARB	SUGAR	FIBER	CALCI	SOD	POTAS	FOLIC	VIT C
ALTERNATIVE BAKING														
Vegan Chocolate Chip	1 serv (2.5 oz)	280	10	4	0	3	46	21	1	20	150	—	—	0
Vegan Expresso Chocolate Chip	1 serv (2 oz)	230	9	3	0	3	35	18	1	20	125	—	—	0
Vegan Lemon	1 serv (2.25 oz)	250	7	2	0	3	42	19	1	40	170	—	—	0
Vegan Oatmeal	1 serv (2.25 oz)	250	10	2	0	5	35	15	2	50	105	—	—	5
Vegan Peanut Butter	1 serv (2.25 oz)	270	10	2	0	5	40	17	1	40	115	—	—	0
Vegan Pumpkin	1 serv (2 oz)	200	6	2	0	2	35	17	1	20	120	—	—	0
Vegan Wheat Free Choco Cherry Chunk	1 serv (1.75 oz)	190	6	2	0	3	32	18	1	20	30	—	—	0
Vegan Wheat Free Hula Nut	1 serv (1.75 oz)	190	6	2	0	6	29	10	2	20	65	—	—	1
Vegan Wheat Free P-nut Fudge Fusion	1 serv (1.75 oz)	190	7	2	0	4	29	15	1	20	75	—	—	0
Vegan Wheat Free Snickerdoodle	1 serv (1.75 oz)	170	3	0	0	3	35	17	1	20	70	—	—	0
AMAY'S														
Chinese Style Almond	1 (0.5 oz)	80	4	2	4	1	10	4	0	10	13	—	—	0
ARCHWAY														
Alpine Fudge	1 (1.3 oz)	160	6	4	<5	1	24	15	tr	0	80	—	—	0
Carrot Cake	1 (1 oz)	130	5	2	5	1	19	11	0	0	200	—	—	0
Chocolate Chip	1 (0.9 oz)	120	6	2	5	tr	16	9	0	0	85	—	—	0
Chocolate Chip Sugar Free	1 (0.8 oz)	110	5	2	0	1	16	0	0	60	65	—	—	0
Coconut Macaroon	2 (1.4 oz)	180	11	9	0	1	21	16	1	0	500	—	—	0
Devils Food Chocolate Drop Fat Free	1 (0.7 oz)	60	0	0	0	1	15	9	0	0	70	—	—	0
Dutch Cocoa	1 (0.9 oz)	100	4	1	0	1	18	10	0	0	65	—	—	0
Frosty Lemon	1 (0.9 oz)	100	4	2	0	tr	16	10	0	0	100	—	—	0
Fruit & Honey Bar	1 (0.9 oz)	110	3	1	5	1	19	10	0	0	100	—	—	0
Fruit Bar Fat Free	1 (0.9 oz)	90	0	0	0	tr	21	11	0	0	90	—	—	0
Fruit Filled Apricot	1 (0.8 oz)	90	3	1	<5	1	15	7	0	0	75	—	—	0
Fruit Filled Raspberry	1 (0.8 oz)	90	3	1	<5	1	15	7	0	0	80	—	—	0
Ginger Snaps	5 (1 oz)	120	5	1	0	1	20	9	0	0	150	—	—	0
Homestyle Chocolate Chip	3 (1 oz)	130	7	2	5	1	17	9	1	0	60	—	—	0
Iced Spice	1 (1 oz)	120	5	2	0	1	19	10	0	20	140	—	—	0

FOOD	PORTION	CALS	FAT	SAT FAT	CHOL	PROT	CARB	SUGAR	FIBER	CALCI	SOD	POTAS	FOLIC	VIT C
ARCHWAY (CONT.)														
Oatmeal	1 (0.9 oz)	100	4	1	5	1	16	8	0	0	100	—	—	0
Oatmeal Apple Filled	1 (0.9 oz)	90	3	1	<5	1	16	8	0	0	70	—	—	0
Oatmeal Pecan	1 (0.9 oz)	110	4	1	5	1	16	8	1	0	120	—	—	0
Oatmeal Raisin	1	120	4	1	<5	2	20	11	tr	20	100	—	—	0
Oatmeal Raspberry Fat Free	1 (1.1 oz)	100	0	0	0	1	23	13	1	0	170	—	—	0
Oatmeal Sugar Free	1 (0.8 oz)	110	5	1	0	1	16	0	0	0	75	—	—	0
Oatmeal Raisin Fat Free	1 (1.1 oz)	100	0	0	0	1	24	14	1	0	60	—	—	0
Old Dutch Apple	1 (0.9 oz)	110	4	1	5	1	18	11	0	0	115	—	—	0
Peanut Butter	1 (1 oz)	150	9	2	5	2	16	8	0	0	110	—	—	0
Peanut Butter Fudge	1 (1.3 oz)	220	13	5	<5	3	23	13	1	0	135	—	—	0
Peanut Butter Sugar Free	1 (0.8 oz)	110	6	2	0	2	14	0	0	0	85	—	—	0
Pecan Crunch	3 (1.2 oz)	180	10	2	5	2	20	9	0	0	140	—	—	0
Rocky Road	1 (0.8 oz)	110	5	2	10	1	16	9	0	0	70	—	—	0
Rocky Road Sugar Free	1 (0.8 oz)	100	5	1	0	1	15	0	tr	40	65	—	—	0
Shortbread Sugar Free	1 (0.8 oz)	110	5	2	0	1	16	0	0	0	45	—	—	0
Windmill	1	90	4	1	0	1	14	7	0	0	95	—	—	0
ARNOTT'S														
Raspberry Tartlets	2	100	4	2	0	1	17	6	tr	40	70	—	—	0
ATKINS														
Endulge Wafer Bars Chocolate Creme	2 bars (1 oz)	120	9	5	0	4	15	0	3	—	115	—	—	—
Endulge Wafer Bars Mint	2 bars (1 oz)	120	9	5	0	4	15	0	3	—	115	—	—	—
Endulge Wafer Bars Peanut Butter	2 bars (1 oz)	120	9	4	0	4	14	0	3	—	125	—	—	—
BAHLSEN														
Afrika	8 (1.1 oz)	170	10	6	5	2	17	11	2	20	20	—	—	0
Butter Leaves	7 (1 oz)	140	7	4	15	2	19	7	tr	0	50	—	—	0
Choco Leibniz	2 (1 oz)	140	7	4	5	2	18	10	tr	0	50	—	—	0
Choco Star Dark Chocolate	3 (1.1 oz)	170	12	6	0	2	16	10	1	0	10	—	—	0
Choco Star Milk Chocolate	3 (1.1 oz)	180	12	6	<5	2	16	12	1	20	25	—	—	0
Chocolate Hearts	4 (1 oz)	160	9	6	5	2	18	8	1	0	25	—	—	0
Delice	6 (1 oz)	140	6	2	0	2	19	5	tr	0	100	—	—	0
Deloba	4 (0.9 oz)	130	5	2	0	2	19	8	tr	0	80	—	—	0

FOOD	PORTION	CALS	FAT	SAT FAT	CHOL	PROT	CARB	SUGAR	FIBER	CALCI	SOD	POTAS	FOLIC	VIT C
BAHLSEN (CONT.)														
Hanover Waffelin	5 (1 oz)	160	10	9	0	1	16	8	0	0	35	—	—	0
Hit Chocolate Vanilla Filled	2 (1 oz)	140	8	6	0	2	18	9	tr	0	75	—	—	0
Hit Vanilla Chocolate Filled	2 (1 oz)	140	7	5	0	2	19	9	tr	0	65	—	—	0
Kipferl	4 (1 oz)	150	9	3	5	2	16	6	0	0	10	—	—	0
Leibniz	6 (1 oz)	130	4	2	10	2	23	7	1	0	125	—	—	0
Nuss Dessert	3 (1.1 oz)	180	11	5	10	2	19	9	tr	20	60	—	—	0
Probiers	6 (1.1 oz)	150	6	3	0	2	21	9	tr	0	60	—	—	0
Twingo	6 (1.1 oz)	170	11	9	0	2	18	11	1	0	15	—	—	0
Waffeletten	4 (1 oz)	160	9	6	<5	2	18	10	1	0	40	—	—	0
BAKER'S BREAKFAST COOKIE														
Apple Pie	1 (3 oz)	204	2	tr	0	8	44	22	6	60	220	—	—	0
Banana Walnut	1 (3 oz)	274	8	1	0	8	52	20	5	0	200	—	—	0
Chocolate Chunk Raisin	1 (3 oz)	260	5	1	0	8	54	24	5	0	200	—	—	0
Double Chocolate Chunk	1 (3 oz)	250	5	1	0	8	50	22	5	40	200	—	—	0
Fruit & Nut	1 (3 oz)	270	5	1	0	8	54	26	5	40	210	—	—	0
Lemon Poppy Seed	1 (3 oz)	230	3	1	0	8	52	22	5	80	200	—	—	0
Mocha Chocolate Chunk	1 (3 oz)	250	5	1	0	8	50	22	5	40	230	—	—	0
Oatmeal Raisin	1 (3 oz)	250	4	1	0	8	54	24	5	40	200	—	—	0
Peanut Butter	1 (3 oz)	290	8	2	0	10	48	20	6	0	230	—	—	0
Peanut Butter & Jelly	1 (3 oz)	320	9	1	0	10	64	34	6	40	340	—	—	5
Pumpkin Spice	1 (3 oz)	230	3	1	0	8	52	22	5	180	200	—	—	2
Vegan Chocolate Chunk	1 (3 oz)	260	6	2	0	8	52	22	5	0	200	—	—	0
Vegan Peanut Butter Chocolate Chunk	1 (3 oz)	310	10	2	0	10	58	24	6	0	240	—	—	0
BAKER'S HARVEST														
Animal	12 (0.9 oz)	130	3	1	—	2	22	5	—	—	80	—	—	—
Chocolate Graham	2 (0.9 oz)	130	3	1	—	2	24	7	1	—	120	—	—	—
Cinnamon Graham	2 (0.9 oz)	130	5	1	—	1	19	7	tr	—	85	—	—	—
Cinnamon Graham Low Fat	2 (0.9 oz)	110	2	0	0	2	22	6	1	—	120	—	—	—
Fig Bars	2 (1.2 oz)	120	3	0	—	tr	23	14	1	—	55	—	—	—
Graham	2 (0.9 oz)	120	4	1	—	1	21	6	tr	—	95	—	—	—
Graham Low Fat	2 (0.9 oz)	110	2	0	0	2	22	6	1	—	120	—	—	—
Iced Oatmeal	1 (0.6 oz)	70	3	1	0	1	11	6	0	—	65	—	—	—
Pecan Shortbread	1 (0.5 oz)	80	5	1	<5	1	10	4	0	0	55	—	—	0
Vanilla Wafers	7 (1.1 oz)	150	6	1	—	1	22	10	1	—	115	—	—	—

FOOD	PORTION	CALS	FAT	SAT FAT	CHOL	PROT	CARB	SUGAR	FIBER	CALCI	SOD	POTAS	FOLIC	VIT C
BARBARA'S BAKERY														
Apple Cinnamon Bars Fat Free Whole Wheat	1 (0.7 oz)	60	0	0	0	1	14	10	2	—	20	—	—	—
Chocolate Chip	1 (0.6 oz)	80	4	2	5	1	10	5	1	—	60	—	—	—
Double Dutch Chocolate	1 (0.6 oz)	80	4	2	5	1	10	5	1	—	60	—	—	—
Fig Bars Fat Free Wheat Free	1 (0.7 oz)	60	0	0	0	tr	15	11	1	—	20	—	—	—
Fig Bars Fat Free Whole Wheat	1 (0.7 oz)	60	0	0	0	tr	16	11	2	—	20	—	—	—
Nature's Choice Coconut Almond	1 bar (1 oz)	120	5	3	0	2	20	8	1	—	10	—	—	—
Nature's Choice Expresso Bean	1 bar (1 oz)	120	3	3	0	2	22	9	1	—	10	—	—	—
Nature's Choice Lemon Yogurt	1 bar (1 oz)	120	4	3	0	2	22	9	1	—	10	—	—	—
Nature's Choice Roasted Peanut	1 bar (1 oz)	130	5	2	0	3	20	8	1	—	50	—	—	—
Old Fashioned Oatmeal	1 (0.6 oz)	70	3	1	5	1	11	5	1	—	65	—	—	—
Raspberry Bars Fat Free Wheat Free Raspberry	1 (0.7 oz)	60	0	0	0	1	15	11	1	—	25	—	—	—
Snackimals Chocolate Chip	8 (1 oz)	120	5	1	0	2	18	8	1	—	85	—	—	—
Snackimals Oatmeal Wheat Free	8 (1 oz)	120	5	0	0	2	19	6	2	—	75	—	—	—
Snackimals Vanilla	8 (1 oz)	120	5	0	0	2	19	7	1	—	55	—	—	—
Traditional Blueberry Low Fat	1 (0.7 oz)	60	1	0	0	1	14	9	1	—	25	—	—	—
Traditional Fig Low Fat	1 (0.7 oz)	60	1	0	0	1	14	9	1	—	25	—	—	—
Traditional Shortbread	1 (0.6 oz)	80	4	3	10	1	10	3	1	—	40	—	—	—
BED & BREAKFAST														
Cranberry Orange Oatmeal	1 (0.8 oz)	110	5	2	10	1	17	9	1	0	75	—	—	0
Enrobed Shortbread	2 (1.4 oz)	190	9	4	15	2	24	10	1	20	125	—	—	0
Fruit Center Key Lime	2 (1.1 oz)	140	6	2	<5	1	22	12	0	0	55	—	—	0
Fruit Center Raspberry	2 (1.1 oz)	140	6	2	<5	1	22	11	0	0	55	—	—	0

FOOD	PORTION	CALS	FAT	SAT FAT	CHOL	PROT	CARB	SUGAR	FIBER	CALCI	SOD	POTAS	FOLIC	VIT C
BEIGEL'S														
Black & White	1 (1 oz)	100	3	1	0	1	18	15	0	0	20	—	—	0
BP GOURMET														
Biscotti Fat Free Cinnamon Crunch	6 (1 oz)	110	0	0	0	2	24	15	0	0	75	—	—	0
Biscotti Fat Free Vanilla Crunch	4 (1 oz)	80	0	0	0	2	18	6	0	20	25	—	—	0
Chocolate Fudge Chip Sugar Free	5 (1 oz)	100	6	3	0	1	13	0	0	0	80	—	—	0
Dreams Chocolate	7 (1 oz)	120	3	2	0	2	21	20	0	0	35	—	—	0
Dreams Fat Free Chocolate Fudge	13 (1 oz)	100	0	0	0	2	25	25	0	0	35	—	—	0
Dreams Fat Free Vanilla	19 (1 oz)	100	0	0	0	2	25	25	0	0	35	—	—	0
Tangos Fat Free Chocolate Fudge Chip	4 (1 oz)	100	0	0	0	2	23	18	0	0	95	—	—	0
BREAKTIME														
Chocolate Chip	1 (0.3 oz)	37	2	tr	0	tr	5	2	tr	—	37	1	—	—
Coconut	1 (0.3 oz)	35	1	tr	0	1	5	3	tr	—	15	3	—	—
Ginger	1 (0.3 oz)	34	1	tr	0	tr	6	3	—	—	<15	—	—	—
Oatmeal	1 (0.3 oz)	35	1	tr	0	1	5	3	tr	—	27	2	—	—
Sprinkles	1 (0.3 oz)	36	2	tr	0	tr	5	3	—	—	46	5	—	—
BRENT & SAM'S														
Chocolate Chip Pecan	2 (0.5 oz)	80	5	1	<5	1	9	6	0	0	60	—	—	0
Chocolate Chip Raspberry	2 (0.5 oz)	70	4	1	<5	tr	10	7	0	0	60	—	—	0
Chocolate Chip	2 (0.5 oz)	70	4	1	<5	1	10	7	0	0	65	—	—	0
Key Lime White Chocolate	2 (0.5 oz)	70	4	2	<5	tr	10	8	0	0	65	—	—	0
Oatmeal Raisin Pecan	2 (0.5 oz)	70	7	1	<5	tr	9	6	1	0	70			0
Toffee Pecan	2 (0.5 oz)	80	5	1	5	tr	9	5	0	0	75	—	—	0
White Chocolate Macadamia	2 (0.5 oz)	80	5	2	<5	tr	9	6	0	0	65	—	—	0
BUD'S BEST														
Cocoa Creme	7 (1 oz)	140	6	2	0	2	21	9	2	20	110	—	—	0
Chocolate Chip	6 (1 oz)	140	6	2	0	2	19	9	1	0	65	—	—	0
French Vanilla	7 (1 oz)	150	6	2	0	2	20	9	2	0	70	—	—	0
Oatmeal	6 (1 oz)	130	5	2	0	2	20	9	tr	0	65	—	—	0
CAFE														
Cinnamony Twists Chocolate Chip	1 (0.5 oz)	40	2	0	0	0	7	4	0	0	25	—	—	0

FOOD	PORTION	CALS	FAT	SAT FAT	CHOL	PROT	CARB	SUGAR	FIBER	CALCI	SOD	POTAS	FOLIC	VIT C
CAFE (CONT.)														
Sugar Free California Almond	4 (1 oz)	110	4	1	0	2	17	0	0	0	60	—	—	0
Twists Cinnamony	1 (0.3 oz)	40	2	0	0	0	7	4	0	0	25	—	—	0
CARBOLITE														
Chocolate Chip	1 (1 oz)	120	9	2	11	4	12	0	4	—	71	—	—	—
Peanut Butter	1 (1 oz)	120	9	2	11	4	12	0	4	—	71	—	—	—
Shortbread	1 (1 oz)	180	9	2	2	4	14	0	5	—	100	—	—	—
CARRIAGE TRADE														
Finnish Ginger Snaps	3	60	7	—	—	2	21	9	tr	0	135	—	—	0
CARR'S														
Ginger Lemon Cremes	2 (1 oz)	140	7	4	<5	1	19	11	tr	—	105	—	—	—
CHORTLES														
Cookies	½ pkg. (1 oz)	125	3	1	0	2	23	11	1	<10	109	—	—	tr
COOKIE LOVER'S														
Chocolate Chip	1 (0.8 oz)	90	4	2	10	1	16	9	0	20	90	—	—	0
Creme Supremes	2 (0.9 oz)	120	5	0	0	1	18	10	1	20	90	—	—	0
Creme Supremes Mint	2 (0.9 oz)	120	5	0	0	1	18	10	1	20	90	—	—	0
Grahams	2 (1 oz)	100	1	0	0	2	22	5	1	0	130	—	—	0
Grahams Cinnamon	2 (1 oz)	110	1	0	0	2	24	6	1	0	130	—	—	0
Peanut Butter	1 (0.8 oz)	100	4	2	15	2	16	7	0	20	55	—	—	0
Shortbread	1 (0.8 oz)	120	7	4	15	2	13	5	0	20	70	—	—	0
COUNTRY CHOICE														
Chocolate Chip Walnut	1	100	4	1	5	1	16	10	tr	0	65	—	—	0
Double Fudge Brownie	1	90	3	1	5	1	16	10	tr	0	85	—	—	0
Ginger	1	90	2	0	5	1	17	10	tr	0	75	—	—	0
Ginger Snaps	5	120	5	0	0	1	19	9	2	0	85	—	—	0
Lemon	1	90	3	0	5	1	17	10	tr	0	75	—	—	0
Oatmeal Chocolate Chip	1	100	4	1	5	2	15	8	1	0	70	—	—	0
Oatmeal Raisin	1	100	3	1	5	1	16	9	1	0	70	—	—	0
Old Fashioned Oatmeal	1	100	3	0	5	2	16	8	1	0	90	—	—	0
Peanut Butter	1	100	5	1	5	2	13	8	tr	0	75	—	—	0
Sandwich Cremes Chocolate	1	130	5	1	0	1	19	11	0	0	100	—	—	0
Sandwich Cremes Duplex	2	130	5	1	0	1	19	11	0	0	115	—	—	0
Sandwich Cremes Ginger Lemon	2	130	5	1	0	1	19	11	0	0	130	—	—	0

FOOD	PORTION	CALS	FAT	SAT FAT	CHOL	PROT	CARB	SUGAR	FIBER	CALCI	SOD	POTAS	FOLIC	VIT C
COUNTRY CHOICE (CONT.)														
Sandwich Cremes Mint Creme	2	130	5	1	0	1	19	11	0	0	100	—	—	0
Vanilla Wafers	7	120	5	0	5	1	19	8	2	0	100	—	—	0
COUNTRY NATURALS														
Sandwich Cremes Vanilla	2	130	5	1	0	1	19	11	0	0	125	—	—	0
DARE														
Blueberry Cheesecake	1 (0.6 oz)	90	5	1	4	1	11	7	tr	—	56	27	—	—
Butter Shortbread	1 (0.5 oz)	63	4	2	6	1	7	2	tr	—	45	2	—	—
Butter Creme	1 (0.6 oz)	85	4	1	2	1	11	4	1	—	96	36	—	—
Carrot Cake	1 (0.6 oz)	92	5	1	3	1	11	7	tr	—	61	39	—	—
Chocolate Chip	1 (0.5 oz)	77	4	1	2	1	9	6	tr	—	42	24	—	—
Chocolate Fudge	1 (0.7 oz)	97	5	3	1	1	13	5	1	—	36	11	—	—
Cinnamon Danish	1 (0.4 oz)	47	2	tr	2	1	7	2	tr	—	25	8	—	—
Coconut Creme	1 (0.7 oz)	99	5	3	1	1	12	7	tr	—	42	17	—	—
French Creme	1 (0.5 oz)	80	5	3	1	1	8	4	tr	—	21	10	—	—
Harvest from the Rain Forest	1 (0.5 oz)	70	4	1	2	1	7	3	tr	—	39	19	—	—
Key Lime Creme	1 (0.6 oz)	86	4	1	0	1	12	5	tr	—	69	25	—	—
Lemon Creme	1 (0.7 oz)	95	5	1	1	1	13	6	tr	—	66	9	—	—
Maple Leaf Creme	1 (0.6 oz)	83	4	1	0	1	12	5	tr	—	53	13	—	—
Maple Walnut Fudge	1 (0.7 oz)	99	5	3	0	1	13	6	tr	—	36	9	—	—
Milk Chocolate Fudge	1 (0.7 oz)	99	5	3	1	1	12	5	tr	—	32	11	—	—
Oatmeal Raisin	1 (0.4 oz)	59	3	1	4	1	8	3	tr	—	22	6	—	—
Social Tea	1 (0.2 oz)	26	1	tr	0	tr	4	—	tr	—	25	5	—	—
Sun Maid Raisin Oatmeal	1 (0.5 oz)	52	3	1	5	1	8	5	tr	—	30	33	—	—
DE BEUKELAER														
Pirouline	8 (1 oz)	130	4	3	15	3	23	13	tr	0	50	—		0
Pirouline Viennese Wafers	1 (1 oz)	150	7	5	30	1	20	9	tr	0	25	—	—	0
DELARCE														
Chocosprits	1 (0.6 oz)	90	5	3	9	1	11	3	tr	0	50	—	—	0
Marquisettes	3 (0.9 oz)	140	7	4	5	2	17	7	1	0	45	—	—	0
Roules d'Or	4 (1 oz)	180	8	6	0	1	19	11	0	40	35	—	—	0
DUNKAROOS														
Chocolate Graham	1 pkg	120	5	1	0	1	20	14	—	—	120	—	—	—
Cinnamon Graham	1 pkg	130	5	2	0	1	21	14	—	—	75	—	—	—
Honey Graham	1 pkg	120	5	1	0	1	20	13	tr	—	100	—	—	—

FOOD	PORTION	CALS	FAT	SAT FAT	CHOL	PROT	CARB	SUGAR	FIBER	CALCI	SOD	POTAS	FOLIC	VIT C
DUTCH MILL														
Chocolate Chip	3 (1.1 oz)	160	10	3	0	1	18	10	1	0	85	—	—	0
Coconut Macaroons	3 (1 oz)	120	7	6	0	1	14	12	0	20	115	—	—	0
Oatmeal Raisin	3 (1 oz)	130	6	2	0	2	18	10	1	0	75	—	—	0
EDDYLEON														
Jelly Graham Raspberry	1 (0.9 oz)	134	8	5	2	1	15	13	tr	30	44	—	—	1
Pudding Cookies	1 (0.9 oz)	134	6	5	2	1	15	13	tr	30	44	—	—	1
ELITE														
Tea Biscuits Chocolate	4	80	2	1	0	1	14	4	0	0	55	—	—	0
ENGLISH BAY														
Strawberry Fruit Bar	1 (1.2 oz)	120	3	1	5	1	22	14	1	0	100	—	—	0
ENTENMANN'S														
Little Bites Chocolate Chip	8 (1.8 oz)	240	12	3	10	2	33	19	1	0	120	—	—	0
Soft Baked Chocolate Chip	1 (0.7 oz)	100	5	2	10	1	13	8	tr	0	60	—	—	0
Soft Baked Double Chocolate Chip	1 (0.7 oz)	100	5	2	10	1	14	8	tr	0	65	—	—	0
Soft Baked Original Chocolate Chip	3 (1 oz)	150	7	2	10	1	20	11	tr	0	90	—	—	0
Soft Baked White Chocolate Macadamia Nut	1 (0.7 oz)	100	6	2	10	1	12	7	tr	0	65	—	—	0
Soft Baked Light Chocolately Chip	2 (1 oz)	120	4	2	0	1	21	13	tr	0	80	—	—	0
Soft Baked Light Oatmeal Raisin	2 (1 oz)	100	0	0	0	2	23	14	1	0	150	—	—	0
ESTEE														
Chocolate Chip	4	150	7	2	0	2	21	5	tr	—	30	55	—	—
Coconut	4	140	6	2	0	2	19	5	tr	—	25	25	—	—
Fig Bars	2	100	1	0	0	1	23	13	3	—	20	80	—	—
Fudge	4	150	7	2	0	2	19	5	1	—	45	55	—	—
Lemon Thins	4	140	6	1	0	2	19	5	tr	—	25	15	—	—
Oatmeal Raisin	4	130	5	1	0	2	19	6	1	—	25	45	—	—
Sandwich Chocolate	3	160	6	2	0	2	24	9	1	—	60	45	—	—
Sandwich Original	3	160	6	2	0	2	24	10	1	—	45	25	—	—
Sandwich Peanut Butter	3	160	7	1	0	4	22	7	1	—	55	85	—	—
Sandwich Vanilla	3	160	5	1	0	2	25	7	tr	—	35	20	—	—
Shortbread	4	130	4	1	0	2	22	5	tr	—	150	30	—	—

FOOD	PORTION	CALS	FAT	SAT FAT	CHOL	PROT	CARB	SUGAR	FIBER	CALCI	SOD	POTAS	FOLIC	VIT C
ESTEE (CONT.)														
Sugar Free Chocolate Chip	3	110	4	1	0	2	22	0	1	—	70	0	—	—
Sugar Free Chocolate Walnut	3	110	4	0	0	2	22	0	1	—	95	0	—	—
Sugar Free Coconut	3	110	4	1	0	2	22	0	1	—	110	0	—	—
Sugar Free Grahams Chocolate	2	110	2	0	0	3	27	0	3	—	110	0	—	—
Sugar Free Grahams Cinnamon	2	90	2	0	0	3	18	0	2	—	90	0	—	—
Sugar Free Grahams Old Fashion	2	90	2	0	0	3	17	0	2	—	115	0	—	—
Sugar Free Lemon	3	110	3	0	0	2	22	0	1	—	90	0	—	—
Sugar Free Wafer Banana Split	5	155	9	2	0	1	22	0	0	—	10	15	—	—
Sugar Free Wafer Chocolate	5	150	9	2	0	1	19	0	0	—	10	80	—	—
Sugar Free Wafer Chocolate Peanut Butter Caramel	5	150	8	2	0	1	22	0	0	—	45	15	—	—
Sugar Free Wafer Lemon Creme	5	150	8	2	0	1	22	0	0	—	10	15	—	—
Sugar Free Wafer Peanut Butter Creme	5	150	8	2	0	1	22	0	0	—	40	15	—	—
Sugar Free Wafer Vanilla	5	150	8	2	0	1	21	0	0	—	10	15	—	—
Sugar Free Wafer Vanilla Strawberry	5	150	8	2	0	1	22	0	0	—	10	15	—	—
Vanilla Thins	4	140	6	1	0	2	19	5	tr	—	25	15	—	—
FALCONE'S														
Sorrentini	1 (1 oz)	100	4	1	10	2	16	6	2	40	55	—	—	0
FAMOUS AMOS														
Butter Shortie	1 (0.5 oz)	80	5	2	10	1	9	3	tr	20	65	—	—	0
Chocolate Chip	4 (1 oz)	140	7	2	0	2	18	10	tr	20	105	—	—	0
Chocolate Chip & Pecan	4 (1 oz)	140	8	2	0	1	18	10	tr	0	100	—	—	0
Chocolate Chip Toffee	4 (1 oz)	130	6	3	0	1	18	10	0	0	115	—	—	0
Chocolate Creme Sandwich	3 (1.2 oz)	140	6	2	0	2	22	13	tr	20	90	—	—	0
Chunky Chocolate Chip	1 (0.5 oz)	70	4	2	0	1	9	5	0	20	80	—	—	0
Fat Free Fig Bar	2 (1 oz)	90	0	0	0	1	21	9	1	20	60	—	—	0

FOOD	PORTION	CALS	FAT	SAT FAT	CHOL	PROT	CARB	SUGAR	FIBER	CALCI	SOD	POTAS	FOLIC	VIT C
FAMOUS AMOS (CONT.)														
Fat Free Strawberry Fruit Bar	2 (1 oz)	90	0	0	0	1	22	11	0	0	50	—	—	0
Fig Bar	2 (1.1 oz)	120	3	1	0	1	22	12	tr	0	150	—	—	0
Oatmeal Chocolate Chip Walnut	4 (1 oz)	140	7	2	0	2	16	9	tr	0	120	—	—	0
Oatmeal Raisin	4 (1 oz)	130	6	1	5	2	20	10	tr	20	135	—	—	0
Oatmeal Macaroon Creme Sandwich	3 (1.2 oz)	160	7	2	0	2	23	12	1	0	—	—	—	0
Peanut Butter Chocolate Chunk	1 (0.5 oz)	80	5	2	0	1	9	5	tr	20	70	—	—	0
Peanut Butter Creme Sandwich	3 (1.2 oz)	160	8	2	0	4	19	9	1	20	115	—	—	0
Pecan Shortie	1 (0.5 oz)	80	5	1	0	1	9	3	tr	20	55	—	—	0
Vanilla Creme Sandwich	3 (1.2 oz)	160	7	2	0	2	24	13	0	0	85	—	—	0
FROOKIE														
Animal Frackers	14 (1 oz)	130	5	0	0	2	18	10	1	0	90	—	—	0
Chocolate Chip Wheat & Gluten Free	3 (1.1 oz)	140	5	2	0	1	23	12	1	40	100	—	—	0
Double Chocolate Wheat & Gluten Free	3 (1.1 oz)	130	4	1	0	1	23	13	1	60	105	—	—	0
Dream Creams Strawberry	4 (1 oz)	140	8	2	0	2	18	7	4	20	55	—	—	0
Dream Creams Vanilla	4 (1 oz)	140	8	2	0	2	18	7	4	20	55	—	—	0
Funky Monkeys Chocolate	16 (1 oz)	120	4	1	0	2	20	9	1	0	120	—	—	0
Funky Monkeys Vanilla	16 (1 oz)	120	4	1	0	2	20	9	1	0	120	—	—	0
Graham Cinnamon	2 (1 oz)	100	3	0	0	2	17	2	1	0	105	—	—	0
Graham Honey	2 (1 oz)	110	3	0	0	2	18	2	1	0	120	—	—	0
Lemon Wafers	8 (1 oz)	110	0	0	0	2	26	18	tr	20	130	—	—	0
Old Fashioned Ginger Snaps	8 (1 oz)	120	2	0	0	1	24	12	tr	0	110	—	—	0
Organic Chocolate Chip	3 (1.1 oz)	150	7	2	0	2	20	9	1	60	115	—	—	1
Organic Double Chocolate Chip	3 (1.1 oz)	140	6	2	0	2	20	11	1	40	95	—	—	1
Organic Iced Lemon	3 (1.3 oz)	165	6	1	0	2	27	14	0	40	115	—	—	1

FOOD	PORTION	CALS	FAT	SAT FAT	CHOL	PROT	CARB	SUGAR	FIBER	CALCI	SOD	POTAS	FOLIC	VIT C
FROOKIE (CONT.)														
Organic Oatmeal Raisin	3 (1.1 oz)	140	5	1	0	2	22	12	1	40	110	—	—	0
Peanut Butter Chunk Wheat & Gluten Free	3 (1.1 oz)	140	5	1	0	3	21	12	0	80	140	—	—	0
Sandwich Chocolate	2 (0.7 oz)	100	4	0	0	1	14	7	1	0	60	—	—	0
Sandwich Lemon	2 (0.7 oz)	100	4	0	0	1	14	7	1	0	60	—	—	0
Sandwich Peanut Butter	2 (0.7 oz)	100	4	0	0	1	14	7	1	0	60	—	—	0
Sandwich Vanilla	2 (0.7 oz)	100	4	0	0	1	14	7	1	0	60	—	—	0
Shortbread	5 (1 oz)	130	5	3	15	2	20	7	tr	0	95	—	—	0
Vanilla Wafers	8 (1 oz)	110	0	0	0	2	26	18	0	20	120	—	—	0
GENERAL HENRY														
Fruit Bars Apple	1 (0.6 oz)	60	1	0	0	1	13	6	tr	—	70	—	—	—
Fruit Bars Blueberry	1 (0.6 oz)	60	1	0	0	1	12	6	tr	—	75	—	—	—
Fruit Bars Fig	1 (0.6 oz)	60	1	0	0	1	12	6	tr	—	70	—	—	—
GIRL SCOUT														
Apple Cinnamon Reduced Fat	3 (1 oz)	120	5	1	0	2	18	6	tr	0	140	—	—	0
Lemon Drops	3 (1.2 oz)	160	8	2	0	2	20	6	0	0	150	—	—	0
Samoas	2 (1 oz)	160	9	6	0	2	17	12	2	0	45	—	—	2
Striped Chocolate Chip	3 (1.2 oz)	180	10	4	0	2	20	11	tr	0	100	—	—	0
Tagalongs	2 (0.9 oz)	150	10	4	0	3	13	8	2	0	85	—	—	0
Thin Mints	4 (1 oz)	140	8	2	0	1	18	10	tr	20	80	—	—	0
Trefoils	5 (1.1 oz)	160	8	1	0	2	20	7	1	0	90	—	—	0
GLENNY'S														
Soy Fudgies All Flavors	3	70	2	0	0	3	14	0	1	—	10	—	—	—
GODIVA														
Biscotti Dipped In Milk Chocolate	1 (0.9 oz)	120	6	3	20	2	15	6	0	20	45	—	—	0
GOL D LITE														
Low Carb Pizzelle	1 (0.3 oz)	46	2	0	0	1	6	0	1	—	0	—	—	—
GOLDEN GRAHAMS TREATS														
Chocolate Chunk	1 bar (0.8 oz)	90	3	1	0	1	17	9	0	0	110	25	40	6
Honey Graham	1 bar (0.8 oz)	90	2	0	0	1	17	9	0	0	120	25	40	6
King Size Chocolate Chunk	1 bar (1.6 oz)	190	5	1	0	2	35	18	1	0	220	50	100	15
King Size Honey Graham	1 bar (1.6 oz)	180	4	1	0	1	36	18	1	0	240	45	100	15

FOOD	PORTION	CALS	FAT	SAT FAT	CHOL	PROT	CARB	SUGAR	FIBER	CALCI	SOD	POTAS	FOLIC	VIT C
GOLIGHTLY														
Fabulous Tastes Caramel Dulce De Leche	4	100	6	4	0	2	14	0	5	20	65	—	—	0
GOODY MAN														
Marshmallow Crispy Squares	1 (1.17 oz)	130	3	1	0	1	24	10	0	0	170	—	—	0
GOURMET														
Chocolate Chip	2 (1.1 oz)	160	9	6	15	2	19	13	1	20	85	—	—	1
Lemon Creme	2 (1.4 oz)	210	10	5	0	1	27	17	0	0	60	—	—	0
Oatmeal Raisin	2 (0.9 oz)	120	6	4	15	2	15	7	1	0	105	—	—	9
Peanut Butter Chip	2 (1 oz)	150	8	4	10	3	17	8	tr	20	135	—	—	0
Raspberry Center	2 (1.1 oz)	140	5	3	10	1	21	12	tr	0	60	—	—	0
GRANDMA'S														
Chocolate Chip	1 (1.4 oz)	190	9	3	0	2	25	13	tr	—	135	—	—	—
Fudge Chocolate Chip	1 (1.4 oz)	170	7	3	<5	1	26	13	1	—	160	—	—	—
Fudge Sandwich	3	180	5	2	0	2	31	15	tr	—	200	—	—	—
Fudge Vanilla Sandwich	3	120	4	1	0	1	21	10	tr	—	130	—	—	—
Mini Fudge	9	150	7	2	0	2	21	12	1	—	180	—	—	—
Mini Peanut Butter	9	150	7	2	0	2	21	10	1	—	140	—	—	—
Mini Vanilla	9	150	7	2	<5	2	22	10	tr	—	85	—	—	—
Oatmeal Raisin	1 (1.4 oz)	160	6	2	5	1	26	15	1	—	250	—	—	—
Old Time Molasses	1 (1.4 oz)	160	4	2	<5	2	29	18	tr	—	230	—	—	—
Peanut Butter	1 (1.4 oz)	190	9	2	5	2	22	12	1	—	200	—	—	—
Peanut Butter Chocolate Chip	1 (1.4 oz)	190	9	3	<5	4	23	15	1	—	170	—	—	—
Peanut Butter Sandwich	5	210	10	3	0	3	28	13	1	—	200	—	—	—
Rich N'Chewy	1 pkg	270	12	4	10	2	39	23	1	—	130	—	—	—
Vanilla Sandwich	5	210	10	3	5	2	30	15	tr	—	125	—	—	—
Vanilla Sandwich	3	180	5	2	0	2	32	17	tr	—	160	—	—	—
GRANNY OATS														
Low Carb Oatmeal	4	98	6	4	25	1	10	0	3	—	140	—	—	—
HANDI-SNACK														
Cookie Jammers Cookies & Fruit Spread	1 pkg (1.3 oz)	130	3	0	0	1	26	14	tr	0	125	15	—	0
HEALTH VALLEY														
Apple Spice	3	100	0	0	0	2	24	11	3	20	50	—	—	1
Apricot Delight	3	100	0	0	0	2	24	11	3	20	50	—	—	1
Biscotti Amaretto	2	120	3	—	0	3	23	7	3	0	50	—	—	0
Biscotti Chocolate	2	120	3	—	0	3	23	7	3	0	50	—	—	0
Biscotti Fruit & Nut	2	120	3	—	0	3	23	7	3	0	50	—	—	0

FOOD	PORTION	CALS	FAT	SAT FAT	CHOL	PROT	CARB	SUGAR	FIBER	CALCI	SOD	POTAS	FOLIC	VIT C
HEALTH VALLEY (CONT.)														
Cheesecake Bars Blueberry	1 bar	160	2	—	0	3	34	17	3	20	30	—	—	1
Cheesecake Bars Raspberry	1 bar	160	2	—	0	3	34	17	3	20	30	—	—	1
Cheesecake Bars Strawberry	1 bar	160	2	—	0	3	34	17	3	20	30	—	—	1
Chips Double Chocolate	3	100	0	0	0	3	24	10	4	20	40	—	—	1
Chips Old Fashioned	3	100	0	0	0	3	24	10	4	20	40	—	—	1
Chips Original	3	100	0	0	0	3	24	10	4	20	40	—	—	1
Chocolate Fudge Center	2	70	0	0	0	2	25	10	3	20	25	—	—	1
Chocolate Sandwich Bars Bavarian Creme	1 bar	150	0	0	0	3	35	18	3	20	30	—	—	1
Chocolate Sandwich Bars Caramel Creme	1 bar	150	0	0	0	3	35	18	3	20	30	—	—	1
Chocolate Sandwich Bars Vanilla Creme	1 bar	150	0	0	0	3	35	18	3	20	30	—	—	1
Date Delight	3	100	0	0	0	2	24	11	3	20	50	—	—	1
Graham Amaranth	8	100	0	0	0	4	23	5	3	20	30	—	—	0
Graham Oat Bran	8	100	0	0	0	4	30	5	3	20	30	—	—	0
Graham Original Amaranth	6	120	3	—	0	3	22	4	3	40	80	—	—	0
Hawaiian Fruit	3	100	0	0	0	2	24	11	3	20	50	—	—	1
Jumbo Apple Raisin	1	80	0	0	0	2	19	9	3	20	35	—	—	1
Jumbo Raisin Raisin	1	80	0	0	0	2	19	9	3	20	35	—	—	1
Jumbo Raspberry	1	80	0	0	0	2	19	9	3	20	35	—	—	1
Marshmallow Bars Chocolate Chip	1	90	0	0	0	1	22	11	1	20	20	—	—	1
Marshmallow Bars Old Fashioned	1	90	0	0	0	1	22	11	1	20	20	—	—	1
Marshmallow Bars Tropical Fruit	1	90	0	0	0	1	22	11	1	20	20	—	—	1
Oat Bran Fruit Bars Raisin Cinnamon	1 bar	160	1	—	0	3	34	18	2	0	10	—	—	0
Raisin Oatmeal	3	100	0	0	0	2	24	11	3	20	50	—	—	1
Raspberry Fruit Center	1	70	0	0	0	2	18	9	2	20	20	—	—	1
Tarts Baked Apple Cinnamon	1	150	0	0	0	3	35	18	3	20	40	—	—	1

FOOD	PORTION	CALS	FAT	SAT FAT	CHOL	PROT	CARB	SUGAR	FIBER	CALCI	SOD	POTAS	FOLIC	VIT C
HEALTH VALLEY (CONT.)														
Tarts California Strawberry	1	150	0	0	0	3	35	18	3	20	40	—	—	1
Tarts Chocolate Fudge	1	150	0	0	0	3	35	18	3	20	50	—	—	1
Tarts Cranberry Apple	1	150	0	0	0	3	35	18	3	20	40	—	—	1
Tarts Mountain Blueberry	1	150	0	0	0	3	35	18	3	20	40	—	—	1
Tarts Red Raspberry	1	150	0	0	0	3	35	18	3	20	40	—	—	1
Tarts Sweet Red Cherry	1	150	0	0	0	3	35	18	3	20	40	—	—	1
HEAVENLY														
Meringues All Flavors Sugar Free Fat Free	1	0	0	0	0	2	1	0	0	—	0	—	—	—
HELLEMA														
Almond	1 pkg (0.6 oz)	90	5	1	0	1	9	4	tr	0	35	—	—	0
HERSHEY'S														
Cripsy Rice Snacks Peanut Butter	1 (0.6 oz)	70	3	1	0	1	10	5	tr	60	130	—	—	1
JACQUES GOURMET														
Palmier Cinnamon	3 (1 oz)	140	9	4	0	1	15	5	0	—	65	—	—	—
Palmier Vanilla	3 (1 oz)	140	9	4	0	1	15	5	0	—	65	—	—	—
JOSEPH'S														
Almond Sugar Free	2 (0.9 oz)	100	5	1	0	1	14	0	0	0	20	—	—	0
Chocolate Chip Sugar Free	2 (0.9 oz)	100	5	1	0	1	15	0	0	0	40	—	—	1
Chocolate Walnut Sugar Free	2 (0.9 oz)	100	6	1	0	1	14	0	1	0	40	—	—	0
Coconut Sugar Free	2 (0.9 oz)	105	5	1	0	1	14	0	0	0	40	—	—	0
Lemon Sugar Free	2 (0.9 oz)	95	4	1	0	1	15	0	0	0	30	—	—	0
Oatmeal Raisin Sugar Free	2 (0.9 oz)	100	5	1	0	2	15	0	0	0	40	—	—	0
Peanut Butter Sugar Free	2 (0.9 oz)	95	5	1	0	2	13	0	1	0	40	—	—	0
Pecan Shortbread Sugar Free	2 (0.9 oz)	100	5	1	0	1	14	0	0	0	40	—	—	0
KAREN'S														
Fabulous Tastes Heavenly Chocolate Chip	4	90	5	4	0	2	16	0	5	20	65	—	—	0
Fabulous Tastes Luscious Raspberry Almond	4	110	6	2	0	3	15	0	5	20	65	—	—	0

FOOD	PORTION	CALS	FAT	SAT FAT	CHOL	PROT	CARB	SUGAR	FIBER	CALCI	SOD	POTAS	FOLIC	VIT C
KAREN'S (CONT.)														
Fabulous Tastes Pecan Vanilla Pralines	4	120	8	3	0	2	15	0	6	10	75	—	—	0
KEDEM														
Tea Biscuits Chocolate	2	32	1	tr	0	1	6	2	tr	0	29	—	—	0
Tea Biscuits Orange	2	32	1	tr	0	1	6	2	tr	0	29	—	—	0
KEEBLER														
Animal Crackers Chocolate Chip	7 (1 oz)	130	5	1	0	2	22	6	0	0	120	—	—	0
Animal Crackers Ernie's	1 box	250	9	2	0	<4	41	14	1	0	290	—	—	0
Animal Crackers Iced	6 (1.1 oz)	150	5	1	0	2	24	9	0	0	110	—	—	0
Animal Crackers Sprinkled	6 (1.1 oz)	150	5	1	0	<2	24	10	0	20	105	—	—	0
Butter	5 (1.1 oz)	150	6	2	10	<2	22	6	tr	0	170	—	—	0
Chips Deluxe	1 (0.5 oz)	80	5	2	0	tr	9	5	tr	0	50	—	—	0
Chips Deluxe Chocolate Lovers	1 (0.6 oz)	90	5	3	5	tr	11	6	0	0	80	—	—	0
Chips Deluxe Coconut	1 (0.5 oz)	80	5	2	0	tr	10	5	tr	0	50	—	—	0
Chips Deluxe Rainbow	1 (0.6 oz)	80	4	2	<5	tr	10	5	tr	0	45	—	—	0
Chips Deluxe Soft 'n Chewy	1 (0.6 oz)	80	4	1	5	tr	11	5	0	0	60	—	—	0
Chips Deluxe w/ Peanut Butter Cups	1 (0.6 oz)	90	5	2	0	tr	9	5	0	0	45	—	—	0
Classic Collection Chocolate Fudge Creme	1 (0.6 oz)	80	4	1	0	tr	12	6	0	0	75	—	—	0
Classic Collection French Vanilla Creme	1 (0.6 oz)	80	4	1	0	tr	12	6	0	0	65	—	—	0
Cookie Stix Butter	5 (1.2 oz)	160	6	3	10	<2	22	8	1	0	150	—	—	0
Cookie Stix Chocolate Chip	4 (0.9 oz)	130	5	2	5	<2	19	9	tr	0	100	—	—	0
Cookie Stix Rainbow	5 (1.2 oz)	150	6	2	5	<2	23	9	tr	0	110	—	—	0
Danish Wedding	4 (0.9 oz)	120	5	2	0	tr	20	11	tr	0	80	—	—	0
Droxies	3 (1.1 oz)	140	6	1	0	<2	21	12	tr	0	95	—	—	0
Droxies Reduced Fat	3 (1.1 oz)	140	5	2	0	<2	23	13	1	0	150	—	—	0
E.L. Fudge Butter w/ Fudge Filling	2 (0.9 oz)	120	6	1	<5	tr	17	7	tr	0	70	—	—	0

FOOD	PORTION	CALS	FAT	SAT FAT	CHOL	PROT	CARB	SUGAR	FIBER	CALCI	SOD	POTAS	FOLIC	VIT C
KEEBLER (CONT.)														
E.L. Fudge Fudge w/ Fudge Filling	2 (0.9 oz)	120	6	1	0	<2	17	7	tr	0	70	—	—	0
E.L. Fudge w/ Peanut Butter Filling	2 (0.9 oz)	120	6	1	0	<2	16	7	tr	0	150	—	—	0
Fudge Shoppe Deluxe Grahams	3 (1 oz)	140	7	5	0	tr	19	10	tr	0	105	—	—	0
Fudge Shoppe Double Fudge 'n Caramel	2 (1 oz)	140	7	4	0	tr	20	12	tr	20	65	—	—	0
Fudge Shoppe Fudge Sticks	3 (1 oz)	150	8	5	0	tr	20	15	tr	0	55	—	—	0
Fudge Shoppe Fudge Sticks Peanut Butter	3 (1 oz)	150	8	4	0	<2	18	14	tr	0	45	—	—	0
Fudge Shoppe Fudge Stripes	3 (1.1 oz)	160	8	5	0	tr	21	10	tr	0	140	—	—	0
Fudge Shoppe Fudge Stripes Reduced Fat	3 (1 oz)	140	5	3	0	tr	21	12	0	20	120	—	—	0
Fudge Shoppe Grasshoppers	4 (1 oz)	150	7	5	0	tr	20	12	tr	0	70	—	—	0
Fudge Shoppe S'mores	3 (1.2 oz)	160	8	5	0	tr	22	12	tr	0	95	—	—	0
Ginger Snaps	5 (1.1 oz)	150	6	1	0	<2	24	10	0	20	120	—	—	0
Golden Fruit Cranberry	1 (0.7 oz)	80	2	0	0	tr	14	6	tr	0	55	—	—	0
Golden Fruit Raisin	1 (0.7 oz)	80	2	1	0	tr	15	9	tr	0	50	—	—	0
Graham Cinnamon Crisp	8 (1 oz)	140	5	1	0	2	22	9	1	0	170	—	—	0
Graham Cinnamon Crisp Low Fat	8 (1 oz)	110	2	1	0	2	24	9	1	0	190	—	—	0
Graham Honey	8 (1.1 oz)	140	4	1	0	2	23	7	0	100	140	—	—	0
Graham Honey Low Fat	8 (1.1 oz)	120	2	1	0	2	26	9	1	0	210	—	—	0
Graham Original	8 (1 oz)	130	3	1	0	2	23	7	tr	0	135	—	—	0
Lemon Coolers	5 (1 oz)	140	6	2	0	tr	21	10	tr	0	100	—	—	0
Oatmeal Country Style	2 (0.8 oz)	120	5	1	0	<2	17	8	tr	0	115	—	—	0
Sandies Almond Shortbread	1 (0.5 oz)	80	5	1	5	tr	9	3	0	0	50	—	—	0
Sandies Pecan Shortbread	1 (0.5 oz)	80	5	1	<5	tr	9	3	tr	0	75	—	—	0
Sandies Simply Shortbread	1 (0.5 oz)	80	5	2	10	tr	9	3	0	0	70	—	—	0

FOOD	PORTION	CALS	FAT	SAT FAT	CHOL	PROT	CARB	SUGAR	FIBER	CALCI	SOD	POTAS	FOLIC	VIT C
KEEBLER (CONT.)														
Snack Size Chips Deluxe	1 pkg (2 oz)	300	16	5	5	3	36	18	tr	0	170	—	—	0
Snack Size Chips Deluxe Chocolate Lovers	1 pkg (2 oz)	280	15	7	20	3	36	20	1	20	170	—	—	0
Snack Size Mini Fudge Stripes	1 pkg (2 oz)	280	14	9	0	3	38	16	2	20	150	—	—	0
Snack Size Rainbow Chips Deluxe	1 pkg (2 oz)	290	16	4	5	3	36	18	1	20	170	—	—	0
Snack Size Sandies w/ Pecans	1 pkg (2 oz)	300	17	4	10	3	33	13	1	0	190	—	—	0
Snackin' Grahams Cinnamon	21 (1 oz)	130	3	1	0	<2	23	9	1	20	210	—	—	0
Snackin' Grahams Honey	23 (1 oz)	130	4	1	0	<2	22	8	tr	20	120	—	—	0
Soft Batch Chocolate Chip	1 (0.6 oz)	80	4	1	0	tr	10	6	tr	0	70	—	—	0
Soft Batch Homestyle Chocolate Chunk	1 (0.9 oz)	130	7	3	0	1	17	10	1	20	80	—	—	0
Soft Batch Homestyle Double Chocolate	1 (0.9 oz)	130	7	2	0	1	17	9	1	20	90	—	—	0
Soft Batch Homestyle Oatmeal Raisin	1 (0.9 oz)	130	5	1	0	1	20	11	tr	20	150	—	—	0
Soft Batch Oatmeal Raisin	1 (0.5 oz)	70	3	1	0	tr	10	6	tr	0	65	—	—	0
Sugar Wafers Creme	3 (0.9 oz)	130	6	2	0	tr	18	13	tr	0	20	—	—	0
Sugar Wafers Lemon	3 (0.9 oz)	130	6	1	0	tr	19	14	0	0	20	—	—	0
Sugar Wafers Peanut Butter	4 (1.1 oz)	170	9	2	0	<3	19	10	1	0	75	—	—	0
Vanilla Wafers	8 (1.1 oz)	150	7	2	0	tr	20	9	tr	0	120	—	—	0
Vanilla Wafers Reduced Fat	8 (1.1 oz)	130	4	1	0	<2	25	11	tr	0	140	—	—	0
Vienna Fingers	2 (1 oz)	140	6	2	0	2	21	8	tr	0	105	—	—	0
Vienna Fingers Lemon	2 (1 oz)	140	6	2	0	2	21	9	0	0	90	—	—	0
KETO														
Low Carb Biscotti Chocolate	1 (1.2 oz)	157	9	9	200	13	6	0	3	—	80	—	—	—
Low Carb Biscotti Lemon Nut	1 (1.2 oz)	157	9	4	200	13	6	0	3	—	80	—	—	—

FOOD	PORTION	CALS	FAT	SAT FAT	CHOL	PROT	CARB	SUGAR	FIBER	CALCI	SOD	POTAS	FOLIC	VIT C
KETO (CONT.)														
Low Carb Biscotti Vanilla Almond	1 (1.2 oz)	157	9	9	200	13	6	0	3	—	80	—	—	—
KNOTT'S BERRY FARM														
Shortbread Apricot	3 (1 oz)	120	5	1	4	2	17	7	0	0	70	—	—	0
Shortbread Boysenberry	3 (1 oz)	120	5	1	4	2	17	7	0	0	60	—	—	0
Shortbread Raspberry	3 (1 oz)	120	5	1	4	2	17	8	0	0	60	—	—	0
LA CHOY														
Fortune	4 (1 oz)	112	tr	tr	0	2	26	11	1	4	11	—	—	0
LA DOLCE VITA														
Biscotti Chocolate Passion	1 (1.2 oz)	130	8	5	45	2	11	8	1	40	135	—	—	0
LANCE														
Apple Bar Fat Free	1 (1.75 oz)	160	0	0	0	1	38	29	tr	0	80	—	—	0
Apple Oatmeal Bar	1 (1.8 oz)	190	6	2	10	2	32	10	1	20	180	30	—	0
Big Town Banana	1 pkg (2 oz)	250	10	3	0	3	37	21	1	20	160	80	—	0
Big Town Chocolate	1 pkg (2 oz)	250	8	3	0	3	40	21	1	0	160	90	—	0
Big Town Vanilla	1 pkg (2 oz)	250	11	3	0	3	37	26	1	0	120	75	—	0
Choc-O-Lunch	1 pkg (1.5 oz)	200	8	2	0	3	31	17	1	0	190	85	—	0
Choc-O-Mint	1 pkg (1.25 oz)	190	9	4	0	2	24	17	1	0	100	80	—	0
Coated Graham	1 pkg (1.3 oz)	190	8	2	0	3	25	13	1	0	95	90	—	0
Fig Bar	1 (1.75 oz)	180	4	1	0	2	34	23	2	20	150	110	—	1
Fudge Chocolate Chip	1 (2 oz)	130	5	2	<5	2	19	5	1	0	75	—	—	0
Gourmet Chocolate Chip	1 (2 oz)	130	6	3	5	2	18	10	1	0	75	—	—	0
Lem-O-Lunch	1 pkg (3.4 oz)	240	11	3	0	3	32	11	1	0	150	75	—	0
Lemon Nekot	1 pkg (1.5 oz)	210	10	2	0	3	28	13	1	0	125	75	—	0
Nut-O-Lunch	1 pkg (3.3 oz)	240	11	3	0	6	29	8	3	0	150	140	—	0
Oatmeal	1 (2 oz)	130	6	1	0	2	18	4	1	0	90	0	—	0
Oatmeal Creme	1 (2 oz)	240	10	3	0	3	35	9	1	20	220	5	—	0
Peanut Butter	1 (2 oz)	140	8	2	<5	4	14	10	1	0	65	105	—	0
Peanut Butter Creme Wafer	1 pkg (1.5 oz)	230	12	3	0	4	26	16	2	60	80	25	—	0
Van-O-Lunch	1 pkg (1.5 oz)	210	8	2	0	2	31	13	0	0	130	45	—	0
LANDIES CANDIES														
Sugar Free Dark Royal Pecan Shortbread	2	167	9	4	0	1	16	0	1	0	27	—	—	0
Sugar Free Milk Chocolate Chip	2	173	11	5	<5	4	17	0	tr	0	91	—	—	1

FOOD	PORTION	CALS	FAT	SAT FAT	CHOL	PROT	CARB	SUGAR	FIBER	CALCI	SOD	POTAS	FOLIC	VIT C
LANDIES CANDIES (CONT.)														
Sugar Free Milk Chocolate Peanut Butter	2	171	8	5	<5	4	17	0	tr	0	91	—	—	0
Sugar Free White Chocolate Lemon	2	177	11	8	<5	3	20	0	0	0	67	—	—	0
LARZARONI														
Arancelli	8 (1 oz)	160	8	tr	8	3	19	8	tr	20	36	—	—	0
Calypso	3 (1 oz)	150	8	6	0	2	18	11	1	0	30	—	—	0
Limonelli	5 (1 oz)	140	8	5	5	2	16	7	2	0	30	—	—	0
Malaika	5 (1 oz)	158	9	tr	17	3	17	10	1	20	36	—	—	0
Nanette	4 (1.2 oz)	170	9	6	<5	3	20	20	tr	40	30	—	—	0
Okla	3 (1 oz)	186	10	tr	6	3	21	18	1	40	43	—	—	0
Oskar	10 (1 oz)	150	9	5	0	2	18	11	tr	0	10	—	—	0
Samba	5 (1 oz)	160	10	9	0	3	14	6	2	0	150	—	—	0
Velieri	3 (0.9 oz)	120	5	3	10	2	17	10	tr	20	60	—	—	0
LINDEN'S														
Lemon	1 (1 oz)	120	5	1	10	—	—	—	—	—	135	—	—	—
LITTLE DEBBIE														
Apple Flips	1 (1.2 oz)	150	5	2	5	1	24	13	tr	0	115	—	—	0
Caramel Bars	1 (1.2 oz)	160	8	2	0	1	22	16	0	13	85	32	—	tr
Cherry Cordials	1 (1.3 oz)	170	8	2	0	1	23	15	tr	0	95	34	—	0
Coconut Rounds	1 (1.2 oz)	150	7	3	0	1	23	13	tr	3	90	31	—	tr
Cookie Wreaths	1 (0.6 oz)	100	5	1	0	1	12	7	0	2	60	10	—	0
Easter Puffs	1 (1.2 oz)	140	6	2	0	1	24	18	0	4	65	22	—	0
Fig Bars	1 (1.5 oz)	150	4	1	0	1	31	20	1	17	110	85	—	tr
Fudge Delights	1 (1.1 oz)	110	2	0	0	1	24	14	tr	11	170	48	—	0
Fudge Rounds	1 (1.2 oz)	140	6	2	0	1	23	14	tr	6	85	48	—	0
German Chocolate Ring	1 (1 oz)	140	8	4	0	1	18	11	1	1	65	63	—	tr
Ginger	1 (0.7 oz)	90	3	1	5	1	15	8	0	12	60	81	—	0
Jelly Creme Pies	1 (1.2 oz)	160	7	2	0	1	23	15	0	4	160	22	—	0
Marshmallow Crispy Bar	1 (1.3 oz)	140	4	1	0	1	26	13	0	0	170	—	—	0
Marshmallow Supremes	1 (1.1 oz)	130	5	1	0	1	22	15	tr	6	65	48	—	0
Marshmallow Pie Banana	1 pkg (1.5 oz)	180	6	2	0	2	30	18	0	6	110	19	—	tr
Marshmallow Pie Chocolate	1 (1.4 oz)	160	6	3	0	1	27	16	1	8	95	47	—	0
Nutty Bar	1 (2 oz)	310	18	3	0	5	32	20	1	10	110	82	—	0
Oatmeal Raisin	1 (1.3 oz)	160	7	2	0	2	25	14	tr	12	170	92	—	tr
Oatmeal Creme Pie	1 (1.3 oz)	170	7	2	0	1	26	14	tr	9	190	55	—	0
Oatmeal Delights	1 (1.1 oz)	110	2	0	0	2	24	15	tr	11	135	62	—	tr
Oatmeal Lights	1 (1.3 oz)	130	3	1	0	2	29	16	tr	10	180	68	—	tr
Peanut Butter Bars	1 (1.9 oz)	270	15	3	0	4	32	19	1	11	140	118	—	0

FOOD	PORTION	CALS	FAT	SAT FAT	CHOL	PROT	CARB	SUGAR	FIBER	CALCI	SOD	POTAS	FOLIC	VIT C
LITTLE DEBBIE (CONT.)														
Peanut Butter & Jelly Oatmeal Pie	1 (1.1 oz)	130	5	1	0	2	22	12	tr	8	100	48	—	0
Peanut Clusters	1 (1.4 oz)	190	11	2	0	3	23	16	tr	23	120	89	—	tr
Pumpkin Delights	1 (1.2 oz)	150	5	2	5	1	24	13	0	7	140	49	—	tr
Raisin Creme Pie	1 (1.2 oz)	140	5	1	0	1	23	16	0	5	120	32	—	tr
Star Crunch	1 (1.1 oz)	140	6	2	0	0	22	12	0	11	70	51	—	0
Sugar Free Chocolate Chip	3 (1.1 oz)	140	7	3	0	2	21	0	tr	20	100	—	—	0
Yo-Yo's	1 (1.2 oz)	130	6	2	0	1	21	12	tr	7	125	59	—	0
LOW CARB CREATIONS														
Chocolate Chip	1 (1 oz)	140	10	4	25	4	11	tr	1	—	40	—	—	—
Coconut	1 (1 oz)	140	10	5	30	5	9	tr	1	—	50	—	—	—
Lemon	1 (1 oz)	140	11	5	30	5	9	tr	1	—	50	—	—	—
Snickerdoodle	1 (1 oz)	140	11	4	30	5	9	tr	1	—	50	—	—	—
LU														
Chocolatier	3 (1 oz)	150	9	7	0	1	17	12	1	0	5	—	—	0
Le Bastogne	2 (0.8 oz)	120	5	3	0	1	18	10	0	0	50	—	—	0
Le Dore	4 (1 oz)	140	6	3	<5	2	21	7	0	0	55	—	—	0
Le Fondant	4 (1.1 oz)	170	10	9	0	1	19	9	1	0	5	—	—	0
Le Palmier	4 (1.2 oz)	180	10	5	0	2	20	7	tr	0	140	—	—	0
Le Petit Beurre	4 (1.2 oz)	150	4	3	10	3	26	7	tr	0	160	—	—	0
Le Petit Ecolier Dark Chocolate	2 (0.9 oz)	130	6	4	<5	2	17	10	1	0	50	—	—	0
Le Petit Ecolier Extra Dark Chocolate	2	120	7	4	<5	2	15	7	2	0	50	—	—	0
Le Petit Ecolier Hazelnut Milk Chocolate	2 (0.9 oz)	130	7	3	5	2	16	8	0	0	55	—	—	0
Le Petit Ecolier Milk Chocolate	2 (0.9 oz)	130	6	4	5	1	17	10	tr	0	55	—	—	0
Le Petit Fruit Strawberry	5 (1.2 oz)	110	1	0	30	1	26	19	0	0	10	—	—	0
Le Raisin Dore	4 (1.2 oz)	160	7	5	20	2	23	11	tr	0	130	—	—	0
Le Truffe Coconut	4 (1.2 oz)	190	12	11	0	1	17	12	1	0	15	—	—	0
Le Truffe Praline Chocolate	4 (1.2 oz)	170	9	7	0	2	20	15	2	0	15	—	—	0
Pim's Orange	2 (0.9 oz)	90	3	2	10	1	16	12	tr	0	25	—	—	0
Pim's Raspberry	2 (0.9 oz)	90	3	1	5	1	17	14	tr	0	25	—	—	0
Pim's Sensation Bar Chocolate	1	110	6	3	0	1	13	8	tr	0	30	—	—	0
Pim's Sensation Bar Hazelnut	1	110	6	3	0	1	13	8	tr	0	30	—	—	0
M&M'S														
Cookies & Milky Way	1 bar (1.20 oz)	180	11	3	0	2	21	13	1	0	95	—	—	0

FOOD	PORTION	CALS	FAT	SAT FAT	CHOL	PROT	CARB	SUGAR	FIBER	CALCI	SOD	POTAS	FOLIC	VIT C
MAMMA SAYS'														
Biscotti Almond Pistachio	1 (0.5 oz)	50	3	1	7	1	7	3	1	10	26	—	—	0
Biscotti Chocolate Macadamia	1 (0.5 oz)	45	3	1	10	1	5	3	1	10	23	—	—	0
Biscotti Orange Citrine	1 (0.5 oz)	60	2	1	10	2	8	4	1	10	40	—	—	0
MAUNA LOA														
Macadamia Nut Chocolate Chip	2	130	6	1	5	2	18	14	1	—	55	—	—	—
Macadamia Nut Hawaiian Crunch	2	150	8	2	10	2	15	8	1	—	30	—	—	—
Macadamia Nut White Chocolate Chip	2	130	6	1	6	2	18	14	1	—	55	—	—	—
MILK LUNCH BRAND														
New England Biscuits	4 (1.1 oz)	140	5	1	<5	2	74	3	1	0	220	—	—	0
MISS MERINGUE														
Minis Chocolate Raspberry	13 (1 oz)	80	0	0	0	1	20	19	0	—	15	—	—	—
Minis Chocolate Chip	13 (1 oz)	120	2	1	0	2	27	26	1	—	20	—	—	—
Minis Mint Chocolate Chip	13 (1 oz)	120	2	1	0	2	26	25	1	—	20	—	—	—
Minis Mochaccino	13 (1 oz)	80	0	0	0	1	20	19	0	—	15	—	—	—
Minis Orange	13 (1 oz)	80	0	0	0	1	20	20	0	—	15	—	—	6
Minis Rainbow Vanilla	13 (1 oz)	110	0	0	0	1	27	27	0	—	25	—	—	—
Minis Toasted Coconut	13 (1 oz)	90	2	1	0	1	19	19	0	—	15	—	—	—
Minis Very Chocolate	13 (1 oz)	80	0	0	0	1	20	19	0	—	15	—	—	—
Minis Very Minty	13 (1 oz)	80	0	0	0	1	20	19	0	—	15	—	—	—
Minis Very Vanilla	13 (1 oz)	80	0	0	0	1	20	19	0	—	15	—	—	—
MOONPIE														
Chocolate	1 (2.75 oz)	330	10	6	0	4	56	24	0	0	256	—	—	0
Mini Banana	1 (1.2 oz)	152	5	3	0	3	26	8	0	0	120	—	—	0
Mini Chocolate	1 (1.2 oz)	152	5	3	0	3	26	8	0	0	120	—	—	0
Mini Vanilla	1 (1.2 oz)	152	5	3	0	3	26	8	0	0	120	—	—	0
MOTHER'S														
Almond Shortbread	3	180	11	4	0	2	19	6	1	—	115	—	—	—
Checkerboard Wafers	8	150	8	5	0	1	20	10	1	—	40	—	—	—
Chocolate Chip	2	160	8	3	10	2	20	11	0	—	105	—	—	—

FOOD	PORTION	CALS	FAT	SAT FAT	CHOL	PROT	CARB	SUGAR	FIBER	CALCI	SOD	POTAS	FOLIC	VIT C
MOTHER'S (CONT.)														
Chocolate Chip Angel	3	180	9	4	0	2	21	8	1	—	70	—	—	—
Chocolate Chip Parade	4	130	5	2	0	1	19	8	1	—	100	—	—	—
Circus Animals	6	140	6	5	0	1	20	12	0	—	55	—	—	—
Classic Assortments	2	140	7	4	0	1	18	9	1	—	105	—	—	—
Cocadas	5	150	7	3	5	2	20	6	2	—	140	—	—	—
Cookie Parade	4	140	7	3	0	1	18	9	2	—	95	—	—	—
Dinosaur Grrrahams	2	130	3	1	0	2	24	7	2	—	130	—	—	—
Double Fudge	2	180	9	5	0	2	24	12	2	—	110	—	—	—
English Tea	2	180	7	4	0	2	26	12	1	—	100	—	—	—
Flaky Flix Fudge	2	140	7	5	0	1	17	12	2	—	50	—	—	—
Flaky Flix Vanilla	2	140	8	5	0	1	17	14	1	—	40	—	—	—
Gaucho Peanut Butter	2	190	10	3	0	3	22	7	2	—	200	—	—	—
Iced Oatmeal	2	130	4	2	0	2	22	10	1	—	160	—	—	—
Iced Raisin	2	180	8	7	0	1	24	12	1	—	110	—	—	—
Macaroon	2	150	8	4	0	1	18	8	2	—	80	—	—	—
Marias	3	170	6	2	5	2	28	9	1	—	150	—	—	—
MLB Double Header Duplex	3	170	8	4	5	2	23	12	1	—	130	—	—	—
Oatmeal	2	110	5	2	0	1	17	14	1	—	150	—	—	—
Oatmeal Chocolate Chip	2	120	5	2	0	2	19	9	1	—	140	—	—	—
Oatmeal Raisin	5	150	7	2	5	2	20	9	2	—	125	—	—	—
Oatmeal Walnut Chocolate Chip	2	130	6	2	0	2	17	9	1	—	135	—	—	—
Rainbow Wafers	8	150	8	5	0	1	20	10	1	—	40	—	—	—
Striped Shortbread	3	170	8	5	0	2	22	8	1	—	75	—	—	—
Sugar	2	140	6	2	0	1	19	8	1	—	75	—	—	—
Taffy	2	180	8	2	0	2	25	11	2	—	160	—	—	—
Triplet Assortment	2	140	7	3	0	1	18	11	1	—	112	—	—	—
Vanilla Wafers	6	150	6	2	4	2	24	14	1	—	85	—	—	—
Wallops Boysenberry	1	80	2	1	0	1	15	9	1	—	40	—	—	—
Wallops Honey Crust Fig	1	80	2	5	0	1	15	9	0	—	55	—	—	—
Wallops Honey Graham Fig	1	80	2	1	0	1	15	9	1	—	55	—	—	—
Wallops Mixed Berry	1	80	2	1	0	1	15	9	1	—	40	—	—	—
Wallops Peach Apricot	1	80	2	1	0	1	15	9	1	—	40	—	—	—
Wallops Raspberry	1	80	2	1	0	1	15	9	1	—	40	—	—	—

FOOD	PORTION	CALS	FAT	SAT FAT	CHOL	PROT	CARB	SUGAR	FIBER	CALCI	SOD	POTAS	FOLIC	VIT C
MOTHER'S (CONT.)														
Wallops Strawberry	1	80	2	1	0	1	15	9	1	—	40	—	—	—
Walnut Fudge	2	130	7	3	0	1	16	7	1	—	90	—	—	—
Zoo Pals	14	140	5	2	0	2	23	6	1	—	120	—	—	—
MRS. ALISON'S														
Coconut Bar	2 (1 oz)	130	6	1	0	2	19	6	0	0	85	—	—	0
Creme Wafers	5 (1.1 oz)	170	10	2	0	1	21	13	tr	0	35	—	—	0
Duplex Sandwich	3 (1 oz)	130	5	2	0	1	20	8	0	0	105	—	—	0
Fudge Fingers	3 (1 oz)	160	10	6	0	tr	19	16	0	0	20	—	—	0
Ginger Snaps	4 (1 oz)	130	3	1	<2	2	23	10	tr	20	170	—	—	0
Jelly Tops	5 (1 oz)	140	7	2	0	2	18	8	0	0	45	—	—	0
Lemon Creme	3 (1 oz)	130	5	2	0	1	21	9	0	0	115	—	—	0
Macaroons	2 (1 oz)	140	7	3	0	2	18	8	tr	0	95	—	—	0
Pecan	2 (1 oz)	140	7	2	0	2	19	7	0	0	75	—	—	0
Shortbread	5 (1 oz)	120	5	1	0	2	19	5	0	0	100	—	—	0
Vanilla Sandwich	3 (1 oz)	130	5	1	0	1	21	9	0	0	115	—	—	0
MURRAY'S														
Sugar Free Double Fudge	3 (1.2 oz)	140	6	3	0	2	23	0	3	20	110	—	—	0
Sugar Free Ginger Snap	6 (1 oz)	110	4	2	0	2	21	0	tr	0	100	—	—	0
Sugar Free Oatmeal	6 (1.1 oz)	120	4	1	0	2	23	0	1	0	130	—	—	0
Sugar Free Peanut Butter	6 (1 oz)	130	7	2	0	3	17	0	1	0	85	—	—	0
Sugar Free Vanilla Sandwich Creme	3 (1 oz)	120	5	2	0	1	21	0	2	0	65	—	—	0
Sugar Free Vanilla Wafers	9 (1.1 oz)	120	4	1	0	2	23	0	tr	0	85	—	—	0
NABISCO														
Barnum's Animal Crackers	10 (1 oz)	130	4	1	0	2	23	7	tr	100	150	—	—	0
Barnum's Animal Crackers Chocolate	10 (1 oz)	130	4	1	0	2	23	8	1	0	160	—	—	0
Biscos Sugar Wafers	8 (1 oz)	140	6	2	0	tr	21	13	0	0	40	—	—	0
Cafe Cremes Cappuccino	2 (1.1 oz)	160	8	2	0	1	22	9	0	20	130	—	—	0
Cafe Cremes Vanilla	2 (1.1 oz)	160	7	2	0	1	22	10	0	20	130	—	—	0
Cafe Cremes Vanilla Fudge	2 (1.1 oz)	200	10	2	0	2	27	14	tr	20	140	—	—	0
Cameo	2 (1 oz)	130	5	1	0	1	21	10	0	0	105	—	—	0
Chips Ahoy!	3 (1.1 oz)	160	8	3	0	2	21	10	1	0	105	—	—	0
Chips Ahoy! Chewy	3 (1.3 oz)	170	8	3	0	1	24	13	tr	0	125	—	—	0

FOOD	PORTION	CALS	FAT	SAT FAT	CHOL	PROT	CARB	SUGAR	FIBER	CALCI	SOD	POTAS	FOLIC	VIT C
NABISCO (CONT.)														
Chips Ahoy! Chunky	1 (0.5 oz)	80	4	2	5	tr	10	6	0	0	35	—	—	0
Chips Ahoy! Munch Size	6 (1.1 oz)	160	8	2	0	2	21	10	1	0	150	—	—	0
Chips Ahoy! Reduced Fat	3 (1.1 oz)	140	5	2	0	2	22	10	tr	0	150	—	—	0
Family Favorites Iced Oatmeal	1 (0.6 oz)	80	3	0	0	1	12	6	0	0	55	—	—	0
Family Favorites Oatmeal	1 (0.6 oz)	80	3	1	0	1	12	5	0	0	65	—	—	0
Famous Chocolate Wafers	5 (1.1 oz)	140	4	2	<5	2	24	11	1	0	230	—	—	0
Grahams	4 (1 oz)	120	3	1	0	2	22	6	1	20	180	—	—	0
Honey Maid Chocolate Grahams	8 (1 oz)	120	3	1	0	2	22	8	1	0	170	—	—	0
Honey Maid Cinnamon Grahams	8 (1 oz)	120	3	0	0	2	23	9	tr	20	180	—	—	0
Honey Maid Honey Grahams	8 (1 oz)	120	3	0	0	2	22	7	1	0	180	—	—	0
Honey Maid Low Fat Cinnamon Grahams	8 (1 oz)	110	2	0	0	2	23	10	tr	20	170	—	—	0
Honey Maid Low Fat Grahams	8 (1 oz)	110	2	0	0	2	23	8	tr	0	200	—	—	0
Honey Maid Oatmeal Crunch	8 (1 oz)	120	3	0	0	2	22	7	1	20	140	—	—	0
Lorna Doone	4 (1 oz)	140	7	1	5	2	19	6	tr	0	130	—	—	0
Mallomars	2	120	5	3	0	1	17	12	tr	0	35	—	—	0
Marshmallow Twirls	1 (1 oz)	130	6	1	0	1	20	14	0	0	75	—	—	0
Mystic Mint	1 (0.5 oz)	90	5	1	0	1	11	8	0	0	65	—	—	0
National Arrowroot	1 (5 g)	20	1	—	—	0	4	1	0	0	15	—	—	0
Newtons Fat Free Fig	2 (1 oz)	90	0	0	0	1	22	12	1	20	115	—	—	0
Newtons Fig	2 (1.1 oz)	110	3	0	0	1	22	14	1	0	125	—	—	0
Newtons Fat Free Apple	2 (1 oz)	90	0	0	0	1	21	12	tr	0	65	—	—	0
Newtons Fat Free Cobblers Apple Cinnamon	1 (0.8 oz)	70	0	0	0	1	17	10	tr	0	40	—	—	0
Newtons Fat Free Cobblers Peach Apricot	1 (0.8 oz)	70	0	0	0	1	17	10	0	0	55	—	—	0

FOOD	PORTION	CALS	FAT	SAT FAT	CHOL	PROT	CARB	SUGAR	FIBER	CALCI	SOD	POTAS	FOLIC	VIT C
NABISCO (CONT.)														
Newtons Fat Free Cranberry	2 (1 oz)	100	0	0	0	1	22	14	tr	0	95	—	—	0
Newtons Fat Free Raspberry	2 (1 oz)	100	0	0	0	1	23	13	tr	0	115	—	—	1
Newtons Fat Free Strawberry	2 (1 oz)	90	0	0	0	1	21	11	0	20	95	—	—	2
Nilla Wafers	8 (1.1 oz)	140	5	1	<5	1	24	12	0	20	100	—	—	0
Nilla Wafers Chocolate Reduced Fat	8 (1 oz)	110	2	0	0	2	23	12	tr	20	120	—	—	0
Nilla Wafers Reduced Fat	8 (1 oz)	120	2	0	0	1	24	12	0	20	105	—	—	0
Nutter Butter Bites	10 (1 oz)	150	7	1	<5	3	20	9	1	0	125	—	—	0
Nutter Butter Chocolate Peanut Butter Sandwich	2 (1 oz)	130	5	1	0	2	19	8	1	0	140	—	—	0
Nutter Butter Peanut Butter Sandwich	2 (1 oz)	130	6	1	<5	2	19	8	tr	20	110	—	—	0
Old Fashioned Ginger Snaps	4 (1 oz)	120	3	1	0	1	22	9	tr	20	230	—	—	0
Oreo	3 (1.2 oz)	160	7	2	0	1	23	13	1	0	220	—	—	0
Oreo Double Stuff	2 (1 oz)	140	7	2	0	1	19	13	tr	0	150	—	—	0
Oreo Mini	1 pkg (0.5 oz)	65	3	1	0	tr	10	6	1	0	75	—	—	0
Oreo Reduced Fat	3 (1.1 oz)	130	4	1	0	—	25	14	1	0	190	—	—	0
Oreo Halloween	2 (1 oz)	140	7	2	0	1	19	13	tr	0	115	—	—	0
Pecanz	1 (0.5 oz)	90	5	1	<5	1	9	3	0	0	50	—	—	0
Pinwheels Chocolate Marshmallow	1 (1 oz)	130	5	3	0	1	21	15	tr	0	35	—	—	0
Rugrats Chocolate Frosted	8 (1.1 oz)	150	5	2	0	1	24	13	tr	0	110	—	—	0
Rugrats Vanilla Frosted	8 (1.1 oz)	150	6	2	0	1	24	13	tr	0	105	—	—	0
Social Tea	6 (1 oz)	120	4	1	5	2	20	7	tr	0	115	—	—	0
Sweet Crispers Chocolate	18 (1.1 oz)	130	3	1	0	2	25	12	1	20	190	—	—	0
Sweet Crispers Chocolate Chip	18 (1.1 oz)	130	3	1	0	2	23	11	tr	0	160	—	—	0
Teddy Grahams Chocolate	24 (1 oz)	130	5	1	0	2	22	9	1	0	170	—	—	0
Teddy Grahams Chocolately Chip	24 (1 oz)	130	5	1	0	2	23	8	tr	0	135	—	—	0
Teddy Grahams Cinnamon	24 (1 oz)	130	4	1	0	2	23	8	1	0	150	—	—	0
Teddy Grahams Honey	24 (1 oz)	130	4	1	0	2	23	8	tr	0	150	—	—	0

FOOD	PORTION	CALS	FAT	SAT FAT	CHOL	PROT	CARB	SUGAR	FIBER	CALCI	SOD	POTAS	FOLIC	VIT C
NATURAL OVENS														
Carob Chip	1	90	4	0	0	2	16	6	3	60	15	—	60	—
Chocolate Raspberry	1	120	5	2	0	2	19	6	3	60	70	—	60	—
Oatmeal Raisin	1	90	3	0	0	3	15	6	3	60	15	—	60	—
NESTLÉ														
Flipz Crunchy Graham White Fudge Chocolate	8 (1 oz)	140	6	5	0	2	19	12	0	40	85	—	—	0
NEWMAN'S OWN														
Fig Newman's Organic	2 (1.3 oz)	120	0	0	0	2	28	15	1	40	140	—	—	0
NONNI'S														
Biscotti Cioccalati	1 (1 oz)	130	5	3	5	2	19	11	1	20	50	—	—	0
Biscotti Decadence	1 (1.1 oz)	130	5	3	25	2	19	11	1	20	65	—	—	0
Biscotti Original	1 (1 oz)	100	4	2	25	2	15	8	1	20	65	—	—	0
Biscotti Paradiso	1 (1.1 oz)	130	6	3	5	2	19	12	0	20	60	—	—	0
NUTRABALANCE														
Fibre Oatmeal Raisin	1 (0.7 oz)	80	4	1	0	1	13	6	3	0	85	—	—	0
Protein Fortified	1 (2 oz)	260	14	5	10	7	28	12	2	60	180	138	—	0
ReNeph Spice	1 (2 oz)	210	7	0	0	9	29	14	0	6	230	125	—	0
OLD BRUSSELS														
Ginger Crisps	2 (0.9 oz)	140	4	1	0	2	23	4	2	0	115	—	—	0
OLD LONDON														
Coffee Toppers Chocolate Creme	3 (0.5 oz)	70	3	2	0	1	9	3	0	0	75	—	—	0
Coffee Toppers Vanilla Creme	3 (0.5 oz)	70	4	3	0	1	9	3	0	0	80	—	—	0
OLDE WORLD														
Pizzelle Almond	3 (1 oz)	90	4	1	45	2	12	4	0	0	15	—	—	0
Pizzelle Anise	3 (1 oz)	90	4	1	45	2	12	4	0	0	15	—	—	0
Pizzelle Chocolate	3 (1 oz)	100	5	1	45	2	11	5	0	0	15	—	—	0
Pizzelle Lemon	3 (1 oz)	90	4	1	45	2	12	4	0	0	15	—	—	0
Pizzelle Vanilla	3 (1 oz)	90	4	1	45	2	12	4	0	0	15	—	—	0
OTIS SPUNKMEYER														
Butter Sugar	1 med (1.3 oz)	160	8	3	15	2	23	14	tr	0	140	0	—	0
Butter Sugar	1 (2 oz)	250	12	5	20	3	35	21	1	0	210	—	—	1
Carnival	1 med (1.3 oz)	170	7	3	10	2	25	16	0	0	80	—	—	0
Chocolate Chip	1 bite size (0.75 oz)	100	5	2	5	1	14	9	0	0	70	—	—	1
Chocolate Chip	1 med (1.3 oz)	170	8	4	10	2	24	16	0	0	120	0	—	0
Chocolate Chip	1 (2 oz)	250	11	6	15	3	36	21	tr	20	210	—	—	1
Chocolate Chip Pecan	1 med (1.3 oz)	170	9	4	10	2	22	14	tr	0	110	0	—	0

FOOD	PORTION	CALS	FAT	SAT FAT	CHOL	PROT	CARB	SUGAR	FIBER	CALCI	SOD	POTAS	FOLIC	VIT C
OTIS SPUNKMEYER (CONT.)														
Chocolate Chip Walnut	1 bite size (0.75 oz)	100	5	3	5	1	13	8	0	0	60	—	—	1
Chocolate Chip Walnut	1 med (1.3 oz)	180	9	4	10	2	22	14	tr	0	105	0	—	0
Chocolate Chip Walnut	1 (2 oz)	270	14	6	15	3	34	21	tr	20	160	—	—	1
Double Chocolate Chip	1 med (1.3 oz)	180	9	5	10	2	23	17	tr	0	130	—	—	0
Double Chocolate Chip	1 bite size (0.75 oz)	100	5	3	5	1	13	10	1	0	75	—	—	1
Oatmeal Raisin	1 med (1.3 oz)	160	7	5	10	2	23	11	1	0	130	—	—	0
Oatmeal Raisin	1 bite size (0.75 oz)	90	4	3	5	1	13	6	tr	0	75	—	—	1
Otis Express Chocolate Chunk	1 (2 oz)	280	13	6	20	3	37	22	1	20	190	—	—	0
Otis Express Double Chocolate Chip	1 (2 oz)	270	14	7	15	3	35	26	1	20	200	—	—	0
Otis Express Oatmeal Raisin	1 (2 oz)	240	10	7	15	3	35	17	2	20	200	—	—	1
Otis Express Peanut Butter	1 (2 oz)	270	15	6	15	5	31	17	2	20	250	—	—	1
Peanut Butter	1 med (1.3 oz)	180	10	4	10	3	20	11	1	0	160	—	—	0
Pinnacle Checkpoint Chocolate Almond Coconut	1 (2.4 oz)	320	18	10	25	4	37	24	2	40	230	—	—	0
Pinnacle Mach One Mocha Chocolate Chunk	1 (2.4 oz)	300	13	6	20	3	43	26	1	40	230	—	—	0
Pinnacle Passport Peanut Butter Chocolate Chunk	1 (2.4 oz)	300	13	5	25	5	42	28	1	20	250	—	—	0
Pinnacle Ripcord Rocky Road	1 (2.4 oz)	310	15	6	15	3	41	27	2	20	230	—	—	0
Pinnacle Takeoff Triple Chocolate	1 (2.4 oz)	300	14	6	20	3	42	26	tr	40	180	—	—	0
Pinnacle Transatlantic Turtle	1 (2.4 oz)	310	16	6	20	3	39	26	2	0	250	—	—	0
Travel Lite Low Fat Apple Cinnamon	1 (1.3 oz)	130	2	0	0	2	26	15	tr	0	90	—	16	0
Travel Lite Low Fat Chocolate Chip	1 (1.3 oz)	130	2	1	0	2	27	16	tr	0	110	—	16	0

FOOD	PORTION	CALS	FAT	SAT FAT	CHOL	PROT	CARB	SUGAR	FIBER	CALCI	SOD	POTAS	FOLIC	VIT C
OTIS SPUNKMEYER (CONT.)														
Travel Lite Low Fat Ginger Spice	1 (1.3 oz)	130	2	0	0	2	26	15	tr	20	90	—	16	0
Travel Lite Low Fat Oatmeal Rum Raisin	1 (1.3 oz)	130	2	0	0	2	26	15	1	0	90	—	16	0
White Chocolate Macadamia Nut	1 med (1.3 oz)	180	10	4	10	2	21	14	tr	0	110	0	—	0
White Chocolate Macadamia Nut	1 (2 oz)	280	15	7	20	3	33	21	tr	20	170	—	—	1
PALLY														
Butter	5 (1 oz)	140	3	2	1	3	23	6	1	0	170	—	—	0
Carnival	5 (1 oz)	130	3	1	0	2	24	9	1	—	130	—	—	—
Cinnamon Biscuit	5 (1 oz)	130	3	1	0	2	23	11	0	0	130	—	—	0
Mariel Biscuit	6 (1 oz)	150	4	1	0	3	23	6	1	0	140	—	—	0
Tea Biscuits	5 (1 oz)	150	4	1	0	2	23	6	1	0	170	—	—	0
PAMELA'S														
Pecan Shortbread Rice Flour	1 (0.8 oz)	130	8	4	20	tr	15	4	tr	0	65	—	—	0
PARMALAT														
Grisbi Lemon	1 (0.6 oz)	90	6	2	5	1	9	5	1	0	0	—	—	0
PEEK FREANS														
Arrowroot	4 (1.2 oz)	150	5	1	0	2	26	7	1	0	80	—	—	0
Assorted Creme	1 (1 oz)	130	6	3	<5	1	19	9	0	0	50	—	—	0
Dream Puffs	2 (0.9 oz)	110	4	3	0	tr	18	12	0	0	50	—	—	0
Fruit Creme	2 (0.9 oz)	130	5	2	0	1	20	10	0	0	35	—	—	0
Ginger Crisp	4 (1.2 oz)	150	4	1	0	2	28	11	tr	20	65	—	—	0
Nice	4 (1.2 oz)	160	6	3	0	2	25	9	1	0	100	—	—	0
Petit Beret Creme Caramel	2 (0.8 oz)	110	5	4	0	tr	15	10	tr	0	120	—	—	0
Petit Beret Fudge Truffle	2 (0.8 oz)	110	5	4	0	tr	15	10	tr	0	100	—	—	0
Petit Beurre	4 (1 oz)	130	4	2	tr	2	22	5	tr	0	115	—	—	0
Rich Tea	4 (1.2 oz)	160	5	2	0	2	25	7	tr	0	150	—	—	0
Shortcake	2 (0.9 oz)	140	7	3	20	1	18	5	0	0	70	—	—	0
Traditional Oatmeal	1 (0.7 oz)	90	3	1	0	1	15	7	tr	0	100	—	—	0
Tropical Cremes Calypso Lime	2 (0.9 oz)	130	5	2	0	1	20	10	0	0	15	—	—	0
PEPPERIDGE FARM														
Biscotti Almond	1 (0.7 oz)	90	4	1	5	2	12	5	0	0	65	—	—	0
Biscotti Chocolate Hazelnut	1 (0.7 oz)	90	5	1	15	2	11	5	2	0	80	—	—	0
Biscotti Cranberry Pistachio	1 (0.7 oz)	90	3	1	5	2	13	7	0	0	65	—	—	0

FOOD	PORTION	CALS	FAT	SAT FAT	CHOL	PROT	CARB	SUGAR	FIBER	CALCI	SOD	POTAS	FOLIC	VIT C
PEPPERIDGE FARM (CONT.)														
Bordeaux	4	130	5	3	10	2	19	12	tr	0	95	—	—	0
Brussels	2	100	5	2	<5	1	13	7	tr	0	55	—	—	0
Chantilly Raspberry	2 (1 oz)	120	3	1	0	1	23	11	tr	0	115	—	—	0
Chessman	3	120	8	3	20	2	18	5	tr	0	80	—	—	0
Chocolate Chunk Soft Baked Double Chocolate	1 (0.9 oz)	130	7	3	0	2	15	9	1	0	60	—	—	0
Chocolate Chip	3	140	7	3	—	2	18	9	tr	0	70	—	—	0
Chocolate Chunk Chesapeake	1 (0.7 oz)	140	8	3	10	2	15	7	0	0	80	—	—	0
Chocolate Chunk Minis Nantucket	1 pkg (1.75 oz)	260	13	5	10	tr	34	17	0	0	115	—	—	0
Chocolate Chunk Minis Sausalito	4 (1 oz)	160	9	4	10	1	18	10	0	0	70	—	—	0
Chocolate Chunk Montauk	1 (0.9 oz)	130	7	3	10	1	17	10	0	0	90	—	—	0
Chocolate Chunk Nantucket	1 (0.9 oz)	140	7	3	10	2	16	9	0	0	80	—	—	0
Chocolate Chunk Sausalito	1 (0.7 oz)	140	8	3	10	2	16	9	0	0	80	—	—	0
Chocolate Chunk Soft Baked	1	140	5	3	<5	1	22	13	1	0	65	—	—	0
Chocolate Chunk Soft Baked Milk Chocolate Macademia	1	130	7	3	10	2	16	9	0	0	75	—	—	0
Chocolate Chunk Soft Baked Reduced Fat	1	110	5	2	15	1	18	8	tr	0	85	—	—	0
Chocolate Chunk Soft Baked White Chocolate Pecan	1	120	5	2	5	1	16	9	1	0	65	—	—	0
Chocolate Chunk Tahoe	1 (0.9 oz)	130	8	3	10	2	15	8	0	0	90	—	—	0
Fruitful Apricot Raspberry Cup	3	140	6	2	—	2	22	10	tr	0	110	—	—	0
Fruitful Strawberry Cup	3	140	5	2	10	2	22	10	tr	0	105	—	—	0
Geneva	3	160	9	4	0	2	19	8	1	0	95	—	—	0
Ginger Man	4 (1 oz)	130	4	1	10	2	21	11	tr	0	100	—	—	0
Goldfish Grahams Cinnamon	1 pkg (1.75 oz)	240	10	4	5	2	37	13	2	0	220	—	—	0
Lemon Nut Crunch	3	170	9	2	15	2	18	7	2	0	60	—	—	0
Lido	1	90	5	2	<5	tr	10	5	0	0	40	—	—	0
Milano	3	180	10	4	—	2	21	11	tr	0	80	—	—	0

FOOD	PORTION	CALS	FAT	SAT FAT	CHOL	PROT	CARB	SUGAR	FIBER	CALCI	SOD	POTAS	FOLIC	VIT C
PEPPERIDGE FARM (CONT.)														
Milano Endless Chocolate	3	180	10	5	<5	2	21	10	1	0	85	—	—	0
Milano Milk Chocolate	3	170	9	4	10	2	21	13	tr	20	110	—	—	0
Milano Double Chocolate	2 (0.7 oz)	140	8	3	10	2	17	10	tr	0	70	—	—	0
Milano Mint	2	130	7	4	<5	1	16	8	1	0	65	—	—	0
Milano Orange	2	130	7	3	—	1	16	8	tr	0	65	—	—	0
Pirouettes Chocolate Laced	5 (1.1 oz)	180	10	3	5	2	20	13	tr	0	90	—	—	0
Pirouettes Traditional	5 (1.2 oz)	170	9	3	5	2	20	13	0	0	90	—	—	0
Shortbread	2	140	7	—	10	2	16	5	tr	0	105	—	—	0
Soft Baked Oatmeal Raisin	1 (0.9 oz)	130	7	3	10	2	16	9	0	0	75	—	—	0
Soft Baked Reduced Fat Oatmeal Raisin	1 (0.9 oz)	100	3	1	10	1	18	8	tr	0	85	—	—	0
Spritzers Cool Key Lime	6 (1.1 oz)	140	7	2	<5	1	21	9	0	40	60	—	—	0
Spritzers Ripe Red Raspberry	5 (1.1 oz)	140	7	2	<5	1	21	9	0	40	60	—	—	0
Spritzers Zesty Lemon	5 (1.1 oz)	140	7	2	<5	1	21	9	0	40	60	—	—	0
Sugar	3	140	6	2	—	2	20	10	tr	0	90	—	—	0
Verona Strawberry	3 (1.1 oz)	140	5	2	10	2	22	10	tr	0	105	—	—	0
PURE DE-LITE														
High Protein Chocolate Fudge	1 (2.2 oz)	210	8	2	10	18	29	0	5	—	260	—	—	—
High Protein Peanut Butter Crunch	1 (2.2 oz)	210	8	2	5	18	28	0	5	—	300	—	—	—
RALSTON														
Animal	12 (0.9 oz)	130	3	1	—	2	22	5	—	—	80	—	—	—
Chocolate Graham	2 (0.9 oz)	130	3	1	—	2	24	7	1	—	120	—	—	—
Cinnamon	2 (0.9 oz)	130	5	1	—	1	19	7	tr	—	85	—	—	—
Cinnamon Low Fat	2 (0.9 oz)	110	2	0	0	2	22	6	1	—	120	—	—	—
Fig Bars	2 (1.2 oz)	120	3	0	—	tr	23	14	1	—	55	—	—	—
Vanilla Wafers	7 (1.1 oz)	150	6	1	—	1	22	10	1	—	115	—	—	—
REAL TORINO														
Lady Fingers	3 (1 oz)	110	1	0	5	2	23	11	0	20	70	—	—	0

FOOD	PORTION	CALS	FAT	SAT FAT	CHOL	PROT	CARB	SUGAR	FIBER	CALCI	SOD	POTAS	FOLIC	VIT C
REKO														
Pizzelle Maple	5 (1 oz)	150	6	1	15	3	20	8	0	0	20	—	—	0
Pizzelle Vanilla	1 (6 g)	30	1	tr	3	1	4	2	0	0	4	—	—	0
ROYAL														
Apple Bars	1 (1.1 oz)	100	2	0	0	1	21	13	1	0	65	—	—	0
Apple Cake	1 (1.1 oz)	110	3	1	0	1	19	8	1	0	50	—	—	0
Brownie Rounds	1 (1.1 oz)	130	6	2	0	1	19	11	0	0	135	—	—	0
Chocolate Chip	1 (1.1 oz)	140	6	2	0	1	20	11	1	0	120	—	—	0
Devilfood	1 (1 oz)	110	5	1	0	1	17	10	0	0	110	—	—	0
Fig Bars	1 (1.1 oz)	100	2	0	0	1	20	13	1	10	65	—	—	0
Oatmeal	1 (1.1 oz)	130	6	1	0	2	19	10	1	0	140	—	—	0
Raisin	1 (1 oz)	110	5	1	0	1	17	10	0	0	115	—	—	0
Strawberry Bars	1 (1.1 oz)	100	2	0	0	1	20	12	1	0	65	—	—	0
SALERNO														
Mini Butter	25 (1 oz)	180	6	3	15	2	20	8	tr	—	125	—	—	—
Mini Dinosaur Chocolate Graham	16 (1 1 oz)	140	5	2	0	2	22	7	1	—	125	—	—	—
Scooter Pie	1 (1.2 oz)	140	5	3	0	1	23	14	0	0	80	—	—	0
SANTA FE FARMS														
Chocolate Chocolate Chip Fat Free	2 (1 oz)	60	0	0	0	2	16	7	3	20	90	—	—	—
Chocolate Mint Fat Free	2 (1 oz)	60	0	0	0	2	16	7	3	20	90	—	—	—
Ginger Fat Free	2 (1 oz)	70	0	0	0	2	17	8	2	20	95	—	—	—
SARGENTO														
MooTown Snackers Honey Graham Sticks & Vanilla Creme w/ Sprinkles	1 pkg (1 oz)	140	7	1	0	2	17	10	0	40	50	—	—	0
MooTown Snackers Vanilla Sticks & Chocolate Fudge Creme	1 pkg (1 oz)	130	6	2	0	1	18	11	tr	0	50	—	—	0
SAVION														
Chocolate Biscuits	5 (1 oz)	120	3	1	0	2	22	6	0	0	45	—	—	0
Tea Biscuits	5 (1 oz)	120	3	1	0	2	22	6	0	0	80	—	—	0
Tea Biscuits Vanilla	5 (1 oz)	120	3	1	0	2	22	6	0	0	80	—	—	0
SCOTTO'S														
Biscotti Fat Free French Vanilla	4 (1 oz)	80	0	0	0	2	18	6	0	20	25	—	—	0

FOOD	PORTION	CALS	FAT	SAT FAT	CHOL	PROT	CARB	SUGAR	FIBER	CALCI	SOD	POTAS	FOLIC	VIT C
SEASON														
Hamantashen Apricot	1 (1 oz)	150	7	4	7	1	20	4	1	—	60	—	—	—
Hamantashen Poppy	1 (1 oz)	150	7	4	7	1	20	4	1	—	60	—	—	—
SIMPLE PLEASURES														
Almond	1 (0.3 oz)	37	2	tr	0	1	5	2	tr	—	9	7	—	—
Cinnamon Snaps	1 (0.2 oz)	31	1	tr	0	1	6	2	tr	—	27	11	—	—
Digestive	1 (0.3 oz)	46	2	tr	0	1	6	2	tr	—	34	13	—	—
Encore Tea Cookie	1 (0.2 oz)	29	1	tr	0	tr	6	1	tr	—	32	5	—	—
Lemon Social Tea	1 (0.2 oz)	29	1	tr	0	tr	6	1	tr	—	32	5	—	—
Oatmeal	1 (0.5 oz)	74	3	1	0	1	5	4	1	—	—	—	—	—
Spice Snaps	1 (0.3 oz)	34	1	tr	0	1	6	2	tr	—	56	18	—	—
Sugar	1 (0.4 oz)	45	2	1	3	1	7	3	tr	—	—	—	—	—
SNACKWELL'S														
Bite Size Chocolate Chip	13 (1 oz)	130	4	2	0	2	22	10	tr	0	160	—	—	0
Bite Size Double Chocolate Chip	13 (1 oz)	130	4	2	0	2	22	10	1	0	190	—	—	0
Chocolate Sandwich	2 (0.8 oz)	110	3	1	0	1	20	11	tr	20	210	—	—	0
Creme Sandwich	1 pkg (1.7 oz)	210	5	1	0	2	38	18	tr	20	230	—	—	0
Fat Free Devil's Food	1 (0.5 oz)	50	0	0	0	1	12	7	0	0	30	—	—	0
Golden Devil's Food	1 (0.5 oz)	50	1	0	0	1	11	7	0	0	25	—	—	0
Mint Creme	2	110	4	1	0	1	19	13	tr	0	70	—	—	0
Oatmeal Raisin	2 (0.9 oz)	110	3	0	<5	2	20	9	tr	0	130	—	—	0
Sugar Free Chocolate Chip	3 (1.2 oz)	150	8	3	<5	2	23	0	tr	0	160	—	—	0
Sugar Free Oatmeal	1 (0.8 oz)	90	3	1	0	1	17	0	tr	0	80	—	—	0
SOYBITE														
All Flavors	1	79	5	1	0	5	7	0	1	—	3	—	—	—
STELLA D'ORO														
Almond Toast Mandel	2 (1 oz)	110	3	1	30	2	21	10	1	20	85	—	—	0
Angel Wings	2 (0.9 oz)	140	9	3	<5	2	13	3	tr	0	80	—	—	0
Angelica	1 (0.8 oz)	100	4	1	15	2	15	6	0	0	45	—	—	0
Anginetti	4 (1.1 oz)	140	4	1	40	2	23	17	tr	40	10	—	—	0
Anisette Sponge	2 (0.9 oz)	90	1	0	40	2	19	9	tr	20	80	—	—	0
Anisette Toast	3 (1.2 oz)	130	1	0	35	2	27	17	tr	20	150	—	—	0
Biscotti Almond	1 (0.8 oz)	100	3	1	10	2	15	7	tr	0	55	—	—	0
Biscotti Chocolate Almond	1 (0.8 oz)	90	3	1	10	2	15	7	1	0	55	—	—	0

FOOD	PORTION	CALS	FAT	SAT FAT	CHOL	PROT	CARB	SUGAR	FIBER	CALCI	SOD	POTAS	FOLIC	VIT C
STELLA D'ORO (CONT.)														
Biscotti Chocolate Chunk	1 (0.8 oz)	90	3	1	10	2	16	9	0	0	60	—	—	0
Biscotti Hazelnut	1 (0.8 oz)	100	4	1	10	2	15	8	0	0	60	—	—	0
Biscottini Cashews	1 (0.7 oz)	110	6	1	5	1	13	5	0	0	50	—	—	0
Breakfast Treats	1 (0.8 oz)	100	3	1	10	1	16	7	tr	0	80	—	—	0
Breakfast Treats Chocolate	1 (0.8 oz)	100	4	1	10	2	15	7	tr	0	70	—	—	0
Breakfast Treats Viennese Cinnamon	1 (0.8 oz)	100	3	1	10	1	17	8	0	20	65	—	—	0
Chinese Dessert Cookies	1 (1.2 oz)	170	9	2	5	2	21	8	tr	0	90	—	—	0
Chocolate Castelets	2 (1 oz)	130	6	2	<5	2	19	8	1	0	55	—	—	0
Egg Jumbo	2 (0.8 oz)	90	1	0	30	2	18	9	tr	0	60	—	—	0
Fruit Slices Fat Free	1 (0.6 oz)	50	0	0	0	1	12	6	tr	0	45	—	—	0
Kichel Low Sodium	21 (1 oz)	150	9	2	80	4	13	1	0	0	25	—	—	0
Lady Stella	3	130	5	1	5	1	20	9	tr	0	55	—	—	0
Margherite Chocolate	2 (1.1 oz)	140	6	2	10	2	22	9	1	0	75	—	—	0
Margherite Vanilla	2 (1.1 oz)	140	5	1	15	2	22	8	tr	0	90	—	—	0
Roman Egg Biscuits	1 (1.2 oz)	140	5	2	20	2	21	9	1	20	125	—	—	0
Sesame Regina	3 (1.1 oz)	150	6	2	10	2	21	8	1	0	85	—	—	0
Swiss Fudge	2 (0.9 oz)	130	7	2	5	1	16	9	0	0	55	—	—	0
STIEFFENHOFER														
Choco Minis	4 (1 oz)	160	8	5	15	1	19	8	1	0	40	—	—	0
Snaky	3 (1 oz)	160	8	2	0	2	19	10	0	20	20	—	—	0
STREIT'S														
Wafers	3 (1 oz)	160	9	2	0	1	19	12	1	20	35	—	—	0
SUISSETTE														
Swiss Chocolate Hearts	4 (1 oz)	170	10	6	5	2	17	11	—	20	40	—	—	—
Swiss Delight	4 (1 oz)	160	9	4	5	2	19	9	—	20	35	—	—	—
Swiss Praline	4 (1 oz)	150	9	6	15	1	17	13	1	20	15	—	—	—
SUNSHINE														
All American Butter	5 (1.1 oz)	140	6	2	<5	2	21	7	tr	0	135	—	—	0
All American Lemon Coolers	5 (1 oz)	140	6	2	0	1	21	10	tr	0	100	—	—	0
All American Mini Chip A Roos	5 (1.1 oz)	160	8	3	0	1	21	10	1	0	140	—	—	0
Animal Crackers	14 (1.1 oz)	140	4	1	0	2	24	7	tr	0	125	—	—	0
Ginger Snaps	7 (1 oz)	130	5	1	0	2	22	9	tr	0	150	—	—	0

FOOD	PORTION	CALS	FAT	SAT FAT	CHOL	PROT	CARB	SUGAR	FIBER	CALCI	SOD	POTAS	FOLIC	VIT C
SUNSHINE (CONT.)														
Golden Fruit Cranberry	1 (0.7 oz)	80	2	0	0	1	14	7	tr	0	55	—	—	0
Golden Fruit Raisin	1 (0.7 oz)	80	2	1	0	1	15	9	tr	0	50	—	—	0
Hydrox	3 (1.1 oz)	150	7	2	0	2	21	11	1	0	125	—	—	0
Hydrox Reduced Fat	3 (1.1 oz)	140	5	2	0	2	23	13	1	0	150	—	—	0
Oatmeal Country Style	2 (0.8 oz)	120	5	1	0	2	17	8	tr	0	115	—	—	0
Sugar Wafers Peanut Butter Creme	4 (1.1 oz)	170	9	2	0	3	19	10	1	0	75	—	—	0
Sugar Wafers Vanilla Creme	3 (0.9 oz)	130	6	2	0	1	18	13	tr	0	30	—	—	0
Vanilla Wafers	7 (1.1 oz)	150	7	2	3	2	21	9	tr	0	110	—	—	0
Vienna Fingers	2 (1 oz)	140	6	2	0	2	21	8	tr	0	105	—	—	0
Vienna Fingers Lemon	2 (1 oz)	140	6	2	0	2	21	9	0	0	90	—	—	0
Vienna Fingers Reduced Fat	2 (1 oz)	130	5	1	0	1	22	9	tr	0	105	—	—	0
SUPER CHIP														
Chocolate Chip	2 (0.9 oz)	100	7	—	—	1	10	0	3	—	170	—	—	—
SWEET'N LOW														
Sugar Free Amaretto Biscotti	4 (1 oz)	120	6	1	10	2	17	0	tr	0	180	—	—	0
Sugar Free Chocolate Chip	4 (1 oz)	135	8	1	10	2	17	0	tr	0	35	—	—	0
Sugar Free Cinnamon Graham	7 (1 oz)	120	6	1	15	2	19	0	tr	0	90	—	—	0
Sugar Free Morning Crunch Bars	2 (1 oz)	120	6	1	10	2	19	0	tr	0	150	—	—	0
Sugar Free Vanilla Wafers	7 (1 oz)	120	6	1	15	2	19	0	tr	0	80	—	—	0
SWEETZELS														
Chocolate Chip	7 (1 oz)	160	9	4	5	1	18	9	0	0	70	—	—	0
Ginger Snaps	4 (1.2 oz)	140	3	1	0	2	25	11	tr	20	120	—	—	0
Vanilla Wafers	7 (1.1 oz)	137	5	1	0	2	22	8	0	0	94	—	—	0
TASTYKAKE														
Chocolate Chip	1 (1.4 oz)	180	7	2	10	2	26	7	1	20	160	—	—	0
Chocolate Chip Bar	1 (2 oz)	270	12	4	10	2	39	22	tr	0	125	—	—	5
Chocolate Fudge Iced	1 (1.4 oz)	170	7	2	55	4	25	9	1	40	190	—	—	0
Fudge Bar	1 (2 oz)	250	10	2	5	3	37	21	1	0	140	—	—	0

FOOD	PORTION	CALS	FAT	SAT FAT	CHOL	PROT	CARB	SUGAR	FIBER	CALCI	SOD	POTAS	FOLIC	VIT C
TASTYKAKE (CONT.)														
Lemon Bar	1 (2 oz)	260	10	1	5	2	41	23	1	0	125	—	—	5
Oatmeal Raisin Bar	1 (2 oz)	260	10	3	15	4	40	18	2	20	230	—	—	0
Oatmeal Raisin Boxed	3 (0.4 oz)	130	6	2	5	1	14	7	tr	0	70	—	—	0
Oatmeal Raisin Iced	1 (1.4 oz)	170	6	2	25	3	27	13	1	20	150	—	—	0
Strawberry Bar	1 (2 oz)	260	10	1	5	2	41	23	1	0	125	—	—	1
Sugar Boxed	3 (0.4 oz)	120	6	2	10	1	18	6	0	0	85	—	—	0
THE SOURCE														
Barry's Raspberry Palmiers	1 (0.7 oz)	80	3	0	0	1	14	8	0	0	50	—	—	0
TOM'S														
Animal Crackers	½ pkg (1 oz)	120	2	1	0	2	23	6	tr	0	140	—	—	0
Big Cookie Chocolate Chip	1 pkg (2.75 oz)	340	16	5	0	4	49	24	1	0	280	—		0
Big Cookie Peanut Butter Chocolate Chip	1 pkg (2 oz)	280	15	5	0	3	37	18	1	0	180	—	—	0
Chocolate Chip	1 pkg (2 oz)	280	15	5	0	3	37	18	1	0	180	—	—	0
Confetti Chip	1 pkg (2 oz)	300	13	6	0	3	40	23	tr	0	140	—	—	0
Fat Free Apple Bar	1 pkg (1.75 oz)	160	0	0	0	2	38	22	1	40	250	—	—	0
Fat Free Fig Bar	1 pkg (1.75 oz)	160	0	0	0	2	40	20	2	0	180	—	—	0
Vanilla Wafers	½ pkg (1 oz)	130	5	1	0	2	20	9	tr	0	100	30	—	0
TREE OF LIFE														
Fat Free Almond Butter	1 (0.8 oz)	60	0	0	0	1	14	6	1	0	50	—	—	0
Fat Free Carrot Cake	1 (0.8 oz)	60	0	0	0	1	14	6	1	0	50	—	—	0
Fat Free Devil's Food Chocolate	1 (0.8 oz)	70	0	0	0	2	15	7	1	20	80	—	—	0
Fat Free Oatmeal Raisin	1 (0.8 oz)	70	0	0	0	2	16	7	1	0	40	—	—	0
Fruit Bars Fat Free Fig	1 (0.8 oz)	70	0	0	0	1	16	11	2	20	100	—	—	—
Fruit Bars Fat Free Peach Apricot	1 (0.8 oz)	70	0	0	0	1	17	9	1	20	110	—	—	—
Fruit Bars Fat Free Wildberry	1 (0.8 oz)	70	0	0	0	1	16	7	2	20	170	—	—	—
Monster Carob Chip	1 (4.7 oz)	700	35	10	10	10	95	40	5	0	375	—	—	0
Monster Granola	1 (4.7 oz)	700	30	10	10	10	95	45	5	0	475	—	—	0
Monster Macaroon	1 (4.7 oz)	750	45	20	10	5	85	40	5	0	375	—	—	0

FOOD	PORTION	CALS	FAT	SAT FAT	CHOL	PROT	CARB	SUGAR	FIBER	CALCI	SOD	POTAS	FOLIC	VIT C
TREE OF LIFE (CONT.)														
Monster Peanut Butter	1 (4.7 oz)	700	35	10	20	15	85	45	5	0	525	—	—	0
Monster Fat Free Carrot Cake	1 cookie (3.8 oz)	240	0	0	0	4	60	40	4	80	120	—	—	5
Monster Fat Free Devil's Food Chocolate	1 cookie (3.8 oz)	320	0	0	0	8	80	48	8	0	180	—	—	5
Monster Fat Free Gingerbread	1 cookie (3.8 oz)	320	0	0	0	8	76	36	8	0	200	—	—	5
Monster Fat Free Maple Pecan	1 cookie (3.8 oz)	360	0	0	0	8	80	40	8	0	200	—	—	5
Oatmeal	1 (0.8 oz)	100	4	2	15	2	16	7	0	20	55	—	—	0
Sandwich Royal Vanilla	2 (0.9 oz)	120	5	0	0	1	17	10	1	20	115	—	—	0
Wheat Free Carob	1 (0.8 oz)	100	5	0	0	1	14	4	6	0	75	—	—	0
Wheat Free Maple Walnut	1 (0.8 oz)	100	6	0	0	2	13	4	6	60	50	—	—	0
Wheat Free Oatmeal	1 (0.8 oz)	90	5	0	0	1	11	3	1	100	25	—	—	0
Wheat Free Peanut Butter	1 (0.8 oz)	109	6	0	0	2	8	3	1	20	100	—	—	0
TWIX														
Bars Chocolate Caramel	1 (0.9 oz)	140	7	3	0	1	18	13	0	20	55	—	—	—
VOORTMAN														
Almonette	2 (1 oz)	150	8	2	0	1	17	6	tr	0	65	—	—	0
Chocolate Chip	1 (0.7 oz)	100	5	2	0	tr	13	6	0	0	45	—	—	0
Chocolate Wafers Sugar Free	3 (1 oz)	160	11	3	0	tr	18	0	0	0	30	—	—	0
Coconut Delight	1 (0.6 oz)	90	5	3	0	tr	10	6	0	0	25	—	—	0
Peanut Delight	1 (0.9 oz)	130	7	2	<5	2	15	6	tr	0	90	—	—	0
Strawberry Wafers Sugar Free	3 (1 oz)	160	11	3	0	tr	18	0	0	0	30	—	—	0
Sugar	1 (0.6 oz)	80	4	1	0	tr	11	5	0	0	45	—	—	0
Turnovers Blueberry	1 (0.9 oz)	100	3	1	<5	1	16	8	0	0	50	—	—	0
Turnovers Cherry	1 (0.9 oz)	100	3	1	<5	1	16	8	0	0	50	—	—	0
Turnovers Strawberry	1 (0.9 oz)	100	3	1	<5	1	16	8	0	0	50	—	—	0
Vanilla Wafers Sugar Free	3 (1 oz)	160	11	3	0	tr	18	0	0	0	30	—	—	0
Windmill	1 (0.7 oz)	90	4	1	0	tr	13	6	0	0	100	—	—	0
WALKERS														
Shortbread Triangles	2 (0.7 oz)	100	6	4	15	1	12	4	0	0	65	—	—	0

FOOD	PORTION	CALS	FAT	SAT FAT	CHOL	PROT	CARB	SUGAR	FIBER	CALCI	SOD	POTAS	FOLIC	VIT C
WEIGHT WATCHERS														
Apple Raisin Bar	1 (0.75 oz)	70	2	1	0	1	14	4	2	0	60	—	—	0
Chocolate Chip	2 (1.06 oz)	140	5	2	0	2	22	15	1	20	90	—	—	0
Chocolate Sandwich	2 (1.06 oz)	140	4	1	0	2	23	16	1	0	160	—	—	0
Fruit Filled Fig	1 (0.7 oz)	70	0	0	0	1	16	9	0	20	50	—	—	0
Fruit Filled Raspberry	1 (0.7 oz)	70	0	0	0	1	16	7	0	0	45	—	—	0
Oatmeal Raisin	2 (1.06 oz)	120	2	0	0	2	22	13	1	20	90	—	—	0
Vanilla Sandwich	2 (1.06 oz)	140	3	1	0	1	25	10	1	0	80	—	—	0
WHITE EAGLE BAKERY														
Chruscik	2 (1 oz)	140	8	3	45	2	16	5	0	60	95	—	—	0
WORTZ														
Animal	9 (1.1 oz)	140	5	1	—	2	22	17	1	—	140	—	—	—
Chocolate Graham	2 (0.9 oz)	130	3	1	—	2	24	7	1	—	120	—	—	—
Cinnamon	2 (0.9 oz)	130	5	1	—	1	19	7	tr	—	85	—	—	—
Vanilla Wafers	7 (1.1 oz)	150	6	1	—	1	22	10	1	—	115	—	—	—
REFRIGERATED														
chocolate chip	1 (0.42 oz)	59	3	1	3	1	8	—	—	3	28	24	—	0
chocolate chip unbaked	1 oz	126	6	2	7	1	17	—	—	7	59	51	—	0
oatmeal	1 (0.4 oz)	56	3	1	3	1	8	—	—	4	39	20	—	—
oatmeal raisin	1 (0.4 oz)	56	3	1	3	1	8	—	—	4	39	20	—	—
peanut butter	1 (0.4 oz)	60	3	1	4	1	7	—	—	13	52	41	—	0
peanut butter dough	1 oz	130	7	2	8	2	15	—	—	29	112	87	—	0
sugar	1 (0.42 oz)	58	3	1	4	1	8	—	—	11	56	20	—	0
sugar dough	1 oz	124	6	2	8	1	17	—	—	23	120	42	—	0
PILLSBURY														
Bunny	2	130	7	2	<5	1	17	7	0	0	100	—	—	0
Chocolate Chip	1 (1 oz)	130	6	3	<5	1	17	12	tr	0	85	—	—	0
Chocolate Chip Reduced Fat	1 (1 oz)	110	3	2	<5	1	19	12	tr	0	85	—	—	0
Chocolate Chip w/ Walnuts	1 (1 oz)	140	7	2	<5	1	17	10	tr	0	90	—	—	0
Chocolate Chunk	1 (1 oz)	130	6	2	<5	1	17	11	tr	0	90	—	—	0
Christmas Tree	2	130	7	2	<5	1	17	7	0	0	100	—	—	0
Double Chocolate	1 (1 oz)	130	6	2	<5	1	17	11	tr	0	90	—	—	0
Flag	2	130	7	2	<5	1	17	7	0	0	100	—	—	0
Frosty	2	130	7	2	<5	1	17	7	0	0	100	—	—	0
M&M's	1 (1 oz)	130	6	2	<5	1	18	11	tr	0	75	—	—	0
Oatmeal Chocolate Chip	1 (1 oz)	120	6	2	<5	1	16	10	tr	0	95	—	—	0
One Step Pan Chocolate Chip	⅛ pan (1 oz)	130	6	2	<5	1	19	13	tr	0	100	—	—	0

FOOD	PORTION	CALS	FAT	SAT FAT	CHOL	PROT	CARB	SUGAR	FIBER	CALCI	SOD	POTAS	FOLIC	VIT C
PILLSBURY (CONT.)														
One Step Pan M&M's	⅛ pan (1 oz)	130	6	2	<5	1	19	12	tr	0	85	—	—	0
Peanut Butter	1 (1 oz)	120	6	2	<5	2	15	10	tr	0	130	—	—	0
Pumpkin	2	130	7	2	<5	1	17	7	0	0	100	—	—	0
Reeses	1 (1 oz)	130	6	3	<5	3	15	10	tr	0	105	—	—	0
Shamrock	2	130	7	2	<5	1	17	7	0	0	100	—	—	0
Sugar	2	130	3	2	<5	1	19	10	0	0	125	—	—	0
Sugar Holiday Red & Green	2	130	6	2	<5	1	19	10	0	0	125	—	—	0
Valentine	2	130	7	2	<5	1	17	7	0	0	100	—	—	0
White Chocolate Chunk	1 (1 oz)	130	6	2	<5	1	17	11	0	0	100	—	—	0
TAKE-OUT														
biscotti w/ nuts chocolate dipped	1 (1.3 oz)	117	6	3	18	2	16	11	1	10	33	—	—	1
black & white	1 lg (3 oz)	302	9	5	58	4	52	31	1	32	72	68	11	tr
finikia	1 (1.2 oz)	171	5	5	27	2	16	5	1	8	26	26	6	tr
koulourakia butter cookie twist	1 (0.9 oz)	113	6	3	32	2	14	5	tr	15	59	16	5	0
linzer tart	1 (2.4 oz)	280	14	4	40	2	34	12	0	20	130	—	—	1
CORIANDER														
leaf dried	1 tsp	2	tr	—	0	tr	tr	—	—	7	1	27	—	3
leaf fresh	¼ cup	1	tr	—	0	tr	tr	—	—	4	1	22	—	—
seed	1 tsp	5	tr	tr	0	tr	1	—	—	13	1	23	—	—
INSTANT INDIA														
Tomato Coriander Paste	2 tbsp (1 oz)	90	6	1	0	1	8	6	0	0	570	—	—	0
CORN														
CANNED														
cream style	½ cup	93	1	tr	0	2	23	—	—	4	365	172	57	6
w/ red & green peppers	½ cup	86	1	tr	0	3	21	—	—	5	396	174	—	10
white	½ cup	66	1	tr	0	2	15	—	—	—	—	—	—	—
yellow	½ cup	66	1	tr	0	2	15	—	1	—	—	—	—	—
DEL MONTE														
Cream Style Golden	½ cup (4.4 oz)	90	1	0	0	2	20	5	2	0	360	—	—	2
Cream Style Golden No Salt Added	½ cup (4.4 oz)	60	1	0	0	1	14	7	2	0	10	—	—	2
Cream Style White	½ cup (4.4 oz)	100	1	0	0	2	21	6	2	0	360	—	—	2
Fiesta	½ cup (4.4 oz)	50	1	0	0	2	12	5	2	0	310	—	—	4

FOOD	PORTION	CALS	FAT	SAT FAT	CHOL	PROT	CARB	SUGAR	FIBER	CALCI	SOD	POTAS	FOLIC	VIT C
DEL MONTE (CONT.)														
Gold & White Supersweet	½ cup (4.4 oz)	80	1	0	0	2	18	6	2	0	360	—	—	4
Whole Kernel Golden	½ cup (4.4 oz)	90	1	0	0	2	18	6	3	0	360	—	—	4
Whole Kernel Golden Supersweet No Salt Added	½ cup (4.4 oz)	60	1	0	0	2	11	7	3	0	10	—	—	4
Whole Kernel Golden Supersweet No Sugar	½ cup (4.4 oz)	60	1	0	0	2	11	7	3	0	360	—	—	4
Whole Kernel Golden Supersweet Vacuum Packed	½ cup (3.7 oz)	70	1	0	0	2	13	4	3	0	270	—	—	4
Whole Kernel White Sweet	½ cup (4.4 oz)	60	1	0	0	2	11	7	3	0	360	—	—	4
GREEN GIANT														
Cream Style	½ cup (4.5 oz)	100	1	0	0	2	22	11	1	0	430	—	—	2
Mexicorn	⅓ cup	60	0	0	0	2	14	4	1	0	250	—	—	4
Niblets	⅓ cup (2.7 oz)	70	0	0	0	2	15	4	2	0	230	—	—	0
Niblets 50% Less Sodium	⅓ cup (2.7 oz)	60	0	0	0	2	14	3	1	0	115	—	—	2
Niblets Extra Sweet	⅓ cup (2.6 oz)	50	1	0	0	2	10	4	2	0	200	—	—	0
Niblets No Added Sugar or Salt	⅓ cup (2.7 oz)	60	0	0	0	2	13	3	2	0	0	—	—	2
White Shoepeg	⅓ cup	80	1	0	0	2	16	3	1	0	220	—	—	4
Whole Sweet	½ cup (4.3 oz)	80	1	0	0	2	18	6	2	0	360	—	—	2
Whole Sweet 50% Less Sodium	½ cup (4.2 oz)	80	1	0	0	2	17	4	2	0	180	—	—	2
S&W														
Cream Style	½ cup (4.4 oz)	60	1	0	0	1	14	7	2	0	360	—	—	2
Whole Kernel	⅓ cup (3 oz)	70	2	0	0	2	12	6	2	0	170	—	—	2
VEG-ALL														
Whole Kernel	½ cup	80	1	0	0	2	16	6	2	0	340	—	—	4
FRESH														
on-the-cob w/ butter cooked	1 ear	155	3	2	6	4	32	—	—	5	30	360	44	7
white cooked	½ cup	89	1	tr	0	3	21	—	—	2	14	204	38	5
white raw	½ cup	66	1	tr	0	2	15	—	—	2	12	208	35	5
yellow cooked	1 ear (2.7 oz)	83	1	tr	0	3	19	—	—	2	13	192	36	5
yellow cooked	½ cup	89	1	tr	0	3	21	—	—	2	14	204	38	5
yellow raw	½ cup	66	1	tr	0	2	15	—	—	2	12	208	35	5
yellow raw	1 ear (3 oz)	77	1	tr	0	3	17	—	—	2	14	243	41	6

FOOD	PORTION	CALS	FAT	SAT FAT	CHOL	PROT	CARB	SUGAR	FIBER	CALCI	SOD	POTAS	FOLIC	VIT C
FROZEN														
cooked	½ cup	67	tr	tr	0	2	17	—	—	2	4	114	19	2
on-the-cob cooked	1 ear (2.2 oz)	59	tr	tr	0	2	14	—	—	2	3	158	19	3
BIRDS EYE														
Baby Gold & White	⅔ cup	100	1	0	0	3	21	3	3	0	0	—	—	9
Cob Big Ear	1 ear	120	1	0	0	—	—	—	3	0	0	—	—	2
Cut	⅓ cup	70	1	0	0	—	—	—	2	0	0	—	—	4
FRESH LIKE														
Cut	3.5 oz	85	1	—	—	3	21	—	1	5	5	196	—	5
On The Cob	1 ear (3 in)	96	1	—	—	3	24	—	1	4	4	304	—	6
GREEN GIANT														
Butter Sauce Niblets	⅔ cup (4.3 oz)	130	3	2	<5	3	23	5	3	0	350	—	—	4
Butter Sauce Shoepeg White	¾ cup (4 oz)	120	3	2	<5	3	21	5	3	0	320	—	—	1
Cream Corn	½ cup (4.1 oz)	110	1	0	0	2	23	6	2	0	330	—	—	2
Extra Sweet Niblets	⅔ cup (3.1 oz)	70	1	0	0	2	13	6	2	0	0	—	—	0
Harvest Fresh Niblets	⅔ cup (3.4 oz)	80	1	0	0	3	17	3	3	0	60	—	—	1
Harvest Fresh Shoepeg White	½ cup (2.6 oz)	70	1	0	0	2	14	3	2	0	45	—	—	2
Niblets	⅔ cup (2.9 oz)	80	1	0	0	2	17	3	2	0	5	—	—	2
On The Cob Extra Sweet	1 ear (4.4 oz)	120	2	0	0	4	22	13	3	0	0	—	—	4
On The Cob Nibblers	1 ear (2.1 oz)	70	1	0	0	2	14	2	1	0	0	—	—	2
On The Cob Niblets	1 ear (5 oz)	160	2	0	0	4	32	6	3	0	10	—	—	6
Select Extra Sweet White	⅔ cup (2.9 oz)	50	1	0	0	2	10	3	3	0	0	—	—	5
Select Shoepeg White	¾ cup (3.2 oz)	100	1	0	0	3	20	2	3	0	0	—	—	6
STOUFFER'S														
Soufflé	½ cup (6 oz)	170	7	2	65	5	21	7	1	40	490	230	—	2
TREE OF LIFE														
Corn	⅔ cup (3.2 oz)	80	1	0	0	3	19	5	1	0	10	—	—	2
TAKE-OUT														
fritters	1 (1 oz)	62	2	tr	12	2	9	—	1	21	126	47	3	1
scalloped	½ cup	258	7	1	47	7	43	—	—	64	246	162	12	14

CORN CHIPS

(*see* CHIPS)

FOOD	PORTION	CALS	FAT	SAT FAT	CHOL	PROT	CARB	SUGAR	FIBER	CALCI	SOD	POTAS	FOLIC	VIT C
CORNISH HEN														
(*see* CHICKEN)														
CORNMEAL														
corn grits cooked	1 cup	146	tr	tr	0	4	31	—	—	1	0	54	1	—
corn grits uncooked	1 cup	579	2	tr	0	14	124	—	—	3	1	213	7	—
white	1 cup (4.8 oz)	505	2	tr	0	12	107	—	10	7	4	224	258	0
whole grain	1 cup (4.3 oz)	442	4	1	0	10	94	—	9	7	43	350	31	0
yellow	1 cup (4.8 oz)	505	2	tr	0	12	107	—	10	7	4	224	258	0
yellow self-rising	1 cup (4.3 oz)	407	4	1	0	10	86	—	8	440	1521	311	228	0
ALBERS														
White	3 tbsp	110	0	0	0	2	24	0	tr	0	0	—	—	0
Yellow	3 tbsp	110	0	0	0	2	24	0	tr	0	0	—	—	0
EXPERT FOODS														
Low Carb Grits Mix	1½ tsp	15	0	0	0	2	2	—	2	—	34	—	—	—
HODGSON MILL														
Cornbread Mix Jalapeño Mexican	¼ cup (1 oz)	100	1	0	0	4	21	1	1	—	310	—	—	—
Yellow Organic	¼ cup (1 oz)	100	1	0	0	3	22	0	3	0	0	—	—	0
Yellow Self Rising	¼ cup (1 oz)	90	1	0	0	3	21	0	3	100	260	—	—	0
INDIAN HEAD														
Stone Ground	¼ cup	100	1	—	0	3	20	0	2	—	0	—	40	—
KENTUCKY KERNAL														
Sweet Cornbread Mix	¼ cup (1 oz)	120	2	0	0	2	24	6	0	—	310	—	—	—
MCKENZIE'S														
Hush Puppies	1 serv (1.9 oz)	190	10	3	0	2	23	2	2	—	470	—	—	—
QUAKER														
Old Fashioned Grits not prep	¼ cup	140	1	—	—	3	32	0	2	—	0	—	60	—
Yellow	3 tbsp (1 oz)	90	1	—	0	2	21	—	2	—	0	—	40	—
TAKE-OUT														
hush puppies	1 (0.75 oz)	74	3	tr	10	3	10	—	1	61	147	32	4	0
CORNSTARCH														
cornstarch	1 cup (4.5 oz)	488	tr	tr	0	tr	117	—	1	3	12	4	0	0
ARGO														
Cornstarch	1 tbsp (8 g)	30	0	0	0	tr	7	—	—	—	0	—	—	—
Cornstarch	1 cup (128 g)	460	tr	0	0	tr	115	—	—	—	tr	—	—	—
ARMOUR														
Cream Cornstarch	1 tbsp (0.4 oz)	40	0	0	0	0	9	0	0	0	0	—	—	0
COTTAGE CHEESE														
creamed	4 oz	117	5	3	17	14	3	—	—	68	457	95	14	tr
creamed	1 cup (7.4 oz)	217	9	6	31	26	6	—	—	126	850	177	26	tr
creamed w/ fruit	4 oz	140	4	2	13	11	15	—	—	54	457	76	11	tr

FOOD	PORTION	CALS	FAT	SAT FAT	CHOL	PROT	CARB	SUGAR	FIBER	CALCI	SOD	POTAS	FOLIC	VIT C
dry curd	1 cup (5.1 oz)	123	1	tr	10	25	3	—	—	46	19	47	21	0
dry curd	4 oz	96	tr	tr	8	20	2	—	—	36	14	37	17	0
lowfat 1%	1 cup (7.9 oz)	164	2	1	10	28	6	—	—	138	918	193	28	tr
lowfat 1%	4 oz	82	1	1	5	14	3	—	—	69	459	97	14	tr
lowfat 2%	4 oz	101	2	1	9	16	4	—	—	77	459	109	15	tr
lowfat 2%	1 cup (7.9 oz)	203	4	3	19	31	8	—	—	155	918	217	30	tr
BREAKSTONE'S														
2% Fat Large Curd	½ cup (4.2 oz)	90	3	2	15	13	4	3	0	80	390	110	—	0
2% Fat Small Curd	½ cup (4.2 oz)	90	3	2	15	13	4	3	0	80	390	110	—	0
4% Fat Large Curd	½ cup (4.2 oz)	120	5	3	25	13	5	4	0	80	400	120	—	0
4% Fat Small Curd	½ cup (4.2 oz)	120	5	3	25	13	5	4	0	80	400	125	—	0
Cottage Doubles Peach	1 pkg (5.5 oz)	140	3	2	15	12	16	13	tr	60	390	—	—	1
Dry Curd	¼ cup (1.9 oz)	45	0	0	<5	8	3	3	0	80	30	95	—	0
Fat Free	½ cup	90	0	0	10	12	8	6	0	80	450	—	—	0
Snack 2% Fat Small Curd	1 pkg (4 oz)	90	2	2	15	12	4	3	0	80	370	105	—	0
Snack 4% Fat Small Curd	1 pkg (4 oz)	110	5	3	25	12	4	4	0	80	380	115	—	0
Snack Free	1 pkg (4 oz)	70	0	0	5	12	6	4	0	80	400	135	—	0
CABOT														
Cottage Cheese	½ cup	100	5	3	15	13	4	4	0	100	400	—	—	0
No Fat	½ cup	70	0	0	5	13	5	5	0	100	410	—	—	0
HORIZON ORGANIC														
Cottage Cheese	½ cup (3.9 oz)	110	5	3	15	13	4	3	0	150	340	—	—	1
KNUDSEN														
1.5% Fat Small Curd Pineapple	½ cup (4.6 oz)	120	2	1	10	11	14	12	0	80	330	110	—	0
2% Fat Small Curd	½ cup (4.2 oz)	100	3	2	15	14	5	4	0	100	400	115	—	0
4% Fat Large Curd	½ cup (4.5 oz)	130	5	4	30	16	4	3	0	80	330	90	—	0
4% Fat Small Curd	½ cup (4.3 oz)	120	5	4	25	14	4	3	0	80	400	95	—	0
Free	½ cup (4.2 oz)	80	0	0	5	14	4	3	0	80	380	90	—	0
On The Go! 1.5% Fat Peach	1 pkg (4 oz)	110	2	1	10	10	13	12	0	60	300	105	—	0
On The Go! 1.5% Fat Pineapple	1 pkg (4 oz)	110	2	1	10	10	13	11	0	60	300	100	—	0
On The Go! 1.5% Fat Strawberry	1 pkg (4 oz)	110	2	1	10	10	13	11	0	60	290	105	—	0
On The Go! 1.5% Fat Tropical Fruit	1 pkg (4 oz)	110	2	2	10	10	13	11	0	60	300	110	—	0

FOOD	PORTION	CALS	FAT	SAT FAT	CHOL	PROT	CARB	SUGAR	FIBER	CALCI	SOD	POTAS	FOLIC	VIT C
KNUDSEN (CONT.)														
On The Go! 2% Fat	1 pkg (4 oz)	90	2	2	15	13	5	3	0	100	370	110	—	0
On The Go! Free	1 pkg (4 oz)	70	0	0	5	13	4	3	0	80	350	85	—	0
LIGHT N'LIVELY														
1% Fat Garden Salad	½ cup (4.2 oz)	80	2	1	10	12	5	5	0	200	390	150	—	0
1% Fat Peach & Pineapple	½ cup (4.3 oz)	110	1	1	10	11	15	14	0	200	340	140	—	0
Fat Free	½ cup (4.4 oz)	80	0	0	5	13	6	4	0	200	440	140	—	0
Lowfat	½ cup	80	2	1	10	12	6	5	0	200	420	—	—	0
COTTONSEED														
kernels roasted	1 tbsp	51	4	1	0	3	2	—	—	10	3	135	—	1
COUSCOUS														
cooked	1 cup (5.5 oz)	176	tr	tr	0	6	36	—	2	13	8	91	24	0
dry	1 cup (6.1 oz)	650	1	tr	0	22	134	—	9	42	17	287	35	0
MELTING POT														
Calypso Cranberry	1 cup	200	0	0	0	7	42	6	1	20	220	—	—	0
Lentil Curry	1 cup	170	0	0	0	7	35	3	1	0	290	—	—	0
Lucky Seven	1 cup	190	1	0	0	7	38	5	1	0	300	—	—	1
Mango Salsa	1 cup	190	0	0	0	6	40	6	1	20	270	—	—	0
Roasted Garlic	1 cup	170	0	0	0	7	34	3	1	0	370	—	—	0
Sesame Ginger	1 cup	180	1	0	0	7	36	5	0	20	350	—	—	0
Sun-Dried Tomatoes	1 cup	190	1	0	0	8	36	3	1	20	230	—	—	0
Wild Mushroom	1 cup	190	0	0	0	8	38	3	1	0	370	—	—	0
NEAR EAST														
Broccoli & Cheese as prep	1 cup	230	3	2	9	7	41	2	3	60	670	—	—	9
Curry as prep	1 cup	220	4	tr	0	7	42	3	3	20	550	—	—	1
Herbed Chicken as prep	1 cup	220	3	tr	0	7	42	2	3	20	510	—	—	0
Original as prep	1 cup	230	5	0	0	8	46	1	2	0	5	—	—	0
Parmesan as prep	1 cup	220	5	2	9	8	41	3	2	60	580	—	—	0
Roasted Garlic Olive Oil as prep	1 cup	230	5	1	0	7	41	1	2	0	570	—	—	0
Toasted Pine Nut as prep	1 cup	230	6	1	27	7	40	2	2	0	510	—	—	0
Tomato Lentil as prep	1 cup	220	3	tr	0	8	42	3	3	20	670	—	—	1
Wild Mushroom Herb as prep	1 cup	230	4	2	9	8	42	2	3	20	590	—	—	0
COWPEAS														
catjang dried cooked	1 cup (2.9 oz)	200	1	tr	0	14	35	—	—	44	32	641	242	1
common canned	1 cup	184	1	tr	0	11	33	—	—	48	718	413	123	7

FOOD	PORTION	CALS	FAT	SAT FAT	CHOL	PROT	CARB	SUGAR	FIBER	CALCI	SOD	POTAS	FOLIC	VIT C
frozen cooked	½ cup	112	tr	tr	0	7	20	—	—	20	5	319	120	2
leafy tips chopped cooked	1 cup	12	tr	tr	0	2	1	—	—	36	3	186	—	10
leafy tips raw chopped	1 cup	10	tr	tr	0	1	2	—	—	23	2	164	—	13

CRAB

CANNED

blue	1 cup	133	2	tr	120	28	0	—	—	137	5	450	—	—
blue	3 oz	84	1	tr	76	17	0	—	—	86	283	318	—	—

BUMBLE BEE

Fancy Lump Meat	½ can (1.9 oz)	40	1	0	50	8	0	0	0	—	300	—	—	—
Fancy White Meat	½ can (1.9 oz)	28	0	0	43	6	1	0	0	—	403	—	—	—

FRESH

alaska king cooked	1 leg (4.7 oz)	129	2	tr	72	26	0	—	—	80	1436	350	—	—
alaska king cooked	3 oz	82	1	tr	45	16	0	—	—	50	911	222	—	—
alaska king raw	1 leg (6 oz)	144	1	—	72	32	0	—	—	80	1438	351	—	—
alaska king raw	3 oz	71	1	—	35	16	0	—	—	39	711	173	—	—
blue cooked	1 cup	138	2	tr	135	27	0	—	—	140	376	437	—	—
blue cooked	3 oz	87	2	tr	85	17	0	—	—	88	237	275	—	—
blue raw	3 oz	74	1	tr	66	15	tr	—	—	76	249	280	—	—
blue raw	1 crab (7 oz)	18	tr	tr	16	4	tr	—	—	19	62	69	—	—
dungeness raw	3 oz	73	1	tr	50	15	1	—	—	39	251	301	—	—
dungeness raw	1 crab (5.7 oz)	140	2	tr	97	28	1	—	—	75	481	577	—	—
queen steamed	3 oz	98	1	tr	60	20	0	—	—	28	587	170	—	—

TAKE-OUT

baked	1 (3.8 oz)	160	2	tr	184	29	4	—	—	415	550	598	20	3
cake	1 (2 oz)	160	10	2	82	11	5	—	—	202	492	162	10	tr
kenagi korean crab cooked	1 serv (3 oz)	71	tr	—	—	16	0	0	0	60	204	170	—	0
mousse	¼ cup	364	20	—	136	—	—	—	—	272	—	—	—	—
soft-shell fried	1 (4.4 oz)	334	18	4	45	11	31	—	—	55	1118	163	20	tr

CRACKER CRUMBS

chocolate wafer cookie crumbs	½ cup (5.9 oz)	728	25	6	0	11	120	—	—	56	980	364	—	—
cracker meal	1 cup (4 oz)	440	2	tr	0	11	93	—	—	27	32	132	—	0
graham cracker crumbs	½ cup (4.4 oz)	540	13	3	0	9	97	—	3	36	756	162	18	0

BAKER'S HARVEST

Graham	⅓ cup (1 oz)	130	4	1	0	2	23	7	1	0	110	—	—	0

KELLOGG'S

Corn Flake Crumbs	2 tbsp (0.4 oz)	40	0	0	0	1	9	1	0	0	105	15	10	0

CRACKERS

cheese	1 (1 in sq) (1 g)	5	tr	tr	0	tr	1	—	—	2	10	1	0	0
cheese	14 (½ oz)	71	4	1	2	1	8	—	—	21	141	21	4	0

FOOD	PORTION	CALS	FAT	SAT FAT	CHOL	PROT	CARB	SUGAR	FIBER	CALCI	SOD	POTAS	FOLIC	VIT C
cheese low sodium	1 (1 in sq) (1 g)	5	tr	tr	0	tr	1	—	—	2	5	1	0	0
cheese low sodium	14 (½ oz)	71	4	1	2	1	8	—	—	21	68	15	4	0
cheese w/ peanut butter filling	1 (0.24 oz)	34	2	tr	0	1	4	—	tr	6	69	17	2	0
crispbread	3	61	2	—	—	1	9	—	1	12	—	—	—	0
crispbread rye	1 (0.35 oz)	37	tr	tr	0	1	8	—	2	3	26	32	2	0
crispbread rye	3	77	1	—	—	2	17	—	3	11	—	—	—	0
melba toast plain	1 (5 g)	19	tr	tr	0	1	4	—	tr	5	41	10	1	0
melba toast pumpernickel	1 (5 g)	19	tr	tr	0	1	4	—	tr	4	45	10	1	—
melba toast rye	1 (5 g)	19	tr	tr	0	1	4	—	tr	4	45	10	1	—
melba toast wheat	1 (5 g)	19	tr	tr	0	1	4	—	tr	2	42	7	1	0
milk	1 (0.42 oz)	55	2	tr	—	1	8	—	—	21	71	14	—	—
oyster cracker	1 (1 g)	4	tr	tr	0	tr	1	—	tr	1	13	1	tr	0
peanut butter sandwich	1 (7 g)	34	2	tr	—	1	4	—	—	7	66	16	—	—
rusk toast	1 (0.35 oz)	41	1	tr	—	1	7	—	—	3	25	25	—	0
rye w/ cheese filling	1 (0.24 oz)	34	2	tr	1	1	4	—	—	16	73	24	—	—
rye wafers plain	1 (0.9 oz)	84	tr	tr	0	2	20	—	—	10	199	124	11	—
rye wafers seasoned	1 (0.8 oz)	84	2	tr	0	2	16	—	—	10	195	100	12	—
saltines	1 (3 g)	13	tr	tr	0	tr	2	—	tr	4	38	4	1	0
saltines fat free low sodium	6 (1 oz)	118	tr	tr	0	3	25	—	—	7	191	34	4	0
saltines fat free low sodium	3 (0.5 oz)	59	tr	tr	0	2	12	—	—	3	95	17	2	0
saltines low salt	1 (3 g)	13	tr	tr	0	tr	2	—	tr	4	19	22	1	0
snack cracker	1 (3 g)	15	1	tr	0	tr	2	—	tr	4	25	4	0	0
snack cracker low salt	1 (3 g)	15	1	tr	0	tr	2	—	tr	4	11	11	0	0
snack cracker w/ cheese filling	1 (7 g)	33	2	tr	0	1	4	—	—	18	98	30	—	—
soup cracker	1 (1 g)	4	tr	tr	0	tr	1	—	tr	1	13	1	tr	0
water biscuits	3	92	3	—	—	2	16	—	1	25	—	—	—	0
wheat w/ cheese filling	1 (0.24 oz)	35	2	tr	1	1	4	—	—	14	64	21	—	tr
wheat w/ peanut butter filling	1 (0.24 oz)	35	2	tr	0	1	4	—	—	12	57	21	—	0
wheat thins	7 (0.5 oz)	67	3	1	0	1	9	—	1	7	113	26	3	0
wheat thins	1 (2 g)	9	tr	tr	0	tr	1	—	—	1	16	4	0	0
wheat thins low salt	7 (0.5 oz)	67	3	1	0	1	9	—	1	7	40	28	3	0
whole wheat	1 (4 g)	18	1	tr	0	tr	3	—	—	2	26	12	1	0
whole wheat low salt	1 (4 g)	18	1	tr	0	tr	3	—	—	2	10	12	1	0
zwieback	1 oz	107	1	—	—	3	21	—	1	12	75	46	—	—

FOOD	PORTION	CALS	FAT	SAT FAT	CHOL	PROT	CARB	SUGAR	FIBER	CALCI	SOD	POTAS	FOLIC	VIT C
AK-MAK														
100% Whole Wheat	5 (1 oz)	116	2	tr	0	5	19	2	4	0	214	—	—	0
Armenian Cracker Bread	1 sheet (1 oz)	100	2	1	0	4	19	2	2	0	200	—	—	0
Armenian Cracker Bread Whole Wheat	1 sheet (1 oz)	116	2	tr	0	5	19	2	4	0	214	—	—	0
Round Cracker Bread No Seeds	1 (1 oz)	100	1	1	0	4	20	2	1	0	170	—	—	0
Round Cracker Bread Seeded	1 (1 oz)	100	2	1	0	4	19	2	2	0	200	—	—	0
Round Cracker Bread Whole Wheat	1 (1 oz)	116	2	tr	0	5	19	2	4	0	214	—	—	0
AMERICAN VINTAGE														
Wine Biscuits All Flavors	5	140	7	1	1	1	17	5	tr	20	190	—	—	—
ANDRE'S														
CarboSave Crackerbread All Flavors	1 oz	140	8	1	0	10	8	2	4	—	120	—	—	—
AUSTIN														
Cracker Sandwich Cheese On Cheese	6 (1.3 oz)	170	7	2	0	3	25	4	tr	40	310	—	—	0
Cracker Sandwich Cheese Peanut Butter	6 (1.3 oz)	170	7	2	0	5	24	3	1	0	320	—	—	0
Cracker Sandwich Toasty Peanut Butter	6 (1.3 oz)	170	7	2	0	5	24	4	1	0	340	—	—	0
Cracker Sandwich Whole Wheat Cheese	6 (1.3 oz)	170	7	2	0	3	25	4	tr	40	280	—	—	2
BAKER'S HARVEST														
Cheese	23 (1 oz)	150	6	2	0	3	18	0	tr	—	370	—	—	—
Cheese Reduced Fat	29 (1 oz)	130	4	1	0	3	21	0	tr	—	310	—	—	—
Oyster	35 (0.5 oz)	70	2	0	—	1	11	0	1	—	150	—	—	—
Saltines Unsalted	5 (0.5 oz)	70	2	—	—	1	11	—	—	—	110	—	—	—
Saltines Deluxe	5 (0.5 oz)	60	2	—	—	1	10	—	—	—	130	—	—	—
Snackers	9 (1.1 oz)	160	8	2	—	2	19	2	tr	—	250	—	—	—
Snackers Reduced Fat	10 (1.1 oz)	140	4	1	0	3	23	2	tr	—	260	—	—	—
Snackers Unsalted	9 (1.1 oz)	160	8	2	—	2	19	2	tr	—	80	—	—	—
Wheat Snacks	16 (1 oz)	140	6	1	—	3	20	2	2	—	120	—	—	—

FOOD	PORTION	CALS	FAT	SAT FAT	CHOL	PROT	CARB	SUGAR	FIBER	CALCI	SOD	POTAS	FOLIC	VIT C
BAKER'S HARVEST (CONT.)														
Wheat Snacks Reduced Fat	16 (1.1 oz)	140	4	1	0	2	23	4	1	—	220	—	—	—
Woven Wheats	7 (1.1 oz)	140	5	1	0	3	21	0	4	—	170	—	—	—
Woven Wheats Reduced Fat	8 (1.1 oz)	130	3	1	0	3	24	0	4	—	180	—	—	—
BARBARA'S BAKERY														
Cheese Bites	26 (1 oz)	120	2	0	0	3	24	0	1	—	290	—	—	—
Right Lite Rounds Original	5 (0.5 oz)	55	5	tr	0	1	12	1	0	—	150	—	—	—
Rite Lite Rounds Savory Poppy	5 (0.5 oz)	70	2	0	0	tr	11	tr	0	—	135	—	—	—
Rite Lite Rounds Tamari Sesame	5 (0.5 oz)	70	2	0	0	1	12	tr	0	—	160	—	—	—
Wheatines All Flavors	1 lg sq (0.5 oz)	50	2	0	0	1	10	tr	1	—	110	—	—	—
BLUE DIAMOND														
Nut Thins Almond	16 (1 oz)	130	5	0	0	3	19	0	tr	20	75	—	—	0
Nut Thins Hazelnut	16 (1 oz)	120	4	0	0	2	20	0	1	0	75	—	—	0
Nut Thins Pecan	16 (1 oz)	130	5	0	0	2	20	0	tr	0	75	—	—	0
BRAN-A-CRISP														
Low Carb Wheat Bran	1	20	0	0	0	1	6	tr	2	—	0	—	—	—
BRETON														
Cabaret	3 (5 g)	70	4	2	0	1	9	1	0	0	160	—	—	0
Garden Vegetable	3	60	3	2	0	1	8	1	1	0	190	—	—	0
Light	1 (5 g)	20	1	tr	0	1	3	tr	tr	—	39	16	—	—
Minis	20 (0.6 oz)	89	4	2	0	2	11	1	tr	—	169	30	—	—
Minis Cheddar Cheese	20 (0.6 oz)	87	4	3	3	3	11	—	—	—	211	34	—	—
Minis Garden Vegetable	20 (0.6 oz)	87	4	3	0	2	12	—	1	—	144	40	—	—
Multi Grain	3	70	4	2	0	2	8	2	1	0	170	—	—	0
Original	3	60	3	2	0	2	8	1	0	0	140	—	—	0
Reduced Fat & Sodium	3	60	2	1	0	2	9	1	tr	0	75	—	—	0
Sesame	3	60	3	2	0	2	7	1	tr	0	100	—	—	0
CHEETERS														
Low Carb All Flavors	1 pkg (1 oz)	104	8	1	0	4	4	1	2	—	110	—	—	—
CHEETOS														
Bacon Cheddar	1 pkg	190	9	3	<5	3	25	3	1	—	410	—	—	—
Cheddar Cheese	1 pkg	210	11	3	<5	3	23	5	1	—	340	—	—	—
Golden Toast	1 pkg	240	14	4	5	4	25	5	1	—	440	—	—	—

FOOD	PORTION	CALS	FAT	SAT FAT	CHOL	PROT	CARB	SUGAR	FIBER	CALCI	SOD	POTAS	FOLIC	VIT C
CHEEZ IT														
Big	13 (1 oz)	150	8	2	0	4	16	tr	tr	40	230	—	—	0
Big Reduced Fat	15 (1 oz)	140	5	1	0	4	20	tr	tr	40	280	—	—	0
Heads & Tails	37 (1 oz)	140	6	2	0	1	18	1	1	20	330	—	—	0
Hot & Spicy	26 (1 oz)	150	8	2	0	4	17	1	tr	0	300	—	—	0
Low Sodium	27 (1 oz)	160	8	2	0	4	16	tr	tr	40	70	—	—	0
Nacho	28 (1 oz)	150	7	2	0	3	18	0	tr	20	280	—	—	0
Original	27 (1 oz)	160	8	2	0	4	16	tr	tr	40	240	—	—	0
Party Mix	½ cup (1 oz)	140	5	1	0	4	19	1	1	20	270	—	—	0
Party Mix Nacho	½ cup (1 oz)	130	5	1	0	3	20	0	1	20	330	—	—	0
Party Mix Reduced Fat	½ cup (1 oz)	130	3	1	0	4	21	1	1	20	300	—	—	0
Peanut Butter	1 pkg (1.3 oz)	190	10	2	0	4	22	3	1	20	400	—	—	0
Reduced Fat	29 (1 oz)	140	5	1	0	4	20	tr	tr	40	280	—	—	0
Snack Mix	½ cup (1 oz)	130	5	1	0	3	21	2	2	20	330	—	—	0
Snack Mix Big Crunch	¾ cup (1 oz)	110	6	1	0	3	20	1	tr	20	360	—	—	0
Snack Mix Double Cheese	¾ cup (1 oz)	110	5	1	0	3	19	1	tr	20	450	—	—	0
White Cheddar	26 (1 oz)	150	7	2	<5	3	18	tr	tr	0	280	—	—	0
COURTNEY'S														
Sun-Dried Tomato Organic	4 (0.5 oz)	60	1	0	0	1	10	0	0	20	130	—	—	0
DARE														
Cabaret	3	70	4	2	0	1	9	1	0	0	160	—	—	0
Vinta	1 (6 g)	30	1	1	0	1	4	1	1	—	—	—	—	—
DORITOS														
Jalapeño Cheese	1 pkg	230	14	4	<5	3	26	5	1	—	450	—	—	—
Nacho Cheddar	1 pkg	240	14	3	<5	4	25	6	1	—	340	—	—	—
EDEN														
Nori Nori Rice	15 (1 oz)	110	0	0	0	3	24	0	2	40	160	25	0	0
ESTEE														
Sugar Free Cracked Pepper	18	120	2	0	0	3	24	0	1	—	200	0	—	—
Sugar Free Golden	10	130	2	0	0	3	28	0	1	—	200	0	—	—
Sugar Free Wheat	17	100	2	0	0	3	18	0	2	—	200	0	—	—
FRITO LAY														
Cheddar Snacks	1 pkg	200	10	3	<5	5	27	tr	1	—	530	—	—	—
FROOKIE														
Cheddar	17 (1 oz)	140	4	1	0	4	23	1	1	20	420	—	—	0
Cracked Pepper	8 (0.7 oz)	70	0	0	0	2	15	1	1	0	85	—	—	0
Garden Vegetable	13 (1 oz)	130	4	0	0	3	19	1	2	0	380	—	—	0
Garlic & Herb	8 (0.7 oz)	70	0	0	0	2	16	1	1	0	170	—	—	0
Pizza	17 (1 oz)	130	3	0	0	3	24	1	1	0	420	—	—	0
Snack & Party	10 (1 oz)	140	5	0	0	2	20	3	1	20	260	—	—	0

FOOD	PORTION	CALS	FAT	SAT FAT	CHOL	PROT	CARB	SUGAR	FIBER	CALCI	SOD	POTAS	FOLIC	VIT C
FROOKIE (CONT.)														
Water Crackers	8 (0.7 oz)	70	0	0	0	2	16	1	1	0	135	—	—	0
Wheat & Onion	12 (1 oz)	120	4	0	0	3	18	0	2	0	400	—	—	0
Wheat & Rye	13 (1 oz)	120	4	0	0	3	18	1	3	0	380	—	—	0
GOLD'N KRACKLE														
Cheese	½ oz	65	2	1	2	2	9	0	0	0	85	—	—	0
Cheese & Oregano	½ oz	65	2	1	2	2	9	0	0	0	85	—	—	0
Hot & Spicy	½ oz	58	1	0	0	2	11	0	0	0	15	—	—	0
Onion & Garlic	½ oz	58	1	0	0	2	11	0	0	0	15	—	—	0
Plain	½ oz	58	1	0	0	2	11	0	0	0	15	—	—	0
HEALTH VALLEY														
Healthy Pizza Garlic & Herb	6	50	0	0	0	2	11	1	2	0	140	—	—	1
Healthy Pizza Italiano	6	50	0	0	0	2	11	1	2	0	140	—	—	1
Healthy Pizza Zesty Cheese	6	50	0	0	0	2	11	1	2	0	140	—	—	1
Low Fat Mild Jalapeño	6	60	2	—	0	2	10	1	2	20	90			1
Low Fat Mild Ranch	6	60	2	—	0	2	10	1	2	20	90	—	—	1
Low Fat Roasted Garlic	6	60	2	—	0	2	10	1	2	20	90	—	—	1
Original Oat Bran	6	120	3	—	0	3	22	3	3	40	80	—	—	0
Original Rice Bran	6	110	3	—	0	3	19	4	3	20	70	—	—	1
Whole Wheat	5	50	0	0	0	2	11	1	2	20	80	—	—	0
Whole Wheat Cheese	5	50	0	0	0	2	11	1	2	20	100	—	—	0
Whole Wheat Herb	5	50	0	0	0	2	11	1	2	20	100	—	—	0
Whole Wheat No Salt Vegetable	5	50	0	0	0	2	11	1	2	0	15	—	—	1
Whole Wheat Onion	5	50	0	0	0	2	11	1	2	20	80	—	—	0
Whole Wheat Vegetable	5	50	0	0	0	3	11	1	2	20	80	—	—	1
HEAVENLY														
All Flavors Cholesterol Free Sugar Free	1	16	4	1	0	1	3	0	0	—	19	—	—	—
KASHI														
TLC Country Cheddar	15 (1 oz)	130	3	0	0	3	21	1	0	40	220	—	—	0
TLC Honey	15 (1 oz)	130	3	0	0	3	22	5	2	20	190	—	—	0
TLC Natural Ranch	15 (1 oz)	130	3	0	0	3	22	3	2	20	200	—	—	0

FOOD	PORTION	CALS	FAT	SAT FAT	CHOL	PROT	CARB	SUGAR	FIBER	CALCI	SOD	POTAS	FOLIC	VIT C
KASHI (CONT.)														
TLC Original 7 Grain	15 (1 oz)	130	3	0	0	3	22	3	2	20	200	—	—	0
KEEBLER														
Club 33% Reduced Fat	5 (0.6 oz)	70	2	0	0	1	12	2	0	0	200	—	—	0
Club 50% Reduced Sodium	4 (0.5 oz)	70	3	1	0	1	9	1	tr	0	80	—	—	0
Club Original	4 (0.5 oz)	70	3	1	0	1	9	1	tr	0	160	—	—	0
Elfin	23 (1 oz)	130	2	0	0	2	24	8	tr	0	140	—	—	0
Export Soda	3 (0.5 oz)	60	2	1	0	1	10	0	tr	0	80	—	—	0
Harvest Bakery Multigrain	2 (0.6 oz)	70	3	1	0	1	10	2	tr	0	80	—	—	0
Munch'ems Cheddar	30 (1 oz)	130	4	1	0	3	21	2	tr	20	320	—	—	0
Munch'ems Cheddar	39 (1 oz)	140	5	1	0	3	20	1	1	20	320	—	—	5
Munch'ems Chili Cheese	28 (1.1 oz)	130	4	2	0	2	23	4	1	0	470	—	—	0
Munch'ems Mexquite BBQ	40 (1 oz)	140	5	1	0	2	22	1	1	20	290	—	—	5
Munch'ems Ranch	33 (1 oz)	130	4	1	0	3	21	2	tr	20	310	—	—	0
Munch'ems Ranch	40 (1 oz)	140	5	2	0	3	20	1	1	20	260	—	—	5
Munch'ems Salsa	28 (1.1 oz)	130	4	1	0	2	23	3	1	0	260	—	—	0
Munch'ems Seasoned Original	30 (1 oz)	130	5	1	0	3	20	1	tr	0	350	—	—	0
Munch'ems Sour Cream & Onion	39 (1 oz)	140	5	2	0	3	20	1	1	20	280	—	—	5
Munch'ems Sour Cream & Onion 55% Reduced Fat	33 (1 oz)	130	4	1	0	2	22	2	0	0	390	—	—	0
Paks Cheese & Peanut Butter	1 pkg	190	9	2	<5	6	22	4	tr	0	420	—	—	0
Paks Club & Cheddar	1 pkg	190	11	3	10	3	20	4	tr	40	320	—	—	0
Paks Toast & Peanut Butter	1 pkg	190	9	2	0	5	23	5	1	0	300	—	—	0
Sandwich Cracker Wheat & Cheddar	1 pkg	200	10	2	<5	3	23	5	tr	40	310	—	—	0
Toasteds Buttercrisp	9 (1 oz)	140	7	2	<5	2	19	2	tr	0	280	—	—	0
Toasteds Buttercrisp	5 (0.6 oz)	80	4	1	0	1	10	1	0	0	150	—	—	0
Toasteds Onion	9 (1 oz)	140	6	1	0	2	19	3	tr	0	310	—	—	0
Toasteds Sesame	9 (1 oz)	140	6	1	0	3	19	1	tr	0	320	—	—	0
Toasteds Sesame	5 (0.6 oz)	80	4	1	0	1	10	1	tr	0	135	—	—	0

FOOD	PORTION	CALS	FAT	SAT FAT	CHOL	PROT	CARB	SUGAR	FIBER	CALCI	SOD	POTAS	FOLIC	VIT C
KEEBLER (CONT.)														
Toasteds Sesame Reduced Fat	10 (1 oz)	120	3	1	0	3	21	2	2	20	310	—	—	0
Toasteds Wheat	9 (1 oz)	140	6	2	0	2	19	3	tr	0	270	—	—	0
Toasteds Wheat	5 (0.6 oz)	80	4	1	0	1	10	2	tr	0	150	—	—	0
Toasteds Wheat Reduced Fat	10 (1 oz)	120	3	1	0	3	22	2	1	0	300	—	—	0
Toasteds Wheat Reduced Fat	5 (0.5 oz)	60	2	0	0	1	10	2	tr	0	160	—	—	0
Town House	5 (0.6 oz)	80	5	1	0	1	9	1	tr	0	150	—	—	0
Town House 50% Reduced Sodium	5 (0.6 oz)	80	5	1	0	1	10	1	tr	0	75	—	—	0
Town House Reduced Fat	6 (0.6 oz)	70	2	1	0	1	11	2	tr	0	180	—	—	0
Town House Wheat	5 (0.6 oz)	80	4	1	0	1	10	1	tr	0	140	—	—	0
Wheatables Honey Wheat	12 (1 oz)	140	6	2	0	2	20	5	1	0	200	—	—	0
Wheatables Original	12 (1 oz)	140	6	2	0	2	10	4	1	0	210	—	—	0
Wheatables Seven Grain	12 (1 oz)	140	6	2	0	2	20	3	1	20	250	—	—	0
Zesta Saltine 50% Reduced Sodium	5 (0.5 oz)	60	2	1	0	1	11	0	tr	0	95	—	—	0
Zesta Saltine Fat Free	5 (0.5 oz)	50	0	0	0	1	11	0	0	0	150	—	—	0
Zesta Saltine Original	5 (0.5 oz)	60	2	1	0	1	10	0	tr	0	190	—	—	0
Zesta Saltine Unsalted Top	5 (0.5 oz)	70	2	1	0	1	10	0	tr	0	90	—	—	0
Zesta Soup & Oyster	42 (0.5 oz)	80	3	1	0	1	10	0	tr	0	160	—	—	0
LANCE														
Bonnie	6 (1⅛ oz)	160	7	3	10	3	23	7	0	0	160	45	—	0
Captain Wafers w/ Cream Cheese & Chives	1 pkg (1.3 oz)	190	9	2	0	4	22	6	0	60	250	135	—	0
Cheese-on-Wheat	1 pkg (1.3 oz)	190	10	2	<5	4	21	4	2	60	280	105	—	0
Cranberry Bar Fat Free	1 (1.75 oz)	160	0	0	0	1	38	30	1	20	55	—	—	0
Lanchee	1 pkg (1¼ oz)	190	11	2	0	5	18	3	1	40	120	125	—	0
Malt	1 pkg (1¼ oz)	190	10	2	0	6	18	2	1	40	130	45	—	0
Nekot	1 pkg (1.5 oz)	210	10	2	0	6	25	12	1	0	130	150	—	0
Nip-Chee	1 pkg (1.3 oz)	190	10	2	<5	4	21	3	1	40	330	120	—	0
Peanut Butter Wheat	1 pkg (1.3 oz)	190	11	2	0	5	20	4	1	40	240	125	—	0
Rye-Chee	1 pkg (1.4 oz)	210	11	3	<5	4	22	5	1	80	340	140	—	0

FOOD	PORTION	CALS	FAT	SAT FAT	CHOL	PROT	CARB	SUGAR	FIBER	CALCI	SOD	POTAS	FOLIC	VIT C
LANCE (CONT.)														
Sour Dough w/ Cheddar & Sour Cream	1 pkg (1.6 oz)	240	15	4	5	4	23	4	1	80	430	90	—	0
Toastchee	1 pkg (1.4 oz)	200	12	2	0	7	19	0	1	0	260	150	—	0
Toasty	1 pkg (1¼ oz)	190	11	2	0	6	17	3	1	40	220	135	—	0
Wheat Italian	¾ cup (1.4 oz)	200	11	2	0	3	23	3	1	60	430	70	—	0
Wheat Pizza	¾ cup (1.4 oz)	200	10	2	0	3	23	3	1	60	390	85	—	0
LITTLE DEBBIE														
Cheese Crackers w/ Peanut Butter	1 (0.9 oz)	140	8	2	0	3	16	2	tr	—	210	—	—	—
Cheese on Cheese Crackers	1 (0.9 oz)	140	8	2	<5	2	15	2	0	—	220	—	—	—
Cream Cheese & Chive	1 (0.9 oz)	140	7	2	0	2	17	4	0	—	220	—	—	—
Toasty Crackers w/ Peanut Butter	1 (0.9 oz)	140	7	2	0	3	16	3	tr	—	210	—	—	—
Wheat Crackers w/ Cheddar Cheese	1 (0.9 oz)	140	8	2	<5	3	15	2	0	—	230	—	—	—
NABISCO														
Royal Lunch	1 (0.4 oz)	60	2	0	0	tr	8	1	0	20	70	—	—	0
Zwieback	1 (8 g)	35	1	—	0	1	6	1	0	0	10	—	—	0
NO-CARB KITCHEN														
Cheese	1	25	3	1	5	3	0	0	0	—	90	—	—	—
NO-NO														
Flatbreads Tortilla Corn Low Fat Sugar Free Everything	3 (1 oz)	95	1	0	0	3	18	0	1	0	140	—	—	0
OLD LONDON														
Mediterranean Toast	3	60	2	1	0	2	9	1	0	0	190	—	—	0
PEPPERIDGE FARM														
Butter Thins	4 (0.5 oz)	70	3	1	10	1	10	1	0	0	95	—	—	0
English Water Biscuits	4 (0.5 oz)	70	2	0	0	2	13	1	0	0	95	—	—	0
Giant Goldfish Peanut Butter Sandwich	1 pkg (1.4 oz)	190	9	2	<5	5	22	3	1	150	310	—	—	0
Giant Goldfish Wheat	14	140	5	1	0	2	21	3	1	20	260	—	—	0
Goldfish Cheddar	55	140	6	2	10	4	19	0	tr	80	250	—	—	0
Goldfish Cheddar 30% Less Sodium	60 (1.1 oz)	150	6	2	10	3	18	0	tr	40	175	—	—	0

FOOD	PORTION	CALS	FAT	SAT FAT	CHOL	PROT	CARB	SUGAR	FIBER	CALCI	SOD	POTAS	FOLIC	VIT C
PEPPERIDGE FARM (CONT.)														
Goldfish Cheese Trio	58	140	6	2	<5	4	19	0	1	40	280	—	—	0
Goldfish Colors On The Go	1 pkg	170	7	2	5	4	24	1	1	40	320	—	—	0
Goldfish Original	55	140	6	2	0	3	19	0	tr	0	230	—	—	0
Goldfish Pizza Flavored	55 (1 oz)	140	6	2	0	3	19	0	1	0	160	—	—	0
Goldfish Pretzel	43 (1 oz)	120	3	1	0	3	22	tr	tr	0	430	—	—	0
Hearty Wheat	3 (0.6 oz)	80	4	0	0	2	10	2	1	0	100	—	—	0
Sesame	3 (0.5 oz)	70	3	0	0	1	9	0	2	0	95	—	—	0
Snack Mix Fat Free Goldfish	⅔ cup (0.9 oz)	90	0	0	0	3	20	0	0	100	380	—	—	0
PETER PAN														
Cheese Peanut Butter	1 pkg	210	10	3	0	5	23	3	1	—	350	—	—	—
Toast Peanut Butter	1 pkg	210	11	3	0	5	23	3	tr	—	280	—	—	—
PREMIUM														
Saltine Fat Free	5	60	0	0	0	1	12	0	0	20	170	—	—	0
Saltine Multigrain	5 (0.5 oz)	60	2	0	0	1	10	0	tr	0	150	—	—	0
Saltine Unsalted Tops	5	70	2	0	0	1	11	0	0	0	115	—	—	0
RALSTON														
Cheese	23 (1 oz)	150	6	2	0	3	18	0	tr	—	370	—	—	—
Cheese Reduced Fat	29 (1 oz)	130	4	1	0	3	21	0	tr	—	310	—	—	—
Oyster	35 (0.5 oz)	70	2	0	—	1	11	0	1	—	150	—	—	—
Rich & Crisp	1 (0.5 oz)	70	3	1	—	1	9	1	0	—	105	—	—	—
Saltines Fat Free	5 (0.5 oz)	60	0	0	0	1	13	—	—	—	135	—	—	—
Saltines Deluxe	5 (0.5 oz)	60	2	—	—	1	10	—	—	—	130	—	—	—
Snackers	9 (1.1 oz)	160	8	2	—	2	19	2	tr	—	250	—	—	—
Snackers Reduced Fat	10 (1.1 oz)	140	4	1	0	2	23	3	tr	—	260	—	—	—
Snackers Unsalted	9 (1.1 oz)	160	8	2	—	2	19	2	tr	—	80	—	—	—
Wheat Snacks	16 (1 oz)	140	6	1	—	3	20	2	2	—	120	—	—	—
Wheat Snacks Reduced Fat	16 (1.1 oz)	140	4	1	0	2	23	4	1	—	220	—	—	—
Woven Wheats	7 (1.1 oz)	140	5	1	0	3	21	0	4	—	170	—	—	—
Woven Wheats Reduced Fat	8 (1.1 oz)	130	3	1	0	3	24	0	4	—	180	—	—	—
REDOVAL FARMS														
Stoned Wheat Thins Cracked Pepper	4 (0.6 oz)	70	3	1	0	1	10	0	tr	0	190	—	—	0
RITZ														
Reduced Fat	5	70	2	0	0	1	11	1	0	20	150	—	—	0

FOOD	PORTION	CALS	FAT	SAT FAT	CHOL	PROT	CARB	SUGAR	FIBER	CALCI	SOD	POTAS	FOLIC	VIT C
RYKRISP														
Seasoned	2	60	2	0	0	1	10	0	3	0	90	—	—	0
SAVORY THINS														
Toasted Onion & Garlic	15 (1 oz)	110	1	0	0	3	23	2	2	0	90	—	—	0
SMUCKER'S														
Snackers Grape	1 pkg (3.3 oz)	410	20	5	0	11	47	23	3	20	480	—	—	1
Snackers Strawberry	1 pkg (3.3 oz)	410	20	5	0	11	47	23	3	20	480	—	—	1
SNACKWELL'S														
Cracked Pepper	5	60	2	0	0	1	10	1	0	20	115	—	—	0
SUNSHINE														
Hi Ho	4 (0.5 oz)	70	4	1	0	1	8	1	tr	0	130	—	—	0
Hi Ho Reduced Fat	5 (0.5 oz)	70	3	1	0	1	10	1	tr	0	140	—	—	0
Krispy	5 (0.5 oz)	60	2	0	0	2	10	tr	tr	0	180	—	—	0
Krispy Fat Free	5 (0.5 oz)	50	0	0	0	1	11	0	0	0	150	—	—	0
Krispy Mild Cheddar	5 (0.5 oz)	60	2	1	0	2	10	0	tr	0	180	—	—	0
Krispy Soup & Oyster	17 (0.5 oz)	60	2	0	0	2	11	tr	tr	0	200	—	—	0
Krispy Unsalted Tops	5 (0.5 oz)	60	2	0	0	2	10	tr	tr	0	120	—	—	0
Krispy Whole Wheat	5 (0.5 oz)	60	2	0	0	2	10	tr	tr	0	130	—	—	0
TREE OF LIFE														
Bite Size Fat Free Cracked Pepper	12 (0.5)	55	0	0	0	1	12	1	0	0	80	—	—	0
Bite Size Fat Free Garden Vegetable	12 (0.5 oz)	55	0	0	0	2	12	1	0	0	80	—	—	0
Bite Size Fat Free Garlic & Herb	12 (0.5 oz)	55	0	0	0	2	12	1	0	0	80	—	—	0
Bite Size Fat Free Toasted Onion	12 (0.5 oz)	55	0	0	0	2	12	1	0	0	80	—	—	0
Oyster	40 (0.5 oz)	60	0	0	0	2	13	0	0	0	130	—	—	0
Saltine Cracked Pepper Fat Free	4 (0.5 oz)	60	0	0	0	2	13	0	1	0	130	—	—	0
Saltine Fat Free	4 (0.5 oz)	50	0	0	0	2	11	0	0	—	140	—	—	—
VENUS														
Fat Free Cracked Pepper	11 (0.5 oz)	60	0	0	0	1	12	1	0	0	80	—	—	0
Fat Free Garden Vegetable	5 (0.5 oz)	60	0	0	0	2	12	1	0	0	80	—	—	0
Fat Free Garlic & Herb	11 (0.5 oz)	60	0	0	0	2	12	1	0	0	90	—	—	0
Fat Free Multi-Grain	5 (0.5 oz)	60	0	0	0	1	12	1	tr	0	100	—	—	0

FOOD	PORTION	CALS	FAT	SAT FAT	CHOL	PROT	CARB	SUGAR	FIBER	CALCI	SOD	POTAS	FOLIC	VIT C
VENUS (CONT.)														
Fat Free Spicy Chili	10 (0.5 oz)	60	0	0	0	1	12	1	tr	0	100	—	—	0
Fat Free Toasted Onion	5 (0.5 oz)	60	0	0	0	1	12	1	0	0	120	—	—	0
Fat Free Toasted Wheat	5 (0.5 oz)	60	0	0	0	2	12	1	tr	0	140	—	—	0
Fat Free Tomato & Basil	10 (0.5 oz)	60	0	0	0	1	12	1	tr	0	100	—	—	0
Fat Free Zesty Italian	10 (0.5 oz)	60	0	0	0	1	12	1	tr	0	120	—	—	0
Garden Vegetable	6 (1 oz)	150	8	2	0	2	20	3	1	0	230	—	—	0
Honey Wheat	1 oz	140	5	0	0	2	21	3	1	0	200	—	—	0
Low Fat Cracker Bread	5 (0.5 oz)	60	2	0	0	1	10	tr	tr	0	105	—	—	0
Low Fat Water Crackers	4 (0.5 oz)	60	1	0	0	1	12	0	0	0	75	—	—	0
Sesame & Flaxseed	1 oz	130	3	0	0	3	23	1	1	0	240	—	—	0
Soup Original	0.5 oz	60	2	0	0	1	11	1	0	0	90	—	—	0
Toasted Wheat	6 (1 oz)	150	7	2	0	3	18	2	tr	20	240	—	—	0
Wine Cheese Caviar Original	0.5 oz	60	2	0	0	1	11	1	0	0	90	—	—	0
Wine Cheese Caviar Pepper & Poppy	0.5 oz	60	2	0	0	1	11	1	0	0	90	—	—	0
WASA														
Crispbread Fiber Rye	1 (0.4 oz)	30	1	0	0	1	7	0	2	20	60	—	—	0
Crispbread Hearty Rye	1 (0.5 oz)	45	0	0	0	1	9	0	2	0	40	—	—	0
WHEAT THINS														
Harvest Crisps Five-Grain	13	140	4	1	0	3	23	4	1	20	240	—	—	0
WHEATSWORTH														
Crackers	5	80	4	1	0	2	10	1	tr	0	170	—	—	0
WISECRACKERS														
Low Fat Poblano Chili & Sweet Onion	4 (0.5 oz)	45	1	0	0	1	8	1	tr	0	89	—	—	0
WORTZ														
Cheese	23 (1 oz)	150	6	2	0	3	18	0	tr	—	370	—	—	—
Oyster	35 (0.5 oz)	70	2	0	—	1	11	0	1	—	150	—	—	—
Rich & Crisp	1 (0.5 oz)	70	3	1	—	1	9	1	0	—	105	—	—	—
Saltines Fat Free	5 (0.5 oz)	60	0	0	0	1	13	—	—	—	135	—	—	—
Saltines Deluxe	5 (0.5 oz)	60	2	—	—	1	10	—	—	—	130	—	—	—
Wheat Snacks	16 (1 oz)	140	6	1	—	3	20	2	2	—	120	—	—	—

FOOD	PORTION	CALS	FAT	SAT FAT	CHOL	PROT	CARB	SUGAR	FIBER	CALCI	SOD	POTAS	FOLIC	VIT C
WORTZ (CONT.)														
Wheat Snacks Reduced Fat	16 (1.1 oz)	140	4	1	0	2	23	4	1	—	220	—	—	—
Woven Wheats	7 (1.1 oz)	140	5	1	0	3	21	0	4	—	170	—	—	—

CRANBERRIES

FOOD	PORTION	CALS	FAT	SAT FAT	CHOL	PROT	CARB	SUGAR	FIBER	CALCI	SOD	POTAS	FOLIC	VIT C
cranberry sauce sweetened	½ cup	209	tr	—	0	tr	54	—	—	5	40	35	—	3
fresh chopped	1 cup	54	tr	—	0	tr	14	—	—	8	1	78	2	15
JOK'N'AL														
Cranberry Sauce	1 tbsp	8	0	0	0	0	2	1	—	—	0	—	—	—
OCEAN SPRAY														
Craisins	⅓ cup	130	0	0	0	0	33	31	2	—	2	16	—	0
Cranberry Sauce Jellied	¼ cup	110	0	0	0	0	27	26	tr	—	35	0	—	0
Cranorange	¼ cup	120	0	0	0	0	30	29	1	—	35	0	—	0
Whole Berry Sauce	¼ cup	110	0	0	0	0	28	27	1	—	35	0	—	0
STEEL'S														
Spiced Cranberry Sauce	⅓ cup	20	0	0	0	0	5	4	1	—	0	—	—	—
WILD THYME FARMS														
Cranberry Sauce	1 tbsp	19	0	0	0	0	5	4	—	—	0	—	—	2

CRANBERRY BEANS

FOOD	PORTION	CALS	FAT	SAT FAT	CHOL	PROT	CARB	SUGAR	FIBER	CALCI	SOD	POTAS	FOLIC	VIT C
canned	1 cup	216	1	tr	0	14	39	—	16	67	863	675	201	2
dried cooked	1 cup	241	1	tr	0	17	43	—	18	44	1	685	366	0

CRANBERRY JUICE

FOOD	PORTION	CALS	FAT	SAT FAT	CHOL	PROT	CARB	SUGAR	FIBER	CALCI	SOD	POTAS	FOLIC	VIT C
cocktail	1 cup	147	tr	—	0	tr	38	—	—	8	10	61	1	108
cranberry juice cocktail	6 oz	108	tr	—	0	0	27	—	—	7	4	34	1	67
cranberry juice cocktail low calorie	6 oz	33	0	0	0	0	9	—	—	16	6	39	—	57
cranberry juice cocktail frzn	12 oz can	821	0	0	0	tr	210	—	—	48	13	213	0	148
cranberry juice cocktail frzn as prep	6 oz	102	0	0	0	0	26	—	—	9	6	27	0	18
CRYSTAL LIGHT														
Cranberry Breeze Drink	1 serv (8 oz)	5	0	0	0	0	0	0	0	0	20	150	—	0
Cranberry Breeze Drink Mix as prep	1 serv (8 oz)	5	0	0	0	0	0	0	0	0	0	10	—	6
EVERFRESH														
Cranberry Cocktail	1 can (8 oz)	140	0	0	0	0	36	36	0	—	0	—	—	—
KETO														
Kooler	½ tsp	0	0	0	0	0	0	0	0	—	0	—	—	—

FOOD	PORTION	CALS	FAT	SAT FAT	CHOL	PROT	CARB	SUGAR	FIBER	CALCI	SOD	POTAS	FOLIC	VIT C
LANGERS														
Cocktail	8 oz	140	0	0	0	0	35	32	—	—	10	—	—	60
Diet	8 oz	30	0	0	0	0	9	9	—	20	10	—	—	60
White	8 oz	120	0	0	0	0	28	28	—	—	10	—	—	60
MOTT'S														
Cocktail	8 fl oz	150	0	0	0	0	37	—	—	—	5	—	—	—
NANTUCKET NECTARS														
Big Cran	8 oz	140	0	0	0	0	34	32	0	0	5	—	—	60
OCEAN SPRAY														
Cocktail	8 oz	140	0	0	0	0	34	34	0	—	35	—	—	60
Cocktail Reduced Calorie	8 oz	50	0	0	0	0	13	13	0	—	35	45	—	60
Cocktail Light Low Calorie	8 oz	40	0	0	0	0	10	10	0	—	35	45	—	60
Cranberry Spritzer	8 oz	160	0	0	0	0	41	40	—	—	50	—	—	—
Cranberry Drink	8 oz	130	0	0	0	—	32	32	—	—	35	0	—	60
Crantastic	8 oz	100	0	0	0	0	32	32	0	—	35	0	—	60
White Cranberry	8 oz	120	0	0	0	0	29	29	—	—	35	0	—	60
White Cranberry Peach	8 oz	120	0	0	0	0	30	30	—	—	35	0	—	60
White Cranberry Strawberry	8 oz	120	0	0	0	0	31	31	—	—	35	0	—	60
TROPICANA														
Twister Ruby Red	1 bottle (10 oz)	160	0	0	0	tr	42	—	—	—	40	—	—	60
VERYFINE														
Cocktail	1 bottle (10 oz)	180	0	0	0	0	45	44	0	0	30	—	—	36
CRAYFISH														
cooked	3 oz	97	1	tr	151	20	0	—	—	26	58	298	—	3
raw	3 oz	76	1	tr	118	16	0	—	—	20	45	233	—	3
raw	8	24	tr	tr	37	5	0	—	—	6	14	74	—	1
CREAM														
(*see also* WHIPPED TOPPINGS)														
clotted cream	2 tbsp (1 oz)	164	18	—	48	tr	1	—	0	10	18	15	2	0
crème fraîche	2 tbsp (1 oz)	100	11	—	40	1	1	—	0	20	10	—	—	0
half & half	1 tbsp (0.5 oz)	20	2	1	6	tr	1	—	—	16	6	19	tr	tr
half & half	1 cup (8.5 oz)	315	28	17	89	7	10	—	—	254	98	314	6	2
heavy whipping	1 tbsp (0.5 oz)	52	6	3	21	tr	tr	—	—	10	6	11	1	tr
heavy whipping whipped	1 cup (4.1 oz)	411	44	27	163	5	7	—	—	77	89	179	9	1
light coffee	1 tbsp (0.5 oz)	29	3	2	10	tr	1	—	—	14	6	18	tr	tr
light coffee	1 cup (8.4 oz)	496	46	29	159	6	9	—	—	14	95	292	6	2
light whipping	1 tbsp (0.5 oz)	44	5	3	17	tr	tr	—	—	10	5	15	1	tr
light whipping cream whipped	1 cup (4.2 oz)	345	37	23	132	5	7	—	—	83	82	231	9	1

FOOD	PORTION	CALS	FAT	SAT FAT	CHOL	PROT	CARB	SUGAR	FIBER	CALCI	SOD	POTAS	FOLIC	VIT C
CABOT														
Whipped	2 tbsp	30	2	2	10	0	2	1	0	0	0	—	—	0
LAND O LAKES														
Fat Free Half & Half	2 tbsp (1 oz)	20	0	0	0	tr	3	2	0	20	30	—	—	0
Half & Half	2 tbsp (1 oz)	40	4	2	15	1	1	1	0	40	20	—	—	0
Heavy Whipping	1 tbsp (0.5 oz)	50	6	4	20	0	0	0	0	0	10	—	—	0
ORGANIC VALLEY														
Half & Half	2 tbsp (1 oz)	40	3	2	15	1	1	1	0	40	15	—	—	0

CREAM CHEESE

FOOD	PORTION	CALS	FAT	SAT FAT	CHOL	PROT	CARB	SUGAR	FIBER	CALCI	SOD	POTAS	FOLIC	VIT C
cream cheese	1 oz	99	10	6	31	2	1	—	—	23	84	34	4	0
cream cheese	1 pkg (3 oz)	297	30	19	93	6	2	—	—	68	251	101	11	0
ALPINE LACE														
Reduced Fat Roasted Garlic & Herbs	1 tsp (1 oz)	60	4	3	10	4	2	1	0	40	190	—	—	0
Reduced Fat Sundried Tomato & Basil	2 tsp (1 oz)	70	5	4	15	4	2	1	0	20	300	—	—	0
BOAR'S HEAD														
Cream Cheese	2 tbsp (1 oz)	100	10	7	30	2	2	2	0	20	100	—	—	0
BREAKSTONE'S														
Temp-Tee Whipped	2 tbsp (0.8 oz)	80	8	5	25	2	tr	tr	0	0	70	25	—	0
GALAXY														
Slices	1 slice (1 oz)	50	3	2	10	4	2	1	0	100	190	—	—	0
HORIZON ORGANIC														
Spreadable	2 tbsp	100	10	7	30	2	1	0	0	20	100	—	—	0
ORGANIC VALLEY														
Cream Cheese	1 oz	100	9	6	30	2	1	tr	0	20	100	—	—	0
PHILADELPHIA														
⅓ Less Fat	1 oz	70	6	4	20	3	tr	tr	0	20	120	—	—	0
Fat Free	1 oz	30	0	0	5	4	2	1	0	150	200	—	—	0
Regular	1 oz	100	10	6	30	2	tr	tr	0	0	90	25	—	0
Soft	2 tbsp (1 oz)	100	10	7	30	2	1	1	0	20	100	40	—	0
Soft Apple Cinnamon	2 tbsp (1.1 oz)	100	8	5	25	1	5	5	0	20	100	40	—	0
Soft Cheesecake	2 tbsp (1 oz)	110	9	6	25	2	4	4	0	20	95	35	—	0
Soft Chives & Onions	2 tbsp (1.1 oz)	110	10	7	30	1	2	2	0	40	135	60	—	0
Soft Garden Vegetable	2 tbsp (1.1 oz)	110	11	7	30	1	1	tr	0	20	170	35	—	0
Soft Honey Nut	2 tbsp (1.1 oz)	110	10	6	30	2	4	3	0	20	150	35	—	0
Soft Pineapple	2 tbsp (1.1 oz)	100	9	6	25	1	4	4	0	40	100	60	—	0
Soft Salmon	3 tbsp (1.1 oz)	100	9	6	30	2	2	1	0	20	200	45	—	0
Soft Strawberry	2 tbsp (1.1 oz)	100	9	6	25	1	5	5	0	40	100	55	—	0

FOOD	PORTION	CALS	FAT	SAT FAT	CHOL	PROT	CARB	SUGAR	FIBER	CALCI	SOD	POTAS	FOLIC	VIT C
PHILADELPHIA (CONT.)														
Soft Free	2 tbsp (1.2 oz)	30	0	0	<5	5	2	1	0	150	200	75	—	0
Soft Free Garden Vegetable	2 tbsp (1.2 oz)	30	0	0	<5	5	2	1	0	150	220	80	—	0
Soft Free Strawberries	2 tbsp (1.2 oz)	45	0	0	<5	4	6	5	0	100	180	70	—	0
Soft Light Jalapeño	2 tbsp (1.1 oz)	60	5	3	15	3	2	2	0	40	210	55	—	0
Soft Light Raspberry	2 tbsp (1.1 oz)	70	5	3	15	3	6	5	0	40	125	50	—	0
Soft Light Roasted Garlic	2 tbsp (1.1 oz)	70	5	3	15	3	2	2	0	40	180	550	—	0
Whipped	2 tbsp (0.7 oz)	70	7	5	25	1	tr	tr	0	0	85	25	—	0
Whipped Chives	2 tbsp (0.7 oz)	70	6	4	20	1	tr	tr	0	20	130	30	—	0
Whipped Smoked Salmon	2 tbsp (0.7 oz)	70	6	4	20	2	1	tr	0	20	140	35	—	0
With Chives	1 oz	90	9	6	30	2	tr	tr	0	0	135	25	—	0
CREAM OF TARTAR														
cream of tartar	1 tsp	8	0	0	0	0	2	—	—	0	2	495	0	0
CREAM SUBSTITUTES														
EXPERTEXTRAS														
RealCream	1 tsp	14	1	1	6	tr	tr	—	—	—	3	—	—	—
CREPES														
basic crepe unfilled	1	75	2	—	55	—	—	—	—	38	—	—	—	—
FRIEDA'S														
Ready-To-Use	2 (0.8 oz)	50	1	0	5	1	9	4	0	0	90	—	—	0
CROAKER														
atlantic breaded & fried	3 oz	188	11	3	71	15	6	—	—	27	296	289	—	—
atlantic raw	3 oz	89	3	1	52	15	0	—	—	13	47	293	—	—
CROCODILE														
cooked	3 oz	78	1	—	—	17	0	0	0	9	—	—	—	0
CROISSANT														
apple	1 (2 oz)	145	5	3	—	4	21	—	1	17	156	51	7	—
cheese	1 (2 oz)	236	12	5	—	5	27	—	2	30	316	76	19	—
plain	1 (2 oz)	232	12	7	—	5	26	—	2	21	424	67	16	—
plain	1 mini (1 oz)	115	6	3	—	2	13	—	1	10	211	34	8	—
SARA LEE														
Broccoli & Cheese	1 (3.7 oz)	280	13	4	30	11	30	0	2	60	430	—	—	0
French Style	1 (1.5 oz)	170	8	3	<5	4	20	0	1	20	200	—	—	—
Ham & Swiss	1 (3.7 oz)	300	16	5	45	12	27	1	2	150	570	—	—	1
Petite	2 (2 oz)	230	11	4	<5	6	26	0	1	40	260	—	—	—
TAKE-OUT														
w/ egg & cheese	1 (4.5 oz)	368	25	14	216	13	24	—	—	244	551	174	47	tr

FOOD	PORTION	CALS	FAT	SAT FAT	CHOL	PROT	CARB	SUGAR	FIBER	CALCI	SOD	POTAS	FOLIC	VIT C
w/ egg cheese & bacon	1 (4.5 oz)	413	28	15	215	16	24	—	—	151	889	201	45	2
w/ egg cheese & ham	1 (5.3 oz)	474	34	17	213	19	24	—	—	144	1081	272	46	11
w/ egg cheese & sausage	1 (5.6 oz)	523	38	18	216	20	25	—	—	144	1115	283	43	tr

CROUTONS

FOOD	PORTION	CALS	FAT	SAT FAT	CHOL	PROT	CARB	SUGAR	FIBER	CALCI	SOD	POTAS	FOLIC	VIT C
plain	1 cup (1 oz)	122	2	tr	0	4	22	—	2	23	209	37	7	0
seasoned	1 cup (1.4 oz)	186	7	2	—	4	25	—	2	38	495	72	16	—
PEPPERIDGE FARM														
Garlic	6 (0.2 oz)	30	1	0	0	1	5	0	0	0	80	—	—	0
Homestyle	6 (0.2 oz)	30	1	0	0	1	5	0	0	0	80	—	—	0
Sourdough	6 (0.2 oz)	35	2	1	0	1	4	0	0	0	70	—	—	0
UP COUNTRY NATURALS														
Organic Whole Wheat Garlic & Herb	¼ cup (0.3 oz)	35	2	0	0	1	5	0	tr	0	110	—	—	0

CUCUMBER

FOOD	PORTION	CALS	FAT	SAT FAT	CHOL	PROT	CARB	SUGAR	FIBER	CALCI	SOD	POTAS	FOLIC	VIT C
fresh raw	1 (11 oz)	38	tr	tr	0	2	8	—	3	43	6	434	38	16
fresh raw sliced	½ cup (1.8 oz)	7	tr	tr	0	tr	1	—	1	7	1	76	7	3
CHIQUITA														
Cucumber	⅓ med (3.5 oz)	15	0	0	0	1	3	2	1	20	0	—	—	6
TAKE-OUT														
cucumber salad	3.5 oz	50	tr	tr	0	1	11	—	—	—	480	—	—	9
kimchee	½ cup (1.8 oz)	36	2	tr	0	tr	4	3	tr	10	173	79	6	6
tzatziki	½ cup (3.4 oz)	72	6	1	5	2	4	3	1	59	197	146	10	3

CUMIN

FOOD	PORTION	CALS	FAT	SAT FAT	CHOL	PROT	CARB	SUGAR	FIBER	CALCI	SOD	POTAS	FOLIC	VIT C
seed	1 tsp	8	tr	—	0	tr	1	—	—	20	4	38	—	tr

CURRANT JUICE

FOOD	PORTION	CALS	FAT	SAT FAT	CHOL	PROT	CARB	SUGAR	FIBER	CALCI	SOD	POTAS	FOLIC	VIT C
black currant nectar	7 oz	110	0	—	—	tr	26	—	—	30	10	196	tr	60
red currant nectar	7 oz	108	tr	—	—	tr	26	—	—	14	tr	220	tr	12

CURRANTS

FOOD	PORTION	CALS	FAT	SAT FAT	CHOL	PROT	CARB	SUGAR	FIBER	CALCI	SOD	POTAS	FOLIC	VIT C
black fresh	½ cup	36	tr	tr	0	1	9	—	—	31	1	180	—	101
zante dried	½ cup	204	tr	tr	0	3	53	—	—	62	6	642	7	3
SUN-MAID														
Zante	¼ cup	130	0	0	0	1	31	29	2	20	10	310	—	—

CUSK

FOOD	PORTION	CALS	FAT	SAT FAT	CHOL	PROT	CARB	SUGAR	FIBER	CALCI	SOD	POTAS	FOLIC	VIT C
fillet baked	3 oz	106	1	—	50	23	0	—	—	12	38	477	—	—

CUSTARD

FOOD	PORTION	CALS	FAT	SAT FAT	CHOL	PROT	CARB	SUGAR	FIBER	CALCI	SOD	POTAS	FOLIC	VIT C
MIX														
as prep w/ 2% milk	½ cup (4.7 oz)	148	4	2	74	7	24	—	—	197	200	287	10	1
as prep w/ whole milk	½ cup (4.7 oz)	163	5	3	—	6	23	—	—	194	—	—	—	1

FOOD	PORTION	CALS	FAT	SAT FAT	CHOL	PROT	CARB	SUGAR	FIBER	CALCI	SOD	POTAS	FOLIC	VIT C
flan as prep w/ 2% milk	½ cup (4.7 oz)	135	2	1	9	4	26	—	—	153	68	194	3	1
flan as prep w/ whole milk	½ cup (4.7 oz)	150	4	3	17	4	25	—	—	150	65	191	5	1
BETTY CROCKER														
Flan w/ Caramel Sauce as prep	1 serv	330	7	4	24	0	60	23	—	250	25	65	—	—
JELL-O														
Americana Custard Dessert as prep w/ 2% milk	½ cup (5 oz)	140	3	2	10	5	25	23	0	200	190	300	—	0
Flan as prep w/ 2% milk	½ cup (5.1 oz)	140	3	2	10	4	26	25	0	150	65	200	—	0
READY-TO-EAT														
SWISS MISS														
Egg Custard	1 pkg (4 oz)	153	5	1	4	5	22	21	0	120	138	—	—	0
TAKE-OUT														
baked	½ cup (5 oz)	148	7	3	123	7	15	—	—	158	109	216	44	1
flan	½ cup (5.4 oz)	220	6	3	140	7	35	—	—	132	86	185	—	1
zabaione	½ cup (57.2 g)	135	5	2	213	3	13	—	0	23	9	16	24	0
CUTTLEFISH														
steamed	3 oz	134	1	tr	190	28	1	—	—	153	632	542	—	7
DANDELION GREENS														
fresh cooked	½ cup	17	tr	—	0	1	3	—	—	73	23	121	—	9
raw chopped	½ cup	13	tr	—	0	1	3	—	—	52	21	111	—	10
DANISH PASTRY														
FROZEN														
MORTON														
Honey Buns	1 (2.28 oz)	270	13	3	0	3	35	16	1	0	160	—	—	0
Honey Buns Mini	1 (1.3 oz)	160	8	2	0	2	19	6	1	0	100	—	—	0
READY-TO-EAT														
plain ring	1 (12 oz)	1305	71	22	292	21	152	—	—	360	1302	316	—	tr
DOLLY MADISON														
Danish Rollers	3 (2.8 oz)	290	10	2	0	3	46	21	1	80	130	—	—	0
TASTYKAKE														
Cheese	1 (3 oz)	290	14	3	20	5	44	22	tr	20	290	—	—	0
Lemon	1 (3 oz)	290	14	3	20	5	44	22	1	20	280	—	—	0
Raspberry	1 (3 oz)	290	14	3	20	5	44	22	1	20	260	—	—	0
TAKE-OUT														
almond	1 (4¼ in) (2.3 oz)	280	16	4	30	5	30	—	2	61	236	62	—	1
apple	1 (4¼ in) (2.5 oz)	264	13	3	—	4	34	—	1	33	251	59	12	3
cheese	1 (4¼ in) (2.5 oz)	266	16	5	—	6	26	—	—	25	319	70	—	—

FOOD	PORTION	CALS	FAT	SAT FAT	CHOL	PROT	CARB	SUGAR	FIBER	CALCI	SOD	POTAS	FOLIC	VIT C
cinnamon	1 (4¼ in) (2.3 oz)	262	15	4	—	5	29	—	1	46	241	81	—	—
cinnamon nut	1 (4¼ in) (2.3 oz)	280	16	4	30	5	30	—	2	61	236	62	—	1
lemon	1 (4¼ in) (2.5 oz)	264	13	3	—	4	34	—	1	33	251	59	12	3
raisin	1 (4¼ in) (2.5 oz)	264	13	3	—	4	34	—	1	33	251	59	12	3
raisin nut	1 (4¼ in) (2.3 oz)	280	16	4	30	5	30	—	2	61	236	62	—	1
raspberry	1 (4¼ in) (2.5 oz)	264	13	3	—	4	34	—	1	33	251	59	12	3
strawberry	1 (4¼ in) (2.5 oz)	264	13	3	—	4	34	—	1	33	251	59	12	3

DATES

FOOD	PORTION	CALS	FAT	SAT FAT	CHOL	PROT	CARB	SUGAR	FIBER	CALCI	SOD	POTAS	FOLIC	VIT C
deglet noor dried	10	240	0	—	0	—	—	—	—	40	—	—	—	—
dried chopped	1 cup	489	1	—	0	4	131	—	—	58	5	1161	22	0
dried whole	10	228	tr	—	0	2	61	—	—	27	2	541	10	0
jujube dried	1 oz	75	tr	—	—	1	19	—	2	18	2	149	—	4
jujube fresh	1 oz	30	tr	—	0	tr	7	—	—	9	1	80	—	17
jujube preserved in sugar	1 oz	91	tr	—	—	tr	22	—	—	7	2	18	tr	tr
medjool	2–3 (1.4 oz)	120	0	0	0	1	31	25	3	20	10	—	—	0
CALAVO														
Dried Pitted	5–6 (1.4 oz)	120	0	0	0	1	31	20	3	20	0	240	—	0
CALIFORNIA REDI-DATE														
Deglet Noor Dried	5–6 (1.4 oz)	120	0	0	0	1	31	29	3	20	0	240	8	0
DROMEDARY														
Chopped Dried	¼ cup	130	0	0	0	1	31	—	—	20	0	190	—	—
SUNDATE														
Fancy Medjool	3	120	0	0	0	1	31	25	3	0	0	170	—	0

DEER

(*see* VENISON)

DELI MEATS/COLD CUTS

(*see also* BEEF, CHICKEN, HAM, MEAT SUBSTITUTES, TURKEY)

FOOD	PORTION	CALS	FAT	SAT FAT	CHOL	PROT	CARB	SUGAR	FIBER	CALCI	SOD	POTAS	FOLIC	VIT C
barbecue loaf pork & beef	1 slice	40	2	1	9	4	1	—	0	13	307	76	2	0
beerwurst beef	1 slice (4 in × ⅛ in)	75	7	3	13	3	tr	—	—	2	214	42	1	3
beerwurst beef	1 slice (2¾ in × 1/16 in)	20	2	1	4	1	tr	—	—	1	62	10	0	1
beerwurst pork	1 slice (4 in × ⅛ in)	55	4	1	13	4	tr	—	—	2	285	58	1	7
beerwurst pork	1 slice (2¾ in × 1/16 in)	14	1	tr	4	1	tr	—	—	0	74	15	0	2

FOOD	PORTION	CALS	FAT	SAT FAT	CHOL	PROT	CARB	SUGAR	FIBER	CALCI	SOD	POTAS	FOLIC	VIT C
berliner pork & beef	1 oz	65	4	2	13	4	1	—	—	3	368	80	—	2
blood sausage	1 oz	95	9	3	30	4	tr	—	—	—	—	—	—	—
bologna beef	1 oz	88	8	3	16	4	tr	—	—	3	278	44	1	6
bologna beef & pork	1 oz	89	8	3	16	3	1	—	—	3	289	51	1	6
bologna pork	1 oz	70	6	2	17	4	tr	—	—	3	336	80	1	10
braunschweiger pork	1 oz	102	9	3	44	4	1	—	—	2	324	57	—	3
braunschweiger pork	1 slice (2½ in × ¼ in)	65	6	2	28	2	1	—	—	2	206	36	—	2
corned beef loaf	1 oz	43	2	1	13	7	0	—	—	3	270	29	—	2
dried beef	1 oz	47	1	—	—	—	tr	—	—	2	—	—	—	—
dutch brand loaf pork & beef	1 oz	68	5	2	13	4	2	—	—	24	354	107	—	5
headcheese pork	1 oz	60	5	1	23	5	tr	—	—	5	356	9	1	6
honey loaf pork & beef	1 oz	36	1	tr	10	4	2	—	—	5	374	97	—	6
honey roll sausage beef	1 oz	42	2	1	12	4	1	—	—	2	304	67	—	4
lebanon bologna beef	1 oz	60	4	2	20	6	1	—	—	4	379	85	—	6
liver cheese pork	1 oz	86	7	3	49	4	1	—	—	2	347	64	—	1
liverwurst pork	1 oz	92	8	3	45	4	1	—	—	7	—	—	9	—
luncheon meat beef	1 oz	87	7	3	18	4	1	—	—	3	377	59	—	4
luncheon meat pork & beef	1 oz	100	9	3	15	4	1	—	—	5	367	57	2	4
luncheon meat pork canned	1 oz	95	9	3	18	4	1	—	—	2	365	61	2	0
luncheon sausage pork & beef	1 oz	74	6	2	18	4	tr	—	—	3	335	70	—	5
luxury loaf pork	1 oz	40	1	tr	10	5	1	—	—	10	347	107	—	6
mortadella beef & pork	1 oz	88	7	3	16	5	1	—	—	5	353	46	—	7
mother's loaf pork	1 oz	80	6	2	13	3	2	—	—	12	320	64	—	0
new england sausage pork & beef	1 oz	46	2	1	14	5	1	—	—	2	346	91	2	6
olive loaf pork	1 oz	67	5	2	11	3	3	—	—	31	421	84	—	2
peppered loaf pork & beef	1 oz	42	2	1	13	5	1	—	—	15	432	112	—	7
pepperoni pork & beef	1 slice (0.2 oz)	27	2	1	—	1	tr	—	—	1	112	19	—	—
pepperoni pork & beef	1 (9 oz)	1248	110	40	—	53	7	—	—	25	5120	871	—	—

FOOD	PORTION	CALS	FAT	SAT FAT	CHOL	PROT	CARB	SUGAR	FIBER	CALCI	SOD	POTAS	FOLIC	VIT C
pickle & pimiento loaf pork	1 oz	74	6	2	10	3	2	—	—	27	394	96	—	4
picnic loaf pork & beef	1 oz	66	5	2	11	4	1	—	—	13	330	76	—	5
salami cooked beef & pork	1 oz	71	6	2	18	4	1	—	—	4	302	56	1	3
salami hard pork	1 pkg (4 oz)	460	38	13	—	26	2	—	—	15	2554	—	—	—
salami hard pork	1 slice (⅓ oz)	41	4	1	—	2	3	—	—	1	226	—	—	—
salami hard pork & beef	1 slice (0.3 oz)	42	3	1	8	2	tr	—	—	1	186	38	—	3
salami hard pork & beef	1 pkg (4 oz)	472	39	14	89	26	3	—	—	8	2101	427	—	29
sandwich spread pork & beef	1 tbsp	35	3	1	6	1	2	—	—	2	152	16	—	0
sandwich spread pork & beef	1 oz	67	5	2	11	2	3	—	—	3	287	31	—	0
summer sausage thuringer cervelat	1 oz	98	8	3	19	5	1	—	—	2	412	65	—	7
BOAR'S HEAD														
Bologna Beef	2 oz	150	13	4	35	7	0	0	0	0	520	—	—	0
Bologna Garlic	2 oz	150	13	5	35	7	1	1	0	0	530	—	—	0
Bologna Lowered Sodium	2 oz	150	13	5	30	8	0	0	0	0	410	—	—	0
Bologna Pork & Beef	2 oz	150	13	5	35	7	tr	tr	0	0	530	—	—	0
Braunschweiger Lite	2 oz	120	8	5	50	9	1	0	0	0	450	—	—	0
Head Cheese	2 oz	90	5	3	65	10	tr	0	0	0	420	—	—	0
Liverwurst Strassburger	2 oz	170	15	6	85	8	1	1	0	0	560	—	—	0
Olive Loaf	2 oz	130	12	5	20	6	tr	tr	0	20	630	—	—	0
Pastrami	2 oz	90	4	2	30	12	2	0	0	0	620	—	—	0
Prosciutto	1 oz	60	3	1	15	8	0	0	0	0	770	—	—	0
Red Pastrami	2 oz	90	4	2	30	12	2	0	0	0	620	—	—	0
Salami Beef	2 oz	120	9	4	25	10	0	0	0	0	470	—	—	0
Salami Cooked	2 oz	130	11	5	40	8	0	0	0	0	550	—	—	0
Salami Genoa	2 oz	180	14	5	55	12	1	0	0	0	970	—	—	0
Salami Hard	1 oz	110	9	4	25	6	tr	0	0	0	490	—	—	0
Spiced Ham	2 oz	120	10	5	30	7	1	0	0	0	570	—	—	0
CARL BUDDIG														
Beef	1 pkg (2.5 oz)	100	5	2	50	14	1	1	—	—	1020	—	—	—
Corned Beef	1 pkg (2.5 oz)	100	5	2	50	14	tr	tr	—	—	980	—	—	—
Pastrami	1 pkg (2.5 oz)	100	5	2	50	14	1	1	—	—	750	—	—	—
HORMEL														
Liverwurst Spread	4 tbsp (2 oz)	130	10	4	70	8	2	1	0	0	650	—	—	1
Pepperoni Chunk	1 oz	140	13	6	35	5	0	0	0	0	470	—	—	0

FOOD	PORTION	CALS	FAT	SAT FAT	CHOL	PROT	CARB	SUGAR	FIBER	CALCI	SOD	POTAS	FOLIC	VIT C
Pepperoni Sliced	16 slices (1 oz)	140	13	5	25	6	1	—	—	—	490	—	—	—
Pepperoni Twin	1 oz	140	13	5	35	5	0	0	0	0	500	—	—	6
Pillow Pack Genoa Salami	2 oz	160	18	7	50	12	0	0	0	0	940	—	—	0
Pillow Pack Pepperoni	16 slices (1 oz)	140	13	6	35	5	0	0	0	0	470	—	—	0
OSCAR MAYER														
Bologna	1 slice (1 oz)	90	8	3	30	3	1	tr	0	0	290	—	—	0
Bologna Beef	1 slice (1 oz)	90	8	4	20	3	1	tr	0	0	310	—	—	0
Bologna Garlic	1 slice (1.4 oz)	110	12	5	40	4	1	tr	0	20	420	—	—	0
Bologna Wisconsin Made Ring	2 oz	180	16	6	35	6	2	1	0	0	460	—	—	0
Braunschweiger Spread	2 oz	190	17	6	90	8	2	tr	0	0	630	—	—	5
Brunschweiger	1 slice (1 oz)	100	9	3	40	4	1	0	0	0	320	—	—	2
Free Bologna	1 slice (1 oz)	20	0	0	5	4	2	tr	0	0	280	—	—	0
Light Bologna	1 slice (1 oz)	60	4	2	15	3	2	tr	0	0	310	—	—	0
Light Bologna Beef	1 slice (1 oz)	60	4	2	15	3	2	tr	0	0	310	—	—	0
Liver Cheese	1 slice (1.3 oz)	120	10	4	80	6	1	0	0	0	420	—	—	0
Luncheon Loaf Spiced	1 slice (1 oz)	70	5	2	20	4	2	1	0	40	340	—	—	0
Old Fashioned Loaf	1 slice (1 oz)	70	5	2	15	4	2	1	0	40	330	—	—	0
Olive Loaf	1 slice (1 oz)	70	6	2	20	3	2	tr	0	40	370	—	—	0
Pepperoni	15 slices (1 oz)	140	13	5	25	6	0	0	0	0	550	—	—	0
Salami Cotto	1 slice (1 oz)	70	5	2	25	3	1	0	0	0	280	—	—	0
Salami Cotto Beef	1 slice (1 oz)	60	5	2	25	4	1	tr	0	0	370	—	—	0
Salami For Beer	1 slices (1.6 oz)	110	9	3	30	6	1	tr	0	0	580	—	—	0
Salami Hard	3 slices (1 oz)	100	9	3	25	6	0	0	0	0	510	—	—	0
Sandwich Spread	2 oz	130	10	4	25	4	8	4	0	0	460	—	—	0
Summer Sausage	2 slices (1.6 oz)	140	13	5	40	7	0	0	0	0	650	—	—	0
Summer Sausage Beef	2 slices (1.6 oz)	140	12	5	35	7	1	tr	0	0	640	—	—	0
SPAM														
Less Salt	2 oz	170	16	6	40	7	0	0	0	0	560	—	—	18
Lite	2 oz	110	8	3	45	9	0	0	0	0	560	—	—	18
Original	2 oz	170	16	6	40	7	0	0	0	0	750	—	—	0
Smoked	2 oz	170	16	6	40	7	0	0	0	0	750	—	—	0
TAKE-OUT														
corned beef	2 oz	70	2	1	40	12	0	—	—	—	390	—	—	12
corned beef brisket	2 oz	90	5	2	35	11	0	—	—	—	370	—	—	12
DILL														
seed	1 tsp	6	tr	tr	0	tr	1	—	—	32	tr	25	—	—
sprigs fresh	1 cup	4	tr	tr	0	tr	1	—	—	18	5	66	13	—

FOOD	PORTION	CALS	FAT	SAT FAT	CHOL	PROT	CARB	SUGAR	FIBER	CALCI	SOD	POTAS	FOLIC	VIT C
sprigs fresh	5	0	tr	tr	0	tr	tr	—	—	2	1	7	1	—
weed dry	1 tsp	3	tr	—	0	tr	1	—	—	18	2	33	—	—

DINNER

(*see also* ASIAN FOOD, PASTA DINNERS, POT PIE, SPANISH FOOD)

AMY'S

FOOD	PORTION	CALS	FAT	SAT FAT	CHOL	PROT	CARB	SUGAR	FIBER	CALCI	SOD	POTAS	FOLIC	VIT C
Country Dinner Vegetable Salisbury Steak	1 pkg (11 oz)	380	12	4	15	11	60	14	9	—	570	—	—	—

BANQUET

FOOD	PORTION	CALS	FAT	SAT FAT	CHOL	PROT	CARB	SUGAR	FIBER	CALCI	SOD	POTAS	FOLIC	VIT C
Beef Patty w/ Country Style Vegetables	1 meal (9.5 oz)	310	20	8	40	11	22	6	2	40	1090	—	—	1
Boneless Pork Rib	1 meal (10 oz)	400	19	8	45	17	40	22	4	80	1070	—	—	2
Boneless White Fried Chicken	1 meal (8.25 oz)	540	34	9	60	16	41	10	3	40	1180	—	—	6
Chicken Parmigiana	1 meal (9.5 oz)	320	18	7	50	10	29	7	3	60	900	—	—	30
Chicken Fingers Meal	1 meal (7.1 oz)	740	43	11	70	22	67	24	6	40	1070	—	—	0
Chicken Fried Beef Steak	1 pkg (10 oz)	420	23	12	35	15	39	9	4	100	1200	—	—	0
Chicken Nuggets Meal	1 meal (6.75 oz)	430	23	8	50	14	42	11	4	20	650	—	—	6
Extra Helping Boneless Pork Riblet	1 meal (15.25 oz)	720	40	15	80	27	62	18	7	100	1590	—	—	0
Extra Helping Fried Beef Steak	1 meal (16 oz)	820	50	23	70	29	63	13	6	150	2260	—	—	0
Extra Helping Fried Chicken	1 meal (14.7 oz)	910	55	13	160	34	70	8	5	80	2400	—	—	1
Extra Helping Meatloaf	1 meal (16 oz)	610	40	15	110	29	34	12	6	60	1940	—	—	6
Extra Helping Salisbury Steak	1 meal (16.5 oz)	740	54	21	130	27	37	7	7	100	2200	—	—	0
Extra Helping Turkey & Gravy w/ Dressing	1 meal (17 oz)	620	32	8	80	28	54	11	10	60	2250	—	—	0
Extra Helping White Fried Chicken	1 meal (13 oz)	690	48	12	70	24	40	3	8	60	1900	—	—	6
Extra Helping Yankee Pot Roast	1 meal (14.5 oz)	410	20	7	50	25	33	25	3	60	1660	—	—	1
Family Size Brown Gravy & Salisbury Steak	1 serv	240	20	10	40	9	7	2	1	0	900	—	—	0
Family Size Brown Gravy & Sliced Beef	1 serv	140	8	4	40	13	5	2	tr	0	850	—	—	0

FOOD	PORTION	CALS	FAT	SAT FAT	CHOL	PROT	CARB	SUGAR	FIBER	CALCI	SOD	POTAS	FOLIC	VIT C
BANQUET (CONT.)														
Family Size Chicken & Broccoli Alfredo	1 serv	270	12	7	40	11	28	3	3	100	540	—	—	6
Family Size Country Style Chicken & Dumplings	1 serv	290	14	5	40	12	30	6	7	40	1270	—	—	0
Family Size Creamy Broccoli Chicken Cheese & Rice	1 serv	280	14	7	45	14	25	6	2	150	980	—	—	0
Family Size Hearty Beef Stew	1 cup	170	7	3	30	10	18	4	4	20	1120	—	—	4
Family Size Homestyle Gravy & Sliced Turkey	2 slices	140	10	4	40	7	5	1	1	0	600	—	—	0
Family Size Mushroom Gravy Charbroiled Beef Patties	1 patty	250	20	9	35	11	6	2	2	20	750	—	—	0
Family Size Potato Ham & Broccoli Au Gratin	⅔ cup	210	13	5	30	7	16	6	2	80	970	—	—	18
Family Size Savory Gravy & Meatloaf	1 slice	120	13	7	35	10	7	2	1	0	750	—	—	0
Fish Sticks	1 meal (6.6 oz)	290	13	5	30	11	33	14	4	60	820	—	—	4
Grilled Chicken	1 meal (9.9 oz)	330	13	3	50	16	37	18	2	40	1210	—	—	5
Honey Roast Turkey Breast	1 meal (9 oz)	270	12	3	30	11	29	8	4	60	1310	—	—	0
Meatloaf	1 meal (9.5 oz)	280	16	6	60	12	23	9	3	40	1020	—	—	0
Our Original Fried Chicken	1 meal (9 oz)	470	27	9	90	21	35	4	2	40	1500	—	—	1
Pork Cutlet Meal	1 meal (10.25 oz)	420	25	7	35	11	36	21	4	60	1060	—	—	0
Salisbury Steak	1 meal (9.5 oz)	340	20	8	50	13	26	5	4	40	1050	—	—	0
Sliced Beef	1 meal (9 oz)	270	10	5	70	26	19	12	4	40	740	—	—	1
Turkey Meal	1 meal (9.25 oz)	290	13	3	35	15	28	6	6	60	1050	—	—	0
Veal Parmagiana	1 meal (8.75 oz)	330	14	5	20	13	37	7	2	20	860	—	—	42
Western Style Beef Patty	1 meal (9.5 oz)	360	21	10	40	14	28	4	3	40	1400	—	—	0

FOOD	PORTION	CALS	FAT	SAT FAT	CHOL	PROT	CARB	SUGAR	FIBER	CALCI	SOD	POTAS	FOLIC	VIT C
BANQUET (CONT.)														
White Meat Fried Chicken	1 meal (8.75 oz)	460	28	11	100	18	40	4	2	40	1100	—	—	2
Yankee Pot Roast	1 meal (9.4 oz)	230	10	4	60	14	20	8	4	40	1130	—	—	4
BIRDS EYE														
Easy Recipe Creations Sweet & Sour w/ Pineapple Tidbits	1⅔ cups	200	1	0	0	2	45	41	3	40	330	—	—	30
Voilà! Beef Sirloin Steak And Garlic Potatoes	1 cup	240	9	2	25	13	26	5	3	40	650	—	—	4
Voilà! Chicken Alfredo	1 cup	230	8	2	20	15	26	5	2	80	660	—	—	21
Voilà! Garden Herb Chicken	1 cup	310	15	5	40	16	28	8	2	100	540	—	—	4
Voilà! Grilled Salsa Chicken w/ Rice	1 cup	240	5	1	25	14	35	5	3	20	1180	—	—	9
Voilà! Homestyle Turkey w/ Roasted Potatoes	1 cup	200	6	2	10	12	24	4	3	40	830	—	—	9
Voilà! Teriyaki	2 cups (6.4 oz)	240	9	5	25	13	26	7	2	40	700	—	—	18
Voilà! Zesty Garlic Chicken	2 cups (6.2 oz)	260	11	3	25	15	28	6	1	60	550	—	—	12
FILLO FACTORY														
Fillo Pie Broccoli & Cheese	¼ pie (4 oz)	350	12	5	20	14	50	1	3	—	370	—	—	—
Fillo Pie Spinach & Cheese	⅕ pie (4.8 oz)	210	7	3	15	12	27	1	2	—	270	—	—	—
GREEN GIANT														
Create A Meal Broccoli Stir Fry as prep	1⅓ cups (9.9 oz)	290	13	3	60	27	16	7	4	60	1160	—	—	54
Create A Meal Cheese & Herb Primavera as prep	1¼ cups (10 oz)	330	11	4	65	30	27	3	4	150	920	—	—	30
Create A Meal Garlic Herb as prep	1¼ cups (10 oz)	340	14	6	145	24	30	4	4	150	670	—	—	24
Create A Meal Hearty Vegetable Stew as prep	1¼ cups (10 oz)	280	9	2	55	23	25	5	3	40	1000	—	—	15
Create A Meal Lemon Herb as prep	1½ cups (10 oz)	360	11	4	65	28	37	12	3	100	830	—	—	24
Create A Meal Mushroom & Wine as prep	1¼ cups (10 oz)	390	16	6	75	28	31	5	4	40	910	—	—	6

FOOD	PORTION	CALS	FAT	SAT FAT	CHOL	PROT	CARB	SUGAR	FIBER	CALCI	SOD	POTAS	FOLIC	VIT C
GREEN GIANT (CONT.)														
Create A Meal Vegetable Almond Stir Fry as prep	1⅓ cups (10 oz)	320	11	2	65	32	22	9	6	80	1190	—	—	9
HEALTHY CHOICE														
Beef Pepper Steak Oriental	1 meal (9.5 oz)	260	5	3	35	19	34	5	2	20	520	—	—	9
Beef Pot Roast	1 meal (11 oz)	300	6	2	40	20	41	24	6	20	600	—	—	18
Beef Stoganoff	1 meal (11 oz)	320	8	3	60	22	40	14	7	60	600	—	—	12
Beef Teriyaki	1 meal (9.5 oz)	310	7	3	40	16	44	17	5	20	600	—	—	2
Beef Tips Français	1 meal (9.5 oz)	300	7	3	40	20	40	6	4	20	520	—	—	0
Beef Tips Portabello	1 meal (11.25 oz)	270	5	3	40	23	34	14	7	40	600	—	—	12
Bowls Chicken Teriyaki w/ Rice	1 meal (9.5 oz)	270	4	1	30	17	41	7	4	20	570	—	—	12
Bowls Country Chicken Bake	1 meal (9.5 oz)	230	8	3	50	18	22	9	4	100	600	—	—	2
Bowls Fiesta Chicken	1 meal (9.5 oz)	220	2	1	30	15	34	6	3	40	550	—	—	0
Bowls Garlic Lemon Chicken w/ Rice	1 meal (9.5 oz)	300	4	2	40	18	48	6	4	20	400	—	—	15
Bowls Roasted Potatoes w/ Ham	1 meal (8.5 oz)	210	4	2	30	17	26	10	6	100	600	—	—	24
Bowls Southwestern Chicken & Pasta	1 meal (9.5 oz)	320	4	2	40	31	39	2	6	40	350	—	—	24
Bowls Turkey Divan	1 meal (9.5 oz)	250	6	2	30	18	31	7	4	100	600	—	—	9
Charbroiled Beef Patty	1 meal (11 oz)	310	9	3	45	16	40	8	4	20	550	—	—	0
Chicken Cantonese	1 meal (10.75 oz)	280	6	3	50	22	34	15	2	40	480	—	—	6
Chicken Parmigiana	1 meal (11.5 oz)	330	8	3	40	19	46	23	3	80	490	—	—	9
Chicken & Vegetables Marsala	1 meal (11.5 oz)	240	4	2	30	20	32	4	3	40	440	—	—	4
Chicken Broccoli Alfredo	1 meal (11.5 oz)	300	7	3	50	25	34	5	2	100	530	—	—	12
Chicken Dijon	1 meal (11 oz)	270	5	2	40	23	33	6	6	60	470	—	—	18
Chicken Teriyaki	1 meal (11 oz)	270	6	2	40	16	37	14	6	20	600	—	—	27
Country Glazed Chicken Breast	1 meal (8.5 oz)	250	5	2	30	19	31	6	3	20	600	—	—	0
Country Herb Chicken	1 meal (12.15 oz)	320	8	3	45	16	44	23	3	40	540	—	—	0

FOOD	PORTION	CALS	FAT	SAT FAT	CHOL	PROT	CARB	SUGAR	FIBER	CALCI	SOD	POTAS	FOLIC	VIT C
HEALTHY CHOICE (CONT.)														
Country Inn Roast Turkey	1 meal (10 oz)	250	6	2	40	20	28	16	4	40	530	—	—	0
Garlic Chicken Milano	1 meal (9.5 oz)	260	6	3	35	18	34	4	3	100	510	—	—	18
Grilled Chicken Sonoma	1 meal (9 oz)	230	4	1	45	16	30	9	3	20	530	—	—	12
Grilled Chicken w/ Mashed Potatoes	1 meal (8 oz)	180	4	2	45	16	18	3	3	0	600	—	—	1
Herb Baked Fish	1 meal (10.9 oz)	340	7	2	35	16	54	11	5	40	480	—	—	0
Herb Breaded Pork Patty	1 meal (8 oz)	280	6	3	30	18	38	4	4	100	570	—	—	5
Homestyle Chicken & Pasta	1 meal (9 oz)	270	6	3	35	21	32	6	5	60	570	—	—	4
Honey Glazed Chicken	1 meal (10 oz)	270	7	3	45	21	32	11	4	40	600	—	—	6
Honey Mustard Chicken	1 meal (9.5 oz)	290	6	3	40	21	38	7	1	0	520	—	—	0
Lemon Pepper Fish	1 meal (10.7 oz)	280	5	2	35	11	49	14	5	20	580	—	—	30
Mandarin Chicken	1 meal (10 oz)	280	3	0	35	20	44	9	4	20	520	—	—	15
Mesquite Beef w/ Barbecue Sauce	1 meal (11 oz)	320	9	3	55	21	36	16	5	40	490	—	—	9
Mesquite Chicken Barbecue	1 meal (10.5 oz)	310	5	2	55	18	48	15	6	40	480	—	—	9
Oriental Style Chicken & Vegetable Stir Fry	1 meal (11.9 oz)	360	6	2	25	19	57	16	5	40	600	—	—	5
Oven Roasted Beef	1 meal (10.15 oz)	280	8	3	50	18	35	10	4	0	600	—	—	12
Roast Turkey Breast	1 meal (8.5 oz)	220	5	2	25	18	28	0	5	20	600	—	—	1
Roasted Chicken	1 meal (11 oz)	230	5	3	50	20	23	9	4	20	560	—	—	4
Sesame Chicken	1 meal (10.8 oz)	360	7	2	20	19	54	17	4	60	600	—	—	6
Shrimp & Vegetables	1 meal (11.8 oz)	270	6	3	50	15	39	6	6	150	560	—	—	30
Sweet & Sour Chicken	1 meal (11 oz)	340	7	2	25	15	54	21	3	20	580	—	—	30
Traditional Meatloaf	1 meal (12 oz)	330	7	4	35	15	52	17	6	40	460	—	—	42
Traditional Salisbury Steak	1 meal (11.5 oz)	330	7	3	50	18	48	24	6	40	470	—	—	12
Traditional Turkey Breast	1 meal (10.5 oz)	330	5	2	35	21	50	26	4	40	600	—	—	0
Tuna Casserole	1 meal (8 oz)	240	5	2	25	16	33	7	4	150	560	—	—	0

FOOD	PORTION	CALS	FAT	SAT FAT	CHOL	PROT	CARB	SUGAR	FIBER	CALCI	SOD	POTAS	FOLIC	VIT C
KID CUISINE														
Circus Show Corn Dog	1 meal (8.8 oz)	490	20	7	30	8	70	46	5	80	800	—	—	12
Cosmic Chicken Nuggets	1 meal (9.1 oz)	500	25	10	45	18	50	19	5	100	1070	—	—	0
Futuristic Fish Sticks	1 meal (8.25 oz)	410	16	4	20	9	57	30	4	60	550	—	—	0
Game Time Taco Roll Up	1 meal (7.35 oz)	420	18	7	25	9	55	25	4	100	740	—	—	0
High Flying Fried Chicken	1 meal (10.1 oz)	440	20	9	70	18	48	20	3	80	940	—	—	0
Parachuting Pork Ribettes	1 meal (7.55 oz)	390	19	8	50	16	39	16	3	60	760	—	—	0
LAURA'S LIFESTYLE														
Carb Conscious Chicken Puttanesca	1 pkg (9 oz)	270	10	2	—	34	7	0	3	—	830	—	—	—
Carb Conscious Chicken Chow Mein	1 pkg (9 oz)	260	8	4	—	34	9	2	3	—	870	—	—	—
Carb Conscious Thai Chicken	1 pkg (9 oz)	280	8	2	—	35	11	2	3	—	840	—	—	—
Carb Conscious Chicken Santa Fe	1 pkg (9 oz)	280	9	2	—	40	9	1	2	—	850	—	—	—
LEAN CUISINE														
Cafe Classics Baked Chicken	1 pkg (8.6 oz)	240	5	2	30	17	33	4	3	80	550	480	—	0
Cafe Classics Baked Fish	1 pkg (9 oz)	290	6	3	40	20	40	6	2	150	590	500	—	9
Cafe Classics Beef Peppercorn	1 pkg (8.75 oz)	260	7	2	25	16	32	5	4	100	590	1060	—	5
Cafe Classics Beef Portobello	1 pkg (9 oz)	220	7	4	35	14	24	6	2	40	590	760	—	0
Cafe Classics Beef Pot Roast	1 pkg (9 oz)	210	6	2	30	13	25	4	6	40	570	630	—	2
Cafe Classics Chicken Carbonara	1 pkg (9 oz)	280	7	2	30	17	36	5	4	100	560	710	—	12
Cafe Classics Chicken Medallions w/ Creamy Cheese Sauce	1 pkg (9.37 oz)	300	7	3	35	19	40	5	2	200	690	580	—	12
Cafe Classics Chicken Mediterranean	1 pkg (10.5 oz)	260	4	1	20	17	38	6	4	60	690	860	—	5
Cafe Classics Chicken & Vegetables	1 pkg (10.5 oz)	240	5	3	30	19	30	5	4	150	690	730	—	4

FOOD	PORTION	CALS	FAT	SAT FAT	CHOL	PROT	CARB	SUGAR	FIBER	CALCI	SOD	POTAS	FOLIC	VIT C
LEAN CUISINE (CONT.)														
Cafe Classics Chicken In Peanut Sauce	1 pkg (9 oz)	260	6	1	30	20	32	7	4	100	690	670	—	6
Cafe Classics Chicken In Wine Sauce	1 pkg (8.1 oz)	220	5	3	45	20	23	7	2	150	690	760	—	1
Cafe Classics Chicken L'Orange	1 pkg (9 oz)	230	2	1	40	20	33	9	2	20	300	430	—	9
Cafe Classics Chicken Parmesan	1 pkg (10.9 oz)	300	6	2	35	21	41	8	5	100	600	920	—	9
Cafe Classics Chicken Piccata	1 pkg (9 oz)	300	9	3	30	14	41	9	2	100	590	290	—	12
Cafe Classics Chicken w/ Basil Cream Sauce	1 pkg (8.5 oz)	260	7	2	35	17	33	4	2	150	650	330	—	5
Cafe Classics Country Vegetables & Beef	1 pkg (9 oz)	210	4	1	25	11	33	9	3	40	590	610	—	6
Cafe Classics Fiesta Chicken	1 pkg (9.25 oz)	270	5	1	30	17	40	3	3	40	690	680	—	24
Cafe Classics Glazed Chicken	1 pkg (8.5 oz)	240	6	1	55	22	25	7	0	0	480	340	—	4
Cafe Classics Glazed Turkey Tenderloins	1 pkg (9 oz)	260	5	1	25	14	41	20	4	100	640	560	—	0
Cafe Classics Grilled Chicken	1 pkg (9.4 oz)	250	5	2	40	22	29	6	3	100	690	700	—	18
Cafe Classics Grilled Chicken Salsa	1 pkg (8.9 oz)	270	7	3	45	15	36	6	4	100	570	480	—	5
Cafe Classics Herb Roasted Chicken	1 pkg (8 oz)	190	4	1	35	17	22	6	4	60	690	630	—	27
Cafe Classics Honey Mustard Chicken	1 pkg (8 oz)	270	4	1	35	19	40	8	1	60	690	400	—	6
Cafe Classics Honey Roasted Chicken	1 pkg (8.5 oz)	270	6	2	25	13	41	13	5	20	550	730	—	9
Cafe Classics Honey Roasted Pork	1 serv (9.5 oz)	250	6	3	45	17	32	11	3	20	590	890	—	15
Cafe Classics Meatloaf w/ Whipped Potatoes	1 pkg (9.4 oz)	260	7	4	45	20	28	5	4	80	600	920	—	0

FOOD	PORTION	CALS	FAT	SAT FAT	CHOL	PROT	CARB	SUGAR	FIBER	CALCI	SOD	POTAS	FOLIC	VIT C
LEAN CUISINE (CONT.)														
Cafe Classics Oriental Beef	1 pkg (9.25 oz)	210	4	2	25	14	30	8	2	20	530	650	—	4
Cafe Classics Oven Roasted Beef	1 pkg (9.25 oz)	260	8	3	50	18	28	7	4	150	590	670	—	15
Cafe Classics Roasted Turkey Breast	1 pkg (9.75 oz)	270	2	1	25	13	49	27	3	40	590	350	—	54
Cafe Classics Salisbury Steak	1 pkg (9.5 oz)	280	8	4	60	24	29	2	4	150	590	600	—	0
Cafe Classics Sirloin Beef Peppercorn	1 pkg (8.75 oz)	220	7	2	35	15	23	6	2	80	580	770	—	0
Cafe Classics Southern Beef Tips	1 pkg (8.75 oz)	270	6	3	35	16	37	10	4	40	480	1080	—	4
Everyday Favorites Chicken Florentine	1 pkg (8 oz)	220	5	2	25	13	32	3	3	100	640	510	—	0
Everyday Favorites Chicken Chow Mein	1 pkg (9 oz)	240	4	1	35	14	37	3	3	40	590	300	—	0
Everyday Favorites Homestyle Turkey	1 pkg (9.4 oz)	240	5	1	40	22	27	6	3	150	590	590	—	1
Everyday Favorites Hunan Beef & Broccoli	1 pkg (8.5 oz)	240	4	1	20	11	40	9	2	20	690	580	—	6
Everyday Favorites Mandarin Chicken	1 pkg (9 oz)	260	5	1	35	15	38	9	2	20	570	370	—	18
Everyday Favorites Roasted Chicken	1 pkg (8.1 oz)	260	7	3	20	14	34	3	4	80	640	410	—	1
Everyday Favorites Stuffed Cabbage	1 pkg (9.5 oz)	210	8	4	20	9	25	4	5	60	590	460	—	4
Everyday Favorites Swedish Meatballs	1 pkg (9.1 oz)	290	7	3	45	22	35	4	4	80	590	600	—	0
Everyday Favorites Vegetable Lasagna	1 pkg (10.5 oz)	260	7	3	20	15	36	9	5	350	590	530	—	9
Hearty Portions Cheese & Spinach Manicotti	1 serv	370	8	2	35	25	50	14	8	400	850	990	—	48
Hearty Portions Chicken & Barbecue Sauce	1 serv	370	6	1	40	20	60	31	6	40	840	1190	—	12
Hearty Portions Homestyle Beef Stroganoff	1 serv	350	9	3	30	23	44	12	9	200	850	1160	—	12

FOOD	PORTION	CALS	FAT	SAT FAT	CHOL	PROT	CARB	SUGAR	FIBER	CALCI	SOD	POTAS	FOLIC	VIT C
LEAN CUISINE (CONT.)														
Hearty Portions Jumbo Rigatoni w/ Meatballs	1 serv	440	9	4	35	25	64	12	7	200	820	1150	—	24
Hearty Portions Oriental Glazed Chicken	1 serv	370	2	1	35	21	66	12	4	60	850	870	—	27
Hearty Portions Roasted Chicken w/ Mushrooms	1 serv	330	4	1	40	23	49	5	4	100	740	720	—	48
Skillet Sensations Beef Teriyaki & Rice	1 serv	280	3	1	25	14	48	11	5	40	700	—	—	18
Skillet Sensations Chicken Primavera	1 serv	320	5	2	30	20	50	7	4	100	790	—	—	51
Skillet Sensations Chicken Oriental	1 serv	280	3	1	15	17	46	10	6	60	790	—	—	24
Skillet Sensations Fiesta Beef & Rice	1 serv	300	4	2	25	19	48	6	6	60	760	—	—	30
Skillet Sensations Garlic Chicken	1 serv	340	5	2	20	20	56	6	4	40	730	—	—	54
Skillet Sensations Herb Chicken & Roasted Potatoes	1 serv	270	5	2	40	18	39	10	5	150	790	—	—	18
Skillet Sensations Roasted Turkey	1 serv	220	2	1	25	14	37	10	6	60	790	—	—	60
Skillet Sensations Savory Beef & Vegetables	1 serv	290	7	3	35	18	38	9	9	100	1440	—	—	9
Skillet Sensations Three Cheese Chicken	1 serv	370	10	4	50	26	45	9	3	250	820	—	—	3
LUZIANNE														
Cajun Creole Dirty Rice	1 serv	160	1	0	0	4	35	0	0	40	680	—	—	0
Cajun Creole Etouffee	1 serv	200	1	0	0	5	42	2	1	20	1030	—	—	2
Cajun Creole Gumbo	1 serv	160	1	0	0	4	33	3	1	20	760	—	—	2
Cajun Creole Jambalaya	1 serv	200	1	0	0	5	43	0	1	20	690	—	—	2
MARIE CALLENDER'S														
Beef Stroganoff w/ Noodles	1 meal (13 oz)	600	27	11	70	20	59	9	4	60	1140	—	—	0
Beef Tips In Mushroom Sauce	1 meal (13 oz)	430	19	7	50	25	39	11	6	60	1020	—	—	9

FOOD	PORTION	CALS	FAT	SAT FAT	CHOL	PROT	CARB	SUGAR	FIBER	CALCI	SOD	POTAS	FOLIC	VIT C
MARIE CALLENDER'S (CONT.)														
Breaded Chicken Parmigiana	1 meal (16 oz)	860	32	8	50	30	63	18	5	20	920	—	—	4
Breaded Fish w/ Mac & Cheese	1 meal (12 oz)	550	28	9	60	22	53	12	3	300	1400	—	—	24
Cheesy Rice w/ Chicken & Broccoli	1 meal (12 oz)	390	13	9	55	24	44	8	6	350	1220	—	—	30
Chicken & Dumplings	1 meal (14 oz)	390	20	10	130	17	34	14	4	60	1650	—	—	5
Chicken & Noodles	1 meal (13 oz)	520	30	11	80	21	42	7	5	100	1320	—	—	9
Chicken Cordon Bleu	1 meal (13 oz)	610	28	9	75	23	58	9	6	200	1920	—	—	18
Chicken Fried Beef Steak & Gravy	1 meal (15 oz)	650	37	13	50	20	50	9	7	100	2260	—	—	24
Chicken Teriyaki	1 meal (13 oz)	510	12	3	55	24	71	22	2	60	1510	—	—	42
Country Fried Chicken & Gravy	1 meal (16 oz)	620	30	9	75	24	63	16	6	40	2300	—	—	4
Country Fried Pork Chop	1 meal (15 oz)	540	28	9	65	23	50	23	8	100	2240	—	—	6
Escalloped Noodles & Chicken	1 meal (13 oz)	740	46	16	90	21	60	10	5	150	1600	—	—	0
Glazed Chicken	1 meal (13 oz)	490	25	11	90	25	40	2	1	40	2130	—	—	2
Grilled Southwestern Style Chicken	1 meal (14 oz)	410	11	6	80	24	43	9	6	150	2020	—	—	4
Grilled Chicken & Mashed Potatoes	1 meal (10 oz)	340	16	6	90	24	20	2	1	20	1090	—	—	0
Grilled Chicken Breast & Rice Pilaf	1 meal (11.75 oz)	360	14	4	10	20	36	14	4	20	1070	—	—	1
Grilled Chicken In Mushroom Sauce	1 meal (14 oz)	480	15	6	65	32	54	0	7	80	1030	—	—	54
Grilled Turkey Breast & Rice Pilaf	1 meal (11.75 oz)	310	10	4	40	22	34	8	4	60	940	—	—	0
Herb Roasted Chicken & Mashed Potatoes	1 meal (14 oz)	580	34	16	205	42	26	16	7	60	2100	—	—	36
Homestyle Turkey & Noodles	1 meal (12 oz)	600	35	18	90	18	52	12	5	100	1570	—	—	0
Honey Roasted Chicken	1 meal (14 oz)	440	17	7	110	45	27	7	7	100	1170	—	—	12

FOOD	PORTION	CALS	FAT	SAT FAT	CHOL	PROT	CARB	SUGAR	FIBER	CALCI	SOD	POTAS	FOLIC	VIT C
MARIE CALLENDER'S (CONT.)														
Honey Smoked Ham Steak w/ Macaroni & Cheese	1 meal (14 oz)	490	13	7	80	29	63	32	5	40	2310	—	—	12
Meatloaf & Gravy w/ Mashed Potatoes	1 meal (14 oz)	540	30	12	95	23	42	30	5	60	1570	—	—	0
Old Fashioned Beef Pot Roast & Gravy	1 meal (15 oz)	500	17	6	110	23	55	13	3	40	1460	—	—	0
Roast Beef	1 meal (14.5 oz)	390	19	8	70	24	30	7	11	80	1240	—	—	12
Sirloin Salisbury Steak & Gravy	1 meal (14 oz)	550	25	11	85	30	51	14	6	250	1660	—	—	4
Skillet Meal Au Gratin Potatoes	⅔ cup (5 oz)	190	10	7	30	7	19	4	2	150	400	—	—	4
Skillet Meal Beef Pot Roast	½ pkg	290	9	4	60	20	33	5	5	40	1200	—	—	0
Skillet Meal Beef Stroganoff	½ pkg	310	11	7	60	21	31	7	5	60	1290	—	—	0
Skillet Meal Chicken & Rice w/ Broccoli & Cheese	½ pkg	440	14	10	70	30	47	5	8	300	1450	—	—	18
Skillet Meal Chicken Teriyaki	½ pkg	340	1	1	30	21	61	14	5	40	1140	—	—	12
Skillet Meal Herb Chicken	½ pkg	290	4	2	35	22	42	1	5	40	1030	—	—	12
Skillet Meal Roasted Chicken & Vegetables	½ pkg	260	6	2	40	21	30	1	7	40	1020	—	—	12
Skillet Meal White & Wild Rice In Cheese Sauce	1 cup	300	13	8	35	11	35	7	2	200	750	—	—	12
Swedish Meatballs	1 meal (12.5 oz)	520	26	12	65	28	44	3	3	40	1020	—	—	0
Sweet & Sour Chicken	1 meal (14 oz)	570	15	3	40	23	66	55	7	40	700	—	—	0
Turkey w/ Gravy & Dressing	1 meal (14 oz)	500	19	9	80	31	52	11	4	100	2040	—	—	24
MORTON														
Breaded Chicken Pattie	1 meal (6.75 oz)	290	17	4	35	10	24	12	4	20	840	—	—	0
Chicken Nuggets	1 meal (7 oz)	340	19	5	30	12	31	12	2	40	470	—	—	2

FOOD	PORTION	CALS	FAT	SAT FAT	CHOL	PROT	CARB	SUGAR	FIBER	CALCI	SOD	POTAS	FOLIC	VIT C
MORTON (CONT.)														
Chili Gravy w/ Beef Enchilada & Tamale	1 meal (10 oz)	270	9	4	10	7	40	3	7	80	1000	—	—	6
Fried Chicken	1 meal (9 oz)	470	30	10	90	20	30	4	3	40	1100	—	—	6
Gravy & Charbroiled Beef Patty	1 meal (9 oz)	310	18	9	20	10	26	3	5	40	1210	—	—	2
Gravy & Salisbury Steak	1 meal (9 oz)	310	20	8	30	7	24	7	3	40	1100	—	—	1
Gravy & Turkey w/ Stuffing	1 meal (9 oz)	240	10	4	40	10	27	5	4	40	1200	—	—	0
Tomato Sauce w/ Meat Loaf	1 meal (9 oz)	250	13	5	20	9	24	17	3	40	1200	—	—	0
Veal Parmagiana w/ Tomato Sauce	1 meal (8.75 oz)	290	15	5	25	8	30	8	4	40	950	—	—	18
NATURE'S CHOICE														
Broccoli Parmesan Alfredo	1 pkg (12 oz)	270	9	3	10	20	29	4	5	250	960	—	—	36
NATURE'S ENTREE														
Hearty Stew	1 pkg (12 oz)	290	9	3	10	18	34	6	3	40	960	—	—	2
Tuscany White Bean	1 pkg (12 oz)	330	8	2	5	21	42	4	4	450	920	—	—	9
PATIO														
Ranchera	1 pkg (13 oz)	470	22	10	35	13	55	4	9	100	2470	—	—	1
STOUFFER'S														
Baked Chicken Breast w/ Mashed Potatoes	1 serv (12.2 oz)	330	14	5	60	25	25	2	3	20	1070	716	—	2
Beef Stroganoff	1 pkg (9.75 oz)	390	20	7	85	23	30	2	2	40	1100	610	—	0
Chicken À La King	1 pkg (9.5 oz)	350	13	4	40	17	41	5	2	100	800	310	—	6
Creamed Chicken	1 pkg (6.5 oz)	260	19	10	80	15	8	5	0	60	680	290	—	0
Creamed Chipped Beef	½ cup (5.5 oz)	160	11	3	40	10	6	5	1	100	690	240	—	0
Creamy Chicken & Broccoli	1 pkg (8.9 oz)	320	15	5	60	19	26	7	2	200	820	400	—	9
Escalloped Chicken & Noodles	1 pkg (10 oz)	430	27	5	50	17	30	4	3	100	1120	330	—	0
Fish w/ Macaroni & Cheese	1 serv (9.5 oz)	460	20	6	55	22	47	8	2	250	970	379	—	4
Glazed Chicken w/ Rice	1 serv (11.8 oz)	290	6	1	45	21	39	9	2	20	810	349	—	0
Green Pepper Steak	1 pkg (10.5 oz)	330	9	3	35	17	45	4	3	20	650	680	—	12

FOOD	PORTION	CALS	FAT	SAT FAT	CHOL	PROT	CARB	SUGAR	FIBER	CALCI	SOD	POTAS	FOLIC	VIT C
STOUFFER'S (CONT.)														
Homestyle Baked Chicken & Gravy & Whipped Potatoes	1 pkg (8.9 oz)	270	12	3	75	22	19	1	2	20	750	570	—	1
Homestyle Beef Pot Roast & Browned Potatoes	1 pkg (8.9 oz)	250	8	3	35	16	29	3	4	20	780	730	—	21
Homestyle Fish Filet w/ Macaroni & Cheese	1 pkg (9 oz)	430	21	5	70	24	37	7	2	150	930	450	—	0
Homestyle Fried Chicken & Whipped Potatoes	1 pkg (7.5 oz)	310	12	4	45	17	33	1	5	20	680	430	—	1
Homestyle Meatloaf & Whipped Potatoes	1 pkg (9.9 oz)	330	16	6	70	20	26	4	3	40	850	510	—	0
Homestyle Roast Turkey w/ w/ Gravy Stuffing & Whipped Potatoes	1 pkg (9.6 oz)	320	13	4	50	19	31	4	3	40	950	410	—	0
Homestyle Salisbury Steak & Gravy & Macaroni & Cheese	1 pkg (9.6 oz)	350	16	7	70	24	27	2	2	150	1290	320	—	0
Meatloaf	1 serv (5.5 oz)	210	12	4	60	16	9	1	1	40	520	250	—	0
Meatloaf w/ Whipped Potatoes	1 serv (11.5 oz)	380	18	7	70	22	33	3	4	60	950	551	—	4
Stuffed Pepper	1 pkg (10 oz)	200	5	2	20	11	27	8	3	20	820	470	—	48
Swedish Meatballs	1 pkg (10.25 oz)	480	24	9	60	24	43	2	3	60	960	330	—	0
SWANSON														
Beef Pot Roast	1 pkg (14 oz)	320	8	3	35	19	44	15	4	60	1200	—	—	15
Chicken Parmigiana w/ Spaghetti	1 pkg (11 oz)	380	17	4	25	17	41	18	5	250	700	—	—	24
Turkey Breast & Stuffing Dinner	1 pkg (11.7 oz)	350	11	3	35	15	43	18	4	40	1080	—	—	6
TAMARIND TREE														
Alu Chole	1 pkg (9.2 oz)	350	6	1	0	12	63	3	9	80	620	—	—	12
Channa Dal Masala	1 pkg (9.2 oz)	340	5	1	0	13	62	4	10	80	700	—	—	12
Dal Makhini	1 pkg (9.2 oz)	330	6	2	5	14	55	3	14	100	670	—	—	2

FOOD	PORTION	CALS	FAT	SAT FAT	CHOL	PROT	CARB	SUGAR	FIBER	CALCI	SOD	POTAS	FOLIC	VIT C
TAMARIND TREE (CONT.)														
Dhingri Mutter	1 pkg (9.2 oz)	290	5	1	0	8	53	6	7	60	680	—	—	9
Navratan Korma	1 pkg (9.2 oz)	430	15	4	5	12	60	7	7	100	700	—	—	9
Palak Paneer	1 pkg (9.2 oz)	380	15	6	35	14	46	6	6	350	640	—	—	9
Saag Chole	1 pkg (9.2 oz)	370	10	2	0	14	55	2	13	200	800	—	—	12
Vegetable Jalfrazi	1 pkg (9.2 oz)	310	6	1	0	8	57	7	7	80	600	—	—	9
TYSON														
BBQ Chicken Potato & Vegetable Medley	1 pkg (14.7 oz)	560	21	5	30	19	73	23	9	60	1190	—	—	6
Beef Stir Fry	1 pkg (14 oz)	430	5	2	45	26	70	25	4	40	1560	—	—	24
Blackened Chicken Spanish Rice & Corn	1 pkg (8.8 oz)	260	5	1	30	17	36	5	4	60	480	—	—	6
Chicken Primavera	1 pkg (11.3 oz)	350	6	3	30	25	48	4	5	150	610	—	—	24
Chicken Divan Candied Carrots & Pasta	1 pkg (9.8 oz)	370	15	4	50	20	38	8	2	100	530	—	—	6
Chicken Français Sliced Potatoes & Green Beans	1 pkg (8.8 oz)	260	10	3	45	19	23	5	6	150	790	—	—	18
Chicken Kiev Rice Pilaf & Broccoli Carrots	1 pkg (9.1 oz)	440	25	11	85	18	36	4	2	40	900	—	—	9
Chicken Marsala Carrots & Red Potatoes	1 pkg (8.8 oz)	180	5	2	30	15	19	6	4	40	520	—	—	1
Chicken Mesquite Corn & Pea Medley & Au Gratin Potatoes	1 pkg (8.8 oz)	320	8	3	25	18	44	11	4	100	780	—	—	0
Chicken Picatta	1 pkg (8.8 oz)	190	6	2	35	17	18	1	5	40	500	—	—	9
Chicken Stir Fry Kit	2¾ cups (14 oz)	430	5	1	45	24	73	24	5	40	1700	—	—	30
Chicken w/ Broccoli & Cheese Carrots & Pasta	1 pkg (8.8 oz)	270	12	5	40	20	19	5	3	100	690	—	—	0
Chicken w/ Mushroom Sauce Rice Pilaf & Candied Carrots	1 pkg (8.8 oz)	220	6	2	30	15	27	8	2	80	510	—	—	4
Chicken w/ Tabasco BBQ Sauce	1 pkg (8.8 oz)	260	7	2	25	13	37	11	5	100	610	—	—	0

FOOD	PORTION	CALS	FAT	SAT FAT	CHOL	PROT	CARB	SUGAR	FIBER	CALCI	SOD	POTAS	FOLIC	VIT C
TYSON (CONT.)														
Fried Chicken & Gravy w/ Mashed Potatoes & Corn	1 pkg (10.8 oz)	360	15	3	30	16	39	4	4	60	840	—	—	5
Grilled Chicken Corn O'Brien & Ranch Beans	1 pkg (8.8 oz)	230	4	1	30	19	30	4	7	40	590	—	—	6
Grilled Italian Chicken Pasta & Vegetable Medley	1 pkg (8.8 oz)	190	4	2	30	21	19	3	3	80	440	—	—	2
Honey Dijon Chicken Pasta & Pea Medley	1 pkg (11.3 oz)	340	7	2	25	20	49	5	6	100	900	—	—	2
Roasted Chicken w/ Garlic Sauce Pasta & Vegetable Medley	1 pkg (8.8 oz)	210	7	2	25	17	20	2	3	40	460	—	—	15
WEIGHT WATCHERS														
Smart One Grilled Salisbury Steak	1 pkg (8.5 oz)	250	9	4	40	18	24	3	3	150	620	—	—	0
Smart Ones Chicken Mirabella	1 pkg (9.2 oz)	180	2	1	20	11	30	4	4	60	480	—	—	9
Smart Ones Fiesta Chicken	1 pkg (8.5 oz)	210	2	1	25	13	35	5	5	40	570	—	—	12
Smart Ones Honey Mustard Chicken	1 pkg (8.5 oz)	200	2	1	30	11	35	10	3	40	370	—	—	12
Smart Ones Lemon Herb Chicken Piccata	1 pkg (8.5 oz)	190	2	1	25	11	33	5	3	20	460	—	—	1
Smart Ones Pepper Steak	1 pkg (10 oz)	240	5	2	35	18	32	4	4	40	690	—	—	12
Smart Ones Risotto w/ Cheese & Mushrooms	1 pkg (10 oz)	290	7	3	20	11	47	7	4	200	540	—	—	12
Smart Ones Roast Turkey Medallions & Mushrooms	1 pkg (8.5 oz)	180	2	1	20	11	30	3	2	20	530	—	—	5
Smart Ones Shrimp Marinara	1 pkg (9 oz)	180	2	1	40	9	31	4	4	100	570	—	—	4
Smart Ones Stuffed Turkey Breast	1 pkg (10 oz)	260	7	2	30	13	37	14	5	80	680	—	—	6
Smart Ones Swedish Meatballs	1 pkg (9 oz)	280	70	4	30	19	34	2	3	150	690	—	—	1
YVES														
Veggie Country Stew	1 pkg (10.5 oz)	170	0	0	0	17	24	2	7	50	1020	510	—	18

DIP

FOOD	PORTION	CALS	FAT	SAT FAT	CHOL	PROT	CARB	SUGAR	FIBER	CALCI	SOD	POTAS	FOLIC	VIT C
BREAKSTONE'S														
Bacon & Onion	2 tbsp (1.1 oz)	60	5	3	20	2	2	1	0	20	180	50	—	0
Chesapeake Clam	2 tbsp (1.1 oz)	50	4	3	20	1	1	tr	0	20	180	30	—	0
Free Creamy Salsa	2 tbsp (1.1 oz)	20	0	0	<5	1	3	2	0	60	240	85	—	0
Free French Onion	2 tbsp (1.1 oz)	25	0	0	<5	2	4	2	0	40	260	85	—	0
Free Ranch	2 tbsp (1.1 oz)	25	0	0	<5	2	4	2	0	60	330	85	—	0
French Onion	2 tbsp (1.1 oz)	50	5	3	20	1	2	1	0	20	160	45	—	0
Toasted Onion	2 tbsp (1.1 oz)	50	5	3	20	1	2	1	0	20	170	45	—	0
CABOT														
Bac'n Horseradish	2 tbsp	50	5	3	15	1	1	tr	0	40	190	—	—	0
Clam	2 tbsp	50	5	3	15	1	1	0	0	20	120	—	—	0
French Onion	2 tbsp	50	5	—	15	1	1	1	0	20	190	—	—	0
Ranch	1 tbsp	50	5	3	15	1	1	1	0	40	160	—	—	0
Salsa Grande	2 tbsp	50	5	3	15	1	1	1	0	40	130	—	—	1
Veggie	2 tbsp	50	5	3	15	1	2	1	0	20	125	—	—	0
CHEEZ WHIZ														
Medium Cheese & Salsa	2 tbsp (1.2 oz)	100	8	5	20	3	3	2	0	80	490	95	—	0
Mild Cheese & Salsa	2 tbsp (1.2 oz)	100	8	5	20	3	3	2	0	80	490	95	—	0
CHI-CHI'S														
Fiesta Bean	2 tbsp (0.9 oz)	35	2	1	0	1	4	0	1	0	140	—	—	0
Fiesta Cheese	2 tbsp (0.9 oz)	40	3	1	10	1	3	1	0	20	270	—	—	0
FRITOS														
Bean	2 tbsp (1.2 oz)	40	1	1	0	2	6	0	0	—	140	—	—	—
Chili Cheese	1.2 oz	45	3	1	<5	1	3	1	0	—	310	—	—	—
French Onion	2 tbsp (1.1 oz)	60	5	3	15	1	4	1	0	—	230	—	—	—
Hot Bean	2 tbsp (1.2 oz)	40	1	0	0	2	5	0	1	—	170	—	—	—
Jalapeño & Cheddar Cheese	2 tbsp (1.2 oz)	50	4	1	5	1	4	2	0	—	300	—	—	—
GRINGO BILLY'S														
Guacamole Mix	1 tsp	10	0	0	0	0	2	0	1	—	40	—	—	—
GUILTLESS GOURMET														
Black Bean Mild	2 tbsp	30	0	0	0	2	5	1	2	30	115	—	—	0
Black Bean Spicy	2 tbsp	30	0	0	0	2	5	0	2	20	110	—	—	0
KNUDSEN														
Free Creamy Salsa	2 tbsp (1.1 oz)	20	0	0	<5	1	3	2	0	60	240	85	—	0
Free French Onion	2 tbsp (1.1 oz)	25	0	0	<5	2	4	2	0	40	260	85	—	0
Free Ranch	2 tbsp (1.1 oz)	25	0	0	<5	2	4	2	0	60	330	85	—	0
KRAFT														
Avocado	2 tbsp (1.1 oz)	60	4	3	0	1	4	tr	0	0	240	25	—	0
Bacon & Horseradish	2 tbsp (1.1 oz)	60	5	3	0	1	3	tr	0	0	220	25	—	0

FOOD	PORTION	CALS	FAT	SAT FAT	CHOL	PROT	CARB	SUGAR	FIBER	CALCI	SOD	POTAS	FOLIC	VIT C
KRAFT (CONT.)														
Clam	2 tbsp (1.1 oz)	60	4	3	0	1	3	tr	0	0	250	20	—	0
Free French Onion	2 tbsp (1.1 oz)	25	0	0	<5	2	4	2	0	40	260	85	—	0
Free Ranch	2 tbsp (1.1 oz)	25	0	0	<5	2	4	2	0	60	330	85	—	0
Free Salsa	2 tbsp (1.1 oz)	20	0	0	<5	1	3	2	0	60	240	85	—	0
French Onion	2 tbsp (1.1 oz)	60	4	3	0	1	4	tr	0	0	230	25	—	0
Green Onion	2 tbsp (1.1 oz)	60	4	3	0	1	4	tr	0	0	190	20	—	0
Jalapeño Cheese	2 tbsp (1.1 oz)	60	4	3	0	1	3	tr	0	0	260	25	—	0
Premium Sour Cream	2 tbsp (1.1 oz)	50	4	3	20	1	1	1	0	20	180	30	—	0
Premium Sour Cream Bacon & Horseradish	2 tbsp (1.1 oz)	60	5	3	15	2	2	1	0	20	240	45	—	0
Premium Sour Cream Bacon & Onion	2 tbsp (1.1 oz)	60	5	3	20	2	2	1	0	20	180	50	—	0
Premium Sour Cream Creamy Onion	2 tbsp (1.1 oz)	45	4	3	15	1	2	1	0	20	160	40	—	0
Premium Sour Cream French Onion	2 tbsp (1.1 oz)	45	4	3	15	tr	2	1	0	20	160	40	—	0
Premium Sour Cream Ranch	2 tbsp (1.1 oz)	50	4	3	15	tr	2	1	0	20	230	40	—	0
Ranch	2 tbsp (1.1 oz)	60	5	3	0	1	3	tr	0	0	210	20	—	0
RACQUET														
Hot Cheddar Jalapeño	2 tbsp	30	3	1	0	0	1	0	0	—	270	—	—	—
RUFFLES														
French Onion	2 tbsp	70	5	1	0	1	4	tr	1	—	240	—	—	—
Ranch	2 tbsp (1.2 oz)	70	6	1	0	1	4	0	0	—	300	—	—	—
SNYDER'S OF HANOVER														
Microwavable Hot Nacho	2 tbsp	48	3	1	3	1	5	2	0	20	270	—	—	0
Microwavable Mild Cheese	2 tbsp	45	3	2	5	2	2	1	0	40	250	—	—	0
Mustard Pretzel	2 tbsp	60	2	0	0	1	12	11	0	0	0	—	—	0
Sour Cream & Onion	2 tbsp	60	5	3	15	1	2	1	0	20	220	—	—	0
TACO BELL														
Fat Free Black Bean	2 tbsp (1.2 oz)	30	0	0	0	2	6	tr	2	0	220	—	—	0
Salsa Con Queso Medium	2 tbsp (1.2 oz)	45	3	1	<5	tr	5	tr	tr	20	270	—	—	0
Salsa Con Queso Mild	2 tbsp (1.2 oz)	45	3	1	<5	tr	5	tr	tr	20	270	—	—	0

FOOD	PORTION	CALS	FAT	SAT FAT	CHOL	PROT	CARB	SUGAR	FIBER	CALCI	SOD	POTAS	FOLIC	VIT C
TYSON														
Bleu Cheese For Dipping Wings	2 tbsp (1.4 oz)	140	14	3	25	1	3	1	1	40	370	—	—	0
UTZ														
Fat Free Sour Cream & Onion	2 tbsp (1.1 oz)	30	0	0	0	1	7	3	0	0	210	—	—	0
Jalapeño & Cheddar	2 tbsp (1 oz)	30	3	1	0	0	2	0	0	0	250	—	—	0
Low Fat Desert Garden	2 tbsp (1.1 oz)	40	2	0	0	1	5	2	0	0	210	—	—	0
Low Fat Salsa Con Queso	2 tbsp (1 oz)	40	2	0	0	1	5	2	0	20	240	—	—	0
Mild Cheddar	2 tbsp (1 oz)	45	3	2	5	2	2	1	0	40	250	—	—	0
Sour Cream & Onion	2 tbsp (1 oz)	60	5	3	15	1	2	1	0	20	220	—	—	0
WALDEN FARMS														
Low Carb Bruschetta	2 tbsp	35	3	—	0	0	0	1	0	—	90	—	—	—
Low Carb Pesto Bruschetta	1 tsp	10	1	—	0	0	9	9	0	—	20	—	—	—
DOCK														
fresh cooked	3½ oz	20	1	—	0	2	3	—	—	38	3	321	—	26
raw chopped	½ cup	15	tr	—	0	1	2	—	—	29	3	261	—	32
DOLPHINFISH														
fresh baked	3 oz	93	1	tr	80	20	0	—	—	—	96	453	—	—
fresh fillet baked	5.6 oz	174	1	tr	149	38	0	—	—	—	179	848	—	—
DOUGHNUTS														
cake type unsugared	1 (1.6 oz)	198	11	2	18	2	23	—	1	21	257	60	4	—
chocolate glazed	1 (1.5 oz)	175	8	3	—	2	24	—	1	89	143	—	—	—
chocolate sugared	1 (1.5 oz)	175	8	3	—	2	24	—	1	89	143	—	—	—
chocolate coated	1 (1.5 oz)	204	13	4	—	2	21	—	1	15	185	—	—	—
creme filled	1 (3 oz)	307	21	6	20	6	26	—	—	22	262	68	—	—
french cruller glazed	1 (1.4 oz)	169	8	2	5	1	24	—	—	11	142	32	—	—
frosted	1 (1.5 oz)	204	13	4	—	2	21	—	1	15	185	—	—	—
honey bun	1 (2.1 oz)	242	14	3	4	4	27	—	1	26	205	65	13	—
jelly	1 (3 oz)	289	16	4	22	5	33	—	—	21	249	67	—	—
old fashioned	1 (1.6 oz)	198	11	2	18	2	23	—	1	21	257	60	4	—
sugared	1 (1.6 oz)	192	10	3	14	2	23	—	1	27	181	46	—	—
wheat glazed	1 (1.6 oz)	162	9	1	9	3	19	—	—	22	160	66	—	—
wheat sugared	1 (1.6 oz)	162	9	1	9	3	19	—	—	22	160	66	—	—
yeast glazed	1 (2.1 oz)	242	14	3	4	4	27	—	1	26	205	65	13	—

FOOD	PORTION	CALS	FAT	SAT FAT	CHOL	PROT	CARB	SUGAR	FIBER	CALCI	SOD	POTAS	FOLIC	VIT C
DOLLY MADISON														
Chocolate Frosted	1 (1.1 oz)	140	8	5	5	1	15	9	1	0	130	—	—	0
Donut Gems Chocolate	4 (2 oz)	260	15	9	10	3	28	17	1	20	230	—	—	0
Donut Gems Crunch	3 (2 oz)	220	10	4	10	3	31	21	0	40	250	—	—	0
Donut Gems Powdered	4 (2 oz)	230	11	5	15	3	30	14	0	20	260	—	—	0
English Cruller	1 (2 oz)	250	14	6	30	2	31	11	1	40	190	—	—	0
Glazed Whirl	1 (1.6 oz)	210	11	5	25	2	25	9	0	40	150	—	—	0
Glazed Yeast	1 (1.5 oz)	190	9	5	10	2	23	6	0	0	130	—	—	0
Old Fashioned	1 (2.1 oz)	280	16	8	20	4	28	23	0	40	360	—	—	0
Plain	1 (1.2 oz)	140	7	3	10	2	15	3	0	0	190	—	—	0
Powdered	1 (1 oz)	120	6	3	10	1	14	7	0	0	140	—	—	0
DUTCH MILL														
Cider	1 (2.1 oz)	240	10	2	15	3	35	23	1	20	220	—	—	0
Cinnamon	1 (1.8 oz)	210	11	5	15	3	26	12	1	20	250	—	—	0
Donut Holes Double-Dipped Chocolate	3 (1.4 oz)	220	16	6	5	2	19	5	0	20	140	—	—	0
Donut Holes Shootin' Stars	3 (1.4 oz)	190	10	3	5	2	23	12	0	40	110	—	—	0
Double-Dipped Chocolate	1 (2.1 oz)	280	17	7	15	3	31	9	1	40	360	—	—	0
Glazed	1 (2.1 oz)	250	12	3	15	3	34	23	1	20	220	—	—	0
Glazed Chocolate	1 (2.4 oz)	270	11	3	15	3	40	10	1	20	380	—	—	0
Plain	1 (1.8 oz)	210	12	5	15	3	25	9	1	20	270	—	—	0
Sugared	1 (1.8 oz)	220	11	5	15	3	27	12	1	20	260	—	—	0
ENTENMANN'S														
Frosted Mini	1 (1 oz)	150	11	3	<5	1	12	7	tr	0	90	—	—	0
HOSTESS														
Blueberry	1 (1.7 oz)	210	13	6	10	2	21	11	0	0	120	—	—	0
Donettes Crumb	3 (1.5 oz)	170	8	3	10	2	23	16	0	40	190	—	—	0
Donettes Frosted	3 (1.5 oz)	200	12	7	10	2	21	13	0	20	170	—	—	0
Donettes Powdered	3 (1.5 oz)	180	9	3	10	2	23	10	0	20	190	—	—	0
Frosted	1 (1.4 oz)	180	11	7	5	2	19	12	0	0	170	—	—	0
Old Fashioned Glazed	1 (2.1 oz)	260	13	6	25	2	33	14	1	80	220	—	—	0
O's Raspberry Filled	1 (2.2 oz)	230	10	4	5	3	34	17	1	0	230	—	—	0
Plain	1 (1.1 oz)	140	7	3	10	2	15	3	0	0	190	—	—	0
Powdered	1 (1.3 oz)	150	8	4	10	2	19	9	0	0	180	—	—	0
LITTLE DEBBIE														
Donut Sticks	1 (1.6 oz)	210	12	3	10	2	24	15	0	13	150	12	—	0
Mini Powdered	1 pkg (2.5 oz)	290	14	4	10	3	38	19	2	—	290	—	—	—

FOOD	PORTION	CALS	FAT	SAT FAT	CHOL	PROT	CARB	SUGAR	FIBER	CALCI	SOD	POTAS	FOLIC	VIT C
SNACK & SMILE														
Mini Donuts Chocolate	6	370	19	10	10	4	45	23	2	20	350	—	40	0
Mini Donuts Glazed	6	340	16	40	20	3	46	28	tr	80	220	—	40	0
Mini Donuts Powdered Sugar	6	320	13	4	10	4	46	22	1	20	360	—	40	0
SUPER														
Donut Chocolate	1 (2.2 oz)	210	11	3	10	4	26	14	1	150	240	—	200	27
Donut Honey Wheat	1 (2.2 oz)	230	11	2	10	5	29	13	tr	150	260	—	180	18
TASTYKAKE														
Mini Plain Glaze	1 pkg (2.5 oz)	260	11	2	25	3	40	23	1	20	330	—	—	0
Mini Powdered Sugar	1 pkg (2.5 oz)	260	12	2	30	3	38	21	tr	20	360	—	—	0
Mini Rich Frosted	1 pkg (3 oz)	370	22	10	25	5	43	23	3	20	340	—	—	0
TOM'S														
Chocolate Gem	1 pkg (2.5 oz)	320	18	5	10	4	37	19	1	0	430	—	—	0
Dunkin' Sticks	1 pkg (2.5 oz)	370	22	7	10	2	43	20	tr	80	300	—	—	0
Powdered Gems	1 pkg (2.5 oz)	320	18	5	10	3	41	23	1	0	430	—	—	0
DRINK MIXERS														
whiskey sour mix not prep	1 pkg (0.6 oz)	64	0	0	0	tr	16	—	—	45	46	3	0	1
whiskey sour mix	2 oz	55	0	0	0	0	14	—	0	1	66	18	0	2
BAJA BOB'S														
Bloody Mary Mix Lean & Mean	4 oz	20	0	0	0	0	4	3	0	—	420	—	—	—
Piña Colada	4 oz	30	1	0	0	1	4	3	1	0	80	—	—	60
Sugar Free Margarita Mix	4 oz	10	0	0	0	0	tr	0	—	—	80	—	—	—
Sugar Free Margarita Mix Desert Lime	4 oz	10	0	0	0	0	tr	0	0	—	45	—	—	—
Sugar Free Margarita Mix Wild Strawberry	4 oz	10	0	0	0	0	tr	0	—	—	80	—	—	—
Sweet-n-Sour Mix	4 oz	10	0	0	0	0	tr	0	—	—	80	—	—	—
DAILY'S														
Bloody Mary Original	1 serv (6 oz)	50	0	0	0	0	14	14	—	—	1040	—	—	—
Margarita Daiquiri Strawberry	1 serv (4 oz)	180	0	0	0	0	47	45	2	—	65	—	—	—
Margarita Green Demon	1 serv (3 oz)	80	0	0	0	0	19	19	—	—	45	—	—	—
Piña Colada	1 serv (3 oz)	160	2	1	0	0	37	36	1	0	115	—	—	0

FOOD	PORTION	CALS	FAT	SAT FAT	CHOL	PROT	CARB	SUGAR	FIBER	CALCI	SOD	POTAS	FOLIC	VIT C
OCEAN SPRAY														
Bloody Mary Mix	4 oz	40	0	0	0	0	10	4	—	—	950	—	—	0
Margarita Mix	4 oz	160	0	0	0	0	40	28	—	—	35	—	—	0
Sour Mix	4 oz	140	0	0	0	0	34	34	—	—	35	—	—	0
TABASCO														
Bloody Mary Mix	1 serv (8.4 oz)	56	tr	tr	0	2	11	8	1	69	1548	—	—	0
Bloody Mary Mix Extra Spicy	1 serv (8.4 oz)	58	tr	tr	0	3	11	10	2	76	1645	—	—	0

DRUM

FOOD	PORTION	CALS	FAT	SAT FAT	CHOL	PROT	CARB	SUGAR	FIBER	CALCI	SOD	POTAS	FOLIC	VIT C
freshwater fillet baked	5.4 oz	236	10	2	126	35	0	—	—	118	148	543	—	—
freshwater baked	3 oz	130	5	1	70	19	0	—	—	65	82	300	—	—

DUCK

FOOD	PORTION	CALS	FAT	SAT FAT	CHOL	PROT	CARB	SUGAR	FIBER	CALCI	SOD	POTAS	FOLIC	VIT C
w/ skin roasted	1 cup (4.9 oz)	472	40	14	118	27	0	—	0	15	83	286	8	0
w/ skin w/ bone leg roasted	3 oz	184	10	3	97	23	0	—	—	9	94	—	—	1
w/ skin w/o bone breast roasted	3 oz	172	9	2	116	21	0	—	—	7	71	—	—	2
w/o skin roasted	1 cup (4.9 oz)	281	16	6	125	33	0	—	0	17	91	353	14	0
w/o skin w/ bone leg braised	1 cup (6.1 oz)	310	10	2	183	51	0	—	—	17	188	—	—	4
w/o skin w/o bone breast broiled	1 cup (6.1 oz)	244	4	1	249	48	0	—	—	16	183	—	—	6
wild w/ skin raw	½ duck (9.5 oz)	571	41	14	216	47	0	—	—	12	152	672	—	14
wild w/o skin breast raw	½ breast (2.9 oz)	102	4	1	—	16	0	—	—	3	47	222	—	5
GRIMAUD FARMS														
Muscovy Duck Confit	1 serv (3 oz)	170	10	4	95	20	tr	—	—	0	140	—	—	0
MAPLE LEAF FARMS														
Breast Filet	4 oz	360	33	9	60	17	0	0	0	—	370	—	—	—
Leg Quarters	4 oz	420	33	11	90	15	0	0	0	—	95	—	—	—
Orange Breast Filet	4 oz	320	28	8	75	15	1	1	—	—	280	—	—	—

DUMPLING

FOOD	PORTION	CALS	FAT	SAT FAT	CHOL	PROT	CARB	SUGAR	FIBER	CALCI	SOD	POTAS	FOLIC	VIT C
HEALTH IS WEALTH														
Potstickers Chicken Free	2 (1.6 oz)	80	4	1	0	4	11	1	1	20	300	—	—	4
Potstickers Pork Free	2 (1.6 oz)	80	4	1	0	4	11	1	1	20	300	—	—	4
Potstickers Vegetable	2 (1.6 oz)	90	3	1	0	7	11	0	5	20	190	—	—	2
Steamed Dumpling	2 (1.6 oz)	50	2	0	0	7	12	0	1	20	310	—	—	4

FOOD	PORTION	CALS	FAT	SAT FAT	CHOL	PROT	CARB	SUGAR	FIBER	CALCI	SOD	POTAS	FOLIC	VIT C
PEPPERIDGE FARM														
Apple	1 (3 oz)	230	11	3	0	3	30	11	1	0	180	—	—	0
Peach	1 (3 oz)	320	11	3	0	3	50	15	4	0	150	—	—	2
DURIAN														
fresh	3.5 oz	141	2	—	0	3	29	—	—	12	1	601	—	42
EEL														
fresh cooked	1 fillet (5.6 oz)	375	24	5	257	38	0	—	—	41	104	555	—	—
fresh cooked	3 oz	200	13	3	137	20	0	—	—	22	55	297	—	—
raw	3 oz	156	10	2	107	16	0	—	—	17	43	232	—	—
smoked	3.5 oz	330	28	7	—	19	0	0	0	—	—	—	—	—
EGG														
(*see also* EGG DISHES, EGG SUBSTITUTES)														
CHICKEN														
fresh	1	75	5	2	213	6	1	—	—	25	63	60	23	0
frozen	1	75	5	2	213	6	1	—	—	25	63	60	23	0
frozen	1 cup	363	24	8	1033	30	3	—	—	120	307	293	114	0
hard cooked	1	77	5	2	213	6	1	—	—	25	62	63	22	0
hard cooked chopped	1 cup	210	14	4	578	17	2	—	—	68	169	172	60	0
poached	1	74	5	2	212	6	1	—	—	25	140	60	18	0
white only	1 cup	121	0	0	0	26	2	—	—	15	399	346	7	0
white only	1	17	0	0	0	4	tr	—	—	2	55	48	1	0
EGGOLOGY														
100% Organic Egg Whites	¼ cup	30	0	0	0	7	1	—	—	—	100	—	—	—
GOLD CIRCLE FARMS														
Cage Free	1 large	70	5	2	215	6	tr	—	—	20	70	—	—	0
HORIZON ORGANIC														
Medium	1 (1.5 oz)	70	4	2	190	6	1	—	—	20	55	—	—	0
LAND O LAKES														
Brown Extra Large	1 (2 oz)	80	5	2	240	7	1	—	—	20	70	—	—	0
ORGANIC VALLEY														
Brown Extra Large	1 (2.2 oz)	90	6	5	225	8	tr	—	—	20	330	—	—	0
Brown Large	1 (2 oz)	80	6	4	200	7	tr	—	—	20	380	—	—	0
Brown Medium	1 (1.8 oz)	70	5	3	175	6	tr	—	—	0	260	—	—	0
OTHER POULTRY														
duck	1 (2.5 oz)	130	10	3	619	9	1	—	0	45	102	156	56	0
duck 100 year old	1 (1 oz)	49	3	—	173	4	1	—	—	18	154	43	—	—
duck preserved hard core	1 (1.8 oz)	80	6	2	220	6	1	0	0	0	350	—	—	0
duck preserved soft core	1 (1.8 oz)	80	6	2	220	7	1	0	0	0	350	—	—	0
duck salted	1 (1 oz)	54	4	—	184	4	2	—	—	34	769	52	—	—
goose	1 (5 oz)	267	19	5	—	20	2	—	—	—	—	—	—	0

FOOD	PORTION	CALS	FAT	SAT FAT	CHOL	PROT	CARB	SUGAR	FIBER	CALCI	SOD	POTAS	FOLIC	VIT C
quail	1 (9 g)	14	1	tr	76	1	tr	—	—	6	—	—	—	0
turkey	1 (2.7 oz)	135	9	3	737	9	1	—	—	78	—	—	—	0

EGG DISHES

FROZEN

WEIGHT WATCHERS

Handy Ham & Cheese Omelet	1 (4 oz)	220	5	3	30	13	30	7	2	100	440	—	—	2

TAKE-OUT

cheese omelette as prep w/ 2 eggs	1 (6.8 oz)	519	44	—	—	31	tr	—	0	546	—	—	—	tr
deviled	2 halves	145	13	3	280	6	1	—	—	31	180	70	25	0
omelette plain	1 serv (3.5 oz)	172	13	4	350	15	tr	tr	0	63	245	146	30	0
salad	½ cup	307	28	6	562	13	2	—	—	189	565	140	49	0
scotch egg	1 (4.2 oz)	301	21	—	—	14	16	—	2	60	—	—	—	—
scrambled plain	2 (3.3 oz)	199	15	6	400	13	2	—	0	54	211	138	53	3
scrambled w/ whole milk & margarine	1 serv	365	27	8	774	24	5	—	—	157	616	304	66	1
sunny side up	1	91	7	2	211	6	1	—	—	25	162	61	18	0

EGG ROLLS

egg roll wrapper fresh	1	83	tr	tr	3	3	16	—	—	13	162	23	5	0

CHUN KING

Chicken Mini	6	210	9	3	15	6	25	3	2	20	650	—	—	0
Chicken Restaurant Style	1 (3 oz)	190	9	5	20	6	22	4	2	20	550	—	—	1
Pork & Shrimp Mini	6	210	9	3	15	6	27	4	2	20	540	—	—	0
Shrimp Mini	6	190	6	2	10	5	28	3	2	20	730	—	—	0
Shrimp Restaurant Style	1 (3 oz)	180	7	3	15	5	25	6	2	40	490	—	—	0

HEALTH IS WEALTH

Broccoli	1 (3 oz)	150	5	1	5	4	23	0	2	60	560	—	—	9
Oriental Vegetable	1 (3 oz)	160	4	1	0	4	23	0	2	40	390	—	—	4
Oriental Chicken Free	1 (3 oz)	120	4	1	0	8	21	0	2	100	390	—	—	6
Pizza	1 (3 oz)	200	9	1	0	7	23	0	3	100	470	—	—	6
Spinach	1 (3 oz)	180	8	1	0	7	20	0	3	100	300	—	—	9
Spring Rolls	1 (1.6 oz)	70	2	1	0	2	10	0	5	20	200	—	—	2
Veggie	1 (3 oz)	130	4	0	0	4	21	0	3	20	550	—	—	9

LA CHOY

Chicken Mini	6	210	9	3	15	6	25	3	2	20	650	—	—	0
Chicken Restaurant Style	1 (3 oz)	210	9	5	15	6	25	4	2	20	550	—	—	1
Pork Restaurant Style	1 (3 oz)	220	11	3	10	5	24	6	2	20	390	—	—	0

FOOD	PORTION	CALS	FAT	SAT FAT	CHOL	PROT	CARB	SUGAR	FIBER	CALCI	SOD	POTAS	FOLIC	VIT C
LA CHOY (CONT.)														
Pork & Shrimp Bite Size	12	210	10	3	10	6	25	3	2	20	540	—	—	0
Pork & Shrimp Mini	6	210	9	3	15	6	27	4	2	20	540	—	—	0
Shrimp Mini	6	190	6	2	10	5	28	3	2	20	730	—	—	0
Shrimp Restaurant Style	1 (3 oz)	180	7	2	15	5	25	6	2	40	490	—	—	0
Sweet & Sour Chicken Restaurant Style	1 (3 oz)	220	9	2	15	6	29	10	2	20	550	—	—	2
Vegetable w/ Lobster Mini	6	190	7	2	5	5	27	3	2	0	440	—	—	1
LOOMPYA														
Lumpia Chicken & Vegetables	2	170	1	0	10	8	31	1	2	20	150	—	—	4
PAGODA														
Sweet & Sour Chicken	1 (2.7 oz)	170	6	2	5	6	25	5	2	40	260	—	—	6
WORTHINGTON														
Vegetarian Egg Rolls	1 (3 oz)	180	8	2	0	6	20	tr	2	0	380	100	—	0
TAKE-OUT														
chicken	1 (3 oz)	140	4	2	15	7	20	5	4	40	510	—	—	1
lobster	1 (4.8 oz)	270	7	2	0	8	43	4	6	20	460	—	—	2
lumpia vegetable & shrimp	2 (3 oz)	120	0	0	10	4	26	1	2	0	300	—	—	2
meat & shrimp	1 (4.8 oz)	320	12	3	10	10	41	3	4	20	470	—	—	5
pork & shrimp	1 (5 oz)	300	10	4	15	13	41	6	7	40	890	—	—	0
shrimp	1 (3 oz)	170	5	1	<5	6	24	5	5	20	420	—	—	0
spicy pork	1 (3 oz)	200	9	2	5	6	23	3	3	20	410	—	—	0
vegetable	1 (3 oz)	170	4	1	0	5	28	4	4	20	520	—	—	0
EGG SUBSTITUTES														
frozen	¼ cup	96	7	1	1	7	2	—	—	44	120	128	—	—
frozen	1 cup	384	27	5	5	27	8	—	—	175	479	512	—	—
liquid	1 cup (8.8 oz)	211	8	2	3	30	2	—	—	133	444	828	—	0
liquid	1½ oz	40	2	tr	tr	6	tr	—	—	25	83	155	—	0
powder	0.7 oz	88	3	1	113	11	4	—	—	32	158	147	—	tr
powder	0.35 oz	44	1	tr	57	5	2	—	—	32	79	74	—	tr
BETTER'N EGGS														
Fat Free Cholesterol Free	¼ cup (2 oz)	30	0	0	0	6	1	1	0	100	100	55	—	0
DEB-EL														
Just Whites	2 tsp	12	0	0	—	3	0	—	0	—	51	—	—	—
EGG BEATERS														
Egg Substitute	¼ cup	30	0	0	0	6	1	tr	0	20	115	—	60	0

FOOD	PORTION	CALS	FAT	SAT FAT	CHOL	PROT	CARB	SUGAR	FIBER	CALCI	SOD	POTAS	FOLIC	VIT C
MORNINGSTAR FARMS														
Breakfast Sandwich Bagel Scramblers Pattie Cheese	1 (5.9 oz)	320	5	1	10	28	40	6	4	250	900	360	—	0
Breakfast Sandwich English Muffin Scramblers Pattie	1 (5.1 oz)	240	3	1	5	22	32	3	5	150	700	350	—	0
Breakfast Sandwich English Muffin Scramblers Pattie Cheese	1 (6 oz)	280	3	1	10	28	35	5	5	300	1000	400	—	0
Scramblers	¼ cup (2 oz)	35	0	0	0	6	2	2	0	20	95	60	—	0
QUICK EGGS														
Fat Free Cholesterol Free	¼ cup	30	0	0	0	6	1	1	0	100	80	—	40	0

EGGNOG

FOOD	PORTION	CALS	FAT	SAT FAT	CHOL	PROT	CARB	SUGAR	FIBER	CALCI	SOD	POTAS	FOLIC	VIT C
eggnog	1 cup	342	19	11	149	10	34	—	—	330	138	420	2	4
eggnog	1 qt	1368	76	45	596	39	138	—	—	1321	553	1678	9	15
eggnog flavor mix as prep w/ milk	9 oz	260	8	5	33	8	39	—	—	291	163	369	12	2
OBERWEIS														
Egg Nog	½ cup	240	15	7	40	3	25	21	0	100	70	—	—	0
TAKE-OUT														
eggnog	1 cup	306	22	14	63	5	16	—	0	49	95	93	3	tr

EGGNOG SUBSTITUTES

FOOD	PORTION	CALS	FAT	SAT FAT	CHOL	PROT	CARB	SUGAR	FIBER	CALCI	SOD	POTAS	FOLIC	VIT C
SILK														
Nog	½ cup	90	2	0	0	3	15	12	0	20	75	—	—	0

EGGPLANT

FOOD	PORTION	CALS	FAT	SAT FAT	CHOL	PROT	CARB	SUGAR	FIBER	CALCI	SOD	POTAS	FOLIC	VIT C
cubed cooked	1 cup	28	tr	tr	0	1	7	1	3	6	3	246	14	1
raw cut up	½ cup (1.4 oz)	11	tr	tr	0	tr	2	—	—	3	1	89	8	1
slices grilled	4 (7 oz)	38	0	0	0	2	0	—	—	22	—	—	—	6
whole peeled raw	1 (1 lb)	117	1	tr	0	5	28	—	—	34	14	992	67	8
PROGRESSO														
Caponata	2 tbsp (1 oz)	25	2	0	0	0	2	2	2	0	130	—	—	0
TASTYBITE														
Punjab Eggplant	½ pkg (5 oz)	130	8	1	0	5	9	3	4	50	780	—	—	0
TAKE-OUT														
baba ghannouj	¼ cup	55	4	—	0	2	5	—	—	—	95	—	—	—
caponata	2 tbsp (1 oz)	30	2	—	0	1	3	2	—	—	115	—	—	4
iman bayildi eggplant w/ onion & tomato	1 serv (15.6 oz)	345	28	4	0	3	25	6	2	43	552	773	59	29

FOOD	PORTION	CALS	FAT	SAT FAT	CHOL	PROT	CARB	SUGAR	FIBER	CALCI	SOD	POTAS	FOLIC	VIT C
indian eggplant runi	1 serv	180	14	4	0	2	13	1	1	30	228	527	13	15
moussaka	1 cup	237	13	5	97	—	—	—	—	—	432	—	—	—
papoutsakis little shoes	1 serv (15.5 oz)	245	16	7	40	12	15	1	1	144	751	669	37	12

ELDERBERRIES

FOOD	PORTION	CALS	FAT	SAT FAT	CHOL	PROT	CARB	SUGAR	FIBER	CALCI	SOD	POTAS	FOLIC	VIT C
fresh	1 cup	105	1	—	0	1	27	—	—	55	—	406	—	52

ELDERBERRY JUICE

FOOD	PORTION	CALS	FAT	SAT FAT	CHOL	PROT	CARB	SUGAR	FIBER	CALCI	SOD	POTAS	FOLIC	VIT C
elderberry	7 oz	76	0	0	0	4	16	—	—	10	2	576	12	52

ELK

FOOD	PORTION	CALS	FAT	SAT FAT	CHOL	PROT	CARB	SUGAR	FIBER	CALCI	SOD	POTAS	FOLIC	VIT C
roasted	3 oz	124	2	1	62	26	0	—	—	4	52	279	—	—

EMU

FOOD	PORTION	CALS	FAT	SAT FAT	CHOL	PROT	CARB	SUGAR	FIBER	CALCI	SOD	POTAS	FOLIC	VIT C
cooked	3 oz	130	—	—	111	—	—	—	—	6	97	270	—	tr

ENDIVE

FOOD	PORTION	CALS	FAT	SAT FAT	CHOL	PROT	CARB	SUGAR	FIBER	CALCI	SOD	POTAS	FOLIC	VIT C
fresh	3.5 oz	9	tr	—	0	2	tr	—	2	54	53	346	tr	—
raw chopped	½ cup	4	tr	tr	0	tr	1	—	—	13	6	79	36	2

ENERGY BARS

(*see also* CEREAL BARS, NUTRITION SUPPLEMENTS)

ALLGOODE ORGANICS

FOOD	PORTION	CALS	FAT	SAT FAT	CHOL	PROT	CARB	SUGAR	FIBER	CALCI	SOD	POTAS	FOLIC	VIT C
Amazin' Peanut Raisin	1 bar	210	11	2	0	7	25	15	3	40	80	250	40	0
Banana Nut Nirvana	1 bar	190	8	4	0	5	30	21	3	20	5	450	—	6
Cashew Almond Passion	1 bar	210	9	1	0	7	25	16	3	60	50	210	—	5
Chocolate Peanut Pleasure	1 bar	200	9	3	5	5	29	22	3	40	15	440	—	6
Honey Nut Harvest	1 bar	210	9	1	0	7	29	17	3	40	50	220	—	0
Nutty Chocolate Apricot	1 bar	200	10	5	5	6	26	19	5	60	15	530	—	12

ATKINS

FOOD	PORTION	CALS	FAT	SAT FAT	CHOL	PROT	CARB	SUGAR	FIBER	CALCI	SOD	POTAS	FOLIC	VIT C
Advantage Almond Brownie	1 bar (1.6 oz)	220	8	4	5	21	21	0	7	300	105	330	100	15
Advantage Chocolate Coconut	1 bar (1.6 oz)	230	11	8	2	19	21	0	9	300	100	230	100	15
Advantage Chocolate Decadence	1 bar (1.6 oz)	220	11	7	2	17	25	0	11	300	65	320	100	15
Advantage Chocolate Mocha Crunch	1 bar (1.6 oz)	220	10	6	2	20	22	0	10	350	120	340	100	15
Advantage Chocolate Peanut Butter	1 bar (1.6 oz)	240	12	6	2	19	21	1	10	300	125	260	100	15

FOOD	PORTION	CALS	FAT	SAT FAT	CHOL	PROT	CARB	SUGAR	FIBER	CALCI	SOD	POTAS	FOLIC	VIT C
ATKINS (CONT.)														
Advantage Cookies 'N Creme	1 bar (1.6 oz)	220	11	7	2	18	22	0	11	300	200	230	100	15
Advantage S'mores	1 bar (1.6 oz)	220	10	5	0	17	26	0	11	350	130	190	100	15
Morning Start Apple Crisp	1 bar	170	9	4	—	11	13	1	6	—	70	—	—	—
Morning Start Blueberry Muffin	1 bar	160	7	4	—	12	16	1	7	—	80	—	—	—
Morning Start Chocolate Chip Crisp	1 bar	160	7	3	—	12	14	tr	5	—	110	—	—	—
BACK TO NATURE														
10th Tee Chocolate Fudge	1 bar	200	6	4	0	7	31	18	1	40	40	—	120	18
10th Tee Peanut Honey	1 bar	260	6	4	0	6	32	16	2	40	64	—	100	15
1st Tee Chocolate Peanut	1 bar	290	8	5	0	9	44	16	1	150	105	—	160	60
1st Tee Oatmeal Raisin	1 bar	280	7	4	0	9	44	16	1	200	150	—	160	60
BALANCE														
Big Bar Honey Peanut	1 bar	310	10	4	5	22	33	27	tr	150	270	180	140	90
Chocolate Banana + Antioxidants	1 bar	200	6	4	5	14	22	17	1	100	135	95	100	120
Chocolate Mint + Antioxidants	1 bar	200	6	4	<5	14	23	18	0	100	200	80	100	120
Gold Caramel Nut Blast	1 bar	210	7	4	0	15	22	13	tr	100	110	115	100	60
Gold Chocolate Peanut Butter	1 bar	210	7	4	0	15	22	11	tr	100	125	125	100	60
Gold Rocky Road	1 bar	210	7	4	0	15	23	13	1	100	70	135	100	60
Gold Triple Chocolate Chaos	1 bar	200	6	4	0	15	22	12	tr	100	85	90	100	60
Gold Crunch Chocolate Chocolate	1 bar	210	6	4	0	15	23	15	tr	100	150	105	100	60
Gold Crunch Chocolate Mint Cookie	1 bar	210	6	4	0	15	23	14	tr	100	160	90	100	60
Gold Crunch S'mores	1 bar	210	7	4	0	15	23	12	0	100	160	100	100	60
Honey Peanut + Ginseng	1 bar	200	6	3	<5	15	22	18	tr	100	190	110	100	60
Lemon Meringue + Calcium	1 bar	190	6	3	0	14	22	17	0	400	150	80	100	60

FOOD	PORTION	CALS	FAT	SAT FAT	CHOL	PROT	CARB	SUGAR	FIBER	CALCI	SOD	POTAS	FOLIC	VIT C
BALANCE (CONT.)														
Original Almond Brownie	1 bar	200	6	2	<5	14	23	18	2	100	115	220	100	60
Original Chocolate	1 bar	200	6	4	<5	14	22	18	tr	100	180	160	100	60
Original Chocolate Raspberry Fudge	1 bar	200	6	3	0	14	22	19	1	100	90	170	100	60
Original Honey Peanut	1 bar	200	6	3	<5	14	24	20	tr	100	180	115	100	60
Original Mocha Chip	1 bar	200	6	4	0	14	23	19	tr	100	125	70	100	60
Original Peanut Butter	1 bar	200	6	3	<5	14	22	17	1	100	230	130	100	60
Original Yogurt Honey Peanut	1 bar	200	6	3	<5	15	22	19	tr	100	190	150	100	60
Outdoor Chocolate Crisp	1 bar	200	6	2	<5	15	21	12	3	80	140	260	—	—
Outdoor Crunchy Peanut	1 bar	200	6	1	<5	15	21	12	2	80	140	250	—	—
Outdoor Honey Almond	1 bar	200	6	1	<5	15	21	12	3	100	140	250	—	—
Outdoor Nut Berry	1 bar	200	6	1	<5	15	21	12	2	100	75	250	—	—
Satisfaction Apple Cinnamon Oatmeal	1 bar	280	5	4	0	12	47	23	6	150	260	140	100	60
Satisfaction Chocolate Crisp	1 bar	280	6	4	0	12	47	22	6	150	270	210	100	60
Satisfaction Chocolate Peanut	1 bar	280	6	4	0	11	48	22	6	150	320	120	100	60
Satisfaction Peanut Butter Crisp	1 bar	280	6	4	0	12	47	21	6	150	350	140	100	60
Yogurt Berry + Antioxidants	1 bar	200	6	3	5	14	22	17	0	100	120	160	100	120
BE NATURAL														
Almond & Apricot	1 bar	218	14	7	0	4	21	15	4	40	34	—	—	1
Almond & Coconut	1 bar	248	18	6	0	4	19	15	1	60	40	—	—	0
Banana & Wheat Bran	1 bar	201	9	8	0	2	29	19	4	0	35	—	—	0
Fruit & Nut Delight	1 bar	225	14	2	0	6	21	14	3	40	72	—	—	0
Macadamia & Apricot	1 bar	224	15	8	0	2	21	16	3	10	37	—	—	0
Nut Delight	1 bar	266	20	3	0	8	20	10	3	50	86	—	—	0
Sesame Nut Split	1 bar	256	17	2	0	7	20	15	2	40	110	—	—	0
Walnut & Date	1 bar	147	9	1	0	2	29	10	1	10	55	—	—	0

FOOD	PORTION	CALS	FAT	SAT FAT	CHOL	PROT	CARB	SUGAR	FIBER	CALCI	SOD	POTAS	FOLIC	VIT C
BE NATURAL (CONT.)														
Yogurt Coated Almond & Apricot	1 bar	233	14	3	0	4	23	20	2	90	60	—	—	0
Yogurt Coated Fruit & Nut	1 bar	190	12	1	0	4	19	15	1	60	40	—	—	0
BENECOL														
Chocolate Crisp	1 bar (1.2 oz)	130	3	2	5	3	23	14	2	20	60	—	—	—
Chocolate Crisp	1 bar (1.2 oz)	130	3	2	5	3	23	14	2	20	60	—	—	—
Peanut Crisp	1 bar (1.2 oz)	140	4	2	5	3	23	14	1	20	105	—	—	—
BETTER BAR														
Chocolate Coated Caramel Pecan	1 bar (1.8 oz)	180	4	2	0	18	15	10	0	200	35	30	80	12
Chocolate Coated Peanut	1 bar (1.8 oz)	180	4	2	0	18	15	10	0	200	35	30	80	12
Yogurt Coated Raspberry	1 bar (1.8 oz)	180	3	2	0	18	15	11	0	200	35	30	80	12
BOOST														
Chocolate Crunch	1 bar (1.5 oz)	190	7	4	<5	4	29	19	tr	150	90	105	60	9
BREAKTHRU														
Organic Chocolate Fudge	1 bar (2.1 oz)	230	3	2	0	10	39	17	3	300	120	210	200	30
Organic Cinnamon Crunch	1 bar (2.1 oz)	220	3	1	0	12	37	16	3	300	160	210	200	30
Organic Honey Graham	1 bar (2.1 oz)	220	3	1	0	12	37	16	3	300	160	210	200	30
Organic Mocha Fudge	1 bar (2.1 oz)	230	3	2	0	10	39	17	3	300	120	210	200	30
CARB OPTIONS														
Chocolate Chip	1 bar	200	8	4	<5	16	17	0	tr	300	200	400	140	21
Chocolate Peanut	1 bar	200	8	4	<5	16	17	tr	tr	300	240	400	140	21
Cinnamon Delight	1 bar	200	8	4	<5	16	17	0	0	300	200	400	60	21
CARBOLITE														
Chocolate Peanut Butter Sugar Free	1 bar (1 oz)	144	12	4	4	tr	2	0	0	120	28	—	—	0
CARBWISE														
Chocolate S'Mores Crunch	1 bar	240	9	6	0	20	24	0	1	250	330	40	120	15
CENTRUM														
Energy Chocolate Nougat	1 (1.98 oz)	220	5	4	0	8	34	25	tr	300	185	135	40	1
Energy Chocolate Peanut Butter	1 (1.98 oz)	220	5	4	0	8	34	25	tr	300	185	135	40	1

FOOD	PORTION	CALS	FAT	SAT FAT	CHOL	PROT	CARB	SUGAR	FIBER	CALCI	SOD	POTAS	FOLIC	VIT C
CHOICE														
Berry Almond Crispy	1 bar	50	1	0	0	2	10	3	0	100	25	15	—	60
Fudge Brownie	1 bar	140	5	3	<5	6	19	3	3	150	80	105	60	30
Peanut Butter Crispy	1 bar	60	2	2	0	1	10	2	tr	60	35	30	—	—
Peanutty Chocolate	1 bar	140	5	3	<5	6	19	9	3	150	80	105	60	30
CLIF BAR														
Apricot	1 bar (2.4 oz)	220	3	0	0	8	43	21	5	300	90	280	80	60
Carrot Cake	1 bar (2.4 oz)	240	4	2	0	10	43	21	5	250	150	250	80	60
Chocolate Brownie	1 bar (2.4 oz)	240	4	1	0	10	41	20	6	250	150	260	80	60
Chocolate Almond Fudge	1 bar (2.4 oz)	230	5	1	0	10	36	20	5	300	140	230	80	60
Chocolate Chip	1 bar (2.4 oz)	240	4	1	0	10	41	21	5	250	170	200	80	60
Chocolate Chip Peanut Crunch	1 bar (2.4 oz)	240	5	1	0	12	39	20	5	250	290	300	8	60
Cookies'N Cream	1 bar (2.4 oz)	230	4	2	0	10	39	21	5	300	180	210	80	60
Cranberry Apple Cherry	1 bar (2.4 oz)	220	2	0	0	8	44	22	5	250	135	240	80	60
Crunchy Peanut Butter	1 bar (2.4 oz)	240	5	1	0	12	39	18	5	250	290	300	80	60
GingerSnap	1 bar (2.4 oz)	230	4	1	0	10	42	20	6	300	140	400	80	60
DELICIOUSLY SLIM														
Chocolate Fudge Cake	1 bar (2.1 oz)	200	6	3	0	20	22	0	tr	100	220	100	60	9
DRSOY														
Double Chocolate	1 bar (1.76 oz)	180	3	3	0	12	27	9	1	350	170	80	400	60
ENSURE														
All Flavors	1 bar (2.1 oz)	230	6	4	<5	9	35	23	1	300	135	—	—	30
EXTEND														
Chocolate Chip Crunch	1 bar (1.4 oz)	160	3	2	0	3	31	8	tr	—	80	—	—	—
Peanut Butter Crunch	1 bar (1.4 oz)	160	3	0	0	4	30	10	0	—	85	—	—	—
FAST FUEL UP														
Natural Chocolate Espresso	1 bar (2.3 oz)	300	19	7	0	8	32	13	3	40	55	—	—	1
Natural Chocolate Crunch	1 bar (2.3 oz)	300	19	7	0	8	32	13	3	40	55	—	—	1
Organic Chocolate Espresso	1 bar (1.8 oz)	230	15	5	0	6	24	10	2	20	40	—	—	0

FOOD	PORTION	CALS	FAT	SAT FAT	CHOL	PROT	CARB	SUGAR	FIBER	CALCI	SOD	POTAS	FOLIC	VIT C
FAST FUEL UP (CONT.)														
Organic Chocolate Crunch	1 bar (1.8 oz)	230	15	6	0	6	24	10	2	20	40	—	—	0
GATORADE														
All Flavors	1 bar (2.3 oz)	260	5	1	0	8	46	20	2	20	160	—	—	18
GENISOY														
Soy Protein Artic Frost Crispy Chocolate Mint	1 bar (2.2 oz)	230	5	4	0	14	33	27	2	250	150	290	400	15
Soy Protein Dutch Crunch Sour Apple Crisp	1 bar (2.2 oz)	230	5	3	0	14	33	26	1	250	160	160	400	15
Soy Protein Fair Trade Arabica Cafe Mocha Fudge	1 bar (2.2 oz)	220	4	3	0	14	33	27	1	250	150	200	400	15
Soy Protein New York Style Blueberry Cheesecake	1 bar (2.2 oz)	220	4	3	0	14	34	28	1	250	160	130	400	15
Soy Protein Obsession Fudge Cookies & Cream	1 bar (2.2 oz)	230	5	3	0	14	33	27	2	250	250	170	400	15
Soy Protein Pure Golden Honey Creamy Peanut Yogurt	1 bar (2.2 oz)	230	5	3	0	14	33	28	1	250	160	200	400	15
Soy Protein Southern Style Chunky Peanut Butter Fudge	1 bar (2.2 oz)	240	6	3	0	14	32	24	1	250	130	270	400	15
Soy Protein Ultimate Chocolate Fudge Brownie	1 bar (2.2 oz)	230	5	3	0	14	33	27	2	250	210	250	400	15
Xtreme Carrot Cake Quake	1 bar (1.6 oz)	190	7	3	0	9	24	18	1	150	90	150	100	15
Xtreme Peanut Butter Fix	1 bar (1.6 oz)	200	8	3	0	9	23	16	2	200	190	190	100	15
Xtreme Raspberry Rush	1 bar (1.6 oz)	190	7	4	0	9	24	18	2	100	90	190	100	15
Xtreme Rocky Roadtrip	1 bar (1.6 oz)	190	7	3	0	9	23	16	2	150	130	180	100	15
GLUCERNA														
All Flavors	1 bar (1.3 oz)	140	4	1	<5	6	24	7	4	250	75	60	—	60
HANSEN'S														
Chocolate Banana Crunch	1 bar	180	3	2	0	3	37	19	2	20	45	—	—	60

FOOD	PORTION	CALS	FAT	SAT FAT	CHOL	PROT	CARB	SUGAR	FIBER	CALCI	SOD	POTAS	FOLIC	VIT C
HANSEN'S (CONT.)														
Chocolate Orchard Crunch	1 bar	170	3	2	0	2	37	19	2	20	30	—	—	60
Natural Bar Tropical Fruit Crunch	1 bar	170	3	2	0	3	35	20	1	20	60	—	—	60
Natural Bar Yogurt Strawberry Crunch	1 bar	190	3	2	0	2	38	21	1	20	60	—	—	60
HEARTBAR														
Cranberry	1 bar (1.8 oz)	190	3	1	0	13	27	21	3	30	95	200	200	250
Original	1 bar (1.76 oz)	180	3	1	0	14	26	15	3	30	140	270	200	250
HI-LO														
Chocolate Caramel	1 bar (1.76 oz)	200	8	5	<5	16	20	tr	0	100	150	—	80	12
Chocolate Mint	1 bar (2.1 oz)	200	6	4	0	20	23	0	tr	100	210	90	60	9
Chocolate Peanut Butter	1 bar (2.1 oz)	210	7	4	0	20	22	0	0	100	250	80	60	9
Chocolate Raspberry	1 bar (2.1 oz)	200	6	3	0	20	22	0	tr	100	220	100	60	9
IDEAL														
Mixed Berry Tart	1 bar (1.7 oz)	200	7	3	0	15	20	13	0	300	240	20	120	15
JENNY CRAIG														
Meal Bar Chocolate Peanut	1 bar (2 oz)	220	5	4	0	10	33	20	1	300	240	170	100	60
Meal Bar Lemon Meringue	1 bar (2 oz)	210	5	3	0	10	31	23	0	300	130	60	100	60
Meal Bar Milk Chocolate	1 bar (2 oz)	210	5	4	0	10	33	20	1	300	180	200	100	60
Meal Bar Oatmeal Raisin	1 bar (1.97 oz)	210	3	0	0	10	35	22	3	300	75	80	100	60
Meal Bar Yogurt Peanut	1 bar (2 oz)	220	5	3	0	10	33	20	0	300	270	170	100	60
KASHI														
GoLean Chocolate Almond Toffee	1 (2.7 oz)	290	6	5	0	13	45	31	—	80	250	250	—	0
GoLean Cookies 'N Cream	1 (2.7 oz)	290	6	4	0	13	50	35	6	80	200	250	—	0
GoLean Frosted Spice Cake	1 (2.7 oz)	290	5	3	0	13	49	33	6	80	200	250	—	0
GoLean Honey Vanilla Yogurt	1 (2.7 oz)	290	5	4	0	13	49	32	6	80	160	280	—	0
GoLean Malted Chocolate Chip	1 (2.7 oz)	290	6	4	20	13	49	35	6	80	200	270	—	1
GoLean Mocha Java	1 (2.7 oz)	290	6	4	0	13	50	35	6	100	190	290	—	0

FOOD	PORTION	CALS	FAT	SAT FAT	CHOL	PROT	CARB	SUGAR	FIBER	CALCI	SOD	POTAS	FOLIC	VIT C
KASHI (CONT.)														
GoLean Oatmeal Raisin Cookie	1 (2.7 oz)	280	5	3	0	13	49	33	6	100	140	250	—	0
GoLean Peanut Butter & Chocolate	1 (2.7 oz)	290	6	5	0	13	48	31	5	80	280	250	—	0
GoLean Strawberries 'N Cream	1 (2.7 oz)	290	5	4	0	13	50	33	6	80	200	230	—	0
GoLean Strawberry Vanilla Yogurt	1 (2.7 oz)	280	4	—	0	11	53	28	6	40	75	—	—	1
GoLean Crunchy Chocolate Caramel Karma	1 (1.6 oz)	140	3	2	20	8	26	15	5	200	180	110	100	9
GoLean Crunchy Chocolate Peanut Bliss	1 (1.8 oz)	270	4	2	0	9	30	13	5	200	220	140	100	9
GoLean Crunchy Sublime Lemon Lime	1 (1.8 oz)	670	3	2	0	9	32	13	5	200	220	140	100	9
LEAN BODY FOR HER														
Chocolate Honey Peanut	1 bar (1.76 oz)	190	7	4	0	16	10	6	tr	250	135	150	200	30
LUNA														
Chai Tea	1 bar (1.7 oz)	180	4	3	0	10	27	12	2	350	125	115	400	60
Chocolate Pecan Pie	1 bar (1.7 oz)	180	5	3	0	10	24	12	2	350	125	105	400	60
LemonZest	1 bar (1.7 oz)	180	4	3	0	10	24	12	2	350	50	90	140	60
Nutz Over Chocolate	1 bar (1.7 oz)	180	5	3	0	10	24	12	2	350	100	105	400	60
Sesame Raisin Crunch	1 bar (1.7 oz)	170	3	1	0	10	26	13	2	350	125	130	400	60
S'Mores	1 bar (1.7 oz)	180	4	3	0	10	26	12	2	350	125	125	400	60
Toasted Nuts 'n Cranberry	1 bar (1.7 oz)	170	3	0	0	10	26	12	2	350	130	100	400	60
Tropical Crisp	1 bar (1.7 oz)	180	5	4	0	10	24	11	2	350	135	120	400	60
MET-RX														
Big 100 Gram Bar Peanut Butter	1 bar (3.5 oz)	340	4	2	15	26	52	38	2	700	135	—	400	60
Source/One Chocolate Cheesecake	1 bar (2.1 oz)	160	5	4	5	15	21	4	tr	600	50	400	400	78
MOMENTUM														
Chocolate Caramel Nut	1 bar	150	6	3	0	12	16	2	3	250	110	—	120	4

FOOD	PORTION	CALS	FAT	SAT FAT	CHOL	PROT	CARB	SUGAR	FIBER	CALCI	SOD	POTAS	FOLIC	VIT C
MOMENTUM (CONT.)														
Chocolate Peanut Butter	1 bar	150	6	4	0	12	16	1	2	250	150	—	120	4
Double Chocolate	1 bar	150	6	4	0	12	17	1	2	250	160	—	120	4
MOTO BAR														
Bodacious Banana Split	1 bar	300	6	2	0	8	54	16	6	40	240	—	—	0
Charming Cherry Almond	1 bar (2.9 oz)	300	6	1	0	8	54	18	3	20	200	—	—	1
Cozy Pumpkin Pie	1 bar	300	6	1	0	8	54	16	6	40	200	—	—	0
Jazzy Peanut Butter & Jelly	1 bar	300	3	1	0	10	52	20	4	40	200	—	—	0
Kooky Cappuccino	1 bar	300	6	1	0	8	54	16	8	40	200	—	—	0
Luscious Lemon Blueberry	1 bar	300	5	1	0	10	54	16	4	20	280	—	—	1
Saucy Apple Cinnamon	1 bar	280	4	1	0	8	54	18	6	20	300	—	—	0
Zany Cranberry Orange	1 bar	300	5	1	0	8	54	18	4	20	250	—	—	0
NEW YOU														
Chocolate Crisp	1 bar (1.65 oz)	180	4	3	0	10	25	11	3	380	170	90	400	100
NUGO														
Banana Chocolate Protein	1 bar	190	3	1	0	11	26	13	3	300	220	—	160	24
Blue Berry Boom	1 bar	180	3	2	0	11	26	13	3	300	250	—	160	24
Chocolate Blast	1 bar	180	3	2	0	11	26	13	3	300	250	—	160	24
Coffee Break	1 bar	180	3	2	0	11	26	13	3	300	250	—	160	24
Orange Smoothie Protein	1 bar	190	3	2	0	17	25	13	1	300	220	—	160	24
Peanut Butter Pleaser	1 bar	180	3	2	0	11	26	13	3	300	250	—	160	24
NUTIVA														
Flaxseed & Raisin Organic	1 bar (1.1 oz)	280	19	2	0	14	12	5	6	0	10	—	—	—
Hempseed Bar Organic	1 bar (1.4 oz)	210	14	2	0	9	11	5	5	0	5	—	—	—
NUTRIBAR														
Chocolate Covered Belgian Chocolate	1 bar (2.3 oz)	252	8	3	—	13	33	—	2	350	255	375	140	15
Chocolate Covered Caramel	1 bar (2.3 oz)	261	8	3	—	13	34	—	tr	350	280	375	140	15
Chocolate Covered Chocolate Fudge	1 bar (2.3 oz)	267	8	3	5	14	35	—	2	350	300	380	140	15

FOOD	PORTION	CALS	FAT	SAT FAT	CHOL	PROT	CARB	SUGAR	FIBER	CALCI	SOD	POTAS	FOLIC	VIT C
NUTRIBAR (CONT.)														
Chocolate Covered Hazelnut	1 bar (2.3 oz)	261	8	3	—	13	34	—	1	350	295	400	140	15
Chocolate Covered Mocha Almond	1 bar (2.3 oz)	261	8	3	—	13	34	—	tr	350	280	375	140	15
Chocolate Covered Peanut	1 bar (2.3 oz)	262	9	3	—	13	34	—	1	350	255	375	140	15
Yogurt Covered Peach Apricot	1 bar (2.3 oz)	261	8	3	—	13	34	—	tr	350	260	375	140	15
Yogurt Covered Raspberry	1 bar (2.3 oz)	261	8	3	—	13	34	—	tr	350	260	375	140	15
Yogurt Covered Wildberry	1 bar (2.3 oz)	261	8	3	—	13	34	—	tr	350	260	375	140	15
ODWALLA BAR!														
Peanut Crunch	1 bar (2.2 oz)	260	7	2	0	8	40	17	3	250	180	—	400	60
PEACEKEEPER														
Nuts About Peace All Flavors	1 bar (1.4 oz)	180	10	1	0	4	17	8	2	60	0	—	—	0
PERMALEAN														
Protein Crunch Chocoholic Chocolate	1 bar (1.8 oz)	170	3	2	0	21	10	1	tr	200	65	100	400	90
Protein Crunch Chocolate Raspberry	1 bar (1.8 oz)	180	2	2	10	21	9	1	0	200	35	90	400	90
Protein Crunch Stark Raving Peanutz	1 bar (1.8 oz)	180	4	2	0	21	9	2	0	200	75	80	400	90
POWERBAR														
Apple Cinnamon	1 bar (2.3 oz)	230	3	1	0	10	45	20	3	300	90	110	400	60
Banana	1 bar (2.3 oz)	230	2	1	0	9	45	20	3	300	90	200	400	60
Chocolate	1 bar (2.3 oz)	230	2	1	0	10	45	14	3	300	90	145	400	60
Essentials Chocolate	1 bar (1.9 oz)	180	4	2	0	10	28	20	3	500	105	—	200	60
Harvest Apple Crisp	1 bar (2.3 oz)	240	4	—	—	7	—	—	—	—	—	—	—	—
Harvest Blueberry	1 bar (2.3 oz)	240	4	1	0	7	45	18	4	150	80	—	200	60
Harvest Strawberry	1 bar (2.3 oz)	240	4	1	0	7	45	18	4	—	80	—	—	—
Malt-Nut	1 bar (2.3 oz)	230	3	1	0	10	45	18	3	300	90	110	400	60
Mocha	1 bar (2.3 oz)	230	3	1	0	10	45	17	3	300	90	145	400	60
Oatmeal Raisin	1 bar (2.3 oz)	230	3	1	0	10	45	20	3	300	120	180	400	60
Peanut Butter	1 bar (2.3 oz)	230	3	1	0	10	45	20	3	300	110	150	400	60
Power Gel Strawberry Banana	1 pkg	110	0	0	0	0	28	5	—	—	50	40	—	—

FOOD	PORTION	CALS	FAT	SAT FAT	CHOL	PROT	CARB	SUGAR	FIBER	CALCI	SOD	POTAS	FOLIC	VIT C
POWERBAR (CONT.)														
Pria Chocolate Honey Graham	1 bar (1 oz)	110	3	2	—	5	16	10	—	300	80	—	240	36
Pria Chocolate Peanut Crunch	1 bar (1 oz)	110	4	2	—	5	16	10	—	300	80	—	240	36
Pria Double Chocolate Cookie	1 bar (1 oz)	110	3	3	—	5	16	10	—	300	90	—	240	36
Pria French Vanilla Crisp	1 bar (1 oz)	110	3	3	—	5	16	10	—	300	80	—	240	36
Vanilla Crisp	1 bar (2.3 oz)	230	3	1	0	9	45	20	3	300	90	110	400	60
Wild Berry	1 bar (2.3 oz)	230	3	1	0	10	45	14	3	300	90	110	400	60
PURE PROTEIN														
Blueberry Cheesecake	1 bar	190	3	2	5	20	23	3	0	500	40	130	200	30
REVIVAL														
Soy Apple Cinnamon Celebration	1 bar	200	5	4	0	21	28	2	1	60	260	40	—	—
Soy Autumn Frost Low Carb	1 bar	200	5	4	0	21	28	2	1	60	260	40	—	—
Soy Chocolate Raspberry Zing Low Carb	1 bar	200	5	3	0	19	28	tr	2	40	240	30	—	—
Soy Chocolate Temptation	1 bar	220	3	1	0	16	30	16	tr	40	270	60	—	—
Soy Marshmallow Krunch	1 bar	220	3	1	0	17	33	21	tr	40	270	40	—	—
Soy Peanut Butter Chocolate Pal	1 bar	240	5	1	0	16	32	18	1	40	260	35	—	—
Soy Peanut Butter Pal	1 bar	240	5	1	0	17	31	19	tr	40	280	35	—	—
SLIM-FAST														
Crispy Peanut Caramel	1 bar	120	4	3	<5	1	21	13	tr	150	80	—	60	6
Dutch Chocolate	1 bar	140	5	2	5	5	20	13	2	40	80	150	40	15
Meal On-The-Go Apple Cobbler	1 bar	220	5	4	<5	8	33	23	2	300	150	125	120	21
Meal On-The-Go Chocolate Cookie Dough	1 bar	220	5	4	<5	8	35	22	2	350	180	90	120	21
Meal On-The-Go Honey Peanut	1 bar	220	5	4	<5	8	34	23	2	300	160	170	120	21
Meal On-The-Go Milk Chocolate Peanut	1 bar	220	5	3	<5	8	36	24	2	300	120	160	120	21
Meal On-The-Go Oatmeal Raisin	1 bar	220	5	4	<5	8	36	19	2	300	100	170	120	21

FOOD	PORTION	CALS	FAT	SAT FAT	CHOL	PROT	CARB	SUGAR	FIBER	CALCI	SOD	POTAS	FOLIC	VIT C
SLIM-FAST (CONT.)														
Meal On-The-Go Rich Chocolate Brownie	1 bar	220	5	3	<5	8	34	23	2	300	150	180	120	21
Meal On-The-Go Toasted Oat & Spice	1 bar	220	5	4	<5	8	35	20	2	300	140	70	120	21
Peanut Butter	1 bar	150	5	3	5	6	19	10	2	40	80	150	40	15
Peanut Butter Crunch	1 bar	130	4	2	0	1	21	20	tr	150	80	750	60	9
Rich Chewy Caramel	1 bar	120	4	3	5	tr	22	11	2	250	65	—	60	60
SNICKERS														
Marathon Chewy Chocolate Peanut	1	220	7	2	5	13	27	18	2	450	240	—	400	60
Marathon Multi Grain Crunch	1	220	7	2	5	9	32	18	2	450	210	—	400	60
SOBE														
Milk Chocolate	1 bar (1.75 oz)	240	14	9	15	2	28	24	tr	60	50	—	—	—
STRIVE														
Crunchy Chocolate Smores	1 bar (2.1 oz)	200	9	5	0	20	25	0	0	250	320	—	140	15
SWEET SUCCESS														
Chewy Chocolate Brownie	1 bar (1.2 oz)	120	4	2	3	2	23	12	3	150	35	—	60	9
THINK!														
Apple Spice	1 bar (2 oz)	205	3	1	62	5	40	15	7	61	36	—	—	14
Chocolate Almond Coconut Raisin	1 bar (2 oz)	243	7	2	9	6	39	13	2	200	160	—	—	12
Chocolate Fruit Harvest	1 bar (2 oz)	217	3	1	38	5	43	18	7	60	42	—	—	12
ZOE														
Flax & Soy Apple Crisp	1 bar (1.83 oz)	180	6	—	—	8	—	—	—	—	—	—	—	—
ZONEPERFECT														
Honey Peanut	1 bar (1.8 oz)	200	7	4	0	14	22	20	1	400	150	130	160	120
ENERGY DRINKS														
AMP														
Energy Drink	1 can (8.4 oz)	120	0	0	0	0	32	30	0	—	75	—	—	—
ARIZONA														
Extreme Energy Shot	1 bottle (8.3 oz)	130	0	0	0	0	34	33	—	—	25	—	—	60
ATKINS														
Cafe Au Lait	1 can (11 oz)	170	9	2	15	20	5	1	3	—	170	680	—	18
Chocolate	1 can (11 oz)	170	9	2	15	20	5	2	3	300	140	550	120	18
Chocolate Royale	1 can (11 oz)	170	9	2	15	20	6	4	1	400	170	850	120	18

FOOD	PORTION	CALS	FAT	SAT FAT	CHOL	PROT	CARB	SUGAR	FIBER	CALCI	SOD	POTAS	FOLIC	VIT C
ATKINS (CONT.)														
Strawberry	1 can (11 oz)	170	9	2	15	20	4	2	2	300	140	440	120	18
Vanilla	1 can (11 oz)	170	9	2	15	20	4	2	2	300	140	440	120	18
BALANCE														
Chocolate as prep w/ 2% milk	1 serv	310	11	4	25	22	32	26	2	600	420	870	120	60
Vanilla as prep w/ 2% milk	1 serv	310	11	4	25	22	32	27	2	600	420	850	120	60
BAWLS														
Guarana	1 bottle (10 oz)	120	0	0	0	0	32	32	—	—	35	—	—	—
Guaranexx Sugar Free	1 bottle (10 oz)	0	0	0	0	0	0	0	0	—	15	—	—	—
BOOKOO														
Energy Drink	8 oz	110	0	0	0	—	27	27	—	—	200	—	—	—
Zero Carb	8 oz	0	0	0	0	0	0	0	0	—	200		—	—
BOOST														
High Protein Vanilla	1 can (8 oz)	240	6	1	10	15	33	16	0	330	170	380	140	60
Vanilla	8 oz	240	4	1	5	10	41	23	0	300	130	400	140	60
BRAIN TWIST														
Flu & Cold Defense All Flavors	8 oz	70	0	0	0	—	16	15	—	—	—	—	—	84
CALIFORNIA JOE														
All Natural Protein Drink Mix as prep	1 serv (8 oz)	165	4	2	0	12	21	18	0	240	166	21	—	—
CHOICE														
Chocolate	1 can (8 oz)	220	10	2	0	9	24	10	3	350	200	430	100	60
Chocolate Fudge Sugar Free	1 pkg (11 oz)	125	3	1	<5	10	11	0	9	250	150	340	80	—
French Vanilla Sugar Free	1 pkg (11 oz)	100	3	0	<5	10	7	0	6	250	130	110	80	—
Strawberries'n Cream Sugar Free	1 pkg (11 oz)	100	3	0	<5	10	7	0	6	250	130	110	80	—
Vanilla	1 can (8 oz)	220	10	2	0	9	24	9	3	350	200	430	100	60
CRUNK														
Energy Drink	1 can	120	0	0	0	0	29	29	—	50	120	—	—	—
FAT BURNER														
Diet Fruit Punch	8 fl oz	0	0	0	0	8	0	—	—	—	—	40	—	0
FUZE														
Energize Blackberry Grape	8 oz	100	0	0	0	0	26	24	—	—	15	—	—	60
Energize Exotic Punch	8 oz	100	0	0	0	0	26	24	—	—	15	—	—	60

FOOD	PORTION	CALS	FAT	SAT FAT	CHOL	PROT	CARB	SUGAR	FIBER	CALCI	SOD	POTAS	FOLIC	VIT C
FUZE (CONT.)														
Energize Mojo Mango	8 oz	100	0	0	0	0	28	24	—	—	15	—	—	60
Essential Cranberry Grapefruit	8 oz	90	0	0	0	0	25	24	—	—	5	—	—	30
Focus Orange Carrot	8 oz	90	0	0	0	0	24	23	—	—	20	—	—	30
Refresh Banana Colada	8 oz	90	0	0	0	0	24	22	—	250	15	—	—	30
Refresh Mixed Berry	8 oz	90	0	0	0	0	25	23	—	10	15	—	—	30
Refresh Peach Mango	8 oz	90	0	0	0	0	24	22	—	100	15	—	—	30
Replenish Agave Cactus	8 oz	90	0	0	0	0	24	23	—	—	25	—	—	60
Slenderize Tropical Punch	8 oz	10	0	0	0	0	2	2	—	—	5	—	—	60
Stamina Grape & Aronia Punch	8 oz	80	0	0	0	0	23	23	—	—	10	—	—	60
Vitaboost Citrus Starfruit Punch	8 oz	90	0	0	0	0	24	21	—	—	10	—	—	90
GATORADE														
All Flavors	1 cup (8 oz)	50	0	0	0	0	14	14	—	—	110	30	—	—
Nutrition Shake All Flavors	1 can (11 oz)	370	6	1	0	18	62	43	1	300	290	740	—	60
X-Factor All Flavors	8 oz	50	0	0	0	0	14	14	—	—	110	20	—	—
GENISOY														
Soy Protein Shake Chocolate	1 scoop (1.2 oz)	120	0	0	0	14	17	15	2	250	170	230	100	15
Soy Protein Shake Vanilla	1 scoop (1.2 oz)	130	0	0	0	14	18	13	0	250	180	70	100	15
Soy Protein Shake Strawberry Banana	1 scoop	130	0	0	0	14	17	14	1	250	170	70	100	15
GUARAVITON														
Energy Drink	8 oz	98	0	0	0	0	20	19	—	—	—	—	—	—
HANSEN'S														
Energy Kiwi Strawberry	8 oz	120	0	0	0	0	30	30	—	100	15	—	—	60
Energy Peach	8 oz	130	0	0	0	0	33	30	—	100	15	—	—	60
Energy Punch	8 oz	120	0	0	0	0	30	30	—	100	15	—	—	60
Healthy Start Carrot Orange Antioxidant Blend	8 oz	130	0	0	0	1	30	29	—	20	25	—	—	120

FOOD	PORTION	CALS	FAT	SAT FAT	CHOL	PROT	CARB	SUGAR	FIBER	CALCI	SOD	POTAS	FOLIC	VIT C
HANSEN'S (CONT.)														
Healthy Start Citrus Punch Focus Blend	8 oz	130	0	0	0	0	34	30	—	—	25	—	—	—
Healthy Start Cranberry Grape Defense Blend	8 oz	110	0	0	0	0	28	26	—	100	26	—	—	60
Healthy Start Tropical Orange Vitamix Blend	8 oz	110	0	0	0	0	30	26	—	100	30	100	—	60
HAPPY BUNNY														
Spaz Juice	1 can (8.4 oz)	110	0	0	0	0	28	27	0	—	10	—	—	—
HEALTHY PLEASURES														
Chocolate Irish Cream	1 bottle (10.5 oz)	260	2	1	6	12	45	45	0	500	320	480	140	30
HIGH VOLTAGE														
Sugar Free	8 oz	5	0	0	0	0	2	0	—	—	55	—	—	60
HYPE														
Classic Energy	1 can (8.3 oz)	110	0	0	0	0	26	26	—	—	0	—	100	9
IMPULSE														
Energy Drink	1 can (8.3 oz)	110	0	0	0	1	28	27	—	—	200	—	—	60
Sugar Free	1 can (8.3 oz)	5	0	0	0	tr	1	0	—	—	—	—	—	60
INVIGOR8														
Energy Boost	1 can	110	0	0	0	0	27	20	1	100	50	—	—	60
Nutrition Boost	1 can	110	0	0	0	0	27	20	1	100	50	—	—	60
JONES SODA														
Big Energy	8 oz	120	0	0	0	1	29	27	—	—	20	—	—	—
Lemon Lime Energy	1 can (8.4 oz)	140	0	0	0	1	33	31	0	—	220	—	—	—
Mixed Berry Energy	1 can (8.4 oz)	140	0	0	0	1	33	31	0	—	220	—	—	—
Orange Energy	1 can (8.4 oz)	140	0	0	0	1	33	31	0	—	220	—	—	—
Sugar Free Energy	1 can (8.4 oz)	10	0	0	0	1	2	0	—	—	135	—	—	—
JUGULAR														
Energy Drink	1 can (8.3 oz)	49	0	0	0	3	9	9	—	0	46	25	—	60
KABOOM														
All Flavors	8 oz	105	0	0	0	0	26	25	0	0	3	—	240	48
KASHI														
GoLean Shake Mix Vanilla	2 scoops	220	0	0	0	22	32	22	7	400	105	470	120	30
GoLean Shake Mix Woman Chocolate	2 scoops	220	1	0	0	22	31	22	7	400	100	630	120	30
Shake Chocolate	1 can	230	3	0	0	15	38	30	7	400	310	590	130	60
Shake Vanilla	1 can	220	3	0	0	15	36	29	7	400	330	600	120	60

FOOD	PORTION	CALS	FAT	SAT FAT	CHOL	PROT	CARB	SUGAR	FIBER	CALCI	SOD	POTAS	FOLIC	VIT C
KINDERCAL														
Vanilla	1 can (8 oz)	250	11	3	5	7	32	—	0	240	88	310	38	58
KRANK'D														
All Flavors	1 bottle (16 oz)	80	0	0	0	0	18	13	—	—	48	44	—	16
LOLLI'S POP														
Cheery Energy Drink	1 bottle	170	0	0	0	0	45	44	—	—	10	—	—	60
Passion Stimulating Elixir	1 bottle	140	0	0	0	0	35	35	—	—	10	—	—	60
NANTUCKET NECTARS														
Super Nectars Ginkgo Mango	8 oz	150	0	0	0	0	38	37	—	0	15	—	—	60
Super Nectars Green Angel	8 oz	140	0	0	0	tr	35	29	—	0	15	—	—	60
Super Nectars Protein Smoothie	8 oz	170	1	—	0	2	38	34	—	0	45	—	—	60
Super Nectars Red Guarana Tea	8 oz	110	0	0	0	0	26	25	—	0	5	—	—	60
Super Nectars Vital C	8 oz	130	0	0	0	tr	32	27	—	20	10	—	—	210
NATURAL OVENS														
Ultra Omega Balance	1 tbsp	75	5	0	3	3	5	1	4	50	10	—	200	30
Zesty Flax Energy Mix	1 tbsp	40	2	1	0	2	5	2	3	60	2	—	40	0
NEW YORK MINUTE														
Energy Drink	1 can (8.4 oz)	130	0	0	0	0	33	33	—	—	215	—	100	105
NITRO2GO														
High Energy	1 can	110	0	0	0	0	28	27	—	—	190	—	—	60
High Energy Lite	1 can	20	0	0	0	0	5	4	0	—	180	—	—	60
NOS														
High Performance	8 oz	110	0	0	0	1	28	27	—	—	115	—	100	60
NUTRASHAKE														
Citrus	1 pkg (4 oz)	200	0	0	0	6	44	—	—	200	30	10	—	—
Citrus Free	1 serv (4 oz)	200	0	0	0	6	44	4	0	200	110	60	—	60
Vanilla	1 serv (8 oz)	400	12	—	36	12	62	—	—	250	120	444	—	—
Vanilla No Added Sugar	1 serv (4 oz)	200	8	—	18	7	25	—	—	—	75	222	—	—
ODWALLA														
Blueberry B Monster	8 fl oz	140	0	0	0	0	33	26	2	—	15	—	16	48
C Monster	8 fl oz	150	1	—	0	2	33	30	2	150	25	—	—	600
Femme Vitale	8 fl oz	130	0	0	0	1	29	28	1	100	10	360	400	180
Glorious Morning	8 fl oz	130	0	0	0	2	31	22	3	300	20	370	—	282
Mango Tango	8 fl oz	150	2	1	0	1	31	28	0	20	55	—	—	60

FOOD	PORTION	CALS	FAT	SAT FAT	CHOL	PROT	CARB	SUGAR	FIBER	CALCI	SOD	POTAS	FOLIC	VIT C
ODWALLA (CONT.)														
Mo Beta	8 fl oz	140	0	0	0	1	34	26	1	40	40	370	—	300
Serious Energy	8 fl oz	150	0	0	0	1	36	21	1	0	35	—	—	9
Strawberry C Monster	8 fl oz	150	0	0	0	2	34	27	tr	20	40	330	—	600
Super Protein	8 fl oz	170	1	—	0	9	33	28	2	350	90	460	—	90
Superfood	8 fl oz	140	1	—	0	2	32	26	2	0	50	440	—	36
Wellness	8 fl oz	150	1	—	0	2	33	—	1	20	35	350	—	150
ORANGE COUNTY CHOPPERS														
High Octane Fuel	1 can (8.4 oz)	110	0	0	0	0	28	27	—	—	10	—	—	—
PEEP ONE														
Erotic Drink	1 can (8.3)	109	tr	—	0	1	27	—	—	24	112	10	—	—
PIMP JUICE														
Energy Drink	1 can	140	0	0	0	0	35	34	—	—	5	—	—	60
PINK														
Diet	1 can	10	0	0	0	0	2	0	—	—	135	—	—	—
PIRANHA														
Phunky Fruit Punch	1 can (8.4 oz)	140	0	0	0	0	35	35	0	0	10	—	—	0
PIT BULL														
Energy Drink	1 can (8.4 oz)	110	0	0	0	tr	28	—	—	—	200	—	—	60
Sugar Free	1 can (8.4 oz)	0	0	0	0	0	0	0	0	—	210	—	—	60
POUNDS OFF														
Dark Chocolate Ecstasy	1 can (11 oz)	200	3	0	0	11	39	32	6	400	220	590	140	27
French Vanilla	1 can (11 oz)	220	3	1	0	12	41	35	5	400	460	440	140	27
POWERADE														
Fruit Punch	8 fl oz	70	0	0	0	0	19	15	—	—	55	30	—	—
Lemon Lime	8 fl oz	70	0	0	0	0	19	15	—	—	55	30	—	—
Mountain Blast	8 fl oz	70	0	0	0	0	19	15	—	—	55	30	—	—
PURE POWER														
Energy Drink	1 can (8.4 oz)	110	0	0	0	0	28	—	—	—	210	—	—	—
Shotz	1 can (5.75 oz)	80	0	0	0	1	19	19	0	—	150	—	—	—
RAW DAWG														
Energy Drink	8 oz	110	0	0	0	0	27	27	—	—	110	—	—	60
Sugar Free	8 oz	0	0	0	0	0	0	0	0	—	110	—	—	60
RED BULL														
Energy Drink	1 can (8.3 oz)	110	0	0	0	0	28	27	—	—	200	—	—	—
Sugar Free	1 can	10	0	0	0	tr	3	0	—	—	200	—	—	—
RED EYE														
Classic	1 bottle (12 oz)	208	0	0	0	0	50	49	—	—	0	—	—	—
Extreme	1 bottle (12 oz)	140	0	0	0	0	37	36	—	—	0	—	—	—
Gold	1 bottle (12 oz)	208	0	0	0	0	49	49	—	—	0	—	—	—
Passion	1 bottle (12 oz)	149	0	0	0	0	37	36	—	—	0	—	—	—
Platinum	1 bottle (12 oz)	149	0	0	0	0	37	36	—	—	0	—	—	—

FOOD	PORTION	CALS	FAT	SAT FAT	CHOL	PROT	CARB	SUGAR	FIBER	CALCI	SOD	POTAS	FOLIC	VIT C
RESQ														
Energy Drink	1 can (8 oz)	126	0	0	0	1	30	—	—	—	—	—	100	—
RIP IT														
Energy Fuel	8 oz	130	0	0	0	1	32	32	—	—	130	—	400	60
Energy Lite	8 oz	0	0	0	0	1	0	0	—	—	130	—	400	60
ROCKSTAR														
Energy Cola	8 oz	120	0	0	0	0	30	29	—	—	35	—	—	30
Energy Drink	8 oz	110	0	0	0	0	29	27	—	—	35	—	—	60
SLIM-FAST														
Chocolate as prep w/ fat free milk	1 serv	190	1	1	9	14	32	29	2	450	240	660	120	21
Chocolate Malt as prep w/ fat free milk	1 serv	190	1	1	8	14	32	29	2	450	250	650	120	21
JumpStart Chocolate as prep w/ fat free milk	1 serv	240	2	1	14	18	39	33	5	400	280	620	160	24
Strawberry as prep w/ fat free milk	1 serv	190	1	1	9	14	32	30	2	450	260	610	120	21
Vanilla as prep w/ fat free milk	1 serv	190	1	1	9	14	32	30	2	450	260	610	120	21
SNAPPLE														
Meal Replacement All Flavors	1 bottle (11.5 oz)	210	0	0	0	7	43	36	5	250	110	400	240	60
SOBE														
Adrenaline Rush	1 can (8.3 oz)	140	0	0	0	1	36	34	—	—	60	22	400	60
Black & Blue Berry Brew	8 oz	120	0	0	0	0	31	31	—	—	24	—	—	60
Courage Cherry Citrus	8 oz	110	0	0	0	0	33	30	—	—	25	—	—	60
Drive	8 oz	120	0	0	0	0	32	31	—	—	15	—	—	—
Elixir Cranberry Grapefruit	8 oz	110	0	0	0	0	29	28	—	40	10	—	—	60
Elixir Orange Carrot 3C	8 oz	90	0	0	0	0	24	23	—	—	20	—	—	—
Elixir Pomegranate Cranberry	8 oz	100	0	0	0	0	26	25	—	40	27	—	—	60
Energy	8 oz	120	0	0	0	0	32	30	—	—	5	—	—	—
Fuerte	8 oz	130	0	0	0	0	35	33	—	—	10	—	—	60
Karma	8 oz	120	0	0	0	0	33	31	—	—	5	—	—	—
Long John Lizard's Grape Grog	8 oz	120	0	0	0	0	31	30	—	—	25	—	—	60
Power	8 oz	120	0	0	0	0	32	31	—	—	5	—	—	60

FOOD	PORTION	CALS	FAT	SAT FAT	CHOL	PROT	CARB	SUGAR	FIBER	CALCI	SOD	POTAS	FOLIC	VIT C
SOBE (CONT.)														
Synergy All Flavors	1 can (11.5 oz)	120	0	0	0	32	29	—	—	140	20	—	—	60
Tsunami	8 oz	110	0	0	0	0	29	27	—	—	20	—	—	60
Wisdom	8.5 oz	110	0	0	0	0	30	29	—	—	5	—	—	60
Zen Blend	8.5 oz	90	0	0	0	0	24	23	—	—	5	—	—	60
SOURCE BURN														
Energy Drink	8 oz	140	0	0	0	0	36	28	—	—	20	—	—	—
Sugar Free	8 oz	10	0	0	0	1	0	0	0	—	15	—	—	60
STEVITA														
All Flavors	2 tsp	0	0	0	0	0	0	0	0	—	0	0	—	—
SWEET SUCCESS														
Creamy Milk Chocolate	1 can	200	3	1	4	10	36	30	3	350	230	—	100	15
Creamy Milk Chocolate as prep w/ skim milk	1 serv	180	1	1	6	11	36	8	6	350	240	—	100	15
TORNADO														
Energy Drink	8 oz	110	0	0	0	1	30	27	—	—	130	—	—	1
TWINLAB														
Hydra Fuel	16 oz	132	0	0	0	0	33	—	—	—	50	99	—	60
Nitro Fuel	16 oz	460	0	0	0	15	100	—	—	—	—	99	—	—
Ultra Fuel	16 oz	400	0	0	0	0	100	30	—	—	55	—	—	60
VIPA														
Energy Drink	1 can (12 oz)	0	0	0	0	0	0	0	0	0	30	—	—	132
WIRED														
Energy Drink	8 oz	110	0	0	0	0	29	27	—	—	225	—	—	—
Sugar Free	8 oz	5	0	0	0	2	2	0	—	—	210	—	—	—
X 3000 Taurine	8 oz	110	0	0	0	2	26	25	—	—	210	—	—	—
XO														
Balance	8 oz	50	0	0	0	0	13	12	—	>20	—	—	—	24
Berry	1 bottle	90	0	0	0	tr	22	19	—	—	140		—	18
Citrus	1 bottle	90	0	0	0	tr	22	19	—	—	135	—	—	15
Defense	8 oz	40	0	0	0	0	9	8	—	—	0	—	—	60
Diet	1 bottle	15	0	0	0	tr	2	0	—	—	125	—	—	18
Endurance	8 oz	50	0	0	0	0	14	12	—	—	0	—	—	36
Energy	8 oz	40	0	0	0	0	9	8	—	—	0	—	—	60
Essential	8 oz	40	0	0	0	0	9	8	—	20	0	50	9	—
Focus	8 oz	40	0	0	0	0	9	8	—	—	0	—	—	60
Grape	1 bottle	90	0	0	0	tr	21	18	—	—	130	—	—	18
Multi-V	8 oz	40	0	0	0	0	9	8	—	20	0	—	—	60
Original	1 bottle	110	0	0	0	tr	28	28	—	—	85	—	—	60
Peach	1 bottle	90	0	0	0	tr	21	19	—	—	130	—	—	18
Power-C	8 oz	40	0	0	0	0	9	8	—	—	0	—	—	150
Rescue	8 oz	40	0	0	0	0	9	8	—	—	0	—	—	60

FOOD	PORTION	CALS	FAT	SAT FAT	CHOL	PROT	CARB	SUGAR	FIBER	CALCI	SOD	POTAS	FOLIC	VIT C
XO (CONT.)														
Revive	8 oz	50	0	0	0	0	13	12	—	—	0	—	—	36
Stress-B	8 oz	40	0	0	0	0	9	8	—	—	0	—	—	36
Vanilla	1 bottle	90	0	0	0	tr	21	20	—	—	65	—	—	15
XS ENERGY														
Citrus Blast	1 can (8.4 oz)	8	0	0	0	2	0	0	0	—	24	25	—	—
Cranberry Grape	1 can (8.4 oz)	8	0	0	0	2	0	0	0	—	24	25	—	—
Electric Lemon Blast	1 can (8.4 oz)	16	0	0	0	2	2	2	—	0	24	25	—	0
Tropical Blast	1 can (8.4 oz)	8	0	0	0	2	0	0	0	—	24	25	—	—
YET														
Your Energy Drink	1 can	8	0	0	0	2	0	0	—	0	46	25	—	60

ENGLISH MUFFIN

FOOD	PORTION	CALS	FAT	SAT FAT	CHOL	PROT	CARB	SUGAR	FIBER	CALCI	SOD	POTAS	FOLIC	VIT C
FROZEN														
WEIGHT WATCHERS														
Sandwich	1 (4 oz)	210	5	3	20	13	28	1	2	100	420	—	—	2
READY-TO-EAT														
apple cinnamon	1	138	2	tr	0	4	28	—	—	84	255	119	—	—
crumpets	1 (1.5 oz)	80	0	0	0	3	16	1	tr	20	270	—	—	0
granola	1	155	1	tr	0	6	31	—	—	129	275	103	—	0
mixed grain	1	155	1	tr	0	6	31	—	—	129	275	103	—	0
plain	1	134	1	tr	0	4	26	—	—	99	265	75	—	—
plain toasted	1	133	1	tr	0	4	26	—	—	99	262	74	—	—
raisin cinnamon	1	138	2	tr	0	4	28	—	—	84	255	119	—	—
sourdough	1	134	1	tr	0	4	26	—	—	99	265	75	—	—
wheat	1	127	1	tr	0	5	26	—	—	101	218	106	—	—
whole wheat	1	134	1	tr	0	6	27	—	4	175	420	139	—	0
MILTON'S														
Multi-Grain	1 (2 oz)	150	1	0	0	4	33	7	3	20	180	—	—	4
PEPPERIDGE FARM														
Original	1	130	1	0	0	5	26	tr	2	20	250	—	32	0
THOMAS'														
Blueberry	1	140	1	0	0	4	29	5	1	60	210	—	—	0
Carb Consider	1	100	2	0	<5	7	23	0	9	150	220	—	—	0
Hearty Grains Honey Wheat	1	130	1	0	0	5	27	3	2	60	190	—	—	0
Original	1	120	1	0	0	4	25	1	1	80	200	—	—	0
Raisin Bran	1	150	2	0	0	4	30	7	2	40	200	—	—	0
Raisin Cinnamon	1	140	1	0	0	4	30	8	1	20	180	—	—	0
Sourdough	1	120	1	0	0	4	25	2	1	80	190	—	—	0
Super Size	1 (3.2 oz)	200	2	0	0	7	41	2	2	150	310	—	—	0
WONDER														
Cinnamon Raisin	1 (2.1 oz)	140	2	1	0	5	26	11	2	60	260	—	—	0
Original	1 (2 oz)	130	1	0	0	4	25	4	1	150	290	—	—	0
Sourdough	1 (2 oz)	130	1	0	0	4	25	1	1	200	290	—	—	0

FOOD	PORTION	CALS	FAT	SAT FAT	CHOL	PROT	CARB	SUGAR	FIBER	CALCI	SOD	POTAS	FOLIC	VIT C
TAKE-OUT														
w/ butter	1 (2.2 oz)	189	6	2	13	5	30	—	—	103	386	69	57	1
w/ cheese & sausage	1 (4 oz)	393	24	10	59	15	29	—	—	168	1036	215	67	1
w/ egg cheese & canadian bacon	1 (4.8 oz)	289	13	5	234	17	28	—	2	151	729	199	44	2
w/ egg cheese & sausage	1 (5.8 oz)	487	31	12	274	22	31	—	—	196	1135	294	54	2

EPAZOTE

FOOD	PORTION	CALS	FAT	SAT FAT	CHOL	PROT	CARB	SUGAR	FIBER	CALCI	SOD	POTAS	FOLIC	VIT C
fresh	1 tbsp (1 g)	tr	0	—	0	0	tr	—	tr	2	tr	5	2	0
fresh sprig	1 (2 g)	1	tr	—	0	tr	tr	—	tr	6	1	13	4	tr

EPPAW

FOOD	PORTION	CALS	FAT	SAT FAT	CHOL	PROT	CARB	SUGAR	FIBER	CALCI	SOD	POTAS	FOLIC	VIT C
raw	½ cup	75	1	—	0	2	16	—	—	55	6	170	—	7

FALAFEL

NEAR EAST

FOOD	PORTION	CALS	FAT	SAT FAT	CHOL	PROT	CARB	SUGAR	FIBER	CALCI	SOD	POTAS	FOLIC	VIT C
Falafel as prep	2½ patties	230	16	2	0	10	18	3	5	40	560	—	—	0
TAKE-OUT														
falafel	1 (1.2 oz)	57	3	tr	0	2	5	—	—	9	50	99	13	tr

FAT

(*see also* BUTTER, BUTTER SUBSTITUTES, MARGARINE, OIL)

FOOD	PORTION	CALS	FAT	SAT FAT	CHOL	PROT	CARB	SUGAR	FIBER	CALCI	SOD	POTAS	FOLIC	VIT C
beef cooked	1 oz	193	20	8	27	3	0	—	—	4	12	34	1	0
beef suet	1 oz	242	27	15	19	tr	0	—	—	—	—	5	—	—
beef tallow	1 tbsp (13 g)	115	13	6	14	0	0	—	—	—	0	0	—	—
chicken	1 cup	1846	205	61	174	0	0	—	—	—	—	—	—	—
chicken	1 tbsp	115	13	4	11	0	0	—	—	—	—	—	—	—
cocoa butter	1 tbsp	120	14	8	0	0	0	0	0	—	—	—	—	—
duck	1 tbsp (13 g)	115	13	4	13	0	0	—	0	0	0	0	0	0
goose	1 tbsp	115	13	4	13	0	0	—	—	—	—	—	—	—
goose	1 oz	257	29	2	—	0	0	—	—	—	—	—	—	—
lamb new zealand	1 oz	182	19	10	25	2	0	—	—	6	6	15	—	—
lard	1 tbsp (13 g)	115	13	5	12	0	0	—	—	tr	0	0	—	—
lard	1 cup (205 g)	1849	205	80	195	0	0	—	—	tr	tr	tr	—	—
nutmeg butter	1 tbsp	120	14	12	—	0	0	0	0	—	—	—	—	—
pork backfat	1 oz	230	25	9	16	1	0	—	0	1	3	—	tr	tr
pork cooked	1 oz	178	18	7	26	3	0	—	0	15	10	—	1	0
salt pork	1 oz	212	23	8	25	23	0	—	—	2	404	19	0	—
shortening	1 cup	1812	205	41	0	0	0	0	0	—	—	—	—	—
shortening	1 tbsp	113	13	3	0	0	0	0	0	—	—	—	—	—
turkey	1 tbsp	115	13	4	13	0	0	—	—	—	—	—	—	—
ucuhuba butter	1 tbsp	120	14	12	—	0	0	0	0	—	—	—	—	—

FAT SUBSTITUTES

SMUCKER'S

FOOD	PORTION	CALS	FAT	SAT FAT	CHOL	PROT	CARB	SUGAR	FIBER	CALCI	SOD	POTAS	FOLIC	VIT C
Baking Healthy 100% Fat Free	1 tbsp	30	0	0	0	0	7	4	0	0	7	—	—	6

FOOD	PORTION	CALS	FAT	SAT FAT	CHOL	PROT	CARB	SUGAR	FIBER	CALCI	SOD	POTAS	FOLIC	VIT C
FAVA BEANS														
PROGRESSO														
Fava Beans	½ cup (4.6 oz)	110	1	0	0	6	20	0	5	20	250	—	—	0
FEIJOA														
fresh	1 (1.75 oz)	25	tr	—	0	1	5	—	—	8	2	78	19	7
puree	1 cup	119	2	—	0	3	26	—	—	41	7	378	93	32
FENNEL														
fresh bulb	1 (8.2 oz)	72	tr	—	0	3	17	—	—	116	122	969	62	28
fresh sliced	1 cup	27	tr	—	0	1	6	—	—	43	45	360	23	11
leaves	1 oz	7	tr	—	—	tr	1	—	1	31	25	—	29	27
seed	1 tsp	7	tr	tr	0	tr	1	—	—	24	2	34	—	—
FENUGREEK														
seed	1 tsp	12	tr	—	0	1	2	—	—	6	2	28	2	tr
FIBER														
APPLE FIBER														
Pure	2 tbsp (7 g)	16	0	0	0	—	7	—	4	—	—	—	—	—
BENEFIBER														
Supplement	1 pkg (4 g)	20	0	0	0	0	4	—	3	—	20	—	—	—
CHOICE														
Fiber Burst Lemon Lime	3 pieces	45	1	0	0	1	12	0	3	—	0	—	—	—
Fiber Burst Tropical Fruit	3 pieces	45	1	0	0	1	11	0	3	—	0	—	—	—
METAMUCIL														
Fiber Wafers Apple Crisp	2	120	5	1	0	2	17	—	6	—	20	—	—	—
ND LABS														
Pure Apple Fiber	1 tbsp (7 g)	16	0	0	0	0	7	—	4	—	—	—	—	—
FIDDLEHEAD FERNS														
fresh	3.5 oz	34	tr	—	0	5	6	—	—	32	1	370	—	27
FIGS														
calimyrna	3 (5.4 oz)	120	0	0	0	1	28	11	4	60	0	—	—	4
canned in heavy syrup	3	75	tr	tr	0	tr	19	—	—	23	1	85	—	1
canned in light syrup	3	58	tr	tr	0	tr	15	—	—	23	1	86	—	1
canned water pack	3	42	tr	—	0	tr	11	—	—	22	1	83	—	1
dried california	½ cup (3.5 oz)	200	1	—	0	4	58	—	17	150	11	710	24	2
dried cooked	½ cup	140	1	tr	0	2	16	—	—	79	6	391	1	6
dried whole	10	477	2	tr	0	6	122	—	17	269	20	1332	14	2
fresh	1 med	50	tr	tr	0	tr	10	—	—	18	1	116	—	1
JENNY														
Sundried Kalamata	4	120	0	0	0	1	28	21	5	60	5	—	—	—

FOOD	PORTION	CALS	FAT	SAT FAT	CHOL	PROT	CARB	SUGAR	FIBER	CALCI	SOD	POTAS	FOLIC	VIT C
FIREWEED														
leaves chopped	1 cup (0.8 oz)	24	1	—	0	1	4	—	2	99	8	114	26	tr
FISH														
FROZEN														
breaded fillet	1 (2 oz)	155	7	2	64	9	14	—	—	11	332	149	10	—
sticks	1 stick (1 oz)	76	3	1	31	4	7	—	—	6	163	73	5	—
GORTON'S														
Baked Au Gratin	1 piece (4.6 oz)	130	5	2	50	14	7	1	—	80	400	—	—	—
Baked Broccoli Cheddar	1 piece (4.6 oz)	130	5	2	50	14	7	1	—	80	310	—	—	—
Baked Primavera	1 piece (4.6 oz)	120	5	3	50	15	4	2	—	100	340	—	—	5
Batter Dipped Portions	1 piece (2.5 oz)	170	11	1	20	6	12	2	—	—	390	—	—	—
Crunchy Golden Fillets Breaded	2 (3.8 oz)	250	14	4	35	10	21	3	—	20	480	—	—	—
Crunchy Golden Sticks	6 (3.8 oz)	250	13	4	30	12	21	3	—	20	340	—	—	—
Garlic & Herb	2 pieces (3.6 oz)	220	11	3	30	10	21	6	—	20	670	—	—	—
Garlic Butter Crumb	1 piece (4.6 oz)	170	9	2	55	17	5	1	—	—	350	—	—	—
Grilled Cajun Blackened	1 piece (3.8 oz)	120	6	1	60	16	1	1	—	—	240	—	—	—
Grilled Garlic Butter	1 piece (3.8 oz)	120	6	1	60	16	1	1	—	—	200	—	—	—
Grilled Italian Herb	1 piece (3.8 oz)	130	6	1	60	17	2	2	—	—	330	—	—	—
Grilled Lemon Butter	1 piece (3.8 oz)	120	6	1	60	16	1	1	—	—	380	—	—	—
Grilled Lemon Pepper	1 piece (3.8 oz)	120	6	1	60	16	1	1	—	—	160	—	—	—
Parmesan	2 pieces (3.6 oz)	260	15	4	30	10	20	4	—	40	650	—	—	—
Ranch	1 piece (3.6 oz)	240	13	4	30	9	22	3	—	20	650	—	—	—
Southern Fried Country Style	2 pieces (3.6 oz)	230	14	4	30	10	16	3	—	20	660	—	—	—
Tenders	3.5 pieces (4 oz)	250	14	4	30	11	20	2	—	20	530	—	—	—
Tenders Extra Crunchy	3.5 pieces (4 oz)	270	12	4	30	11	29	4	—	20	640	—	—	—
TAKE-OUT														
fish cake	1 (4.7 oz)	166	7	2	—	18	6	—	—	179	—	—	—	5
jamaican brown fish stew	1 serv	426	22	5	84	48	9	—	2	—	419	—	—	—
kedgeree	5.6 oz	242	11	—	—	21	15	—	1	58	—	—	—	0

FOOD	PORTION	CALS	FAT	SAT FAT	CHOL	PROT	CARB	SUGAR	FIBER	CALCI	SOD	POTAS	FOLIC	VIT C
mousse	1 serv (3.5 oz)	185	14	—	—	13	3	tr	tr	40	540	250	—	tr
stew	1 cup (7.9 oz)	157	4	2	—	19	10	—	—	32	—	—	—	11
taramasalata	2 tbsp	124	14	—	10	1	1	—	—	6	182	16	2	0

FISH OIL

cod liver	1 tbsp	123	14	3	78	0	0	—	—	—	—	—	—	—
herring	1 tbsp	123	14	3	104	0	0	—	—	—	—	—	—	—
menhaden	1 tbsp	123	14	4	71	0	0	—	—	—	—	—	—	—
salmon	1 tbsp	123	14	3	66	0	0	—	—	—	—	—	—	—
sardine	1 tbsp	123	14	4	97	0	0	—	—	—	—	—	—	—
shark	1 oz	270	29	—	—	0	0	0	0	—	—	—	—	—
whale	1 oz	270	29	—	—	0	0	0	0	—	—	—	—	—

FISH PASTE

fish paste	2 tsp	15	1	—	—	1	tr	—	0	25	—	—	—	0

FISH SUBSTITUTES

LOMA LINDA

Ocean Platter not prep	⅓ cup (0.9 oz)	90	1	0	0	14	8	0	4	0	450	450	—	0

WORTHINGTON

Fillets	2 (3 oz)	180	10	2	0	16	8	tr	4	0	750	130	—	0
Tuno	½ cup (1.9 oz)	80	6	1	0	6	2	0	1	20	290	35	—	0

FLAXSEED

ARROWHEAD

Organic Flax Seeds	¼ cup	140	9	—	0	5	10	0	6	—	0	—	—	—

BITE ME

Flax Bar	1 bar (1.8 oz)	242	11	2	0	7	30	5	12	—	79	236	—	—

BOB'S RED MILL

Flax Seed Meal	2 tbsp	60	5	—	0	3	4	0	4	—	0	—	—	—

CRACKER FLAX

Organic Apple Raisin	1 oz	130	5	0	5	6	16	4	9	40	55	—	—	0

HODGSON MILL

Milled	2 tbsp	60	1	0	0	3	4	0	4	20	0	30	16	—

FLOUNDER

FRESH

cooked	3 oz	99	1	tr	58	21	0	—	—	16	89	292	—	—
cooked	1 fillet (4.5 oz)	148	2	tr	86	31	0	—	—	23	133	436	—	—

TAKE-OUT

battered & fried	3.2 oz	211	11	3	31	13	15	—	—	17	484	292	51	0
breaded & fried	3.2 oz	211	11	3	31	13	15	—	—	17	484	292	51	0

FLOUR

buckwheat whole groat	1 cup (4.2 oz)	402	4	1	0	15	85	—	12	49	13	692	65	0
corn masa	1 cup (4 oz)	416	4	1	0	11	87	—	11	161	6	340	213	0

FOOD	PORTION	CALS	FAT	SAT FAT	CHOL	PROT	CARB	SUGAR	FIBER	CALCI	SOD	POTAS	FOLIC	VIT C
cottonseed lowfat	1 oz	94	tr	tr	0	14	10	—	—	135	10	500	—	1
peanut defatted	1 cup	196	tr	tr	0	31	21	—	—	84	108	774	149	0
peanut lowfat	1 cup	257	13	2	0	20	19	—	—	78	0	815	—	—
potato	1 cup (6.3 oz)	628	1	tr	0	14	143	—	—	59	61	2843	—	34
rice brown	1 cup (5.5 oz)	574	4	tr	0	11	121	—	7	17	13	457	25	0
rice white	1 cup (5.5 oz)	578	2	1	0	9	127	—	4	16	1	120	6	0
rye dark	1 cup (4.5 oz)	415	3	tr	0	18	88	—	29	72	2	934	77	0
rye light	1 cup (3.6 oz)	374	1	tr	0	9	82	—	15	21	2	238	22	0
rye medium	1 cup (3.6 oz)	361	2	tr	0	10	79	—	15	24	3	347	19	0
sesame lowfat	1 oz	95	tr	tr	0	14	10	—	—	42	11	113	8	—
triticale whole grain	1 cup (4.6 oz)	439	2	tr	0	17	95	—	19	46	3	606	96	0
white all-purpose	1 cup (4.4 oz)	455	1	tr	0	13	95	—	2	19	3	134	193	0
white bread	1 cup (4.8 oz)	495	2	tr	0	16	99	—	3	21	3	137	211	0
white cake unsifted	1 cup (4.8 oz)	496	1	tr	0	11	107	—	2	19	3	144	211	0
white self-rising	1 cup (4.4 oz)	443	1	tr	0	12	93	—	3	423	1588	155	193	0
white unbleached	1 cup (4.4 oz)	455	1	tr	0	13	95	—	3	19	3	134	193	0
whole wheat	1 cup (4.2 oz)	407	2	tr	0	16	87	—	15	41	6	486	53	0
ALL TRUMP														
Flour	¼ cup (1 oz)	100	0	0	0	4	22	tr	tr	—	0	30	—	—
ARROWHEAD														
Whole Grain Oat	⅓ cup	120	3	—	0	5	18	0	3	—	0	—	—	—
BETTY CROCKER														
Softasilk Velvet Cake Flour	¼ cup (1 oz)	100	0	0	0	2	23	tr	tr	0	0	35	—	0
GOLD MEDAL														
All Purpose	¼ cup (1 oz)	100	0	0	0	3	22	tr	tr	0	0	40	40	0
Better For Bread	¼ cup (1 oz)	100	0	0	0	4	22	0	tr	0	0	35	40	0
Organic All Purpose	¼ cup (1 oz)	100	0	0	0	3	22	—	tr	—	0	40	40	—
Self Rising	¼ cup (1 oz)	100	0	0	0	3	22	—	tr	60	400	35	40	0
Unbleached	¼ cup (1 oz)	100	0	0	0	3	22	tr	tr	0	0	40	40	0
Wondra	¼ cup	100	0	0	0	3	23	—	tr	—	0	35	—	—
HECKERS														
All Purpose Unbleached	¼ cup	100	0	0	0	3	22	tr	tr	0	0	35	40	0
Whole Wheat	¼ cup	100	1	0	0	4	21	0	3	0	0	—	—	0
HODGSON MILL														
White Unbleached Organic	¼ cup (1 oz)	100	0	0	0	3	23	0	3	0	0	—	—	0
Whole Wheat Graham Organic	¼ cup (1 oz)	100	1	0	0	3	22	0	3	0	0	—	—	0
LA PINA														
Flour	¼ cup (1 oz)	100	0	0	0	2	23	tr	1	0	0	35	100	0

FOOD	PORTION	CALS	FAT	SAT FAT	CHOL	PROT	CARB	SUGAR	FIBER	CALCI	SOD	POTAS	FOLIC	VIT C
RED BAND														
All Purpose	¼ cup (1 oz)	100	0	0	0	2	23	—	tr	0	0	40	—	0
Self-Rising	¼ cup (1 oz)	100	0	0	0	2	22	—	tr	60	400	40	—	0
ROBIN HOOD														
All Purpose	¼ cup (1 oz)	100	0	0	0	3	22	tr	tr	0	0	40	—	0
Self-Rising	¼ cup (1 oz)	100	0	0	0	3	22	tr	tr	0	0	35	—	0
Unbleached	¼ cup (1 oz)	100	0	0	0	3	22	tr	tr	0	0	40	—	0
Whole Wheat	¼ cup (1 oz)	90	1	—	0	4	21	—	3	0	0	110	—	0
FRENCH BEANS														
dried cooked	1 cup	228	1	tr	0	12	43	—	17	111	11	655	132	2

FRENCH FRIES

(*see* POTATOES)

FRENCH TOAST

FOOD	PORTION	CALS	FAT	SAT FAT	CHOL	PROT	CARB	SUGAR	FIBER	CALCI	SOD	POTAS	FOLIC	VIT C
FROZEN														
french toast	1 slice (2 oz)	126	4	1	48	4	19	—	2	63	292	79	14	—
TAKE-OUT														
plain	1 slice	151	7	2	75	7	16	—	—	64	311	86	15	tr
sticks	5 (4.9 oz)	513	29	5	75	8	58	—	3	78	499	127	82	0
w/ butter	2 slices (4.7 oz)	356	19	8	116	10	36	—	—	73	513	177	73	tr

FROG'S LEGS

FOOD	PORTION	CALS	FAT	SAT FAT	CHOL	PROT	CARB	SUGAR	FIBER	CALCI	SOD	POTAS	FOLIC	VIT C
TAKE-OUT														
as prep w/ seasoned flour & fried	1 (0.8)	70	5	—	12	4	15	—	—	5	—	—	tr	0

FRUCTOSE

FOOD	PORTION	CALS	FAT	SAT FAT	CHOL	PROT	CARB	SUGAR	FIBER	CALCI	SOD	POTAS	FOLIC	VIT C
ESTEE														
Fructose	1 tsp	15	0	0	0	0	4	4	0	—	0	0	—	—
Packet	1 pkg	10	0	0	0	0	3	3	0	—	0	0	—	—

FRUIT DRINKS

(*see also individual names*)

FOOD	PORTION	CALS	FAT	SAT FAT	CHOL	PROT	CARB	SUGAR	FIBER	CALCI	SOD	POTAS	FOLIC	VIT C
FROZEN														
TREE OF LIFE														
Organic Smoothie Banana Raspberry Strawberry	⅔ cup (5 oz)	90	0	0	0	1	23	15	3	0	0	—	—	36
Organic Smoothie Mango Strawberry Raspberry	⅔ cup (5 oz)	70	0	0	0	1	18	15	4	20	0	—	—	42
Organic Smoothie Strawberry Banana	⅔ cup (5 oz)	90	0	0	0	7	23	15	3	0	0	—	—	36

FOOD	PORTION	CALS	FAT	SAT FAT	CHOL	PROT	CARB	SUGAR	FIBER	CALCI	SOD	POTAS	FOLIC	VIT C
TREE OF LIFE (CONT.)														
Organic Smoothie Strawberry Blueberry Banana	⅔ cup (5 oz)	90	0	0	0	1	22	12	3	0	0	—	—	24
MIX														
CRYSTAL LIGHT														
Fruit Punch as prep	1 serv (8 oz)	5	0	0	0	0	0	0	0	0	0	45	—	6
Lemon-Lime Drink as prep	1 serv (8 oz)	5	0	0	0	0	0	0	0	0	0	5	—	6
Passion Fruit Pineapple Drink as prep	1 serv (8 oz)	5	0	0	0	0	tr	0	0	0	0	10	—	0
Pineapple Orange Drink as prep	1 serv (8 oz)	5	0	0	0	0	0	0	0	0	0	0	—	0
Strawberry Orange Banana as prep	1 serv (8 oz)	5	0	0	0	0	0	0	0	0	0	35	—	0
Strawberry Kiwi as prep	1 serv (8 oz)	5	0	0	0	0	0	0	0	0	0	0	—	0
Watermelon Strawberry as prep	1 serv (8 oz)	5	0	0	0	0	0	0	0	0	0	15	—	0
KOOL-AID														
Grape Berry Splash Drink as prep	1 serv (8 oz)	70	0	0	0	0	17	17	0	0	0	0	—	6
Grape Berry Splash Drink as prep w/ sugar	1 serv (8 oz)	100	0	0	0	0	25	25	0	0	0	0	—	6
Kickin' Kiwi Lime Drink as prep	1 serv (8 oz)	60	0	0	0	0	16	16	0	0	0	0	—	6
Kickin' Kiwi Lime Drink as prep w/ sugar	1 serv (8 oz)	100	0	0	0	0	25	25	0	0	10	0	—	6
Lemon-Lime Drink as prep w/ sugar	1 serv (8 oz)	100	0	0	0	0	25	25	0	0	5	0	—	6
Man-O-Mango Berry Drink as prep	1 serv (8 oz)	60	0	0	0	0	16	16	0	0	0	0	—	6
Man-O-Mango Berry Drink as prep w/ sugar	1 serv (8 oz)	100	0	0	0	0	25	25	0	0	0	0	—	6
Oh Yeah Orange Pineapple Drink as prep	1 serv (8 oz)	60	0	0	0	0	16	16	0	0	0	0	—	6

FOOD	PORTION	CALS	FAT	SAT FAT	CHOL	PROT	CARB	SUGAR	FIBER	CALCI	SOD	POTAS	FOLIC	VIT C
KOOL-AID (CONT.)														
Oh Yeah Orange Pineapple Drink as prep w/ sugar	1 serv (8 oz)	100	0	0	0	0	25	25	0	0	0	0	—	6
Pina-Pineapple Drink as prep	1 serv (8 oz)	60	0	0	0	0	17	17	0	0	0	0	—	6
Piña-Pineapple Drink as prep w/ sugar	1 serv (8 oz)	100	0	0	0	0	25	25	0	0	0	0	—	6
Roarin' Raspberry Cranberry Drink as prep	1 serv (8 oz)	70	0	0	0	0	17	17	0	0	20	0	—	6
Roarin' Raspberry Cranberry Drink as prep w/ sugar	1 serv (8 oz)	100	0	0	0	0	25	25	0	0	10	0	—	6
Slammin' Strawberry Kiwi Drink as prep	1 serv (8 oz)	70	0	0	0	0	17	17	0	0	15	0	—	6
Slammin' Strawberry Kiwi Drink as prep w/ sugar	1 serv (8 oz)	100	0	0	0	0	25	25	0	0	15	0	—	6
Strawberry Raspberry Drink as prep	1 serv (8 oz)	60	0	0	0	0	16	16	0	0	0	0	—	6
Strawberry Raspberry Drink as prep w/ sugar	1 serv (8 oz)	100	0	0	0	0	25	25	0	0	0	0	—	6
Sugar Free Tropical Punch as prep	1 serv (8 oz)	5	0	0	0	0	0	0	0	0	10	10	—	6
Tropical Punch as prep	1 serv (8 oz)	60	0	0	0	0	16	16	0	0	0	0	—	6
Tropical Punch as prep w/ sugar	1 serv (8 oz)	100	0	0	0	0	25	25	0	0	15	0	—	6
Watermelon Cherry Drink as prep	1 serv (8 oz)	60	0	0	0	0	16	16	0	0	0	0	—	6
Watermelon Cherry Drink as prep w/ sugar	1 serv (8 oz)	100	0	0	0	0	25	25	0	0	10	0	—	6
TANG														
Orange Pineapple as prep	1 serv (8 oz)	100	0	0	0	0	24	24	0	60	45	0	—	60
READY-TO-DRINK														
fruit punch	6 fl oz	87	tr	0	0	tr	22	—	—	14	41	47	2	55
pineapple & orange drink	8 fl oz	125	0	0	0	3	29	—	—	13	9	116	27	56

FOOD	PORTION	CALS	FAT	SAT FAT	CHOL	PROT	CARB	SUGAR	FIBER	CALCI	SOD	POTAS	FOLIC	VIT C
APPLE & EVE														
Apple Cranberry	8 oz	120	0	0	0	1	30	26	—	100	20	—	—	60
CAPRI SUN														
Fruit Punch	1 pkg (7 oz)	100	0	0	0	0	26	26	0	0	20	25	—	0
Maui Punch	1 pkg (7 oz)	100	0	0	0	0	27	27	0	0	20	20	—	0
Mountain Cooler	1 pkg (7 oz)	90	0	0	0	0	24	24	0	0	25	25	—	0
Pacific Cooler	1 pkg (7 oz)	100	0	0	0	0	26	26	0	0	20	25	—	0
Red Berry	1 pkg (7 oz)	100	0	0	0	0	26	26	0	0	20	25	—	0
Safari Punch	1 pkg (7 oz)	100	0	0	0	0	25	25	0	0	20	25	—	0
Strawberry Kiwi Drink	1 pkg (7 oz)	100	0	0	0	0	26	26	0	0	20	25	—	0
Surfer Cooler Drink	1 pkg (7 oz)	100	0	0	0	0	27	27	0	0	20	30	—	0
CERES														
Cranberry & Kiwi	8 oz	110	0	0	0	0	28	24	0	30	14	252	—	60
Medley	8 oz	130	0	0	0	0	31	29	2	20	10	248	—	60
Youngberry	8 oz	120	0	0	0	0	30	25	0	20	10	190	—	30
CHAMPION LYTE														
All Flavors	1 bottle	0	0	0	0	0	0	0	0	0	55	25	—	0
CITRUS SQUEEZE														
California Punch	8 oz	130	0	0	0	0	33	33	—	—	85	—	—	—
Florida Punch	8 oz	120	0	0	0	0	30	30	—	—	100	—	—	—
COCO LOPEZ														
Mango Kiwi	8 fl oz	130	0	0	0	0	33	33	—	—	0	—	—	—
CRYSTAL LIGHT														
Fruit Punch	1 serv (8 oz)	5	0	0	0	0	0	0	0	0	20	105	—	0
Kiwi Strawberry	1 serv (8 oz)	5	0	0	0	0	0	0	0	0	20	110	—	0
Orange Strawberry Banana Drink	1 serv (8 oz)	5	0	0	0	0	0	0	0	0	20	95	—	0
DEL MONTE														
Peach Raspberry	5.5 fl oz	160	0	0	0	1	40	33	3	20	10	—	—	60
Pineapple Banana Orange	5.5 fl oz	170	0	0	0	1	44	34	1	20	10	—	—	60
Strawberry Peach Banana	5.5 fl oz	150	0	0	0	1	39	30	1	20	10	—	—	60
DOLE														
Apple Berry Burst	8 fl oz	120	0	0	0	0	31	—	—	—	20	—	—	60
Cranberry Apple	8 fl oz	120	0	0	0	0	30	—	—	—	35	200	—	60
Fruit Fiesta	8 fl oz	140	0	0	0	0	34	—	—	—	20	—	—	60
Fruit Punch	1 carton (10 oz)	160	0	0	0	0	39	—	—	—	25	—	—	—
Mountain Cherry	8 fl oz	150	0	0	0	0	30	28	—	—	30	—	—	60
Orange Peach Mango	8 oz	120	0	0	0	1	28	—	—	—	35	340		60

FOOD	PORTION	CALS	FAT	SAT FAT	CHOL	PROT	CARB	SUGAR	FIBER	CALCI	SOD	POTAS	FOLIC	VIT C
DOLE (CONT.)														
Orange Strawberry Banana	8 oz	120	0	0	0	1	28	—	—	—	30	290	—	60
Orchard Peach	8 oz	140	0	0	0	1	34	28	—	20	35	240	—	60
Pineapple Orange	8 oz	120	0	0	0	2	27	—	—	—	20	350	—	60
Pineapple Orange Strawberry	8 oz	130	0	0	0	0	32	—	—	40	20	400	—	60
Tropical Fruit	8 oz	160	0	0	0	0	38	—	0	—	30	250	—	60
EDEN														
Organic Apple Cherry Juice	8 oz	120	0	0	0	0	30	29	1	14	15	330	—	0
EVERFRESH														
Cranberry-Apple Drink	1 can (8 oz)	120	0	0	0	0	31	31	0	—	0	—	—	—
Grape-Strawberry	1 can (8 oz)	120	0	0	0	0	31	31	0	—	0	—	—	—
Kiwi-Strawberry	1 can (8 oz)	120	0	0	0	0	30	30	0	—	0	—	—	—
Mandarin Orange Mango Drink	1 can (8 oz)	120	0	0	0	0	29	29	0	—	0	—	—	—
Orange Banana Strawberry Drink	1 can (8 oz)	120	0	0	0	0	30	30	0	—	19	—	—	—
Tropical Fruit Punch	1 can (8 oz)	120	0	0	0	0	30	30	0	—	0	—	—	—
Wild Blackberry Lime Drink	1 can (8 oz)	120	0	0	0	0	29	29	0	—	0	—	—	—
FRESH SAMANTHA														
Banana Strawberry	1 cup (8 oz)	130	0	0	0	4	11	—	6	20	24	130	24	30
Carrot Orange	1 cup (8 oz)	100	0	0	0	4	8	—	4	40	24	150	40	72
Desperately Seeking C	1 cup (8 oz)	110	0	0	0	4	9	—	7	0	0	120	40	600
Protein Blast	1 cup (8 oz)	160	1	0	—	9	10	—	8	40	24	150	32	48
Super Juice	1 cup (8 oz)	140	1	0	—	4	11	—	8	20	0	160	40	48
The Big Bang	1 cup (8 oz)	100	0	0	0	2	8	—	8	0	0	70	24	21
FRUITOPIA														
Fruit Integration	8 fl oz	110	0	0	0	0	29	29	—	—	80	—	—	60
GUZZLER														
Citrus Punch	8 fl oz	140	0	0	0	tr	25	25	—	—	10	—	—	60
Island Punch	8 fl oz	140	0	0	0	0	29	22	0	—	30	—	—	—
HANSEN'S														
Fruit Punch 100% Juice	1 box (4.23 oz)	60	0	0	0	0	15	14	—	100	5	—	—	60
Juice Slam Wild Berry	1 box	120	0	0	0	0	29	25	—	20	15	143	—	15
Smoothie Apricot Nectar	1 can	170	0	0	0	1	43	43	—	20	50	250	—	60

FOOD	PORTION	CALS	FAT	SAT FAT	CHOL	PROT	CARB	SUGAR	FIBER	CALCI	SOD	POTAS	FOLIC	VIT C
HANSEN'S (CONT.)														
Smoothie Cranberry Twist	1 can	180	0	0	0	0	45	44	—	20	50	—	—	60
Smoothie Energy Island Blast	1 can	170	0	0	0	1	40	40	—	40	40	230	—	60
Smoothie Guava Strawberry	1 can	170	0	0	0	0	43	43	—	30	50	130	—	60
Smoothie Mango Pineapple	1 can	170	0	0	0	0	43	43	—	40	50	130	—	60
Smoothie Peach Berry	1 can	170	0	0	0	0	43	43	—	30	50	150	—	60
Smoothie Pineapple Coconut	1 can	180	0	0	0	0	43	43	—	30	50	120	—	60
Smoothie Strawberry Banana	1 can	180	0	0	0	0	44	43	—	30	50	140	—	60
Smoothie Tropical Passion	1 can	170	0	0	0	0	44	43	—	30	50	150	—	60
Smoothie Whipped Orange	1 can	180	0	0	0	0	44	44	—	30	50	180	—	60
Smoothie Lite Cranberry Raspberry	1 can	50	0	0	0	0	13	13	—	10	45	130	—	60
JUICY JUICE														
Apple Grape	1 box (8.45 oz)	140	0	0	0	0	34	32	0	0	15	190	—	78
Berry	1 box (8.45 oz)	130	0	0	0	0	37	31	0	0	15	190	—	78
Punch	1 box (8.45 oz)	140	0	0	0	0	34	32	0	0	15	—	—	78
Punch	1 box (4.23 oz)	70	0	0	0	0	17	15	0	0	10	100	—	60
Tropical	1 box (8.45 oz)	140	0	0	0	0	34	31	0	0	15	200	—	78
KOOL-AID														
Bursts Great Bluedini	1 (7 oz)	100	0	0	0	0	24	24	0	0	30	15	—	0
Bursts Kickin' Kiwi Lime	1 (7 oz)	100	0	0	0	0	24	24	0	0	30	15	—	0
Bursts Oh Yeah Orange Pineapple	1 (7 oz)	100	0	0	0	0	24	24	0	0	30	15	—	0
Bursts Slammin' Strawberry Kiwi	1 (7 oz)	100	0	0	0	0	24	24	0	0	30	15	—	0
Bursts Tropical Punch	1 (7 oz)	100	0	0	0	0	24	24	0	0	30	15	—	0
Splash Grape Berry Punch	1 serv (8 oz)	120	0	0	0	0	31	31	0	0	35	15	—	0
Splash Kiwi Strawberry Drink	1 serv (8 oz)	110	0	0	0	0	29	29	0	0	35	15	—	0
Splash Tropical Punch	1 serv (8 oz)	120	0	0	0	0	31	31	0	0	35	15	—	0

FOOD	PORTION	CALS	FAT	SAT FAT	CHOL	PROT	CARB	SUGAR	FIBER	CALCI	SOD	POTAS	FOLIC	VIT C
LANGERS														
100% Juice Pineapple Coconut	8 oz	140	3	3	0	0	28	27	1	40	55	—	—	30
Blueberry Cranberry	8 oz	135	0	0	0	0	34	34	—	—	10	—	—	60
Cranberry Berry	8 oz	135	0	0	0	0	34	31	—	—	10	—	—	60
Cranberry Fuji	8 oz	160	0	0	0	0	39	35	—	—	10	—	—	60
Cranberry Grape	8 oz	165	0	0	0	0	41	37	—	0	10	—	—	60
Cranberry Grape Cocktail	8 oz	165	0	0	0	0	41	37	—	—	10	—	—	60
Cranberry Orange	8 oz	130	0	0	0	0	33	30	—	—	10	—	—	60
Diet Cranberry Berry	8 oz	30	0	0	0	0	8	8	—	20	10	—	—	60
Diet Cranberry Grape	8 oz	30	0	0	0	0	8	8	—	20	10	—	—	60
Fruit Punch Cocktail	8 oz	120	0	0	0	0	30	30	—	—	14	—	—	—
Kiwi Raspberry Cocktail	8 oz	120	0	0	0	0	29	26	—	—	0	—	—	60
Kiwi Strawberry Cocktail	8 oz	120	0	0	0	0	29	26	—	—	0	—	—	—
Mango Orange	8 oz	130	0	0	0	0	33	30	—	—	0	—	—	60
Mixed Berry 100% Juice	8 oz	120	0	0	0	0	30	27	—	20	15	—	—	6
Pineapple Orange Guava	8 oz	130	0	0	0	0	30	30	—	—	0	—	—	60
Ruby Orange	8 oz	130	0	0	0	0	33	30	—	0	10	—	—	60
Tropical Ruby	8 oz	135	0	0	0	0	34	34	—	0	10	—	—	60
White Cranberry Raspberry	8 oz	120	0	0	0	0	28	28	—	—	10	—	—	60
MOTT'S														
Berry	1 box (8 oz)	100	0	0	0	0	26	—	—	—	10	—	—	—
Fruit Punch	8 fl oz	130	0	0	0	0	32	—	—	—	0	—	—	—
Fruit Punch	1 box (8 oz)	110	0	0	0	0	27	—	—	—	15	—	—	—
NAKED JUICE														
Berry Blast	8 oz	120	0	0	0	1	30	26	1	20	10	330	—	126
Blue Machine	8 oz	150	1	—	—	1	40	29	8	20	30	380	400	102
Green Machine	8 oz	130	0	0	0	1	33	27	1	20	15	440	—	36
Power C	8 oz	120	1	—	—	1	29	23	3	20	15	—	—	60
Protein Zone	8 oz	210	4	2	20	17	27	25	tr	60	135	460	—	126
Red Machine	8 oz	160	3	—	—	2	32	25	4	40	15	290	400	6
Strawberry Banana C	8 oz	120	0	0	0	2	28	23	3	20	5	—	—	300
Very Berry	8 oz	130	0	0	0	2	30	24	1	20	10	370	—	300
Well Being	8 oz	210	4	—	—	17	29	26	1	60	130	—	—	132

FOOD	PORTION	CALS	FAT	SAT FAT	CHOL	PROT	CARB	SUGAR	FIBER	CALCI	SOD	POTAS	FOLIC	VIT C
NANTUCKET NECTARS														
California Melonberry	8 oz	110	0	0	0	0	28	28	—	0	15	—	—	60
Cranberry Apple	8 oz	140	0	0	0	0	36	34	—	0	5	—	—	60
Fruit Punch	8 oz	130	0	0	0	0	32	30	—	0	5	—	—	60
Kiwi Berry	8 oz	120	0	0	0	0	30	26	—	0	5	—	—	60
Organic Banana Mango Carrot	8 oz	120	0	0	0	0	30	28	—	—	30	—	—	—
Organic Blueberry Banana	8 oz	120	0	0	0	0	30	28	—	—	30	—	—	—
Organic Cranberry Orange	8 oz	130	0	0	0	0	31	30	—	—	30	—	—	—
Peach Orange	8 oz	130	0	0	0	0	31	26	1	0	25	—	—	15
Pineapple Orange Guava	8 oz	120	0	0	0	0	31	28	—	0	0	—	—	60
Pomegranate Pear	8 oz	110	0	0	0	0	28	27	0	—	30	—	—	—
Watermelon Strawberry	8 oz	120	0	0	0	0	30	27	—	0	5	—	—	60
OBERWEIS														
Fruit Punch	8 oz	120	0	0	0	0	30	29	0	0	5	—	—	1
OCEAN SPRAY														
Citrus Splash Spritzer	8 oz	160	0	0	0	0	40	40	—	—	50	—	—	—
Cran*Grape	8 oz	170	0	0	0	0	41	41	0	—	35	—	—	60
Cran*Raspberry	8 oz	140	0	0	0	0	36	36	0	—	35	—	—	60
Cran*Strawberry	8 oz	140	0	0	0	0	36	35	tr	—	35	—	—	60
Cranapple	8 oz	160	0	0	0	0	41	40	tr	—	35	—	—	60
Grape Cranberry	8 oz	170	0	0	0	—	41	41	—	—	35	0	—	60
Kiwi Strawberry	8 oz	120	0	0	0	0	31	31	0	—	35	0	—	60
Mandarin Magic	8 oz	120	0	0	0	0	31	31	0	—	60	0	—	60
Orange Citrus Spritzer	8 oz	160	0	0	0	0	41	40	—	—	50	—	—	—
Ruby Tangerine Spritzer	8 oz	160	0	0	0	0	41	40	—	—	50	—	—	—
White Cranberry Apple Juice	8 oz	120	0	0	0	—	30	30	—	—	35	30	—	60
Wildberry Spritzer	8 oz	160	0	0	0	0	41	40	—	—	50	—	—	—
ODWALLA														
Blackberry Fruit Shake	8 fl oz	140	0	0	0	1	35	30	1	20	0	400	—	36
Carrot Orange Apple	8 fl oz	100	0	0	0	2	23	21	1	40	80	410	—	60
Orange Piña Smoothie	8 fl oz	140	0	0	0	0	33	33	1	20	10	—	—	72

FOOD	PORTION	CALS	FAT	SAT FAT	CHOL	PROT	CARB	SUGAR	FIBER	CALCI	SOD	POTAS	FOLIC	VIT C
ODWALLA (CONT.)														
Rooty Fruity	8 fl oz	110	1	—	0	0	24	21	0	20	90	—	—	48
Strawberry Banana	8 fl oz	120	1	—	0	1	31	26	3	20	0	510	—	66
PURITY ORGANIC														
Citrus Punch	8 oz	123	tr	—	—	tr	33	—	tr	—	tr	—	—	60
SHASTA PLUS														
Apple-Strawberry	1 can (11.5 oz)	160	0	0	0	0	41	41	0	—	45	—	—	60
Fruit Punch	1 can (11.5 oz)	160	0	0	0	0	39	39	0	—	45	—	—	60
Pineapple-Cherry	1 can (11.5 oz)	160	0	0	0	0	40	40	0	—	45	—	—	60
SNAPPLE														
Diet Cranberry Raspberry	8 fl oz	10	0	0	0	0	2	2	—	—	10	—	—	—
Final Fruit Fireworks	8 oz	120	0	0	0	0	29	29	—	—	10	—	—	—
Fruit Punch	8 fl oz	110	0	0	0	0	29	27	—	—	10	—	—	—
Go Bananas	8 oz	120	0	0	0	0	30	26	—	—	10	—	—	—
Kiwi Strawberry	8 fl oz	110	0	0	0	0	28	26	—	—	10	—	—	—
Pie	8 oz	120	0	0	0	0	31	29	—	—	35	—	—	—
Snapricot Orange	8 oz	120	0	0	0	0	30	28	—	—	10	—	—	—
SOY20														
All Flavors	1 bottle (12 oz)	90	0	0	0	0	22	22	—	—	10	—	—	—
SQUEEZIT														
Berry B. Wild	1 bottle (7 oz)	110	0	0	0	0	28	27	0	0	0	—	—	0
Lemon Lime	1 bottle (7 oz)	110	0	0	0	0	28	25	0	0	0	—	—	0
Rockin' Red Puncher	1 bottle (7 oz)	110	0	0	0	0	24	23	0	0	0	—	—	0
Tropical Punch	1 bottle (7 oz)	110	0	0	0	0	28	26	0	0	0	—	—	0
TROPICANA														
Berry Punch	8 fl oz	130	0	0	0	0	32	—	—	—	15	—	—	—
Citrus Punch	8 fl oz	140	0	0	0	0	36	33	—	—	15	—	—	—
Fruit Punch	8 oz	130	0	0	0	0	32	—	—	—	15	—	—	—
Tangerine Orange Juice	8 fl oz	110	0	0	0	2	25	—	—	20	0	450	60	72
Tropics Orange Strawberry Banana	8 fl oz	110	0	0	0	tr	27	23	—	20	5	380	—	36
Tropics Orange Kiwi Passion	8 fl oz	100	0	0	0	tr	26	23	—	20	15	300	—	6
Tropics Orange Peach Mango	8 fl oz	110	0	0	0	tr	28	24	—	20	15	300	—	36
Tropics Orange Pineapple	8 fl oz	110	0	0	0	tr	27	24	—	20	15	340	—	6
Twister Apple Raspberry Blackberry	1 bottle (10 fl oz)	160	1	—	0	0	38	—	—	—	20	—	—	60

FOOD	PORTION	CALS	FAT	SAT FAT	CHOL	PROT	CARB	SUGAR	FIBER	CALCI	SOD	POTAS	FOLIC	VIT C
TROPICANA (CONT.)														
Twister Citrus Punch	1 bottle (10 oz)	180	0	0	0	0	45	—	—	—	15	—	—	—
Twister Cranberry Punch	1 bottle (10 oz)	170	0	0	0	0	43	—	—	—	20	—	—	—
Twister Fruit Punch	1 bottle (10 oz)	170	0	0	0	0	43	—	—	—	40	—	—	60
Twister Light Orange Strawberry Banana	1 bottle (10 oz)	45	0	0	0	tr	11	—	—	—	25	—	—	60
Twister Orange Cranberry	1 bottle (10 fl oz)	160	0	0	0	tr	40	—	—	—	60	—	—	60
Twister Orange Strawberry Banana	1 bottle (10 oz)	160	0	0	0	tr	40	—	—	—	60	—	—	60
Twister Ruby Red Tangerine	1 bottle (10 oz)	160	0	0	0	0	40	—	—	—	25	—	—	60
Twister Strawberry Kiwi	1 bottle (10 oz)	160	0	0	0	0	42	—	—	—	25	—	—	60
V8														
Splash Berry Blend	8 oz	110	0	0	0	0	28	26	—	—	40	125	—	60
VERYFINE														
Apple Cranberry	1 bottle (10 oz)	190	0	0	0	0	48	48	0	0	10	—	—	60
Apple Quenchers Black Cherry White Grape	8 fl oz	120	0	0	0	0	30	30	0	0	10	—	—	60
Apple Quenchers Cranberry Tangerine	8 fl oz	120	0	0	0	0	31	31	0	0	10	—	—	60
Apple Quenchers Peach Kiwi	8 fl oz	130	0	0	0	0	33	31	0	0	25	—	—	60
Apple Quenchers Peach Plum	8 fl oz	130	0	0	0	0	32	31	0	0	25	—	—	60
Apple Quenchers Pear Passionfruit	8 fl oz	120	0	0	0	0	31	29	0	0	15	—	—	60
Apple Quenchers Raspberry Cherry	8 fl oz	120	0	0	0	0	31	30	0	0	25	—	—	60
Apple Quenchers Raspberry Lime	8 fl oz	120	0	0	0	0	30	30	0	0	25	—	—	60
Apple Quenchers Strawberry Banana	8 fl oz	120	0	0	0	0	30	29	0	0	20	—	—	60
Chillers Artic Mango Tangerine	8 fl oz	110	0	0	0	0	27	24	tr	0	5	—	—	60
Chillers Freezing Fruit Punch	8 fl oz	130	0	0	0	0	33	33	0	0	20	—	—	60

FOOD	PORTION	CALS	FAT	SAT FAT	CHOL	PROT	CARB	SUGAR	FIBER	CALCI	SOD	POTAS	FOLIC	VIT C
VERYFINE (CONT.)														
Chillers Lemon Lime Blizzard	8 fl oz	120	0	0	0	0	29	29	0	0	5	—	—	60
Chillers Shivering Strawberry Melon	1 can (11.5 oz)	160	0	0	0	0	41	40	0	0	10	—	—	60
Cranberry Raspberry	8 fl oz	160	0	0	0	0	41	41	0	0	10	—	—	60
Fruit Punch	1 bottle (10 oz)	170	0	0	0	0	42	41	0	0	25	—	—	60
Juice-Ups Berry	8 fl oz	140	0	0	0	0	34	34	0	0	15	—	—	60
Juice-Ups Fruit Punch	8 fl oz	140	0	0	0	0	34	34	0	0	15	—	—	60
Orange Strawberry	8 fl oz	120	0	0	0	0	31	31	0	0	30	—	—	60
Papaya Punch	1 bottle (10 oz)	160	0	0	0	0	39	38	0	0	25	—	—	60
Pineapple Orange	1 bottle (10 oz)	160	0	0	0	0	39	38	0	0	20	—	—	60
Strawberry Banana	1 can (11.5 oz)	160	0	0	0	0	40	40	0	0	15	—	—	60
Strawberry Banana Punch	1 can (11.5 oz)	190	0	0	0	0	48	47	0	0	30	—	—	60
FRUIT MIXED														
(*see also individual names*)														
CANNED														
fruit cocktail in heavy syrup	½ cup	93	tr	tr	0	1	24	—	—	8	7	112	—	2
fruit cocktail juice pack	½ cup	56	tr	tr	0	1	15	—	—	10	4	118	—	3
fruit cocktail water pack	½ cup	40	tr	tr	0	1	10	—	—	6	5	115	—	3
fruit salad in heavy syrup	½ cup	94	tr	tr	0	tr	24	—	—	8	7	103	—	3
fruit salad in light syrup	½ cup	73	tr	tr	0	tr	19	—	—	8	7	104	—	3
fruit salad juice pack	½ cup	62	tr	tr	0	1	16	—	—	14	7	144	—	4
fruit salad water pack	½ cup	37	tr	tr	0	tr	10	—	—	8	4	95	—	2
mixed fruit in heavy syrup	½ cup	92	tr	tr	0	tr	24	—	—	1	5	108	—	88
tropical fruit salad in heavy syrup	½ cup	110	tr	—	0	1	29	—	—	17	3	168	—	22
DEL MONTE														
Cherry Mixed Light Syrup	½ cup (4.4 oz)	90	0	0	0	1	22	19	1	0	10	—	—	5
Chunky Mixed Fruit Naturals	½ cup (4.4 oz)	60	0	0	0	0	15	14	1	0	10	—	—	2
Chunky Mixed In Extra Light Syrup	½ cup (4.4 oz)	60	0	0	0	0	15	14	1	0	10	—	—	2

FOOD	PORTION	CALS	FAT	SAT FAT	CHOL	PROT	CARB	SUGAR	FIBER	CALCI	SOD	POTAS	FOLIC	VIT C
DEL MONTE (CONT.)														
Chunky Mixed In Heavy Syrup	½ cup (4.5 oz)	100	0	0	0	0	24	23	1	0	10	—	—	2
Citrus Salad	½ cup (4.4 oz)	80	0	0	0	0	20	17	0	0	20	—	—	42
Fruit Cocktail Fruit Naturals	½ cup (4.4 oz)	60	0	0	0	0	15	14	1	0	10	—	—	2
Fruit Cocktail In Extra Light Syrup	½ cup (4.4 oz)	60	0	0	0	0	15	14	1	0	10	—	—	2
Fruit Cocktail In Heavy Syrup	½ cup (4.5 oz)	100	0	0	0	0	24	23	1	0	10	—	—	2
Fruit Cup Fruit Naturals Mixed	1 pkg (4 oz)	50	0	0	0	0	13	12	1	0	10	—	—	12
Fruit Cup Mixed In Extra Light Syrup	1 pkg (4 oz)	50	0	0	0	0	13	12	1	0	10	—	—	12
Fruit Salad In Extra Light Syrup	½ cup (4.5 oz)	70	0	0	0	1	22	13	2	0	5	—	—	36
Fruit To Go Fruity Combo	1 pkg (4 oz)	70	0	0	0	1	18	16	1	0	10	—	—	60
Fruit To Go Wild Berry Jumble	1 pkg (4 oz)	80	0	0	0	1	20	17	1	0	10	—	—	60
Orchard Select California Mixed	½ cup (4.5 oz)	80	0	0	0	1	19	18	1	0	10	—	—	48
Orchard Select Premium Mixed	½ cup (4.4 oz)	80	0	0	0	tr	20	18	tr	0	10	—	—	60
Snack Cups Strawberry Banana Peaches	1 pkg	70	0	0	0	tr	17	16	tr	0	10	—	—	60
Snack Cups Tropical Fruit	1 pkg	70	0	0	0	tr	18	16	tr	0	5	—	—	60
SunFresh Ambrosia Salad	½ cup	70	0	0	0	0	16	13	1	0	25	—	—	60
Tropical Fruit Salad	½ cup (4.3 oz)	60	0	0	0	0	16	14	1	40	15	—	—	30
Tropical Fruit Salad In Light Syrup	½ cup (4.4 oz)	80	0	0	0	0	21	20	1	0	10	—	—	48
Very Cherry Mixed Fruit	½ cup (4.4 oz)	90	0	0	0	1	22	19	1	0	10	—	—	5
DOLE														
FruitBowls Tropical Fruit	1 pkg (4 oz)	60	0	0	0	tr	16	14	2	—	10	160	—	24
Tropical Fruit Salad	½ cup (4.3 oz)	80	0	0	0	tr	20	18	1	—	10	—	—	—
MOTT'S														
Fruitsations Banana	1 pkg (4 oz)	90	0	0	0	0	23	—	—	—	0	—	—	—

FOOD	PORTION	CALS	FAT	SAT FAT	CHOL	PROT	CARB	SUGAR	FIBER	CALCI	SOD	POTAS	FOLIC	VIT C
MOTT'S (CONT.)														
Fruitsations Cherry	1 pkg (4 oz)	70	0	0	0	0	19	—	—	—	0	—	—	—
Fruitsations Mango Peach	1 pkg (4 oz)	70	0	0	0	0	22	—	—	—	0	—	—	—
Fruitsations Mixed Berry	1 pkg (4 oz)	90	0	0	0	0	22	20	1	20	0	—	—	1
Fruitsations Pear	1 pkg (4 oz)	90	0	0	0	0	23	—	—	—	0	—	—	—
Fruitsations Strawberry	1 pkg (4 oz)	80	0	0	0	0	19	—	—	—	10	—	—	—
Fruitsations Tropical Fruit	1 pkg (4 oz)	70	0	0	0	0	19	—	—	—	0	—	—	—
Healthy Harvest Peach Medley	1 pkg (3.9 oz)	50	0	0	0	0	13	11	1	0	0	—	—	15
SUNFRESH														
Ambrosia Salad	½ cup (4.5 oz)	70	0	0	0	0	16	13	1	0	25	—	—	43
Mixed Fruit In Light Syrup	½ cup (4.6 oz)	90	0	0	0	1	20	12	2	0	25	—	—	60
Tropical Salad In Extra Light Syrup	½ cup (4.5 oz)	80	0	0	0	1	20	16	0	0	10	—	—	48
WHITE HOUSE														
Apple Banana Sauce	1 pkg (4 oz)	100	0	0	0	0	23	21	1	—	25	—	—	60
Apple Mixed Berry Sauce	1 pkg (4 oz)	110	0	0	0	0	23	23	1	—	25	—	—	60
Apple Peach Sauce	1 pkg (4 oz)	100	0	0	0	0	23	21	1	—	20	—	—	60
DRIED														
mixed	11 oz pkg	712	1	tr	0	7	188	—	—	110	52	2332	—	11
PARADISE														
Old English Fruit & Peel Mix	1 tbsp (0.8 oz)	70	0	0	0	06	18	11	1	20	15	—	—	1
SUN-MAID														
Tropical Medley	¼ cup (1.4 oz)	130	0	0	0	1	32	29	1	20	10	—	—	1
FROZEN														
mixed fruit sweetened	1 cup	245	tr	tr	0	4	61	—	—	18	8	327	—	188
BIRDS EYE														
Mixed Fruit	½ cup	90	0	0	0	1	23	21	—	—	5	—	—	42
TREE OF LIFE														
Organic Mixed Berries	¾ cup (5 oz)	60	0	0	0	0	16	6	3	20	0	—	—	42
FRUIT SNACKS														
fruit leather	1 bar (0.8 oz)	81	1	1	0	tr	18	—	—	7	18	32	—	16
fruit leather pieces	1 oz	97	2	tr	0	tr	22	—	—	5	114	48	—	16
fruit leather pieces	1 pkg (0.9 oz)	92	2	tr	0	tr	21	—	—	5	109	44	—	15

FOOD	PORTION	CALS	FAT	SAT FAT	CHOL	PROT	CARB	SUGAR	FIBER	CALCI	SOD	POTAS	FOLIC	VIT C
fruit leather rolls	1 sm (0.5 oz)	49	tr	tr	0	tr	12	—	—	4	8	41	—	1
fruit leather rolls	1 lg (0.7 oz)	73	1	tr	0	tr	18	—	—	7	13	62	—	1
BETTY CROCKER														
Fruit By The Foot All Flavors	1 roll	80	2	—	—	0	17	10	—	—	50	—	—	15
COOLFRUITS														
Apple Grape	1 bar (0.5 oz)	51	tr	0	0	tr	12	9	1	20	0	100	—	0
Apple Strawberry	1 bar (0.5 oz)	51	tr	0	0	tr	12	9	1	20	0	—	—	0
Wild Blueberry	1 bar (0.5 oz)	51	tr	0	0	tr	12	9	1	20	0	100	—	0
FAVORITE BRANDS														
Cherry Fruit Snack	1 pkg (0.9 oz)	80	0	0	0	1	19	14	—	—	15	—	—	15
Creepy Crawler Fruit Snacks	1 pkg (0.9 oz)	80	0	0	0	1	19	14	—	—	15	—	—	15
Dinosaur Fruit Snack	1 pkg (0.9 oz)	80	0	0	0	1	19	14	—	—	15	—	—	15
Grape Fruit Snack	1 pkg (0.9 oz)	80	0	0	0	1	19	13	—	—	15	—	—	15
Space Alien Fruit Snack	1 pkg (0.9 oz)	80	0	0	0	1	19	14	—	—	15	—	—	15
Sports Fruit Snacks	1 pkg (0.9 oz)	80	0	0	0	1	19	14	—	—	15	—	—	15
Strawberry Fruit Snack	1 pkg (0.9 oz)	80	0	0	0	1	19	14	—	—	15	—	—	15
Teenage Mutant Ninja Turtle Fruit Snacks	1 pkg (0.9 oz)	80	0	0	0	1	19	14	—	—	15	—	—	15
The Mega Roll Strawberry	1 pkg (1 oz)	110	3	2	—	0	22	14	2	—	15	—	—	15
The Roll Cherry	1 pkg (0.75 oz)	80	2	1	—	0	16	10	1	—	10	—	—	15
The Roll Strawberry	1 pkg (0.75 oz)	80	2	1	—	0	16	10	1	—	10	—	—	15
Troll Fruit Snacks	1 pkg (0.9 oz)	80	0	0	0	1	19	14	0	—	15	—	—	15
Zoo Animal Fruit Snacks	1 pkg (0.9 oz)	80	0	0	0	1	19	14	—	—	15	—	—	15
HEALTH VALLEY														
Bakes Apple	1 bar	70	0	0	0	2	19	11	2	0	30	—	—	2
Bakes Date	1 bar	70	0	0	0	2	19	11	2	0	30	—	—	2
Bakes Raisin	1 bar	70	0	0	0	2	19	11	2	0	30	—	—	2
Fruit Bars Apple	1	140	0	0	0	3	35	13	3	0	0	—	—	0
Fruit Bars Apricot	1	140	0	0	0	3	35	12	4	0	5	—	—	0
Fruit Bars Date	1	140	0	0	0	3	34	12	3	0	5	—	—	0
Fruit Bars Raisin	1	140	0	0	0	2	35	17	3	0	5	—	—	0
SENSIBLE FOODS														
Crackin' Fruit Cherry Berry	1 pkg (0.6 oz)	51	0	0	0	1	13	14	1	10	85	—	—	10
Crackin' Fruit Tropical Fruit	1 pkg (0.6 oz)	65	1	0	0	tr	16	14	1	10	61	—	—	10

FOOD	PORTION	CALS	FAT	SAT FAT	CHOL	PROT	CARB	SUGAR	FIBER	CALCI	SOD	POTAS	FOLIC	VIT C
SUNBELT														
Fruit Jammers	1 pkg (1 oz)	100	1	1	0	0	23	13	0	—	15	—	—	—
SUNKIST														
100% Fruit Roll All Flavors	1 (0.5 oz)	50	0	0	0	0	12	5	1	0	10	—	—	15
WEIGHT WATCHERS														
Apple & Cinnamon	1 pkg (0.5 oz)	50	0	0	0	0	13	9	2	0	125	—	—	0
Apple Chips	1 pkg (0.75 oz)	70	0	0	0	0	18	13	3	0	125	—	—	0
Peach & Strawberry	1 pkg (0.5 oz)	50	0	0	0	0	13	11	2	0	125	—	—	0
GARLIC														
clove	1	4	tr	tr	0	tr	1	—	—	5	1	12	tr	1
fresh chopped	1 tsp	4	tr	tr	0	tr	tr	tr	1	5	0	11	0	1
powder	1 tsp	9	tr	—	0	tr	2	—	—	2	1	31	—	—
DOROT														
Frozen Crushed Cubes	1 cube (4 g)	5	0	0	0	0	1	0	0	0	40	—	—	0
MCCORMICK														
Garlic Salt	¼ tsp	0	0	0	0	0	0	0	0	—	250	—	—	—
GEFILTE FISH														
sweet	1 piece (1.5 oz)	35	1	tr	12	4	3	—	—	10	220	38	1	—
GELATIN														
MIX														
low calorie	½ cup	8	0	0	0	2	0	—	0	tr	9	45	0	0
mix as prep	½ cup (4.7 oz)	80	0	0	0	2	19	11	—	3	57	1	—	0
mix not prep	1 pkg (3 oz)	324	0	0	0	7	77	—	—	—	216	6	—	0
mix w/ fruit	½ cup (3.7 oz)	73	tr	—	0	1	18	—	—	5	30	110	—	4
powder unsweetened	1 pkg (7 g)	23	0	tr	—	6	0	—	—	4	14	1	—	0
JELL-O														
1-2-3-Brand Strawberry as prep	⅔ cup (5.2 oz)	130	2	1	0	2	26	22	0	0	50	0	—	0
Apricot as prep	½ cup (5 oz)	80	0	0	0	2	19	19	0	0	80	0	—	0
Berry Black as prep	½ cup (5 oz)	80	0	0	0	2	19	19	0	0	80	0	—	0
Berry Blue as prep	½ cup (5 oz)	80	0	0	0	2	19	19	0	0	80	0	—	0
Black Cherry as prep	½ cup (5 oz)	80	0	0	0	2	19	19	0	0	80	0	—	0
Cherry as prep	½ cup (5 oz)	80	0	0	0	2	19	19	0	0	100	0	—	0
Cranberry as prep	½ cup (5 oz)	80	0	0	0	0	19	19	0	0	75	0	—	0
Cranberry Raspberry as prep	½ cup (5 oz)	80	0	0	0	2	19	19	0	0	75	0	—	0

FOOD	PORTION	CALS	FAT	SAT FAT	CHOL	PROT	CARB	SUGAR	FIBER	CALCI	SOD	POTAS	FOLIC	VIT C
JELL-O (CONT.)														
Cranberry Strawberry as prep	½ cup (5 oz)	80	0	0	0	2	19	19	0	0	75	0	—	0
Grape as prep	½ cup (5 oz)	80	0	0	0	2	19	19	0	0	80	0	—	0
Lemon as prep	½ cup (5 oz)	80	0	0	0	2	19	19	0	0	120	0	—	0
Lime as prep	½ cup (5 oz)	80	0	0	0	2	19	19	0	0	90	0	—	0
Mango as prep	½ cup (5 oz)	80	0	0	0	2	19	19	0	0	80	0	—	0
Mixed Fruit as prep	½ cup (5 oz)	80	0	0	0	2	19	19	tr	0	80	0	—	0
Orange as prep	½ cup (5 oz)	80	0	0	0	2	19	19	0	0	80	0	—	0
Peach as prep	½ cup (5 oz)	80	0	0	0	2	19	19	0	0	80	0	—	0
Peach Passion Fruit as prep	½ cup (5 oz)	80	0	0	0	2	19	19	0	0	80	0	—	0
Pineapple as prep	½ cup (5 oz)	80	0	0	0	2	19	19	0	0	80	0	—	0
Raspberry as prep	½ cup (5 oz)	80	0	0	0	2	19	19	0	0	80	0	—	0
Sparkling White Grape as prep	½ cup (5 oz)	80	0	0	0	2	19	19	0	0	80	0	—	0
Strawberry as prep	½ cup (5 oz)	80	0	0	0	2	19	19	0	0	90	0	—	0
Strawberry Banana as prep	½ cup (5 oz)	80	0	0	0	2	19	19	0	0	80	0	—	0
Strawberry Kiwi as prep	½ cup (5 oz)	80	0	0	0	2	19	19	0	0	80	0	—	0
Sugar Free Cherry as prep	½ cup (4.2 oz)	10	0	0	0	1	0	0	0	0	70	0	—	0
Sugar Free Cranberry as prep	½ cup (4.2 oz)	10	0	0	0	1	0	0	0	0	80	0	—	0
Sugar Free Lemon	½ cup (4.2 oz)	10	0	0	0	1	0	0	0	0	55	0	—	0
Sugar Free Lime as prep	½ cup (4.2 oz)	10	0	0	0	1	0	0	0	0	60	0	—	0
Sugar Free Mixed Fruit as prep	½ cup (4.2 oz)	10	0	0	0	1	0	0	0	0	50	0	—	0
Sugar Free Orange as prep	½ cup (4.2 oz)	10	0	0	0	1	0	0	0	0	65	0	—	0
Sugar Free Raspberry as prep	½ cup (4.2 oz)	10	0	0	0	1	0	0	0	0	55	0	—	0
Sugar Free Strawberry as prep	½ cup (4.2 oz)	10	0	0	0	1	0	0	0	0	55	0	—	0
Sugar Free Strawberry Banana as prep	½ cup (4.2 oz)	10	0	0	0	1	0	0	0	0	50	0	—	0
Sugar Free Strawberry Kiwi as prep	½ cup (4.2 oz)	10	0	0	0	1	0	0	0	0	60	0	—	0

FOOD	PORTION	CALS	FAT	SAT FAT	CHOL	PROT	CARB	SUGAR	FIBER	CALCI	SOD	POTAS	FOLIC	VIT C
JELL-O (CONT.)														
Sugar Free Watermelon as prep	½ cup (4.2 oz)	10	0	0	0	1	0	0	0	0	55	0	—	0
Watermelon as prep	½ cup (5 oz)	80	0	0	0	2	19	19	0	0	80	0	—	0
Wild Strawberry as prep	½ cup (5 oz)	80	0	0	0	2	19	19	0	0	120	0	—	0
READY-TO-EAT														
HANDI-SNACKS														
Gels Blue Raspberry	1 serv (4 oz)	80	0	0	0	0	20	20	0	0	45	30	—	0
Gels Cherry	1 serv (4 oz)	80	0	0	0	0	20	20	0	0	45	30	—	0
Gels Orange	1 serv (3.5 oz)	80	0	0	0	0	20	20	0	0	45	30	—	0
Gels Strawberry	1 serv (3.5 oz)	80	0	0	0	0	20	20	0	0	40	30	—	0
HUNT'S														
Snack Pack Gels Cherry	1 serv (3.5 oz)	100	0	0	0	0	25	24	0	15	42	—	—	2
Snack Pack Gels Raspberry Berry	1 serv (3.5 oz)	100	0	0	0	0	25	24	0	15	42	—	—	2
Snack Pack Gels Strawberry	1 serv (3.5 oz)	100	0	0	0	0	25	24	0	15	42	—	—	2
Snack Pack Gels Strawberry Orange	1 serv (3.5 oz)	100	0	0	0	0	25	24	0	15	42	—	—	2
JELL-O														
Berry Black	1 serv (3.5 oz)	70	0	0	0	1	17	17	0	0	40	0	—	0
Berry Blue	1 serv (3.5 oz)	70	0	0	0	1	17	17	0	0	40	0	—	0
Cherry	1 serv (3.5 oz)	70	0	0	0	1	17	17	0	0	40	0	—	0
Orange	1 serv (3.5 oz)	70	0	0	0	1	17	17	0	0	40	0	—	0
Orange Strawberry Banana	1 serv (3.5 oz)	70	0	0	0	1	17	17	0	0	40	0	—	0
Raspberry	1 serv (3.5 oz)	70	0	0	0	1	17	17	0	0	40	0	—	0
Rhymin' Lymon	1 serv (3.5 oz)	70	0	0	0	1	17	17	0	0	40	0	—	0
Strawberry	1 serv (3.5 oz)	70	0	0	0	1	17	17	0	0	40	0	—	0
Strawberry Kiwi	1 serv (3.5 oz)	10	0	0	0	1	0	0	0	0	45	0	—	0
Sugar Free Orange	1 serv (3.2 oz)	10	0	0	0	1	0	0	0	0	45	0	—	0
Sugar Free Raspberry	1 serv (3.2 oz)	10	0	0	0	1	0	0	0	0	45	0	—	0
Sugar Free Strawberry	1 serv (3.2 oz)	10	0	0	0	1	0	0	0	0	45	0	—	0
Tropical Berry	1 serv (3.5 oz)	10	0	0	0	1	0	0	0	0	45	0	—	0
Tropical Fruit Punch	1 serv (3.5 oz)	70	0	0	0	1	17	17	0	0	40	0	—	0
Wild Watermelon	1 serv (3.5 oz)	70	0	0	0	1	17	17	0	0	40	0	—	0

FOOD	PORTION	CALS	FAT	SAT FAT	CHOL	PROT	CARB	SUGAR	FIBER	CALCI	SOD	POTAS	FOLIC	VIT C
SWISS MISS														
Gels Berry Strawberry	1 pkg (3.5 oz)	79	0	0	0	1	18	18	0	3	38	—	—	tr
Gels Berry Lemon	1 pkg (3.5 oz)	79	0	0	0	1	18	18	0	3	38	—	—	tr
Gels Raspberry Orange	1 pkg (3.5 oz)	79	0	0	0	1	18	18	0	3	38	—	—	tr
Gels Strawberry Raspberry	1 pkg (3.5 oz)	79	0	0	0	1	18	18	0	3	38	—	—	tr
GIBLETS														
capon simmered	1 cup (5 oz)	238	8	3	629	38	0	—	—	19	80	222	601	13
chicken floured & fried	1 cup (5 oz)	402	19	6	647	47	6	—	—	26	164	478	550	13
chicken simmered	1 cup (5 oz)	228	7	2	570	37	1	—	—	18	85	229	545	12
turkey simmered	1 cup (5 oz)	243	7	2	606	39	3	—	—	18	85	291	501	3
GINGER														
ground	1 tsp (1.8 g)	6	tr	tr	0	tr	1	—	—	2	1	24	—	—
pickled	0.5 oz	5	0	0	0	tr	1	—	tr	3	52	4	—	—
root fresh	5 slices	8	tr	tr	0	tr	2	—	—	2	1	46	—	1
root fresh	¼ cup	17	tr	tr	0	tr	4	—	—	4	3	100	—	1
root fresh sliced	¼ cup	17	tr	tr	0	tr	4	—	—	4	3	100	—	1
EDEN														
Pickled w/ Shiso Leaves	1 tbsp	15	0	0	0	0	3	1	1	20	340	0	0	0
MCCORMICK														
Crystallized	¼ tsp	15	0	0	0	0	3	—	—	—	0	—	—	—
GINKGO NUTS														
canned	1 oz	32	tr	tr	0	1	6		—	1	87	51	—	—
dried	1 oz	99	tr	tr	0	3	21	—	—	6	4	283	—	8
raw	1 oz	52	tr	tr	0	1	11	—	—	1	1	145	—	4
GINSENG														
dried	1 oz	90	tr	—	—	5	20	—	2	64	16	296	—	2
fresh	1 oz	28	tr	—	—	1	6	—	tr	32	5	92	—	4
GIZZARDS														
chicken simmered	1 cup (5 oz)	222	5	2	281	5	2	—	—	14	97	259	77	2
turkey simmered	1 cup (5 oz)	236	6	2	336	43	1	—	—	22	79	306	75	2
SHADY BROOK														
Turkey	4 oz	130	4	1	180	22	—	—	—	—	90	—	—	—
GNOCCHI														
BELLINO														
w/ Potato	1 cup	240	1	0	0	5	55	2	2	0	550	—	—	0
GOAT														
roasted	3 oz	122	3	1	64	23	0	—	—	15	73	344	5	—
GOOSE														
w/ skin roasted	6.6 oz	574	41	13	172	47	0	—	—	25	132	618	4	0

FOOD	PORTION	CALS	FAT	SAT FAT	CHOL	PROT	CARB	SUGAR	FIBER	CALCI	SOD	POTAS	FOLIC	VIT C
w/ skin roasted	½ goose (1.7 lbs)	2362	170	53	708	195	0	—	—	104	543	2546	17	0
w/o skin roasted	½ goose (1.3 lbs)	1406	75	27	569	171	0	—	—	84	447	2291	—	—
w/o skin roasted	5 oz	340	18	7	138	41	0	—	—	20	108	554	—	—

GOOSEBERRIES

FOOD	PORTION	CALS	FAT	SAT FAT	CHOL	PROT	CARB	SUGAR	FIBER	CALCI	SOD	POTAS	FOLIC	VIT C
canned in light syrup	½ cup	93	tr	tr	0	1	24	—	—	20	3	97	4	13
fresh	1 cup	67	1	tr	0	1	15	—	—	38	1	297	—	42

GRAPE JUICE

FOOD	PORTION	CALS	FAT	SAT FAT	CHOL	PROT	CARB	SUGAR	FIBER	CALCI	SOD	POTAS	FOLIC	VIT C
bottled	1 cup	155	tr	tr	0	1	38	—	—	22	7	334	7	tr
frzn sweetened as prep	1 cup	128	tr	tr	0	tr	32	—	—	9	5	53	3	60
frzn sweetened not prep	6 oz	386	1	tr	0	1	96	—	—	28	15	159	9	180
grape drink	6 oz	84	0	0	0	0	22	—	—	—	12	10	1	64
CAPRI SUN														
Drink	1 pkg (7 oz)	100	0	0	0	0	25	25	0	0	20	20	—	0
CERES														
Hanepoot White Grape	8 oz	130	0	0	0	0	33	30	0	40	10	190	—	27
DAILY														
Drink	8 oz	110	0	0	0	0	27	27	—	—	30	—	—	—
EVERFRESH														
Juice	1 can (8 oz)	150	0	0	0	0	38	38	0	—	10	—	—	—
HANSEN'S														
White Grape 100% Juice	1 box (4.23 oz)	90	0	0	0	0	22	21	—	0	10	—	—	60
JUICY JUICE														
Drink	1 box (8.45 oz)	140	0	0	0	0	34	32	0	0	15	180	—	78
Drink	1 box (4.23 oz)	70	0	0	0	0	17	16	—	0	10	90	—	60
KETO														
Kooler	½ tsp	0	0	0	0	0	0	0	0	—	0	—	—	—
KOOL-AID														
Bursts Grape Drink	1 (7 oz)	100	0	0	0	0	25	25	0	0	30	15	—	9
Drink as prep w/ sugar	1 serv (8 oz)	100	0	0	0	0	25	25	0	0	10	0	—	6
Drink Mix as prep	1 serv (8 oz)	60	0	0	0	0	16	16	0	0	0	0	—	6
Sugar Free Drink Mix as prep	1 serv (8 oz)	5	0	0	0	0	0	0	0	0	0	0	—	6
LANGERS														
Cocktail	8 oz	160	0	0	0	0	40	36	—	—	15	—	—	—
MOTT'S														
100% Juice	1 box (8 oz)	130	0	0	0	0	33	—	—	—	15	—	—	—
Grape Juice	8 fl oz	130	0	0	0	0	31	—	—	—	10	—	—	—

FOOD	PORTION	CALS	FAT	SAT FAT	CHOL	PROT	CARB	SUGAR	FIBER	CALCI	SOD	POTAS	FOLIC	VIT C
NANTUCKET NECTARS														
Grapeade	8 oz	130	0	0	0	0	33	29	—	0	5	—	—	60
Organic Concord Grape	8 oz	130	0	0	0	0	33	32	—	—	30	—	—	—
SHASTA PLUS														
Grape Drink	1 can (11.5 oz)	160	0	0	0	0	39	39	0	—	45	—	—	60
SQUEEZIT														
Grumpy Grape	1 bottle (7 oz)	110	0	0	0	0	28	27	0	0	0	—	—	0
VERYFINE														
100% Juice	1 bottle (10 oz)	200	0	0	0	0	47	43	0	0	35	—	—	2
Chillers Glacial Grape	1 can (11.5 oz)	160	0	0	0	0	41	41	0	0	10	—	—	60
Grape Drink	1 bottle (10 oz)	160	0	0	0	0	41	37	0	0	10	—	—	36
Juice-Ups	8 fl oz	130	0	0	0	0	32	32	0	0	10	—	—	60
WELCH'S														
100% Juice	8 oz	170	0	0	0	0	42	40	—	—	20	—	—	72
100% White	8 oz	160	0	0	0	0	39	37	—	—	20	—	—	72
GRAPE LEAVES														
canned	1 (4 g)	3	tr	tr	0	tr	tr	—	0	12	114	1	3	0
fresh raw	1 (3 g)	3	tr	tr	0	tr	1	—	tr	11	tr	8	2	tr
TAKE-OUT														
dolmas	5 (4.2 oz)	200	11	1	0	2	23	3	2	20	570	—	—	1
GRAPEFRUIT														
CANNED														
juice pack	½ cup	46	tr	tr	0	1	11	—	—	19	9	209	—	42
unsweetened	1 cup	93	tr	tr	0	1	22	—	—	18	3	378	26	72
water pack	½ cup	44	tr	tr	0	1	11	—	—	18	2	161	11	27
SUNFRESH														
Red & White	½ cup (4.4 oz)	45	0	0	0	1	9	8	2	20	15			60
FRESH														
pink	½	37	tr	tr	0	1	9	—	1	13	0	158	15	47
pink sections	1 cup	69	tr	tr	0	1	18		1	25	1	296	28	88
red	½	37	tr	tr	0	1	9	—	—	13	0	158	15	47
red sections	1 cup	69	tr	tr	0	1	18	—	—	25	1	296	28	88
white	½	39	tr	tr	0	1	10	—	1	17	0	175	12	39
white sections	1 cup	76	tr	tr	0	2	19	—	1	28	0	340	23	77
GRAPEFRUIT JUICE														
fresh	1 cup	96	tr	tr	0	1	23	—	—	22	2	400	—	94
frzn as prep	1 cup	102	tr	tr	0	1	24	—	—	19	2	337	9	83
frzn not prep	6 oz	302	1	tr	0	4	72	—	—	18	6	1002	26	248
sweetened	1 cup	116	tr	tr	0	1	28	—	—	20	4	405	26	67
APPLE & EVE														
Made In The Shade Ruby Red	8 fl oz	130	0	0	0	0	32	32	—	—	35	—	—	60

FOOD	PORTION	CALS	FAT	SAT FAT	CHOL	PROT	CARB	SUGAR	FIBER	CALCI	SOD	POTAS	FOLIC	VIT C
EVERFRESH														
Juice	1 can (8 oz)	90	0	0	0	0	22	22	0	—	0	—	—	—
Ruby Red Cocktail	1 can (8 oz)	130	0	0	0	0	32	32	0	—	0	—	—	—
FRESH SAMANTHA														
Juice	1 cup (8 oz)	90	0	0	0	1	7	—	0	0	0	110	24	72
LANGERS														
Diet Ruby Red	8 oz	40	0	0	0	0	9	9	—	200	10	—	—	60
Ruby Red	8 oz	130	0	0	0	0	33	30	—	0	10	—	—	60
MOTT'S														
100% Juice	8 fl oz	110	0	0	0	2	27	—	—	—	10	—	—	—
NANTUCKET NECTARS														
100% Ruby Red	8 oz	100	0	0	0	0	25	20	—	20	5	—	—	48
OCEAN SPRAY														
100% Juice Pink	8 oz	110	0	0	0	tr	28	28	0	—	35	280	—	60
100% Juice White	8 oz	100	0	0	0	1	24	24	tr	—	35	240	—	60
Ruby Drink	8 oz	120	0	0	0	—	30	30	—	—	35	10	—	60
Ruby Red Drink	8 oz	130	0	0	0	0	33	33	0	—	35	50	—	60
ODWALLA														
Juice	8 fl oz	90	0	0	0	2	20	16	0	20	5	0	—	78
TROPICANA														
Golden	8 oz	90	0	0	0	1	22	—	—	20	0	370	16	60
Ruby Red	8 oz	90	0	0	0	1	22	—	—	20	0	300	16	72
Season's Best	8 oz	90	0	0	0	tr	22	—	—	20	15	280	—	60
Twister Pink	1 bottle (10 oz)	140	0	0	0	0	34	—	—	—	20	—	—	5
With Double Vitamin C	8 fl oz	110	0	0	0	1	27	—	—	20	15	430	60	144
VERYFINE														
100% Juice	1 bottle (10 oz)	110	0	0	0	0	25	21	0	0	20	—	—	60
Pink	1 bottle (10 oz)	150	0	0	0	0	38	34	0	0	35	—	—	60
Ruby Red	8 fl oz	120	0	0	0	0	29	27	0	0	25	—	—	60
GRAPES														
fresh	10	36	tr	tr	0	tr	9	—	tr	5	1	93	2	5
thompson seedless in heavy syrup	½ cup	94	tr	tr	0	1	25	—	—	13	7	132	—	1
thompson seedless water pack	½ cup	48	tr	tr	0	1	13	—	—	13	7	131	—	1
CHIQUITA														
Grapes	1½ cups (4.8 oz)	90	1	0	0	1	24	23	1	20	0	—	—	15

GRAVY

FOOD	PORTION	CALS	FAT	SAT FAT	CHOL	PROT	CARB	SUGAR	FIBER	CALCI	SOD	POTAS	FOLIC	VIT C
CANNED														
au jus	1 cup	38	tr	tr	1	3	6	—	—	10	—	—	—	2
beef	1 cup	124	6	3	7	9	11	—	—	14	1305	189	—	0
beef	1 can (10 oz)	155	7	3	9	11	14	—	—	17	1630	236	—	0
chicken	1 cup	189	14	3	5	5	13	—	—	48	1375	260	—	0
mushroom	1 cup	120	6	1	0	3	13	—	—	17	1259	253	—	0
turkey	1 cup	122	5	1	5	6	12	—	—	10	—	—	—	0
CAMPBELL'S														
Beef	¼ cup	29	1	tr	1	1	4	1	tr	5	421	18	—	tr
Brown	¼ cup	46	3	tr	tr	1	4	1	1	4	350	31	—	tr
Chicken	¼ cup	42	2	1	3	1	4	tr	1	17	244	33	—	0
Turkey	¼ cup	29	1	tr	2	1	3	tr	tr	5	289	38	—	tr
HEINZ														
Home Style Chicken	¼ cup	25	1	0	0	0	4	0	0	0	340	—	—	0
MIX														
au jus as prep w/ water	1 cup	32	1	1	1	1	4	—	—	23	964	—	—	—
brown as prep w/ water	1 cup	75	2	1	2	2	13	—	—	66	1076	57	—	—
chicken as prep	1 cup	83	2	1	3	3	14	—	—	39	1133	—	—	—
mushroom as prep	1 cup	70	1	1	1	2	14	—	—	49	1402	—	—	—
onion as prep w/ water	1 cup	77	1	tr	tr	2	16	—	—	72	1013	—	—	—
pork as prep	1 cup	76	2	1	3	2	13	—	—	32	1235	—	—	—
turkey as prep	1 cup	87	2	1	3	3	15	—	—	50	1498	—	—	—
BOURNVITA														
Extract	2 heaping tsp	34	1	—	—	1	7	—	—	8	—	—	—	0
BOVRIL														
Extract	1 heaping tsp	9	0	—	—	2	tr	—	0	2	—	—	—	0
DURKEE														
Au Jus as prep	¼ cup	5	0	0	0	0	1	0	0	0	320	—	—	0
Brown as prep	¼ cup	10	1	0	0	0	3	0	0	0	250	—	—	0
Brown Mushroom as prep	¼ cup	15	0	0	0	1	3	0	0	0	300	—	—	0
Brown Onion as prep	¼ cup	15	0	0	0	1	4	0	0	0	290	—	—	0
Chicken as prep	¼ cup	20	1	0	0	1	4	0	0	0	350	—	—	0
Country as prep	¼ cup	35	2	1	0	1	5	1	0	0	370	—	—	0
Homestyle as prep	¼ cup	15	1	0	0	1	3	0	0	40	240	—	—	0
Onion as prep	¼ cup	10	0	0	0	1	3	0	0	0	310	—	—	0
Pork as prep	¼ cup	10	0	0	0	1	3	0	0	0	240	—	—	0
Sausage as prep	¼ cup	35	2	1	0	1	5	1	0	0	570	—	—	0
Swiss Steak as prep	¼ cup	15	0	0	0	0	4	0	0	0	370	—	—	0
Turkey as prep	¼ cup	20	0	0	0	1	4	1	0	0	270	—	—	0

FOOD	PORTION	CALS	FAT	SAT FAT	CHOL	PROT	CARB	SUGAR	FIBER	CALCI	SOD	POTAS	FOLIC	VIT C
FRENCH'S														
Au Jus as prep	¼ cup	5	0	0	0	0	1	0	0	0	220	—	—	0
Brown as prep	¼ cup	10	1	0	0	0	3	0	0	0	250	—	—	0
Chicken as prep	¼ cup	25	1	0	0	1	4	0	0	0	250	—	—	0
Country as prep	¼ cup	35	2	1	0	1	5	1	0	0	370	—	—	0
Herb Brown as prep	¼ cup	15	1	0	0	1	3	0	0	0	350	—	—	0
Homestyle as prep	¼ cup	10	1	0	0	0	3	0	0	0	230	—	—	0
Mushroom as prep	¼ cup	10	1	0	0	0	3	0	0	0	250	—	—	0
Onion	¼ cup	15	1	0	0	0	4	0	0	0	260	—	—	0
Pork as prep	¼ cup	10	1	0	0	0	3	0	0	0	250	—	—	0
Turkey as prep	¼ cup	20	0	0	0	1	4	1	0	0	270	—	—	0
LOMA LINDA														
Gravy Quik Brown	1 tbsp (5 g)	20	0	0	0	tr	4	0	0	0	370	5	—	0
Gravy Quik Chicken	1 tbsp (5 g)	20	0	0	0	1	3	0	0	0	410	30	—	0
Quik Gravy Country	1 tbsp (5 g)	25	1	0	0	tr	4	0	0	0	250	5	—	0
Quik Gravy Mushroom	1 tbsp (5 g)	15	0	0	0	tr	3	0	tr	0	300	30	—	0
Quik Gravy Onion	1 tbsp (5 g)	20	0	0	0	tr	3	0	tr	0	230	20	—	0
MARMITE														
Extract	1 heaping tsp	9	0	—	—	2	tr	—	—	5	—	—	—	0
MCCORMICK														
Au Jus Natural as prep	¼ cup	5	0	0	—	0	1	—	—	—	310	—	—	—
Beef & Herb as prep	¼ cup	30	1	—	<5	1	3	1	—	—	290	—	—	—
Brown as prep	¼ cup	20	1	—	—	tr	3	—	—	—	340	—	—	—
Chicken as prep	¼ cup	20	0	0	—	0	4	1	—	—	330	—	—	—
Onion as prep	¼ cup	20	1	—	—	tr	3	—	—	—	340	—	—	—
Pork as prep	¼ cup	20	—	—	—	0	4	1	—	—	320	—	—	—
Turkey as prep	¼ cup	20	0	—	—	0	3	1	—	—	350	—	—	—
GREAT NORTHERN BEANS														
canned	1 cup	299	1	tr	0	19	55	—	13	139	11	919	213	3
dried cooked	1 cup	209	1	tr	0	15	37	—	12	121	4	692	181	2
EDEN														
Organic	½ cup (4.6 oz)	110	1	0	0	5	20	1	8	73	65	270	25	0
GREEN GIANT														
Great Northern	½ cup (4.4 oz)	100	1	0	0	6	18	0	6	100	290	—	—	0
HURST														
HamBeens w/ Ham	3 tbsp (1.2 oz)	120	1	0	0	7	22	1	11	60	63	—	—	0

GREEN BEANS

FOOD	PORTION	CALS	FAT	SAT FAT	CHOL	PROT	CARB	SUGAR	FIBER	CALCI	SOD	POTAS	FOLIC	VIT C
CANNED														
green beans	½ cup	13	tr	tr	0	1	3	—	1	18	170	74	22	3
italian	½ cup	13	tr	tr	0	1	3	—	1	18	170	74	22	3
italian low sodium	½ cup	13	tr	tr	0	1	3	—	1	18	1	74	22	3
low sodium	½ cup	13	tr	tr	0	1	3	—	1	18	1	74	22	3
DEL MONTE														
Cut	½ cup (4.2 oz)	20	0	0	0	1	4	2	2	20	390	—	—	2
Cut Italian	½ cup (4.2 oz)	30	0	0	0	1	6	2	3	20	390	—	—	2
Cut No Salt Added	½ cup (4.2 oz)	20	0	0	0	1	4	2	2	20	10	—	—	2
French Style	½ cup (4.2 oz)	20	0	0	0	1	4	2	2	20	390	—	—	2
French Style No Salt Added	½ cup (4.2 oz)	20	0	0	0	1	4	2	2	20	10	—	—	2
French Style Seasoned	½ cup (4.2 oz)	20	0	0	0	1	4	2	2	20	360	—	—	2
Whole	½ cup (4.2 oz)	20	0	0	0	1	4	2	2	20	390	—	—	2
GREEN GIANT														
Cut	½ cup (4.2 oz)	20	0	0	0	tr	4	2	1	20	400	—	—	2
Cut 50% Less Sodium	½ cup (4.2 oz)	20	0	0	0	tr	4	2	1	20	200	—	—	1
French Style	½ cup (4.1 oz)	20	0	0	0	tr	4	2	1	20	390	—	—	2
Kitchen Sliced	½ cup (4.2 oz)	20	0	0	0	tr	4	2	1	20	400	—	—	4
Whole	½ cup (4.1 oz)	25	0	0	0	tr	5	2	2	20	330	—	—	2
S&W														
Blue Lake Cut	½ cup (4.2 oz)	20	0	0	0	1	4	2	2	20	340	—	—	4
French Style	½ cup (4.2 oz)	20	0	0	0	1	4	2	2	20	340	—	—	4
Whole Small	½ cup (4.2 oz)	20	0	0	0	1	4	2	2	20	390	—	—	4
VEG-ALL														
French Style	½ cup	20	0	0	0	tr	4	2	2	20	400	—	—	2
FRESH														
cooked	½ cup	22	tr	tr	0	1	5	—	—	29	2	185	21	6
raw	½ cup	17	tr	tr	0	1	4	—	1	21	3	115	20	9
FROZEN														
cooked	½ cup	18	tr	tr	0	1	4	—	—	31	9	76	—	6
italian cooked	½ cup	18	tr	tr	0	1	4	—	—	31	9	76	—	6
BIRDS EYE														
Cut	½ cup	25	0	0	0	—	—	—	2	20	0	—	—	6
Italian	½ cup	35	0	0	0	—	—	—	3	40	0	—	—	12
FRESH LIKE														
Cut	3.5 oz	29	tr	—	—	1	7	—	1	41	6	149	—	11
French Cut	3.5 oz	29	tr	—	—	1	7	—	1	46	6	174	—	9
GREEN GIANT														
Cut	¾ cup (2.8 oz)	25	0	0	0	1	5	2	2	20	0	—	—	6

FOOD	PORTION	CALS	FAT	SAT FAT	CHOL	PROT	CARB	SUGAR	FIBER	CALCI	SOD	POTAS	FOLIC	VIT C
GREEN GIANT (CONT.)														
Harvest Fresh & Almonds	⅔ cup (2.8 oz)	60	3	0	0	2	5	2	2	40	95	—	—	5
Harvest Fresh Cut	⅔ cup (2.9 oz)	25	0	0	0	tr	5	2	2	40	95	—	—	6
STOUFFER'S														
Green Bean Mushroom Casserole	1 serv (4 oz)	130	8	2	2	3	12	5	2	60	450	190	—	2
TREE OF LIFE														
Cut	⅔ cup (2.8 oz)	25	0	0	0	1	4	2	2	20	10	—	—	1
GREENS														
READY PAC														
Microwave Leafy Greens as prep	½ cup	15	0	0	0	2	2	1	2	80	100	—	—	0
GROUNDCHERRIES														
fresh	½ cup	37	tr	—	0	1	8	—	—	6	—	—	—	8
GROUPER														
cooked	3 oz	100	1	tr	40	21	0	—	—	18	45	403	—	—
cooked	1 fillet (7.1 oz)	238	3	1	95	50	0	—	—	42	107	959	—	—
raw	3 oz	78	1	tr	31	16	0	—	—	23	45	410	—	—
GUAR GUM														
BOB'S RED MILL														
Guar Gum	1 tbsp	20	0	0	0	0	6	0	6	—	2	—	—	—
GUAVA														
fresh	1	45	1	tr	0	1	11	—	—	18	2	256	—	165
guava sauce	½ cup	43	tr	tr	0	tr	11	—	—	8	4	268	—	174
GUAVA JUICE														
CERES														
Guava	8 oz	120	0	0	0	0	29	29	0	20	5	140	—	60
NANTUCKET NECTARS														
Guava	8 oz	130	0	0	0	0	33	29	0	0	5	—	—	60
GUINEA HEN														
w/ skin raw	½ hen (12.1 oz)	545	22	—	—	81	0	—	—	—	—	—	—	—
w/o skin raw	½ hen (9.3 oz)	292	7	—	166	55	0	—	—	—	—	—	—	—
HADDOCK														
fresh cooked	1 fillet (5.3 oz)	168	1	tr	110	36	0	—	—	64	131	598	—	—
fresh cooked	3 oz	95	1	tr	63	21	0	—	—	36	74	339	—	—
fresh raw	3 oz	74	1	tr	49	16	0	—	—	28	58	264	—	—
roe raw	1 oz	37	tr	—	103	7	tr	—	—	—	—	—	—	4
smoked	1 oz	33	tr	tr	21	7	0	—	—	14	214	116	—	—
smoked	3 oz	99	1	tr	65	21	0	—	—	41	649	353	—	—

FOOD	PORTION	CALS	FAT	SAT FAT	CHOL	PROT	CARB	SUGAR	FIBER	CALCI	SOD	POTAS	FOLIC	VIT C
TAKE-OUT														
breaded & fried	1 piece (3.5 oz)	187	9	3	63	23	3	0	tr	40	350	325	3	0
HAKE														
raw	3.5 oz	84	1	—	—	17	0	—	—	41	101	294	—	—
HALIBUT														
atlantic & pacific cooked	½ fillet (5.6 oz)	223	5	1	65	42	0	—	—	95	110	916	—	—
atlantic & pacific cooked	3 oz	119	2	tr	35	23	0	—	—	51	59	490	—	—
atlantic & pacific raw	3 oz	93	2	tr	27	18	0	—	—	40	46	382	—	—
greenland baked	3 oz	203	15	2	50	16	0	—	—	3	87	292	1	—
greenland baked	5.6 oz	380	28	5	94	29	0	—	—	6	163	546	2	—
HALVA														
(*see* SESAME)														
HAM														
canned extra lean roasted	3 oz	116	4	1	26	18	tr	—	0	5	965	—	4	0
center slice country style lean roasted	4 oz	220	9	3	80	31	tr	—	0	11	3045	—	6	0
chopped canned	1 oz	68	5	2	14	5	tr	—	—	2	387	81	—	0
ham & cheese loaf	1 oz	73	6	4	16	9	1	—	—	33	762	166	—	14
ham & cheese spread	1 tbsp	37	3	1	9	2	tr	—	—	33	179	24	—	1
ham salad spread	1 tbsp	32	2	1	6	1	2	—	—	1	137	22	—	1
minced	1 oz	75	6	2	20	5	1	—	—	3	353	88	—	8
patty cooked	1 patty (2 oz)	203	18	7	43	8	1	—	0	5	632	—	2	0
prosciutto	1 oz	55	2	—	20	8	tr	—	0	3	765	145	1	0
sliced extra lean 5% fat	1 oz	37	1	tr	13	5	tr	—	—	2	405	99	1	7
sliced regular 11% fat	1 oz	52	3	1	16	5	1	—	—	2	373	94	1	8
steak boneless extra lean	1 (2 oz)	69	2	1	26	11	0	—	0	2	720	—	2	18
westphalian smoked	1 oz	105	10	—	—	5	0	—	—	3	398	70	—	—
ALPINE LACE														
Boneless Cooked 98% Fat Free	2 slices (2 oz)	60	1	1	25	9	2	1	0	0	530	—	—	0
Honey Ham 98% Fat Free	2 slices (2 oz)	60	1	1	25	9	2	1	0	0	530	—	—	0
Smoked Virginia 98% Fat Free	2 slices (2 oz)	60	1	1	25	9	2	1	0	0	400	—	—	0

FOOD	PORTION	CALS	FAT	SAT FAT	CHOL	PROT	CARB	SUGAR	FIBER	CALCI	SOD	POTAS	FOLIC	VIT C
ARMOUR														
Chopped Ham canned	2 oz	130	11	4	35	8	1	1	0	0	880	—	—	0
Deviled Ham Spread	1 pkg (3 oz)	210	18	6	60	13	0	0	0	0	700	—	—	0
Lean Slices Brown Sugar	1 pkg (2.5 oz)	90	2	1	35	13	4	1	—	—	700	—	—	—
Star Canned	1 oz	34	1	—	11	—	—	—	—	—	—	—	—	—
BOAR'S HEAD														
Black Forest Smoked	2 oz	60	1	0	30	10	2	2	0	0	580	—	—	0
Cappy	2 oz	60	2	1	15	10	3	2	0	0	530	—	—	0
Deluxe	2 oz	60	1	0	25	9	2	2	0	0	590	—	—	0
Deluxe Lowered Sodium	2 oz	50	1	0	20	10	tr	0	0	0	460	—	—	0
Maple Glazed Honey	2 oz	60	1	0	20	10	3	3	0	0	570	—	—	0
Pepper	2 oz	60	1	0	20	10	2	1	0	0	610	—	—	0
Rosemary & Sundried Tomato	2 oz	70	3	1	10	10	2	0	0	0	590	—	—	0
Sweet Slices Smoked	3 oz	100	3	2	30	15	1	0	0	0	780	—	—	0
Virginia	2 oz	60	1	0	25	9	3	3	0	0	590	—	—	0
Virginia Smoked	2 oz	60	1	0	25	9	2	2	0	0	590	—	—	0
CARL BUDDIG														
Ham Sliced w/ Natural Juices	1 pkg (2.5 oz)	120	7	3	40	12	1	1	—	—	980	—	—	—
Honey Ham Sliced w/ Natural Juice	1 pkg (2.5 oz)	120	7	3	40	12	3	3	—	—	760	—	—	—
Lean Slices Oven Roasted Honey Ham	1 pkg (2.5 oz)	90	2	1	35	13	4	4	—	—	850	—	—	—
Lean Slices Smoked	1 pkg (2.5 oz)	80	2	1	35	14	1	1	—	—	850	—	—	—
HILLSHIRE														
Deli Select Honey Ham	6 slices (2 oz)	60	2	1	25	10	2	2	0	0	600	—	—	4
HORMEL														
Black Label Canned (refrigerated)	3 oz	100	5	2	40	14	1	1	0	0	1020	—	—	0
Black Label Canned (self stable)	3 oz	110	5	2	45	14	0	0	0	0	970	—	—	0
Cure 81 Half Ham	3 oz	100	5	2	45	16	0	1	0	0	890	—	—	0
Curemaster	3 oz	80	3	1	40	14	0	0	0	0	940	—	—	0
Deviled Ham	4 tbsp (2 oz)	150	12	4	40	9	2	2	0	0	430	—	—	0

FOOD	PORTION	CALS	FAT	SAT FAT	CHOL	PROT	CARB	SUGAR	FIBER	CALCI	SOD	POTAS	FOLIC	VIT C
HORMEL (CONT.)														
Ham & Cheese Patties	1 patty (2 oz)	190	17	6	45	7	0	0	0	20	470	—	—	0
Ham Patties	1 (2 oz)	180	17	6	35	7	1	1	0	0	550	—	—	0
Light & Lean 97 Sliced	1 slice (1 oz)	25	1	0	15	4	0	0	0	0	340	—	—	0
Primissimo Prosciutti	2 oz	120	7	3	50	15	0	0	0	0	1080	—	—	0
Spiral Cure 81	3 oz	150	9	5	50	15	1	1	0	0	1090	—	—	0
LOUIS RICH														
Carving Board Baked	2 slices (1.6 oz)	50	2	1	25	8	1	tr	0	0	550	—	—	0
Carving Board Honey Glazed Thin	6 slices (2.1 oz)	70	2	1	30	11	2	2	0	0	750	—	—	0
Carving Board Honey Glazed Traditional	2 slices (1.6 oz)	50	2	1	25	8	1	1	0	0	560			0
Carving Board Smoked	1 slice (1.6 oz)	45	2	1	20	8	0	0	0	0	570	—	—	0
Dinner Slices Baked	1 slice (3.3 oz)	80	2	1	40	16	1	1	0	0	1150	—	—	0
OSCAR MAYER														
Baked	3 slices (2.2 oz)	70	3	1	30	11	2	2	0	0	790	—	—	0
Boiled	3 slices (2.2 oz)	60	3	1	30	10	0	0	0	0	820	—	—	0
Chopped	1 slice (1 oz)	50	3	2	15	4	1	tr	0	0	340	—	—	0
Dinner Slice	3 oz	80	3	1	40	14	0	0	0	0	1010	—	—	0
Dinner Steaks	1 (2 oz)	60	2	1	30	10	0	0	0	0	750	—	—	0
Free Baked	3 slices (1.6 oz)	35	0	0	15	7	1	1	0	0	520	—	—	0
Free Honey	3 slices (1.6 oz)	35	0	0	15	7	2	1	0	0	580	—	—	0
Free Smoked	3 slices (1.6 oz)	35	0	0	15	7	1	tr	0	0	550	—	—	0
Honey	3 slices (2.2 oz)	70	3	1	30	10	2	2	0	0	760	—	—	0
Lower Sodium	3 slices (2.2 oz)	70	3	1	30	10	2	1	0	0	520	—	—	0
Lunchables Ham Bagels	1 pkg	410	10	5	40	16	64	27	2	250	890	—	—	60
Lunchables Ham Wraps	1 pkg	430	13	5	35	15	64	25	2	300	1050	—	—	60
Smoked	3 slices (2.2 oz)	60	3	1	30	11	0	0	0	0	760	—	—	0
SPAM														
Spread	4 tbsp (2 oz)	140	12	4	40	8	1	1	0	0	570	—	—	0
WAMPLER														
Black Forest	2 oz	60	2	—	25	10	2	—	—	—	650	—	—	—
HAM DISHES														
TAKE-OUT														
croquettes	1 (3.1 oz)	217	14	5	77	12	11	—	tr	50	475	180	11	tr
salad	½ cup	287	23	5	237	16	5	—	tr	33	671	232	22	1

FOOD	PORTION	CALS	FAT	SAT FAT	CHOL	PROT	CARB	SUGAR	FIBER	CALCI	SOD	POTAS	FOLIC	VIT C
HAM SUBSTITUTES														
YVES														
Veggie Ham Deli Slices	1 serv (2.2 oz)	80	0	0	0	14	6	2	1	40	480	140	—	0
HAMBURGER														
KID CUISINE														
Buckaroo Beef Patty Sandwich w/ Cheese	1 meal (8.5 oz)	410	15	7	30	12	58	27	4	150	600	—	—	0
TAKE-OUT														
double patty w/ bun	1 reg	544	28	10	99	30	43	—	—	87	554	363	38	0
double patty w/ cheese & bun	1 reg	457	28	13	110	28	22	—	—	232	635	308	29	0
double patty w/ cheese & double bun	1 reg	461	22	10	80	22	44	—	—	224	892	285	36	0
double patty w/ cheese ketchup mayonnaise onion pickle tomato & bun	1 reg	416	21	8	60	21	35	—	—	171	1051	335	23	2
double patty w/ ketchup mayonnaise onion pickle tomato & bun	1 reg	649	35	13	94	30	53	—	—	169	920	389	34	3
double patty w/ ketchup cheese mayonnaise mustard pickle tomato & bun	1 lg	706	44	18	141	38	40	—	—	240	1149	596	48	tr
double patty w/ ketchup mustard mayonnaise onion pickle tomato & bun	1 lg	540	27	11	122	34	40	—	—	102	791	569	27	1
double patty w/ ketchup mustard onion pickle & bun	1 reg	576	32	12	102	32	39	—	—	92	742	527	45	1
single patty w/ bacon ketchup cheese mustard onion pickle & bun	1 lg	609	37	16	112	32	37	—	—	162	1044	331	33	2
single patty w/ bun	1 reg	275	12	4	36	12	31	—	—	63	387	145	25	0
single patty w/ bun	1 lg	400	23	8	71	23	25	—	—	74	474	268	32	0

FOOD	PORTION	CALS	FAT	SAT FAT	CHOL	PROT	CARB	SUGAR	FIBER	CALCI	SOD	POTAS	FOLIC	VIT C
single patty w/ cheese & bun	1 lg	608	33	15	96	30	47	—	—	91	1589	644	38	0
single patty w/ cheese & bun	1 reg	320	15	6	50	15	32	—	—	140	500	165	26	0
single patty w/ ketchup cheese ham mayonnaise pickle tomato & bun	1 lg	745	48	21	122	40	38	—	—	301	1713	539	50	7
single patty w/ ketchup mustard mayonnaise onion pickle tomato & bun	1 reg	279	13	4	26	13	27	—	—	63	504	227	18	2
triple patty w/ cheese & bun	1 lg	769	51	22	161	56	27	—	—	282	1211	821	51	3
triple patty w/ ketchup mustard pickle & bun	1 lg	693	41	16	142	50	29	—	—	65	713	785	31	1

HAMBURGER SUBSTITUTES

(*see also* MEAT SUBSTITUTES)

AMY'S

FOOD	PORTION	CALS	FAT	SAT FAT	CHOL	PROT	CARB	SUGAR	FIBER	CALCI	SOD	POTAS	FOLIC	VIT C
All American Burger	1 (2.5 oz)	120	3	0	0	10	15	2	3	—	390	—	—	—
California Burger	1 (2.5 oz)	130	5	1	0	6	19	2	5	—	430	—	—	—
Chicago Burger	1 (2.5 oz)	160	5	2	5	10	20	2	3	—	390	—	—	—
BOCA BURGERS														
Flamed Grilled	1	120	4	1	<5	14	6	0	4	150	370	—	—	0
Hint of Garlic	1 patty (2.5 oz)	110	2	1	3	14	9	0	4	—	296	316	—	—
Vegan Original	1 patty (2.5 oz)	84	0	0	0	12	9	0	5	—	269	338	—	—
DR. PRAEGER'S														
California Burger	1 (2.7 oz)	100	3	0	0	8	10	0	4	50	190	—	—	4
FRANKLIN FARMS														
Veggiburger Portabella	1 (3 oz)	120	2	0	0	15	11	3	4	60	460	—	—	54
GARDENBURGER														
Classic Greek	1 (2.5 oz)	120	3	2	10	6	17	2	2	80	310	—	—	1
Fire Roasted Vegetable	1 (2.5 oz)	120	3	2	10	7	17	2	2	100	270	—	—	6
Hamburger Style	1 (2.5 oz)	90	0	0	0	16	7	0	3	80	370	—	—	6
Hamburger Style w/ Cheese	1 (2.5 oz)	110	3	2	5	16	7	0	3	100	380	—	—	6
Savory Mushroom	1 (2.5 oz)	120	3	2	10	6	18	1	4	100	270	—	—	0
GARDENVEGAN														
Fat-Free Patty	1 patty (2.5 oz)	140	0	0	0	11	23	tr	4	20	250	—	—	0

FOOD	PORTION	CALS	FAT	SAT FAT	CHOL	PROT	CARB	SUGAR	FIBER	CALCI	SOD	POTAS	FOLIC	VIT C
GREEN GIANT														
Southwestern Style	1 patty (3.2 oz)	140	4	2	0	18	9	1	5	80	370	—	—	0
HARMONY FARMS														
Soy Burgers Onion	1 (2.5 oz)	90	3	0	0	10	7	1	3	40	230	—	—	0
Soy Burgers Garlic	1 (2.5 oz)	110	3	0	0	12	10	1	23	40	240	—	—	0
Soy Burgers Mushroom	1 (2.5 oz)	110	3	0	0	11	9	1	3	40	320	—	—	0
Soy Burgers Original	1 (2.5 oz)	110	3	0	0	12	7	1	4	40	250	—	—	0
LIGHTLIFE														
Barbecue Grilles	1 patty (2.7 oz)	120	4	2	0	10	11	3	0	—	180	—	—	—
Lemon Grilles	1 patty (2.7 oz)	140	6	2	0	11	11	2	0	—	280	—	—	—
Light Burgers	1 (3 oz)	130	1	0	0	16	12	2	2	—	410	—	—	—
Tamari Grilles	1 patty (2.7 oz)	120	5	2	0	11	9	2	0	—	260	—	—	—
LOMA LINDA														
Patty Mix not prep	⅓ cup (0.9 oz)	90	1	0	0	14	7	0	5	20	480	400	—	0
Redi-Burger	⅝ in slice (3 oz)	120	3	1	0	18	7	1	4	0	450	140	—	0
Vege-Burger	¼ cup (1.9 oz)	70	2	1	0	11	2	0	2	0	115	30	—	0
MORNINGSTAR FARMS														
Better'n Burger	1 (2.7 oz)	80	0	0	0	13	8	tr	3	20	360	390	—	0
Garden Grille	1 patty (2.5 oz)	120	3	1	<5	6	18	1	4	60	280	130	—	0
Garden Veggie Patties	1 patty	100	3	1	0	10	9	1	4	40	350	180	—	0
Hard Rock Cafe Veggie Burger	1 (3 oz)	170	8	1	0	6	18	3	3	0	340	180	—	2
Harvest Burger	1	140	4	2	0	18	8	tr	5	80	390	380	—	0
Harvest Burger Italian Style	1 patty (3.2 oz)	140	5	2	0	17	8	tr	5	80	370	440	—	0
Harvest Burger Southwestern	1 (3.2 oz)	140	4	2	0	16	9	1	5	80	370	450	—	0
Spicy Black Bean Burger	1 (2.7 oz)	110	1	0	0	11	16	2	5	40	470	350	—	0
NATURAL TOUCH														
Garden Veggie Pattie	1 (2.4 oz)	110	3	1	0	10	8	0	3	0	280	160	—	0
Okara Pattie	1 (2.2 oz)	110	5	1	0	11	4	0	3	40	360	170	—	0
Original Veggie Burger Kit not prep	¼ pkg (0.8 oz)	80	0	0	0	14	6	0	4	60	360	150	—	0
Southwestern Veggie Burger Kit not prep	¼ pkg (0.9 oz)	90	0	0	0	12	9	tr	4	60	360	300	—	0
Spicy Black Bean Burger	1 (2.7 oz)	100	1	0	0	11	15	2	5	60	330	230	—	0
Vegan Burger	1 (2.7 oz)	70	0	0	0	11	6	0	3	60	370	390	—	0

FOOD	PORTION	CALS	FAT	SAT FAT	CHOL	PROT	CARB	SUGAR	FIBER	CALCI	SOD	POTAS	FOLIC	VIT C
SUPERBURGERS														
Vegan Organic Original	1 (3 oz)	98	2	1	0	10	14	0	2	60	350	—	—	0
Vegan Organic Smoked	1 (3 oz)	98	2	1	0	10	14	0	2	60	350	—	—	0
Vegan Organic TexMex	1 (3 oz)	110	1	1	0	10	14	0	3	80	195	—	—	0
V'DORA														
Vegetable BurgerLites	1 (3.3 oz)	58	0	0	0	4	4	1	0	50	98	—	—	35
WORTHINGTON														
Granburger not prep	3 tbsp (0.6 oz)	60	1	0	0	10	3	0	2	40	410	220	—	0
Prosage Patties	1 (1.3 oz)	80	3	1	0	9	3	0	2	0	300	100	—	0
Vegetarian Burger	¼ cup (1.9 oz)	60	2	0	0	9	2	0	1	0	270	25	—	0
YVES														
Black Bean & Mushroom Burgers	1 (3 oz)	100	0	0	0	12	13	1	7	60	450	380	—	0
Garden Vegetable Patties	1 (3 oz)	90	0	0	0	11	11	1	7	40	470	290	—	0
Veggie Burgers	1 (3 oz)	119	2	0	0	16	9	2	4	60	480	350	—	1
HAZELNUTS														
dried blanched	1 oz	191	19	1	0	4	5	—	—	55	1	131	—	—
dried unblanched	1 oz	179	18	1	0	4	4	—	—	53	1	125	20	tr
dry roasted unblanched	1 oz	188	19	1	0	3	5	—	—	55	1	131	—	—
oil roasted unblanched	1 oz	187	18	1	0	4	5	—	2	56	1	132	—	—
LOW CARB CREATIONS														
Soft Hazelnut Brittle	2 pieces (1 oz)	160	12	2	0	5	16	1	1	—	160	—	—	—
TORRAS														
Hazelnut Chocolate Spread	1 tsp	27	2	2	1	tr	3	0	0	—	3	—	—	—
TWIST														
Sugar Free Chocolate Hazelnut Spread	2 tbsp	180	14	4	0	1	2	0	0	—	0	—	—	—
HEART														
beef simmered	3 oz	148	5	1	164	24	tr	—	—	5	54	198	2	1
chicken simmered	1 cup (5 oz)	268	11	3	350	11	tr	—	—	27	69	192	116	3
lamb braised	3 oz	158	7	3	212	21	2	—	—	12	54	160	2	6
pork braised	1 cup	215	7	2	320	34	1	—	0	10	51	—	6	3
pork braised	1	191	7	2	285	30	1	—	0	9	45	—	5	3

FOOD	PORTION	CALS	FAT	SAT FAT	CHOL	PROT	CARB	SUGAR	FIBER	CALCI	SOD	POTAS	FOLIC	VIT C
turkey simmered	1 cup (5 oz)	257	9	3	327	39	3	—	—	19	79	265	114	3
veal braised	3 oz	158	6	2	150	25	tr	—	—	7	50	169	—	—

HEARTS OF PALM
canned	1 (1.2 oz)	9	tr	tr	0	1	2	—	—	19	141	58	13	3
canned	1 cup (5.1 oz)	41	1	tr	0	4	7	—	—	84	622	259	57	12

HEMP
HEMPNUT
Shelled Hempseed	1 oz	162	13	1	0	9	3	1	2	21	3	—	—	—

NUTIVA
Hempseed	1½ tbsp (0.5 oz)	70	5	1	0	4	3	0	2	0	0	—	—	—

HERBAL TEA
(*see* TEA/HERBAL TEA)

HERBS/SPICES
(*see also individual names*)
cajun seasoning	1 tbsp	19	1	—	—	1	3	—	1	—	5	—	—	—
chinese five spice	1 tsp	7	tr	—	—	0	2	—	tr	4	1	23	—	—
curry powder	1 tsp	6	tr	—	0	tr	1	—	—	10	1	31	—	tr
garam masala	1 tsp	8	tr	—	0	tr	1	—	—	15	2	29	0	0
poultry seasoning	1 tsp	5	tr	—	0	tr	1	—	—	15	tr	10	—	tr
pumpkin pie spice	1 tsp	6	tr	—	0	tr	1	—	—	12	1	11	—	tr

CHI-CHI'S
Seasoning Mix	1 tsp (3 g)	10	0	0	0	0	1	0	0	0	290	—	—	2

EDEN
Furikake Seasoning	½ tsp	5	0	0	0	0	1	0	1	14	25	10	—	0

GRINGO BILLY'S
Meat Rubs Chipotle	¼ tsp	0	0	0	0	0	0	0	0	—	151	—	—	—
Meat Rubs Ultimate	¼ tsp	0	0	0	0	0	0	0	0	—	155	—	—	—
Tuna Seasoning	1 tsp	5	1	0	0	0	1	0	1	—	92	—	—	—

INSTANT INDIA
Curry Paste Cilantro Garlic	2 tbsp (1 oz)	110	3	1	0	2	4	2	0	0	140	—	—	0
Curry Paste Ginger Garlic	2 tbsp (1 oz)	90	3	1	0	1	8	6	0	0	570	—	—	0

MCCORMICK
Big'n Season Buffalo Wings	1 tbsp (8 g)	30	0	0	—	0	5	3	—	—	710	—	—	—
Big'n Season Chicken	1 tbsp (6 g)	20	0	0	—	tr	3	—	—	—	460	—	—	—
Big'n Season Pot Roast	1 tsp	10	0	0	—	tr	1	—	—	—	390	—	—	—

FOOD	PORTION	CALS	FAT	SAT FAT	CHOL	PROT	CARB	SUGAR	FIBER	CALCI	SOD	POTAS	FOLIC	VIT C
MCCORMICK (CONT.)														
Blends Bon Appetit	¼ tsp	0	0	0	0	0	0	0	0	—	300	—	—	—
Cajun Seasoning	¼ tsp	0	0	0	0	0	0	0	0	—	80	—	—	—
Greek Seasoning	¼ tsp	0	0	0	0	0	0	0	0	—	20	—	—	—
Jamaican Jerk Seasoning	¼ tsp	0	0	0	0	0	0	0	0	—	125	—	—	—
Meat Loaf Seasoning	1 tsp (4 g)	15	0	0	—	0	2	2	—	—	350	—	—	—
Seafood Seasoning	¼ tsp	0	0	0	0	0	0	0	0	—	110	—	—	—
MRS. DASH														
Classic Italian	¼ tsp	0	0	0	0	0	0	0	0	—	0	10	—	—
Extra Spicy	¼ tsp	0	0	0	0	0	0	0	0	—	0	10	—	—
Garlic & Herb	¼ tsp	0	0	0	0	0	0	0	0	—	0	10	—	—
Grilling Blend Mesquite	¼ tsp	0	0	0	0	0	0	0	0	—	0	5	—	—
Grilling Blend Original Chicken	¼ tsp	0	0	0	0	0	0	0	0	—	0	5	—	—
Grilling Blend Original Steak	¼ tsp	0	0	0	0	0	0	0	0	—	0	5	—	—
Lemon Pepper	¼ tsp	0	0	0	0	0	0	0	0	—	0	10	—	—
Minced Onion Medley	¼ tsp	0	0	0	0	0	0	0	0	—	0	15	—	—
Original Blend	¼ tsp	0	0	0	0	0	0	0	0	—	0	10	—	—
Table Blend	¼ tsp	0	0	0	0	0	0	0	0	—	0	10	—	—
Tomato Basil Garlic	¼ tsp	0	0	0	0	0	0	0	0	—	0	5	—	—

HERRING

FOOD	PORTION	CALS	FAT	SAT FAT	CHOL	PROT	CARB	SUGAR	FIBER	CALCI	SOD	POTAS	FOLIC	VIT C
atlantic cooked	3 oz	172	10	2	65	20	0	—	—	63	98	356	—	1
atlantic cooked	1 fillet (5 oz)	290	17	4	110	33	0	—	—	105	165	599	—	1
atlantic raw	3 oz	134	8	2	51	15	0	—	—	49	76	278	—	1
pacific baked	3 oz	213	15	4	84	18	0	—	—	—	81	461	—	—
pacific fillet baked	5.1 oz	360	26	6	142	30	0	—	—	—	137	781	—	—
roe canned	1 oz	34	1	—	—	6	tr	—	—	4	—	—	—	—
roe raw	1 oz	37	tr	—	103	7	tr	—	—	—	—	—	—	4
smoked	3.5 oz	210	14	3	70	22	0	0	0	67	550	435	10	0
TAKE-OUT														
atlantic kippered	1 fillet (1.4 oz)	87	5	1	33	10	0	—	—	33	367	179	—	tr
atlantic pickled	½ oz	39	3	tr	2	2	1	—	—	12	131	10	tr	—
fried	1 serv (3.5 oz)	233	15	—	69	23	2	—	0	35	100	400	10	0

HICKORY NUTS

FOOD	PORTION	CALS	FAT	SAT FAT	CHOL	PROT	CARB	SUGAR	FIBER	CALCI	SOD	POTAS	FOLIC	VIT C
dried	1 oz	187	18	2	0	4	5	—	—	17	0	124	—	—

FOOD	PORTION	CALS	FAT	SAT FAT	CHOL	PROT	CARB	SUGAR	FIBER	CALCI	SOD	POTAS	FOLIC	VIT C
HOMINY														
CANNED														
white	1 cup (5.6 oz)	482	1	tr	0	2	23	—	4	16	336	14	2	0
VAN CAMP														
Golden	½ cup (4.3 oz)	80	1	0	0	4	17	0	1	0	540	—	—	0
White	½ cup (4.3 oz)	80	1	0	0	1	16	0	1	0	530	—	—	0
HONEY														
honey	1 tbsp (0.7 oz)	64	0	0	0	tr	17	17	—	1	1	11	0	tr
honey	1 cup (11.9 oz)	1031	0	0	0	1	279	270	—	20	12	176	5	2
orange blossom	1 tbsp	60	0	0	0	0	17	16	0	0	0	—	—	0
wild honey	1 tbsp	60	0	0	0	0	17	16	—	—	0	—	—	—
STEEL'S														
Sugar Free	1 tbsp	24	0	0	0	0	6	0	0	—	0	—	—	—
SUEBEE														
Clover	1 tbsp	60	0	0	0	0	17	16	—	—	0	—	—	—
HONEYDEW														
FRESH														
cubed	1 cup	60	tr	—	0	1	16	—	—	10	17	461	—	42
wedge	⅒ melon	46	tr	—	0	1	12	—	—	8	13	350	—	32
CHIQUITA														
Wedge	⅒ melon (4.7 oz)	50	0	0	0	1	13	12	1	0	35	—	—	27
HORSE														
roasted	3 oz	149	5	2	58	24	0	—	—	7	47	322	—	2
HORSERADISH														
japanese wasabi	¼ tsp	1	—	—	0	—	tr	—	0	2	0	5	tr	1
wasabi root raw	1 (5.9 oz)	184	1	—	0	8	40	—	12	216	29	960	30	71
wasabi root raw sliced	1 cup (4.6 oz)	142	1	—	0	6	31	—	10	166	22	738	23	71
BOAR'S HEAD														
Horseradish	1 tsp (5 g)	5	0	0	0	0	0	0	0	0	30	—	—	0
EDEN														
Wasabi Powder	1 tsp	10	0	0	0	0	1	0	1	2	0	—	—	1
KRAFT														
Cream Style	1 tsp (5 g)	0	0	0	0	0	0	0	0	0	50	10	—	1
Horseradish Sauce	1 tsp (5 g)	20	2	0	<5	0	tr	tr	0	0	35	0	—	0
Prepared	1 tsp (5 g)	0	0	0	0	0	0	0	0	0	50	10	—	1
HOT CHOCOLATE														
mix as prep w/ water	7 oz	103	1	1	—	3	23	—	—	96	149	203	tr	1
mix w/ equal as prep w/ water	7 oz	48	tr	tr	—	4	9	—	—	90	173	405	2	0

FOOD	PORTION	CALS	FAT	SAT FAT	CHOL	PROT	CARB	SUGAR	FIBER	CALCI	SOD	POTAS	FOLIC	VIT C
CARNATION														
Hot Cocoa 70 Calorie	1 pkg (0.7 oz)	70	0	0	0	3	15	15	tr	80	140	210	—	0
Hot Cocoa Double Chocolate Meltdown	1 pkg (1.2 oz)	150	4	3	0	2	27	24	1	40	170	260	—	0
Hot Cocoa Fat Free Raspberry	1 pkg (0.3 oz)	30	0	0	0	2	4	3	1	60	150	—	—	0
Hot Cocoa Fat Free w/ Marshmallows	1 pkg (0.4 oz)	45	0	0	0	7	10	7	tr	40	100	—	—	0
Hot Cocoa Lactose Free	1 pkg (1 oz)	120	2	0	0	1	25	19	1	0	115	—	—	0
Hot Cocoa Marshmallow Blizzard	1 pkg (1.5 oz)	180	2	0	<5	2	39	33	tr	60	140	210	—	0
Hot Cocoa Milk Chocolate	3 tbsp (1 oz)	110	1	0	<5	2	24	20	tr	40	95	250	—	0
Hot Cocoa Rich Chocolate as prep w/ 2% milk	1 pkg	200	8	4	21	tr	27	12	tr	300	288	—	—	0
Hot Cocoa Rich Chocolate Fat Free	1 pkg (0.3 oz)	25	0	0	0	2	4	3	1	60	135	210	—	0
Hot Cocoa Rich Chocolate No Sugar Added	3 tbsp (0.5 oz)	50	0	0	<5	4	8	7	tr	100	140	—	—	0
Hot Cocoa Rich Chocolate w/ Marshmallows	3 tbsp (1 oz)	110	1	0	<5	1	24	21	tr	40	95	240	—	0
COUNTRY CHOICE														
Irish Chocolate Mint	1 pkg	100	0	0	0	3	23	20	tr	100	160	—	—	0
Royal Chocolate	1 pkg	100	0	0	0	3	23	20	tr	100	160	—	—	0
Soy Cocoa Irish Chocolate Mint	1 pkg	100	1	0	0	2	23	17	1	60	130	—	—	0
Soy Cocoa Royal Chocolate	1 pkg	100	1	0	0	2	23	17	1	60	130	—	—	0
KETO														
Hot Cocoa	1 tsp	12	0	0	0	1	2	0	1	—	—	—	—	—
LOW CARB CREATIONS														
Cocoa as prep	1 cup	30	2	0	0	0	3	tr	0	0	70	—	—	0
White Hot Chocolate	1 cup	25	2	0	0	0	3	tr	0	0	50	—	—	0
NESTLÉ														
Hot Cocoa Rich Chocolate	1 pkg (1 oz)	110	1	1	0	1	24	19	tr	40	60	200	—	0

FOOD	PORTION	CALS	FAT	SAT FAT	CHOL	PROT	CARB	SUGAR	FIBER	CALCI	SOD	POTAS	FOLIC	VIT C
NESTLÉ (CONT.)														
Hot Cocoa Rich w/ Marshmallows	1 pkg (1 oz)	110	1	1	0	1	24	19	tr	60	60	200	—	0
SIPPER SWEETS														
Sugar Free Low Carb Mix	1 serv	50	3	0	0	1	3	0	0	—	80	—	—	—
SWISS MISS														
Caramel Cream	1 serv	110	3	0	0	1	21	18	tr	40	140	—	—	0
Hot Cocoa And Cream	1 serv	153	5	3	6	2	25	21	1	49	159	—	—	0
Hot Cocoa Chocolate Sensation	1 serv	148	4	2	tr	2	27	23	1	35	171	—	—	0
Hot Cocoa Diet	1 serv	22	tr	tr	tr	2	4	2	1	49	185	—	—	0
Hot Cocoa Fat Free	1 serv	52	tr	0	0	4	9	7	1	110	185	—	—	0
Hot Cocoa Fat Free Marshmallow Lovers	1 serv	65	tr	0	0	3	13	10	1	92	155	—	—	0
Hot Cocoa Lite	1 serv	76	1	tr	0	2	18	15	2	36	177	—	—	0
Hot Cocoa Marshmallow Lovers	1 serv	142	3	1	2	2	27	22	1	39	152	—	—	0
Hot Cocoa Milk Chocolate No Sugar Added	1 serv	55	1	1	1	2	10	6	1	74	164	—	—	0
Hot Cocoa Rich Chocolate	1 serv	110	2	tr	1	2	23	21	1	47	140	—	—	0
Hot Cocoa w/ Marshmallows No Sugar Added	1 serv	56	1	0	1	3	10	6	1	62	146	—	—	0
Hot Cocoa White Chocolate	1 serv	109	1	tr	1	3	21	21	tr	33	128	—	—	0
Milk Chocolate	1 pkg	120	3	1	0	1	22	17	1	40	160	—	—	0
Milk Chocolate w/ Marshmallows	1 pkg	120	3	1	tr	1	23	17	tr	40	150	—	—	0
Premiere Hot Cocoa Almond Mocha	1 serv	144	3	1	1	2	28	26	1	39	207	—	—	0
Premiere Hot Cocoa Raspberry Truffle	1 serv	144	3	1	1	2	28	26	1	42	220	—	—	—
Premiere Hot Cocoa Suisse Truffle	1 serv	142	2	1	1	2	28	26	1	43	225	—	—	0
Rich Hot Cocoa No Sugar Added	1 serv	54	1	1	1	2	10	6	1	72	165	—	—	0

FOOD	PORTION	CALS	FAT	SAT FAT	CHOL	PROT	CARB	SUGAR	FIBER	CALCI	SOD	POTAS	FOLIC	VIT C
SWISS MISS (CONT.)														
Sidewalk Cafe Cappuccino	1 serv	119	4	1	1	3	18	17	1	91	35	—	—	0
Sidewalk Cafe Cinnamon	1 serv	126	4	1	1	3	21	20	1	100	46	—	—	0
Sidewalk Cafe French Vanilla	1 serv	121	4	1	1	3	19	15	tr	83	32	—	—	0
Sidewalk Cafe Mocha	1 serv	120	4	1	1	3	20	19	1	96	43	—	—	0
WEIGHT WATCHERS														
Hot Cocoa Mix as prep	1 pkg	70	0	0	0	6	7	6	1	250	160	—	—	0
TAKE-OUT														
hot cocoa	1 cup	218	9	6	33	9	26	—	—	298	123	480	12	2
mexican hot chocolate	1 cup	173	6	4	18	10	20	—	1	306	150	442	13	2
HOT DOG														
beef	1 (1.5)	142	13	5	27	5	1	—	—	6	462	75	2	11
beef	1 (2 oz)	180	16	7	35	7	1	—	—	11	585	95	2	14
beef & pork	1 (1.5 oz)	144	13	5	22	5	1	—	—	6	504	75	2	12
beef & pork	1 (2 oz)	183	17	6	29	6	1	—	—	6	639	95	2	15
chicken	1 (1.5 oz)	116	9	2	45	6	3	—	—	43	617	—	—	—
pork cheesefurter smokie	1 (1.5 oz)	141	12	5	29	6	1	—	—	25	465	89	—	8
turkey	1 (1.5 oz)	102	8	—	48	6	1	—	—	48	642	80	—	—
APPLEGATE FARMS														
Chicken Natural Uncured	1 (1.5 oz)	120	5	2	40	14	1	0	0	20	450	—	—	0
Natural Turkey	1 (1.5 oz)	120	5	2	40	14	1	0	0	20	450	—	—	0
ARMOUR														
Star Jumbo Beef	1	190	18	—	30	6	—	—	—	—	590	—	—	—
BOAR'S HEAD														
Beef	1 (2 oz)	160	14	6	30	7	1	0	0	0	440	—	—	0
Beef Lite	1 (1.6 oz)	90	6	3	25	7	0	0	0	0	270	—	—	0
Pork & Beef	1 (2 oz)	150	14	5	25	7	0	0	0	0	460	—	—	0
HEALTH IS WEALTH														
Uncured Beef	1 (1.5 oz)	80	6	3	20	6	1	—	—	—	340	—	—	—
Uncured Chicken	1 (1.5 oz)	100	8	2	30	8	1	—	—	—	320	—	—	1
HEALTHY CHOICE														
Beef Low Fat	1 (1.8 oz)	70	3	1	15	6	7	2	0	0	440	—	—	2
Turkey Low Fat Pork Beef	1 (1.4 oz)	60	2	1	10	5	5	1	—	40	350	—	—	4
HORMEL														
Fat Free	1 (1.8 oz)	45	0	0	15	5	5	3	0	0	580	—	—	6
Fat Free Beef	1 (1.8 oz)	45	0	0	10	6	5	2	0	0	590	—	—	6

FOOD	PORTION	CALS	FAT	SAT FAT	CHOL	PROT	CARB	SUGAR	FIBER	CALCI	SOD	POTAS	FOLIC	VIT C
KID CUISINE														
Mystical Mini Corn Dogs	4 pieces	230	14	4	35	8	18	7	0	0	600	—	—	0
LOUIS RICH														
Bun Length	1 (2 oz)	110	8	3	55	6	3	1	0	80	650	—	—	0
Cheese	1 (1.6 oz)	90	6	3	40	6	2	tr	0	100	480	—	—	0
Franks	1 (1.6 oz)	80	6	2	40	5	2	tr	0	60	510	—	—	0
ORGANIC VALLEY														
All-Natural Beef	1 (1.6 oz)	90	6	3	25	7	1	—	—	—	310	—	—	12
OSCAR MAYER														
Beef	1 (1.6 oz)	140	13	6	30	5	1	tr	0	0	460	—	—	0
Big & Juicy Franks Deli Style	1 (2.7 oz)	230	22	10	50	9	1	0	0	0	680	—	—	0
Big & Juicy Franks Original	1 (2.7 oz)	240	22	9	45	9	1	1	0	0	700	—	—	0
Big & Juicy Franks Quarter Pound	1 (4 oz)	350	32	13	65	13	2	2	0	20	1050	—	—	0
Big & Juicy Weiners Hot 'N Spicy	1 (2.7 oz)	220	20	8	45	10	1	tr	0	0	750	—	—	0
Big & Juicy Weiners Smokie Links	1 (2.7 oz)	220	19	7	50	10	1	tr	0	0	770	—	—	0
Big & Juicy Weiners Original	1 (2.7 oz)	240	22	9	45	9	1	tr	0	0	690	—	—	0
Bun-Length Beef	1 (2 oz)	180	17	7	35	6	2	1	0	0	580	—	—	0
Cheese	1 (1.6 oz)	140	13	5	35	5	1	tr	0	80	510	—	—	0
Fat Free Beef	1 (1.8 oz)	40	0	0	15	7	3	2	0	0	460	—	—	0
Fat Free Turkey & Beef	1 (1.8 oz)	40	0	0	15	6	3	1	0	0	490	—	—	0
Jumbo Beef	1 (2 oz)	180	17	7	35	6	2	1	0	0	580	—	—	0
Light Beef	1 (1.6 oz)	90	6	3	20	5	2	tr	—	—	490	—	—	—
Wieners	1 (1.6 oz)	150	13	5	35	5	1	tr	0	20	430	—	—	0
Wieners Bun-Length	1 (2 oz)	190	17	6	40	6	2	1	0	40	550	—	—	0
Wieners Jumbo	1 (2 oz)	180	17	6	40	6	2	1	0	40	550	—	—	0
Wieners Light	1 (2 oz)	110	8	4	35	7	2	1	0	20	590	—	—	0
Wieners Little	6 (2 oz)	180	17	6	35	6	2	1	0	0	570	—	—	0
WAMPLER														
Chicken	1 (2 oz)	120	11	3	60	7	0	0	1	80	480	—	—	0
TAKE-OUT														
corndog	1	460	19	5	79	17	56	—	—	101	972	262	60	0
w/ bun chili	1	297	13	5	51	14	31	—	—	19	480	166	50	3
w/ bun plain	1	242	15	5	44	10	18	—	—	24	671	143	30	tr

FOOD	PORTION	CALS	FAT	SAT FAT	CHOL	PROT	CARB	SUGAR	FIBER	CALCI	SOD	POTAS	FOLIC	VIT C
HOT DOG SUBSTITUTES														
LIGHTLIFE														
Smart Deli Jumbo's	1 link (2.7 oz)	80	0	0	0	16	4	1	1	—	590	—	—	—
Smart Dogs	1 (1.5 oz)	45	0	0	0	9	2	0	0	—	230	—	—	—
Tofu Pups	1 (1.4 oz)	60	3	1	0	8	2	0	0	—	140	—	—	—
Wonder Dogs	1 (1.5 oz)	60	2	1	0	9	2	0	0	—	320	—	—	—
LOMA LINDA														
Big Franks	1 (1.8 oz)	110	7	1	0	10	2	0	2	0	240	50	—	0
Big Franks Low Fat	1 (1.8 oz)	80	3	1	0	11	3	0	2	0	220	50	—	0
Corn Dogs	1 (2.5 oz)	150	4	1	0	7	22	4	3	0	500	60	—	0
MORNINGSTAR FARMS														
America's Original Veggie Dog	1 (2 oz)	80	1	0	0	11	6	2	1	0	580	60	—	0
Meatfree Corn Dog	1 (2.5 oz)	150	4	1	0	7	22	4	3	0	500	60	—	0
Meatfree Mini Corn Dog	4 (2.7 oz)	170	5	1	0	11	21	6	1	0	580	90	—	0
NATURAL TOUCH														
Vege Frank	1 (1.6 oz)	100	6	1	0	10	2	0	2	0	470	50	—	0
QUORN														
Meat-Free Dogs	1 (1.5 oz)	70	4	0	5	5	3	0	2	20	250	—	—	0
WORTHINGTON														
Veja Links Low Fat	1 (1.1 oz)	40	2	0	0	5	1	0	0	0	190	20	—	0
YVES														
Good Dogs	1 (1.8 oz)	70	2	0	0	13	2	1	1	40	460	170	—	0
Tofu Dogs	1 (1.3 oz)	45	1	0	0	9	2	0	0	0	240	90	—	1
Veggie Dogs	1 (1.6 oz)	60	0	0	0	11	1	0	1	20	400	130	—	0
Veggie Dogs Chili	1 (1.6 oz)	50	0	0	0	10	3	1	2	20	360	105	—	0
Veggie Dogs Jumbo	1 (2.7 oz)	100	2	0	0	16	7	1	2	20	480	170	—	0
Veggie Dogs Jumbo Hot N' Spicy	1 (2.7 oz)	106	2	0	0	19	4	2	2	40	480	190	—	1
HUMMUS														
hummus	1 cup	420	21	3	0	12	50	—	—	124	599	427	146	19
ATHENOS														
Travelers Hummus & Pita	1 pkg	325	13	3	0	8	48	5	3	100	750	—	—	3
GUILTLESS GOURMET														
Original	2 tbsp	35	2	0	0	1	4	0	1	0	115	—	—	0
Roasted Garlic	2 tbsp	35	2	0	0	1	4	0	1	0	115	—	—	0

FOOD	PORTION	CALS	FAT	SAT FAT	CHOL	PROT	CARB	SUGAR	FIBER	CALCI	SOD	POTAS	FOLIC	VIT C
TAKE-OUT														
hummus	⅓ cup	140	7	1	0	4	17	—	—	41	200	142	49	6

HYACINTH BEANS

FOOD	PORTION	CALS	FAT	SAT FAT	CHOL	PROT	CARB	SUGAR	FIBER	CALCI	SOD	POTAS	FOLIC	VIT C
dried cooked	1 cup	228	1	—	0	16	40	—	—	77	13	653	—	0

ICE CREAM AND FROZEN DESSERTS

(*see also* ICES AND ICE POPS, PUDDING POPS, SHERBET, YOGURT FROZEN)

FOOD	PORTION	CALS	FAT	SAT FAT	CHOL	PROT	CARB	SUGAR	FIBER	CALCI	SOD	POTAS	FOLIC	VIT C
chocolate	½ cup (4 fl oz)	143	7	4	22	3	19	13	—	72	50	164	10	1
dixie cup chocolate	1 (3.5 fl oz)	125	6	4	20	2	16	11	—	63	44	145	9	tr
dixie cup strawberry	1 (3.5 fl oz)	112	5	—	17	2	16	9	—	70	35	109	7	5
dixie cup vanilla	1 (3.5 fl oz)	116	6	4	25	2	14	9	—	74	46	115	3	tr
strawberry	½ cup (4 fl oz)	127	6	—	19	2	18	10	—	79	40	124	8	5
vanilla	½ cup (4 fl oz)	132	7	4	29	2	16	10	—	85	53	131	3	tr
vanilla soft serve	½ cup	111	2	1	10	4	19	—	—	138	62	194	6	1
ATKINS														
Endulge Butter Pecan	½ cup	170	15	7	40	2	12	1	4	60	40	—	—	0
Endulge Chocolate	½ cup	140	12	7	45	2	13	1	5	60	20	—	—	0
Endulge Chocolate Peanut Butter Swirl	½ cup	170	14	7	40	3	14	1	5	60	70	—	—	0
Endulge Vanilla	½ cup	140	12	7	45	2	13	1	4	60	30	—	—	0
Endulge Vanilla Fudge	½ cup	140	10	6	40	2	14	1	4	60	30	—	—	0
Endulge Bars Chocolate Fudge	1 bar	130	11	6	40	2	12	1	5	60	20	—	—	0
Endulge Bars Chocolate Fudge Swirl	1 bar	180	16	12	30	3	12	1	4	60	25	—	—	0
Endulge Bars Peanut Butter Swirl	1 bar	180	17	12	30	2	12	1	4	60	25	—	—	0
Endulge Bars Vanilla Fudge Swirl	1 bar	180	16	12	30	2	12	1	4	60	25	—	—	0
BETTER THAN ICE CREME														
Soy Vanilla as prep	½ cup	110	3	tr	0	1	21	8	0	300	83	45	—	0
BON BONS														
Dark Chocolate	5 pieces	190	13	8	15	2	16	12	0	60	35	—	—	0
Milk Chocolate	5 pieces	200	14	8	10	2	17	13	0	40	35	—	—	0

FOOD	PORTION	CALS	FAT	SAT FAT	CHOL	PROT	CARB	SUGAR	FIBER	CALCI	SOD	POTAS	FOLIC	VIT C
BREYERS														
Almond Joy	½ cup	140	5	3	30	4	20	16	tr	80	75	—	—	0
Banana Fudge Chunk	½ cup	170	9	5	20	2	21	19	tr	60	40	—	—	0
Butter Almond	½ cup	160	10	5	20	4	14	14	tr	100	85	—	—	0
Butter Pecan	½ cup	170	11	5	20	3	14	14	0	100	115	—	—	0
Butter Pecan Homemade	½ cup	170	11	5	50	3	18	13	0	100	70	—	—	0
Butter Pecan No Sugar Added	½ cup	120	7	3	10	3	15	4	tr	80	115	—	—	0
Caramel Praline Crunch	½ cup	180	9	5	20	2	22	19	0	80	75	—	—	1
Caramel Toffee Crunch	½ cup	180	9	6	50	3	22	20	0	80	100	—	—	1
CarbSmart Chocolate	½ cup	130	10	6	25	2	10	4	3	60	50	—	—	0
CarbSmart Strawberry	½ cup	130	9	6	25	2	10	4	3	60	25	—	—	0
CarbSmart Vanilla	½ cup	130	9	6	25	2	10	4	3	60	25	—	—	0
Cherry Chocolate Chip	½ cup	150	8	5	20	3	18	17	0	100	45	—	—	0
Cherry Vanilla	½ cup	140	8	5	20	2	16	16	0	80	30	—	—	0
Chocolate	½ cup	150	8	5	20	3	17	16	tr	80	35	—	—	0
Chocolate 98% Fat Free	½ cup	90	2	1	5	3	21	14	4	80	50	—	—	0
Chocolate Caramel No Sugar Added	½ cup	110	4	3	10	3	16	4	tr	80	55	—	—	0
Chocolate Chip	½ cup	160	9	5	20	3	17	17	0	100	40	—	—	0
Chocolate Chip Cookie Dough	½ cup	170	9	6	25	3	20	17	0	100	55	—	—	0
Chocolate Rainbow	½ cup	140	7	5	20	3	16	14	0	100	40	—	—	0
Coffee	½ cup	140	8	5	20	3	15	15	0	100	40	—	—	0
Cookies & Cream	½ cup	160	8	5	20	3	18	16	tr	100	50	—	—	0
Creamsicle	½ cup	130	5	3	15	2	20	16	0	60	35	—	—	0
Deep Chocolate Fudge	½ cup	200	12	8	30	3	21	19	1	80	60	—	—	1
Dulce De Leche	½ cup	150	7	4	20	3	20	19	0	100	105	—	—	0
French Vanilla	½ cup	150	8	5	50	3	15	15	0	100	45	—	—	0
French Vanilla Light	½ cup	120	4	2	35	3	18	14	0	100	50	—	—	0
French Vanilla No Sugar Added	½ cup	110	5	3	35	3	14	5	0	100	60	—	—	0
Fresa Banana	½ cup	140	5	4	15	2	20	16	0	80	35	—	—	12
Heath English Toffee	½ cup	190	9	5	20	2	22	20	0	80	120	—	—	0

FOOD	PORTION	CALS	FAT	SAT FAT	CHOL	PROT	CARB	SUGAR	FIBER	CALCI	SOD	POTAS	FOLIC	VIT C
BREYERS (CONT.)														
Hershey w/ Almonds	½ cup	170	8	5	15	3	24	21	tr	80	65	—	—	0
Ice Cream Cake Oreo	1 slice	190	10	5	30	3	21	17	tr	80	100	—	—	0
Ice Cream Cake Vanilla	1 slice	190	11	7	40	3	19	16	0	100	40	—	—	0
Klondike Sandwich	½ cup	160	7	4	20	3	21	15	0	80	70	—	—	0
Mint Chocolate Chip	½ cup	160	9	5	20	3	17	17	0	100	40	—	—	0
Mint Chocolate Chip Light	½ cup	130	5	3	10	3	20	18	0	100	45	—	—	0
Mint Oreo	½ cup	170	7	4	15	2	23	17	0	80	75	—	—	0
Mocha Almond Fudge	½ cup	170	9	4	15	4	18	15	2	80	45	—	—	0
Oreo	½ cup	160	6	5	20	3	20	16	0	80	80	—	—	0
Peach	½ cup	130	6	4	15	2	17	16	0	60	25	—	—	0
Peanut Butter & Fudge	½ cup	170	10	5	20	4	17	15	tr	100	80	—	—	0
Reese's Peanut Butter Cups	½ cup	180	9	5	15	3	22	18	0	80	75	—	—	0
Rocky Road	½ cup	160	8	5	20	3	20	19	tr	80	60	—	—	0
SpongeBob Cookie Dough	½ cup	160	7	4	15	2	21	17	0	80	95	—	—	0
Strawberry	½ cup	120	6	4	15	2	15	15	0	80	30	—	—	6
Strawberry Shortcake	½ cup	160	6	4	15	2	23	18	0	60	40	—	—	0
Turtle Sundae	½ cup	190	11	6	30	3	20	17	tr	80	70	—	—	1
Vanilla	½ cup	140	8	5	20	3	15	15	0	100	40	—	—	0
Vanilla Calcium Rich	½ cup	130	7	4	20	3	14	14	0	300	40	—	—	0
Vanilla Fudge Twirl	½ cup	140	7	5	20	3	18	15	tr	100	45	—	—	0
Vanilla Homemade	½ cup	140	8	5	40	2	16	14	0	100	60	—	—	0
Vanilla Lactose Free	½ cup	130	7	5	20	2	14	14	0	80	35	—	—	0
Vanilla Light	½ cup	110	3	2	10	3	17	15	0	100	50	—	—	0
Vanilla Light 2% Milk	½ cup	130	5	3	30	3	18	15	0	100	60	—	—	0
Vanilla No Sugar Added	½ cup	100	5	3	15	3	15	4	0	100	45	—	—	0
Vanilla Caramel Brownie	½ cup	170	9	5	50	3	20	17	0	80	90	—	—	1
Vanilla Fudge Brownie	½ cup	180	9	5	25	3	19	16	tr	80	80	—	—	0

FOOD	PORTION	CALS	FAT	SAT FAT	CHOL	PROT	CARB	SUGAR	FIBER	CALCI	SOD	POTAS	FOLIC	VIT C
BREYERS (CONT.)														
Vanilla Fudge Twirl No Sugar Added	½ cup	110	4	3	10	3	19	4	tr	80	50	—	—	0
Wild Berry Swirl	½ cup	140	8	5	20	2	16	16	0	80	35	—	—	0
BUTTERFINGER														
Bar	1 (2.5 oz)	190	13	8	15	2	16	14	0	60	35	—	—	0
CALIFORNIA JOE														
Soft Serve Chocolate	½ cup (2.5 oz)	72	0	0	0	5	11	10	1	150	60	—	—	0
Soft Serve Vanilla	½ cup (2.5 oz)	70	0	0	0	5	11	10	1	150	60	—	—	0
CARNATION														
Cup Chocolate	1 (3 oz)	140	8	5	25	2	16	14	0	60	40	—	—	0
Cup Chocolate Malt	1 (12 oz)	270	6	1	20	7	48	36	1	200	130	—	—	0
Cup Strawberry	1 (3 oz)	100	5	3	20	1	12	10	0	40	25	—	—	2
Cup Vanilla	1 (5 oz)	170	10	5	35	2	19	16	0	60	50	—	—	0
Cup Vanilla	1 (3 oz)	100	6	3	20	1	11	9	0	40	30	—	—	0
Cup Vanilla Malt	1 (12 oz)	260	6	0	20	6	48	37	0	200	130	—	—	0
Sundae Cup Strawberry	1 (5 oz)	200	8	5	30	2	29	23	0	40	55	—	—	2
Sundae Cup Chocolate	1 (5 oz)	210	9	6	30	2	30	22	1	40	55	—	—	0
COOL CREATIONS														
Cookies & Cream Sandwich	1 (3.5 oz)	240	11	4	15	2	34	18	1	60	250	—	—	0
Mickey Mouse Bar	1 (2.5 oz)	120	8	4	15	2	10	9	0	40	25	—	—	0
Mini Sandwich	1 (2.3 oz)	110	5	2	10	1	16	8	0	20	70	—	—	0
DIPPIN' DOTS														
Chocolate	⅝ cup (3 oz)	190	9	6	40	4	22	22	0	100	70	—	—	0
DRUMSTICK														
Cone Chocolate	1 (4.6 oz)	320	17	10	25	6	36	20	2	100	90	—	—	0
Cone Chocolate Dipped	1 (4.6 oz)	320	16	10	25	5	40	20	1	100	90	—	—	0
Cone Vanilla	1 (4.6 oz)	340	19	11	20	6	35	20	2	100	90	—	—	0
Cone Vanilla Caramel	1 (4.6 oz)	360	20	13	25	6	38	24	2	100	100	—	—	0
Cone Vanilla Fudge	1 (4.6 oz)	360	20	10	20	5	39	25	2	100	100	—	—	0
EDY'S														
3 Musketeers	½ cup	160	7	4	20	3	22	19	—	60	50	—	—	—
Dreamery Banana Split	½ cup	240	11	7	60	3	31	27	1	80	45	—	—	5
Dreamery Black Raspberry Avalanche	½ cup	270	16	10	80	4	27	23	1	80	50	—	—	0

FOOD	PORTION	CALS	FAT	SAT FAT	CHOL	PROT	CARB	SUGAR	FIBER	CALCI	SOD	POTAS	FOLIC	VIT C
EDY'S (CONT.)														
Dreamery Caramel Toffee Bar Heaven	½ cup	290	16	9	75	4	32	29	0	100	90	—	—	0
Dreamery Cashew Praline Parfait	½ cup	280	16	9	75	4	30	26	0	80	75	—	—	0
Dreamery Chocolate Truffle Explosion	½ cup	280	15	55	8	5	31	27	1	100	85	—	—	0
Dreamery Chocolate Peanut Butter Chunk	½ cup	310	18	9	50	7	29	25	2	100	110	—	—	0
Dreamery Coney Island Waffle Cone	½ cup	310	18	12	70	4	32	28	1	80	55	—	—	0
Dreamery Cool Mint	½ cup	300	17	11	75	4	32	29	1	80	55	—	—	0
Dreamery Deep Dish Apple Pie	½ cup	280	15	9	75	3	34	28	0	80	95	—	—	0
Dreamery Dulce De Leche	½ cup	270	14	9	70	4	32	30	0	100	70	—	—	0
Dreamery Grandma's Cookie Dough	½ cup	300	17	9	75	4	32	25	0	80	80	—	—	0
Dreamery Harvest Peach	½ cup	230	13	7	70	3	25	22	0	80	35	—	—	8
Dreamery New York Strawberry Cheesecake	½ cup	260	15	9	80	4	27	23	0	80	70	—	—	4
Dreamery Nothing But Chocolate	½ cup	280	14	8	65	5	34	28	1	100	70	—	—	0
Dreamery Nuts About Malt	½ cup	290	17	9	70	5	29	24	1	80	65	—	—	0
Dreamery Raspberry Brownie A La Mode	½ cup	270	14	7	75	3	34	27	1	80	60	—	—	0
Dreamery Strawberry Fields	½ cup	220	12	7	65	3	26	23	1	80	35	—	—	6
Dreamery Tiramisù	½ cup	260	13	8	75	4	31	25	0	80	150	—	—	0

FOOD	PORTION	CALS	FAT	SAT FAT	CHOL	PROT	CARB	SUGAR	FIBER	CALCI	SOD	POTAS	FOLIC	VIT C
EDY'S (CONT.)														
Dreamery Vanilla	½ cup	260	15	9	70	5	25	24	0	150	55	—	—	0
Grand Black Cherry Vanilla	½ cup	140	7	4	25	2	17	15	—	60	25	—	—	—
Grand Blue Ribbon Chocolate Cake	½ cup	180	10	5	25	3	20	15	—	60	60	—	—	—
Grand Butter Pecan	½ cup	170	10	5	25	3	16	13	—	60	70	—	—	—
Grand Cherry Chocolate Chip	½ cup	160	8	5	25	2	19	16	—	60	40	—	—	—
Grand Chocolate	½ cup	150	8	5	25	3	16	15	—	60	35	—	—	—
Grand Chocolate Caramel Swirl	½ cup	170	9	6	25	2	19	16	—	60	45	—	—	—
Grand Chocolate Chips	½ cup	170	9	6	25	3	18	15	—	60	45	—	—	—
Grand Chocolate Fudge Mousse	½ cup	160	8	5	25	2	19	15	—	60	45	—	—	—
Grand Chocolate Fudge Sundae	½ cup	170	9	5	20	3	20	16	—	60	50	—	—	—
Grand Coffee	½ cup	140	8	5	25	2	15	13	—	60	40	—	—	—
Grand Cookie Dough	½ cup	180	9	5	25	3	21	15	—	60	65	—	—	—
Grand Cookies 'N Cream	½ cup	160	8	5	25	3	19	14	—	60	50	—	—	—
Grand Double Fudge Brownie	½ cup	170	9	5	30	2	19	15	—	60	45	—	—	—
Grand Espresso Chip	½ cup	150	8	5	25	2	17	14	—	60	50	—	—	—
Grand French Vanilla	½ cup	160	9	5	50	2	17	11	—	60	40	—	—	—
Grand French Vanilla Fudge Pie	½ cup	160	8	5	45	2	20	14	—	40	55	—	—	—
Grand Mint Chocolate Chips	½ cup	170	9	6	25	3	18	15	—	60	45	—	—	—
Grand Neapolitan	½ cup	140	7	5	25	2	16	14	—	60	35	—	—	—
Grand Nutty Cone Crunch	½ cup	180	10	6	25	3	19	15	—	60	45	—	—	—
Grand Real Strawberry	½ cup	130	6	4	20	2	16	15	—	60	30	—	—	—
Grand Rocky Road	½ cup	170	10	5	25	3	17	13	—	60	30	—	—	—
Grand Spumoni	½ cup	150	8	5	25	3	16	13	—	60	40	—	—	—
Grand Strawberry Cupcake	½ cup	140	6	4	25	2	19	15	—	60	40	—	—	—
Grand Tin Roof Sundae	½ cup	170	9	5	25	3	18	15	—	60	50	—	—	—

FOOD	PORTION	CALS	FAT	SAT FAT	CHOL	PROT	CARB	SUGAR	FIBER	CALCI	SOD	POTAS	FOLIC	VIT C
EDY'S (CONT.)														
Grand Utimate Caramel Cup	½ cup	170	8	5	20	2	22	19	—	60	55	—	—	—
Grand Vanilla	½ cup	140	8	5	25	2	15	13	—	60	30	—	—	—
Grand Vanillaberry Bar	½ cup	130	5	3	20	2	19	16	—	40	25	—	—	—
Grand Light Butter Pecan	½ cup	120	5	2	20	3	16	12	—	60	60	—	—	—
Grand Light Chocolate Raspberry Escape	½ cup	130	5	3	15	3	19	14	—	6	45	—	—	—
Grand Light Chocolate Fudge Mousse	½ cup	120	4	2	20	3	17	13	—	60	45	—	—	—
Grand Light Cookie Dough	½ cup	130	5	3	20	3	19	13	—	60	65	—	—	—
Grand Light Cookies'N Cream	½ cup	120	4	2	15	3	18	12	—	60	60	—	—	—
Grand Light Crazy For Caramel	½ cup	120	4	3	15	3	19	15	—	60	55	—	—	—
Grand Light French Silk	½ cup	130	5	3	15	3	19	14	—	60	50	—	—	—
Grand Light Mint Chocolate Chips	½ cup	120	5	3	20	3	17	13	—	60	50	—	—	—
Grand Light Peanut Butter Cups	½ cup	120	5	3	20	3	17	13	—	60	50	—	—	—
Grand Light Rocky Road	½ cup	120	4	2	20	3	17	12	—	60	40	—	—	—
Grand Light S'Mores & More	½ cup	130	4	2	15	3	22	13	—	40	60	—	—	—
Grand Light Strawberry Shortcake	½ cup	110	4	2	20	2	18	14	—	40	40	—	—	—
Grand Light Vanilla	½ cup	100	3	2	20	3	15	11	—	60	45	—	—	—
Homemade All Natural Vanilla	½ cup	130	7	5	30	3	14	14	—	60	55	—	—	—
Homemade Brownies A La Mode	½ cup	150	7	4	30	3	18	16	—	60	65	—	—	—
Homemade Chocolate Chip Cookie Jar	½ cup	180	10	7	25	3	19	16	—	60	90	—	—	—

FOOD	PORTION	CALS	FAT	SAT FAT	CHOL	PROT	CARB	SUGAR	FIBER	CALCI	SOD	POTAS	FOLIC	VIT C
EDY'S (CONT.)														
Homemade Chocolate Chip Mousse	½ cup	170	9	6	30	3	19	18	—	60	60	—	—	—
Homemade Double Chocolate Chunk	½ cup	170	9	6	30	3	19	18	—	60	55	—	—	—
Homemade Mint Chocolate Chunk	½ cup	170	9	6	25	3	18	17	—	60	65	—	—	—
Homemade Old Fashioned Butter Pecan	½ cup	160	10	5	30	3	15	14	—	60	90	—	—	—
Homemade Strawberries & Cream	½ cup	120	6	4	25	2	15	15	—	60	45	—	—	—
Homemade Vanilla Custard	½ cup	150	8	5	55	4	15	15	—	100	55	—	—	—
M&M's Almond	½ cup	180	10	5	25	3	21	17	—	60	55	—	—	—
M&M's Chocolate Brownie Sundae	½ cup	180	9	5	25	3	22	18	—	80	55	—	—	—
M&M's Mint	½ cup	200	11	6	25	3	21	19	—	60	60	—	—	—
M&M's Vanilla	½ cup	180	9	5	25	3	22	18	—	60	50	—	—	—
Milky Way	½ cup	160	7	4	25	3	21	17	—	80	70	—	—	—
Snickers	½ cup	180	9	5	25	3	21	15	—	60	70	—	—	—
Snickers Cruncher	½ cup	190	10	6	25	3	21	17	—	60	65	—	—	—
Twix	½ cup	190	9	5	25	3	23	18	—	60	70	—	—	—
Twix Peanut Butter	½ cup	190	11	5	25	3	20	15	—	60	80	—	—	—
FLINTSTONES														
Cool Cream	1 (2.75 oz)	90	2	1	5	1	18	14	0	40	30	—	—	12
Push-Up Pebbles Treats	1 (2.75 oz)	120	6	4	20	1	15	14	0	60	25	—	—	0
GOOD HUMOR														
Bar Oreo	1 (4 oz)	250	15	8	15	3	28	18	tr	60	160	—	—	0
Bar Reese's Peanut Butter	1 (4 oz)	310	21	13	20	4	27	23	tr	100	90	—	—	0
Bar Toasted Almond	1 (3 oz)	180	10	3	5	2	22	16	tr	40	35	—	—	0
Bar Vanilla Dark Chocolate	1 (3 oz)	190	13	9	10	2	15	12	tr	60	35	—	—	0
Bar Vanilla Milk Chocolate	1 (3 oz)	180	13	9	15	2	15	12	0	80	45	—	—	0
Bar Candy Center Crunch	1 (4 oz)	310	23	17	15	3	24	19	tr	100	85	—	—	0
Bar Strawberry Shortcake	1 (4 oz)	230	12	4	10	2	30	17	tr	40	90	—	—	0

FOOD	PORTION	CALS	FAT	SAT FAT	CHOL	PROT	CARB	SUGAR	FIBER	CALCI	SOD	POTAS	FOLIC	VIT C
GOOD HUMOR (CONT.)														
Chocolate Eclair Bar	1 (4 oz)	220	11	5	10	2	30	16	tr	40	85	—	—	0
Cone Premium Sundae	1 (4.3 oz)	270	15	8	15	4	29	18	tr	60	95	—	—	0
Cone Strawberry Shortcake	1 (4.3 oz)	230	10	5	5	2	34	19	tr	20	85	—	—	0
Giant Sandwich Neapolitan	1 (6 oz)	250	10	5	20	4	37	20	tr	100	210	—	—	0
Giant Sandwich Vanilla	1 (6 oz)	250	10	5	20	4	36	20	0	100	210	—	—	0
King Cone	1 (4.6 fl oz)	250	13	6	15	4	30	19	tr	80	100	—	—	0
King Cone Giant	1 (8 oz)	190	21	11	40	7	44	30	tr	150	160	—	—	1
Number 1 Bar	1 (4 oz)	200	11	8	10	2	21	15	tr	60	50	—	—	0
Sandwich Chocolate Chip Cookie	1 (4.5 oz)	290	13	6	20	3	41	24	1	60	210	—	—	0
Sandwich Vanilla	1 (3.5 oz)	160	6	3	10	3	25	12	0	40	160	—	—	0
Sundae Twist Cup	1 (6 oz)	160	3	2	10	2	33	29	0	150	100	—	—	0
HAAGEN-DAZS														
Bars Chocolate & Almonds	1 (3.7 oz)	380	27	14	90	6	27	24	2	150	65	—	—	0
Bars Chocolate & Dark Chocolate	1 (3.6 oz)	350	24	15	65	5	28	24	2	100	45	—	—	0
Bars Chocolate Peanut Butter Swirl	1 (3 oz)	320	23	11	60	6	21	19	2	100	65	—	—	0
Bars Coffee & Almond Crunch	1 (3.7 oz)	370	27	15	90	5	27	26	tr	150	80	—	—	0
Bars Cookies & Cream Crunch	1 (3.6 oz)	370	26	15	85	5	30	26	tr	150	100	—	—	0
Bars Dulce De Leche Caramel	1 (3.7 oz)	370	24	15	75	4	34	33	0	150	90	—	—	0
Bars Tropical Coconut	1 (3.5 oz)	340	24	15	90	5	25	25	0	150	70	—	—	2
Bars Vanilla & Almonds	1 (3.7 oz)	380	28	14	90	6	26	24	1	150	70	—	—	0
Bars Vanilla & Dark Chocolate	1 (3.6 oz)	350	24	15	85	5	27	24	1	100	50	—	—	0
Bars Vanilla & Milk Chocolate	1 (3.5 oz)	340	24	14	90	5	25	24	tr	150	65	—	—	0
Butter Pecan	½ cup	310	23	11	110	5	21	18	tr	100	110	—	—	0
Cappuccino Commotion	½ cup	310	21	12	100	5	25	23	1	—	90	—	—	—
Cherry Vanilla	½ cup	240	15	9	100	4	23	22	0	100	60	—	—	1
Chocolate	½ cup	270	18	11	115	5	22	21	1	150	60	—	—	0

FOOD	PORTION	CALS	FAT	SAT FAT	CHOL	PROT	CARB	SUGAR	FIBER	CALCI	SOD	POTAS	FOLIC	VIT C
HAAGEN-DAZS (CONT.)														
Chocolate Brownie w/ Walnuts	½ cup	290	19	9	100	5	25	20	1	—	75	—	—	—
Chocolate Chocolate Fudge	½ cup	290	18	12	100	5	27	24	tr	100	90	—	—	0
Chocolate Chocolate Chip	½ cup	300	20	12	105	5	26	24	2	100	55	—	—	0
Chocolate Swiss Almond	½ cup	300	20	11	100	4	24	21	2	—	55	—	—	—
Cinnamon	½ cup	250	17	10	110	4	20	20	0	—	65	—	—	—
Coffee	½ cup	270	18	11	120	5	21	21	0	150	70	—	—	0
Coffee Mocha Chip	½ cup	290	19	12	110	5	25	22	tr	100	75	—	—	0
Cookie Dough Chip	½ cup	310	20	12	95	4	29	24	0	100	125	—	—	0
Cookies & Cream	½ cup	270	17	10	105	5	23	21	0	150	90	—	—	0
Creme Caramel Pecan	½ cup	320	20	10	95	5	29	26	0	100	120	—	—	0
Dulce De Leche Caramel	½ cup	290	17	10	100	5	28	26	0	150	95	—	—	0
Low Fat Chocolate	½ cup	170	3	2	30	7	29	15	tr	200	50	—	—	0
Low Fat Coffee Fudge	½ cup	170	3	2	25	5	32	22	0	150	95	—	—	0
Low Fat Strawberry	½ cup	150	2	1	15	5	28	18	0	150	40	—	—	5
Low Fat Vanilla	½ cup	170	3	2	20	7	29	15	0	200	50	—	—	0
Macadamia Brittle	½ cup	300	20	12	110	4	25	24	0	150	110	—	—	0
Mango	½ cup	250	14	6	85	4	28	27	tr	100	50	—	—	5
Mint Chip	½ cup	300	19	12	105	5	26	23	tr	100	85	—	—	0
Pineapple Coconut	½ cup	230	12	8	90	4	25	24	0	100	55	—	—	0
Pistachio	½ cup	290	20	11	110	5	22	19	tr	100	80	—	—	0
Rum Raisin	½ cup	270	17	10	110	4	22	21	0	100	60	—	—	0
Strawberry	½ cup	250	16	10	95	4	23	22	tr	150	65	—	—	6
Vanilla	½ cup	270	18	11	120	5	21	21	0	150	70	—	—	0
Vanilla Chocolate Chip	½ cup	310	20	12	105	5	26	22	tr	100	75	—	—	0
Vanilla Fudge	½ cup	290	18	12	100	5	25	24	0	150	95	—	—	0
Vanilla Swiss Almond	½ cup	300	20	11	105	5	24	21	tr	100	75	—	—	0
HEALTHY CHOICE														
Butter Pecan Crunch	½ cup	120	2	1	5	3	22	21	tr	100	60	—	—	0

FOOD	PORTION	CALS	FAT	SAT FAT	CHOL	PROT	CARB	SUGAR	FIBER	CALCI	SOD	POTAS	FOLIC	VIT C
HEALTHY CHOICE (CONT.)														
Cappuccino Chocolate Chunk	½ cup	120	2	1	10	3	22	19	1	100	60	—	—	0
Cappuccino Mocha Crunch	½ cup	120	2	1	5	3	22	19	tr	100	55	—	—	0
Cherry Chocolate Chunk	½ cup	110	2	1	<5	3	19	19	tr	100	55	—	—	0
Chocolate Chocolate Chunk	½ cup	120	2	1	5	3	21	18	2	100	45	—	—	0
Coconut Cream Pie	½ cup	120	2	1	5	3	23	17	1	100	75	—	—	0
Cookies Creme De Mint	½ cup	130	2	1	5	3	24	20	tr	100	60	—	—	0
Cookies 'N Cream	½ cup	120	2	1	5	3	21	19	tr	100	90	—	—	0
Fudge Brownie	½ cup	120	2	1	5	3	22	20	tr	100	55	—	—	0
Mint Chocolate Chip	½ cup	120	2	1	5	3	21	20	tr	100	50	—	—	0
Old Fashioned Blueberry Hill	½ cup	120	2	1	<5	2	23	17	1	100	50	—	—	0
Old Fashioned Butterscotch Blonde	½ cup	140	2	1	10	3	26	22	tr	100	75	—	—	0
Old Fashioned Cherry Vanilla	½ cup	120	2	1	5	2	22	17	tr	100	50	—	—	0
Old Fashioned Strawberry	½ cup	110	2	1	0	2	20	17	1	100	35	—	—	4
Peanut Butter Cup	½ cup	110	2	1	5	3	19	18	tr	100	65	—	—	0
Praline & Caramel	½ cup	130	2	1	5	3	25	24	tr	100	70	—	—	0
Praline Caramel Cluster	½ cup	130	2	1	<5	3	25	24	tr	100	70	—	—	0
Rocky Road	½ cup	140	2	1	5	3	28	19	tr	100	60	—	—	0
Turtle Fudge Cake	½ cup	130	2	1	<5	3	25	23	2	100	60	—	—	0
Vanilla	½ cup	100	2	1	5	3	18	17	tr	100	50	—	—	0
Vanilla Bean	½ cup	110	2	1	5	3	19	18	tr	100	45	—	—	0
Wild Raspberry Truffle	½ cup	120	2	1	6	3	22	15	tr	100	55	—	—	0
HERSHEY'S														
Butter Pecan	½ cup	170	9	6	35	3	15	14	0	80	80	—	—	0
French Vanilla	½ cup	170	10	6	70	3	17	16	0	100	90	—	—	0
Vanilla Chocolate Strawberry	½ cup	160	9	5	35	3	18	16	0	100	60	—	—	5
KLONDIKE														
Bar Almond	1	300	21	14	20	4	24	21	0	100	70	—	—	1
Bar Cappuccino	1	280	19	14	20	3	24	21	0	100	70	—	—	1

FOOD	PORTION	CALS	FAT	SAT FAT	CHOL	PROT	CARB	SUGAR	FIBER	CALCI	SOD	POTAS	FOLIC	VIT C
KLONDIKE (CONT.)														
Bar Caramel & Peanut	1	290	19	12	15	4	25	21	tr	80	150	—	—	0
Bar Caramel Crunch	1	270	17	13	25	3	26	24	0	100	80	—	—	0
Bar Chocolate	1	280	19	14	20	3	23	21	tr	80	55	—	—	0
Bar Dark Chocolate	1	280	19	13	20	3	24	20	tr	100	55	—	—	0
Bar Heath	1	300	20	14	20	3	26	24	0	100	100	—	—	1
Bar Krunch	1	280	19	14	20	3	25	21	0	100	90	—	—	1
Bar Oreo	1	160	10	3	10	2	17	9	tr	40	95	—	—	0
Bar Original	1	280	19	14	20	3	24	22	0	100	75	—	—	1
Bar Peppermint Patty	1	280	19	13	20	3	24	20	tr	100	55	—	—	0
Bar Reese's	1	220	15	9	15	3	20	17	tr	60	65	—	—	0
Big Bear Sandwich Neapolitan	1	300	12	6	25	5	42	25	1	100	230	—	—	0
Big Bear Sandwich Vanilla	1	300	12	6	25	5	42	25	tr	100	240	—	—	0
Big Bear Cone Vanilla	1	330	20	8	15	6	33	23	1	100	95	—	—	0
Big Bear Cone Vanilla Caramel	1	360	21	9	15	6	36	27	1	100	120	—	—	0
Big Bear Cone Vanilla Fudge	1	380	20	9	15	6	38	28	1	100	90	—	—	0
CarbSmart Fudge Bar	1	60	7	5	20	2	9	3	1	60	45	—	—	0
CarbSmart Ice Cream Bar	1	130	15	11	15	2	9	5	2	400	40	—	—	0
Choco Taco	1	290	16	8	10	4	35	24	1	80	115	—	—	0
Cone Oreo	1	250	12	6	15	3	32	21	1	60	95	—	—	0
Cone Reese's	1	290	15	7	15	4	33	24	tr	80	140	—	—	0
Cookie Sandwich Chips	1	470	20	9	30	7	66	38	2	100	65	—	—	1
Cookie Sandwich Oreo	1	230	9	4	10	3	34	18	2	60	310	—	—	0
Minis	2 pieces	170	11	8	15	2	15	13	0	80	45	—	—	0
Sandwich Double Decker	1	370	14	7	30	6	54	30	1	150	330	—	—	1
Slim-A-Bear 98% Fat Free Sandwich Vanilla	1	130	2	0	5	4	28	14	3	100	120	—	—	0
Slim-A-Bear No Sugar Added Cone Vanilla	1	270	15	5	5	8	31	6	4	250	110	—	–	0

FOOD	PORTION	CALS	FAT	SAT FAT	CHOL	PROT	CARB	SUGAR	FIBER	CALCI	SOD	POTAS	FOLIC	VIT C
KLONDIKE (CONT.)														
Slim-A-Bear No Sugar Added Fudge Bar	1	90	2	1	5	3	22	5	4	100	90	—	—	0
Slim-A-Bear No Sugar Added Reduced Fat Bar Vanilla	1	160	9	7	5	4	21	6	4	250	75	—	—	0
Slim-A-Bear No Sugar Added Sandwich Vanilla	1	120	3	1	5	4	25	3	2	150	230	—	—	0
Sundae Cup	1	280	17	10	35	6	26	22	tr	150	75	—	—	0
NESTLÉ CRUNCH														
Chocolate	1 bar (3 oz)	200	14	11	15	2	17	14	0	60	40	—	—	0
Crunch King	1 (4 oz)	270	19	14	20	3	21	16	0	80	45	—	—	0
Nuggets	8 pieces	310	21	10	20	4	25	19	0	80	60	—	—	0
Reduced Fat	1 (2.5 oz)	130	7	5	5	3	14	6	0	40	40	—	—	0
Vanilla	1 bar (3 oz)	200	14	11	15	2	16	13	0	60	40	—	—	0
NUTRASHAKE														
High Calorie High Protein All Flavors	1 serv (4 oz)	200	10	—	60	6	24	—	—	206	217	225	—	—
PERRY'S														
No Fat No Sugar Added Caramel	½ cup (2.8 oz)	90	0	0	0	4	25	5	1	150	90	—	—	1
No Fat No Sugar Added Chocolate	½ cup (2.6 oz)	80	0	0	0	5	21	5	2	150	80	—	—	1
No Fat No Sugar Added Peach	½ cup (2.9 oz)	90	0	0	0	3	24	6	tr	100	70	—	—	12
No Fat No Sugar Added Strawberry	½ cup (2.8 oz)	90	0	0	0	4	23	6	tr	150	75	—	—	1
No Fat No Sugar Added Vanilla	½ cup (2.6 oz)	80	0	0	0	4	21	5	tr	150	80	—	—	1
POPSICLE														
Bar Col Crunch Chocolate Eclair	1 (3 oz)	160	8	3	5	2	20	12	tr	40	70	—	—	0
Bar Col Crunch Strawberry Shortcake	1 (3 oz)	170	9	3	5	1	21	12	0	40	60	—	—	0
Bar Snoopy	1 (3.5 oz)	150	8	6	15	2	16	13	0	80	45	—	—	0
Bar Sprinklers	1 (2.1 oz)	130	6	3	10	1	18	14	0	40	25	—	—	0
Cone Crispy	1 (2.5 oz)	150	7	4	5	2	20	12	0	40	60	—	—	0

FOOD	PORTION	CALS	FAT	SAT FAT	CHOL	PROT	CARB	SUGAR	FIBER	CALCI	SOD	POTAS	FOLIC	VIT C
POPSICLE (CONT.)														
Creamsicle Pop	1 (1.75 oz)	70	2	1	5	1	13	10	0	20	20	—	—	0
Cup Cookies & Cream	1 (10 oz)	310	13	8	30	5	45	29	1	200	160	—	—	1
Fruit Juicee Cups	1 (4 oz)	80	0	0	0	0	20	19	—	—	0	—	—	—
Ice Cream Bar Vanilla	1 (3 oz)	160	11	9	15	2	15	15	1	60	35	—	—	0
Ice Cream Pops Minis	2 (2.8 oz)	190	13	9	15	2	18	15	0	60	35	—	—	0
Sandwich Cookie Rugrats	1 (2.5 oz)	140	6	4	10	2	20	10	tr	40	80	—	—	0
Sandwiches Minis	1 (2 oz)	100	4	2	5	2	15	7	0	20	95	—	—	0
Scribblers Ice Cream Pops	2 (2.4 oz)	130	5	4	15	3	17	13	0	100	45	—	—	0
Swirl Bar Bubble Gum	1 (2.6 oz)	60	0	0	0	0	13	10	—	—	0	—	—	—
WWE Bar	1 (3.6 oz)	180	8	5	10	2	23	13	tr	60	95	—	—	0
X-Men Wolverine Bar	1 (4 oz)	100	0	0	0	0	25	20	—	—	15	—	—	—
RICE DREAM														
Cappuccino	½ cup (3.2 oz)	150	6	1	0	tr	23	17	1	20	100	60	—	1
Carob	½ cup (3.2 oz)	150	6	1	0	1	24	17	2	20	100	70	—	1
Carob Almond	½ cup (3.2 oz)	170	8	1	0	1	24	17	2	20	95	100	—	1
Cherry Vanilla	½ cup (3.2 oz)	150	6	1	0	tr	24	18	1	20	90	60	—	1
Cocoa Marble Fudge	½ cup (3.2 oz)	150	6	1	0	1	25	15	2	20	100	100	—	1
Cookies N' Dream	½ cup (3.2 oz)	170	7	1	0	1	26	17	1	0	100	90	—	1
Mint Chocolate Chip	½ cup (3.2 oz)	170	8	2	0	1	26	19	1	20	95	70	—	1
Neapolitan	½ cup (3.2 oz)	150	6	1	0	1	24	18	2	20	100	80	—	1
Orange Vanilla Swirl	½ cup (3.2 oz)	250	6	1	0	tr	23	17	1	20	100	60	—	1
Strawberry	½ cup (3.2 oz)	140	5	0	0	tr	24	19	1	20	85	110	—	5
Vanilla Swiss Almond	½ cup (3.2 oz)	180	8	2	0	1	25	18	1	20	95	60	—	1
RICE DREAM SUPREME														
Cappuccino Almond Fudge	½ cup (3.2 oz)	170	8	1	0	1	24	15	2	20	95	100	—	1
Cherry Chocolate Chunk	½ cup (3.2 oz)	170	7	2	0	1	27	19	1	20	85	70	—	1
Chocolate Almond Chunk	½ cup (3.2 oz)	170	8	2	0	2	25	18	2	20	95	80	—	1
Chocolate Fudge Brownie	½ cup (3.2 oz)	170	7	1	0	1	28	16	2	20	95	120	—	1
Double Espresso Bean	½ cup (3.2 oz)	160	7	1	0	1	24	17	1	20	100	60	—	1

FOOD	PORTION	CALS	FAT	SAT FAT	CHOL	PROT	CARB	SUGAR	FIBER	CALCI	SOD	POTAS	FOLIC	VIT C
RICE DREAM SUPREME (CONT.)														
Mint Chocolate Cookie	½ cup (3.2 oz)	170	8	1	0	1	26	18	1	20	100	90	—	1
Peanut Butter Cup	½ cup (3.2 oz)	180	8	2	0	3	25	18	2	20	105	70	—	1
Pralines N' Dream	½ cup (3.2 oz)	180	9	1	0	1	25	16	1	20	95	80	—	1
SILHOUETTE														
The Skinny Cow Low Fat Ice Cream Sandwich Vanilla	1	130	2	1	0	5	23	22	2	80	145	—	—	0
SLIM-FAST														
Chocolate Fudge Bar	1 bar	110	2	1	10	3	22	17	tr	250	80	—	—	9
Ice Cream Sandwich Chocolate	1	130	2	1	<5	3	27	14	tr	250	150	—	—	9
Ice Cream Sandwich Vanilla	1	130	1	1	<5	3	27	14	tr	250	150	—	—	9
STARBUCKS														
Caramel Cappuccino Swirl	½ cup	240	12	7	65	4	30	28	0	100	100	—	—	0
Classic Coffee	½ cup	230	12	7	65	5	26	24	0	100	50	—	—	0
Coffee Almond Fudge	½ cup	250	13	7	60	5	29	25	1	100	65	—	—	0
Frappuccino Bar Java Fudge	1 bar	130	2	1	5	4	25	16	4	100	50	—	—	0
Frappuccino Bar Mocha	1 bar	120	2	1	10	4	22	15	3	100	50	—	—	0
Java Chip	½ cup	250	13	8	60	4	29	26	0	100	55	—	—	0
Low Fat Latte	½ cup	170	3	2	10	5	30	23	0	100	60	—	—	0
Mud Pie	½ cup	240	11	6	55	4	32	27	1	100	85	—	—	0
White Chocolate Latte	½ cup	280	15	6	60	5	31	29	0	100	60	—	—	0
TOFUTTI														
Cuties Chocolate	1 (1.4 oz)	130	5	1	0	2	16	9	0	—	110	2	—	—
Cuties Vanilla	1 (1.4 oz)	121	5	1	0	2	17	9	0	—	121	1	—	—
Monkey Bars Peanut Butter	1 bar (2.5 oz)	220	13	8	0	3	22	18	tr	—	105	—	—	—
TURKEY HILL														
Black Cherry	½ cup	140	7	5	25	2	18	16	0	80	30	—	—	0
Black Raspberry	½ cup	140	7	—	30	—	18	—	—	—	35	—	—	—
Butter Pecan	½ cup	170	11	5	30	2	16	15	0	80	50	—	—	0
Chocolate Marshmallow	½ cup	160	7	—	30	—	24	—	—	—	30	—	—	—
Chocolate Mint Chip	½ cup	180	11	—	30	—	18	—	—	—	40	—	—	—

FOOD	PORTION	CALS	FAT	SAT FAT	CHOL	PROT	CARB	SUGAR	FIBER	CALCI	SOD	POTAS	FOLIC	VIT C
TURKEY HILL (CONT.)														
Chocolate Peanut Butter Cup	½ cup	180	11	—	30	—	18	—	—	—	60	—	—	—
Colombian Coffee	½ cup	140	8	—	30	—	16	—	—	—	35	—	—	—
Cookies 'N Cream	½ cup	160	9	5	30	2	19	17	0	80	60	—	—	0
Death By Chocolate	½ cup	160	8	—	30	—	21	—	—	—	35	—	—	—
Dutch Chocolate	½ cup	150	8	—	30	—	19	—	—	—	30	—	—	—
Egg Nog	½ cup	150	8	—	45	—	17	—	—	—	35	—	—	—
Fat Free No Sugar Added Caramel Fudge Decadence	½ cup	100	0	0	0	—	23	—	—	—	75	—	—	—
Fat Free No Sugar Added Cherry Vanilla Fudge	½ cup	90	0	0	0	—	20	—	—	—	80	—	—	—
Fat Free No Sugar Added Dutch Chocolate	½ cup	90	0	0	0	—	20	—	—	—	70	—	—	—
Fat Free No Sugar Added Vanilla Bean	½ cup	90	0	0	0	—	20	—	—	—	60	—	—	—
Fudge Ripple	½ cup	140	7	—	30	—	20	—	—	—	70	—	—	—
Light Butter Pecan	½ cup	130	6	3	15	3	17	16	0	100	80	—	—	0
Light Choco Mint Chip	½ cup	140	5	4	15	3	19	18	0	100	75	—	—	0
Light Tin Lizzie Sundae	½ cup	140	5	—	10	—	21	—	—	—	120	—	—	—
Light Vanilla & Chocolate	½ cup	110	3	2	15	3	18	18	0	100	60	—	—	0
Light Vanilla Bean	½ cup	110	3	2	15	3	18	17	0	100	65	—	—	0
Neapolitan	½ cup	150	8	5	30	2	18	17	0	80	30	—	—	0
Orange Swirl	½ cup	140	6	—	20	—	19	—	—	—	25	—	—	—
Original Vanilla	½ cup	140	8	—	30	—	16	—	—	—	35	—	—	—
Peanut Butter Ripple	½ cup	170	11	—	30	—	16	—	—	—	60	—	—	—
Philadelphia Style Butter Almond	½ cup	180	12	—	35	—	15	—	—	—	105	—	—	—
Philadelphia Style Chocolate	½ cup	170	10	—	35	—	18	—	—	—	40	—	—	—
Philadelphia Style Mint Chocolate Chip	½ cup	180	11	—	35	—	18	—	—	—	50	—	—	—
Philadelphia Style Sweet Cherry Vanilla	½ cup	160	8	—	30	—	18	—	—	—	50	—	—	—

FOOD	PORTION	CALS	FAT	SAT FAT	CHOL	PROT	CARB	SUGAR	FIBER	CALCI	SOD	POTAS	FOLIC	VIT C
TURKEY HILL (CONT.)														
Philadelphia Style Vanilla Bean	½ cup	170	10	—	35	—	16	—	—	—	50	—	—	—
Rocky Road	½ cup	170	8	4	30	3	23	19	0	80	40	—	—	0
Rum Raisin	½ cup	150	7	—	30	—	19	—	—	—	30	—	—	—
Sandwich Choco Mint Chip	1	200	8	—	25	—	27	—	—	—	180			
Sandwich Vanilla	1	190	8	—	25	—	26				180			
Strawberries 'N Cream	½ cup	140	6	—	25	—	19				30			
Sundae Cones Rocky Road	1	340	19	—	25	—	37	—	—	—	110	—		
Sundae Cones Tin Roof Sundae	1	290	17	—	25	—	30	—	—	—	135	—	—	—
Tin Roof Sundae	½ cup	160	9	5	30	2	19	18	0	80	70	—	—	0
Vanilla & Chocolate	½ cup	150	8	5	30	2	17	16	0	80	35	—	—	0
Vanilla Bean	½ cup	140	8	5	30	2	16	16	0	80	35	—	—	0
WEIGHT WATCHERS														
Chocolate Chip Cookie Dough Sundae	1 (2.64 oz)	190	5	2	5	3	35	15	1	80	120	—	—	0
Chocolate Mousse	1 bar	40	1	1	5	2	9	3	1	80	20	—	—	0
Chocolate Treat	1 bar	100	1	0	0	3	20	17	1	100	25	—	—	0
English Toffee Crunch	1 bar	110	6	3	5	2	12	10	1	80	30	—	—	0
Orange Vanilla Treat	1 bar	40	1	0	5	2	10	3	0	60	15	—	—	0
Vanilla Sandwich	1 bar	150	3	1	5	3	28	14	1	150	150	—	—	0
TAKE-OUT														
cone vanilla light soft serve	1 (4.6 oz)	164	6	4	28	4	24	—	—	153	92	169	5	1
gelato chocolate hazelnut	½ cup (5.3 oz)	370	29	4	92	9	26	21	2	179	49	352	35	1
gelato vanilla	½ cup (3 oz)	211	15	8	151	3	18	18	0	67	78	77	15	tr
sundae caramel	1 (5.4 oz)	303	9	5	25	7	49	—	—	189	195	318	12	3
sundae hot fudge	1 (5.4 oz)	284	9	5	21	6	48	—	—	207	182	395	9	2
sundae strawberry	1 (5.4 oz)	269	8	4	21	6	45	—	—	161	92	270	18	2

ICE CREAM CONES AND CUPS

sugar cone	1	40	tr	tr	0	1	8	—	tr	4	32	14	1	0
wafer cone	1	17	tr	tr	0	tr	3	—	tr	1	6	4	0	0
DUTCH MILL														
Chocolate Covered Wafer Cups	1 (0.5 oz)	80	5	2	0	1	8	6	0	0	—	—	—	0

FOOD	PORTION	CALS	FAT	SAT FAT	CHOL	PROT	CARB	SUGAR	FIBER	CALCI	SOD	POTAS	FOLIC	VIT C
FROOKIE														
Chocolate Crunch	1 (0.4 oz)	50	1	0	0	1	10	4	tr	0	10	—	—	0
Honey Crunch	1 (0.4 oz)	45	1	0	0	1	9	1	tr	0	20	—	—	0
KEEBLER														
Chocolatey Cone	1 (0.4 oz)	50	1	0	0	tr	10	4	0	0	40	—	—	0
Fudge Dipped Cup	1 (0.3 oz)	35	2	1	0	0	6	2	0	0	20	—	—	0
Ice Creme Cup	1 (0.2 oz)	15	0	0	0	0	4	0	0	0	20	—	—	0
Sugar Cone	1 (0.4 oz)	50	1	0	0	tr	10	4	0	0	15	—	—	0
Waffle Bowl	1 (0.4 oz)	50	1	0	0	tr	10	4	0	0	25	—	—	0
Waffle Cone	1 (0.4 oz)	50	1	0	0	tr	10	4	0	0	25	—	—	0

ICE CREAM TOPPINGS

FOOD	PORTION	CALS	FAT	SAT FAT	CHOL	PROT	CARB	SUGAR	FIBER	CALCI	SOD	POTAS	FOLIC	VIT C
butterscotch	2 tbsp (1.4 oz)	103	tr	tr	—	1	27	—	—	22	143	—	—	—
caramel	2 tbsp (1.4 oz)	103	tr	tr	—	1	27	—	—	22	143	—	—	—
marshmallow cream	1 jar (7 oz)	615	tr	—	0	3	157	—	—	6	90	9	2	—
marshmallow cream	1 oz	88	tr	—	0	1	23	—	—	1	13	1	0	—
pineapple	2 tbsp (1.5 oz)	106	0	—	0	tr	28	—	—	9	26	133	1	25
pineapple	1 cup (11.5 oz)	861	—	—	0	1	226	—	—	75	214	1078	9	199
strawberry	2 tbsp (1.5 oz)	107	tr	—	0	tr	28	—	—	10	9	31	1	11
strawberry	1 cup (11.5 oz)	863	1	—	0	1	225	—	—	81	73	248	5	85
walnuts in syrup	2 tbsp (1.4 oz)	167	9	1	0	2	22	—	—	—	—	—	—	—
COLAC														
Passion Fruit	1 tbsp	31	0	0	0	0	13	0	0	—	0	—	—	—
Strawberry	1 tbsp	31	0	0	0	0	13	0	0	—	0	—	—	—
HERSHEY'S														
Chocolate Shoppe Caramel	2 tbsp	100	0	0	0	tr	25	—	—	—	95	—	—	—
Chocolate Shoppe Double Chocolate	1 tbsp	60	1	1	0	tr	12	—	—	—	30	—	—	—
Chocolate Shoppe Hot Fudge	1 tbsp	70	3	1	<5	tr	10	—	—	—	80	—	—	—
Chocolate Shoppe Hot Fudge Fat Free	2 tbsp	100	0	0	0	1	23	—	—	—	135	—	—	—
Sprinkles Candy Coated Milk Chocolate	1 tbsp	70	3	2	<5	tr	10	—	—	—	10	—	—	—
KRAFT														
Butterscotch	2 tbsp (1.4 oz)	130	2	1	<5	tr	28	18	0	0	150	40	—	0
Caramel	2 tbsp (1.4 oz)	120	0	0	0	2	28	20	0	60	90	90	—	0

FOOD	PORTION	CALS	FAT	SAT FAT	CHOL	PROT	CARB	SUGAR	FIBER	CALCI	SOD	POTAS	FOLIC	VIT C
KRAFT (CONT.)														
Chocolate	2 tbsp (1.4 oz)	110	0	0	0	2	26	20	1	20	30	190	—	0
Hot Fudge	2 tbsp (1.4 oz)	140	5	2	0	1	24	17	tr	40	100	85	—	0
Pineapple	2 tbsp (1.4 oz)	110	0	0	0	0	28	19	0	0	15	15	—	5
Strawberry	2 tbsp (1.4 oz)	110	0	0	0	0	29	22	0	0	15	25	—	4
REESE'S														
Sprinkles Peanut Butter & Milk Chocolate	1 tbsp	70	4	2	0	1	10	—	—	—	25	—	—	—
SMUCKER'S														
Plate Scapers Caramel	2 tbsp	100	0	0	0	1	25	18	—	—	105	—	—	—
STEEL'S														
Sugar Free Butterscotch	2 tbsp	60	0	0	0	0	21	0	0	—	10	—	—	—
Sugar Free Chocolate Fudge	2 tbsp	45	3	2	10	2	5	0	2	—	15	—	—	—
Sugar Free Hot Fudge	2 tbsp	65	3	0	0	1	18	0	1	—	13	—	—	—
Sugar Free Peanut Butter Fudge	2 tbsp	75	6	2	7	2	5	0	2	—	41	—	—	—

ICED TEA

FOOD	PORTION	CALS	FAT	SAT FAT	CHOL	PROT	CARB	SUGAR	FIBER	CALCI	SOD	POTAS	FOLIC	VIT C
MIX														
instant artifically sweetened lemon flavored as prep w/ water	8 oz	5	0	0	0	tr	1	—	—	5	24	41	5	0
instant sweetened lemon flavor as prep w/ water	9 oz	87	tr	tr	0	tr	22	—	—	6	—	50	10	0
instant unsweetened lemon flavor as prep w/ water	8 oz	4	0	0	0	tr	0	—	—	5	14	49	—	0
ATKINS														
Sugar Free Lemon not prep	2 tbsp	0	0	0	0	0	0	0	0	—	5	—	—	—
CARB OPTIONS														
Lemon as prep	1 serv	0	0	0	0	0	0	0	0	—	0	—	—	—
CRYSTAL LIGHT														
Decaffeinated as prep	1 serv (8 oz)	5	0	0	0	0	tr	0	0	0	0	20	—	0
Iced Tea as prep	1 serv (8 oz)	5	0	0	0	0	0	0	0	0	0	15	—	0
Peach Tea as prep	1 serv (8 oz)	5	0	0	0	0	0	0	0	0	0	15	—	0
Raspberry Tea as prep	1 serv (8 oz)	5	0	0	0	0	0	0	0	0	0	15	—	0

FOOD	PORTION	CALS	FAT	SAT FAT	CHOL	PROT	CARB	SUGAR	FIBER	CALCI	SOD	POTAS	FOLIC	VIT C
LIPTON														
100% Tea as prep	1 serv	0	0	0	0	0	0	0	—	—	0	—	—	0
100% Tea Decaffeinated as prep	1 serv	0	0	0	0	0	0	0	—	—	0	—	—	0
100% Tea Unsweetened as prep	1 serv	0	0	0	0	0	0	0	—	—	0	—	—	0
Calorie Free as prep	1 serv	0	0	0	0	0	0	0	—	—	0	—	—	0
Decaffeinated Ice Tea Brew as prep	1 serv (8 oz)	0	0	0	0	0	0	0	0	0	0	—	—	0
Decaffeinated Lemon as prep	1 serv	90	0	0	0	0	22	22	—	—	0	—	—	0
Diet Decaffeinated Lemon as prep	1 serv	5	0	0	0	0	1	0	—	—	0	—	—	0
Diet Lemon as prep	1 serv	5	0	0	0	0	1	0	—	—	0	—	—	0
Diet Peach as prep	1 serv	5	0	0	0	0	1	0	—	—	0	—	—	0
Diet Raspberry as prep	1 serv	5	0	0	0	0	1	0	—	—	0	—	—	0
Diet Tea & Lemonade as prep	1 serv	10	0	0	0	0	2	0	—	—	5	—	—	0
Herbal Iced Collection	1 tea bag	0	0	0	0	0	tr	0	—	—	0	—	—	0
Ice Tea Brew as prep	1 serv (8 oz)	0	0	0	0	0	0	0	0	0	0	—	—	0
Lemon as prep	1 pkg (0.5 oz)	50	0	0	0	0	13	13	—	—	0	—	—	0
Lemon as prep	1 serv	90	0	0	0	0	22	22	—	—	0	—	—	0
Natural Brew 100% Tea as prep	1 serv	0	0	0	0	0	0	0	—	—	0	—	—	0
Natural Brew 100% Tea Decaffeinated as prep	1 serv	0	0	0	0	0	0	0	—	—	0	—	—	0
Natural Brew Diet Lemon as prep	1 serv	5	0	0	0	0	1	0	—	—	0	—	—	0
Natural Brew Diet Peach as prep	1 serv	5	0	0	0	0	1	0	—	—	0	—	—	0
Natural Brew Diet Tropical as prep	1 serv	5	0	0	0	0	1	0	—	—	0	—	—	0
Natural Brew Tropical as prep	1 serv	90	0	0	0	0	22	22	—	—	0	—	—	0

FOOD	PORTION	CALS	FAT	SAT FAT	CHOL	PROT	CARB	SUGAR	FIBER	CALCI	SOD	POTAS	FOLIC	VIT C
LIPTON (CONT.)														
Natural Brew Unsweetened Lemon as prep	1 serv	0	0	0	0	0	tr	0	—	—	0	—	—	0
Peach as prep	1 serv	90	0	0	0	0	22	22	—	—	0	—	—	0
Rasberry as prep	1 serv	90	0	0	0	0	22	22	—	—	0	—	—	0
Tea & Lemonade as prep	1 serv	90	0	0	0	0	22	22	—	—	0	—	—	0
NESTEA														
100% Tea	2 tsp (1 g)	0	0	0	0	0	tr	0	0	0	0	45	—	0
100% Tea Decafe	2 tsp (1 g)	0	0	0	0	0	tr	0	0	0	0	45	—	0
Ice Teasers Lemon	1 serv (0.5 oz)	5	0	0	0	0	1	0	0	0	0	35	—	0
Ice Teasers Orange	1 serv (0.5 oz)	5	0	0	0	0	1	0	0	0	0	35	—	0
Ice Teasers Wild Cherry	1 serv (0.5 oz)	5	0	0	0	0	1	0	0	0	0	30	—	0
Lemon	2 tsp (1 g)	5	0	0	0	0	1	0	0	0	0	30	—	0
Lemon & Sugar	2 tbsp (0.7 oz)	80	0	0	0	0	19	19	0	0	0	30	—	0
Lemonade Tea	2 tbsp (0.7 oz)	80	0	0	0	0	19	17	0	0	0	95	—	0
Sugar Free	2 tbsp (0.7 oz)	5	0	0	0	0	1	0	0	0	0	25	—	0
Sugar Free Decafe	1 tbsp (0.7 oz)	5	0	0	0	0	1	0	0	0	0	35	—	0
Sun Tea	1 tsp (1 g)	0	0	0	0	0	tr	0	0	0	0	45	—	0
READY-TO-DRINK														
APPLE & EVE														
Lemon Fruit	8 fl oz	100	0	0	0	0	25	22	—	—	20	—	—	—
Peach Fruit	8 fl oz	100	0	0	0	0	25	22	—	—	20	—	—	—
Raspberry Fruit	8 fl oz	100	0	0	0	0	25	22	—	—	20	—	—	—
Tangerine Fruit	8 fl oz	100	0	0	0	0	25	22	—	—	20	—	—	—
CRYSTAL LIGHT														
Lemon	1 serv (8 oz)	5	0	0	0	0	0	0	0	0	40	50	—	0
Peach Tea	1 serv (8 oz)	5	0	0	0	0	0	0	0	0	40	35	—	0
Raspberry Tea	1 serv (8 oz)	5	0	0	0	0	0	0	0	0	40	35	—	0
FUZE														
LemonAID	8 oz	70	0	0	0	0	19	17	—	—	15	—	—	60
Slenderize Cranberry Raspberry	8 oz	7	0	0	0	0	2	—	—	—	10	—	—	60
Vitamin Tea Diet Peach	8 oz	5	0	0	0	0	1	0	0	—	5	—	—	30
Vitamin Tea Green Tea w/ Ginseng	8 oz	60	0	0	0	0	16	16	—	—	5	—	—	30
Vitamin Tea Lemon	8 oz	70	0	0	0	0	18	17	—	—	5	—	—	30
White Tea	8 oz	60	0	0	0	0	15	15	—	—	0	—	100	60
White Tea No Carb Diet Pomegranate	8 oz	0	0	0	0	0	0	0	0	—	0	—	100	60

FOOD	PORTION	CALS	FAT	SAT FAT	CHOL	PROT	CARB	SUGAR	FIBER	CALCI	SOD	POTAS	FOLIC	VIT C
GLACEAU VITAMIN WATER														
Determination	8 oz	50	0	0	0	0	13	12	—	—	0	—	—	24
Leadership	8 oz	50	0	0	0	0	13	12	—	—	0	—	—	30
Perseverance	8 oz	50	0	0	0	0	13	12	—	—	0	—	—	30
Vital-T	8 oz	50	0	0	0	0	13	13	—	—	0	—	—	—
HANSEN'S														
Chai	8 oz	150	0	0	0	0	38	32	—	—	15	—	—	60
China Black	8 oz	90	0	0	0	0	25	24	—	—	15	—	—	60
Green	8 oz	70	0	0	0	0	18	18	—	—	15	—	—	60
Green Diet Lemon	8 oz	0	0	0	0	0	0	0	—	—	15	—	—	60
Green Diet Peach	8 oz	0	0	0	0	0	0	0	—	—	15	—	—	60
Green Lemon	8 oz	70	0	0	0	0	18	17	—	—	15	—	—	60
Green Peach	8 oz	70	0	0	0	0	18	17	—	—	15	—	—	60
Oolong	8 oz	70	0	0	0	0	25	24	—	—	15	—	—	60
Spice	8 oz	90	0	0	0	25	24	—	—	—	15	—	—	60
HAWAIIAN														
Iced Tea	1 can	120	0	0	0	0	35	35	0	0	50	—	—	60
HONEST TEA														
Assam	8 oz	17	0	0	0	0	5	4	—	—	10	—	—	12
Black Forest Berry	8 oz	25	0	0	0	0	8	8	—	—	5	—	—	—
Gold Rush	8 oz	9	0	0	0	0	3	2	—	—	10	—	—	—
Green Dragon	8 oz	30	0	0	0	0	9	9	—	—	5	—	—	—
Kashmiri Chai	8 oz	17	0	0	0	0	6	5	—	—	0	—	—	—
Lori's Lemon	8 oz	30	0	0	0	0	9	9	—	—	5	—	—	—
Moroccan Mint	8 oz	17	0	0	0	0	5	5	—	—	5	—	—	—
Peach Oo-La-Long	8 oz	30	0	0	0	0	9	9	—	—	5	—	—	—
INKO'S														
White Tea	1 bottle (16 oz)	56	0	0	0	0	14	14	—	—	tr	—	—	—
White Tea Hint O'Mint	1 bottle	0	0	0	0	0	0	0	—	—	tr	—	—	—
LIPTON														
Carribean Cooler	1 can (12 oz)	130	0	0	0	0	34	34	—	—	75	—	—	0
Diet Lemon	1 bottle (16 oz)	10	0	0	0	0	0	0	—	—	10	—	—	0
Diet Lemon	8 oz	0	0	0	0	0	0	0	—	—	10	—	—	0
Green Tea & Passion Fruit	1 bottle (16 oz)	160	0	0	0	0	38	38	—	—	10	—	—	0
Lemon	1 bottle (16 oz)	180	0	0	0	0	42	42	—	—	10	—	—	0
Lemon	1 can (12 oz)	120	0	0	0	0	33	33	—	—	75	—	—	0
Lemon	8 oz	80	0	0	0	0	20	20	—	—	15	—	—	15
Natural Lemon	1 box (8 oz)	100	0	0	0	0	25	24	—	—	10	—	—	60
Peach	1 bottle (16 oz)	220	0	0	0	0	52	52	—	—	10	—	—	0
Peach	8 oz	80	0	0	0	0	20	20	—	—	15	—	—	0
Raspberry	1 bottle (16 oz)	220	0	0	0	0	52	52	—	—	10	—	—	0
Raspberry	8 oz	80	0	0	0	0	20	20	—	—	15	—	—	0

FOOD	PORTION	CALS	FAT	SAT FAT	CHOL	PROT	CARB	SUGAR	FIBER	CALCI	SOD	POTAS	FOLIC	VIT C
LIPTON (CONT.)														
Raspberry Blast	1 can (12 oz)	130	0	0	0	0	35	35	—	—	75	—	—	0
Southern Style Extra Sweet No Lemon	1 bottle (16 oz)	240	0	0	0	0	58	58	—	—	10	—	—	0
Southern Style Lemon	1 bottle (16 oz)	200	0	0	0	0	50	50	—	—	10	—	—	0
Southern Style Sweetened No Lemon	1 bottle (16 oz)	200	0	0	0	0	48	48	—	—	10	—	—	0
Sweet	8 oz	80	0	0	0	0	20	20	—	—	15	—	—	0
Sweetened No Lemon	1 bottle (16 oz)	140	0	0	0	0	36	36	—	—	10	—	—	0
Sweetened Lemon	8 oz	80	0	0	0	0	20	20	—	—	15	—	—	15
Tangerine Twist	1 can (12 oz)	120	0	0	0	0	33	33	—	—	75	—	—	0
Tea & Lemonade	1 bottle (16 oz)	220	0	0	0	0	52	52	—	—	10	—	—	0
Unsweetened No Lemon	1 bottle (16 oz)	0	0	0	0	0	0	0	—	—	10	—	—	0
MAD RIVER														
Red Tea w/ Guarana	8 oz	90	0	0	0	0	24	23	—	—	10	—	—	—
NANTUCKET NECTARS														
Diet	8 oz	5	0	0	0	0	1	0	—	0	25	—	—	0
Diet Green Tea	8 oz	5	0	0	0	0	1	0	—	0	5	—	—	0
Half & Half	8 oz	90	0	0	0	0	23	21	—	0	0	—	—	60
Iced Tea	8 oz	80	0	0	0	0	20	19	—	0	0	—	—	60
Matt Fee	8 oz	80	0	0	0	0	20	18	—	0	0	—	—	0
Raspberry	8 oz	90	0	0	0	0	23	22	—	0	20	—	—	60
Savannah	8 oz	80	0	0	0	0	20	18	—	0	0	—	—	60
NEW LEAF														
All Flavors	8 oz	75	0	0	0	0	19	19	—	—	0	—	—	—
OREGON CHAI														
Original Latte	1 bottle (9.5 oz)	150	4	3	15	2	26	25	0	80	50	—	—	0
REPUBLIC OF TEA														
No Carb Unsweetened All Flavors	1 bottle (12 oz)	0	0	0	0	0	0	0	0	—	0	—	—	—
SNAPPLE														
Diet Lemon	8 fl oz	0	0	0	0	0	1	0	—	—	10	—	—	—
Diet Peach	8 fl oz	0	0	0	0	0	1	0	—	—	10	—	—	—
Diet Raspberry	8 fl oz	0	0	0	0	0	1	0	—	—	10	—	—	—
Diet Lime Green Tea	8 oz	0	0	0	0	0	1	0	—	—	10	—	—	—
Kiwi Teawi	8 oz	100	0	0	0	0	26	24	—	—	10	—	—	—
Lemon	8 fl oz	100	0	0	0	0	25	23	—	—	10	—	—	—
Lime Green Tea	8 fl oz	100	0	0	0	0	25	23	—	—	10	—	—	—

FOOD	PORTION	CALS	FAT	SAT FAT	CHOL	PROT	CARB	SUGAR	FIBER	CALCI	SOD	POTAS	FOLIC	VIT C
SNAPPLE (CONT.)														
Peach	8 fl oz	100	0	0	0	0	26	24	—	—	10	—	—	—
Raspberry	8 fl oz	100	0	0	0	0	26	25	—	—	10	—	—	—
Very Cherry	8 oz	100	0	0	0	0	25	23	—	—	10	—	—	—
SOBE														
Lemon	8 oz	90	0	0	0	0	25	24	—	—	5	—	—	—
SOY20														
Lemon Green Tea	1 bottle (12 oz)	90	0	0	0	0	22	22	—	—	10	—	—	—
SWEET LEAF TEA														
Diet Sweet	8 oz	0	0	0	0	0	0	0	—	—	10	—	—	—
Hibiscus Herbal	8 oz	25	0	0	0	0	8	8	—	—	10	—	—	72
Lemon & Lime	8 oz	0	0	0	0	0	0	0	—	—	0	—	—	—
Mint & Honey Green	8 oz	60	0	0	0	0	15	15	—	—	0	—	—	—
Peach	8 oz	75	0	0	0	0	19	19	—	—	10	—	—	—
Raspberry & Tangerine	8 oz	75	0	0	0	0	19	19	—	—	0	—	—	—
Sweet Tea	8 oz	75	0	0	0	0	19	19	—	—	0	—	—	—
T42														
A Classic Earl Grey	8 oz	60	0	0	0	0	14	14	—	—	5	—	—	—
Herbal All Flavors	8 oz	70	0	0	0	0	18	17	—	—	5	—	—	—
Jamaican Ginger Green Tea	8 oz	70	0	0	0	0	16	16	—	—	6	—	—	—
Lemon And Honey Green Tea	8 oz	60	0	0	0	0	12	12	—	—	6	—	—	—
Wake-Up Blend English Breakfast	8 oz	45	0	0	0	0	11	11	—	—	5	—	—	—
With Lemon	8 oz	60	0	0	0	0	14	14	—	—	0	—	—	—
TRADEWINDS														
Diet Green Tea	8 oz	0	0	0	0	0	0	0	0	0	0	—	—	0
Diet Raspberry	8 oz	0	0	0	0	0	0	0	0	0	0	—	—	0
Mango Green Tea	8 oz	80	0	0	0	0	20	20	—	0	0	—	—	0
TURKEY HILL														
Blueberry Oolong w/ Vitamins C & E	1 cup	100	0	0	0	—	24	24	—	—	—	—	—	—
Decaffeinated	1 cup	80	0	0	0	—	20	20	—	—	—	—	—	—
Decaffeinated Orange	1 cup	10	0	0	0	—	2	2	—	—	—	—	—	—
Diet	1 cup	0	0	0	0	0	0	0	—	—	—	—	—	—
Diet Decaffeinated	1 cup	0	0	0	0	0	0	0	—	—	0	—	—	—
Diet Green Tea w/ Ginseng & Honey	1 cup	5	0	0	0	—	tr	tr	—	—	—	—	—	—

FOOD	PORTION	CALS	FAT	SAT FAT	CHOL	PROT	CARB	SUGAR	FIBER	CALCI	SOD	POTAS	FOLIC	VIT C
TURKEY HILL (CONT.)														
Green Tea w/ Ginseng & Honey	1 cup	70	0	0	0	17	17	—	—	—	—	—	—	—
Lemon	1 cup	100	0	0	0	—	24	24	—	—	—	—	—	—
Mint Tea w/ Chamomile	1 cup	90	0	0	0	—	21	21	—	—	—	—	—	—
Oolong w/ Ginkgo Biloba & Ginseng	1 cup	100	0	0	0	—	25	25	—	—	—	—	—	—
Orange	1 cup	100	0	0	0	—	25	25	—	—	—	—	—	—
Peach	1 cup	110	0	0	0	—	28	28	—	—	—	—	—	—
Raspberry Tea	1 cup	110	0	0	0	0	28	28	—	—	0	—	—	—
Regular	1 cup	90	0	0	0	0	22	22	—	—	0	—	—	—
XS ENERGY														
Energy Tea Berry Typhoon	1 can (8.4 oz)	12	0	0	0	2	1	0	—	0	30	25	—	0
ICES AND ICE POPS														
fruit & juice bar	1 (3 fl oz)	75	tr	—	0	1	19	17	—	5	3	48	5	1
gelatin pop	1 (1.5 oz)	31	0	0	0	1	7	7	—	—	20	1	0	—
ice coconut pineapple	½ cup (4 fl oz)	109	3	—	0	0	23	—	—	0	34	—	—	13
ice fruit w/ Equal	1 bar (1.7 oz)	12	0	0	0	tr	3	—	—	1	3	13	0	0
ice lime	½ cup (4 fl oz)	75	0	0	0	tr	31	—	—	—	—	3	—	1
ice pop	1 (2 fl oz)	42	0	0	0	0	11	—	—	0	7	2	—	0
BREYERS														
Fruit Bars No Sugar Added	1 (1.75 oz)	25	0	0	0	0	5	2	0	0	0	—	—	2
Juice Bar Strawberry	1 (3.75 oz)	120	0	0	0	0	30	23	tr	—	10	—	—	4
Soft Frozen Cup Lemonade	1 pkg (12 oz)	290	0	0	0	0	74	56	—	—	25	—	—	—
Soft Frozen Cup Strawberry	1 pkg (12 oz)	260	0	0	0	0	66	51	—	—	25	—	—	—
CARNATION														
Cup Orange Sherbet	1 (5 oz)	150	2	1	5	1	32	28	0	20	30	—	—	0
Cup Orange Sherbet	1 (3 oz)	90	1	0	5	1	19	17	0	20	20	—	—	0
COLD FUSION														
Protein Juice Bar All Flavors	1 bar (3.8 oz)	130	0	0	0	11	23	23	0	30	0	—	—	60

FOOD	PORTION	CALS	FAT	SAT FAT	CHOL	PROT	CARB	SUGAR	FIBER	CALCI	SOD	POTAS	FOLIC	VIT C
COOL CREATIONS														
Ice Pop	1 pop (2 oz)	50	0	0	0	0	13	13	0	0	5	—	—	0
Mickey Mouse Bar	1 (4 oz)	170	11	4	15	2	17	10	0	60	40	—	—	0
Surprise Pops	1 (2 oz)	60	0	0	0	0	14	13	0	0	5	—	—	0
COOLFRUITS														
Fruit Juice Freezer Pops Grape & Cherry	3 pops (3 oz)	70	0	0	0	0	18	18	0	—	10	100	—	—
DOLE														
Fruit'n Juice Coconut	1 bar (4 oz)	210	7	5	10	3	33	30	0	80	50	—	—	1
Fruit'n Juice Lemonade	1 bar (4 oz)	120	0	0	0	1	28	24	0	0	55	—	—	6
Fruit'n Juice Lime	1 bar (4 oz)	110	0	0	0	0	28	24	0	0	55	—	—	1
Fruit'n Juice Peach Passion	1 bar (2.5 oz)	70	0	0	0	0	17	15	0	0	5	—	—	6
Fruit'n Juice Pineapple Coconut	1 bar (4 oz)	150	4	4	0	1	27	24	0	0	5	—	—	1
Fruit'n Juice Pineapple Orange Banana	1 bar (4 oz)	110	0	0	0	0	26	24	0	0	5	—	—	15
Fruit'n Juice Pineapple Orange Banana	1 bar (2.5 oz)	70	0	0	0	0	16	15	0	0	5	—	—	6
Fruit'n Juice Raspberry	1 bar (2.5 oz)	70	0	0	0	0	16	13	0	0	5	—	—	1
Fruit'n Juice Strawberry	1 bar (4 oz)	110	0	0	0	0	26	24	0	0	5	—	—	15
Fruit'n Juice Strawberry	1 bar (2.5 oz)	70	0	0	0	0	17	15	0	0	5	—	—	15
Grape No Sugar Added	1 bar (1.75 oz)	25	0	0	0	0	6	3	0	0	5	—	—	15
Raspberry	1 bar (1.75 oz)	45	0	0	0	0	11	10	0	0	5	—	—	1
Raspberry No Sugar Added	1 bar (1.75 oz)	25	0	0	0	0	6	3	0	0	5	—	—	2
Strawberry	1 bar (1.75 oz)	45	0	0	0	0	11	10	0	0	5	—	—	6
Strawberry No Sugar Added	1 bar (1.75 oz)	25	0	0	0	0	6	3	0	0	5	—	—	5
EDY'S														
Fruit Bars Strawberry	1 (3 oz)	80	0	0	0	0	21	20	0	0	0	—	—	15
Sherbet Berry Rainbow	½ cup	130	1	1	5	1	29	23	—	40	35	—	—	—
Sherbet Lime	½ cup	130	2	1	5	1	28	23	—	40	35	—	—	—
Sherbet Orange Cream	½ cup	120	2	1	10	2	23	19	—	40	40	—	—	—
Sherbet Raspberry	½ cup	130	1	1	5	1	28	22	—	40	35	—	—	—

FOOD	PORTION	CALS	FAT	SAT FAT	CHOL	PROT	CARB	SUGAR	FIBER	CALCI	SOD	POTAS	FOLIC	VIT C
EDY'S (CONT.)														
Sherbet Starburst Orange & Cherry	½ cup	150	2	1	5	1	33	25	—	40	40	—	—	—
Sherbet Starburst Strawberry	½ cup	160	3	2	5	1	33	25	—	40	40	—	—	—
Sherbet Swiss Orange	½ cup	150	3	3	5	1	30	25	—	40	40	—	—	—
Sherbet Tropical Rainbow	½ cup	130	1	1	5	1	29	24	—	40	35	—	—	—
Sorbet Coconut	½ cup	140	3	3	5	1	28	21	0	0	20	—	—	0
Sorbet Lemon	½ cup	140	0	0	0	0	35	25	0	0	20	—	—	9
Sorbet Mandarin Orange	½ cup	130	0	0	0	0	32	24	0	0	25	—	—	2
Sorbet Peach	½ cup	130	0	0	0	0	32	28	1	0	10	—	—	18
Sorbet Raspberry	½ cup	130	0	0	0	0	33	23	1	0	15	—	—	9
Sorbet Strawberry	½ cup	120	0	0	0	0	31	27	0	0	10	—	—	18
Whole Fruit Bars Creamy Coconut	1 bar	120	3	3	0	3	21	16	—	80	40	—	—	—
Whole Fruit Bars Lemonade	1 bar	80	0	0	0	0	20	19	—	0	0	—	—	—
Whole Fruit Bars Lime	1 bar	80	0	0	0	0	20	19	—	0	0	—	—	—
Whole Fruit Bars Tangerine	1 bar	80	0	0	0	0	20	19	—	0	0	—	—	—
Whole Fruit Bars Wild Berry	1 bar	80	0	0	0	0	21	20	—	0	0	—	—	—
FLINTSTONES														
Push-Up Sherbet Treats	1 (2.75 oz)	100	2	1	5	1	20	14	0	40	25	—	—	12
FROZFRUIT														
Banana Cream	1 bar (4 oz)	150	7	5	25	1	20	18	1	40	20	—	—	2
Cantaloupe	1 bar (4 oz)	60	0	0	0	0	35	14	0	0	5	—	—	15
Cappuccino Cream	1 bar (3 oz)	140	6	4	25	1	18	13	0	40	20	—	—	0
Cherry	1 bar (4 oz)	70	0	0	0	1	18	17	1	0	0	—	—	2
Coconut Cream	1 bar (4 oz)	170	11	8	20	2	17	15	2	40	25	—	—	0
Kiwi Strawberry	1 bar (4 oz)	90	0	0	0	0	23	21	2	20	0	—	—	36
Lemon	1 bar (4 oz)	90	0	0	0	0	22	20	0	0	10	—	—	6
Lemon Iced Tea	1 bar (4 oz)	80	0	0	0	0	19	14	0	0	10	—	—	0
Lime	1 bar (4 oz)	90	0	0	0	0	21	19	0	0	10	—	—	2
Orange	1 bar (4 oz)	90	0	0	0	0	21	19	0	0	15	—	—	12
Piña Colada Cream	1 bar (4 oz)	170	8	6	20	2	23	21	1	40	20	—	—	4
Pineapple	1 bar (4 oz)	80	0	0	0	0	19	18	0	0	0	—	—	6
Raspberry	1 bar (4 oz)	80	0	0	0	0	20	18	1	0	5	—	—	6
Strawberry	1 bar (4 oz)	80	0	0	0	0	20	18	1	0	20	—	—	21

FOOD	PORTION	CALS	FAT	SAT FAT	CHOL	PROT	CARB	SUGAR	FIBER	CALCI	SOD	POTAS	FOLIC	VIT C
FROZFRUIT (CONT.)														
Strawberry Banana Cream	1 bar (4 oz)	140	6	3	20	1	22	19	1	40	20	—	—	9
Strawberry Cream	1 bar (4 oz)	130	5	3	20	1	21	20	1	40	20	—	—	15
Tropical	1 bar (4 oz)	90	0	0	0	0	23	22	1	0	0	—	—	9
Watermelon	1 bar (4 oz)	50	0	0	0	0	13	12	0	0	0	—	—	1
GOOD HUMOR														
Great White	1 (3 oz)	70	0	0	0	0	18	14	—	—	0	—	—	—
Hyper Stripe	1 (2.7 oz)	80	0	0	0	0	19	15	—	—	10	—	—	—
HAAGEN-DAZS														
Sorbet Chocolate	½ cup	120	0	0	0	2	28	20	2	0	70	—	—	0
Sorbet Mango	½ cup	120	0	0	0	0	31	29	tr	0	0	—	—	2
Sorbet Orange	½ cup	120	0	0	0	0	30	24	tr	0	0	—	—	15
Sorbet Orchard Peach	½ cup	130	0	0	0	0	33	29	tr	0	0	—	—	4
Sorbet Raspberry	½ cup	120	0	0	0	0	30	26	2	0	0	—	—	2
Sorbet Strawberry	½ cup	120	0	0	0	0	30	27	1	0	0	—	—	12
Sorbet Zesty Lemon	½ cup	120	0	0	0	0	31	27	tr	0	0	—	—	4
Sorbet Bar Chocolate	1 (2.7 oz)	80	0	0	0	1	20	14	1	0	50	—	—	0
Sorbet Bars Raspberry & Vanilla Yogurt	1 (2.5 oz)	90	0	0	0	2	21	15	tr	60	15	—	—	1
Sorbet Bars Strawberry & Vanilla Ice Cream	1 (2.5 oz)	110	5	4	35	1	15	14	0	40	20	—	—	5
MR. FREEZE														
Assorted	2 bars (3 oz)	45	0	0	0	0	11	11	0	0	20	0	—	0
Tropical	2 bars (3 oz)	45	0	0	0	0	11	11	0	0	20	0	—	0
NATURAL CHOICE														
Organic Banana	½ cup (3.6 oz)	110	0	0	0	0	28	27	tr	0	0	—	—	0
Organic Blueberry	½ cup (3.6 oz)	100	0	0	0	0	27	25	tr	0	0	—	—	9
Organic Kiwi	½ cup (3.6 oz)	110	0	0	0	0	28	27	tr	0	10	—	—	9
Organic Lemon	½ cup (3.6 oz)	110	0	0	0	0	28	27	tr	0	10	—	—	9
Organic Mango	½ cup (3.6 oz)	110	0	0	0	0	28	27	tr	0	10	—	—	9
Organic Strawberry	½ cup (3.6 oz)	110	0	0	0	0	28	27	tr	0	10	—	—	9
Organic Strawberry Kiwi	½ cup (3.6 oz)	110	0	0	0	0	28	27	tr	0	10	—	—	9
POPSICLE														
All Natural Ice Pops	1 (1.75 oz)	50	0	0	0	0	12	9	—	100	5	—	—	—
Bar Bart Simpson	1 (4 oz)	110	1	—	—	0	26	20	—	—	20	—	—	—
Bar Dora The Explorer	1 (4 oz)	100	0	0	0	0	25	20	—	—	15	—	—	—

FOOD	PORTION	CALS	FAT	SAT FAT	CHOL	PROT	CARB	SUGAR	FIBER	CALCI	SOD	POTAS	FOLIC	VIT C
POPSICLE (CONT.)														
Bar Fruti Holanda Lemon Lime	1 (3 oz)	90	0	0	0	0	23	18	—	—	15	—	—	—
Bar Fruti Holanda Strawberry	1 (3 oz)	90	0	0	0	0	23	19	—	—	5	—	—	2
Bar Incredible Hulk	1 (4 oz)	100	0	0	0	0	25	20	—	—	15	—	—	—
Bar Jimmy Neutron	1 (4 oz)	100	0	0	0	0	25	19	—	—	15	—	—	—
Bar Mega Warheads	1 (4 oz)	110	1	0	0	0	26	20	0	20	20	—	—	4
Bar Power Ranger	1 (4 oz)	100	0	0	0	0	23	18	—	—	15	—	—	—
Bar Spider Man	1 (4 oz)	100	0	0	0	0	25	20	—	—	15	—	—	—
Bar SpongeBob	1 (4 oz)	100	0	0	0	0	25	20	—	—	15	—	—	—
Big Stick Pops Big Reds	1 (3.5 oz)	70	0	0	0	0	17	12	—	—	0	—	—	—
Big Stick Pops Cherry Pineapple	1 (3.5 oz)	50	0	0	0	0	12	10	0	—	5	—	—	—
Bubble Play	1 (4 oz)	100	0	0	0	0	28	21	—	—	15	—	—	—
Creamsicle Bar	1 (2.5 oz)	100	3	2	5	1	18	14	0	40	30	—	—	0
Creamsicle Sugar Free	2 (3.3 oz)	40	2	2	0	1	10	0	6	20	0	—	—	—
Creamsicle Pop No Sugar Added	1 (1.75 oz)	25	0	0	0	tr	6	1	0	60	20	—	—	0
Cup Cherry	1 (12 oz)	240	0	0	0	0	62	59	—	—	10	—	—	—
Cup Frostee Fudge	1 (10 oz)	280	11	7	35	7	41	33	2	200	95	—	—	2
Cup Lemon	1 (12 oz)	230	0	0	0	0	60	59	—	—	10	—	—	—
Cup Screwball	1 (3.75 oz)	110	0	0	0	0	27	22	—	—	15	—	—	—
Firecracker	1 (1.6 oz)	35	0	0	0	0	9	7	—	—	0	—	—	—
Fruita Holanda Coconut Bar	1 (3 oz)	120	3	2	—	0	25	21	tr	—	75	—	—	—
Fudgsicle Bar	1 (2.5 oz)	90	2	1	5	3	16	13	tr	80	65	—	—	0
Fudgsicle Bar Fat Free	1 (1.75 oz)	60	0	0	0	3	13	10	tr	80	50	—	—	0
Fudgsicle Pop	1 (1.75 oz)	60	1	1	5	2	11	9	tr	60	45	—	—	0
Fudgsicle Pops No Sugar Added	2 (1.75 oz)	90	1	0	0	3	19	3	1	80	85	—	—	—
Minis Fudge Bar	2 (2.4 oz)	80	2	2	0	3	16	13	tr	80	60	—	—	0
Pop Great White	1 (1.75 oz)	45	0	0	0	0	11	9	—	—	0	—	—	—
Pop Lick-A-Color	1 (2 oz)	50	0	0	0	0	13	12	—	—	0	—	—	—
Pop Sherbet Cyclone	1 (1.8 oz)	50	1	0	0	1	11	10	0	20	10	—	—	30
Pop Towering Tornado	1 (3.5 oz)	90	0	0	0	0	21	10	—	—	0	—	—	—
Pop Ups Orange Burst	1 (2.75 oz)	80	1	0	<5	tr	19	15	0	20	15	—	—	27

FOOD	PORTION	CALS	FAT	SAT FAT	CHOL	PROT	CARB	SUGAR	FIBER	CALCI	SOD	POTAS	FOLIC	VIT C
POPSICLE (CONT.)														
Pop Ups Reckless Rainbow	1 (2.75 oz)	90	1	0	<5	tr	19	15	0	20	15	—	—	27
Pop Ups SpongeBob	1 (2:75 oz)	90	2	1	5	1	17	13	0	20	20	—	—	0
Pops Tropical Sugar Free	1 (1.75 oz)	15	0	0	0	0	3	0	—	—	0	—	—	—
Pops Wild Bunch	2 (2.2 oz)	60	0	0	0	0	14	11	—	—	5	—	—	—
Rainbow Floats	1 (1.75 oz)	60	2	1	5	1	11	8	0	20	15	—	—	0
Rainbow Pops	1 (1.75 oz)	45	0	0	0	0	11	11	—	—	0	—	—	—
Scribblers Juice Pops	2 (2.4 oz)	60	0	0	0	0	16	15	—	—	0	—	—	—
Shots	1 serv (1.7 oz)	40	1	—	—	0	9	9	—	—	0	—	—	—
Snow Cone	1 (7 oz)	30	0	0	0	0	7	5	—	—	5	—	—	—
Sugar Free Pops Orange Cherry Grape	1 (1.75 oz)	15	0	0	0	0	3	0	—	—	0	—	—	6
Super Mario Bros Bar	1 (4 oz)	100	0	0	0	0	25	20	—	—	15	—	—	—
Swirl Bar Cotton Candy	1 (2.6 oz)	60	0	0	0	0	13	10	—	—	0	—	—	—
Tingle Twister Ice Pops	1 (1.75 oz)	45	0	0	0	0	11	9	—	—	0	—	—	—
Torpedo Pop Cherry	1 (1.75 oz)	35	0	0	0	0	8	6	—	—	0	—	—	—
SILHOUETTE														
Fat Free Fudge Bars	1	90	0	0	0	—	—	—	—	100	—	—	—	—
JACKFRUIT														
fresh	3.5 oz	70	tr	—	0	1	4	—	—	27	2	407	—	9
JALAPEÑO														
(*see* PEPPERS)														
JAM/JELLY/PRESERVES														
all flavors jam	1 tbsp (0.7 oz)	48	0	0	0	tr	13	10	tr	—	—	—	—	—
all flavors jam	1 pkg (0.5 oz)	34	0	0	0	tr	9	7	tr	—	—	—	—	—
all flavors jelly	1 tbsp (0.7 oz)	52	0	0	0	tr	14	12	tr	—	—	—	—	—
all flavors jelly	1 pkg (0.5 oz)	38	0	0	0	tr	10	9	tr	—	—	—	—	—
all flavors preserve	1 pkg (0.5 oz)	34	0	0	0	tr	9	7	tr	—	—	—	—	—
all flavors preserve	1 tbsp (0.7 oz)	48	0	0	0	tr	13	10	tr	—	—	—	—	—
apple butter	1 tbsp (0.6 oz)	33	0	0	0	0	9	—	—	1	0	16	—	tr
apple butter	1 cup (9.9 oz)	519	1	—	0	tr	135	—	—	13	1	258	—	5
apple jelly	1 tbsp (0.7 oz)	52	0	0	0	tr	14	12	tr	2	7	12	0	tr
apple jelly	1 pkg (0.5 oz)	38	0	0	0	tr	10	9	tr	1	5	9	0	tr
apricot jam	0.5 oz	36	0	0	0	tr	9	—	—	1	—	15	—	—
blackberry jam	0.5 oz	34	0	0	0	tr	8	—	—	—	—	—	—	—
cherry jam	0.5 oz	36	0	0	0	tr	9	—	—	1	—	13	—	tr

FOOD	PORTION	CALS	FAT	SAT FAT	CHOL	PROT	CARB	SUGAR	FIBER	CALCI	SOD	POTAS	FOLIC	VIT C
lingonberry jam	0.5 oz	23	tr	tr	—	tr	6	4	tr	—	—	—	—	—
orange jam	0.5 oz	35	0	0	0	tr	9	—	—	5	2	8	—	1
orange marmalade	1 tbsp (0.7 oz)	49	0	0	0	tr	13	—	—	8	11	7	7	1
orange marmalade	1 pkg (0.5 oz)	34	0	0	0	0	9	—	—	5	8	5	5	1
plum jam	0.5 oz	34	0	0	0	tr	9	—	—	—	—	—	—	—
quince jam	0.5 oz	43	0	0	0	0	8	—	—	—	—	—	—	—
raspberry jam	0.5 oz	35	0	0	0	tr	9	—	—	—	—	—	—	tr
raspberry jelly	0.5 oz	37	0	0	0	0	9	—	—	—	—	10	—	—
red currant jam	0.5 oz	34	0	0	0	1	8	—	—	—	—	—	—	3
red currant jelly	0.5 oz	38	0	0	0	0	9	—	—	1	1	11	—	—
rose hip jam	0.5 oz	36	0	0	0	tr	9	—	—	10	1	24	—	7
strawberry jam	1 tbsp (0.7 oz)	48	0	0	0	tr	13	10	tr	4	8	15	7	2
strawberry jam	1 pkg (0.5 oz)	34	0	0	0	tr	9	7	tr	3	6	11	5	1
strawberry preserve	1 tbsp (0.7 oz)	48	0	0	0	tr	13	10	tr	4	8	15	7	2
strawberry preserve	1 pkg (0.5 oz)	34	0	0	0	tr	9	7	tr	3	6	11	5	1
COLAC														
Jelly All Flavors	1 tbsp	37	0	0	0	0	15	0	0	—	0	—	—	—
EDEN														
Cherry Butter	1 tbsp	35	0	0	0	0	9	8	1	0	0	110	—	0
Organic Apple Butter	1 tbsp	20	0	0	0	0	5	4	0	0	0	0	0	0
ESTEE														
Fruit Spread Apple Spice	1 tbsp	16	0	0	0	0	4	4	0	—	20	30	—	—
Fruit Spread Apricot	1 tbsp	16	0	0	0	0	4	4	0	—	20	35	—	—
Fruit Spread Grape	1 tbsp	16	0	0	0	0	4	4	0	—	20	35	—	—
Fruit Spread Peach	1 tbsp	16	0	0	0	0	4	4	0	—	20	25	—	—
Fruit Spread Red Raspberry	1 tbsp	16	0	0	0	0	4	4	0	—	25	30	—	—
Fruit Spread Strawberry	1 tbsp	16	0	0	0	0	4	4	0	—	—	20	—	—
JOK'N'AL														
Low Carb Fruit Spreads All Flavors	1 tbsp	10	0	0	0	0	3	2	0	—	0	—	—	—
POLANER														
All Fruit Peach	1 tbsp	40	0	0	0	0	8	—	—	—	0	—	—	4
All Fruit Raspberry	1 tbsp	40	0	0	0	0	10	9	—	—	0	—	—	—
SARABETH'S														
Spreadable Fruit Orange Apricot	1 tbsp	30	0	0	0	0	8	8	—	—	0	—	—	2

FOOD	PORTION	CALS	FAT	SAT FAT	CHOL	PROT	CARB	SUGAR	FIBER	CALCI	SOD	POTAS	FOLIC	VIT C
SARABETH'S (CONT.)														
Spreadable Fruit Peach Apricot	1 tbsp	40	0	0	0	0	99	6	1	—	0	—	—	1
Spreadable Fruit Strawberry Raspberry	1 tbsp	40	0	0	0	0	10	9	tr	—	<5	—	—	1
SMUCKER'S														
Concord Grape Jelly	1 tbsp	50	0	0	0	0	13	12	—	—	5	—	—	—
Peach Preserves	1 tbsp	50	0	0	0	0	13	12	—	—	0	—	—	—
Simply Fruit Red Raspberry	1 tbsp	40	0	0	0	0	10	8	—	—	0	—	—	—
TABASCO														
Spicy Pepper Jelly	1 tbsp (0.6 oz)	50	0	0	0	0	12	11	0	0	40	—	—	0
WELCH'S														
Grape Jam	1 tbsp	50	0	0	0	0	13	13		—	10	—	—	—
WHITE HOUSE														
Apple Butter	1 tbsp (0.6 oz)	35	0	0	0	0	9	7	—	—	5	—	—	—
WILD THYME FARMS														
Fruit Spreads Blackberry Currant Ginger	1 tsp	8	0	0	0	0	2	2	—	—	0	—	—	1
Fruit Spreads Mango Apricot	1 tsp	7	0	0	0	0	2	2	—	—	0	—	—	1
JAPANESE FOOD														
(see ASIAN FOOD, SUSHI)														
JAVA PLUM														
fresh	3	5	tr	—	0	tr	1	—	—	2	1	7	—	1
fresh	1 cup	82	tr	—	0	1	21	—	—	25	18	106	—	19
JELLY														
(see JAM/JELLY/PRESERVES)														
JUTE														
cooked	1 cup	32	tr	tr	0	3	6	1	2	184	10	479	90	29
KALE														
chopped cooked	½ cup	21	tr	tr	0	1	4	—	—	47	15	148	9	27
frzn chopped cooked	½ cup	20	tr	tr	0	2	4	—	—	90	10	209	9	16
raw chopped	½ cup	21	tr	tr	0	1	3	—	—	46	15	152	10	41
scotch chopped cooked	½ cup	18	tr	tr	0	1	4	—	—	86	29	178	9	34
KEFIR														
kefir	7 oz	132	8	—	—	6	10	—	—	—	92	320	—	—
KETCHUP														
banana	1 tsp	10	0	0	0	0	2	2	0	—	75	—	—	—
ketchup	1 tbsp	16	tr	tr	0	tr	4	—	tr	3	178	72	2	2

FOOD	PORTION	CALS	FAT	SAT FAT	CHOL	PROT	CARB	SUGAR	FIBER	CALCI	SOD	POTAS	FOLIC	VIT C
ketchup	1 pkg (0.2 oz)	6	tr	tr	0	tr	2	—	tr	1	71	29	1	1
low sodium	1 tbsp	16	tr	tr	0	tr	4	—	tr	3	3	72	2	2
ATKINS														
Ketch-A-Tomato	1 tbsp	10	0	0	0	0	2	0	1	0	160	—	—	2
DEL MONTE														
Ketchup	1 tbsp (0.5 oz)	15	0	0	0	0	4	4	0	0	190	—	—	1
ESTEE														
Ketchup	1 tbsp	15	0	0	0	0	5	1	0	—	190	0	—	—
HEALTHY CHOICE														
Ketchup	1 tbsp (0.5 oz)	9	tr	0	0	tr	2	2	tr	3	97	—	—	1
HEINZ														
Ketchup	1 tbsp	15	0	0	0	0	4	4	0	0	190	—	—	0
No Salt	1 tbsp	20	0	0	0	0	5	4	0	0	0	—	—	0
One Carb	1 tbsp	5	0	0	0	0	1	1	0	0	190	—	—	0
Organic	1 tbsp	20	0	0	0	0	5	4	0	0	190	—	—	0
HUNT'S														
Ketchup	1 tbsp	15	0	0	0	0	4	4	0	0	180	—	—	0
No Salt	1 tbsp	20	0	0	0	0	4	4	0	0	0	40	—	0
Squeeze	1 tbsp	15	0	0	0	0	4	4	0	0	180	—	—	0
KETO														
Ketchup	1 tbsp	4	0	0	0	0	1	0	0	—	15	—	—	—
MCILHENNY														
Spicy	1 tbsp (0.6 oz)	20	0	0	0	0	5	2	0	0	160	—	—	0
MUIR GLEN														
Organic	1 tbsp (0.6 oz)	15	0	0	0	0	3	3	0	0	190	—	—	1
SMUCKER'S														
Tomato	1 tbsp	25	0	0	0	0	7	6	—	—	110	—	—	—
STEEL'S														
Sugar Free	1 tbsp	10	0	0	0	0	0	0	0	—	40	—	—	—
STOKELYS														
Tomato	1 tbsp	15	0	0	0	0	4	4	—	—	190	—	—	—
TREE OF LIFE														
Ketchup	1 tbsp (0.5 oz)	10	0	0	0	0	3	3	—	0	25	—	—	6
WALDEN FARMS														
Calorie Free	1 tbsp	0	0	0	0	0	0	0	0	—	170	—	—	—
KIDNEY														
beef simmered	3 oz	122	3	1	329	22	0	—	—	15	114	152	83	1
lamb braised	3 oz	117	3	1	481	20	1	—	—	15	128	151	69	10
pork cooked	1 cup	211	7	2	672	36	0	—	0	18	112	—	57	9
pork cooked	3 oz	128	4	1	408	22	0	—	0	11	68	—	35	9
veal braised	3 oz	139	5	1	672	22	0	—	—	25	93	135	18	7
KIDNEY BEANS														
canned	1 cup	207	1	tr	0	13	38	—	9	69	889	658	126	3
dried cooked	1 cup	225	1	tr	0	15	40	—	11	0	4	713	229	2

FOOD	PORTION	CALS	FAT	SAT FAT	CHOL	PROT	CARB	SUGAR	FIBER	CALCI	SOD	POTAS	FOLIC	VIT C
BUSH'S														
Light Red	½ cup	110	0	0	0	7	20	1	7	80	260	—	—	1
EDEN														
Organic Cannellini	½ cup (4.6 oz)	100	1	—	—	6	17	1	5	39	40	250	0	0
GREEN GIANT														
Dark Red	½ cup (4.5 oz)	110	0	0	0	6	18	tr	5	40	400	—	—	0
Light Red	½ cup (4.5 oz)	110	0	0	0	8	20	2	6	60	340	—	—	0
HUNT'S														
Kidney Beans	½ cup (4.5 oz)	94	1	0	0	6	20	6	5	37	484	—	—	tr
PROGRESSO														
Dark Red	½ cup (4.5 oz)	110	0	0	0	8	20	2	6	60	340	—	—	0
Red	½ cup (4.6 oz)	110	1	0	0	7	20	0	8	40	280	—	—	0
S&W														
Dark Red Premium	½ cup (4.6 oz)	100	1	0	0	7	23	7	6	80	460	400	—	5
VAN CAMP														
Dark Red	½ cup (4.6 oz)	90	0	0	0	6	20	2	6	40	760	—	—	0
Light Red	½ cup (4.6 oz)	90	0	0	0	6	20	3	6	40	390	—	—	0
KIWI														
fresh	1 med	46	tr	—	0	1	11	—	3	20	4	252	—	75
CHIQUITA														
Fresh	2 med (5.2 oz)	100	1	0	0	2	24	16	4	60	0	—	—	144
KNISH														
GABILA'S														
Potato	1 (4.5 oz)	170	6	1	0	6	29	2	5	20	440	—	—	0
TAKE-OUT														
cheese & blueberry	1 (7 oz)	378	13	—	40	24	40	—	—	—	—	—	—	—
cheese & cherry	1 (7 oz)	378	13	—	40	24	40	—	—	—	—	—	—	—
everything	1 (7 oz)	221	8	—	0	7	34	—	—	—	—	—	—	—
kashe	1 (7 oz)	270	8	—	0	7	45	—	—	—	—	—	—	—
potato	1 lg (7 oz)	332	12	3	72	8	49	5	1	54	470	358	35	8
potato	1 med (3.5 oz)	166	6	2	36	4	25	2	tr	27	235	179	17	4
potato w/ broccoli & cheese	1 (7 oz)	312	15	—	24	12	33	—	—	—	—	—	—	—
potato w/ spinach & mushroom	1 (7 oz)	214	8	—	0	6	32	—	—	—	—	—	—	—
KOHLRABI														
raw sliced	½ cup	19	tr	tr	0	1	4	—	—	17	14	245	—	43
sliced cooked	½ cup	24	tr	tr	0	1	5	—	—	20	17	279	—	44
KRILL														
fresh	1 oz	22	1	—	—	3	tr	—	0	114	119	81	—	1

FOOD	PORTION	CALS	FAT	SAT FAT	CHOL	PROT	CARB	SUGAR	FIBER	CALCI	SOD	POTAS	FOLIC	VIT C
KUMQUAT														
fresh	1	12	tr	—	0	tr	3	—	—	8	1	37	—	7
LAMB														
cubed lean only braised	3 oz	190	7	3	92	29	0	—	—	13	60	221	18	—
cubed lean only broiled	3 oz	158	6	2	77	24	0	—	—	11	65	285	19	—
ground broiled	3 oz	240	17	7	82	21	0	—	—	19	69	288	16	—
leg lean & fat Choice roasted	3 oz	219	14	6	79	22	14	—	—	9	56	266	17	—
loin chop w/ bone lean & fat Choice broiled	1 chop (2.3 oz)	201	15	6	64	16	0	—	—	13	49	209	12	—
loin chop w/ bone lean only Choice broiled	1 chop (1.6 oz)	100	5	2	44	14	0	—	—	9	39	175	11	—
new zealand lean & fat cooked	3 oz	259	19	9	93	21	0	—	—	14	39	138	—	—
new zealand lean only cooked	3 oz	175	8	3	93	25	0	—	—	11	43	160	—	—
rib chop lean & fat Choice broiled	3 oz	307	25	11	84	19	0	—	—	16	64	230	12	—
rib chop lean only Choice broiled	3 oz	200	11	4	78	24	0	—	—	14	73	266	18	—
shank lean & fat Choice braised	3 oz	206	11	5	90	24	0	—	—	17	61	218	14	—
shank lean & fat Choice roasted	3 oz	191	11	4	77	22	0	—	—	8	55	277	19	—
shoulder chop w/ bone lean & fat Choice braised	1 chop (2.5 oz)	244	17	7	84	21	0	—	—	18	51	216	13	—
shoulder chop w/ bone lean only Choice braised	1 chop (1.9 oz)	152	8	3	66	19	0	—	—	14	41	185	12	—
sirloin lean & fat Choice roasted	3 oz	248	21	7	82	21	0	—	—	10	58	256	14	—
LAMB DISHES														
TAKE-OUT														
couscous lamb	1 serv	275	80	3	8	—	—	—	—	—	460	—	—	—
curry	¾ cup	345	17	3	89	26	22	—	—	24	258	317	16	3
lamb fattoush salad	1 serv	606	31	—	109	—	—	—	—	—	924	—	—	—
lamb tagine casserole	1 serv	261	12	5	57	—	—	—	—	—	381	—	—	—
moroccan pilaf w/ bulgur	1 serv	327	13	2	54	—	—	—	—	—	303	—	—	—
moussaka	5.6 oz	312	21	—	—	15	16	—	1	141	—	—	—	6

FOOD	PORTION	CALS	FAT	SAT FAT	CHOL	PROT	CARB	SUGAR	FIBER	CALCI	SOD	POTAS	FOLIC	VIT C
sambousa lamb & vegetable pocket	1	645	54	9	38	—	—	—	—	—	317	—	—	—
stew	¾ cup	124	5	1	29	10	11	—	2	54	140	364	37	20

LAMBSQUARTERS
chopped cooked	½ cup	29	1	tr	0	3	5	—	—	232	—	—	—	33

LEEKS
chopped cooked	¼ cup	8	tr	tr	0	tr	2	—	—	8	3	23	6	1
cooked	1 (4.4 oz)	38	tr	tr	0	1	9	—	—	37	13	108	30	5
freeze dried	1 tbsp	1	0	0	0	tr	tr	—	—	1	0	5	1	tr
raw	1 (4.4 oz)	76	tr	tr	0	2	18	—	—	73	25	223	80	15
raw chopped	¼ cup	16	tr	tr	0	tr	4	—	—	15	5	47	17	3

LEMON
fresh	1 med	22	tr	tr	0	1	12	—	—	66	3	157	—	83
peel	1 tbsp	0	tr	tr	0	tr	1	—	—	8	0	10	—	8
wedge	1	5	tr	tr	0	tr	3	—	—	16	1	39	—	21

LEMON CURD
lemon curd made w/ egg	2 tsp	29	1	—	—	tr	4	—	0	2	—	—	—	1
lemon curd made w/ starch	2 tsp	28	—	—	—	tr	6	—	0	1	—	—	—	0

LEMON EXTRACT
VIRGINIA DARE
Extract	1 tsp	22	0	—	0	—	—	—	—	0	—	—	—	—

LEMON GRASS
fresh	1 cup (2.4 oz)	66	tr	tr	0	1	17	-	0	44	4	484	50	tr
fresh	1 tbsp (5 g)	5	tr	tr	0	tr	1	—	0	3	tr	35	4	tr

LEMON JUICE
bottled	1 tbsp	3	tr	tr	0	tr	1	—	—	2	3	15	2	4
fresh	1 tbsp	4	0	—	0	tr	1	—	—	1	0	19	2	7
frzn	1 tbsp	3	tr	tr	0	tr	1	—	—	1	0	11	1	5

CANARINO
Italian Hot Lemon Beverage	1 cup	0	0	0	0	0	0	0	0	—	0	—	—	—

REALEMON
Juice	1 tsp (5 ml)	0	0	0	0	0	0	—	—	—	0	—	—	—

LEMONADE
FROZEN
as prep w/ water	1 cup	100	tr	tr	0	tr	26	—	—	8	8	38	6	10
not prep	1 can (6 oz)	397	tr	tr	0	1	103	—	—	15	8	148	22	39
MIX														
powder as prep w/ water	9 fl oz	113	tr	tr	0	0	29	—	—	29	19	1	0	34
powder w/ equal	1 pitcher (67 oz)	40	0	0	0	tr	10	—	—	408	58	6	0	47

FOOD	PORTION	CALS	FAT	SAT FAT	CHOL	PROT	CARB	SUGAR	FIBER	CALCI	SOD	POTAS	FOLIC	VIT C
COUNTRY TIME														
Lem'n Berry Sippers Cranberry Raspberry Lemonade as prep	1 serv (8 oz)	90	0	0	0	0	21	21	0	0	0	0	—	0
Lem'n Berry Sippers Raspberry Lemonade as prep	1 serv (8 oz)	90	0	0	0	0	21	21	0	0	0	0	—	0
Lem'n Berry Sippers Strawberry Lemonade as prep	1 serv (8 oz)	90	0	0	0	0	21	21	0	0	0	0	—	0
Lem'n Berry Sippers Wildberry Lemonade as prep	1 serv (8 oz)	90	0	0	0	0	21	21	0	0	0	0	—	0
Lem'n Berry Sippers Sugar Free Strawberry Lemonade as prep	1 serv (8 oz)	5	0	0	0	0	0	0	0	0	0	0	—	0
Lemonade as prep	1 serv (8 oz)	70	0	0	0	0	17	17	0	0	15	5	—	6
Pink as prep	1 serv (8 oz)	70	0	0	0	0	17	17	0	0	15	5	—	6
Sugar Free as prep	1 serv (8 oz)	5	0	0	0	0	0	0	0	0	0	40	—	6
Sugar Free Pink as prep	1 serv (8 oz)	5	0	0	0	0	0	0	0	0	0	40	—	6
CRYSTAL LIGHT														
Lemonade as prep	1 serv (8 oz)	5	0	0	0	0	0	0	0	0	0	60	—	6
Pink as prep	1 serv (8 oz)	5	0	0	0	0	0	0	0	0	0	40	—	6
KETO														
Kooler Pink	½ tsp	0	0	0	0	0	0	0	0	—	0	—	—	—
KOOL-AID														
Lemonade as prep	1 serv (8 oz)	70	0	0	0	0	17	17	0	0	0	0	—	6
Mix as prep w/ sugar	1 serv (8 oz)	100	0	0	0	0	25	25	0	0	10	0	—	6
Pink as prep w/ sugar	1 serv (8 oz)	100	0	0	0	0	25	25	0	0	10	0	—	6
Soarin' Strawberry Lemonade as prep	1 serv (8 oz)	70	0	0	0	0	17	17	0	0	15	0	—	6
Soarin' Strawberry Lemonade as prep w/ sugar	1 serv (8 oz)	100	0	0	0	0	25	25	0	0	0	0	—	6

FOOD	PORTION	CALS	FAT	SAT FAT	CHOL	PROT	CARB	SUGAR	FIBER	CALCI	SOD	POTAS	FOLIC	VIT C
KOOL-AID (CONT.)														
Sugar Free Soarin' Strawberry Lemonade as prep	1 serv (8 oz)	5	0	0	0	0	0	0	0	0	0	0	—	6
Sugar Free Mix as prep	1 serv (8 oz)	5	0	0	0	0	0	0	0	0	0	0	—	6
LOW CARB CREATIONS														
Lemonade as prep	1 serv	10	0	0	0	0	2	tr	0	0	0	—	—	0
Raspberry as prep	1 serv	10	0	0	0	0	2	0	0	0	0	—	—	0
SIPPER SWEETS														
Sugar Free Low Carb	1 serv	8	0	0	0	0	1	0	0	—	0	—	—	—
READY-TO-DRINK														
CRYSTAL LIGHT														
Lemonade	1 serv (8 oz)	5	0	0	0	0	0	0	0	0	20	160	—	0
Pink	1 serv (8 oz)	5	0	0	0	0	0	0	0	0	20	160	—	0
EVERFRESH														
Lemonade	1 can (8 oz)	120	0	0	0	0	29	29	0	—	0	—	—	—
Ruby Red	1 can (8 oz)	110	0	0	0	0	27	27	0	—	0	—	—	—
HANSEN'S														
Sparkling	8 fl oz	100	0	0	0	0	25	25	—	—	10	6	—	—
Sparkling Pink	8 fl oz	120	0	0	0	0	31	31	—	—	10	6	—	—
LANGERS														
Raspberry Lemonade	8 oz	120	0	0	0	0	29	26	—	—	0	—	—	60
White Cranberry Lemonade	8 oz	120	0	0	0	0	30	28	—	—	15	—	—	60
MINUTE MAID														
Chilled	8 fl oz	110	0	0	0	0	28	26	—	—	25	150	—	—
NANTUCKET NECTARS														
Authentic	8 oz	120	0	0	0	0	30	28	—	0	0	—	—	60
Pink	8 oz	120	0	0	0	0	30	27	—	0	0	—	—	60
NEWMAN'S OWN														
Lemonade	1 bottle (10 oz)	140	0	0	0	0	34	34	0	0	45	—	—	2
Roadside Virginia	8 fl oz	110	0	0	0	0	27	27	0	0	40	—	—	2
OCEAN SPRAY														
Spritzer	8 oz	160	0	0	0	0	41	40	—	—	50	—	—	—
ODWALLA														
Pure Squeezed	8 fl oz	96	0	0	0	0	24	18	0	0	0	—	—	15
Strawberry Quencher	8 fl oz	110	0	0	0	0	28	25	0	0	0	—	—	54
PURITY ORGANIC														
Lemonade	8 oz	123	tr	—	—	tr	33	—	tr	—	tr	—	—	60

FOOD	PORTION	CALS	FAT	SAT FAT	CHOL	PROT	CARB	SUGAR	FIBER	CALCI	SOD	POTAS	FOLIC	VIT C
SHASTA PLUS														
Lemonade	1 can (11.5 oz)	160	0	0	0	0	40	40	0	—	45	—	—	60
SNAPPLE														
Diet Pink	8 fl oz	20	0	0	0	0	4	4	—	—	10	—	—	—
Lemonade	8 fl oz	120	0	0	0	0	30	28	—	—	10	—	—	—
Pink	8 fl oz	120	0	0	0	0	29	28	—	—	10	—	—	—
T42														
Lemonade	8 oz	90	0	0	0	0	25	25	—	—	10	—	—	12
Pink	8 oz	90	0	0	0	0	25	25	—	—	10	—	—	12
THREE DRINKS														
Sparkling	12 oz	12	0	0	0	0	3	2	—	—	20	—	—	—
TURKEY HILL														
Lemonade	1 cup	120	0	0	0	0	29	29	—	—	0	—	—	—
Raspberry	1 cup	120	0	0	0	—	29	29	—	—	—	—	—	—
Strawberry Kiwi	1 cup	120	0	0	0	—	29	29	—	—	—	—	—	—
VERYFINE														
Chillers	1 can (11.5 oz)	190	0	0	0	0	48	48	0	0	15	—	—	60
Chillers Cherry	8 fl oz	120	0	0	0	0	29	29	0	0	15	—	—	60
Chillers Peach	8 fl oz	120	0	0	0	0	31	31	0	0	15	—	—	60
Chillers Pink	1 can (11.5 oz)	180	0	0	0	0	45	45	0	0	15	—	—	60
Chillers Strawberry	1 can (11.5 oz)	170	0	0	0	0	43	42	0	0	20	—	—	60
ZEIGLER'S														
Old Fashioned	8 oz	120	0	0	0	0	30	27	0	0	25	—	—	9

LENTILS

FOOD	PORTION	CALS	FAT	SAT FAT	CHOL	PROT	CARB	SUGAR	FIBER	CALCI	SOD	POTAS	FOLIC	VIT C
dried cooked	1 cup	231	1	tr	0	18	40	—	—	37	4	731	358	3
NATURAL TOUCH														
Lentil Rice Loaf	1 in slice (3.2 oz)	170	9	3	0	8	14	tr	4	20	370	160	—	0
NEAR EAST														
Lentil Pilaf as prep	1 cup	200	3	2	9	11	36	3	8	20	630	—	—	1
SHILOH FARMS														
Organic Green not prep	¼ cup (1.6 oz)	150	0	0	0	11	27	2	7	40	15	—	—	0
TASTYBITE														
Bengal Lentils	½ pkg (5 oz)	190	5	1	0	7	30	2	1	80	150	—	—	0
Jodhpur Lentils	½ pkg (5 oz)	190	9	4	0	6	22	0	2	50	600	—	—	0
Madras Lentils	½ pkg (5 oz)	130	7	3	22	6	12	2	5	50	860	—	—	0
TAKE-OUT														
indian sambar	1 serv	236	5	2	10	15	37	—	9	—	189	—	—	—
middle eastern lentil salad	1 serv (4.5 oz)	158	3	tr	0	—	—	—	—	—	382	—	—	—
yemiser selatta ethopian lentil salad	1 serv (3 oz)	115	7	1	0	4	11	1	2	19	536	234	73	56

FOOD	PORTION	CALS	FAT	SAT FAT	CHOL	PROT	CARB	SUGAR	FIBER	CALCI	SOD	POTAS	FOLIC	VIT C
LETTUCE														
(*see also* SALAD)														
arugula	½ cup (0.4 oz)	3	tr	—	0	tr	tr	—	tr	16	3	37	10	2
bibb	1 head (6 oz)	21	tr	tr	0	2	4	—	2	—	8	416	119	13
boston	1 head (6 oz)	21	tr	tr	0	2	4	—	2	—	8	416	119	13
boston	2 leaves	2	tr	tr	0	tr	tr	—	tr	—	1	39	11	1
cornsalad field salad	1 cup (1.9 oz)	7	tr	—	0	1	1	—	1	19	2	232	80	19
iceberg	1 leaf	3	tr	tr	0	tr	tr	—	tr	4	2	32	11	1
iceberg	1 head (19 oz)	70	1	tr	0	5	11	—	5	102	48	852	302	21
looseleaf shredded	½ cup	5	tr	tr	0	tr	1	—	—	19	3	74	—	5
romaine shredded	½ cup	4	tr	tr	0	tr	1	—	tr	10	2	81	38	7
DOLE														
Iceberg	1 cup (3 oz)	15	0	0	0	1	3	2	1	0	10	—	—	4
Romaine	1½ cups (3 oz)	15	0	0	0	1	2	2	2	40	5	—	—	21
Shredded	1½ cups (3 oz)	15	0	0	0	1	3	2	1	0	10	—	—	4
EARTHBOUND FARM														
Romaine Salad Organic	1½ cups (2.9 oz)	15	0	0	0	3	3	2	1	20	5	—	—	12
GREEN GIANT														
Hearts Of Romaine	6 leaves	20	1	0	0	1	3	2	1	10	140	—	—	2
READY PAC														
Baby Arugula	4 cups	20	1	0	0	2	3	0	2	150	25	—	—	12
Bella Romaine	1½ cups	15	0	0	0	1	2	1	1	20	5	—	—	5
LILY ROOT														
dried	1 oz	89	1	—	—	2	21	—	tr	9	25	195	—	5
fresh	1 oz	32	tr	—	—	1	8	—	tr	1	3	—	—	6
LIMA BEANS														
CANNED														
large	1 cup	191	tr	tr	0	12	36	—	—	50	809	531	121	0
lima beans	½ cup	88	tr	tr	0	5	17	—	5	35	312	353	20	9
DEL MONTE														
Green	½ cup (4.4 oz)	80	0	0	0	4	15	0	4	20	390	—	—	5
EDEN														
Organic Baby	½ cup (4.6 oz)	100	1	0	0	6	17	—	4	20	35	290	8	0
S&W														
Small Green	½ cup (4.4 oz)	80	0	0	0	4	15	0	4	20	390	—	—	5
VEG-ALL														
Baby Green	½ cup	90	1	0	0	4	15	1	3	20	330	—	—	0
DRIED														
baby cooked	1 cup	229	1	tr	0	15	42	—	17	52	5	729	273	0
cooked	½ cup	104	tr	tr	0	6	20	—	—	27	14	485	—	9
large cooked	1 cup	217	1	tr	0	15	39	—	14	32	4	955	156	0

FOOD	PORTION	CALS	FAT	SAT FAT	CHOL	PROT	CARB	SUGAR	FIBER	CALCI	SOD	POTAS	FOLIC	VIT C
HURST														
HamBeens Baby Limas w/ Ham	1 serv	120	1	0	0	7	22	1	9	20	63	—	—	0
HamBeens Large Limas w/ Ham	1 serv	120	1	0	0	7	22	1	9	20	63	—	—	0
FROZEN														
cooked	½ cup	94	tr	tr	0	6	18	—	—	19	26	370	—	5
fordhook cooked	½ cup	85	tr	tr	0	5	16	—	—	19	45	347	—	11
BIRDS EYE														
Baby	½ cup	130	0	0	0	7	24	2	6	20	115	—	—	15
Fordhook	½ cup	100	0	0	0	6	19	3	5	20	10	—	—	15
FRESH LIKE														
Baby	3.5 oz	138	1	—	—	7	25	—	2	34	106	494	—	19
GREEN GIANT														
Butter Sauce	⅔ cup (3.6 oz)	120	3	2	<5	6	18	1	6	20	330	—	—	2
Harvest Fresh Baby	½ cup (2.7 oz)	80	0	0	0	4	15	tr	4	20	130	—	—	5
LIME														
fresh	1	20	tr	tr	0	tr	7	—	—	22	1	68	6	20
LIME JUICE														
bottled	1 tbsp	3	tr	tr	0	tr	1	—	—	2	2	12	1	1
fresh	1 tbsp	4	tr	tr	0	tr	1	—	—	2	0	17	—	5
limeade	1 can (6 oz)	408	tr	tr	0	tr	108	—	—	11	—	129	—	—
ODWALLA														
Summertime Lime	8 fl oz	90	0	0	0	0	23	21	0	0	10	—	—	5
REALIME														
Juice	1 tsp (5 ml)	0	0	0	0	0	0	—	—	—	0	—	—	—
LING														
blue raw	3.5 oz	83	1	—	—	17	0	—	—	—	—	—	—	—
fresh baked	3 oz	95	1	—	—	21	0	—	—	37	147	413	—	—
fresh fillet baked	5.3 oz	168	1	—	—	37	0	—	—	66	261	734	—	—
LINGCOD														
baked	3 oz	93	1	tr	57	19	0	—	—	15	64	476	—	—
fillet baked	5.3 oz	164	2	tr	101	34	0	—	—	27	114	846	—	—
LIQUOR/LIQUEUR														
(_see also_ BEER AND ALE, CHAMPAGNE, WINE)														
7&7	1 serv	178	0	0	0	0	19	—	0	4	21	3	—	—
alabama slammer	1 serv	103	tr	0	0	tr	7	—	tr	1	tr	13	2	3
amaretto sour	1 serv	295	tr	tr	0	2	57	—	4	75	98	362	55	98
angel's kiss	1 serv	85	1	1	5	tr	5	—	0	7	4	12	tr	tr
anisette	1 oz	111	0	0	0	—	11	—	0	—	—	—	—	—
antifreeze	1 serv	177	tr	tr	0	1	31	—	tr	20	2	372	56	93

FOOD	PORTION	CALS	FAT	SAT FAT	CHOL	PROT	CARB	SUGAR	FIBER	CALCI	SOD	POTAS	FOLIC	VIT C
apricot brandy	1 oz	96	0	0	0	—	9	—	0	—	—	—	—	—
apricot sour	1 serv	164	tr	0	0	tr	8	—	tr	3	5	49	4	14
aquavit	1 oz	65	0	0	—	0	0	0	0	—	—	—	—	0
b 52	1 serv	247	4	2	0	1	25	—	0	—	24	7	—	—
b&b	1 serv	75	0	0	0	0	0	0	0	—	tr	—	—	—
bahama breeze	1 serv	70	tr	0	0	tr	9	—	tr	3	2	34	5	6
bahama mama	1 serv	153	tr	tr	0	1	23	—	tr	23	2	207	33	27
bailey's & amaretto	1 serv	184	5	3	0	1	16	—	0	—	29	0	—	—
banana colada	1 serv	376	1	tr	0	2	64	—	3	49	4	736	77	36
bay breeze	1 serv	173	tr	tr	0	1	18	—	tr	17	2	302	19	73
bend me over	1 serv	242	tr	tr	0	1	32	—	tr	18	33	319	47	78
benedictine	1 oz	104	0	0	0	—	11	—	0	—	—	—	—	—
betsy ross	1 serv	206	0	0	0	tr	5	—	0	2	3	44	1	—
black devil	1 serv	220	tr	tr	0	tr	1	—	tr	5	43	6	—	2
black russian	1 serv	184	tr	tr	0	0	12	—	0	—	3	8	—	—
bloody mary	1 serv	150	tr	tr	0	1	5	—	1	11	332	195	21	32
blue whale	1 serv	222	tr	0	0	tr	23	—	0	1	63	18	—	2
bourbon & soda	1 serv (4 oz)	105	0	0	0	0	0	0	0	4	16	2	0	0
bourbon sour	1 serv	166	tr	0	0	tr	8	—	tr	3	5	49	4	14
brandy	2 oz	255	—	—	—	—	—	—	—	—	—	—	—	—
brandy alexander	1 serv	266	6	4	20	1	12	—	0	29	17	48	—	tr
brandy sour	1 serv	164	tr	0	0	tr	8	—	tr	4	5	49	4	14
bushwacher	1 serv	286	5	2	0	tr	27	—	tr	tr	23	18	3	tr
campari	2 oz	245	—	—	—	—	—	—	—	—	—	—	—	—
cherry heering	2 oz	245	—	—	—	—	—	—	—	—	—	—	—	—
coffee liqueur	1 serv (1.5 oz)	175	tr	tr	0	tr	24	—	0	1	4	15	0	0
coffee w/ cream liqueur	1 serv (1.5 oz)	154	7	5	7	1	10	—	0	7	43	15	0	0
cognac	1 oz	67	0	0	0	0	tr	0	0	—	—	—	—	0
cosmopolitan martini	1 serv	126	tr	0	0	tr	7	—	tr	2	1	18	1	7
creme de almonde	1 oz	102	—	—	—	—	—	—	—	—	—	—	—	—
creme de banana	1 oz	99	—	—	—	—	—	—	—	—	—	—	—	—
creme de cassis	1 oz	82	—	—	—	—	—	—	—	—	—	—	—	—
creme de menthe	1 serv (1.5 oz)	186	tr	tr	0	0	21	—	0	0	3	0	0	0
curaçao liqueur	1 oz	81	0	0	0	—	9	—	0	—	—	—	—	—
daiquiri	1 serv	187	0	0	0	0	15	—	0	tr	7	1	—	—
daiquiri banana	1 serv	277	tr	tr	0	1	32	—	1	4	7	235	11	5
dark & stormy	1 serv	64	0	0	0	0	0	0	0	—	tr	1	—	—
doctor pepper	1 serv	95	0	0	0	0	12	—	0	1	1	tr	—	—
drambuie	2 oz	225	—	—	—	—	—	—	—	—	—	—	—	—
frozen daiquiri	1 serv	393	2	—	—	—	—	—	—	—	—	—	—	—
frozen daiquiri pineapple	1 serv	186	tr	tr	0	1	28	—	2	21	3	365	37	123

FOOD	PORTION	CALS	FAT	SAT FAT	CHOL	PROT	CARB	SUGAR	FIBER	CALCI	SOD	POTAS	FOLIC	VIT C
frozen tequila screwdriver	1 serv	159	tr	tr	0	1	17	—	1	16	2	287	39	84
fuzzy navel	1 serv	247	tr	tr	0	1	10	—	tr	10	2	188	28	47
gibson	1 serv (4 oz)	254	—	—	—	—	—	—	—	—	—	—	—	—
gimlet vodka	1 serv	150	tr	0	0	tr	6	—	1	7	3	21	2	6
gin	1 serv (1.5 oz)	110	0	0	0	0	0	—	0	0	1	0	0	0
gin & tonic	1 serv (7.5 oz)	171	0	0	0	0	16	—	—	4	10	12	1	1
gin ricky	1 serv	114	tr	0	0	tr	1	—	tr	10	38	20	1	5
grasshopper	1 serv	275	5	3	15	1	26	—	0	22	13	38	1	tr
happy hawaiian	1 serv	434	8	5	0	2	60	—	tr	32	50	266	43	20
harvey wallbanger	1 serv	198	tr	tr	0	1	16	—	tr	17	2	311	47	78
head banger	1 serv	165	0	0	0	0	4	—	0	—	tr	1	—	—
hot buttered rum	1 serv	219	4	3	10	tr	15	—	4	101	48	49	4	101
hot toddy	1 serv	188	1	tr	0	tr	13	—	5	102	9	33	5	4
hurricane	1 serv	205	tr	0	0	tr	19	—	tr	3	2	43	7	9
kamikaze	1 serv	136	0	0	0	0	2	—	0	—	2	1	—	—
long island iced tea	1 serv	292	tr	0	0	tr	7	—	0	1	33	10	—	1
lynchburg lemonade	1 serv	465	tr	tr	0	tr	85	—	1	11	38	107	15	27
mai tai	1 serv	165	tr	tr	0	tr	17	—	tr	2	51	24	—	1
manhattan	1 serv	171	tr	0	0	tr	3	—	tr	2	9	16	—	—
margarita	1 serv	173	0	0	0	0	11	—	0	—	3	—	—	—
margarita strawberry	1 serv	106	tr	tr	0	tr	11	—	1	11	1	128	13	41
martini apple	1 serv	147	tr	tr	0	tr	4	—	tr	2	2	38	tr	tr
martini rum	1 serv	131	0	0	0	tr	tr	—	tr	1	1	3	—	1
martini vodka	1 serv	135	tr	tr	0	tr	1	—	tr	5	45	7	—	tr
mellow yellow	1 serv	95	0	0	0	0	4	—	0	—	0	0	—	—
mexican grasshopper	1 serv	638	19	12	66	1	52	—	0	42	29	79	2	tr
mint julep	1 serv	136	tr	tr	0	tr	17	—	tr	8	3	19	4	1
mississippi mud	1 serv	496	12	7	45	3	46	—	0	87	46	132	4	1
narragansett	1 serv	168	0	0	0	0	2	—	0	1	5	6	—	—
nutcracker	1 serv	730	10	6	0	2	64	—	0	—	65	20	—	—
old fashioned	1 serv	223	tr	0	0	tr	4	—	tr	1	5	12	—	—
orange crush	1 serv	461	tr	tr	0	0	65	—	tr	8	5	46	1	90
pain killer	1 serv	277	tr	tr	0	1	20	—	tr	26	5	231	38	29
peppermint pattie	1 serv	344	tr	tr	0	tr	37	—	0	1	7	15	—	—
piña colada	1 serv (4.5 oz)	262	3	1	0	1	40	—	tr	11	9	100	14	7
planter's cocktail	1 serv	105	0	0	0	tr	3	—	tr	1	1	19	2	7
planter's punch	1 serv	233	tr	tr	0	2	34	—	4	79	33	447	67	124
presbyterian	1 serv	170	0	0	0	tr	8	—	tr	8	26	5	tr	1
purple passion	1 serv	215	tr	tr	0	tr	22	—	0	11	14	102	6	23
rob roy	1 serv	171	0	0	0	tr	3	—	tr	3	13	15	tr	1
rum	1 serv (1.5 oz)	97	0	0	0	0	0	—	0	0	0	1	0	0

FOOD	PORTION	CALS	FAT	SAT FAT	CHOL	PROT	CARB	SUGAR	FIBER	CALCI	SOD	POTAS	FOLIC	VIT C
rum boogie	1 serv	134	tr	0	0	tr	12	—	tr	5	3	12	1	3
rum cola	1 serv	209	tr	0	0	tr	21	—	tr	7	8	19	1	4
rum highball	1 serv	170	0	0	0	0	11	—	0	4	9	2	—	—
rum punch	1 serv	448	1	tr	0	1	88	—	1	33	12	300	34	217
rusty nail	1 serv	159	0	0	0	0	6	—	0	—	tr	1	—	0
salty dog	1 serv	210	tr	tr	0	1	19	—	tr	18	3	304	19	71
scotch & soda	1 serv	104	0	0	0	tr	tr	—	tr	10	38	5	tr	1
screwdriver rum	1 serv	166	tr	tr	0	1	16	—	tr	17	2	311	47	78
sea breeze	1 serv	207	tr	tr	0	tr	19	—	tr	8	3	118	6	57
sex on the beach	1 serv	190	tr	tr	0	tr	18	—	tr	4	2	58	—	34
singapore sling	1 serv (4 oz)	115	—	—	—	—	—	—	—	—	—	—	—	—
slippery nipple	1 serv	142	2	2	0	tr	11	—	0	—	16	5	—	—
sloe gin fizz	1 serv (2.5 oz)	132	0	0	0	0	4	—	0	2	1	35	tr	11
snake bite	1 serv	362	0	0	0	0	22	—	0	—	7	2	—	—
sour rum	1 serv	156	tr	0	0	tr	8	—	tr	4	5	49	4	14
southern comfort	1 serv (1.5 oz)	184	—	—	—	—	—	—	—	—	—	—	—	—
swizzle rum	1 serv	187	0	0	0	0	15	—	0	9	44	5	—	—
tequila	1 serv (1.5 oz)	117	—	—	—	—	—	—	—	—	—	—	—	—
tequila gimlet	1 serv	150	tr	0	0	tr	6	—	1	7	3	21	2	6
tequila sour	1 serv	156	tr	0	0	tr	8	—	tr	3	5	48	4	14
tequila stinger	1 serv	221	tr	0	0	0	14	—	0	—	2	—	—	—
tequila sunrise	1 serv (6.8 oz)	232	tr	tr	0	1	24	—	0	0	120	21	23	41
tom collins	1 serv (7.5 oz)	121	0	0	0	tr	3	—	—	10	39	18	2	4
vermouth cassis	1 serv	97	tr	0	0	tr	5	—	tr	14	54	31	1	4
vodka	1 serv (1.5 oz)	97	0	0	0	0	0	—	0	0	0	0	0	0
vodka sour	1 serv	138	tr	0	0	tr	3	—	tr	1	1	17	1	4
vodka stinger	1 serv	378	tr	tr	0	0	28	—	0	—	4	1	—	—
whiskey	1 serv (1.5 oz)	105	0	0	0	0	tr	—	0	0	0	1	0	0
whiskey sour	1 serv	159	0	0	0	tr	6	—	tr	9	8	74	8	27
white russian	1 serv	290	8	5	31	tr	17	—	0	14	12	27	1	tr
zombie	1 serv	235	tr	tr	0	tr	10	—	tr	8	5	129	19	31

LITCHI JUICE

CERES

Litchi	8 oz	120	0	0	0	0	30	25	0	0	10	190	—	60

LIVER

(see also PÂTÉ)

beef braised	3 oz	137	4	2	331	21	3	—	—	6	59	200	184	19
beef pan-fried	3 oz	184	7	2	410	23	7	—	—	9	90	309	187	19
chicken stewed	1 cup (5 oz)	219	8	3	883	34	1	—	—	20	71	196	1077	22
duck raw	1 (1.5 oz)	60	2	1	227	8	2	—	—	5	—	—	24	—
goose raw	1 (3.3 oz)	125	4	1	—	15	6	—	—	40	132	216	—	—
lamb braised	3 oz	187	7	3	426	26	2	—	—	7	48	188	62	3
lamb fried	3 oz	202	11	4	419	22	3	—	—	8	105	299	340	11
pork braised	3 oz	140	4	1	302	22	3	—	0	9	42	—	139	20

FOOD	PORTION	CALS	FAT	SAT FAT	CHOL	PROT	CARB	SUGAR	FIBER	CALCI	SOD	POTAS	FOLIC	VIT C
sheep raw	3.5 oz	131	4	—	—	21	0	—	—	4	95	282	tr	31
turkey simmered	1 cup (5 oz)	237	8	3	876	34	5	—	—	15	89	272	932	3
veal braised	3 oz	140	6	2	477	18	2	—	—	6	45	174	645	26
veal fried	3 oz	208	10	4	280	25	3	—	—	10	112	372	272	18
SHADY BROOK														
Turkey	4 oz	160	5	2	530	23	—	—	—	—	110	—	—	—

LIVER SUBSTITUTES

FOOD	PORTION	CALS	FAT	SAT FAT	CHOL	PROT	CARB	SUGAR	FIBER	CALCI	SOD	POTAS	FOLIC	VIT C
SABRA														
Vegetarian Liver	1 oz	70	7	1	14	1	1	1	1	20	87	—	—	0

LOBSTER

FOOD	PORTION	CALS	FAT	SAT FAT	CHOL	PROT	CARB	SUGAR	FIBER	CALCI	SOD	POTAS	FOLIC	VIT C
northern cooked	3 oz	83	1	tr	61	17	1	—	—	52	323	299	9	—
northern cooked	1 cup	142	1	tr	104	30	2	—	—	88	551	510	16	—
northern raw	1 lobster (5.3 oz)	136	1	—	143	28	1	—	—	—	—	—	—	—
northern raw	3 oz	77	1	—	81	77	tr	—	—	—	—	—	—	—
spiny steamed	3 oz	122	2	tr	76	22	3	—	—	53	193	—	—	—
spiny steamed	1 (5.7 oz)	233	3	tr	146	43	5	—	—	102	370	—	—	—
PROGRESSO														
Lobster Sauce	½ cup (4.3 oz)	100	7	1	5	3	6	3	2	20	430	—	—	0
TAKE-OUT														
newburg	1 cup	485	27	—	455	46	13	—	—	218	127	271	—	—

LOGANBERRIES

FOOD	PORTION	CALS	FAT	SAT FAT	CHOL	PROT	CARB	SUGAR	FIBER	CALCI	SOD	POTAS	FOLIC	VIT C
frzn	1 cup	80	tr	—	0	2	19	—	—	38	1	213	38	23

LONGANS

FOOD	PORTION	CALS	FAT	SAT FAT	CHOL	PROT	CARB	SUGAR	FIBER	CALCI	SOD	POTAS	FOLIC	VIT C
fresh	1	2	0	0	0	tr	tr	—	—	0	0	9	—	3

LOQUATS

FOOD	PORTION	CALS	FAT	SAT FAT	CHOL	PROT	CARB	SUGAR	FIBER	CALCI	SOD	POTAS	FOLIC	VIT C
fresh	1	5	tr	tr	0	tr	1	—	—	2	0	26	—	—

LOTUS

FOOD	PORTION	CALS	FAT	SAT FAT	CHOL	PROT	CARB	SUGAR	FIBER	CALCI	SOD	POTAS	FOLIC	VIT C
root raw sliced	10 slices	45	tr	tr	0	2	14	—	—	36	33	450	—	36
root sliced cooked	10 slices	59	tr	tr	0	1	14	—	—	23	40	323	—	24
seeds dried	1 oz	94	1	tr	0	4	18	—	—	46	1	389	—	0
EDEN														
Root	1 serv (0.3 oz)	35	0	0	0	1	8	1	2	11	25	160	0	0

LOX

(*see* SALMON)

LUPINES

FOOD	PORTION	CALS	FAT	SAT FAT	CHOL	PROT	CARB	SUGAR	FIBER	CALCI	SOD	POTAS	FOLIC	VIT C
dried cooked	1 cup	197	5	1	0	26	16	—	—	85	7	407	—	—

LYCHEES

FOOD	PORTION	CALS	FAT	SAT FAT	CHOL	PROT	CARB	SUGAR	FIBER	CALCI	SOD	POTAS	FOLIC	VIT C
fresh	1	6	tr	—	0	tr	2	—	—	0	0	16	—	7

MACADAMIA NUTS

FOOD	PORTION	CALS	FAT	SAT FAT	CHOL	PROT	CARB	SUGAR	FIBER	CALCI	SOD	POTAS	FOLIC	VIT C
dry roasted w/ salt	10–12 nuts (1 oz)	200	22	4	0	2	4	2	1	20	80	100	—	—
oil roasted	1 oz	204	22	3	0	2	4	—	—	13	3	94	—	0

FOOD	PORTION	CALS	FAT	SAT FAT	CHOL	PROT	CARB	SUGAR	FIBER	CALCI	SOD	POTAS	FOLIC	VIT C
HAWAIIAN HOST														
Chocolate Covered	1 piece (0.5 oz)	53	6	3	2	1	8	7	tr	40	15	—	—	0
KETO														
Chocolately Covered	1 oz	171	19	5	—	2	6	0	4	60	—	—	—	0
MACFARMS OF HAWAII														
Chocolate Covered	¼ cup (1.3 oz)	210	16	6	5	3	18	15	2	60	25	—	—	0
Dry Roasted Salted	¼ cup (1.3 oz)	220	23	4	0	3	4	1	3	20	65	—	—	0
Kona Coffee Dark Chocolate Covered	¼ cup (1.3 oz)	210	16	6	5	3	18	15	2	60	25	—	—	0
MARANATHA														
Macadamia Butter	2 tbsp	230	24	—	—	3	5	1	3	—	0	—	—	—
MAUNA LOA														
Chocolate Trio	9 pieces	200	15	7	5	2	19	17	2	—	10	—	—	—
Dry Roasted Salted	¼ cup	200	21	4	0	2	4	1	2	—	60	—	—	—
Dry Roasted Unsalted	¼ cup	200	21	4	0	2	4	1	2	—	0	—	—	—
Honey Roasted	¼ cup	210	21	3	0	2	6	4	2	—	35	—	—	—
Kona Coffee Glazed	¼ cup	190	15	3	<5	2	10	6	1	—	55	—	—	—
Maui Onion & Garlic	¼ cup	200	16	7	0	2	18	14	3	—	0	—	—	—
Milk Chocolate Coated	13 pieces	200	12	5	5	2	25	23	1	—	10	—	—	—
Milk Chocolate Toffee	7 pieces	210	13	5	5	2	23	21	1	40	70	—	—	0
MACE														
ground	1 tsp	8	1	tr	0	tr	1	—	—	4	1	8	—	—
MACKEREL														
CANNED														
jack	1 can (12.7 oz)	563	23	7	285	84	0	—	—	870	1368	700	19	3
jack	1 cup	296	12	4	150	44	0	—	—	458	720	369	10	2
DRIED														
EDEN														
Bonito Flakes	2 tbsp	4	0	0	1	1	0	0	0	tr	4	13	—	0
FRESH														
atlantic cooked	3 oz	223	15	4	64	20	0	—	—	13	71	341	—	tr
atlantic raw	3 oz	174	12	3	60	16	0	—	—	10	76	267	—	tr
jack baked	3 oz	171	9	2	51	22	0	—	—	25	94	442	2	—
jack fillet baked	6.2 oz	354	18	5	106	45	0	—	—	52	194	916	4	—
king baked	3 oz	114	2	tr	58	22	0	—	—	34	172	474	7	—

FOOD	PORTION	CALS	FAT	SAT FAT	CHOL	PROT	CARB	SUGAR	FIBER	CALCI	SOD	POTAS	FOLIC	VIT C
king fillet baked	5.4 oz	207	4	1	105	40	0	—	—	61	312	859	14	—
pacific baked	3 oz	171	9	2	51	22	0	—	—	25	94	442	2	—
pacific fillet baked	6.2 oz	354	18	5	106	45	0	—	—	52	194	916	4	—
spanish cooked	3 oz	134	5	2	62	20	0	—	—	11	56	471	—	—
spanish cooked	1 fillet (5.1 oz)	230	9	3	107	34	0	—	—	19	96	808	—	—
spanish raw	3 oz	118	5	2	65	16	0	—	—	10	50	379	—	—
SMOKED														
atlantic	3.5 oz	296	24	5	93	19	0	—	—	20	384	310	1	0
MALANGA														
fresh	½ cup	137	tr	—	—	2	32	—	—	—	—	—	—	8
MALT														
nonalcoholic	12 fl oz	32	0	0	0	1	5	—	—	25	—	—	—	—
SKYY														
Blue	1 bottle	235	—	—	—	—	35	—	—	—	—	—	—	—
Sport	1 bottle	160	—	—	—	—	15	—	—	—	—	—	—	—
MALTED MILK														
chocolate as prep w/ milk	1 cup	229	9	6	34	9	30	—	—	304	172	499	16	3
chocolate flavor powder	3 heaping tsp (¾ oz)	79	1	tr	1	1	18	—	—	13	53	130	4	tr
natural flavor as prep w/ milk	1 cup	237	10	6	37	10	27	—	—	354	223	529	22	3
natural flavor powder	3 heaping tsp (¾ oz)	87	2	1	4	2	19	—	—	63	103	159	10	1
CARNATION														
Chocolate	3 tbsp (0.7 oz)	90	1	1	0	1	18	14	tr	0	40	115	—	0
Original	3 tbsp (0.7 oz)	90	2	1	5	3	15	10	tr	40	40	115	—	0
MAMMY-APPLE														
fresh	1	431	4	—	0	4	106	—	—	93	127	398	—	118
MANGO														
fresh	1	135	1	tr	0	1	35	—	—	21	4	322	—	57
DEL MONTE														
In Extra Light Syrup	½ cup (4.4 oz)	100	1	0	0	0	25	20	0	—	5	—	—	42
RAINFOREST FARMS														
Slices Dried	6 slices (1.3 oz)	140	1	0	0	1	33	30	2	0	108	—	—	18
TOMORROW'S TROPICALS														
Fresh	½ (3.6 oz)	70	1	0	0	0	17	15	1	0	0	—	—	9
MANGO JUICE														
CERES														
Mango	8 oz	120	0	0	0	0	30	26	1	20	10	190	—	60
FRESH SAMANTHA														
Mango Mama	1 cup (8 oz)	120	0	0	0	2	10	—	8	0	0	110	32	30

FOOD	PORTION	CALS	FAT	SAT FAT	CHOL	PROT	CARB	SUGAR	FIBER	CALCI	SOD	POTAS	FOLIC	VIT C
GUZZLER														
Mango Passion	8 fl oz	140	0	0	0	0	22	0	—	—	30	—	—	—
LANGERS														
Mongo Mango	8 oz	120	0	0	0	0	30	27	—	—	0	—	—	60
NAKED JUICE														
Mighty Mango	8 oz	120	0	0	0	1	30	18	0	20	15	280	—	162
SNAPPLE														
Mango Madness	8 fl oz	110	0	0	0	0	29	27	—	—	10	—	—	—
TANG														
Drink Mix as prep	1 serv (8 oz)	100	0	0	0	0	25	25	0	40	0	0	—	60
MARGARINE														
squeeze	1 tsp	34	4	1	0	tr	0	—	—	3	37	4	tr	tr
stick corn	1 tsp	34	4	1	0	0	0	—	—	1	44	2	tr	tr
stick corn	1 stick (4 oz)	815	91	15	0	1	1	—	—	34	1070	48	1	tr
tub corn	1 tsp	34	4	1	0	0	0	—	—	1	51	2	tr	tr
tub diet	1 tsp	17	2	tr	0	0	0	—	—	1	46	1	tr	tr
BENECOL														
Single Serve Light	1 pkg (0.3 oz)	30	3	0	0	—	—	—	—	tr	65	2	—	—
Tub Light	1 tbsp (0.5 oz)	45	5	1	0	—	—	—	—	tr	110	4	—	—
Tub Regular	1 tbsp (0.5 oz)	80	9	1	0	—	—	—	—	tr	110	4	—	—
BLUE BONNET														
Light Stick	1 tbsp	50	5	1	0	0	tr	—	—	—	90	—	—	—
Soft Spread	1 tbsp	60	7	2	0	0	0	0	0	—	110	—	—	—
Soft Spread Light	1 tbsp	40	5	1	0	0	tr	—	—	—	90	—	—	—
Stick	1 tbsp	80	9	2	0	0	0	0	0	—	110	—	—	—
BRUMMEL & BROWN														
Spread Make With Yogurt	1 tbsp (0.5 oz)	45	5	1	0	0	0	0	0	—	90	—	—	—
I CAN'T BELIEVE IT'S NOT BUTTER														
Spray	5 sprays	0	0	0	0	0	0	0	0	—	0	—	—	—
PROMISE														
Stick	1 tbsp	90	10	2	0	0	0	0	0	—	65	—	—	—
TAKE CONTROL														
Light	1 tbsp	45	5	1	<5	0	0	0	—	—	85	—	—	—
Spread	1 tbsp (0.5 oz)	80	8	1	<5	0	0	0	0	—	85	—	—	—
WEIGHT WATCHERS														
Light	1 tbsp	45	4	1	0	0	2	0	0	0	70	—	—	0
Light Sodium Free	1 tbsp	45	4	1	0	0	2	0	0	0	0	—	—	0
MARINADE														
(*see* SAUCE)														
MARJORAM														
dried	1 tsp	2	tr	—	0	tr	tr	—	—	12	tr	9	—	—

FOOD	PORTION	CALS	FAT	SAT FAT	CHOL	PROT	CARB	SUGAR	FIBER	CALCI	SOD	POTAS	FOLIC	VIT C
MARLIN														
raw	3 oz	110	3	—	—	20	0	0	0	8	—	—	—	1
MARSHMALLOW														
marshmallow	1 cup (1.6 oz)	146	tr	—	0	1	37	—	—	1	22	2	—	0
marshmallow	1 reg (0.3 oz)	23	0	0	0	tr	6	—	—	0	3	0	0	0
GOL D LITE														
Sugar Free	⅓ pkg (0.9 oz)	51	0	0	0	0	19	0	0	—	0	—	—	—
JUST BORN														
Peeps	5 (1.5 oz)	160	0	0	0	1	40	36	—	—	15	—	—	—
MATZO														
egg	1 (1 oz)	111	1	tr	—	4	22	—	1	11	6	43	—	—
egg & onion	1 (1 oz)	111	1	tr	—	3	22	—	1	10	81	24	3	—
plain	1 (1 oz)	112	tr	tr	0	3	24	—	1	4	0	32	4	0
whole wheat	1 (1 oz)	99	tr	tr	0	4	22	—	3	7	1	89	10	0
EDDYLEON														
Dark Chocolate Coated Egg Matzo	1 oz	97	3	2	8	27	17	16	1	—	7	—	—	—
Milk Chocolate Coated Egg Matzo	1 oz	97	4	3	8	3	16	15	1	20	7	—	—	—
MANISCHEWITZ														
Matzo Meal	¼ cup (1 oz)	130	0	0	0	3	23	1	1	0	0	—	—	0
MAYONNAISE														
mayonnaise	1 tbsp	99	11	2	8	tr	tr	—	—	2	78	5	—	—
mayonnaise	1 cup	1577	175	26	130	2	6	—	—	40	1250	75	—	—
reduced calorie	1 tbsp	34	3	1	4	0	2	—	—	—	75	—	—	—
reduced calorie	1 cup	556	46	8	58	1	38	—	—	—	1193	—	—	—
sandwich spread	1 tbsp	60	5	1	12	tr	3	—	—	—	—	—	—	—
BLUE PLATE														
Squeeze	1 tbsp	100	11	2	10	0	0	0	0	0	80	—	—	0
HELLMAN'S														
Mayonnaise	1 tbsp	100	11	2	5	0	0	—	—	—	80	—	—	—
KRAFT														
Fat Free	1 tbsp (0.6 oz)	10	0	0	0	0	2	1	0	0	120	10	—	0
Light	1 tbsp (0.5 oz)	50	5	1	5	0	2	tr	0	0	90	10	—	0
Real	1 tbsp (0.5 oz)	100	11	2	5	0	0	0	0	0	75	0	—	0
WEIGHT WATCHERS														
Fat Free	1 tbsp	10	0	0	0	0	3	2	0	0	105	—	—	0
Light	1 tbsp	25	2	0	5	0	1	1	0	0	130	—	—	0
Light Low Sodium	1 tbsp	25	2	0	5	0	1	0	0	0	40	—	—	0
MAYONNAISE TYPE SALAD DRESSING														
mayonnaise type salad dressing	1 cup	916	78	12	60	2	56	—	—	33	1670	21	—	—

FOOD	PORTION	CALS	FAT	SAT FAT	CHOL	PROT	CARB	SUGAR	FIBER	CALCI	SOD	POTAS	FOLIC	VIT C
mayonnaise type salad dressing	1 tbsp	57	5	1	4	tr	4	—	—	—	—	—	—	—
reduced calorie w/o cholesterol	1 tbsp	68	7	1	0	7	2	—	—	—	49	—	—	—
reduced calorie w/o cholesterol	1 cup	1084	107	17	0	tr	36	—	—	—	794	—	—	—
CARB OPTIONS														
Whipped Dressing	1 tbsp	50	5	1	5	0	0	0	0	—	105	—	—	—
MIRACLE WHIP														
Free	1 tbsp (0.5 oz)	15	0	0	0	0	2	2	0	0	125	10	—	0
Light	1 tbsp (0.5 oz)	35	3	0	<5	0	2	2	0	0	130	0	—	0
Salad Dressing	1 tbsp (0.6 oz)	70	7	1	5	0	2	1	0	0	95	0	—	0
NASOYA														
Nayonnaise	1 tbsp	35	4	1	0	0	1	tr	0	—	115	—	—	—
Nayonnaise Dijon	1 tbsp	30	3	1	0	0	1	0	0	—	140	—	—	—
WEIGHT WATCHERS														
Fat Free Whipped Dressing	1 tbsp	15	0	0	0	0	3	2	0	0	95	—	—	0
MEAT STICKS														
jerky beef	1 oz	96	4	1	32	11	4	—	—	—	815	—	—	—
jerky beef	1 lg piece (0.7 oz)	67	3	1	22	8	3	—	—	—	569	—	—	—
smoked	1 (0.7 oz)	109	10	4	26	4	1	—	—	13	293	—	0	—
smoked	1 oz	156	14	6	38	6	2	—	—	19	420	—	0	—
BIG ONES														
BBQ	1 (1 oz)	130	12	5	35	5	1	1	0	0	680	—	—	0
Hot n'Spicy	1 (1 oz)	130	12	5	35	6	1	1	0	0	580	—	—	0
Original	1 (1 oz)	130	12	5	35	5	1	1	0	0	620	—	—	0
Teriyaki	1 (1 oz)	130	12	5	35	6	2	2	0	0	440	—	—	0
JACK LINK'S														
Kippered Beefsteak Teriyaki	1 oz	80	1	1	25	13	5	4	0	20	440	—	—	0
LANCE														
Beef & Cheese	1 pkg (1.5 oz)	150	11	6	45	9	3	0	0	150	630	—	—	0
Beef Jerky	1 piece (0.25 oz)	30	2	1	<5	2	tr	0	0	0	160	45	—	0
Beef Snack	1 piece (0.63 oz)	100	8	4	10	4	1	0	0	0	290	65	—	0
Hot Sausage	1 piece (0.9 oz)	60	5	2	15	4	1	1	0	0	540	10	—	0
LOWREY'S														
Smokehouse Tender Hickory Smoked	1 pkg (1 oz)	80	2	1	25	10	5	4	0	0	710	—	—	0
Smokehouse Tender Original	1 pkg (1 oz)	60	1	0	25	11	2	1	1	0	750	—	—	0

FOOD	PORTION	CALS	FAT	SAT FAT	CHOL	PROT	CARB	SUGAR	FIBER	CALCI	SOD	POTAS	FOLIC	VIT C
LOWREY'S (CONT.)														
Smokehouse Tender Peppered	1 pkg (1 oz)	60	1	0	25	11	2	1	1	0	720	—	—	0
OBERTO														
Beef Jerky	1 pkg (1.3 oz)	100	1	0	25	15	8	9	—	—	780	—	—	—
PEMMICAN														
Original Tender Kippered Beef Steak	1	110	5	3	35	12	3	0	0	0	1100	—	—	0
Peppered Tender Kippered Beef Steak	1	110	5	3	35	12	3	0	0	0	1170	—	—	0
ROUGH CUT														
Beef Steak Hot	1 pkg (1 oz)	70	1	0	25	10	2	2	0	0	710	—	—	0
Beef Steak Original	1 pkg (1 oz)	60	1	0	25	10	2	2	0	0	730	—	—	0
Beef Steak Peppered	1 pkg (1 oz)	60	1	0	25	10	2	1	0	0	740	—	—	0
RUSTLERS ROUNDUP														
Beef Jerky	1 serv (5 g)	20	2	1	5	2	tr	0	tr	—	115	—	—	—
Flamin' Hot	1 serv (8 g)	40	3	2	10	2	1	tr	tr	—	140	—	—	—
Smoky Steak	1 serv (0.8 oz)	60	2	1	20	8	1	tr	0	—	580	—	—	—
Spicy	1 serv (0.5 oz)	70	6	3	20	3	1	0	tr	—	250	—	—	—
SLIM JIM														
Spicy	1 (4½ in) (0.3 oz)	50	4	2	5	2	0	0	0	0	125	—	—	0
Spicy Big	1 (.44 oz)	70	6	3	10	1	1	0	0	0	190	—	—	0
Spicy Giant	1 (0.97 oz)	150	14	6	15	6	2	0	1	0	410	—	—	0
Spicy Super	1 (0.64 oz)	100	9	4	10	4	1	0	0	0	260	—	—	0
MEAT SUBSTITUTES														
simulated meat product	1 oz	88	1	tr	0	11	11	—	—	57	3	—	—	—
BOCA BURGERS														
Chef Max's Original	1 patty (2.5 oz)	110	2	1	3	14	9	0	4	—	296	316	—	—
FRIEDA'S														
Soyrizo	4 tbsp (1.9 oz)	120	9	1	0	7	5	2	3	60	440	—	—	1
SoyTaco	1 oz	50	3	1	0	4	3	0	2	40	180	—	—	1
KEN & ROBERT'S														
Veggie Pockets	1 (4.5 oz)	250	8	1	0	8	40	3	5	20	490	—	—	5
Veggie Pockets Bar B Que	1 (4.5 oz)	290	8	1	0	10	45	2	5	40	450	—	—	5
Veggie Pockets Broccoli & Cheddar	1 (4.5 oz)	250	8	0	0	9	38	2	4	40	490	—	—	18
Veggie Pockets Greek	1 (4.5 oz)	250	8	0	0	10	37	2	4	60	450	—	—	9

FOOD	PORTION	CALS	FAT	SAT FAT	CHOL	PROT	CARB	SUGAR	FIBER	CALCI	SOD	POTAS	FOLIC	VIT C
KEN & ROBERT'S (CONT.)														
Veggie Pockets Indian	1 (4.5 oz)	260	8	1	0	8	40	2	5	20	490	—	—	6
Veggie Pockets Pizza	1 (4.5 oz)	270	8	1	0	9	41	2	4	40	490	—	—	6
Veggie Pockets Pot Pie	1 (4.5 oz)	250	9	1	0	8	38	2	2	20	410	—	—	2
Veggie Pockets Potato & Cheddar	1 (4.5 oz)	260	8	1	0	6	42	2	2	20	370	—	—	5
Veggie Pockets Santa Fe	1 (4.5 oz)	250	8	1	0	8	39	2	5	20	550	—	—	6
Veggie Pockets Tex Mex	1 (4.5 oz)	260	8	1	0	9	46	2	6	40	490	—	—	5
LIGHTLIFE														
Foney Baloney	3 slices (1.5 oz)	60	3	1	0	8	2	0	0	—	240	—	—	
Gimme Lean Beef	2 oz	70	0	0	0	9	8	1	1	—	240	—	—	—
Smart Deli Bologna	3 slices (1.5 oz)	50	0	0	0	10	2	0	0	—	300	—	—	—
Smart Deli Ham	3 slices (1.5 oz)	50	0	0	0	10	2	0	0	—	300	—	—	—
Smart Deli Peppercorn	3 slices (1.5 oz)	45	0	0	0	10	1	0	0	—	300	—	—	—
Smart Deli Sticks Soylami	1 oz	40	0	0	0	9	1	0	0	—	280	—	—	—
Smart Deli Sticks Pepperoni	1 oz	45	0	0	0	9	2	1	0	—	300	—	—	—
Smart Ground Original	⅓ cup (1.9 oz)	70	0	0	0	12	5	1	3	—	180	—	—	—
Smart Ground Taco	⅓ cup (2 oz)	60	0	0	0	10	6	0	3	—	170	—	—	—
LOMA LINDA														
Dinner Cuts	2 slices (3.2 oz)	90	2	1	0	17	3	0	2	0	500	40	—	0
Nuteena	⅜ in slice (1.9 oz)	160	13	5	0	6	6	tr	2	0	120	170	—	0
Sandwich Spread	¼ cup (1.9 oz)	80	5	1	0	4	7	tr	3	20	260	140	—	0
Savory Dinner Loaf Mix not prep	⅓ cup (0.9 oz)	90	2	0	0	14	7	0	5	20	560	410	—	0
Swiss Stake	1 piece (3.2 oz)	120	6	1	0	9	8	tr	4	20	430	230	—	0
Tender Bits	6 pieces (3 oz)	110	5	1	0	11	7	0	3	0	440	55	—	0
Tender Rounds	6 pieces (2.8 oz)	120	5	1	0	14	5	tr	3	0	330	70	—	0
Vita Burger Chunks not prep	¼ cup (0.7 oz)	70	1	0	0	10	6	1	3	40	350	500	—	0
Vita Burger Granules	3 tbsp (0.7 oz)	70	1	0	0	10	6	1	3	40	350	500	—	0
MORNINGSTAR FARMS														
Burger Style Recipe Crumbles	⅔ cup (1.9 oz)	80	3	0	0	10	4	tr	2	20	210	120	—	0

FOOD	PORTION	CALS	FAT	SAT FAT	CHOL	PROT	CARB	SUGAR	FIBER	CALCI	SOD	POTAS	FOLIC	VIT C
MORNINGSTAR FARMS (CONT.)														
Ground Meatless	½ cup (1.9 oz)	60	0	0	0	10	4	0	2	20	260	100	—	0
Harvest Burger Recipe Crumbles	½ cup (2 oz)	70	0	0	0	12	5	0	3	60	200	460	—	0
Quarter Prime	1 patty (3.4 oz)	140	2	0	0	24	6	1	3	60	370	210	—	9
NATURAL TOUCH														
Dinner Entree	1 patty (3 oz)	220	15	3	0	19	2	0	2	40	380	100	—	0
Loaf Mix not prep	4 tbsp (1 oz)	100	1	0	0	14	10	tr	7	40	700	410	—	0
Stroganoff Mix not prep	4 tbsp (0.8 oz)	90	4	2	10	5	10	1	3	60	610	230	—	0
Taco Mix not prep	3 tbsp (0.6 oz)	60	1	0	0	8	5	tr	3	20	590	380	—	0
Vegan Burger Crumbles	½ cup (1.9 oz)	60	0	0	0	10	4	0	2	20	260	100	—	0
QUORN														
Grounds	⅔ cup (3 oz)	80	3	1	0	13	5	1	4	20	220	—	—	0
SOY7														
Burger Bits as prep	½ cup	60	1	0	0	9	5	tr	2	—	340	—	—	—
Burger Mix as prep	1 serv (3.2 oz)	120	3	0	0	16	9	tr	3	—	400	—	—	—
Recipe Strips as prep	¾ cup	70	1	1	0	11	7	tr	3	—	340	—	—	—
Taco Mix as prep	¼ cup	70	1	0	0	11	6	1	3	—	100	—	—	—
WORTHINGTON														
Beef Style Meatless	⅜ in slice (1.9 oz)	110	7	1	0	9	4	tr	3	0	620	45	—	0
Bolono	3 slices (2 oz)	80	4	1	0	10	2	0	2	40	720	120	—	0
Choplets	2 slices (3.2 oz)	90	2	1	0	17	3	0	2	0	500	40	—	0
Corned Beef Meatless	4 slices (2 oz)	140	9	2	0	10	5	tr	2	0	520	60	—	0
Country Stew	1 cup (8.4 oz)	210	9	2	0	13	20	2	5	60	830	270	—	0
Dinner Roast	¾ in slice (3 oz)	180	12	2	<5	12	5	1	3	40	580	55	—	0
FriPats	1 patty (2.2 oz)	130	6	1	0	14	4	0	3	60	320	125	—	0
Multigrain Cutlets	2 slices (3.2 oz)	100	2	1	0	15	5	0	4	0	390	30	—	0
Numete	⅜ in slice (1.9 oz)	130	10	3	0	6	5	tr	3	0	270	160	—	0
Prime Stakes	1 piece (3.2 oz)	120	7	1	0	10	4	0	4	0	440	80	—	0
Prosage Roll	⅝ in slice (1.9 oz)	140	10	2	0	10	2	0	2	0	390	80	—	0
Protose	⅜ in slice (1.9 oz)	130	7	1	0	13	5	tr	3	0	280	50	—	0
Salami Meatless	3 slices (2 oz)	130	8	1	0	12	2	0	2	20	930	95	—	0
Savory Slices	3 slices (2.9 oz)	150	9	4	0	10	6	0	3	0	540	40	—	0
Smoked Beef Meatless	6 slices (2 oz)	120	6	1	0	11	6	1	3	0	730	150	—	0
Stakelets	1 piece (2.5 oz)	140	8	2	0	12	6	0	2	40	480	95	—	0

FOOD	PORTION	CALS	FAT	SAT FAT	CHOL	PROT	CARB	SUGAR	FIBER	CALCI	SOD	POTAS	FOLIC	VIT C
WORTHINGTON (CONT.)														
Veelets	1 patty (2.5 oz)	180	9	2	0	14	10	tr	5	40	390	120	—	0
Vegetable Skallops	½ cup (3 oz)	90	2	1	0	15	3	0	2	0	410	10	—	0
Vegetable Steaks	2 pieces (2.5 oz)	80	2	1	0	15	3	0	3	0	300	20	—	0
Wham	2 slices (1.6 oz)	80	5	1	0	7	1	1	0	0	430	90	—	0
YVES														
Veggie Bologna	4 slices (2.2 oz)	70	0	0	0	15	2	1	0	20	460	—	—	0
Veggie Ground Italian	⅓ cup (2 oz)	60	0	0	0	10	4	0	3	40	270	240	—	0
Veggie Ground Round Italian	⅓ cup (1.9 oz)	60	0	0	0	10	4	0	3	40	270	240	—	0
Veggie Ground Round Original	2 oz	60	0	0	0	10	4	0	3	40	270	240	—	0
Veggie Pizza Pepperoni Slices	1 serv (1.7 oz)	70	0	0	0	14	4	0	3	40	480	140	—	0
Veggie Salami Deli Slices	1 serv (2.2 oz)	90	0	0	0	17	5	1	1	40	390	150	—	0
MELON														
melon balls frzn	1 cup	55	tr	—	0	1	14	—	—	17	53	484	45	11
SUNFRESH														
Melon Salad In Extra Light Syrup	½ cup (4.5 oz)	45	0	0	0	0	10	8	2	0	15	—	—	30
MEXICAN FOOD														
(see SALSA, SPANISH FOOD, TORTILLA)														
MILK														
CANNED														
condensed sweetened	1 oz	123	3	2	13	3	21	—	—	108	49	142	4	1
condensed sweetened	1 cup	982	27	17	104	24	166	—		868	389	1136	34	8
evaporated	½ cup	169	10	6	37	9	13	—	—	329	122	382	10	2
evaporated skim	½ cup	99	tr	tr	5	10	14	—	—	369	147	423	11	2
CARNATION														
Evaporated	2 tbsp	40	2	2	10	2	3	3	—	80	30	90	—	—
Evaporated Fat Free	2 tbsp	25	0	0	0	2	4	4	—	80	40	110	—	—
Sweetened Condensed	⅓ cup	330	8	5	10	3	22	22	0	250	45	—	—	—
PET														
Evaporated	2 tbsp	40	2	2	10	2	3	3	—	80	30	—	—	—
DRIED														
buttermilk	1 tbsp	25	tr	tr	5	2	3	—	—	77	34	103	3	tr
nonfat instantized	1 pkg (3.2 oz)	244	tr	tr	12	32	47	—	—	837	499	1552	45	5
CARNATION														
Nonfat	⅓ cup	80	0	0	<5	8	12	12	0	300	125	390	—	1

FOOD	PORTION	CALS	FAT	SAT FAT	CHOL	PROT	CARB	SUGAR	FIBER	CALCI	SOD	POTAS	FOLIC	VIT C
SACO														
Cultured Buttermilk	4 tbsp (0.8 oz)	80	tr	0	4	5	13	12	0	220	166	—	—	1
SANALAC														
Powder	¼ cup (0.8 oz)	85	tr	0	6	8	13	12	0	302	117	—	—	2
REFRIGERATED														
1%	1 cup	102	3	2	10	8	12	—	—	300	123	381	12	2
1%	1 qt	409	10	6	39	32	47	—	—	1200	493	1524	50	9
1% protein fortified	1 qt	477	12	7	39	39	54	—	—	1397	574	1774	58	11
1% protein fortified	1 cup	119	3	2	10	10	14	—	—	349	143	444	15	3
2%	1 cup	121	5	3	18	8	12	—	—	297	122	377	12	2
2%	1 qt	485	19	12	73	33	47	—	—	1187	487	1507	50	9
buffalo	7 oz	224	16	—	—	8	10	—	—	390	80	200	—	6
buttermilk	1 cup	99	2	1	9	8	12	—	—	285	257	371	—	2
buttermilk	1 qt	396	9	5	34	32	47	—	—	1141	1028	1483	—	10
camel	7 oz	160	8	—	—	10	10	—	—	264	60	188	—	—
donkey	7 oz	86	2	—	—	4	12	—	—	220	—	—	—	4
goat	1 cup	168	10	7	28	9	11	—	—	326	122	499	1	3
goat	1 qt	672	40	26	111	35	43	—	—	1303	486	1995	6	13
human	1 cup	171	11	5	34	3	17	—	—	79	42	126	13	12
indian buffalo	1 cup	236	17	11	46	9	13	—	—	412	127	434	14	5
low sodium	1 cup	149	8	5	33	8	11	—	—	246	6	617	—	—
mare	7 oz	98	4	—	—	4	12	—	—	220	—	128	—	30
nonfat	1 cup	86	tr	tr	4	8	12	—	—	302	125	406	13	2
nonfat protein fortified	1 qt	400	2	2	20	39	55	—	—	1407	578	1786	59	11
sheep	1 cup	264	17	11	—	15	13	—	—	474	108	334	—	10
whole	1 cup	150	8	5	33	8	11	—	—	291	120	370	12	2
BORDEN														
Fat Free Skim	1 cup	80	0	0	5	8	12	11	0	300	125	—	—	2
COOL COW														
Low Fat	1 cup (8 oz)	110	3	1	<5	9	12	12	0	300	125	—	—	2
FARMLAND														
Skim Plus	1 cup (8 oz)	110	0	0	<5	11	17	16	0	400	170	—	—	4
HOOD														
Carb Countdown	8 oz	138	8	5	35	12	3	3	0	350	210	—	—	0
Carb Countdown 2%	8 oz	100	5	3	20	12	3	2	0	350	210	—	—	0
Carb Countdown Fat Free	8 oz	78	0	0	<5	12	3	3	0	350	210	—	—	0
HORIZON ORGANIC														
Fat Free	1 cup (8 oz)	80	0	0	4	8	12	11	0	300	125	—	—	2

FOOD	PORTION	CALS	FAT	SAT FAT	CHOL	PROT	CARB	SUGAR	FIBER	CALCI	SOD	POTAS	FOLIC	VIT C
LAND O LAKES														
1% Lowfat	1 carton (10 oz)	120	3	2	15	10	13	13	—	300	135	—	—	2
Fat Free	1 carton (10 oz)	100	5	0	5	10	13	13	—	300	140	—	—	2
Whole	1 carton (10 oz)	180	10	7	45	10	13	13	—	300	135	—	—	2
NUTRABALANCE														
LactaCare	1 pkg (8 oz)	500	18	—	0	18	64	—	—	572	240	780	120	20
ORGANIC VALLEY														
Low Fat	1 cup	100	3	2	10	8	12	12	0	300	120	—	—	2
Nonfat	1 cup	80	0	0	5	8	13	12	0	300	125	—	—	2
Reduced Fat	1 cup	130	5	3	20	8	12	11	0	300	120	—	—	2
Whole	1 cup	150	8	5	30	8	12	11	0	300	120	—	—	2
STONYFIELD FARM														
Organic Whole Milk	1 cup (8 oz)	180	10	6	40	9	12	12	0	540	125	447	—	2
Organic Whole Milk Vanilla	1 cup (8 oz)	230	8	5	30	8	30	30	0	450	130	439	—	2
TURKEY HILL														
Cool Moos 2% Reduced Fat	1 cup	130	5	3	20	8	12	11	—	—	120	—	—	1
Cool Moos Whole Milk	1 cup	160	8	5	35	8	12	11	—	—	120	—	—	2

MILK DRINKS

FOOD	PORTION	CALS	FAT	SAT FAT	CHOL	PROT	CARB	SUGAR	FIBER	CALCI	SOD	POTAS	FOLIC	VIT C
chocolate milk	1 cup	208	8	5	30	8	26	—	—	280	149	417	12	2
chocolate milk	1 qt	833	34	21	122	32	103	—	—	1121	596	1669	47	9
chocolate milk 1%	1 cup	158	3	2	7	8	26	—	—	287	152	426	12	2
chocolate milk 1%	1 qt	630	10	6	29	32	104	—	—	1147	607	1702	48	9
chocolate milk 2%	1 cup	179	5	3	17	8	26	—	—	284	150	422	12	2
strawberry flavor mix as prep w/ whole milk	9 oz	234	8	5	33	8	33	—	—	292	128	370	12	2
COCIO														
Chocolate Milk	1 bottle	225	7	—	25	9	32	28	tr	390	130	—	—	5
GARELICK														
Colossal Coffee	1 cup	145	3	2	15	8	23	22	0	300	125	—	—	2
Ultimate Chocolate	1 cup	150	3	2	15	8	29	27	1	300	210	—	—	2
HERSHEY'S														
Chocolate Milk Fat Free	1 bottle	160	0	0	5	10	31	30	tr	500	150	—	—	—
Chocolate Milk Reduced Fat	1 bottle	200	5	3	20	8	31	28	1	500	135	—	—	—

FOOD	PORTION	CALS	FAT	SAT FAT	CHOL	PROT	CARB	SUGAR	FIBER	CALCI	SOD	POTAS	FOLIC	VIT C
HOOD														
Carb Countdown Chocolate Milk	8 oz	100	5	3	25	12	3	2	1	350	350	—	—	0
HORIZON ORGANIC														
Lowfat Chocolate Milk	1 cup (8 oz)	160	3	2	10	9	26	24	1	300	200	—	—	2
KETO														
Chocolate Milk Mix	1 scoop	36	1	—	—	8	3	0	1	—	80	—	—	—
LAND O LAKES														
Chocolate	1 cup (8.4 oz)	200	7	5	30	8	27	26	0	500	180	—	—	2
NESQUIK														
Chocolate Milk Reduced Fat	1 cup	200	5	3	15	8	32	30	tr	400	150	—	—	1
ORGANIC VALLEY														
Chocolate Milk Reduced Fat	1 cup	180	5	3	10	8	26	25	0	300	190	—	—	4
QUIK														
Banana Lowfat	1 cup (8.4 oz)	200	5	3	20	7	31	30	0	250	95	350	—	0
Banana Powder	2 tbsp (0.8 oz)	90	0	0	0	0	27	20	0	0	0	0	—	0
Chocolate	1 cup (8.4 oz)	230	8	5	30	7	33	30	1	250	130	400	—	0
Chocolate Lowfat	1 carton (8.4 oz)	200	5	3	20	8	30	29	0	250	130	440	—	0
Cookies n Cream Powder	2 tbsp (0.8 oz)	100	1	1	0	1	21	14	1	0	190	0	—	0
Strawberry	1 cup (8.4 oz)	230	8	5	30	7	33	30	0	250	100	330	—	0
Strawberry Lowfat	1 carton (8.4 oz)	210	5	3	20	8	35	35	0	250	100	330	—	0
Strawberry Powder	2 tbsp (0.8 oz)	90	0	0	0	0	22	21	0	0	0	0	—	0
ROSA'S ORIGINAL														
Horchata All Flavors	8 oz	160	2	—	5	3	32	29	0	—	60	—	—	—
TURKEY HILL														
Cool Moos Chocolate 1% Lowfat	1 cup	180	3	2	10	8	32	30	—	—	180	—	—	1
Cool Moos Orange Cream 1% Lowfat	1 cup	190	3	2	10	8	33	32	—	—	135	—	—	36
Cool Moos Strawberry 1% Lowfat	1 cup	160	3	2	10	8	27	27	—	—	125	—	—	2
Cool Moos Vanilla 1% Lowfat	1 cup	160	3	2	10	8	26	25	—	—	125	—	—	2

MILK SUBSTITUTES

FOOD	PORTION	CALS	FAT	SAT FAT	CHOL	PROT	CARB	SUGAR	FIBER	CALCI	SOD	POTAS	FOLIC	VIT C
imitation milk	1 cup	150	8	2	tr	4	15	—	—	79	191	279	0	0
imitation milk	1 qt	600	33	7	2	17	60	—	—	317	764	1116	0	0
8TH CONTINENT														
Soymilk Low Fat Chocolate	1 bottle (8 oz)	140	3	1	0	7	23	21	1	300	190	—	—	0
Soymilk Low Fat Original	1 bottle (8 oz)	80	3	0	0	7	8	6	tr	300	170	—	—	0
Soymilk Low Fat Vanilla	1 bottle (8 oz)	90	3	0	0	7	11	10	tr	300	170	—	—	0
BETTER THAN MILK														
Rice Original	2 tbsp (0.66 oz)	78	2	tr	0	0	15	4	1	300	150	6	—	6
Rice Original Light	2 tbsp (0.66 oz)	66	0	0	0	0	17	4	1	300	144	11	—	0
Rice Vanilla	2 tbsp (0.66 oz)	78	2	tr	0	0	15	5	1	300	118	5	—	6
Rice Vanilla Light	2 tbsp (0.66 oz)	66	0	0	0	0	17	5	1	300	141	10	—	0
Soy Carob	2 tbsp (1 oz)	90	2	tr	0	3	18	9	2	300	165	186	—	6
Soy Chocolate	2 tbsp (1.1 oz)	112	2	tr	0	3	21	19	1	300	146	287	—	6
Soy Light	2 tbsp (0.66 oz)	73	2	tr	0	6	8	5	1	300	139	122	—	6
Soy Original	2 tbsp (0.8 oz)	100	3	0	0	2	16	5	0	80	100	250	—	0
Soy Vanilla	2 tbsp (0.7 oz)	77	2	tr	0	6	8	6	1	300	178	164	—	6
BLUE DIAMOND														
Almond Breeze Chocolate	8 oz	120	3	0	0	1	21	20	1	200	160	180	—	0
Almond Breeze Original	8 oz	60	2	0	0	1	8	7	1	200	150	145	—	0
Almond Breeze Vanilla	8 oz	90	3	0	0	1	15	15	1	200	150	150	—	0
EDENBLEND														
Organic	8 oz	120	3	1	0	7	18	8	0	13	85	270	28	0
EDENSOY														
Organic Light	8 oz	93	2	tr	0	5	14	5	0	80	84	215	48	0
Organic Light Vanilla	8 oz	120	2	tr	0	4	21	10	0	75	87	196	69	0
GALAXY														
Veggie Milk Chocolate	1 cup (8 oz)	150	2	0	0	9	26	20	1	400	130	—	100	5
Veggie Milk Original	1 cup (8 oz)	110	3	0	0	9	13	8	2	400	130	—	100	5
HANSEN'S														
Soy Smoothie Lemon Chiffon	8 oz	150	0	0	0	5	33	32	tr	300	41	73	—	60
Soy Smoothie Orange Dream	8 oz	150	0	0	0	5	31	31	tr	300	41	73	—	60
HARMONY FARMS														
Original Rice Beverage	1 cup (8 oz)	90	0	0	0	13	21	14	0	20	100	60	—	0

FOOD	PORTION	CALS	FAT	SAT FAT	CHOL	PROT	CARB	SUGAR	FIBER	CALCI	SOD	POTAS	FOLIC	VIT C
HARMONY HOUSE														
Enriched Rice Beverage	1 cup (8 oz)	90	0	0	0	1	21	14	0	400	100	60	—	15
Enriched Soy Beverage	1 cup (8 oz)	90	0	0	0	13	21	14	0	20	100	60	—	0
Original Soy Beverage	1 cup (8 oz)	90	0	0	0	13	21	14	0	20	100	60	—	0
HEALTH VALLEY														
Soo Moo	1 cup	110	0	—	0	6	22	17	1	40	60	—	—	0
KETO														
Low Carb Mix	1 scoop	54	2	—	30	8	1	—	—	—	80	—	—	—
NUTRABALANCE														
NuTaste	1 pkg (8 oz)	80	2	tr	0	8	7	—	8	300	210	46	—	2
RICE DREAM														
Carob	1 box (8 oz)	150	3	0	0	1	32	24	0	20	100	83	—	1
Chocolate	1 box (8 oz)	170	3	0	0	1	36	25	2	20	115	126	—	1
Chocolate Enriched	1 box (8 oz)	170	3	0	0	1	36	25	0	300	115	—	—	1
Organic Original	1 box (8 oz)	120	2	0	0	1	25	11	0	20	90	54	—	0
Organic Original Enriched	1 box (8 oz)	120	2	0	0	1	25	11	0	300	90	60	—	0
Vanilla	1 box (8 oz)	130	2	0	0	1	28	12	0	20	90	57	—	0
Vanilla Enriched	1 box (8 oz)	130	2	0	0	1	28	12	0	300	90	—	—	0
SILK														
Chocolate	1 cup	140	4	0	0	5	23	19	0	300	75	100	24	0
Organic Plain	1 cup	100	4	0	0	7	8	4	0	300	75	80	24	0
Vanilla	1 bottle (11 oz)	140	5	1	0	8	14	8	0	400	130	110	32	0
SOY DREAM														
Carob	8 oz	210	5	1	—	7	36	22	—	40	150	290	60	0
Chocolate Enriched	8 oz	210	5	1	—	7	35	22	—	300	150	370	60	0
Original	8 oz	140	5	1	—	8	14	8	—	40	140	270	80	0
Original Enriched	8 oz	140	5	1	—	8	14	8	—	300	140	270	80	0
Vanilla	8 oz	170	5	1	—	8	23	18	—	40	140	290	80	0
Vanilla Enriched	8 oz	140	5	1	—	8	23	18	—	300	160	270	80	0
TREE OF LIFE														
Original Rice Beverage	1 cup	90	0	0	0	13	21	14	0	20	100	60	—	0
VITAMITE														
Non-Dairy	1 cup (8 oz)	110	5	2	0	3	14	4	0	300	120	170	—	0
VITASOY														
1% Low Fat Vanilla Delight	8 oz	90	2	0	0	4	13	9	0	300	120	—	—	0
Carob Supreme	8 fl oz	150	5	1	0	8	20	12	tr	40	180	—	—	0
Creamy Unsweetened	8 oz	80	4	1	0	6	5	1	0	20	150	—	—	0

FOOD	PORTION	CALS	FAT	SAT FAT	CHOL	PROT	CARB	SUGAR	FIBER	CALCI	SOD	POTAS	FOLIC	VIT C
VITASOY (CONT.)														
Creamy Original	8 fl oz	110	5	1	0	9	9	4	1	20	150	—	—	0
Enriched Light Original	8 fl oz	60	2	1	0	4	7	4	0	300	115	—	—	0
Enriched Light Vanilla	8 fl oz	90	2	1	0	4	13	10	0	300	105	—	—	0
Green Tea Soymilk	8 oz	130	4	1	0	7	16	7	1	40	180	—	—	0
Original Creamy	8 fl oz	110	4	1	0	7	12	5	1	300	140	—	—	0
Original Light	8 fl oz	60	2	1	0	4	7	4	0	200	115	—	—	0
Rich Chocolate	8 fl oz	160	4	1	0	7	24	16	1	300	180	—	—	0
Rich Cocoa	8 fl oz	150	5	1	0	8	21	10	1	40	180	—	—	0
Vanilla Light	8 fl oz	90	2	1	0	4	14	10	0	20	110	—	—	0
Vanilla Delite	8 fl oz	120	4	1	0	7	14	9	1	20	115	—	—	0
WHITE WAVE														
Mocha	1 cup	140	4	0	0	6	20	15	1	200	50	—	—	0
MILKFISH														
baked	3 oz	162	7	—	57	22	0	—	—	56	—	—	—	—
MILKSHAKE														
chocolate	10 oz	360	11	7	37	10	58	—	—	319	273	567	10	1
strawberry	10 oz	319	8	—	31	10	53	—	—	320	234	516	9	2
thick shake chocolate	10.6 oz	356	8	5	32	9	63	—	—	396	333	672	15	0
thick shake vanilla	11 oz	350	10	6	37	12	56	—	—	457	299	572	21	0
vanilla	10 oz	314	8	5	32	10	51	—	—	344	232	492	9	2
BREYERS														
Quick Vanilla	1 serv (10 oz)	320	17	11	45	6	37	36	0	200	95	—	—	1
CARB OPTIONS														
Chocolate Delite	1 can (11 oz)	190	9	2	15	20	6	1	4	350	200	480	120	60
Creamy Vanilla	1 can (11 oz)	190	9	2	15	20	6	1	4	350	200	350	120	60
HERSHEY'S														
Chocolate	1 bottle	270	8	5	20	10	43	41	tr	350	140	—	—	—
Cookies 'N' Cream	1 bottle	280	7	5	20	10	45	44	0	350	180	—	—	—
Strawberry	1 bottle	280	7	5	20	7	47	46	10	250	180	—	—	0
Vanilla Cream	1 bottle	320	7	5	20	9	55	44	0	350	240	—	—	—
MILLET														
cooked	1 cup (6.1 oz)	207	2	tr	0	6	41	—	2	5	3	108	33	0
MISO														
dried	1 oz	86	3	—	—	7	10	—	1	51	2130	219	—	0
miso	½ cup	284	8	1	0	16	39	—	7	92	5036	226	46	0
EDEN														
Organic Genmai	1 tbsp	25	1	0	0	2	3	1	tr	0	810	80	0	0
Tekka	1 tsp	5	0	0	0	tr	tr	0	0	4	70	17	—	0

FOOD	PORTION	CALS	FAT	SAT FAT	CHOL	PROT	CARB	SUGAR	FIBER	CALCI	SOD	POTAS	FOLIC	VIT C
MOLASSES														
blackstrap	1 cup (11.5 oz)	771	tr	—	0	0	199	—	—	2821	180	8174	2	—
blackstrap	1 tbsp (0.7 oz)	47	0	0	0	0	12	—	—	172	11	498	0	—
molasses	1 cup (11.5 oz)	873	1	—	0	0	226	195	—	671	120	4802	1	—
molasses	1 tbsp (0.7 oz)	53	0	0	0	0	14	12	—	41	7	293	0	—
BRER RABBIT														
Dark	1 tbsp	60	0	0	0	0	16	13	—	20	30	231	—	—
MOTT'S														
Sulphured	1 tbsp	50	0	0	0	0	12	—	—	—	10	—	—	—
Unsulphured	1 tbsp	50	0	0	0	0	14	—	—	—	0	—	—	—
MONKFISH														
baked	3 oz	82	2	—	27	16	0	—	—	7	20	—	—	—
MOOSE														
roasted	3 oz	114	1	tr	66	25	0	—	—	5	58	284	—	4
MOTH BEANS														
dried cooked	1 cup	207	1	tr	0	14	37	—	—	6	17	538	—	2
MOUSSE														
FROZEN														
SARA LEE														
Chocolate	⅕ pkg (4.3 oz)	400	25	20	30	5	37	27	2	60	190	—	—	0
WEIGHT WATCHERS														
Chocolate Mousse	1 (2.75 oz)	190	5	2	5	6	31	14	3	100	150	—	—	0
TAKE-OUT														
chocolate	½ cup (7.1 oz)	447	33	19	299	9	33	—	—	202	87	296	—	—
orange	½ cup	87	5	—	1	3	19	—	—	71	24	—	—	—
MUFFINS														
FROZEN														
PEPPERIDGE FARM														
Blueberry	1 (2 oz)	180	7	1	30	2	28	12	0	20	260	—	—	0
Bran w/ Raisins	1 (2 oz)	180	6	1	25	4	30	17	0	60	310	—	—	0
Corn	1 (2 oz)	190	7	1	30	3	28	8	0	20	270	—	—	0
Orange Cranberry	1 (2 oz)	180	6	1	36	2	29	12	0	20	190	—	—	0
SARA LEE														
Blueberry	1 (2.2 oz)	220	11	2	15	3	27	12	tr	20	170	—	—	1
Corn	1 (2.2 oz)	260	14	3	25	3	30	14	1	20	220	—	—	0
WEIGHT WATCHERS														
Chocolate Chocolate Chip	1 (2.5 oz)	190	2	1	0	3	39	14	4	80	350	—	—	0
Fat Free Banana	1 (2.5 oz)	170	0	0	0	3	41	17	3	80	310	—	—	0
Fat Free Blueberry	1 (2.5 oz)	160	0	0	0	3	38	15	2	60	290	—	—	0

FOOD	PORTION	CALS	FAT	SAT FAT	CHOL	PROT	CARB	SUGAR	FIBER	CALCI	SOD	POTAS	FOLIC	VIT C
MIX														
blueberry	1 (1¼ oz)	149	4	1	23	3	24	—	—	13	219	39	—	—
corn	1 (1.75 oz)	160	5	1	31	4	25	—	—	37	397	65	6	tr
wheat bran as prep	1 (1¼ oz)	138	5	1	34	5	23	—	—	16	233	73	—	0
BETTY CROCKER														
Apple Cinnamon as prep	1	170	7	2	36	1	23	11	—	20	200	15	24	—
Apple Streusel as prep	1	210	8	1	18	2	33	18	—	200	210	30	24	—
Banana Nut as prep	1	170	6	1	18	2	27	12	1	200	240	40	24	—
Cranberry Orange as prep	1	150	5	1	18	2	25	12	—	200	150	—	16	—
Double Chocolate as prep	1	220	11	4	27	2	30	26	—	200	210	—	16	—
Golden Corn as prep	1	160	5	1	36	2	24	6	—	20	210	25	64	—
Lemon Poppyseed as prep	1	180	8	1	36	1	24	13	—	40	180	25	24	—
Sunkist Lemon Poppyseed as prep	1	190	7	1	18	2	29	14	—	200	230	25	24	—
Twice The Blueberries as prep	1	140	3	1	18	2	25	12	1	200	180	20	16	—
Wild Blueberry as prep	1	170	5	1	18	2	28	14	tr	200	270	20	24	—
CARBSENSE														
Honey Bran not prep	1 serv (1.3 oz)	120	4	0	0	9	16	0	12	—	120	—	—	—
GOLD MEDAL														
Corn	1	160	6	2	35	3	25	8	0	20	270	60	—	0
HODGSON MILL														
Bran	¼ cup (1.3 oz)	130	1	0	0	4	27	5	3	0	150	—	—	0
Cornbread	¼ cup (1.3 oz)	130	1	0	0	4	28	3	3	0	240	—	—	0
Whole Wheat	¼ cup (1.3 oz)	130	1	0	0	4	27	6	3	—	560	—	—	—
KETOGENICS														
Apple Cinnamon Bran as prep	1	190	10	0	54	2	10	0	7	—	210	—	—	—
Chocolate Chip as prep	1	215	14	0	36	2	10	0	5	—	210	—	—	—
Wild Blueberry as prep	1	190	14	0	36	13	10	0	4	—	210	—	—	—
MINICARB														
Apple Cinnamon as prep	1	225	16	2	35	12	7	2	4	—	135	—	—	—
Sweet Corn as prep	1	225	16	1	35	12	80	1	6	—	245	—	—	—

FOOD	PORTION	CALS	FAT	SAT FAT	CHOL	PROT	CARB	SUGAR	FIBER	CALCI	SOD	POTAS	FOLIC	VIT C
ROBIN HOOD														
Apple Cinnamon	1	170	8	2	35	3	23	11	0	20	220	55	—	0
Banana Nut	1	170	8	2	35	3	21	9	0	20	190	70	—	0
Blueberry	1	160	6	2	35	3	24	12	0	20	220	45	—	0
Caramel Nut	1	170	7	2	35	3	24	11	0	20	230	50	—	0
SWEET REWARDS														
Low Fat Apple Cinnamon as prep	1	140	2	0	16	2	26	15	—	200	180	25	16	—
READY-TO-EAT														
blueberry	1 (2 oz)	158	4	1	17	3	27	—	2	33	255	70	—	1
corn	1 (2 oz)	174	5	1	—	3	29	—	—	42	297	39	—	—
oat bran wheat free	1 (2 oz)	154	4	1	0	4	28	—	4	36	224	289	10	—
toaster type blueberry	1	103	3	tr	—	2	18	—	—	4	158	27	—	0
toaster type corn	1	114	4	1	—	2	19	—	—	6	142	30	—	0
toaster type wheat bran w/ raisins	1 (1.3 oz)	106	3	1	—	2	19	—	—	13	178	60	—	0
ATKINS														
Blueberry	1 (3.5 oz)	210	10	1	0	14	17	1	6	150	380	—	—	0
DOLLY MADISON														
Blueberry	1 (1.75 oz)	170	7	3	0	2	26	8	0	40	280	—	—	0
Mega Banana Nut	1 (5.9 oz)	620	31	5	75	8	78	39	2	200	540	—	—	1
Mega Blueberry	1 (5.9 oz)	590	28	4	80	8	78	41	1	200	590	—	—	0
Mega Chocolate Chip	1 (5.9 oz)	620	29	5	80	8	78	41	2	200	580	—	—	0
Mega Cranberry Orange	1 (5.9 oz)	590	28	5	90	6	79	41	1	200	580	—	—	0
Mega Cream Cheese	1 (5.9 oz)	620	33	7	90	7	73	41	1	200	630	—	—	0
DUTCH MILL														
Apple Oat Bran	1 (2 oz)	180	5	1	0	3	31	5	1	60	210	—	—	0
Banana Walnut	1 (2 oz)	220	6	2	5	3	33	15	1	40	210	—	—	0
Carrot	1 (2 oz)	190	7	2	30	3	31	19	1	40	230	—	—	0
Corn	1 (2 oz)	190	6	3	40	4	31	14	1	40	280	—	—	0
Cranberry Orange	1 (2 oz)	170	6	3	55	3	26	14	1	40	290	—	—	0
Raisin Bran	1 (2 oz)	230	5	3	30	2	37	12	3	40	330	—	—	0
HOSTESS														
Banana Bran Low Fat	1 (2.7 oz)	240	3	1	0	4	47	24	2	20	270	—	—	0
Blueberry Low Fat	1 (2.7 oz)	230	3	1	0	4	47	23	1	200	350	—	—	0
Hearty Banana Nut	1 (5.9 oz)	620	31	5	75	8	78	39	2	200	540	—	—	1
Hearty Blueberry	1 (5.9 oz)	590	28	4	80	8	78	41	1	200	590	—	—	0

FOOD	PORTION	CALS	FAT	SAT FAT	CHOL	PROT	CARB	SUGAR	FIBER	CALCI	SOD	POTAS	FOLIC	VIT C
HOSTESS (CONT.)														
Hearty Chocolate Chip	1 (5.9 oz)	620	29	2	80	8	78	41	2	200	580	—	—	0
Hearty Cranberry Orange	1 (5.9 oz)	590	28	5	90	6	79	41	1	200	580	—	—	0
Hearty Cream Cheese	1 (5.9 oz)	620	33	7	90	7	73	41	1	200	630	—	—	0
Mini Banana Walnut	3 (1.2 oz)	160	9	1	25	2	16	8	0	0	100	—	—	0
Mini Blueberry	3 (1.2 oz)	150	8	1	25	1	18	8	0	0	110	—	—	0
Mini Chocolate Chip	3 (1.2 oz)	160	9	3	20	2	17	9	0	0	100	—	—	0
Mini Cinnamon Apple	3 (1.2 oz)	160	9	2	25	1	16	8	0	0	110	—	—	0
Mini Cinnamon Bites	3 (1.1 oz)	130	6	1	15	1	18	8	0	0	110	—	—	0
Mini Rocky Road	3 (1.2 oz)	160	9	3	20	2	17	9	0	0	140	—	—	0
Muffin Loaf Apple Spice	1 (3.7 oz)	430	18	4	80	3	61	41	1	60	350	—	—	0
Muffin Loaf Banana Nut	1 (3.8 oz)	460	20	3	60	4	63	29	0	40	300	—	—	0
Muffin Loaf Blueberry	1 (3.8 oz)	440	19	3	80	5	62	34	2	60	460	—	—	0
Muffin Loaf Chocolate Chocolate Chip	1 (3.8 oz)	400	17	4	45	5	58	32	2	20	330	—	—	0
Muffin Loaf Raspberry	1 (3.8 oz)	440	19	3	80	5	62	34	2	60	460	—	—	0
Oat Bran	1 (1.5 oz)	160	8	1	0	2	21	9	1	0	150	—	—	0
NATURAL OVENS														
Blueberry	1 (2.5 oz)	180	5	1	0	4	29	10	2	80	360	—	60	24
Carrot Nut	1 (2.5 oz)	170	6	1	0	4	35	15	2	100	380	—	100	42
Raisin Bran	1 (2.5 oz)	170	3	0	0	4	36	15	5	100	300	—	80	30
OTIS SPUNKMEYER														
Apple Cinnamon	1 (4 oz)	420	22	4	70	6	54	32	tr	40	420	—	—	2
Cheese Streusel	½ muffin (2 oz)	220	10	3	25	3	30	18	tr	20	170	—	32	0
Low Fat Wild Blueberry	1 (2.25 oz)	200	4	1	35	3	38	24	tr	20	160	—	—	0
Mayport Almond Poppy Seed	½ muffin (2 oz)	210	12	3	40	3	23	17	tr	20	230	—	—	0
Mayport Banana Nut	1 (2.25 oz)	270	14	3	30	3	33	20	tr	0	210	—	—	1
Mayport Chocolate Chocolate Chip	1 (2.25 oz)	260	13	3	40	4	33	22	1	20	190	—	—	0
Mayport Chocolate Chip	½ muffin (2 oz)	240	13	3	35	3	28	18	tr	20	210	—	—	0
Mayport Cinnamon Spice	½ muffin (2 oz)	230	13	3	40	3	26	16	1	40	250	—	—	1

FOOD	PORTION	CALS	FAT	SAT FAT	CHOL	PROT	CARB	SUGAR	FIBER	CALCI	SOD	POTAS	FOLIC	VIT C
OTIS SPUNKMEYER (CONT.)														
Mayport Corn	½ muffin (2 oz)	230	13	2	50	3	26	14	0	20	240	—	—	0
Mayport Harvest Bran	1 (2.25 oz)	240	10	2	35	4	34	20	3	40	240	—	32	0
Mayport Lemon	½ muffin (2 oz)	230	13	3	40	3	27	15	1	20	280	—	—	0
Mayport Orange	½ muffin (2 oz)	230	13	3	40	3	27	16	tr	20	230	—	—	0
Mayport Pineapple	½ muffin (2 oz)	210	12	3	40	3	25	17	1	20	270	—	—	1
Mayport Wild Blueberry	1 (2.25 oz)	230	13	3	45	3	27	20	1	20	230	—	—	2
Mayport Low Fat Apple Cinnamon	1 (4 oz)	380	6	1	65	5	75	50	1	60	300	—	60	0
Mayport Low Fat Banana Nut	1 (4 oz)	350	6	1	65	6	70	45	1	60	400	—	60	0
Mayport Low Fat Chocolate Chocolate Chip	1 (4 oz)	370	6	2	65	7	73	47	2	40	290	—	60	0
UNCLE WALLY'S														
Chocolate Passion	1 (2 oz)	130	0	0	0	2	30	18	1	0	210	—	—	0
Cranberry Orange Supreme	1 (2 oz)	130	0	0	0	3	25	12	1	20	230	—	—	1
Fat Free Apple Cinnamon Delight	1 (2 oz)	110	0	0	0	3	28	13	1	20	280	—	—	0
Fat Free Wild Blueberry Bliss	1 (2 oz)	120	0	0	0	30	25	12	1	0	230	—	—	0
Golden Waves Of Corn	1 (2 oz)	120	0	0	0	3	28	12	1	0	260	—	—	0
Honey Raisin Bran	1 (2 oz)	130	0	0	0	3	29	15	1	20	210	—	—	0
No Nut Banana	1 (2 oz)	130	0	0	0	3	27	15	1	0	230	—	—	0
VITAMUFFIN														
Blue Bran	1 (2 oz)	100	0	0	0	3	24	13	4	20	360	—	200	30
Cran Bran	1 (2 oz)	100	0	0	0	3	24	13	4	20	360	—	200	30
Deep Chocolate	1 (4 oz)	200	3	2	0	8	50	24	12	40	460	340	400	60
Multi Bran	1 (2 oz)	100	0	0	0	3	24	13	4	20	360	—	200	30
VitaTops Apple Berry Bran	1 (2 oz)	100	0	0	0	3	25	10	5	20	140	170	200	30
VitaTops Blue Bran	1 (2 oz)	100	0	0	0	3	24	13	4	20	360	—	200	30
VitaTops Cran Bran	1 (2 oz)	100	0	0	0	3	24	13	4	20	360	—	200	30
VitaTops Deep Chocolate	1 (2 oz)	100	2	1	0	4	25	12	6	20	230	170	200	30
VitaTops MultiBran	1 (2 oz)	100	0	0	0	3	24	13	4	20	360	—	200	30
WEIGHT WATCHERS														
Fat Free Apple Crisp	1 (2.5 oz)	160	0	0	0	3	37	16	1	40	290	—	—	0

FOOD	PORTION	CALS	FAT	SAT FAT	CHOL	PROT	CARB	SUGAR	FIBER	CALCI	SOD	POTAS	FOLIC	VIT C
WEIGHT WATCHERS (CONT.)														
Fat Free Cranberry Orange	1 (2.5 oz)	160	0	0	0	3	38	14	1	40	290	—	—	0
Fat Free Double Chocolate	1 (2.5 oz)	180	0	0	0	3	40	26	2	60	300	—	—	0
Fat Free Wild Blueberry	1 (2.5 oz)	160	0	0	0	3	36	15	1	40	280	—	—	0
Low Fat Apple Cinnamon	1 (2.5 oz)	170	3	0	0	4	35	20	2	60	200	—	—	0
Low Fat Blueberry	1 (2.5 oz)	180	3	0	0	4	37	20	2	60	200	—	—	0
Low Fat Carrot	1 (2.5 oz)	160	3	0	0	4	34	16	2	60	200	—	—	0
Low Fat Chocolate Chip	1 (2.5 oz)	180	3	1	0	4	38	21	2	60	200	—	—	0
Low Fat Cranberry Orange	1 (2.5 oz)	180	3	0	0	4	38	20	2	60	190	—	—	0
Low Fat Lemon Poppy	1 (2.5 oz)	190	3	0	0	4	38	20	2	100	200	—	—	0
TAKE-OUT														
raisin bran lowfat	1 (4 oz)	270	1	0	0	5	61	35	5	60	560	—	—	0
MULBERRIES														
fresh	1 cup	61	1	—	0	2	14	—	—	55	14	271	—	51
MULLET														
striped cooked	3 oz	127	4	1	54	21	0	—	—	26	61	389	—	—
striped raw	3 oz	99	3	1	42	16	0	—	—	34	55	304	7	—
MUNG BEANS														
dried cooked	1 cup	213	1	tr	0	14	39	—	—	55	4	536	321	2
MUNGO BEANS														
dried cooked	1 cup	190	1	tr	1	14	33	—	—	95	13	416	170	2
MUSHROOMS														
CANNED														
chanterelle	3.5 oz	12	1	—	0	1	tr	—	6	5	165	155	—	3
pieces	½ cup	19	tr	tr	0	1	4	—	—	—	—	—	10	—
straw	1 cup (6.4 oz)	58	1	tr	0	7	8	—	5	18	699	699	69	0
whole	1 (0.4 oz)	3	tr	tr	0	tr	1	—	—	—	—	—	2	—
BINB														
Pieces & Stems	1 can (4.2 oz)	30	0	0	0	3	4	1	2	0	460	—	—	0
Sliced	1 can (4.2 oz)	30	0	0	0	3	4	1	2	0	460	—	—	0
Sliced With Garlic	1 can (4.2 oz)	35	1	0	0	3	4	1	1	0	410	—	—	0
Whole	1 can (4.2 oz)	30	0	0	0	3	4	1	2	0	460	—	—	0
GREEN GIANT														
Pieces & Stems	½ cup (4.2 oz)	30	0	0	0	3	4	1	2	0	440	—	—	0
Sliced	½ cup (4.2 oz)	30	0	0	0	2	3	1	2	0	440	—	—	0
Whole	½ cup (4.2 oz)	30	0	0	0	3	4	1	2	0	440	—	—	0

FOOD	PORTION	CALS	FAT	SAT FAT	CHOL	PROT	CARB	SUGAR	FIBER	CALCI	SOD	POTAS	FOLIC	VIT C
DRIED														
chanterelle	1 oz	25	tr	—	0	5	tr	—	17	24	9	1	—	tr
cloud ear	1 (5 g)	13	tr	—	0	tr	3	—	3	7	2	34	2	0
cloud ears	1 cup (1 oz)	80	tr	—	0	3	20	—	20	45	10	211	11	0
shiitake	4 (½ oz)	44	tr	tr	0	1	11	—	—	2	2	230	—	—
straw	1 piece (6 g)	2	tr	0	0	tr	tr	—	tr	1	21	21	2	0
tree ear	½ cup (0.4 oz)	36	tr	—	0	1	10	—	—	14	8	85	19	0
wood ear mok yee	½ cup (0.4 oz)	25	tr	—	—	2	8	—	4	30	6	91	—	—
EDEN														
Shitake	6 (0.4 oz)	35	0	0	0	2	7	2	5	8	0	200	—	0
FRESH														
chanterelle	3.5 oz	11	tr	—	0	2	tr	—	6	8	3	507	—	6
enoki raw	1 (4 in)	2	tr	tr	0	tr	tr	—	—	0	0	19	1	1
morel	3.5 oz	9	tr	—	0	2	0	—	7	11	2	390	—	5
oyster raw	1 lg (5.2 oz)	55	1	—	0	6	9	—	4	9	46	764	70	0
oyster raw	1 sm (0.5 oz)	6	tr	—	0	1	1	—	tr	1	5	77	7	0
portabella	1 serv (2 oz)	14	tr	0	0	1	3	—	—	2	2	137	6	0
raw	1 (½ oz)	5	tr	tr	0	tr	1	—	tr	1	1	67	4	1
raw sliced	½ cup	9	tr	tr	0	1	2	—	tr	2	1	130	7	1
shitake cooked	4 (2.5 oz)	40	tr	tr	0	1	10	—	—	2	3	85	—	tr
sliced cooked	½ cup	21	tr	tr	0	2	4	—	1	4	2	277	14	3
whole cooked	1 (0.4 oz)	3	tr	tr	0	tr	1	—	—	1	0	43	2	1
MUSKRAT														
roasted	3 oz	199	10	—	—	26	0	—	—	31	81	272	—	6
MUSSELS														
blue raw	1 cup	129	3	1	42	18	6	—	—	39	429	479	—	—
blue raw	3 oz	73	2	tr	24	10	3	—	—	22	243	272	—	—
fresh blue cooked	3 oz	147	4	1	48	20	6	—	—	28	313	228	—	—
MUSTARD														
dry mustard	1 tsp	15	1	tr	0	1	1	—	—	17	tr	23	—	—
organic yellow	1 tsp	5	0	0	0	0	0	0	0	—	70	—	—	—
yellow ready-to-use	1 tsp	5	tr	tr	0	tr	tr	—	—	4	63	7	—	0
BOAR'S HEAD														
Delicatessen Style	1 tsp (5 g)	0	0	0	0	0	0	0	0	0	40	—	—	0
Honey	1 tsp (5 g)	10	0	0	0	0	2	1	0	0	25	—	—	0
COUNTRY CUPBOARD														
Smokey Garlic or Horseradish	1 tsp	10	0	0	0	0	2	1	0	—	5	—	—	—
EDEN														
Organic Stone Ground	1 tsp	0	0	0	0	0	1	0	0	0	65	0	0	0
FRENCH'S														
Classic Yellow	1 tsp	0	0	0	0	0	0	0	0	—	55	—	—	—

FOOD	PORTION	CALS	FAT	SAT FAT	CHOL	PROT	CARB	SUGAR	FIBER	CALCI	SOD	POTAS	FOLIC	VIT C
GULDEN'S														
Spicy Brown	1 tsp	5	0	0	0	0	0	—	—	—	50	—	—	—
HUNT'S														
Mustard	1 tsp (5 g)	3	tr	0	0	tr	tr	tr	tr	5	64	—	—	0
KOSCIUSZKO														
Spicy Brown	1 tsp	5	tr	—	0	tr	tr	—	—	—	60	—	—	—
KRAFT														
Horseradish Mustard	1 tsp (5 g)	0	0	0	0	0	0	0	0	0	55	5	—	0
Mustard	1 tsp (5 g)	0	0	0	0	0	0	0	0	0	60	5	—	0
LUZIANNE														
Creole Mustard	1 tbsp	10	0	0	0	1	2	0	0	0	320	—	—	0
TREE OF LIFE														
Dijon	1 tsp (5 g)	0	0	0	0	0	0	—	—	—	66	—	—	—
Dijon Imported	1 tsp (5 g)	5	0	0	0	tr	tr	—	—	—	120	—	—	
Stone Ground	1 tsp (5 g)	0	0	0	0	0	0	—	—	—	55	—	—	—
Yellow	1 tsp (5 g)	0	0	0	0	0	0	—	—	—	55	—	—	—
WILD THYME FARMS														
Chili Pepper Garlic	1 tsp	5	0	0	0	0	1	—	—	—	95	—	—	1
Dill Horseradish	1 tsp	5	0	0	0	0	1	—	—	—	50	—	—	—
MUSTARD GREENS														
fresh chopped cooked	½ cup	11	tr	tr	0	2	1	—	—	52	11	141	—	18
fresh raw chopped	½ cup	7	tr	tr	0	1	1	—	—	29	7	99	—	20
frozen chopped cooked	½ cup	14	tr	tr	0	2	2	—	—	75	19	104	—	10
BIRDS EYE														
Chopped	1 cup	30	0	0	0	2	2	1	2	80	20	—	—	15
NATTO														
natto	½ cup	187	10	1	0	16	13	—	—	191	6	642	—	11
NAVY BEANS														
CANNED														
navy	1 cup	296	1	tr	0	20	54	—	—	123	1173	755	163	2
DRIED														
cooked	1 cup	259	1	tr	0	16	48	—	—	128	2	669	255	2
HURST														
HamBeens w/ Ham	3 tbsp (1.2 oz)	120	1	0	0	8	20	1	11	40	63	—	—	2
NECTARINE														
fresh	1	67	1	—	0	1	16	—	2	6	0	288	5	7
CHIQUITA														
Fresh	1 med (4.9 oz)	70	1	0	0	1	16	12	2	0	0	—	—	9

FOOD	PORTION	CALS	FAT	SAT FAT	CHOL	PROT	CARB	SUGAR	FIBER	CALCI	SOD	POTAS	FOLIC	VIT C
NEUFCHATEL														
neufchatel	1 oz	74	7	4	22	3	1	—	—	21	113	32	3	0
neufchatel	1 pkg (3 oz)	221	20	13	65	8	3	—	—	64	339	97	10	0
HORIZON ORGANIC														
Neufchatel	2 tbsp	70	6	4	20	3	tr	tr	0	20	120	—	—	0
ORGANIC VALLEY														
Neufchatel	1 oz	70	6	4	20	2	1	tr	0	20	115	—	—	0
PHILADELPHIA														
Neufchatel	1 oz	70	6	4	20	3	tr	tr	0	20	120	30	—	0
NOODLE DISHES														
(*see also* PASTA DINNERS)														
HORMEL														
Microcup Meals Noodles & Chicken	1 cup (7.5 oz)	200	9	3	40	8	20	2	1	20	1140	—	—	0
HUNT'S														
Noodles & Chicken	1 cup (8.7 oz)	176	6	2	37	12	21	3	2	33	1282	—	—	36
Noodles & Beef	1 cup (8.7 oz)	151	4	2	17	10	22	2	5	22	1241	—	—	33
KRAFT														
Noodle Classics Cheddar Cheese as prep	1 cup (7.4 oz)	400	19	5	70	13	47	8	1	150	760	360	40	0
Noodle Classics Savory Chicken as prep	1 cup (8.5 oz)	340	13	3	55	10	46	5	2	40	1370	360	40	0
LIPTON														
Noodles & Sauce Alfredo as prep	1 cup (2.2 oz)	330	14	6	80	15	42	5	2	150	1040	—	100	0
Noodles & Sauce Alfredo Broccoli as prep	1 cup (2.2 oz)	340	14	6	80	12	43	5	2	150	970	—	100	5
Noodles & Sauce Beef as prep	1 cup (2.1 oz)	280	10	2	60	8	43	2	2	0	910	—	100	0
Noodles & Sauce Butter as prep	1 cup (2.2 oz)	310	14	6	70	8	41	4	2	0	870	—	100	0
Noodles & Sauce Butter & Herb as prep	1 cup (2.2 oz)	300	13	5	65	9	42	4	2	0	780	—	100	0
Noodles & Sauce Chicken as prep	1 cup (2.1 oz)	290	11	3	65	8	42	2	2	0	830	—	100	0
Noodles & Sauce Chicken Broccoli as prep	1 cup (2.1 oz)	310	11	4	70	11	44	4	2	80	840	—	100	4
Noodles & Sauce Chicken Tetrazzini as prep	1 cup (2 oz)	300	12	4	70	10	41	4	2	80	950	—	100	0

FOOD	PORTION	CALS	FAT	SAT FAT	CHOL	PROT	CARB	SUGAR	FIBER	CALCI	SOD	POTAS	FOLIC	VIT C
LIPTON (CONT.)														
Noodles & Sauce Creamy Chicken as prep	1 cup (2.1 oz)	320	13	5	75	11	42	5	2	80	810	—	100	0
Noodles & Sauce Parmesan as prep	1 cup (2.1 oz)	330	15	6	75	14	40	5	2	150	850	—	100	2
Noodles & Sauce Sour Cream & Chives as prep	1 cup (2.2 oz)	310	14	6	70	10	41	4	2	20	870	—	100	1
Noodles & Sauce Stroganoff as prep	1 cup (2 oz)	300	11	4	70	11	40	5	2	80	950	—	100	0
TAKE-OUT														
bami goreng indonesian noodle dish	1 cup	170	3	1	0	5	25	4	4	40	500	—	—	2
noodle pudding	½ cup	132	7	4	27	6	11	—	—	51	222	81	8	1
NOODLES														
cellophane	1 cup	492	tr	tr	0	tr	121	—	—	35	14	14	—	0
chow mein	1 cup (1.6 oz)	237	14	2	0	4	25	—	2	9	189	52	39	0
egg	1 cup (38 g)	145	2	tr	36	5	27	—	—	12	8	89	11	0
egg cooked	1 cup (5.6 oz)	213	2	tr	53	8	40	—	2	19	11	45	102	0
japanese soba cooked	1 cup (4 oz)	113	tr	tr	0	6	24	—	—	5	68	40	8	0
japanese somen cooked	1 cup (6.2 oz)	231	tr	tr	0	7	48	—	—	14	283	51	4	0
korean acorn noodles not prep	2 oz	195	tr	—	—	7	41	—	tr	—	—	—	—	0
rice cooked	1 cup (6.2 oz)	192	tr	tr	0	2	44	—	2	7	33	7	5	0
spinach/egg cooked	1 cup (5.6 oz)	211	3	1	53	8	39	—	4	30	19	59	102	0
ANNIE CHUN'S														
Chow Mein	2 oz	200	1	0	0	8	39	1	3	0	350	—	—	0
Rice	2 oz	210	0	0	0	2	50	0	0	0	75	—	—	0
Rice Hunan	2 oz	210	0	0	0	2	50	0	0	0	75	—	—	0
Rice Pad Thai	2 oz	210	0	0	0	2	50	0	0	0	75	—	—	0
Rice Pad Thai Basil	2 oz	210	0	0	0	2	50	0	0	0	75	—	—	0
AZUMAYA														
Spinach	1 cup	210	1	0	0	8	42	1	2	20	370	—	—	0
Thin Cut	1 cup	210	1	0	0	8	43	1	2	20	400	—	—	0
Wide Cut	1 cup	210	1	0	0	8	43	1	2	20	410	—	—	0
CHUN KING														
Chow Mein	½ cup (1 oz)	137	6	1	0	3	19	0	1	7	217	—	—	0
EDEN														
Kudzu	2 oz	200	0	0	0	0	48	0	2	0	0	0	0	0

FOOD	PORTION	CALS	FAT	SAT FAT	CHOL	PROT	CARB	SUGAR	FIBER	CALCI	SOD	POTAS	FOLIC	VIT C
HODGSON MILL														
Four Color Veggie Egg	2 oz	200	2	1	35	9	37	0	2	20	25	—	—	0
Whole Wheat Egg not prep	2 oz	190	0	0	30	10	34	0	4	20	20	—	28	0
LA CHOY														
Chow Mein	½ cup (1 oz)	137	6	1	0	3	19	0	1	7	217	—	—	0
Chow Mein Crispy Wide	½ cup (1 oz)	148	8	2	0	3	16	0	1	6	289	—	—	0
Rice	½ cup (1 oz)	121	3	1	0	2	21	0	tr	5	378	—	—	0
MANISCHEWITZ														
Fine Yolk Free	1½ cups	210	1	0	0	8	40	2	2	0	20	—	120	0
Fine Egg	1½ cups	220	3	1	65	8	40	2	2	20	15	—	120	0
Wide Yolk Free	1¾ cups	210	1	0	0	8	40	2	2	0	20	—	120	0
NASOYA														
Chinese	1 cup	210	1	0	0	8	43	1	2	20	400	—	—	0
Japanese	1 cup	210	1	0	0	8	43	1	2	20	410	—	—	0
Spinach	1 cup	210	1	0	0	8	42	1	2	20	0	—	—	0
PENNSYLVANIA DUTCH														
Yolk Free Ribbons as prep	1½ cups	210	1	0	0	7	41	2	2	0	15	—	100	0

NOPALES

FOOD	PORTION	CALS	FAT	SAT FAT	CHOL	PROT	CARB	SUGAR	FIBER	CALCI	SOD	POTAS	FOLIC	VIT C
cooked	1 cup (5.2 oz)	23	tr	—	0	2	5	—	—	245	30	290	4	8
raw sliced	1 cup (3 oz)	14	tr	—	0	1	3	—	—	140	19	275	3	12

NUTMEG

FOOD	PORTION	CALS	FAT	SAT FAT	CHOL	PROT	CARB	SUGAR	FIBER	CALCI	SOD	POTAS	FOLIC	VIT C
ground	1 tsp	12	1	1	0	tr	1	—	—	4	tr	8	—	—

NUTRITION SUPPLEMENTS

(*see also* CEREAL BARS, ENERGY BARS, ENERGY DRINKS)

FOOD	PORTION	CALS	FAT	SAT FAT	CHOL	PROT	CARB	SUGAR	FIBER	CALCI	SOD	POTAS	FOLIC	VIT C
BOOST														
High Protein Powder Vanilla as prep w/ water	1 serv (8 oz)	200	1	0	10	13	36	35	0	290	190	560	133	20
ENLIVE!														
Drink All Flavors	1 box (8.1 oz)	300	0	0	<5	10	65	15	0	60	65	40	—	24
ENSURE														
Supplement All Flavors	1 can (8 fl oz)	250	6	1	<5	9	40	18	0	300	200	370	100	30
ESSENTIAL														
Protein Powder	1 serv (0.6 oz)	70	tr	0	0	16	6	5	tr	98	5	750	100	—
GENISOY														
Soy Natural Protein Powder	1 scoop (1 oz)	100	0	0	0	25	0	0	0	250	290	90	100	15
GLUCERNA														
Shakes All Flavors	1 can (8 oz)	220	9	1	<5	10	29	7	3	250	210	60	—	60

FOOD	PORTION	CALS	FAT	SAT FAT	CHOL	PROT	CARB	SUGAR	FIBER	CALCI	SOD	POTAS	FOLIC	VIT C
JUVEN														
Grape w/ Arginine, Glutamine, HMB	1 pkg (0.8 oz)	90	—	—	—	—	2	2	—	200	—	260	—	—
Orange w/ HMB	1 pkg (0.8 oz)	90	0	0	—	—	—	—	—	200	—	260	—	—
MET-RX														
Lite	1 pkg (1.6 oz)	170	1	1	30	25	16	3	1	350	125	160	200	30
Mass Action	1 scoop (0.9 oz)	60	4	—	—	—	15	9	—	200	270	—	—	10
Original	1 pkg (2.5 oz)	250	2	2	15	37	22	3	tr	1000	370	900	400	60
Protein Shake	1 can	200	3	1	10	25	20	1	2	940	110	370	200	78
Ultra	1 pkg (2.6 oz)	250	2	2	50	40	19	5	2	570	230	260	200	30
NATURE MADE														
CalBurst	1 piece	15	—	—	—	—	—	—	—	500	—	—	—	—
NESTLÉ														
Additions	2⅓ tsp (0.7 oz)	100	5	1	0	6	9	1	0	0	90	—	—	0
NUTRABALANCE														
EggPro	1 tbsp (7.5 g)	30	0	0	0	6	1	0	0	0	96	84	tr	0
NUTRIBAR														
Shake Chocolate Supreme as prep w/ 2% milk	1 serv (10 oz)	262	8	4	—	14	34	—	2	370	290	790	140	13
Shake Vanilla as prep w/ 2% milk	1 (10 oz)	259	7	4	—	14	35	—	2	380	285	600	140	13
PERMALEAN														
Protein Powder Bodacious Berry	1 scoop (1 oz)	104	tr	0	0	20	1	3	—	tr	tr	—	—	tr
Protein Powder Chocoholic Chocolate	1 scoop (1 oz)	104	tr	0	0	20	5	3	—	tr	tr	—	—	tr
POUNDS OFF														
All Flavors	1 bar (2.1 oz)	210	5	1	0	11	32	18	2	350	25	—	400	60
VIACTIV														
Calcium Chews	1	20	1	—	—	—	—	—	—	500	—	—	—	—
Chocolate	1	20	1	—	—	—	—	—	—	500	—	—	—	—
NUTS MIXED														
(see also individual names)														
dry roasted w/ peanuts	1 oz	169	15	2	0	5	7	—	—	20	3	169	14	tr
dry roasted w/ peanuts salted	1 oz	169	15	2	0	5	7	—	—	20	223	169	14	tr
mixed nuts chocolate covered	¼ cup (1.5 oz)	240	17	7	5	4	20	17	2	80	25	—	—	0
oil roasted w/ peanuts	1 oz	175	16	2	0	5	6	—	—	31	3	165	24	tr
oil roasted w/ peanuts salted	1 oz	175	16	2	0	5	6	—	—	31	217	165	24	tr

FOOD	PORTION	CALS	FAT	SAT FAT	CHOL	PROT	CARB	SUGAR	FIBER	CALCI	SOD	POTAS	FOLIC	VIT C
oil roasted w/o peanuts	1 oz	175	16	3	0	4	6	—	—	30	3	154	16	tr
oil roasted w/o peanuts salted	1 oz	175	16	3	0	4	6	—	—	30	233	154	0	tr
ESTEE														
Fruit & Nut Mix	¼ cup	210	12	7	<5	6	19	10	2	—	45	270	—	—
HERE'S HOWE														
Royal Mixed Nuts	1 oz	180	17	3	0	5	7	2	2	40	160	—	—	0
JUDY'S														
Sugar Free Mixed Nut Brittle	¼ piece (1 oz)	120	7	2	<5	2	3	0	tr	—	30	—	—	—
MARANATHA														
Cashew Macadamia Butter	2 tbsp	210	20	4	0	4	8	2	2	20	5	—	—	0
Tamari Organic	¼ cup	160	14	2	0	6	7	1	2	20	140	—	—	0
Tamari Roasted	¼ cup	160	14	2	0	6	7	1	2	20	140	—	—	0
MAUNA LOA														
Macadamia Mixed	¼ cup	190	15	2	0	5	8	1	2	—	60	—	—	—
Macadamias & Cashews	¼ cup	180	15	3	0	4	8	1	1	—	65	—	—	—

OCTOPUS

FOOD	PORTION	CALS	FAT	SAT FAT	CHOL	PROT	CARB	SUGAR	FIBER	CALCI	SOD	POTAS	FOLIC	VIT C
fresh steamed	3 oz	140	2	tr	82	25	4	—	—	90	—	—	—	—

OHELOBERRIES

FOOD	PORTION	CALS	FAT	SAT FAT	CHOL	PROT	CARB	SUGAR	FIBER	CALCI	SOD	POTAS	FOLIC	VIT C
fresh	1 cup	39	tr	—	0	1	10	—	—	10	2	54	—	8

OIL

FOOD	PORTION	CALS	FAT	SAT FAT	CHOL	PROT	CARB	SUGAR	FIBER	CALCI	SOD	POTAS	FOLIC	VIT C
almond	1 cup	1927	218	1	0	0	0	0	0	—	—	—	—	—
almond	1 tbsp	120	14	1	0	0	0	0	0	—	—	—	—	—
apricot kernel	1 tbsp	120	14	1	0	0	0	0	0	—	—	—	—	—
apricot kernel	1 cup	1927	218	14	0	0	0	0	0	—	—	—	—	—
avocado	1 tbsp	124	14	2	0	0	0	0	0	—	—	—	—	—
avocado	1 cup	1927	218	25	0	0	0	0	0	—	—	—	—	—
babassu palm	1 tbsp	120	14	11	0	0	0	0	0	—	—	—	—	—
butter oil	1 cup	1795	204	127	524	1	0	—	—	—	—	—	—	—
butter oil	1 tbsp	112	13	8	33	tr	0	—	—	—	—	—	—	—
canola	1 tbsp	124	14	2	0	0	0	0	0	—	—	—	—	—
canola	1 cup	1927	218	15	0	0	0	0	0	—	—	—	—	—
coconut	1 tbsp	117	14	12	0	0	0	0	0	—	—	—	—	—
corn	1 tbsp	120	14	2	0	0	0	0	0	—	—	—	—	—
corn	1 cup	1927	218	28	0	0	0	0	0	—	—	—	—	—
cottonseed	1 tbsp	120	14	4	0	0	0	0	0	—	—	—	—	—
cottonseed	1 cup	1927	218	56	0	0	0	0	0	—	—	—	—	—
cupu assu	1 tbsp	120	14	7	0	0	0	0	0	—	—	—	—	—
grapeseed	1 tbsp	120	14	1	0	0	0	0	0	—	—	—	—	—
hazelnut	1 tbsp	120	14	1	0	0	0	0	0	—	—	—	—	—
hazelnut	1 cup	1927	218	1	0	0	0	0	0	—	—	—	—	—

FOOD	PORTION	CALS	FAT	SAT FAT	CHOL	PROT	CARB	SUGAR	FIBER	CALCI	SOD	POTAS	FOLIC	VIT C
mustard	1 tbsp	124	14	2	0	0	0	0	0	—	—	—	—	—
mustard	1 cup	1927	218	25	0	0	0	0	0	—	—	—	—	—
oat	1 tbsp	120	14	3	0	0	0	0	0	—	—	—	—	—
olive	1 cup	1909	216	26	0	0	0	0	0	tr	tr	—	—	—
olive	1 tbsp	119	14	2	0	0	0	0	0	tr	0	—	—	—
palm	1 cup	1927	218	107	0	0	0	0	0	—	—	—	—	—
palm	1 tbsp	120	14	7	0	0	0	0	0	—	—	—	—	—
palm kernel	1 tbsp	117	14	11	0	0	0	0	0	—	—	—	—	—
palm kernel	1 cup	1879	218	178	0	0	0	0	0	—	—	—	—	—
peanut	1 cup	1909	216	36	0	0	0	0	0	tr	tr	tr	—	—
peanut	1 tbsp	119	14	2	0	0	0	0	0	tr	tr	0	—	—
poppyseed	1 tbsp	120	14	2	0	0	0	0	0	—	—	—	—	—
pumpkin seed	1 oz	217	29	—	—	0	0	0	0	—	—	—	—	—
rice bran	1 tbsp	120	14	3	0	0	0	0	0	—	—	—	—	—
safflower	1 cup	1927	218	20	0	0	0	0	0	—	—	—	—	—
safflower	1 tbsp	120	14	1	0	0	0	0	0	—	—	—	—	—
sesame	1 tbsp	120	14	2	0	0	0	0	0	—	—	—	—	—
sheanut	1 tbsp	120	14	6	0	0	0	0	0	—	—	—	—	—
soybean	1 tbsp	120	14	2	0	0	0	0	0	tr	0	—	—	—
soybean	1 cup	1927	218	31	0	0	0	0	0	tr	tr	—	—	—
soybean organic	1 tbsp	120	14	2	0	0	0	0	0	—	0	—	—	—
sunflower	1 tbsp	120	14	1	0	0	0	0	0	—	—	—	—	—
sunflower	1 cup	1927	218	23	0	0	0	0	0	—	—	—	—	—
teaseed	1 tbsp	120	14	3	0	0	0	0	0	—	—	—	—	—
tomatoseed	1 tbsp	120	14	3	0	0	0	0	0	—	—	—	—	—
vegetable	1 cup	1927	218	2	0	0	0	0	0	—	—	—	—	—
vegetable	1 tbsp	120	14	2	0	0	0	0	0	—	—	—	—	—
walnut	1 tbsp	120	14	1	0	0	0	0	0	—	—	—	—	—
walnut	1 cup	1927	218	20	0	0	0	0	0	—	—	—	—	—
wheat germ	1 tbsp	120	14	3	0	0	0	0	0	—	—	—	—	—
ALPHA														
Hazelnut	1 oz	257	29	2	0	0	0	0	0	tr	—	—	—	—
BERTOLLI														
Classico	1 tbsp	120	14	—	0	—	—	—	—	—	—	—	—	—
Extra Light	1 tbsp	120	14	—	0	—	—	—	—	—	—	—	—	—
Extra Virgin	1 tbsp	120	14	—	0	—	—	—	—	—	—	—	—	—
EDEN														
Olive Spanish Extra Virgin	1 tbsp	120	14	2	0	0	0	0	0	0	0	0	0	0
Safflower	1 tbsp (0.5 oz)	120	14	1	0	0	0	—	—	—	0	—	—	—
ENOVA														
Oil	1 tbsp	120	14	1	0	0	0	0	0	—	0	—	—	—
HOLLYWOOD														
Safflower	1 tbsp	120	14	1	0	0	0	0	0	—	0	—	—	—

FOOD	PORTION	CALS	FAT	SAT FAT	CHOL	PROT	CARB	SUGAR	FIBER	CALCI	SOD	POTAS	FOLIC	VIT C
HOUSE OF TSANG														
Hot Chili Sesame	1 tsp (5 g)	45	5	1	0	0	0	0	0	0	0	—	—	0
Mongolian Fire	1 tsp (5 g)	45	5	1	0	0	0	0	0	0	0	—	—	0
Pure Sesame	1 tsp (5 g)	45	5	1	0	0	0	0	0	0	0	—	—	0
Singapore Curry	1 tsp (5 g)	45	5	1	0	0	0	0	0	0	0	—	—	0
Wok Oil	1 tbsp (0.5 oz)	130	14	3	0	0	0	0	0	0	0	—	—	0
LORIVA														
5 Pepper Hot	1 tbsp	120	14	1	0	—	—	—	—	—	—	—	—	—
Avocado	1 tbsp	120	14	2	0	—	—	—	—	—	—	—	—	—
Basil Flavored	1 tbsp	120	14	1	0	—	—	—	—	—	—	—	—	—
Canola	1 tbsp	120	14	1	0	—	—	—	—	—	—	—	—	—
Canolive	1 tbsp	120	14	1	0	—	—	—	—	—	—	—	—	—
Garlic Flavored	1 tbsp	120	14	1	0	—	—	—	—	—	—	—	—	—
Grapeseed	1 tbsp	120	14	1	0	—	—	—	—	—	—	—	—	—
Olive	1 tbsp	120	14	2	0	—	—	—	—	—	—	—	—	—
Olive Organic Extra Virgin	1 tbsp	120	14	1	0	—	—	—	—	—	—	—	—	—
Peanut	1 tbsp	120	14	2	0	—	—	—	—	—	—	—	—	—
Rice Bran	1 tbsp	120	14	2	0	—	—	—	—	—	—	—	—	—
Safflower	1 tbsp	120	14	1	0	—	—	—	—	—	—	—	—	—
Sesame	1 tbsp	120	14	2	0	—	—	—	—	—	—	—	—	—
Sunflower	1 tbsp	120	14	2	0	—	—	—	—	—	—	—	—	—
Toasted Sesame	1 tbsp	120	14	2	0	—	—	—	—	—	—	—	—	—
Walnut	1 tbsp	120	14	2	0	—	—	—	—	—	—	—	—	—
MAZOLA														
Oil	1 tbsp	120	14	2	0	0	0	0	0	—	0	—	—	—
MONINI														
Olive Extra Virgin	1 tbsp	118	13	2	0	0	0	0	0	—	—	—	—	—
ORVILLE REDENBACHER'S														
Popping	1 tbsp (0.5 oz)	120	14	2	0	0	0	0	0	0	0	—	—	0
PAM														
Butter	⅓ sec spray (0.3 g)	0	0	0	0	0	0	—	—	—	0	—	—	—
Cooking Spray	⅓ sec spray (0.3 g)	0	0	0	0	0	0	—	—	—	0	—	—	—
Olive Oil	⅓ sec spray (0.3 g)	0	0	0	0	0	0	—	—	—	0	—	—	—
POMPEIAN														
Olive	1 tbsp (0.3 g)	130	14	—	0	—	—	—	—	0	—	—	—	—
PROGRESSO														
Olive Extra Mild	1 tbsp (0.5 oz)	120	14	2	0	0	0	0	0	0	0	—	—	0
Olive Extra Virgin	1 tbsp (0.5 oz)	120	14	2	0	0	0	0	0	0	0	—	—	0
Olive Riviera Blend	1 tbsp (0.5 oz)	120	14	2	0	0	0	0	0	0	0	—	—	0

FOOD	PORTION	CALS	FAT	SAT FAT	CHOL	PROT	CARB	SUGAR	FIBER	CALCI	SOD	POTAS	FOLIC	VIT C
TREE OF LIFE														
Olive Extra Virgin Organic	1 tbsp (0.5 g)	130	14	1	0	0	0	—	—	—	0	—	—	—
WEIGHT WATCHERS														
Butter Spray	⅓ sec spray	0	0	0	0	0	0	0	0	0	0	—	—	0
Cooking Spray	⅓ sec spray	0	0	0	0	0	0	0	0	0	0	—	—	0
WESSON														
Canola	1 tbsp	120	14	4	1	0	0	0	0	—	0	—	—	—

OKRA

FOOD	PORTION	CALS	FAT	SAT FAT	CHOL	PROT	CARB	SUGAR	FIBER	CALCI	SOD	POTAS	FOLIC	VIT C
FRESH														
raw	8 pods	36	tr	tr	0	2	7	—	—	77	8	287	83	20
raw sliced	½ cup	19	tr	tr	0	1	4	—	—	41	4	151	44	11
sliced cooked	½ cup	25	tr	tr	0	1	6	—	—	50	4	257	37	13
sliced cooked	8 pods	27	tr	tr	0	2	6	—	—	54	5	273	39	14
FROZEN														
sliced cooked	1 pkg (10 oz)	94	1	tr	0	5	21	—	—	245	8	597	371	31
sliced cooked	½ cup	34	tr	tr	0	2	8	—	—	88	3	215	134	11
BIRDS EYE														
Cut	¾ cup	25	0	0	0	1	5	1	3	60	35	—	—	2
Whole	9 pods	25	0	0	0	1	5	1	3	60	35	—	—	2
MCKENZIE'S														
Breaded Okra	1 serv (2.8 oz)	90	1	0	0	3	—	2	3	—	350	—	—	—

OLIVES

FOOD	PORTION	CALS	FAT	SAT FAT	CHOL	PROT	CARB	SUGAR	FIBER	CALCI	SOD	POTAS	FOLIC	VIT C
green	3 extra lg	15	2	tr	0	tr	tr	—	tr	8	312	7	—	0
green	4 med	15	2	tr	0	tr	tr	—	tr	8	312	7	—	0
green olive tapenade	1 tbsp	25	3	0	0	0	1	1	0	20	210	—	—	2
ripe	1 colossal	12	1	tr	0	tr	1	—	—	14	136	1	—	tr
ripe	1 sm	4	tr	tr	0	tr	tr	—	tr	3	28	0	0	0
ripe	1 lg	5	tr	tr	0	tr	tr	—	tr	4	38	0	0	0
ripe	1 jumbo	7	1	tr	0	tr	tr		—	8	75	1	—	tr
spanish stuffed	5 (0.5 oz)	15	1	0	0	0	1	0	0	20	320	—	—	0
ITALIA IN TAVOLA														
Black Olives Paste	1 tbsp (0.5 oz)	20	2	—	0	0	tr	—	—	—	470	—	—	—
PROGRESSO														
Olive Salad (drained)	2 tbsp (0.8 oz)	25	3	0	0	0	1	tr	tr	0	360	—	—	0
VLASIC														
Ripe Colossal Pitted	2 (0.6 oz)	20	2	0	0	0	1	0	0	0	110	—	—	0
Ripe Jumbo Pitted	3 (0.6 oz)	25	2	0	0	0	1	0	0	0	135	—	—	0
Ripe Large Pitted	4 (0.5 oz)	25	3	0	0	0	1	0	0	0	115	—	—	0

FOOD	PORTION	CALS	FAT	SAT FAT	CHOL	PROT	CARB	SUGAR	FIBER	CALCI	SOD	POTAS	FOLIC	VIT C
VLASIC (CONT.)														
Ripe Medium Pitted	5 (0.5 oz)	25	3	0	0	0	1	0	0	0	115	—	—	0
Ripe Sliced	¼ cup (0.5 oz)	25	3	0	0	0	1	0	0	0	115	—	—	0
Ripe Small Pitted	6 (0.5 oz)	25	3	0	0	0	1	0	0	0	115	—	—	0

ONION

FOOD	PORTION	CALS	FAT	SAT FAT	CHOL	PROT	CARB	SUGAR	FIBER	CALCI	SOD	POTAS	FOLIC	VIT C
CANNED														
chopped	½ cup	21	tr	tr	0	1	5	—	—	51	416	124	—	—
whole	1 (2.2 oz)	12	tr	tr	0	1	3	—	—	29	234	70	—	—
BOAR'S HEAD														
Sweet Vidalia In Sauce	1 tbsp	10	0	0	0	0	2	2	0	0	15	—	—	1
DRIED														
flakes	1 tbsp	16	tr	tr	0	tr	4	—	—	13	1	81	8	4
powder	1 tsp	7	tr	—	0	tr	2	—	—	8	1	20	—	0
shallots	1 tbsp	3	0	0	0	tr	1	—	—	2	1	15	1	tr
FRESH														
chopped cooked	½ cup	47	tr	tr	0	1	11	—	—	23	3	174	16	6
raw chopped	1 tbsp	4	tr	tr	0	tr	1	—	tr	2	0	16	2	1
raw chopped	½ cup	30	tr	tr	0	1	7	—	—	16	2	125	15	5
scallions raw chopped	1 tbsp	2	tr	tr	0	tr	tr	—	tr	4	1	17	4	1
scallions raw sliced	½ cup	16	tr	tr	0	1	4	—	1	30	8	138	32	9
shallots raw chopped	1 tbsp	7	tr	tr	0	tr	2	—	—	4	1	33	—	1
welsh raw	3½ oz	34	tr	tr	0	2	7	—	—	18	—	—	—	27
ANTIOCH FARMS														
Vidalia	1 med	60	0	—	0	1	14	—	3	40	10	200	tr	12
NATURE'S HARVEST														
Onion	1 med (5.2 oz)	60	0	0	0	2	14	9	3	40	5	—	—	12
FROZEN														
chopped cooked	½ cup	30	tr	tr	0	tr	7	—	—	17	12	114	14	3
chopped cooked	1 tbsp	4	tr	tr	0	tr	1	—	—	2	2	16	0	tr
rings	7 (2.5 oz)	285	19	6	0	4	27	—	—	21	263	90	9	1
rings cooked	2 (0.7 oz)	81	5	2	0	1	8	—	—	6	75	26	3	tr
whole cooked	3½ oz	28	tr	0	0	tr	7	—	—	27	8	101	13	5
BIRDS EYE														
Diced	⅔ cup	30	0	0	0	tr	6	5	1	0	30	—	—	0
Pearl Onions In Real Cream Sauce	½ cup	60	2	1	10	2	8	6	1	40	280	—	—	0
Small Whole	17	30	0	0	0	—	—	—	1	20	10	—	—	6
MCKENZIE'S														
Onion Rounds	1 serv (3.2 oz)	220	10	2	0	3	28	3	6	—	210	—	—	—

FOOD	PORTION	CALS	FAT	SAT FAT	CHOL	PROT	CARB	SUGAR	FIBER	CALCI	SOD	POTAS	FOLIC	VIT C
TAKE-OUT														
fried	½ cup (7.5 oz)	176	11	6	—	3	17	—	—	57	—	—	—	20
rings breaded & fried	8 to 9	275	16	7	14	4	31	—	—	73	430	129	11	tr

OPOSSUM

roasted	3 oz	188	9	—	—	26	0	—	—	—	—	—	—	—

ORANGE

CANNED

DEL MONTE

Mandarin In Light Syrup	½ cup (4.5 oz)	80	0	0	0	0	19	19	1	0	10	—	—	4

DOLE

Fruit Bowls Mandarin Oranges	1 pkg	70	0	0	0	0	18	17	0	—	10	75	—	24

FRESH

california navel	1	65	tr	tr	0	1	16	—	3	56	1	250	47	80
california valencia	1	59	tr	tr	0	1	14	—	3	48	0	217	47	59
florida	1	69	tr	tr	0	1	17	—	4	65	1	254	26	68
peel	1 tbsp	6	tr	tr	0	tr	2	—	—	10	0	13	—	8
sections	1 cup	85	tr	tr	0	2	21	—	4	52	0	326	55	96

ORANGE EXTRACT

VIRGINIA DARE

Extract	1 tsp	22	0	—	0	—	—	—	—	0	—	—	—	—

ORANGE JUICE

canned	1 cup	104	tr	tr	0	1	25	—	—	21	6	436	—	86
chilled	1 cup	110	1	tr	0	2	25	—	—	24	2	473	45	82
fresh	1 cup	111	tr	tr	0	2	26	—	—	27	2	496	—	124
frzn as prep	1 cup	112	tr	tr	0	2	27	—	1	22	2	474	109	97
frzn not prep	6 oz	339	tr	tr	0	5	81	—	2	67	7	1435	331	294
mandarin orange	7 oz	94	tr	—	—	2	20	—	—	38	—	—	—	64
orange drink	6 oz	94	0	0	0	0	24	—	—	12	31	33	—	64

BIG JUICY

Drink	8 oz	110	0	0	0	0	28	28	—	—	55	—	—	—

CAPRI SUN

Drink	1 pkg (7 oz)	100	0	0	0	0	25	25	0	0	20	40	—	0

EVERFRESH

Juice	1 can (8 oz)	100	0	0	0	0	24	24	0	—	0	—	—	—
Ruby Red Orange Drink	1 can (8 oz)	130	0	0	0	0	33	33	0	—	0	—	—	—

FRESH SAMANTHA

Juice	1 cup (8 oz)	100	0	0	0	1	8	—	0	0	0	120	40	72

HORIZON ORGANIC

Juice Pulp Free	8 fl oz	110	0	0	0	2	26	22	—	20	0	450	60	72

FOOD	PORTION	CALS	FAT	SAT FAT	CHOL	PROT	CARB	SUGAR	FIBER	CALCI	SOD	POTAS	FOLIC	VIT C
JUICY JUICE														
Punch	1 box (8.45 oz)	130	0	0	0	0	33	28	0	0	15	230	—	78
Punch	1 box (4.23 oz)	60	0	0	0	0	15	14	0	0	5	110	—	60
KOOL-AID														
Drink Mix Orange as prep	1 serv (8 oz)	60	0	0	0	0	16	16	0	0	5	0	—	6
Orange Drink as prep w/ sugar	1 serv (8 oz)	100	0	0	0	0	25	25	0	0	10	0	—	6
MINUTE MAID														
Heart Wise	8 oz	110	0	0	0	2	27	24	—	20	20	450	60	72
Light	8 oz	50	0	0	0	0	13	10	—	350	15	450	24	72
Original	8 fl oz	110	0	0	0	2	27	24	—	20	25	450	60	72
Original Calcium + Vitamin D	8 oz	110	0	0	0	2	27	24	—	350	15	—	60	72
Plus Calcium	8 fl oz	110	0	0	0	2	27	24	—	350	20	450	60	72
Simply Orange 100%	8 fl oz	110	0	0	0	2	26	22	—	20	0	450	60	72
Simply Orange Calcium Fortified	8 fl oz	110	0	0	0	2	26	22	—	320	0	450	60	72
Simply Orange Grove Made	8 fl oz	110	0	0	0	2	26	22	—	20	0	450	60	72
MOTT'S														
100% Juice	1 box (8 oz)	130	0	0	0	2	31	—	—	—	10	—	—	—
100% Juice	8 fl oz	130	0	0	0	2	31	—	—	—	10	—	—	—
NAKED JUICE														
Just OJ	8 oz	110	0	0	0	2	25	25	0	20	0	470	—	108
NUTRASHAKE														
Fortified	1 pkg (4 oz)	50	0	0	0	0	12	—	4	200	0	216	—	150
OCEAN SPRAY														
100% Juice	8 oz	120	0	0	0	0	31	31	0	—	35	300	—	60
ODWALLA														
Organic	8 fl oz	110	0	0	0	2	25	24	—	20	0	450	—	144
SHASTA PLUS														
Orange Drink	1 can (11.5 oz)	160	0	0	0	0	40	40	0	—	45	—	—	60
SIMPLY ORANGE														
Pulp Free w/ Calcium	8 oz	110	0	0	0	2	26	22	—	350	0	450	60	72
SNAPPLE														
Orangeade	8 fl oz	120	0	0	0	0	29	29	—	—	10	—	—	—
SQUEEZIT														
Smarty Arty Orange	1 bottle (7 oz)	110	0	0	0	0	27	26	0	0	45	—	—	0
TANG														
Orange Drink as prep	1 serv (8 oz)	90	0	0	0	0	23	23	0	80	0	50	—	60

FOOD	PORTION	CALS	FAT	SAT FAT	CHOL	PROT	CARB	SUGAR	FIBER	CALCI	SOD	POTAS	FOLIC	VIT C
TANG (CONT.)														
Sugar Free Orange as prep	1 serv (8 oz)	5	0	0	0	0	0	0	0	tr	0	75	—	60
TROPICANA														
Double Vitamin C	8 fl oz	110	0	0	0	2	26	—	—	20	0	450	60	144
HomeStyle	8 oz	110	0	0	0	2	26	22	—	20	0	450	60	72
Light'N Healthy	8 oz	70	0	0	0	1	17	14	—	200	10	450	40	72
Original No Pulp	8 oz	110	0	0	0	2	26	22	—	20	0	450	60	72
Ruby Red	8 oz	110	0	0	0	2	26	—	—	20	0	450	60	72
Season's Best	8 oz	110	0	0	0	1	27	—	—	20	15	430	60	72
With Calcium + Vitamin D	8 oz	110	0	0	0	2	26	22	—	350	0	450	60	72
TURKEY HILL														
Orangeade	1 cup	120	0	0	0	—	30	30	—	—	—	—	—	—
VERYFINE														
100% Juice	1 bottle (10 oz)	150	0	0	0	0	37	35	2	0	45	—	—	60
Chillers Arctic Orange	8 fl oz	130	0	0	0	0	33	32	0	0	10	—	—	60
Juice Blend	1 can (11.5 oz)	160	0	0	0	0	39	34	0	0	10	—	—	42
Juice-Ups Orange Punch	8 fl oz	140	0	0	0	0	35	35	0	0	15	—	—	60
Orange Drink	1 bottle (10 oz)	160	0	0	0	0	41	36	0	0	90	—	—	36
TAKE-OUT														
orange julius	1 serv (24 oz)	443	tr	tr	0	2	118	—	1	40	10	713	92	219
OREGANO														
ground	1 tsp	5	tr	tr	0	tr	1	—	—	24	tr	25	—	—
ORGAN MEATS														
(*see* BRAINS, GIBLETS, GIZZARD, HEART, KIDNEY, LIVER, SWEETBREADS)														
OSTRICH														
cooked	3 oz	120	3	—	74	22	—	—	—	5	57	—	—	—
OYSTERS														
canned eastern	1 cup	170	6	2	136	18	10	—	—	111	277	568	22	—
canned eastern	3 oz	58	2	1	46	6	3	—	—	38	95	195	8	—
eastern cooked	6 med	58	2	1	46	6	3	—	—	38	94	192	8	—
eastern cooked	3 oz	117	4	1	93	12	7	—	—	76	190	389	15	—
eastern raw	6 med	58	2	1	46	6	3	—	—	38	94	192	8	—
eastern raw	1 cup	170	6	2	136	18	10	—	—	111	277	568	25	—
pacific raw	3 oz	69	2	tr	—	8	4	—	—	7	90	143	—	—
pacific raw	1 med	41	1	tr	—	5	2	—	—	4	53	84	—	—
steamed	1 med	41	1	tr	—	5	2	—	—	4	53	76	—	—
steamed	3 oz	138	4	1	—	16	8	—	—	14	180	257	—	—
BUMBLE BEE														
Fancy Whole	2 oz	70	3	1	45	7	3	0	0	—	140	—	—	—
Smoked	½ can (1.9 oz)	120	7	2	35	10	6	0	0	—	210	—	—	—

FOOD	PORTION	CALS	FAT	SAT FAT	CHOL	PROT	CARB	SUGAR	FIBER	CALCI	SOD	POTAS	FOLIC	VIT C
TAKE-OUT														
breaded & fried	6 (4.9 oz)	368	18	5	109	13	40	—	—	27	677	182	13	4
oysters rockefeller	3 oysters	66	2	—	38	7	5	—	—	102	80	—	—	—
stew	1 cup	278	18	10	100	15	15	—	tr	331	928	427	14	4

PANCAKE/WAFFLE SYRUP

FOOD	PORTION	CALS	FAT	SAT FAT	CHOL	PROT	CARB	SUGAR	FIBER	CALCI	SOD	POTAS	FOLIC	VIT C
low calorie	1 tbsp	12	0	0	0	0	3	—	0	—	—	—	0	0
maple	1 tbsp (0.8 oz)	52	0	—	0	0	13	12	—	13	2	41	0	0
maple	1 cup (11.1 oz)	824	1	—	0	tr	212	191	—	211	27	643	1	0
pancake syrup	1 cup (11 oz)	903	0	0	0	0	238	—	—	4	290	7	0	0
pancake syrup	1 tbsp (0.7 oz)	57	0	0	0	0	15	—	—	0	17	0	0	0
pancake syrup light	1 oz	46	0	—	0	0	13	—	—	0	57	1	0	0
pancake syrup w/ butter	1 cup (11 oz)	933	5	3	14	tr	234	—	—	6	307	9	0	0
pancake syrup w/ butter	1 tbsp (0.7 oz)	59	tr	tr	1	0	15	—	—	0	20	1	0	0
ATKINS														
Sugar Free	¼ cup	0	0	0	0	0	0	0	0	—	40	—	—	—
AUNT JEMIMA														
Original	¼ cup	210	0	0	0	0	52	32	—	—	120	—	—	—
COUNTRY CUPBOARD														
Boysenberry	¼ cup	0	0	0	0	1	0	0	0	—	0	—	—	—
Maple Butter	¼ cup	0	0	0	0	1	2	0	0	—	0	—	—	—
Strawberry	¼ cup	0	0	0	0	1	1	0	0	—	0	—	—	—
ESTEE														
Maple	¼ cup	80	0	0	0	0	20	20	0	—	125	0	—	—
KETO														
Maple Butter	¼ cup	0	0	0	0	0	1	1	0	—	20	—	—	—
KETOGENICS														
Zero Carb	¼ cup	0	0	0	0	0	0	0	0	—	40	—	—	—
LOG CABIN														
Lite	¼ cup	100	0	0	0	0	25	24	—	—	130	—	—	—
Original	¼ cup	210	0	0	0	0	53	39	0	—	100	—	—	—
MRS. BUTTER-WORTH'S														
Lite	¼ cup	100	0	0	0	0	25	24	—	—	130	—	—	—
Original	¼ cup (2 oz)	230	0	0	0	0	56	35	—	—	95	—	—	—
SMUCKER'S														
Breakfast Syrup Sugar Free	¼ cup (2 oz)	30	0	0	0	0	8	0	—	—	60	—	—	—
STONEWALL KITCHEN														
Maine Maple	¼ cup	210	0	0	0	0	54	51	0	—	5	—	—	—

PANCAKES

FOOD	PORTION	CALS	FAT	SAT FAT	CHOL	PROT	CARB	SUGAR	FIBER	CALCI	SOD	POTAS	FOLIC	VIT C
FROZEN														
buttermilk	1 (4 in diam)	83	1	tr	3	2	16	—	—	22	183	26	—	—

FOOD	PORTION	CALS	FAT	SAT FAT	CHOL	PROT	CARB	SUGAR	FIBER	CALCI	SOD	POTAS	FOLIC	VIT C
plain	1 (4 in diam)	83	1	tr	3	2	16	—	—	22	183	26	—	—
EGGO														
Buttermilk	3 (4.1 oz)	270	8	2	15	7	44	10	1	40	610	120	60	0
GOLDEN														
Potato	1 (1.3 oz)	70	3	0	5	2	10	2	1	0	190	—	—	0
MIX														
buckwheat	1 (4 in diam)	62	2	1	20	2	9	—	—	77	160	70	—	tr
buttermilk	1 (4 in diam)	74	1	tr	—	2	14	—	tr	48	239	67	—	—
plain	(1–4 in diam)	74	1	tr	—	2	14	—	tr	48	239	67	—	—
sugar free low sodium	1 (3 in diam)	44	tr	tr	0	1	9	—	—	13	58	85	1	0
whole wheat	1 (4 in diam)	92	3	1	27	4	13	—	—	110	252	123	—	tr
ATKINS														
Quick Quisine Buttermilk not prep	⅓ cup	100	0	0	0	14	13	1	5	—	320	—	—	—
Quick Quisine Original not prep	¼ cup	80	2	1	5	13	6	0	3	—	120	—	—	—
AUNT JEMIMA														
Buttermilk Pancake & Waffle Mix not prep	⅓ cup	160	3	1	10	4	31	6	1	150	460	—	40	0
Pancake & Waffle Mix Whole Wheat as prep	3 pancakes	200	7	2	57	4	30	4	3	150	784	170	40	0
AUNT PAULA'S														
Pancake & Waffle Mix as prep	2	132	8	—	0	21	6	0	4	—	0	—	—	—
BETTY CROCKER														
Buttermilk as prep	3	200	3	1	10	5	20	3	1	100	540	130	40	—
Original as prep	3	200	3	1	10	6	39	9	2	100	540	120	40	—
BIG TRAIN														
Low Carb Pancake & Waffle Mix as prep	3	190	10	5	108	11	12	0	5	50	300		—	0
BISQUICK														
Shake 'N Pour Blueberry as prep	3	210	4	1	0	6	40	8	1	80	640	—	40	0
BRUCE														
Sweet Potato Pancakes	2	210	3	1	0	6	39	5	2	100	670	—	40	5
CARBOLITE														
Low Carb Mix not prep	⅓ cup	100	tr	—	—	21	10	0	tr	—	310	—	—	—

FOOD	PORTION	CALS	FAT	SAT FAT	CHOL	PROT	CARB	SUGAR	FIBER	CALCI	SOD	POTAS	FOLIC	VIT C
CARBSENSE														
Buckwheat not prep	½ cup	140	3	0	0	21	10	0	7	—	430	—	—	—
Buttermilk not prep	½ cup	140	3	0	0	21	10	0	7	—	320	—	—	—
ESTEE														
Pancake Mix as prep	4 (4 in diam)	180	0	0	0	4	40	tr	1	—	255	340	—	—
HODGSON MILL														
Buckwheat	⅓ cup (1.8 oz)	160	1	0	0	5	36	2	5	150	590	—	—	0
HUNGRY JACK														
Potato as prep	3 (3 in diam)	90	2	0	50	3	16	tr	1	100	380	—	—	0
KETO														
Banana not prep	⅓ cup	114	2	—	—	19	6	0	2	—	224	—	—	—
Original not prep	⅓ cup	114	2	—	—	19	5	0	2	—	224	—	—	—
KETOGENICS														
Low Carb not prep	⅔ cup	185	4	2	94	23	15	1	6	—	400	—	—	—
MINICARB														
Apple Cinnamon as prep	2	150	6	1	10	12	17	2	13	—	170	—	—	—
ROBIN HOOD														
Buttermilk as prep	3	230	6	2	60	8	35	6	1	150	560	160	—	0
TAKE-OUT														
blueberry	1 (4 in diam)	84	4	1	21	2	11	—	—	78	157	52	5	1
plain	1 (4 in diam)	86	4	1	23	2	11	—	—	83	157	50	5	tr
potato	1 (4 in diam)	78	6	1	60	2	4	—	tr	10	238	88	7	4
w/ butter & syrup	2 (8.1 oz)	520	14	6	58	8	91	—	—	128	1104	251	30	4
PAPAYA														
fresh	1	117	tr	tr	0	2	30	—	—	72	8	780	—	188
fresh cubed	1 cup	54	tr	tr	0	1	14	—	—	33	4	359	—	87
SUNFRESH														
In Extra Light Syrup	½ cup (4.5 oz)	70	0	0	0	1	17	16	1	0	5	—	—	5
PAPAYA JUICE														
nectar	1 cup	142	tr	tr	0	tr	36	—	—	24	14	78	5	8
CERES														
Papaya	8 oz	120	0	0	0	0	30	27	0	20	5	190	—	30
EVERFRESH														
Premium Drink	1 can (8 oz)	140	0	0	0	0	35	35	0	—	0	—	—	—
NANTUCKET NECTARS														
Cocktail	8 oz	120	0	0	0	0	30	27	—	0	0	—	—	60
PAPRIKA														
paprika	1 tsp	6	tr	tr	0	tr	1	—	—	4	1	49	—	1
PARSLEY														
dry	1 tbsp	1	tr	—	0	tr	tr	—	—	1	2	25	6	1

FOOD	PORTION	CALS	FAT	SAT FAT	CHOL	PROT	CARB	SUGAR	FIBER	CALCI	SOD	POTAS	FOLIC	VIT C
dry	1 tsp	1	tr	—	0	tr	tr	—	—	4	1	11	—	tr
fresh chopped	½ cup	11	tr	tr	0	1	2	—	—	41	17	166	46	40

PARSNIPS

fresh cooked	1 (5.6 oz)	130	tr	tr	0	2	31	—	—	59	17	588	93	21
fresh sliced cooked	½ cup	63	tr	tr	0	1	15	—	—	29	8	287	45	10
raw sliced	½ cup	50	tr	tr	0	1	12	—	—	24	7	251	45	11

PASSION FRUIT

purple fresh	1	18	tr	—	0	tr	4	—	—	2	5	63	—	5

PASSION FRUIT JUICE

purple	1 cup	126	tr	—	0	1	34	—	—	9	—	—	—	74
yellow	1 cup	149	tr	—	0	2	36	—	—	9	15	687	—	45
CERES														
Passion Fruit	8 oz	120	0	0	0	0	31	28	0	20	10	190	—	30

PASTA

(*see also* NOODLES, PASTA DINNERS, PASTA SALAD)

DRY														
corn cooked	1 cup (4.9 oz)	176	1	tr	0	4	39	—	7	1	0	43	8	0
corn spaghetti	2 oz	180	2	0	0	4	35	3	3	20	5	—	—	0
elbows	1 cup	389	2	tr	0	13	78	—	—	19	8	170	19	0
elbows cooked	1 cup (4.9 oz)	197	1	tr	0	7	40	—	2	10	1	43	98	0
shells small cooked	1 cup (4 oz)	162	1	tr	0	5	33	—	2	8	1	36	81	0
spaghetti cooked	1 cup (4.9 oz)	197	1	tr	0	7	40	—	2	10	1	43	98	0
spinach spaghetti cooked	1 cup (4.9 oz)	182	1	tr	0	6	37	—	—	42	20	81	17	0
spirals cooked	1 cup (4.7 oz)	189	tr	tr	0	6	38	—	2	9	1	42	94	0
vegetable cooked	1 cup (4.7 oz)	172	tr	tr	0	6	36	—	6	15	8	42	87	0
whole wheat all shapes cooked	1 cup (4.9 oz)	174	tr	tr	0	7	37	—	4	21	4	62	7	0
ANNIE CHUN'S														
Soba Noodles	2 oz	200	1	0	0	8	39	1	3	0	390	—	—	0
ATKINS														
All Shapes not prep	2 oz	230	3	0	0	36	15	2	9	100	270	—	—	0
Quick Quisine All Shapes as prep	¾ cup	210	3	1	0	4	13	2	8	—	280	—	—	—
BARILLA														
Conchiglie Rigate	1 cup (2 oz)	200	1	0	0	6	40	1	2	0	0	—	120	0
Gemelli as prep	1 cup (2 oz)	200	1	0	0	7	42	1	2	0	0	—	—	0
Pastina	2 oz	210	2	1	65	8	40	tr	2	0	20	—	120	0
Tortelloni Porcini Mushroom	¾ cup	240	8	5	50	8	32	3	5	60	335	—	—	0
Tortelloni Ricotta & Asparagus	¾ cup	240	8	5	60	7	32	2	5	60	450	—	—	0

FOOD	PORTION	CALS	FAT	SAT FAT	CHOL	PROT	CARB	SUGAR	FIBER	CALCI	SOD	POTAS	FOLIC	VIT C
BARILLA (CONT.)														
Tortelloni Ricotta & Spinach	¾ cup	240	8	7	50	8	31	3	4	100	450	—	—	0
BELLA VITA														
Low Carb Penne Rigate	2 oz	190	1	0	0	28	18	3	8	150	40	—	—	0
CUORE														
Capellini cooked	1⅓ cups (2 oz)	190	1	0	0	7	39	1	3	0	0	—	120	0
Fusilli cooked	1⅓ cups (2 oz)	190	1	0	0	7	39	1	3	0	0	—	120	0
Tortiglioni cooked	1⅓ cups (2 oz)	190	1	0	0	7	39	1	3	0	0	—	120	0
DARIELLE														
All Shapes not prep	2 oz	160	1	0	0	28	18	3	8	—	40	—	—	—
DAVINCI														
Rotini	1 cup	210	1	0	0	6	43	3	2	20	0	—	140	0
Spaghetti	2 oz	210	1	0	0	6	43	3	2	20	0	—	140	0
DECECCO														
Whole Wheat Linguine cooked	2 oz	180	2	0	<5	8	33	1	7	20	0	—	—	0
DREAMFIELDS														
All Shapes not prep	2 oz	190	1	0	0	7	42	1	4	0	0	—	100	0
DUC AMICI														
Pasta Lite Low Carb Fusilli	2 oz	160	1	0	0	28	10	3	7	150	50	—	—	0
EDEN														
Organic Extra Fine	2 oz	210	2	0	0	9	40	1	3	20	0	180	—	0
Organic Gemelli	2 oz	210	2	0	0	8	40	2	5	20	0	280	21	0
Organic Pesto Gemelli	2 oz	210	1	0	0	8	41	2	4	20	0	220	18	0
Organic Ribbons Saffron	2 oz	210	2	0	0	9	40	1	3	20	0	180	9	0
Organic Spaghetti Semolina	2 oz	200	1	0	0	8	40	1	2	20	0	135	9	0
Organic Spaghetti 50% Whole Grain	2 oz	210	1	0	0	8	41	2	4	20	0	220	18	0
Organic Spirals Kamut Vegetable	2 oz	210	2	0	0	8	40	3	6	20	45	210	24	0
Organic Spirals Sesame Rice	2 oz	200	2	0	0	8	37	1	4	80	0	280	16	0
Organic Spirals Mixed Grain	2 oz	210	2	0	0	8	41	3	7	20	15	210	32	0
Organic Spirals Spinach	2 oz	210	1	0	0	8	41	2	4	20	30	320	18	0

FOOD	PORTION	CALS	FAT	SAT FAT	CHOL	PROT	CARB	SUGAR	FIBER	CALCI	SOD	POTAS	FOLIC	VIT C
EDEN (CONT.)														
Organic Vegetable Alphabets	2 oz	200	1	0	0	8	40	1	2	20	15	135	9	0
Spirals Rye	2 oz	200	0	0	0	6	44	1	8	26	10	300	130	1
GOYA														
Coditos not prep	½ cup	230	1	0	0	8	47	2	3	20	0	—	—	1
HODGSON MILL														
Four Color Veggie Bows	2 oz	200	1	0	0	8	41	0	1	0	15	—	120	0
Four Color Veggie Rotini Spirals	2 oz	200	1	0	0	8	41	0	1	0	15	—	120	0
Pastamania! Durum Wheat Fettuccine	2 oz	200	2	1	30	8	38	0	1	20	20	—	—	0
Pastamania! Fettuccine Garlic & Parsley	2 oz	200	2	1	30	8	38	0	1	20	20	—	—	0
Pastamania! Fettuccine w/ Jerusalem Artichoke	2 oz	210	2	0	0	8	41	0	2	0	10	—	—	0
Pastamania! Fettucine w/ Mushroom	2 oz	210	2	1	35	8	41	1	2	20	15	—	—	0
Pastamania! Fusilli Tre Colore w/ Tomato & Spinach	2 oz	200	1	0	0	7	40	2	2	0	20	—	—	0
Pastamania! Sea Shell Mix	2 oz	200	1	0	0	8	40	0	1	0	10	—	—	0
Pastamania! Spinach Fettuccine	2 oz	200	2	1	40	8	37	0	2	20	35	—	—	0
Pastamania! Thin Linguine	2 oz	200	2	1	30	8	38	0	1	20	20	—	—	0
Pastamania! Tomato Spinach & Durum Wheat	2 oz	210	2	1	35	8	40	1	2	20	29	—	—	0
Spaghetti Whole Wheat not prep	2 oz	190	0	0	0	9	34	0	6	20	10	—	28	0
Whole Wheat Lasagne not prep	2 oz	190	0	0	0	9	34	0	6	20	10	—	28	0
Whole Wheat Spinach Spaghetti not prep	2 oz	190	1	0	0	9	35	0	5	40	25	—	28	0
KETO														
Elbows not prep	1.6 oz	108	0	0	0	22	5	0	1	—	120	—	—	—
Spaghetti not prep	1.3 oz	130	1	0	0	22	7	0	2	—	120	—	—	—

FOOD	PORTION	CALS	FAT	SAT FAT	CHOL	PROT	CARB	SUGAR	FIBER	CALCI	SOD	POTAS	FOLIC	VIT C
LUNDBERG														
Spaghetti Organic Brown Rice	2 oz	210	2	1	0	4	44	3	3	0	5	190	—	0
PASTALIA														
Heart Health Low Carb not prep	2 oz	176	2	—	—	30	10	tr	3	—	180	—	—	—
REAL TORINO														
Tirali not prep	1 cup (2 oz)	210	1	0	0	6	43	3	2	20	0	—	140	0
REVIVAL														
Soy Penne	⅙ box	200	2	0	0	14	34	2	1	25	85	88	—	—
Soy Thin Spaghetti	⅙ box	200	2	0	0	14	34	2	1	25	85	88	—	—
RONZONI														
Elbows not prep	½ cup (2 oz)	210	1	0	0	7	42	2	2	—	0	—	100	—
Healthy Harvest Whole Wheat Blend	2 oz	210	2	0	0	7	42	2	3	—	0	—	100	—
Lasagne	2½ pieces (2 oz)	210	1	0	0	7	42	2	2	—	0	—	100	—
Tradizione D'Italia All Shapes	2 oz	210	1	0	0	7	42	2	2	—	0	—	100	—
SOY7														
Pasta All Shapes	2 oz	200	1	0	0	13	33	2	2	—	120	—	—	—
WHEY COOL														
High Protein Xtreme Rotini	1 serv (2 oz)	210	2	0	5	42	8	4	1	—	270	—	—	—
FRESH														
cooked	2 oz	75	1	tr	33	3	14	—	—	3	3	14	36	0
spinach cooked	2 oz	74	1	tr	19	3	14	—	—	10	3	21	36	0
DI GIORNO														
Linguine	1 cup	200	2	0	0	8	38	1	2	0	140	140	60	0
REFRIGERATED														
BUITONI														
Angel Hair	1¼ cups	230	3	1	50	10	43	1	2	20	20	—	—	0
Fettuccine	1¼ cups	240	3	1	55	10	45	1	2	20	20	—	—	0
Fettuccine Spinach	1¼ cups	260	3	1	75	12	45	1	2	60	110	—	—	1
Linguine	1¼ cups	240	3	1	55	10	45	1	2	20	20	—	—	0
Ravioletti Three Cheese	1 cup	270	6	3	35	12	43	3	2	100	330	—	—	0
Ravioletti Beef	1 cup	300	7	2	35	12	46	3	2	40	370	—	—	0
Ravioli Four Cheese	1 serv (9 oz)	330	14	9	65	12	40	3	3	150	630	—	—	0
Ravioli Beef	1¼ cups	340	10	3	60	15	48	4	2	60	530	—	—	0
Ravioli Chicken Parmesan	1¼ cups	310	8	2	55	14	45	3	2	40	620	—	—	0

FOOD	PORTION	CALS	FAT	SAT FAT	CHOL	PROT	CARB	SUGAR	FIBER	CALCI	SOD	POTAS	FOLIC	VIT C
BUITONI (CONT.)														
Ravioli Garden Vegetable	1 cup	250	5	2	40	11	39	4	2	100	500	—	—	2
Ravioli Light Four Cheese	1¼ cups	230	4	2	35	12	37	3	2	100	390	—	—	0
Ravioli Roasted Chicken & Garlic	1¼ cups	340	11	3	50	14	47	3	2	40	550	—	—	0
Tortellini Herb Chicken	1 cup	340	9	3	40	13	52	3	2	20	410	—	—	0
Tortellini Spinach Cheese	1 cup	330	8	4	55	15	49	3	3	200	510	—	—	0
Tortellini Three Cheese	1 cup	320	7	4	40	15	50	4	3	150	480	—	—	0
Tortelloni Cheese & Roasted Garlic	1 cup	270	8	4	35	12	37	2	2	150	360	—	—	0
Tortelloni Chicken & Prosciutto	1 cup	330	9	3	45	14	47	2	2	40	630	—	—	0
Tortelloni Mozzarella & Herb	1 cup	330	10	5	45	14	46	3	2	150	450	—	—	0
Tortelloni Mozzarella & Pepperoni	1 cup	330	10	5	45	15	45	3	2	150	440	—	—	0
Tortelloni Sun Dried Tomato	1 cup	310	9	2	25	12	46	4	3	80	340	—	—	0
Tortelloni Sweet Italian Sausage	1 cup	330	9	3	35	13	48	5	3	40	280	—	—	0
DI GIORNO														
Angel's Hair	1 cup	160	2	0	0	6	31	1	2	0	115	110	40	0
Beef & Roasted Garlic Tortellini	1 cup	340	11	4	50	14	46	2	1	80	390	200	60	0
Fettuccine	1 cup	200	2	0	0	8	38	1	2	0	140	140	60	0
Four Cheese Raviolo	1 cup	350	15	9	70	14	40	1	2	250	390	200	60	0
Herb Linguine	1 cup	200	2	0	0	8	38	1	2	20	140	150	60	0
Italian Sausage Ravioli In Green Bell Pepper Pasta	1¼ cups	350	12	6	55	14	45	3	3	100	570	250	60	0
Lemon Chicken Tortellini In Cracked Black Pepper Pasta	1 cup	270	5	3	40	13	42	2	1	60	290	150	40	0
Light Cheese Ravioli	1 cup	280	7	4	40	15	40	1	2	250	400	170	60	0
Mozzarella Garlic Tortelloni	1 cup	300	8	5	45	15	42	1	1	250	400	150	60	0
Pesto Tortelloni	1 cup	320	8	5	45	16	46	1	3	250	430	230	60	0

FOOD	PORTION	CALS	FAT	SAT FAT	CHOL	PROT	CARB	SUGAR	FIBER	CALCI	SOD	POTAS	FOLIC	VIT C
DI GIORNO (CONT.)														
Portabello Mushroom Tortelloni	1 cup	310	7	5	40	13	48	1	3	200	490	360	60	0
Red Bell Pepper Fettuccine	1 cup	200	2	0	0	8	38	1	2	0	140	130	60	2
Spinach Fettuccine	1 cup	190	2	0	0	8	38	tr	2	40	160	220	60	0
Sun-Dried Tomato Ravioli	1⅓ cups	380	14	8	55	17	48	5	3	250	600	420	60	1
Three Cheese Tortellini	¾ cup	250	7	4	35	11	37	2	2	150	300	125	40	0

PASTA DINNERS

(*see also* PASTA SALAD)

CANNED

FOOD	PORTION	CALS	FAT	SAT FAT	CHOL	PROT	CARB	SUGAR	FIBER	CALCI	SOD	POTAS	FOLIC	VIT C
CHEF BOYARDEE														
99% Fat Free Beef Ravioli	1 cup (8.6 oz)	210	1	0	15	9	41	6	3	20	1150	—	—	0
99% Fat Free Cheese Ravioli	1 cup (8.8 oz)	210	1	0	<5	7	44	9	4	40	860	—	—	1
Beef Ravioli	1 cup (8.6 oz)	230	5	3	20	9	37	5	4	0	1150	—	—	0
Beefaroni	1 cup (8.7 oz)	260	7	3	25	10	37	9	5	0	870	—	—	0
Macaroni & Cheese	½ can (7.5 oz)	180	2	—	20	8	35	0	2	—	1090	—	—	—
Mini Ravioli	1 cup (8.8 oz)	252	6	3	20	8	37	5	3	0	1180	—	—	0
Spaghetti & Meat Balls	1 cup (8.4 oz)	240	10	4	25	9	32	7	3	0	950	—	—	0
Tortellini Cheese	½ can (7 oz)	230	1	—	15	9	48	12	5	—	770	—	—	—
Tortellini Meat	½ can (7 oz)	260	4	2	30	10	48	12	4	—	810	—	—	—
FRANCO-AMERICAN														
Beef Raviolios	1 can (7.7 oz)	250	5	2	12	9	39	10	4	37	911	387	—	0
Beefy Mac	1 can (7.5 oz)	228	8	3	10	9	30	10	3	38	1144	347	—	1
Elbow Macaroni & Cheese	1 can (7.5 oz)	187	6	3	7	6	25	2	2	96	875	121	—	0
Spaghetti 'N Beef	1 can (7.5 oz)	226	8	4	14	10	30	9	3	38	1063	409	—	0
Spaghetti w/ Meatballs	1 can (7.2 oz)	249	9	4	14	10	33	12	4	33	917	379	—	0
KID'S KITCHEN														
Microwave Meals Cheezy Mac & Beef	1 cup (7.5 oz)	260	7	3	30	15	33	7	1	100	910	—	—	1
Microwave Meals Noodle Rings & Chicken	1 cup (7.5 oz)	150	4	2	30	10	17	2	1	40	1110	—	—	0
Microwave Meals Spaghetti Rings & Franks	1 cup (7.5 oz)	240	9	4	30	9	32	11	1	80	810	—	—	2

FOOD	PORTION	CALS	FAT	SAT FAT	CHOL	PROT	CARB	SUGAR	FIBER	CALCI	SOD	POTAS	FOLIC	VIT C
PROGRESSO														
Beef Ravioli	1 cup (9.1 oz)	260	5	2	5	9	45	9	4	40	940	—	—	4
Cheese Ravioli	1 cup (9.1 oz)	220	2	1	<5	7	43	9	4	40	930	—	—	2
FROZEN														
AMY'S														
Bowl Stuffed Pasta Shells	1 pkg (10 oz)	300	12	7	30	19	30	7	5	—	740	—	—	—
Cannelloni w/ Vegetables	1 pkg (9 oz)	330	12	8	15	16	34	10	6	—	390	—	—	—
Lasagna Cheese	1 pkg (10.25 oz)	330	12	7	35	19	38	6	5	—	680	—	—	—
Lasagna Garden Vegetable	1 pkg (10.25 oz)	290	9	4	20	13	41	7	5	—	720	—	—	—
Macaroni & Cheese	1 pkg (9 oz)	410	16	10	50	16	47	6	3	—	590	—	—	—
Macaroni & Soy Cheese	1 pkg (9 oz)	370	15	2	0	16	42	2	4	—	500	—	—	—
Pasta & Vegetable Alfredo	1 cup	220	8	4	20	11	27	6	4	—	460	—	—	—
Pasta Primavera	1 pkg (9 oz)	300	11	6	45	15	37	7	3	—	670	—	—	—
Ravioli w/ Sauce	1 pkg (8 oz)	340	12	5	25	15	43	3	3	—	580	—	—	—
Rice Mac & Cheese	1 pkg (9 oz)	140	16	10	50	16	47	6	3	—	590	—	—	—
Skillet Meals	1 cup	250	11	3	5	9	27	3	3	—	480	—	—	—
Tofu Vegetable Lasagna	1 pkg (9.5 oz)	300	10	2	0	13	41	6	6	—	630	—	—	—
Vegetable Lasagna	1 pkg (9.5 oz)	280	12	5	20	14	29	5	3	—	680	—	—	—
BANQUET														
Chicken Pasta Primavera	1 meal (9.5 oz)	320	12	6	25	11	40	9	6	60	840	—	—	0
Family Size Egg Noodles w/ Beef & Brown Gravy	1 serv	150	5	3	35	11	16	1	2	0	1120	—	—	0
Family Size Lasagna w/ Meat Sauce	1 cup	270	10	6	45	14	33	3	2	100	900	—	—	54
Family Size Macaroni & Cheese	1 cup	230	7	3	10	8	32	7	3	100	1290	—	—	0
Fettuccine Alfredo	1 meal (9.5 oz)	350	16	7	25	11	40	5	4	100	850	—	—	6
Homestyle Noodles & Chicken	1 meal (12 oz)	390	19	7	50	12	44	5	7	60	1080	—	—	0
Lasagna w/ Meat Sauce	1 meal (9.5 oz)	260	8	3	15	10	38	10	3	80	820	—	—	1

FOOD	PORTION	CALS	FAT	SAT FAT	CHOL	PROT	CARB	SUGAR	FIBER	CALCI	SOD	POTAS	FOLIC	VIT C
BANQUET (CONT.)														
Macaroni & Cheese	1 meal (12 oz)	420	14	8	20	15	57	7	5	150	1330	—	—	0
BIRDS EYE														
Easy Recipe Creations Basil Herb Primavera	2¼ cup	260	11	7	25	9	31	5	3	100	750	—	—	24
Easy Recipe Creations Tortellini Parmigiana	2¼ cups	240	12	7	25	9	25	5	4	150	870	—	—	36
Pasta Secrets Italian Pesto	2⅓ cups	240	9	2	5	9	32	6	2	100	700	—	—	18
Pasta Secrets Primavera	2⅓ cups	230	10	3	10	9	26	4	3	200	430	—	—	30
Pasta Secrets Ranch	2⅓ cups	300	15	6	25	7	29	8	2	200	460	—	—	4
Pasta Secrets Three Cheese	2 cups	230	8	3	5	9	31	8	2	100	590	—	—	21
Pasta Secrets White Cheddar	2 cups	240	10	3	10	7	30	7	2	200	560	—	—	21
Pasta Secrets Zesty Garlic	2 cups	240	10	3	5	7	31	6	2	150	310	—	—	15
GREEN GIANT														
Create A Meal Creamy Alfredo as prep	1¼ cups (10 oz)	380	12	5	75	34	33	9	4	250	990	—	—	27
Create A Meal Creamy Cheddar as prep	1½ cups (10 oz)	290	10	6	45	20	29	8	4	200	1470	—	—	36
Create A Meal Creamy Chicken Noodle as prep	1¼ cups (10 oz)	350	11	5	65	28	34	8	3	150	970	—	—	5
Pasta Accents Alfredo	2 cups (5.6 oz)	210	5	3	15	9	25	5	4	150	480	—	—	12
Pasta Accents Creamy Cheddar	2⅓ cups (6.7 oz)	250	8	3	15	9	36	6	5	150	700	—	—	6
Pasta Accents Florentine	2 cups (7.3 oz)	310	9	3	20	13	44	5	5	300	910	—	—	5
Pasta Accents Garden Herb Seasoning	2 cups (6.8 oz)	230	7	4	15	9	32	4	7	80	750	—	—	9
Pasta Accents Garlic Seasoning	2 cups (6.6 oz)	260	10	5	15	7	36	5	5	60	640	—	—	5
Pasta Accents Primavera	2¼ cups (7 oz)	320	12	5	20	13	40	5	7	150	500	—	—	15

FOOD	PORTION	CALS	FAT	SAT FAT	CHOL	PROT	CARB	SUGAR	FIBER	CALCI	SOD	POTAS	FOLIC	VIT C
GREEN GIANT (CONT.)														
Pasta Accents White Cheddar Sauce	1¾ cups (5.6 oz)	300	12	4	20	10	38	7	4	200	570	—	—	12
HEALTHY CHOICE														
Beef Macaroni	1 meal (8.5 oz)	220	4	2	20	12	34	9	5	40	450	—	—	54
Bowls Cheese & Chicken Tortellini	1 meal (8.7 oz)	250	5	2	20	11	40	5	6	100	600	—	—	36
Breaded Chicken Breast Strips w/ Macaroni & Cheese	1 meal (8 oz)	270	5	3	40	22	34	9	1	150	600	—	—	1
Cheese Ravioli Parmigiana	1 meal (9 oz)	260	5	3	20	11	44	14	6	150	290	—	—	0
Chicken Fettuccine Alfredo	1 meal (8.5 oz)	280	7	3	35	21	30	3	4	100	600	—	—	2
Fettuccine Alfredo	1 meal (8 oz)	240	5	3	20	11	37	4	2	100	560	—	—	0
Lasagna Bake	1 pkg (9 oz)	270	7	3	20	13	38	13	4	100	600	—	—	0
Macaroni & Cheese	1 meal (9 oz)	240	5	3	20	12	36	8	3	200	600	—	—	0
Manicotti w/ Three Cheeses	1 meal (11 oz)	300	9	3	35	15	40	14	5	250	550	—	—	0
Spaghetti & Sauce w/ Seasoned Beef	1 meal (10 oz)	260	8	2	30	14	43	7	5	40	470	—	—	15
Stuffed Pasta Shells	1 meal (10.35 oz)	370	6	3	20	18	60	12	5	250	570	—	—	5
JOSEPH'S PASTA														
Grilled Chicken Ravioli w/ Roasted Red Pepper Sauce	1 pkg (14 oz)	540	15	8	150	36	66	3	6	180	1440	—	—	7
KID CUISINE														
Magical Macaroni & Cheese	1 meal (10.6 oz)	440	13	5	15	10	72	25	4	100	670	—	—	0
LEAN CUISINE														
Cafe Classics Bow Tie Pasta & Chicken	1 pkg (9.5 oz)	220	4	1	40	15	32	6	5	80	690	720	—	15
Cafe Classics Cheese Lasagna w/ Chicken Scaloppini	1 pkg (10 oz)	270	8	3	35	22	27	7	4	150	690	680	—	6
Cafe Classics Shrimp & Angel Hair Pasta	1 pkg (10 oz)	240	5	1	45	15	35	7	2	100	670	480	—	18
Everyday Favorites Alfredo Pasta Primavera	1 pkg (10 oz)	290	7	3	10	11	46	6	3	150	570	300	—	12

FOOD	PORTION	CALS	FAT	SAT FAT	CHOL	PROT	CARB	SUGAR	FIBER	CALCI	SOD	POTAS	FOLIC	VIT C
LEAN CUISINE (CONT.)														
Everyday Favorites Angel Hair Pasta	1 pkg (10 oz)	240	4	1	5	9	43	11	4	80	500	580	—	15
Everyday Favorites Cheese Cannelloni	1 pkg (9.1 oz)	230	4	2	15	21	28	8	4	350	590	560	—	4
Everyday Favorites Cheese Lasagna Casserole	1 pkg (10 oz)	270	6	3	10	13	40	6	5	200	590	420	—	9
Everyday Favorites Cheese Ravioli	1 pkg (8.5 oz)	260	7	4	35	12	38	8	4	150	590	450	—	5
Everyday Favorites Chicken Lasagna	1 pkg (10 oz)	280	7	3	40	20	34	6	2	250	590	650	—	2
Everyday Favorites Classic Cheese Lasagna	1 pkg (11.5 oz)	290	6	4	25	20	38	9	4	300	590	620	—	9
Everyday Favorites Fettucini Alfredo	1 pkg (9.25 oz)	280	7	3	15	13	42	6	3	200	540	250	—	0
Everyday Favorites Fettucini Primavera	1 pkg (10 oz)	270	7	3	15	13	38	8	4	250	580	370	—	0
Everyday Favorites Lasagna w/ Meat Sauce	1 pkg (10.5 oz)	300	8	5	30	23	35	7	4	400	570	590	—	12
Everyday Favorites Macaroni & Cheese	1 pkg (10 oz)	290	7	4	20	15	42	5	2	200	630	470	—	0
Everyday Favorites Macaroni & Beef	1 pkg (10 oz)	270	4	2	25	15	43	9	4	60	590	520	—	0
Everyday Favorites Penne Pasta	1 pkg (10 oz)	260	4	1	0	9	47	13	5	60	390	520	—	6
Everyday Favorites Spaghetti w/ Meat Sauce	1 pkg (11.5 oz)	290	5	2	20	11	50	10	7	60	570	550	—	9
Everyday Favorites Spaghetti w/ Meatballs	1 pkg (9.5 oz)	270	6	3	20	16	37	6	4	80	590	540	—	6
Family Style Favorites Five Cheese Lasagna	1 serv (8 oz)	210	5	3	20	14	27	6	3	250	690	450	—	1
Skillet Sensations Chicken Alfredo	1 serv	280	6	4	30	20	36	6	3	200	590	—	—	48
MARIE CALLENDER'S														
Cheese Ravioli In Marinara Sauce w/ Spirals & Garlic Bread	1 meal (16 oz)	750	29	9	30	25	96	18	11	500	1070	—	—	0
Extra Cheese Lasagna	1 meal (15 oz)	590	27	13	50	27	61	19	7	800	1230	—	—	0

FOOD	PORTION	CALS	FAT	SAT FAT	CHOL	PROT	CARB	SUGAR	FIBER	CALCI	SOD	POTAS	FOLIC	VIT C
MARIE CALLENDER'S (CONT.)														
Fettuccine Alfredo & Garlic Bread	1 meal (14 oz)	920	55	23	90	23	62	5	3	250	1270	—	—	0
Fettuccine Alfredo Supreme	1 meal (13 oz)	450	27	12	80	15	35	1	4	150	680	—	—	1
Fettuccine Primavera w/ Tortellini	1 meal (14 oz)	750	49	21	65	19	57	10	6	200	1130	—	—	6
Fettuccine w/ Broccoli & Chicken	1 meal (13 oz)	710	43	17	85	26	53	7	6	150	910	—	—	9
Lasagna w/ Meat Sauce	1 meal (15 oz)	630	31	15	75	29	59	24	3	500	1230	—	—	0
Macaroni & Cheese	1 meal (12 oz)	540	24	15	50	25	55	12	5	400	1930	—	—	0
Skillet Meal Chicken Alfredo	½ pkg	490	29	14	75	28	32	5	7	150	1220	—	—	30
Skillet Meal Penne Pasta & Meatballs	½ pkg	600	31	11	45	26	53	4	4	150	1360	—	—	0
Skillet Meal Rigatoni Vegetables In Cheese Sauce	1 cup	290	12	7	30	12	32	16	4	200	640	—	—	4
Spaghetti w/ Meat Sauce & Garlic Bread	1 meal (17 oz)	670	25	11	35	27	65	20	9	150	1100	—	—	0
Stuffed Pasta Trio	1 meal (10.5 oz)	380	16	9	50	15	40	26	5	500	950	—	—	1
MORTON														
Macaroni & Cheese	1 serv (8 oz)	240	8	4	20	9	34	10	3	100	1190	—	—	0
Spaghetti w/ Meat Sauce	1 meal (8.5 oz)	200	6	3	5	5	30	13	4	20	750	—	—	0
QUORN														
Fettuccine Alfredo	1 pkg (10.5 oz)	360	16	9	45	17	40	5	4	200	920	—	—	21
Lasagna	1 pkg (10.5 oz)	360	12	4	15	23	43	13	4	200	910	—	—	9
SEEDS OF CHANGE														
Organic Lasagna Creamy Spinach	1 pkg (11 oz)	370	16	11	35	19	36	4	7	300	750	—	—	0
SLIM-FAST														
Fettuccine Alfredo	1 pkg	240	6	3	20	10	41	4	5	400	890	400	120	60
Rotini w/ Tomato & Italian Herb	1 pkg	240	2	1	<5	10	45	7	4	250	890	400	120	60
Shells & Creamy Cheese Sauce	1 pkg	240	6	3	20	10	40	5	5	400	890	400	120	60

FOOD	PORTION	CALS	FAT	SAT FAT	CHOL	PROT	CARB	SUGAR	FIBER	CALCI	SOD	POTAS	FOLIC	VIT C
STOUFFER'S														
Cheddar Pasta w/ Beef & Tomatoes	1 pkg (11 oz)	450	19	10	51	25	45	7	3	350	1130	380	—	5
Cheese Manicotti	1 pkg (9 oz)	380	17	9	45	18	38	10	4	450	880	450	—	2
Cheese Ravioli	1 pkg (10.6 oz)	380	13	6	100	15	51	11	6	250	700	450	—	12
Chicken Lasagna	1 serv (7.8 oz)	320	17	5	30	13	29	5	4	200	750	325	—	5
Fettucini Alfredo	1 pkg (10 oz)	520	28	16	100	16	17	5	4	300	1060	190	—	0
Fettucini Primavera	1 pkg (10 oz)	430	20	12	50	13	49	6	5	250	1100	250	—	0
Five Cheese Lasagna	1 pkg (10.75 oz)	360	13	7	35	21	40	10	6	350	960	470	—	6
Grilled Chicken & Angel Hair Pasta	1 pkg (10.9 oz)	380	13	4	40	25	40	6	5	250	750	320	—	0
Homestyle Chicken Fettucini	1 pkg (10.5 oz)	390	15	4	65	31	32	8	3	300	1250	520	—	1
Homestyle Chicken Parmigiana w/ Spaghetti	1 pkg (12 oz)	460	16	4	45	24	54	9	5	150	1060	670	—	12
Homestyle Veal Parmigiana w/ Spaghetti	1 pkg (11.9 oz)	430	17	5	80	21	49	10	6	150	1120	680	—	12
Lasagna Bake	1 pkg (10.25 oz)	370	12	5	30	18	47	9	6	150	900	440	—	9
Lasagna w/ Meat Sauce	1 cup	250	8	5	30	17	27	5	2	100	720	—	—	2
Macaroni & Cheese	1 cup (6 oz)	320	16	7	30	13	31	5	3	300	990	210	—	0
Macaroni & Cheese w/ Broccoli	1 pkg (10.5 oz)	360	17	8	25	15	37	7	5	300	1050	400	—	9
Macaroni & Beef	1 pkg (11.5 oz)	420	20	8	50	20	40	12	5	60	1530	630	—	9
Noodles Romanoff	1 pkg (12 oz)	490	25	6	60	18	48	7	4	150	1400	280	—	0
Pasta Shells w/ American Cheese	1 cup (6 oz)	260	10	4	20	11	31	8	2	250	1190	280	—	0
Salisbury Steak w/ Macaroni & Cheese	1 serv (11.3 oz)	410	19	8	70	26	34	4	2	250	1230	360	—	2
Spaghetti w/ Meat Sauce	1 pkg (10 oz)	350	12	4	35	15	46	7	5	60	570	430	—	9
Spaghetti w/ Meatballs	1 pkg (12.6 oz)	440	15	5	50	19	56	8	5	60	830	500	—	5
Tuna Noodle Casserole	1 pkg (10 oz)	320	10	4	40	20	37	7	0	200	1130	390	—	0

FOOD	PORTION	CALS	FAT	SAT FAT	CHOL	PROT	CARB	SUGAR	FIBER	CALCI	SOD	POTAS	FOLIC	VIT C
STOUFFER'S (CONT.)														
Turkey Tettrazini	1 pkg (10 oz)	360	17	7	55	19	33	5	1	100	1060	380	—	2
Vegetable Lasagna	1 pkg (10.5 oz)	440	20	8	35	21	43	9	5	500	1110	470	—	0
WEIGHT WATCHERS														
Garden Lasagna	1 pkg (11 oz)	270	7	4	30	14	36	6	5	350	610	—	—	6
Homestyle Macaroni & Cheese	1 pkg (9 oz)	290	7	3	10	12	45	2	2	200	630	—	—	0
Smart Ones Angel Hair Pasta	1 pkg (9 oz)	180	2	0	0	9	32	4	4	100	600	—	—	5
Smart Ones Bowtie Pasta & Mushrooms Marsala	1 pkg (9.65 oz)	270	7	4	40	11	40	3	4	80	520	—	—	5
Smart Ones Chicken Fettucini	1 pkg (10 oz)	300	7	2	70	21	39	4	4	200	590	—	—	2
Smart Ones Creamy Rigatoni w/ Broccoli & Chicken	1 pkg (9 oz)	230	2	1	20	14	40	5	4	150	670	—	—	5
Smart Ones Fettucini Alfredo w/ Broccoli	1 pkg (8.5 oz)	230	6	4	20	13	32	8	3	200	540	—	—	1
Smart Ones Lasagna Florentine	1 pkg (10 oz)	200	2	0	10	11	33	5	5	200	640	—	—	9
Smart Ones Lasagna Alfredo	1 pkg (9 oz)	300	7	4	25	14	46	6	3	250	680	—	—	1
Smart Ones Lasagna w/ Meat Sauce	1 pkg (10.25 oz)	270	6	4	55	18	36	8	6	350	570	—	—	6
Smart Ones Lasagna w/ Meat Sauce	1 pkg (9 oz)	240	2	1	10	13	43	5	4	150	520	—	—	5
Smart Ones Macaroni & Cheese	1 pkg (9 oz)	220	2	1	5	9	42	5	4	100	640	—	—	0
Smart Ones Pasta & Spinach Romano	1 pkg (10.4 oz)	260	8	3	15	12	35	7	4	250	510	—	—	12
Smart Ones Pasta w/ Tomato Basil Sauce	1 pkg (9.6 oz)	260	7	3	10	10	40	4	3	150	360	—	—	9
Smart Ones Penne Pasta w/ Sun-Dried Tomatoes	1 pkg (10 oz)	280	8	5	15	11	40	5	3	200	560	—	—	6

FOOD	PORTION	CALS	FAT	SAT FAT	CHOL	PROT	CARB	SUGAR	FIBER	CALCI	SOD	POTAS	FOLIC	VIT C
WEIGHT WATCHERS (CONT.)														
Smart Ones Penne Pollo	1 pkg (10 oz)	290	6	3	55	22	38	5	3	150	590	—	—	4
Smart Ones Ravioli Florentine	1 pkg (8.5 oz)	220	2	1	5	9	43	5	4	100	490	—	—	9
Smart Ones Spaghetti Marinara	1 pkg (9 oz)	280	7	2	5	9	46	7	4	60	690	—	—	9
Smart Ones Spaghetti w/ Meat Sauce	1 pkg (10 oz)	280	6	2	15	15	41	8	4	0	560	—	—	9
Smart Ones Spicy Penne & Ricotta	1 pkg (10.2 oz)	280	6	2	5	11	45	5	4	150	400	—	—	6
Smart Ones Tuna Noodle Casserole	1 pkg (9.5 oz)	270	7	3	45	13	38	6	4	150	670	—	—	4
Smart Ones Zita Mozzarella	1 pkg (9 oz)	290	7	2	5	11	47	5	5	100	600	—	—	2
YVES														
Veggie Lasagna	1 pkg (10.5 oz)	300	3	0	0	17	51	9	4	150	650	330	—	9
Veggie Macaroni	1 pkg (10.5 oz)	230	2	0	0	14	38	6	3	100	580	260	—	9
Veggie Penne	1 pkg (10.5 oz)	220	2	0	0	12	36	7	4	200	730	230	—	15
MIX														
ANNIE'S HOMEGROWN														
Mac & Cheese Meals	1 pkg	230	5	3	10	9	40	0	tr	100	560	—	100	0
ARAMANA														
Cheddar Cheeseburger as prep	1 cup	260	17	10	55	16	11	2	4	—	840	—	—	—
Creamy Chicken Alfredo as prep	1 cup	260	16	10	55	17	12	2	5	—	720	—	—	—
Mild Mexican as prep	1 cup	260	16	10	55	17	12	2	5	—	840	—	—	—
ATKINS														
Quick Quisine Elbows & Cheese as prep	1 cup	250	7	2	10	32	17	0	9	—	500	—	—	—
Quick Quisine Fettuccine Alfredo as prep	1 cup	210	7	3	10	32	16	1	9	—	620	—	—	—
Quick Quisine Pesto Cream as prep	1 cup	240	6	2	5	32	17	1	10	—	580	—	—	—
HAMBURGER HELPER														
Ravioli as prep	1 cup	280	10	4	50	20	30	5	1	20	840	410	60	0

FOOD	PORTION	CALS	FAT	SAT FAT	CHOL	PROT	CARB	SUGAR	FIBER	CALCI	SOD	POTAS	FOLIC	VIT C
HAMBURGER HELPER (CONT.)														
Ravioli w/ White Cheese Topping as prep	1 cup	310	10	4	50	20	34	7	1	60	960	450	60	0
HODGSON MILL														
Macaroni & Cheese Whole Wheat	1 serv	250	1	1	<5	11	45	8	6	100	570	—	28	0
KETO														
Macaroni & Cheese not prep	1 serv	112	10	—	—	24	5	0	1	—	20	—	—	—
KRAFT														
Deluxe Macaroni & Cheese Four Cheese Blend as prep	1 cup (6.2 oz)	320	10	7	25	14	44	4	1	200	910	170	60	0
Deluxe Macaroni & Cheese Original as prep	1 cup (6.1 oz)	320	10	6	25	14	44	4	1	200	730	190	60	0
Light Deluxe Macaroni & Cheese as prep	1 cup (6.5 oz)	290	5	3	15	14	48	7	1	200	810	310	60	0
Macaroni & Cheese All Shapes as prep	1 cup (6.9 oz)	410	18	5	10	12	49	8	1	100	750	340	60	0
Macaroni & Cheese Original as prep	1 cup (6.9 oz)	410	18	5	10	12	49	8	1	100	750	340	60	0
Macaroni & Cheese Original as prep light recipe	1 cup (6.4 oz)	290	6	2	10	12	48	8	2	150	580	310	60	0
Premium Macaroni & Cheese Cheesy Alfredo as prep	1 cup (6.9 oz)	410	19	5	10	11	49	8	2	150	810	330	60	0
Premium Macaroni & Cheese Mild White Cheddar as prep	1 cup (6.8 oz)	410	19	4	10	12	49	8	1	150	740	330	60	0
Premium Macaroni & Cheese Thick 'N Creamy as prep	1 cup (7.6 oz)	420	19	5	15	13	50	9	2	150	760	360	60	0
Premium Macaroni & Cheese Three Cheese as prep	1 cup (6.9 oz)	410	18	4	10	12	49	8	2	150	790	330	60	0

FOOD	PORTION	CALS	FAT	SAT FAT	CHOL	PROT	CARB	SUGAR	FIBER	CALCI	SOD	POTAS	FOLIC	VIT C
KRAFT (CONT.)														
Spaghetti Classics Mild Italian as prep	1 cup (9.1 oz)	240	3	1	<5	11	46	9	3	60	850	590	40	9
Spaghetti Classics Tangy Italian as prep	1 cup (8.9 oz)	240	2	1	0	11	46	7	3	60	830	590	40	9
Spaghetti Classics w/ Meat Sauce as prep	1 cup (8.2 oz)	330	10	4	15	11	47	7	3	60	810	410	40	4
Spaghetti Classics Zesty Cheese as prep	1 cup (8.6 oz)	240	2	1	5	11	46	9	3	60	800	630	40	9
LIPTON														
Pasta & Sauce Angel Hair Chicken Broccoli as prep	1 cup	260	8	1	0	8	43	2	2	0	810	—	100	4
Pasta & Sauce Angel Hair Parmesan as prep	1 cup	280	11	3	10	8	41	3	2	40	960	—	100	0
Pasta & Sauce Bow Tie Chicken Primavera as prep	1 cup	290	10	4	10	9	43	6	2	100	820	—	100	1
Pasta & Sauce Bow Tie Italian Cheese as prep	1 cup	300	12	5	15	10	41	4	tr	150	900	—	100	0
Pasta & Sauce Butter & Herbs as prep	1 cup	270	10	3	5	7	40	3	2	0	830	—	100	0
Pasta & Sauce Cheddar Broccoli as prep	1 cup	340	11	4	15	11	49	7	1	150	970	—	120	4
Pasta & Sauce Chicken Herb Parmesan as prep	1 cup	80	9	2	5	8	43	3	2	40	910	—	100	0
Pasta & Sauce Chicken Stir-Fry as prep	1 cup	270	8	1	0	8	43	3	2	20	900	—	100	1
Pasta & Sauce Creamy Garlic as prep	1 cup	350	13	5	15	10	50	6	1	100	980	—	100	0
Pasta & Sauce Creamy Mushroom as prep	1 cup	320	11	4	15	10	46	4	0	100	870	—	100	0
Pasta & Sauce Garlic & Butter Linguine as prep	1 cup	260	9	2	5	7	40	3	2	0	850	—	100	0

FOOD	PORTION	CALS	FAT	SAT FAT	CHOL	PROT	CARB	SUGAR	FIBER	CALCI	SOD	POTAS	FOLIC	VIT C
LIPTON (CONT.)														
Pasta & Sauce Mild Cheddar Cheese as prep	1 cup	290	10	4	10	10	41	4	tr	150	930	—	100	0
Pasta & Sauce Roasted Garlic Chicken as prep	1 cup	290	10	3	10	9	43	3	tr	400	880	—	100	0
Pasta & Sauce Roasted Garlic & Olive Oil w/ Tomato as prep	1 cup	270	9	2	0	8	42	3	2	0	880	—	100	2
Pasta & Sauce Rotini Primavera as prep	1 cup	320	12	5	15	10	45	4	2	100	980	—	100	4
Pasta & Sauce Savory Herb w/ Garlic as prep	1 cup	280	9	3	5	8	52	3	2	20	890	—	100	0
Pasta & Sauce Three Cheese Rotini as prep	1 cup	320	12	5	15	11	44	5	tr	150	970	—	100	0
MELTING POT														
Terrazza Black Beans & Penne	1 cup	180	1	0	0	8	36	5	2	20	480	—	—	1
Terrazza Florentine Red Beans & Fusilli	1 cup	220	1	0	<5	10	43	6	2	40	350	—	—	0
Terrazza Red Lentils & Bow Ties	1 cup	240	2	1	40	13	42	7	5	20	390	—	—	0
Terrazza Tuscan White Beans & Gemelli	1 cup	220	1	0	<5	10	44	6	3	40	450	—	—	1
NEAR EAST														
Angel Hair w/ Spicy Tomato as prep	1 cup	240	6	1	0	8	39	3	3	20	630	—	—	12
Radiatore Basil & Herb as prep	1 cup	240	6	1	3	8	39	2	3	20	380	—	—	9
Vermicelli Garlic & Oil as prep	1 cup	310	9	2	3	10	48	3	3	20	510	—	—	4
VELVEETA														
Rotini & Cheese w/ Broccoli as prep	1 cup (7.2 oz)	400	16	10	50	18	47	5	2	300	1230	270	60	4
Shells & Cheese Bacon as prep	1 cup (6.8 oz)	360	14	8	40	17	43	4	1	250	1140	230	60	0
Shells & Cheese Original as prep	1 cup (6.6 oz)	360	13	8	40	16	44	4	1	250	1030	210	60	0
Shells & Cheese Salsa as prep	1 cup (7.5 oz)	380	14	9	40	17	47	5	2	250	1180	300	60	0

FOOD	PORTION	CALS	FAT	SAT FAT	CHOL	PROT	CARB	SUGAR	FIBER	CALCI	SOD	POTAS	FOLIC	VIT C
WHEY COOL														
High Protein Macaroni & Cheese as prep	1 serv	260	5	2	15	46	12	7	1	—	780	—	—	—
SHELF-STABLE														
HORMEL														
Microcup Meals Lasagna	1 cup (7.5 oz)	250	14	7	25	8	24	6	1	40	950	—	—	0
Microcup Meals Macaroni & Cheese	1 cup (7.5 oz)	260	11	6	35	11	30	3	1	100	690	—	—	0
Microcup Meals Ravioli w/ Tomato Sauce	1 cup (7.5 oz)	220	6	2	15	8	34	12	2	60	840	—	—	2
Microcup Meals Spaghetti & Meatballs	1 cup (7.5 oz)	220	7	4	25	11	28	10	1	60	930	—	—	0
IT'S PASTA ANYTIME														
Penne w/ Tomato Italian Sausage Sauce	1 pkg (15.25 oz)	540	8	1	<5	17	100	17	12	80	1100	—	—	9
KID'S KITCHEN														
Microwave Meals Beefy Macaroni	1 cup (7.5 oz)	190	6	3	30	11	23	4	2	40	790	—	—	0
Microwave Meals Macaroni & Cheese	1 cup (7.5 oz)	260	11	6	35	11	30	3	1	100	690	—	—	0
Microwave Meals Mini Ravioli	1 cup (7.5 oz)	240	7	3	20	10	34	6	1	40	950	—	—	1
Microwave Meals Spaghetti & Meatballs	1 cup (7.5 oz)	220	7	4	25	11	28	10	1	60	950	—	—	0
Microwave Meals Spaghetti Ring & Meatballs	1 cup (7.5 oz)	250	7	3	20	11	35	12	3	60	1200	—	—	1
LUNCH BUCKET														
Beef Ravioli In Tomato Sauce	1 pkg (7.5 oz)	180	4	2	5	5	32	8	3	40	740	—	—	0
Italian Pasta w/ Chicken	1 pkg (7.5 oz)	130	2	1	10	5	24	7	2	20	610	—	—	0
Lasagna 'n Meatsauce	1 pkg (7.5 oz)	160	3	2	5	5	29	9	2	20	850	—	—	0
Macaroni 'n Beef in Meatsauce	1 pkg (7.5 oz)	180	5	2	10	0	10	0	8	20	820	—	—	0
Macaroni 'n Cheese	1 pkg (7.5 oz)	190	7	5	20	7	24	0	2	150	930	—	—	0
Pasta 'n Chicken	1 pkg (7.5 oz)	150	5	2	20	5	22	1	2	20	810	—	—	0
Spaghetti 'n Meatsauce	1 pkg (7.5 oz)	160	3	2	5	5	29	9	2	20	850	—	—	0

FOOD	PORTION	CALS	FAT	SAT FAT	CHOL	PROT	CARB	SUGAR	FIBER	CALCI	SOD	POTAS	FOLIC	VIT C
TAKE-OUT														
fettuccini alfredo	1 cup	715	170	36	60	—	—	—	—	—	735	—	—	—
lasagna	1 piece (2.5 in × 2.5 in)	374	21	11	107	22	25	—	2	359	668	354	11	13
lasagna vegetarian	2 cups	720	130	24	43	—	—	—	—	—	1740	—	—	—
macaroni & cheese	1 cup	230	10	5	24	9	26	—	—	199	730	139	—	tr
manicotti	¾ cup (6.4 oz)	273	12	6	77	14	28	—	2	76	414	303	17	12
ravioli cheese w/ tomato sauce	2 cups	530	0	1	75	—	—	—	—	—	1100	—	—	—
rigatoni w/ sausage sauce	¾ cup	260	12	4	59	10	28	—	3	44	106	286	8	16
spaghetti w/ clam sauce	1 serv	395	65	9	16	—	—	—	—	—	310	—	—	—
spaghetti w/ marinara sauce	1 cup	260	0	2	9	—	—	—	—	—	955	—	—	—
spaghetti w/ meatballs & cheese	1 cup	407	19	6	104	21	38	—	—	164	696	913	22	45
tortellini cheese w/ tomato sauce	1 cup	470	15	7	75	—	—	—	—	—	945	—	—	—
PASTA SALAD														
MIX														
KRAFT														
Herb & Garlic as prep	¾ cup (4.9 oz)	280	14	2	0	6	34	5	2	2	670	170	40	2
Pasta Salad Classic Ranch w/ Bacon as prep	¾ cup (4.7 oz)	350	22	4	10	7	32	3	2	0	480	150	40	0
Pasta Salad Creamy Caesar as prep	¾ cup (4.8 oz)	340	21	4	15	7	31	5	2	60	630	320	40	4
Pasta Salad Garden Primavera as prep	¾ cup (5 oz)	240	8	2	<5	8	35	3	2	60	710	190	40	4
Pasta Salad Italian 97% Fat Free as prep	¾ cup (4.9 oz)	190	2	1	<5	8	35	5	2	100	740	220	40	4
Pasta Salad Parmesan Peppercorn as prep	¾ cup (4.9 oz)	360	23	4	15	7	29	3	2	60	570	150	40	1
SUDDENLY SALAD														
Classic Pasta	¾ cup	250	8	1	0	7	38	5	2	40	910	200	—	0
Classic Pasta Reduced Fat Recipe	¾ cup	210	4	1	0	7	38	5	2	0	910	200	—	0
Garden Italian 98% Fat Free	¾ cup	140	1	0	0	5	28	4	2	20	520	130	—	0

FOOD	PORTION	CALS	FAT	SAT FAT	CHOL	PROT	CARB	SUGAR	FIBER	CALCI	SOD	POTAS	FOLIC	VIT C
TAKE-OUT														
elbow macaroni salad	3.5 oz	160	5	2	0	3	26	—	—	—	590	—	—	1
italian style pasta salad	3.5 oz	140	7	1	0	3	15	—	—	20	480	—	—	9
mustard macaroni salad	3.5 oz	190	10	1	0	4	23	—	—	—	560	—	—	4
pasta salad w/ vegetables	3.5 oz	140	4	3	0	4	21	—	—	40	210	—	—	4
PÂTÉ														
antipasto pâté	1 can (2.25 oz)	110	9	2	5	3	3	1	1	20	530	—	—	5
chicken liver canned	1 tbsp (13 g)	109	2	—	—	2	1	—	—	1	—	—	—	—
duck pâté	1 oz	96	8	—	—	4	1	tr	—	—	—	—	—	—
fish pâté	1 oz	76	7	—	—	3	1	—	—	52	286	45	—	—
goose liver smoked canned	1 tbsp (13 g)	60	6	—	20	1	1	—	—	—	—	—	—	—
liver canned	1 tbsp (13 g)	41	4	—	—	5	tr	—	—	9	91	18	8	0
mushroom anchovy pâté	1 can (2.25 oz)	130	11	2	5	2	7	1	1	20	400	—	—	1
pâté foie gras	1 oz	127	13	3	109	3	1	—	—	3	211	49	162	1
pork pâté	1 oz	107	10	4	51	3	1	1	0	11	189	27	29	tr
pork pâté en croute	1 oz	91	7	3	32	3	3	tr	tr	—	214	—	—	—
rabbit pâté	1 oz	66	5	3	21	5	1	—	—	3	97	89	—	tr
salmon pâté	1 can (2.25 oz)	140	10	2	10	6	6	1	0	20	420	—	—	1
shrimp pâté	1 can (2.25 oz)	140	10	2	25	6	7	1	0	20	450	—	—	1
smoked turkey pâté	1 can (2.25 oz)	170	13	3	15	6	7	1	0	20	480	—	—	1
PEACH														
CANNED														
halves in heavy syrup	1 half	60	tr	tr	0	tr	16	—	—	8	5	74	3	2
halves in light syrup	1 half	44	tr	tr	0	tr	12	—	—	3	4	79	3	2
halves juice pack	1 half	34	tr	tr	0	tr	9	—	—	15	3	98	—	3
halves water pack	1 half	18	tr	tr	0	tr	5	—	—	2	3	76	3	2
peach sauce	½ cup	120	0	0	0	tr	32	31	1	0	0	—	—	6
spiced in heavy syrup	1 cup	180	tr	tr	0	1	49	—	—	15	9	206	—	13
spiced in heavy syrup	1 fruit	66	tr	tr	0	tr	18	—	—	5	3	75	—	5
DEL MONTE														
Fruit Cup Diced Extra Light Syrup	1 pkg (4 oz)	50	0	0	0	0	13	12	1	0	10	—	—	12
Fruit Cup Diced In Heavy Syrup	1 serv (4 oz)	80	0	0	0	0	20	19	1	0	10	—	—	12
Fruit Cup Fruit Naturals Diced	1 pkg (4 oz)	50	0	0	0	0	13	12	1	0	10	—	—	12

FOOD	PORTION	CALS	FAT	SAT FAT	CHOL	PROT	CARB	SUGAR	FIBER	CALCI	SOD	POTAS	FOLIC	VIT C
DEL MONTE (CONT.)														
Fruit Pleasures Raspberry Flavor	½ cup (4.5 oz)	80	0	0	0	1	20	19	1	0	10	—	—	4
Fruit To Go Banana Berry Peaches	1 pkg (4 oz)	70	0	0	0	1	17	16	1	0	10	—	—	60
Fruitrageous Peachy Pie	1 pkg (4 oz)	80	0	0	0	1	21	20	1	0	10	—	—	12
Fruitrageous Wild Raspberry Flavor	1 pkg (4 oz)	80	0	0	0	1	20	19	1	0	10	—	—	12
Halves Ginger Flavor	½ cup (4.5 oz)	90	0	0	0	0	22	19	1	0	10	—	—	2
Halves In Extra Light Syrup	½ cup (4.4 oz)	60	0	0	0	0	15	14	1	0	10	—	—	5
Halves In Heavy Syrup	½ cup (4.5 oz)	100	0	0	0	0	24	23	1	0	10	—	—	1
Halves Melba In Heavy Syrup	½ cup (4.5 oz)	100	0	0	0	0	24	23	1	0	10	—	—	5
Orchard Select Sliced Cling	½ cup	80	0	0	0	tr	22	19	tr	0	10	—	—	60
Slice Fruit Natural	½ cup (4.4 oz)	60	0	0	0	0	15	14	1	0	10	—	—	5
Sliced In Extra Light Syrup	½ cup (4.4 oz)	60	0	0	0	0	14	13	1	0	10	—	—	1
Sliced Natural Raspberry Flavor	½ cup (4.4 oz)	80	0	0	0	0	20	19	1	0	10	—	—	4
Sliced Natural Harvest Spice Flavor	½ cup (4.5 oz)	80	0	0	0	1	21	20	1	0	10	—	—	4
Whole Spiced In Heavy Syrup	½ cup (4.2 oz)	100	0	0	0	0	24	23	1	0	10	—	—	5
DOLE														
All Natural Yellow Cling Sliced	½ cup	80	0	0	0	1	17	16	tr	—	10	—	—	24
DRIED														
halves	10	311	1	tr	0	5	80	—	11	37	9	1295	—	6
halves	1 cup	383	1	tr	0	6	98	—	13	45	12	1594	—	8
halves cooked w/ sugar	½ cup	139	tr	tr	0	1	36	—	—	11	3	395	tr	5
halves cooked w/o sugar	½ cup	99	tr	tr	0	1	25	—	—	12	3	413	tr	5
FRESH														
peach	1	37	tr	tr	0	1	10	—	1	5	0	171	3	6
sliced	1 cup	73	tr	tr	0	1	19	—	—	9	1	334	6	11
CHIQUITA														
Peach	1 med (3.4 oz)	40	0	0	0	14	10	9	2	0	0	—	—	6
FROZEN														
slices sweetened	1 cup	235	tr	tr	0	2	60	—	—	6	16	325	—	235

FOOD	PORTION	CALS	FAT	SAT FAT	CHOL	PROT	CARB	SUGAR	FIBER	CALCI	SOD	POTAS	FOLIC	VIT C
PEACH JUICE														
nectar	1 cup	134	tr	tr	0	1	35	—	—	13	17	101	—	13
CERES														
Peach	8 oz	120	0	0	0	0	30	26	0	0	5	240	—	60
NANTUCKET NECTARS														
The Original	8 oz	120	0	0	0	0	30	26	—	20	15	—	—	0
PEANUT BUTTER														
chunky	2 tbsp	188	16	3	0	8	7	—	2	13	156	239	29	0
chunky	1 cup	1520	129	25	0	62	56	—	17	105	1255	1928	237	0
chunky w/o salt	2 tbsp	188	16	3	0	8	7	—	2	13	5	239	29	0
chunky w/o salt	1 cup	1520	129	25	0	62	56	—	17	105	44	1928	237	0
smooth	2 tbsp	188	16	3	0	8	7	—	2	11	153	231	25	0
smooth	1 cup	1517	128	25	0	63	53	—	15	88	1234	1861	202	0
smooth w/o salt	1 cup	1517	129	25	0	63	53	—	15	88	44	1861	201	0
smooth w/o salt	2 tbsp	188	16	3	0	8	7	—	2	11	5	231	25	0
CARB OPTIONS														
Creamy	2 tbsp	190	17	4	0	7	5	tr	2	0	150	—	40	0
ESTEE														
Creamy Low Sodium	2 tbsp (1 oz)	190	15	3	0	7	7	2	2	—	0	200	—	—
JIF														
Apple Cinnamon	2 tbsp (1.3 oz)	200	16	3	0	6	11	8	2	—	115	—	—	—
Berry Blend	2 tbsp (1.2 oz)	200	17	4	0	6	10	7	1	—	115	—	—	—
Chocolate Silk	2 tbsp (1.3 oz)	190	15	3	0	5	14	12	1	—	115	—	—	—
Creamy	2 tbsp	190	16	3	0	8	7	3	2	—	150	—	—	—
Extra Crunchy	2 tbsp (1.1 oz)	190	16	3	0	8	7	3	2	—	130	—	—	—
Reduced Fat Creamy	2 tbsp (1.3 oz)	190	12	3	0	8	15	4	2	—	250	—	24	—
Reduced Fat Crunchy	2 tbsp (1.3 oz)	190	12	3	0	8	15	4	2	—	220	—	24	—
Simply	2 tbsp (1.1 oz)	190	16	3	0	8	6	2	2	—	1	—	—	—
MARANATHA														
Crunchy	2 tbsp	190	16	—	—	8	7	2	2	—	80	—	—	—
Salted	2 tbsp	190	16	3	0	8	7	2	2	20	80	—	—	0
P.B.														
Slices	1 slice (1 oz)	170	14	3	0	6	5	3	1	—	110	—	—	—
PEANUT BUTTER & CO.														
Cinnamon Raisin Swirl	2 tbsp	143	7	1	0	10	10	4	2	10	67	—	—	0
Crunch Time	2 tbsp	200	16	2	0	7	7	2	2	0	120	—	—	0
Dark Chocolate Dreams	2 tbsp	175	12	3	0	8	8	3	2	10	82	—	—	0
Smooth Operator	2 tbsp	200	16	2	0	7	7	2	2	0	120	—	—	0
The Heat Is On	2 tbsp	164	10	2	0	9	9	4	2	10	86	—	—	0

FOOD	PORTION	CALS	FAT	SAT FAT	CHOL	PROT	CARB	SUGAR	FIBER	CALCI	SOD	POTAS	FOLIC	VIT C
PEANUT BUTTER & CO. (CONT.)														
White Chocolate Wonderful	1 tbsp	165	12	3	0	7	8	3	2	10	56	—	—	0
PEANUT WONDER														
Low Sodium	2 tbsp	100	3	0	0	4	13	5	0	40	95	—	—	5
Regular	2 tbsp	100	3	0	0	4	13	5	0	40	220	—	—	5
REESE'S														
Peanut Butter Chips	1 tbsp	80	4	4	0	3	7	—	—	—	35	—	—	—
SKIPPY														
Creamy	2 tbsp	190	17	4	0	7	7	3	2	0	150	—	—	0
Creamy w/ 2 slices white bread	1 sandwich	340	19	3	0	14	33	—	—	40	430	—	—	—
Reduced Fat Creamy	2 tbsp	190	12	3	0	7	15	5	2	0	190	—	24	0
Roasted Honey Nut	2 tbsp	190	17	4	0	7	7	3	2	0	125	—	—	0
Roasted Honey Nut Super Chunk	2 tbsp	190	17	4	0	7	7	3	2	0	125	—	—	0
Squeeze Stix	1 pkg	140	12	3	0	6	5	3	2	0	120	—	—	21
Squeeze Stix Chocolate	1 pkg	140	10	3	0	4	9	7	2	0	85	—	—	0
Squeez'It	2 tbsp	190	17	4	0	7	7	3	2	0	160	—	—	0
Super Chunk	2 tbsp	190	17	4	0	7	7	3	2	0	140	—	—	0
TROPICAL SOURCE														
Chips Dairy Free	13 pieces (1.5 oz)	80	5	3	0	2	9	7	0	0	7	—	—	0
PEANUTS														
chocolate coated	1 cup (5.2 oz)	773	50	22	13	19	74	—	—	155	61	748	12	0
chocolate coated	10 (1.4 oz)	208	13	6	4	5	20	—	—	42	16	201	3	0
cooked	½ cup	102	7	1	0	4	7	—	—	18	240	58	24	0
dry roasted	1 cup	855	73	10	0	35	31	—	12	79	1187	960	212	0
dry roasted w/ salt	30 nuts (1 oz)	170	14	2	0	7	6	2	2	20	230	190	40	—
AT LAST!														
Chocolate Covered	1 pkg (0.9 oz)	150	11	5	0	4	18	0	5	—	15	—	—	—
ESTEE														
Candy Coated	¼ cup	200	9	4	<5	5	23	6	1	—	45	180	—	—
FRITO LAY														
Honey Roasted	1 serv (1.5 oz)	270	21	4	0	10	10	5	3	—	80	—	—	—
Hot	1 serv (1.1 oz)	190	16	3	0	7	6	2	2	—	250	—	—	—
Salted	1 oz	200	16	4	0	7	5	1	2	—	180	—	—	—
JUDY'S														
Sugar Free Coconut Peanut Brittle	¼ piece (1 oz)	90	5	2	0	1	2	0	1	—	0	—	—	—

FOOD	PORTION	CALS	FAT	SAT FAT	CHOL	PROT	CARB	SUGAR	FIBER	CALCI	SOD	POTAS	FOLIC	VIT C
LANCE														
Honey Toasted	1 pkg (1⅛ oz)	220	15	3	0	9	13	5	3	20	170	240	—	0
Roasted	1 pkg (1¼ oz)	190	14	3	0	9	6	1	4	20	0	310	—	0
Salted	1 pkg (1⅛ oz)	200	15	3	0	9	6	0	4	0	150	240	—	0
Salted Long Tube	¼ cup (1 oz)	180	14	3	0	8	5	0	3	0	135	210	—	0
LITTLE DEBBIE														
Salted	¼ cup (1 oz)	160	14	2	0	7	5	1	2	—	130	—	—	—
LOW CARB CREATIONS														
Soft Peanut Brittle	2 pieces (1 oz)	140	10	2	0	6	8	<2	2	—	150	—	—	—
SWEET DELIGHT														
Peanut Roasters	⅓ pkg (1 oz)	160	12	—	0	7	7	tr	3	—	200	—	—	—
TOM'S														
Double Coated	1 pkg (1.35 oz)	220	15	6	0	8	15	10	1	20	60	190	—	0
Toasted	1 pkg (1.4 oz)	240	19	4	0	11	7	1	2	20	160	—	—	0
WEIGHT WATCHERS														
Honey Roasted	1 pkg (0.7 oz)	100	5	1	0	7	7	3	2	0	100	—	—	0
PEAR														
CANNED														
halves in heavy syrup	1 cup	188	tr	tr	0	1	49	—	—	12	13	165	3	3
halves in heavy syrup	1 half	68	tr	tr	0	tr	15	—	—	4	4	51	1	1
halves in light syrup	1 half	45	tr	tr	0	tr	12	—	—	4	4	52	1	1
halves juice pack	1 cup	123	tr	tr	0	1	32	—	—	21	10	238	—	4
halves water pack	1 half	22	tr	tr	0	tr	6	—	—	—	41	5	1	1
DEL MONTE														
Fruit Cup Diced In Heavy Syrup	1 pkg (4 oz)	80	0	0	0	0	20	19	1	0	10	—	—	12
Fruit Cup Diced Extra Light Syrup	1 pkg (4 oz)	50	0	0	0	0	13	12	1	0	10	—	—	12
Fruit To Go Peachy Peaches	1 pkg (4 oz)	70	0	0	0	1	17	16	1	0	10	—	—	60
Halves Fruit Naturals	½ cup (4.4 oz)	60	0	0	0	0	15	14	1	0	10	—	—	5
Halves In Extra Light Syrup	½ cup (4.4 oz)	60	0	0	0	0	15	14	1	0	10	—	—	2
Halves In Heavy Syrup	½ cup (4.5 oz)	100	0	0	0	0	24	33	1	0	10	—	—	2
Orchard Select Sliced Bartlett	½ cup	80	0	0	0	tr	20	19	2	0	10	—	—	60
Sliced In Extra Light Syrup	½ cup (4.5 oz)	60	0	0	0	0	15	14	1	0	10	—	—	2
DRIED														
halves	1 cup	472	1	tr	0	3	125	—	—	60	10	959	—	13
halves	10	459	1	tr	0	3	122	—	—	59	10	932	—	12

FOOD	PORTION	CALS	FAT	SAT FAT	CHOL	PROT	CARB	SUGAR	FIBER	CALCI	SOD	POTAS	FOLIC	VIT C
halves cooked w/ sugar	½ cup	196	tr	tr	0	1	52	—	—	22	4	344	0	5
halves cooked w/o sugar	½ cup	163	tr	tr	0	tr	43	—	—	21	4	331	0	5
FRESH														
asian	1 (4.3 oz)	51	tr	tr	0	1	13	—	—	5	0	148	10	2
pear	1	98	1	tr	0	1	25	—	4	19	1	208	12	7
sliced w/ skin	1 cup	97	1	tr	0	1	25	—	4	19	1	207	12	7
CHIQUITA														
Pear	1 med (5.8 oz)	100	1	0	0	1	25	17	4	20	0	—	—	6

PEAR JUICE

FOOD	PORTION	CALS	FAT	SAT FAT	CHOL	PROT	CARB	SUGAR	FIBER	CALCI	SOD	POTAS	FOLIC	VIT C
nectar	1 cup	149	tr	tr	0	tr	39	—	—	11	9	33	—	3
CERES														
Pear	8 oz	120	0	0	0	0	30	29	0	20	10	190	—	30

PEAS

FOOD	PORTION	CALS	FAT	SAT FAT	CHOL	PROT	CARB	SUGAR	FIBER	CALCI	SOD	POTAS	FOLIC	VIT C
CANNED														
green	½ cup	59	tr	tr	0	4	11	—	—	17	186	147	38	8
green low sodium	½ cup	59	tr	tr	0	4	11	—	—	17	2	147	38	8
DEL MONTE														
Sweet	½ cup (4.4 oz)	60	0	0	0	3	13	6	4	20	390	—	—	9
Sweet No Salt Added	½ cup (4.4 oz)	60	0	0	0	3	11	6	4	20	10	—	—	9
Sweet Very Young Small	½ cup (4.4 oz)	60	0	0	0	3	10	5	4	0	360	—	—	9
GREEN GIANT														
Sweet	½ cup (4.3 oz)	60	0	0	0	4	11	3	4	20	390	—	—	6
Sweet 50% Less Sodium	½ cup (4.3 oz)	60	0	0	0	4	11	2	3	20	195	—	—	6
LESUEUR														
Early Peas	½ cup (4.2 oz)	60	0	0	0	4	12	4	3	20	380	—	—	6
Early Peas 50% Less Sodium	½ cup (4.2 oz)	60	0	0	0	4	11	3	4	20	190	—	—	6
Sweet	½ cup (4.2 oz)	60	0	0	0	4	12	4	3	20	380	—	—	6
Sweet 50% Less Sodium	½ cup (4.2 oz)	60	0	0	0	4	11	3	4	20	190	—	—	6
S&W														
Petite	½ cup (4.4 oz)	70	0	0	0	4	12	4	4	20	330	—	—	9
Small	½ cup (4.4 oz)	70	0	0	0	4	12	4	4	20	330	—	—	9
VEG-ALL														
Tender Sweet	½ cup	60	1	0	0	4	10	4	3	20	370	—	—	9
DRIED														
split cooked	1 cup	231	1	tr	0	16	41	—	—	26	4	710	127	1

FOOD	PORTION	CALS	FAT	SAT FAT	CHOL	PROT	CARB	SUGAR	FIBER	CALCI	SOD	POTAS	FOLIC	VIT C
HURST														
HamBeens Green Split Peas w/ Ham	1 serv	120	1	0	0	8	21	1	4	20	63	—	—	0
FRESH														
green cooked	½ cup	67	tr	tr	0	4	13	—	—	22	2	217	51	11
green raw	½ cup	58	tr	tr	0	4	11	—	—	18	3	176	47	29
snap peas cooked	½ cup	34	tr	tr	0	3	6	—	2	33	3	192	—	38
snap peas raw	½ cup	30	tr	tr	0	2	5	—	2	36	3	144	—	43
FROZEN														
green cooked	½ cup	63	tr	tr	0	4	11	—	—	19	70	134	47	8
snap peas cooked	1 pkg (10 oz)	132	1	tr	0	9	23	—	—	150	12	549	—	56
snap peas cooked	½ cup	42	tr	tr	0	3	7	—	—	48	4	173	—	18
BIRDS EYE														
Butter Peas	½ cup	110	1	0	0	7	20	1	4	20	10	—	—	1
Crowder	½ cup	120	1	0	0	8	22	1	4	20	10	—	—	1
Field Peas w/ Snaps	⅔ cup	130	1	0	0	9	24	1	4	40	15	—	—	2
Green	½ cup	70	0	0	0	—	—	—	5	20	125	—	—	15
Purple Hull Peas	½ cup	110	1	0	0	7	21	1	4	20	10	—	—	1
Sugar Snap	½ cup	40	0	0	0	—	—	—	2	40	10	—	—	15
Tiny Tender	¾ cup	40	0	0	0	—	—	—	2	0	40	—	—	5
FRESH LIKE														
Garden	3.5 oz	85	1	—	—	5	14	—	2	23	79	149	—	20
GREEN GIANT														
Butter Sauce	¾ cup (4 oz)	100	2	2	<5	4	16	4	5	0	400	—	—	5
Butter Sauce LeSueur Baby Peas	¾ cup (4 oz)	100	2	2	<5	5	16	4	4	40	370	—	—	6
Harvest Fresh LeSueur Baby	⅔ cup (3.2 oz)	70	0	0	0	4	13	4	4	20	220	—	—	6
Harvest Fresh Sugar Snap	⅔ cup (3.2 oz)	50	0	0	0	3	10	5	3	60	95	—	—	6
Harvest Fresh Sweet	⅔ cup (3.3 oz)	60	0	0	0	4	12	6	4	0	200	—	—	6
LeSueur Baby Sweet	⅔ cup (2.8 oz)	60	0	0	0	5	11	3	5	20	150	—	—	6
LeSueur Early June	⅔ cup (2.8 oz)	80	0	0	0	5	11	3	5	20	150	—	—	6
LeSueur Early June w/ Mushrooms	¾ cup (3 oz)	60	0	0	0	4	10	2	4	0	105	—	—	5
Select Sugar Snap	¾ cup (2.8 oz)	35	0	0	0	2	7	3	3	60	0	—	—	6
Sweet	⅔ cup (3.1 oz)	70	0	0	0	4	13	2	4	20	135	—	—	12
LA CHOY														
Snow Pea Pods	½ pkg (3 oz)	35	2	0	0	2	4	2	2	20	0	—	—	15

FOOD	PORTION	CALS	FAT	SAT FAT	CHOL	PROT	CARB	SUGAR	FIBER	CALCI	SOD	POTAS	FOLIC	VIT C
TREE OF LIFE														
Peas	⅔ cup (3.1 oz)	70	0	0	0	5	12	6	4	0	100	—	—	9
SHELF-STABLE														
TASTYBITE														
Agra Peas & Greens	½ pkg (5 oz)	260	14	5	0	8	26	1	1	50	380	—	—	0
TAKE-OUT														
pea & potato curry	1 serv (7 oz)	284	22	—	—	5	19	—	6	56	—	—	—	12
pea curry	1 serv (4.4 oz)	438	42	—	—	5	11	—	4	41	—	—	—	14
PECANS														
candied	1 oz	190	17	3	0	tr	10	4	5	0	75	—	—	0
dry roasted	1 oz	187	18	1	0	2	6	—	—	10	0	105	12	—
dry roasted salted	1 oz	187	18	1	0	2	6	—	—	10	260	105	12	—
halves dry roasted w/ salt	20 (1 oz)	200	21	2	0	3	4	1	3	20	110	120	8	—
halves dried	1 cup	721	73	6	0	8	20	—	7	39	1	423	42	2
oil roasted	1 oz	195	20	2	0	2	5	—	—	10	0	102	—	—
oil roasted salted	1 oz	195	20	2	0	2	5	—	—	10	252	102	—	—
KETO														
Chocolately Covered	1 oz	207	19	4	—	3	6	0	5	40	—	—	—	0
SWEET DELIGHTS														
Pecan Roasters	⅓ pkg (1 oz)	210	21	2	0	3	4	1	2	—	100	—	—	—
PECTIN														
powder	1 pkg (1.75 oz)	163	tr	—	0	tr	45	—	—	4	100	4	0	—
powder	¼ pkg (0.4 oz)	39	0	0	0	0	11	—	—	1	24	1	0	—
SLIM SET														
Packet	1 pkg	208	0	0	0	0	44	—	14	—	42	—	—	—
Powder	1 tbsp	3	0	0	0	0	1	—	tr	—	1	—	—	—
SURE JELL														
For Lower Sugar Recipes	1 tsp (2.8 g)	20	0	0	0	0	4	4	0	0	40	0	—	0
Fruit Pectin	1 tsp (3.6 g)	20	0	0	0	0	4	4	0	0	0	0	—	0
PEPEAO														
dried	½ cup	36	tr	—	0	1	10	—	—	14	8	85	—	tr
raw sliced	1 cup	25	tr	—	0	tr	7	—	—	16	9	42	—	1
PEPPER														
black	1 tsp	5	tr	tr	0	tr	1	—	—	9	1	26	—	—
cayenne	1 tsp	6	tr	tr	0	tr	1	—	—	3	1	36	—	1
red	1 tsp	6	tr	tr	0	tr	1	—	—	3	1	36	—	1
white	1 tsp	7	tr	—	0	tr	2	—	—	6	tr	2	—	—
MCCORMICK														
Lemon & Pepper Seasoning Salt	¼ tsp	0	0	0	0	0	0	0	0	—	130	—	—	—

FOOD	PORTION	CALS	FAT	SAT FAT	CHOL	PROT	CARB	SUGAR	FIBER	CALCI	SOD	POTAS	FOLIC	VIT C
PEPPERS														
CANNED														
chili green	1 cup (5.5 oz)	29	tr	tr	0	1	6	—	2	50	552	157	75	0
chili green hot chopped	½ cup	17	tr	tr	0	1	4	—	—	5	—	—	—	46
chili red hot	1 (2.6 oz)	18	tr	tr	0	1	4	—	—	5	—	—	—	50
chili red hot chopped	½ cup	17	tr	tr	0	1	4	—	—	5	—	—	—	46
green halves	½ cup	13	tr	tr	0	1	3	—	—	28	958	102	—	33
jalapeño chopped	½ cup	17	tr	tr	0	1	3	—	—	18	995	92	—	9
red halves	½ cup	13	tr	tr	0	1	3	—	—	28	958	102	—	33
CHI-CHI'S														
Chilies Diced Green	2 tbsp (1.2 oz)	10	0	0	0	0	1	0	0	0	20	—	—	6
Chilies Green Whole	¾ pepper (1 oz)	10	0	0	0	0	1	0	0	0	15	—	—	6
OLD EL PASO														
Green Chiles Chopped	2 tbsp (1 oz)	5	0	0	0	0	1	0	1	40	110	—	—	6
PROGRESSO														
Cherry Sliced & So Hot	2 tbsp (1 oz)	25	2	0	0	0	2	1	1	0	30	—	—	18
Hot Cherry	1 (1 oz)	10	0	0	0	0	2	0	tr	0	150	—	—	0
Pepper Salad (drained)	2 tbsp (1 oz)	15	1	0	0	0	1	tr	tr	20	160	—	—	2
Roasted	1 piece (1 oz)	10	0	0	0	0	3	tr	0	0	55	—	—	0
Sweet Fried w/ Onions	2 tbsp (0.9 oz)	20	2	0	0	0	2	1	1	0	130	—	—	15
Tuscan	3 (1 oz)	10	0	0	0	0	2	0	1	0	450	—	—	0
ROSARITA														
Chilies Diced Green	2 tbsp (1 oz)	6	tr	0	0	tr	1	tr	1	23	85	—	—	6
Chilies Green Strips	¼ cup (1.2 oz)	5	tr	0	0	tr	1	1	1	17	74	—	—	7
Chilies Whole Green	2 tbsp (1.2 oz)	5	tr	0	0	tr	1	1	1	17	74	—	—	7
Jalapeño Whole w/ Escabeche	¼ cup (1.2 oz)	8	tr	0	0	1	1	tr	1	18	430	—	—	9
Jalapeños Diced	2 tbsp (1 oz)	5	tr	0	0	tr	1	tr	1	10	121	—	—	1
Jalapeños Nacho Sliced	2 tbsp (1 oz)	2	tr	0	0	tr	1	tr	tr	20	224	—	—	2
VLASIC														
Hot Sliced Cherry	1 oz	5	0	0	0	0	1	1	—	—	480	—	—	6
Jalapeño Sliced	1 oz	10	0	0	0	0	2	2	—	—	480	—	—	4
Mild Cherry	1 oz	5	0	0	0	0	1	1	—	—	480	—	—	6

FOOD	PORTION	CALS	FAT	SAT FAT	CHOL	PROT	CARB	SUGAR	FIBER	CALCI	SOD	POTAS	FOLIC	VIT C
VLASIC (CONT.)														
Pepper Rings Hot	1 oz	5	0	0	0	0	1	1	—	—	480	—	—	9
Pepper Rings Mild	1 oz	5	0	0	0	0	1	1	—	—	480	—	—	9
DRIED														
ancho	1 (0.6 oz)	48	1	tr	0	2	9	—	4	10	7	410	12	0
green	1 tbsp	1	tr	tr	0	tr	tr	—	—	1	1	13	1	8
pasilla	1 (7 g)	24	1	—	0	1	4	—	2	7	6	156	12	0
red	1 tbsp	1	tr	tr	0	tr	tr	—	—	1	1	13	1	8
FRESH														
banana	1 cup (4.4 oz)	33	1	tr	0	2	7	—	4	17	16	317	36	27
banana	1 (4 in) (1.2 oz)	9	tr	tr	0	1	2	—	1	5	4	84	10	27
chili green hot	1	18	tr	tr	0	1	4	—	—	8	3	153	11	109
chili green hot chopped	½ cup	30	tr	tr	0	2	7	—	—	13	5	255	18	182
chili red chopped	½ cup	30	tr	tr	0	2	7	—	—	13	5	255	18	182
chili red hot	1 (1.6 oz)	18	tr	tr	0	1	4	—	—	8	3	153	11	109
green	1 (2.6 oz)	20	tr	tr	0	1	5	—	1	7	1	131	16	95
green chopped	½ cup	13	tr	tr	0	tr	3	—	1	5	1	89	11	45
green chopped cooked	½ cup	19	tr	tr	0	1	5	—	—	6	1	113	11	51
green cooked	1 (2.6 oz)	20	tr	tr	0	1	5	—	—	7	1	121	11	54
habanero chile	1 tsp	9	tr	—	0	1	2	—	1	5	2	99	7	27
hungarian	1 (0.9 oz)	8	tr	tr	0	tr	2	—	0	3	tr	55	14	0
jalapeño	1 (0.5 oz)	4	tr	tr	0	tr	1	—	tr	1	tr	30	7	6
jalapeño sliced	1 cup (3.2 oz)	27	1	tr	0	1	5	—	3	9	1	197	42	6
red	1 (2.6 oz)	20	tr	tr	0	1	5	—	1	7	1	131	16	141
red chopped	½ cup	13	tr	tr	0	tr	3	—	1	5	1	69	11	95
red chopped cooked	½ cup	19	tr	tr	0	1	5	—	—	6	1	113	11	125
red cooked	1 (2.6 oz)	20	tr	tr	0	1	5	—	—	7	1	121	11	125
serrano	1 (6 g)	2	tr	0	0	tr	tr	—	tr	1	1	19	1	3
serrano chopped	1 cup (3.7 oz)	34	tr	tr	0	2	7	4	4	12	11	320	24	3
yellow	10 strips	14	tr	—	0	1	3	—	—	6	1	110	14	95
yellow	1 (6.5 oz)	50	tr	—	0	2	12	—	—	20	3	393	48	341
CHIQUITA														
Pepper	1 med (5.2 oz)	30	0	0	0	1	7	4	2	20	0	—	—	114
FROZEN														
green chopped	1 oz	6	tr	tr	0	tr	1	—	—	3	1	26	4	16
red chopped	1 oz	6	tr	tr	0	tr	1	—	—	3	1	26	4	16
BIRDS EYE														
Diced Green	¾ cup	20	0	0	0	1	4	3	2	0	10	—	—	18
PERCH														
FRESH														
cooked	1 fillet (1.6 oz)	54	1	tr	53	11	0	—	—	47	36	158	—	—
cooked	3 oz	99	1	tr	98	21	0	—	—	87	67	293	—	—

FOOD	PORTION	CALS	FAT	SAT FAT	CHOL	PROT	CARB	SUGAR	FIBER	CALCI	SOD	POTAS	FOLIC	VIT C
ocean perch atlantic cooked	1 fillet (1.8 oz)	60	1	tr	27	12	0	—	—	69	48	175	—	—
ocean perch atlantic cooked	3 oz	103	2	tr	46	20	0	—	—	117	82	298	—	—
ocean perch atlantic raw	3 oz	80	1	tr	36	16	0	—	—	91	64	232	—	—
raw	3 oz	77	1	tr	76	16	0	—	—	68	52	228	—	—
red raw	3.5 oz	114	4	—	—	18	0	—	—	22	80	308	—	1

PERSIMMON

FOOD	PORTION	CALS	FAT	SAT FAT	CHOL	PROT	CARB	SUGAR	FIBER	CALCI	SOD	POTAS	FOLIC	VIT C
dried japanese	1	93	tr	—	0	tr	25	—	—	8	1	273	—	0
fresh	1	32	tr	—	0	tr	8	—	—	7	0	78	—	17
fresh japanese	1	118	tr	—	0	1	31	—	—	13	3	270	13	13

PHEASANT

FOOD	PORTION	CALS	FAT	SAT FAT	CHOL	PROT	CARB	SUGAR	FIBER	CALCI	SOD	POTAS	FOLIC	VIT C
breast w/o skin raw	½ breast (6.4 oz)	243	6	2	—	44	0	—	—	6	60	440	—	11
leg w/o skin raw	1 (3.6 oz)	143	5	2	—	24	0	—	—	31	48	316	—	—
roasted	3.5 oz	215	9	3	120	33	0	0	0	50	100	400	20	0
w/ skin raw	½ pheasant (14 oz)	723	37	11	—	91	0	—	—	50	161	971	—	21
w/o skin raw	½ pheasant (12.4 oz)	470	13	4	—	83	0	—	—	45	131	921	—	21

PHYLLO

FOOD	PORTION	CALS	FAT	SAT FAT	CHOL	PROT	CARB	SUGAR	FIBER	CALCI	SOD	POTAS	FOLIC	VIT C
phyllo dough	1 oz	85	2	tr	0	2	15	—	—	3	137	21	5	0
sheet	1	57	1	tr	0	1	10	—	—	2	92	14	3	0
EKIZIAN														
Sheets	¼ lb	433	9	4	62	12	76	2	—	24	287	117	31	0
FILLO FACTORY														
Fillo Dough Spelt Vegan	3 sheets (2 oz)	180	1	0	0	0	31	0	4	—	120	—	—	—
Fillo Dough Vegan	3 sheets (2 oz)	170	1	0	0	5	36	1	1	—	220	—	—	—
Fillo Dough Whole Wheat Vegan	3 sheets (2 oz)	190	1	0	0	6	40	0	3	—	135	—	—	—
Pastry Shells Vegan	3 (0.4 oz)	45	2	2	0	1	7	0	0	—	50	—	—	—

PICANTE

(*see* SALSA)

PICKLES

FOOD	PORTION	CALS	FAT	SAT FAT	CHOL	PROT	CARB	SUGAR	FIBER	CALCI	SOD	POTAS	FOLIC	VIT C
dill	1 (2.3 oz)	12	tr	tr	0	tr	3	—	—	6	833	75	1	1
dill low sodium	1 (2.3 oz)	12	tr	tr	0	tr	3	—	1	6	12	75	1	1
dill low sodium sliced	1 slice	1	tr	tr	0	tr	tr	—	tr	1	1	7	0	tr
dill sliced	1 slice	1	tr	tr	0	tr	tr	—	tr	1	77	7	0	tr
gherkins	1 oz	6	tr	—	0	tr	1	—	—	9	274	—	—	tr

FOOD	PORTION	CALS	FAT	SAT FAT	CHOL	PROT	CARB	SUGAR	FIBER	CALCI	SOD	POTAS	FOLIC	VIT C
kosher dill	1 (2.3 oz)	12	tr	tr	0	tr	3	—	1	6	833	75	1	1
polish dill	1 (2.3 oz)	12	tr	tr	0	tr	3	—	1	6	833	75	1	1
quick sour	1 (1.2 oz)	4	tr	tr	0	tr	1	—	—	0	423	8	—	tr
quick sour low sodium	1 (1.2 oz)	4	tr	tr	0	tr	1	—	—	0	6	8	—	tr
quick sour sliced	1 slice	1	tr	tr	0	tr	tr	—	—	0	85	2	—	tr
sweet	1 (1.2 oz)	41	tr	tr	0	tr	11	—	tr	1	328	11	0	tr
sweet gherkin	1 sm (½ oz)	20	tr	tr	0	tr	5	—	—	2	107	30	—	1
sweet low sodium	1 (1.2 oz)	41	tr	tr	0	tr	11	—	tr	1	6	11	0	tr
sweet sliced	1 slice	7	tr	tr	0	tr	2	—	tr	0	56	2	0	tr
CLAUSSEN														
Bread 'N Butter Chips	4 slices (1 oz)	20	0	0	0	0	4	3	0	0	170	—	—	0
Deli Style Hearty Garlic Whole	½ (1 oz)	5	0	0	0	0	1	tr	0	0	260	—	—	0
Kosher Dill Spears	1 spear (1.2 oz)	5	0	0	0	0	1	0	0	0	320	—	—	0
Kosher Dills Halves	1 half (1 oz)	5	0	0	0	0	1	0	0	0	330	—	—	0
Kosher Dills Mini	1 (0.8 oz)	5	0	0	0	0	1	0	0	0	300	—	—	0
Kosher Dills Whole	½ (1 oz)	5	0	0	0	0	1	0	0	20	330	—	—	0
New York Deli Style Half Sours Whole	½ (1 oz)	5	0	0	0	0	1	tr	0	0	260	—	—	0
Sandwich Slices Bread 'N Butter	2 (1.2 oz)	25	0	0	0	0	5	3	0	0	210	—	—	0
Sandwich Slices Deli Style Hearty Garlic	2 (1.2 oz)	5	0	0	0	0	1	tr	0	20	320	—	—	0
Sandwich Slices Kosher Dills	2 (1.2 oz)	5	0	0	0	0	1	tr	0	0	440	—	—	1
Super Slices For Burgers	1 (0.8 oz)	5	0	0	0	0	1	0	0	20	320	—	—	0
MT OLIVE														
Bread & Butter No Sugar Added	1 oz	0	0	0	0	0	tr	0	0	—	105	—	—	—
VLASIC														
Hamburger Dill Chips	1 oz	5	0	0	0	0	1	1	—	—	400	—	—	—
Kosher Cross Cuts	1 oz	5	0	0	0	0	1	1	—	—	220	—	—	—
Kosher Spears	1 oz	5	0	0	0	0	1	1	—	—	220	—	—	—
Kosher Whole	1 oz	5	0	0	0	0	1	1	—	—	220	—	—	—
Sweet Butter Chips	1 oz	30	0	0	0	0	7	7	—	—	190	—	—	—
Sweet Gherkins	1 oz	35	0	0	0	0	9	9	—	—	260	—	—	—
Whole Dills	1 oz	5	0	0	0	0	1	1	—	—	390	—	—	—

PIE

FOOD	PORTION	CALS	FAT	SAT FAT	CHOL	PROT	CARB	SUGAR	FIBER	CALCI	SOD	POTAS	FOLIC	VIT C
FROZEN														
apple	⅛ of 9 in pie (4.4 oz)	297	14	3	0	2	43	—	2	13	333	826	5	4
blueberry	⅛ of 9 in pie (4.4 oz)	289	13	2	0	2	44	—	—	10	406	63	—	—
cherry	⅛ of 9 in pie (4.4 oz)	325	14	3	0	3	50	—	1	15	308	102	10	—
chocolate creme	⅙ of 8 in pie (4 oz)	344	22	6	6	3	38	—	—	41	153	144	8	—
coconut creme	⅙ of 7 in pie (2.2 oz)	191	11	5	0	1	24	—	1	19	163	42	—	0
lemon meringue	⅙ of 8 in pie (4.5 oz)	303	10	2	51	2	53	—	1	63	165	100	10	4
peach	⅙ of 8 in pie (4.1 oz)	261	12	2	0	2	39	—	—	9	316	146	—	—
AMY'S														
Apple	1 serv (4 oz)	240	8	5	25	2	37	15	2	—	135	—	—	—
MRS. SMITH'S														
Apple	1 slice (4.3 oz)	350	19	4	0	3	41	8	3	20	430	—	—	0
Blueberry	1 slice (4.6 oz)	330	17	4	0	3	43	16	3	0	500	—	—	0
Cappuccino	1 slice (4.2 oz)	300	13	8	0	4	45	27	2	80	260	—	—	0
Cherry	1 slice (4.3 oz)	320	17	4	0	3	41	7	2	20	490	—	—	0
Cherry Crumb	1 slice (4.2 oz)	320	12	3	0	3	52	28	1	0	250	—	—	0
Chocolate Cream	1 slice (4.6 oz)	340	18	8	15	3	43	25	2	20	380	—	—	0
Chocolate Mint Cream	1 slice (4.3 oz)	360	15	8	0	3	53	32	2	80	240	—	—	0
Coconut Custard	1 slice (4.4 oz)	260	14	5	70	6	28	16	tr	100	310	—	—	0
Cookies 'N Cream	1 slice (4.3 oz)	360	16	8	0	4	52	32	2	60	290	—	—	0
Dutch Apple	1 slice (4.4 oz)	330	13	3	0	3	50	25	2	0	300	—	—	0
French Silk	1 slice (4.4 oz)	560	40	20	55	4	48	34	1	40	280	—	—	0
Key West Lime	1 slice (4.3 oz)	430	18	11	15	5	62	49	1	150	290	—	—	6
Lemon Cream	1 slice (5 oz)	440	26	17	0	3	49	32	tr	40	180	—	—	4
Lemonade	1 slice (4.3 oz)	340	15	10	0	3	51	31	1	60	280	—	—	5
Mince	1 slice (4.6 oz)	380	17	4	0	3	53	26	2	40	520	—	—	0
Mixed Berry	1 slice (4.2 oz)	300	13	3	0	2	44	24	2	40	360	—	—	0
Peach	1 slice (4.6 oz)	320	17	4	0	3	40	16	2	0	450	—	—	0
Peach Lattice	1 slice (4.2 oz)	290	13	3	0	2	42	23	2	0	280	—	—	0
Peanut Butter Silk	1 slice (4.6 oz)	600	41	19	55	8	51	36	2	40	330	—	—	0
Pecan	1 slice (4.8 oz)	560	27	5	65	6	75	33	2	0	450	—	—	0
Pumpkin Custard	1 slice (4.6 oz)	270	13	3	40	5	35	18	2	80	330	—	—	0
Raspberry	1 slice (4.6 oz)	330	17	4	0	3	44	18	1	20	510	—	—	0
S'Mores Cream	1 slice (4.3 oz)	360	16	8	0	3	53	32	2	60	300	—	—	0
Strawberry Banana	1 slice (4.3 oz)	330	15	9	0	3	48	27	1	60	270	—	—	0

FOOD	PORTION	CALS	FAT	SAT FAT	CHOL	PROT	CARB	SUGAR	FIBER	CALCI	SOD	POTAS	FOLIC	VIT C
MRS. SMITH'S (CONT.)														
Sweet Potato Custard	1 slice (4.6 oz)	340	17	4	40	4	44	25	2	40	240	—	—	0
SARA LEE														
Apple 45% Reduced Fat	⅙ pie (4.5 oz)	290	8	2	<5	4	51	16	2	20	400	—	—	0
Chocolate Silk	⅕ pie (4.8 oz)	500	32	16	<5	4	49	35	<2	40	440	—	—	0
Coconut Cream	⅕ pie (4.8 oz)	480	31	14	0	4	47	35	2	40	430	—	—	0
Homestyle Apple	⅛ pie (4.6 oz)	340	16	4	0	3	46	26	1	—	310	—	—	1
Homestyle Blueberry	⅛ pie (4.6 oz)	360	15	4	0	3	54	26	2	—	340	—	—	2
Homestyle Cherry	⅛ pie (4.6 oz)	320	16	4	0	3	42	27	2	—	290	—	—	—
Homestyle Dutch Apple	⅛ pie (4.6 oz)	350	15	3	0	3	53	30	2	—	320	—	—	1
Homestyle Mince	⅛ pie (4.6 oz)	390	17	4	0	3	56	30	3	20	450	—	—	2
Homestyle Peach	⅛ pie (4.6 oz)	320	14	3	0	3	46	30	2	—	250	—	—	21
Homestyle Pecan	⅛ pie (4.2 oz)	520	24	5	45	5	70	28	3	20	480	—	—	—
Homestyle Pumpkin	⅛ pie (4.6 oz)	260	11	3	30	4	37	18	2	60	460	—	—	0
Homestyle Raspberry	⅛ pie (4.6 oz)	380	19	5	<5	3	48	20	2	—	330	—	—	5
Lemon Meringue	⅙ pie (5 oz)	350	11	3	0	2	59	42	5	—	460	—	—	0
WEIGHT WATCHERS														
Mississippi Mud	1 piece (2.45 oz)	160	5	2	5	4	26	16	1	80	120	—	—	0
MIX														
JELL-O														
No Bake Chocolate Silk as prep	⅙ pie (4.4 oz)	320	16	6	5	5	37	20	tr	150	490	260	—	0
SNACK														
apple	1 (3 oz)	266	14	7	13	2	33	—	—	127	325	51	4	1
cherry	1 (3 oz)	266	14	7	13	2	33	—	—	127	325	51	4	1
lemon	1 (3 oz)	266	14	7	13	2	33	—	—	127	325	51	4	1
DOLLY MADISON														
Apple	1 (4.5 oz)	480	22	9	15	3	67	36	2	60	390	—	—	0
Blueberry	1 (4.5 oz)	480	21	10	20	3	70	31	2	60	460	—	—	0
Cherry	1 (4.5 oz)	470	22	11	20	3	65	35	1	60	470	—	—	0
Chocolate Pudding	1 (4.5 oz)	530	25	11	30	4	71	31	1	150	410	—	—	0
Lemon	1 (4.5 oz)	500	24	11	20	3	66	46	0	60	430	—	—	0
Peach	1 (4.5 oz)	480	21	10	25	3	66	30	1	60	460	—	—	0
Pecan	1 (3 oz)	360	19	8	70	3	44	19	1	60	320	—	—	0
Pecan Fried	1 (4.5 oz)	530	21	9	10	4	80	32	1	100	430	—	—	0
Pineapple	1 (4.5 oz)	460	21	10	15	4	62	29	1	60	340	—	—	0

FOOD	PORTION	CALS	FAT	SAT FAT	CHOL	PROT	CARB	SUGAR	FIBER	CALCI	SOD	POTAS	FOLIC	VIT C
HOSTESS														
Apple	1 (4.5 oz)	480	22	9	15	3	67	36	2	60	390	—	—	0
Blackberry	1 (4.5 oz)	520	21	11	15	3	79	29	2	60	400	—	—	0
Blueberry	1 (4.5 oz)	480	21	10	20	3	70	31	2	60	460	—	—	0
Cherry	1 (4.5 oz)	470	22	11	20	3	65	35	1	60	470	—	—	0
French Apple	1 (4.5 oz)	480	22	9	15	3	67	36	2	60	390	—	—	0
Lemon	1 (4.5 oz)	500	24	11	20	3	66	46	0	60	430	—	—	0
Peach	1 (4.5 oz)	480	21	10	25	3	68	30	1	60	460	—	—	0
Pineapple	1 (4.5 oz)	460	21	10	15	4	62	29	1	60	430	—	—	0
Strawberry	1 (4.5 oz)	510	23	9	15	3	71	35	2	60	360	—	—	0
LANCE														
Pecan	1 (3 oz)	350	17	4	25	4	46	35	3	0	200	50	—	0
TASTYKAKE														
Apple	1 (4 oz)	270	11	1	0	3	41	20	1	20	300	—	—	0
Blueberry	1 (4 oz)	300	11	1	0	3	49	23	1	20	300	—	—	4
Cherry	1 (4 oz)	290	11	1	0	3	46	16	tr	20	300	—	—	0
Coconut Creme	1 (4 oz)	370	21	4	55	5	42	21	1	60	420	—	—	1
French Apple	1 (4.2 oz)	310	11	1	0	3	52	30	1	20	290	—	—	0
Lemon	1 (4 oz)	300	13	2	40	3	44	24	tr	20	320	—	—	1
Peach	1 (4 oz)	280	11	1	0	3	43	21	1	20	300	—	—	2
Pineapple	1 (4 oz)	290	12	1	20	3	45	24	1	20	310	—	—	1
Pineapple Cheese	1 (4 oz)	320	12	3	20	5	50	26	1	60	410	—	—	2
Pumpkin	1 (4 oz)	340	14	2	35	4	47	22	1	40	530	—	—	1
Strawberry	1 (3.5 oz)	320	12	1	0	3	51	29	1	20	300	—	—	9
Tastyklair	1 (4 oz)	400	20	3	90	5	50	26	0	40	290	—	—	0
TOM'S														
Apple	1 pkg (3 oz)	330	17	8	5	2	42	21	1	0	250	—	—	0
Banana Marshmallow	1 pkg (2.75 oz)	320	11	7	0	3	54	33	0	20	190	—	—	0
Cherry	1 pkg (3 oz)	320	18	8	5	2	37	24	1	0	240	—	—	0
Chocolate Marshmallow	1 pkg (2.75 oz)	320	11	6	0	3	53	32	tr	20	190	—	—	0
TAKE-OUT														
apple	⅛ of 9 in pie (5.4 oz)	411	19	5	0	4	58	—	3	11	327	123	7	3
banana cream	⅛ of 9 in pie (5.2 oz)	398	20	6	75	7	49	—	—	110	355	245	17	2
blueberry	⅛ of 9 in pie (5.2 oz)	360	18	4	0	4	49	—	—	10	272	74	7	1
butterscotch	⅛ of 9 in pie (4.5 oz)	355	18	5	78	6	42	—	—	128	335	221	14	1
cherry	⅛ of 9 in pie (6.3 oz)	486	22	5	0	5	69	—	—	18	343	138	12	2
coconut creme	⅛ of 9 in pie (4.7 oz)	396	21	8	77	6	46	—	—	113	356	183	14	1

FOOD	PORTION	CALS	FAT	SAT FAT	CHOL	PROT	CARB	SUGAR	FIBER	CALCI	SOD	POTAS	FOLIC	VIT C
coconut custard	⅙ of 8 in pie (3.6 oz)	271	14	6	36	6	32	—	—	84	348	182	—	—
custard	⅛ of 9 in pie (4.5 oz)	262	11	4	87	7	34	—	2	107	256	159	13	1
lemon meringue	⅛ of 9 in pie (4.5 oz)	362	16	4	68	5	50	—	2	15	307	83	11	4
mince	⅛ of 9 in pie (5.8 oz)	477	18	4	0	18	79	—	—	37	419	335	9	10
pecan	⅙ of 8 in pie (4 oz)	452	21	4	36	5	65	—	4	19	480	84	7	1
pumpkin	⅙ of 8 in pie (3.8 oz)	229	10	2	22	4	30	—	3	66	308	168	17	—
vanilla cream	⅛ of 9 in pie (4.4 oz)	350	18	5	78	6	41	—	—	113	327	158	14	1

PIE CRUST

FROZEN

FOOD	PORTION	CALS	FAT	SAT FAT	CHOL	PROT	CARB	SUGAR	FIBER	CALCI	SOD	POTAS	FOLIC	VIT C
baked	⅛ of 9 in pie (0.6 oz)	82	5	2	—	1	8	—	—	3	104	18	—	—
baked	9 in shell (4.4 oz)	647	41	13	—	6	63	—	—	26	815	138	—	—
puff pastry baked	1 shell (1.4 oz)	223	15	2	0	3	18	—	—	4	101	25	4	0

PEPPERIDGE FARM

FOOD	PORTION	CALS	FAT	SAT FAT	CHOL	PROT	CARB	SUGAR	FIBER	CALCI	SOD	POTAS	FOLIC	VIT C
Puff Pastry Sheets	⅙ sheet (1.4 oz)	170	11	3	0	3	14	1	0	0	200	—	—	0
Puff Pastry Shell	1 (1.6 oz)	190	13	4	0	4	16	2	0	0	230	—	—	0
Puff Pastry Squares	1 sq (2 oz)	240	16	5	0	4	19	2	0	0	250	—	—	0

PET-RITZ

FOOD	PORTION	CALS	FAT	SAT FAT	CHOL	PROT	CARB	SUGAR	FIBER	CALCI	SOD	POTAS	FOLIC	VIT C
Deep Dish	⅛ pie (0.7 oz)	90	5	2	<5	1	10	0	0	0	85	—	—	0
Regular	⅛ pie (0.6 oz)	80	5	2	<5	tr	9	tr	0	0	60	—	—	0
Tart Shells	1 (1 oz)	130	8	2	0	1	13	0	0	0	170	—	—	0

MIX

FOOD	PORTION	CALS	FAT	SAT FAT	CHOL	PROT	CARB	SUGAR	FIBER	CALCI	SOD	POTAS	FOLIC	VIT C
as prep	⅛ of 9 in pie	100	6	2	0	1	10	—	—	12	146	12	—	0
as prep (0.7 oz)	9 in crust (5.6 oz)	801	49	12	0	11	81	—	—	96	1167	99	—	0

BETTY CROCKER

FOOD	PORTION	CALS	FAT	SAT FAT	CHOL	PROT	CARB	SUGAR	FIBER	CALCI	SOD	POTAS	FOLIC	VIT C
Pie Crust as prep	⅛ crust	110	8	2	0	1	9	—	—	—	135	10	16	—

MINICARB

FOOD	PORTION	CALS	FAT	SAT FAT	CHOL	PROT	CARB	SUGAR	FIBER	CALCI	SOD	POTAS	FOLIC	VIT C
Pie Crust Mix	1 slice	105	7	4	40	9	1	0	0	—	320	—	—	—

READY-TO-EAT

FOOD	PORTION	CALS	FAT	SAT FAT	CHOL	PROT	CARB	SUGAR	FIBER	CALCI	SOD	POTAS	FOLIC	VIT C
chocolate cookie crumb	⅛ of 9 in pie (1 oz)	139	9	2	0	1	15	—	—	8	185	48	1	0
chocolate cookie crumb	9 in crust (7.7 oz)	1130	69	15	3	12	122	—	—	68	1502	375	1	tr
graham cracker	9 in crust (8.4 oz)	1181	60	12	0	10	156	—	—	50	1365	210	17	tr
graham cracker	⅛ of 9 in pie (1 oz)	148	8	2	0	1	20	—	—	6	171	26	2	0

FOOD	PORTION	CALS	FAT	SAT FAT	CHOL	PROT	CARB	SUGAR	FIBER	CALCI	SOD	POTAS	FOLIC	VIT C
vanilla wafer cracker crumbs	9 in crust (6.1 oz)	937	64	13	69	7	89	—	—	74	909	140	11	tr
vanilla wafer cracker crumbs	⅛ of 9 in pie (0.8 oz)	119	8	2	9	1	11	—	—	9	116	18	1	0
KEEBLER														
Graham Single Serve	1 (0.8 oz)	120	6	1	0	1	15	6	tr	0	150	—	—	0
Reduced Fat Graham	⅛ pie (0.7 oz)	90	4	0	0	1	14	6	0	0	85	—	—	0
REFRIGERATED														
ALL READY														
Crust	⅛ pie (0.9 oz)	120	7	3	5	tr	13	tr	0	0	100	—	—	0

PIE FILLING

FOOD	PORTION	CALS	FAT	SAT FAT	CHOL	PROT	CARB	SUGAR	FIBER	CALCI	SOD	POTAS	FOLIC	VIT C
apple	1 can (21 oz)	599	1	tr	0	1	156	143	6	27	259	268	0	—
apple	⅛ can (2.6 oz)	74	tr	tr	0	tr	19	18	1	3	32	33	0	—
cherry	1 can (21 oz)	683	1	tr	0	3	175	—	—	65	54	625	24	—
cherry	⅛ can (2.6 oz)	85	tr	tr	0	tr	22	—	—	8	7	78	3	—
pumpkin pie mix	1 cup	282	tr	tr	0	3	71	—	—	99	561	372	—	10
COLAC														
All Flavors	1 tbsp	19	0	0	0	0	7	0	0	—	0	—	—	—
COMSTOCK														
Light Cherry	⅓ cup	60	0	0	0	0	15	14	1	0	15	—	—	0
Red Ruby Cherry	⅓ cup (3.1 oz)	90	0	0	0	0	23	19	1	0	25	—	—	0
LIBBY'S														
Pumpkin Pie Mix	⅓ cup	90	1	0	0	tr	20	17	2	0	115	—	—	0
SMUCKER'S														
Pie Glaze Strawberry	2 oz	80	0	0	0	0	21	20	—	—	0	—	—	—

PIEROGI

FOOD	PORTION	CALS	FAT	SAT FAT	CHOL	PROT	CARB	SUGAR	FIBER	CALCI	SOD	POTAS	FOLIC	VIT C
pierogi	¾ cup (4.4 oz)	307	19	7	49	11	24	—	—	156	369	101	8	1
HEALTH IS WEALTH														
Potato & Cheddar	2 (2.8 oz)	140	2	0	0	5	27	1	3	40	360	—	—	1
Potato & Onion	2 (2.8 oz)	140	2	0	0	4	27	1	3	20	300	—	—	1
MRS. T'S														
Broccoli & Cheddar	3 (4.2 oz)	200	5	1	10	6	34	2	2	40	570	—	—	12
Jalapeño & Cheddar	3 (4.2 oz)	190	3	1	10	6	34	2	2	40	550	—	—	9
Potato & American Cheese	3 (4.2 oz)	220	4	2	15	8	39	1	2	40	420	—	—	6
Potato & Roasted Garlic	3 (4.2 oz)	190	4	1	5	5	36	2	2	20	430	—	—	9
Potato & Cheddar	3 (4.2 oz)	180	3	1	10	7	34	3	2	40	430	—	—	0
Potato & Onion	3 (4.2 oz)	180	2	0	0	5	34	1	2	20	410	—	—	9
Rogies Cheddar & Bacon	7 (3 oz)	140	3	1	5	5	24	1	1	10	430	—	—	4

FOOD	PORTION	CALS	FAT	SAT FAT	CHOL	PROT	CARB	SUGAR	FIBER	CALCI	SOD	POTAS	FOLIC	VIT C
MRS. T'S (CONT.)														
Rogies Jalapeño & Cheddar	7 (3 oz)	120	2	1	5	4	23	1	1	20	350	—	—	5
Rogies Potato & Cheddar	7 (3 oz)	130	2	1	5	4	24	1	1	20	350	—	—	5
PIGEON														
w/ skin & bone	3.5 oz	169	10	—	110	21	0	—	—	45	90	330	—	—
PIGEON PEAS														
dried cooked	1 cup	204	1	tr	0	11	39	—	—	72	9	644	186	0
dried cooked	½ cup	102	tr	tr	0	6	20	—	—	36	5	322	93	0
PIGNOLIA														
(*see* PINE NUTS)														
PIG'S EARS AND FEET														
ear simmered	1	184	12	4	100	18	tr	—	0	20	185	—	0	0
feet pickled	1 lb	921	73	25	417	61	tr	—	0	145	4187	—	18	0
feet pickled	1 oz	58	5	2	26	4	tr	—	0	9	262	—	1	0
feet simmered	3 oz	165	11	4	85	16	0	—	0	38	26	—	1	0
HORMEL														
Pickled Feet	2 oz	80	6	2	45	7	0	0	0	20	530	—	—	0
Pickled Hocks	2 oz	110	8	3	45	9	0	0	0	0	530	—	—	0
PIKE														
northern cooked	½ fillet (5.4 oz)	176	1	tr	78	38	0	—	—	113	76	514	—	6
northern cooked	3 oz	96	1	tr	43	21	0	—	—	62	42	282	3	—
northern raw	3 oz	75	1	tr	33	16	0	—	—	48	33	220	—	3
roe raw	1 oz	37	tr	—	103	7	tr	—	—	—	—	—	—	4
walleye baked	3 oz	101	1	tr	94	21	0	—	—	120	56	424	—	—
walleye fillet bakcd	4.4 oz	147	2	tr	137	30	0	—	—	175	81	618	—	—
PILLNUTS														
canarytree dricd	1 oz	204	23	9	0	3	1	—	—	41	1	144	—	—
PIMIENTOS														
canned	1 tbsp	3	tr	tr	0	tr	1	—	—	1	2	19	1	10
canned	1 slice	0	0	0	0	tr	tr	—	—	0	0	2	0	1
DROMEDARY														
Peeled	½ tsp (4 g)	0	0	0	0	0	0	0	0	0	0	—	—	0
Unpeeled	½ tsp (4 g)	0	0	0	0	0	0	0	0	0	0	—	—	1
PINE NUTS														
pignolia dried	1 tbsp	51	5	1	0	2	1	—	—	3	0	60	—	—
pignolia dried	1 oz	146	14	2	0	7	4	—	—	7	1	170	—	—
pinyon dried	1 oz	161	17	3	0	3	5	—	—	2	20	178	—	1
PROGRESSO														
Pignoli	1 jar (1 oz)	170	13	1	0	10	2	0	0	0	0	—	—	0

PINEAPPLE

FOOD	PORTION	CALS	FAT	SAT FAT	CHOL	PROT	CARB	SUGAR	FIBER	CALCI	SOD	POTAS	FOLIC	VIT C
CANNED														
chunks in heavy syrup	1 cup	199	tr	tr	0	1	52	—	—	35	3	264	12	19
chunks juice pack	1 cup	150	tr	tr	0	1	39	—	—	34	4	304	—	24
crushed in heavy syrup	1 cup	199	tr	tr	0	1	52	—	—	35	3	264	12	19
slices in heavy syrup	1 slice	45	tr	tr	0	tr	12	—	—	8	1	60	3	4
slices in light syrup	1 slice	30	tr	tr	0	tr	8	—	—	8	1	61	3	4
slices juice pack	1 slice	35	tr	tr	0	tr	9	—	—	8	1	70	—	6
slices water pack	1 slice	19	tr	tr	0	tr	5	—	—	9	1	74	3	5
tidbits in heavy syrup	1 cup	199	tr	tr	0	1	52	—	—	35	3	264	12	19
tidbits in juice	1 cup	150	tr	tr	0	1	19	—	—	34	4	304	—	24
tidbits in water	1 cup	79	tr	tr	0	1	20	—	—	37	3	313	12	19
DEL MONTE														
Chunks In Heavy Syrup	½ cup (4.3 oz)	90	0	0	0	0	24	22	1	0	10	—	—	12
Chunks In Its Own Juice	½ cup (4.3 oz)	70	0	0	0	0	17	15	1	0	10	—	—	12
Crushed In Heavy Syrup	½ cup (4.3 oz)	90	0	0	0	0	24	22	1	0	10	—	—	12
Crushed In Its Own Juice	½ cup (4.3 oz)	70	0	0	0	0	17	15	1	0	10	—	—	12
Fruit Cup Tidbits	1 pkg (4 oz)	50	0	0	0	1	15	13	1	0	10	—	—	12
Sliced In Heavy Syrup	2 slices (4.1 oz)	90	0	0	0	0	23	21	1	0	10	—	—	12
Sliced In Its Own Juice	½ cup (4 oz)	60	0	0	0	0	16	14	1	0	10	—	—	12
Spears In Its Own Juice	½ cup (4.3 oz)	70	0	0	0	0	17	15	1	0	10	—	—	12
Tidbits In Its Own Juice	½ cup (4.3 oz)	70	0	0	0	0	17	15	1	0	10	—	—	12
Wedges In Its Own Juice	½ cup (4.3 oz)	70	0	0	0	0	17	15	1	0	10	—	—	12
DOLE														
All Natural Chunks	½ cup	60	0	0	0	0	16	13	tr	—	10	—	—	24
Chunks Juice Pack	½ cup	60	0	0	0	0	15	13	1	—	10	—	—	15
SUNFRESH														
In Lightly Sweetened Juice	½ cup	70	0	0	0	0	18	15	tr	0	10	—	—	60
FRESH														
diced	1 cup	77	tr	tr	0	1	19	—	2	11	1	175	16	24
sliced	1 slice	42	tr	tr	0	tr	10	—	1	6	1	95	9	13

FOOD	PORTION	CALS	FAT	SAT FAT	CHOL	PROT	CARB	SUGAR	FIBER	CALCI	SOD	POTAS	FOLIC	VIT C
BONITA HILL														
Golden Extra Sweet	2 slices (3.9 oz)	60	0	0	0	1	16	13	1	20	10	—	—	15
CALA FRUIT														
Golden Sliced	1 serv (3.5 oz)	50	0	0	0	0	12	11	1	0	0	—	—	15
FROSTY FRESH														
Peeled & Cored	½ cup	60	0	0	0	0	14	13	1	—	0	—	—	18
FROZEN														
chunks sweetened	½ cup	104	tr	tr	0	tr	27	—	—	11	2	122	—	10
PINEAPPLE JUICE														
canned	1 cup	139	tr	tr	0	1	34	—	—	42	2	334	58	27
frzn as prep	1 cup	129	tr	tr	0	1	32	—	—	28	3	340	—	30
frzn not prep	6 oz	387	tr	tr	0	3	96	—	—	84	6	1020	—	91
CERES														
Pineapple	8 oz	120	0	0	0	0	29	25	2	40	5	300	—	60
DEL MONTE														
Juice	6 fl oz	80	0	0	0	1	20	17	0	20	5	—	—	60
DOLE														
Chilled	8 oz	130	0	0	0	0	30	—	—	—	10	310	—	60
PINK BEANS														
dried cooked	1 cup	252	1	tr	0	15	47	—	—	88	3	858	284	0
PINTO BEANS														
CANNED														
pinto	1 cup	186	1	tr	0	11	35	—	—	89	998	723	145	2
CHI-CHI'S														
Pinto Beans	½ cup (4.3 oz)	100	1	0	0	6	18	1	3	20	540	—	—	0
EDEN														
Organic Spicy	½ cup (4.6 oz)	125	0	0	0	6	24	7	2	80	195	380	—	0
GREEN GIANT														
Pinto Beans	½ cup (4.4 oz)	110	1	0	0	6	20	2	5	80	280	—	—	0
PROGRESSO														
Pinto Beans	½ cup (4.6 oz)	110	1	0	0	7	18	tr	7	40	250	—	—	0
DRIED														
cooked	1 cup	235	1	tr	0	14	44	—	—	82	3	800	294	4
HURST														
HamBeens w/ Ham	3 tbsp (1.2 oz)	120	1	0	0	7	20	1	6	40	63	—	—	1
FROZEN														
cooked	3 oz	152	tr	tr	0	9	29	—	—	49	—	—	—	1
PISTACHIOS														
dried	1 cup	739	62	8	0	26	32	—	14	173	7	1399	74	—
dry roasted	1 oz	172	15	2	0	4	8	—	—	20	2	275	—	—
dry roasted salted	1 cup	776	68	9	0	19	35	—	—	90	1040	1242	—	—
dry roasted salted	1 oz	172	15	2	0	4	8	—	—	20	260	275	—	—

FOOD	PORTION	CALS	FAT	SAT FAT	CHOL	PROT	CARB	SUGAR	FIBER	CALCI	SOD	POTAS	FOLIC	VIT C
dry roasted w/ salt	47 nuts (1 oz)	160	13	2	0	6	8	2	3	40	120	290	16	—
with shells dry roasted unsalted	½ cup	180	14	2	0	6	9	3	3	40	10	—	—	0
AMERICAN ALMOND														
Pistachio Paste	2 tbsp	160	11	1	0	4	14	10	2	20	0	—	—	1
LANCE														
Pistachios	1 pkg (1⅛ oz)	90	7	1	0	4	4	0	2	20	105	160	—	0
SWEET DELIGHTS														
Pistachio Roasters	⅓ pkg (1 oz)	190	14	—	0	6	9	3	3	—	220	300	—	—

PITANGA

FOOD	PORTION	CALS	FAT	SAT FAT	CHOL	PROT	CARB	SUGAR	FIBER	CALCI	SOD	POTAS	FOLIC	VIT C
fresh	1 cup	57	1	—	0	1	13	—	—	16	5	178	—	46
fresh	1	2	tr	—	0	tr	1	—	—	1	0	7	—	2

PIZZA

(*see also* PIZZA DOUGH, PIZZA SAUCE)

FOOD	PORTION	CALS	FAT	SAT FAT	CHOL	PROT	CARB	SUGAR	FIBER	CALCI	SOD	POTAS	FOLIC	VIT C
AMY'S														
Cheese	⅓ pie	300	13	4	15	12	38	4	2	—	530	—	—	—
Mushroom & Olive	⅓ pie	250	9	3	10	10	33	3	2	—	560	—	—	—
Pesto	⅓ pie	310	12	4	10	12	39	3	2	—	480	—	—	—
Pocket Sandwich Cheese Pizza	1 (4.5 oz)	300	9	4	15	14	42	5	4	—	450	—	—	—
Pocket Sandwich Vegetarian Pizza	1 (4.5 oz)	250	6	3	10	11	39	4	4	—	360	—	—	—
Roasted Vegetable	⅓ pie	260	8	2	0	6	42	5	2	—	490	—	—	—
Snacks Cheese	5–6 pieces	180	6	3	10	9	22	3	2	—	290	—	—	—
Soy Cheese	⅓ pie	290	11	1	0	12	37	3	2	—	590	—	—	—
Spinach	⅓ pie	300	12	4	15	12	38	4	2	—	590	—	—	—
Veggie Combo	⅓ pie	280	9	3	10	10	36	4	2	—	580	—	—	—
APPIAN WAY														
Pizza Mix Thick Crust	⅓ pie (4.2 oz)	290	5	2	10	10	51	4	2	100	830	—	—	0
Pizza Mix Thin Crust	⅓ pie (4.1 oz)	250	3	1	0	7	48	4	2	40	740	—	—	0
BANQUET														
Pepperoni	1 pie (6.75 oz)	490	23	7	35	11	56	30	5	200	790	—	—	0
Pizza Snack Cheese	6 pieces (7.5 oz)	200	8	4	20	9	24	4	2	100	360	—	—	5
Pizza Snack Pepperoni	6 pieces (7.5 oz)	230	11	5	20	8	23	4	2	60	430	—	—	1
Pizza Snack Pepperoni & Sausage	6 pieces (7.5 oz)	210	9	4	20	8	24	4	2	80	440	—	—	5
DI GIORNO														
Rising Crust 12 inch Four Cheese	⅙ pie (4.9 oz)	320	11	6	25	16	39	6	3	300	870	250	—	0

FOOD	PORTION	CALS	FAT	SAT FAT	CHOL	PROT	CARB	SUGAR	FIBER	CALCI	SOD	POTAS	FOLIC	VIT C
DI GIORNO (CONT.)														
Rising Crust 12 inch Italian Sausage	⅙ pie (5.3 oz)	360	14	7	35	18	40	6	3	250	1000	300	—	0
Rising Crust 12 inch Pepperoni	⅙ pie (5.2 oz)	370	16	8	35	18	40	6	3	250	1080	320	—	0
Rising Crust 12 inch Supreme	⅙ pie (5.8 oz)	380	17	8	40	18	40	7	3	250	1100	340	—	1
Rising Crust 12 inch Three Meat	⅙ pie (5.4 oz)	380	16	8	40	19	40	6	3	250	1100	330	—	0
Rising Crust 12 inch Vegetable	⅙ pie (5.6 oz)	310	10	5	20	15	41	7	3	250	830	290	—	4
Rising Crust 8 inch Chicken Supreme	⅓ pie (4.8 oz)	270	9	5	30	16	33	5	2	200	740	230	—	1
Rising Crust 8 inch Four Cheese	⅓ pie (4 oz)	260	9	5	20	14	33	5	2	250	720	200	—	0
Rising Crust 8 inch Italian Sausage	⅓ pie (4.4 oz)	300	12	6	25	15	33	5	2	200	830	240	—	0
Rising Crust 8 inch Pepperoni	⅓ pie (4.2 oz)	300	13	6	30	15	33	5	2	200	880	253	—	0
Rising Crust 8 inch Spinach	⅓ pie (4.3 oz)	250	8	4	15	15	33	5	3	200	670	240	—	0
Rising Crust 8 inch Supreme	⅓ pie (4.7 oz)	310	14	6	30	15	34	5	2	200	900	270	—	1
Rising Crust 8 inch Three Meat	⅓ pie (4.4 oz)	310	13	6	30	15	34	5	2	200	900	260	—	0
Rising Crust 8 inch Vegetable	⅓ pie (4.6 oz)	250	8	4	15	13	33	6	2	200	680	230	—	2
FRESCHETTA														
Pepperoni	½ pie (5.8 oz)	470	21	9	45	19	51	5	2	200	1350	—	—	0
HEALTH IS WEALTH														
Pizza Munchees	6 (3 oz)	190	5	0	0	2	9	0	1	0	560	—	—	2
HEALTHY CHOICE														
French Bread Cheese	1 piece (6 oz)	340	5	2	15	22	51	9	5	250	480	—	—	0
French Bread Pepperoni	1 piece (6 oz)	340	5	2	20	24	49	6	6	300	580	—	—	0
French Bread Sausage	1 piece (6 oz)	320	5	2	25	21	48	9	5	150	580	—	—	0
French Bread Supreme	1 piece (6.35 oz)	330	5	2	20	21	51	7	6	150	580	—	—	0
French Bread Vegetable	1 piece (6 oz)	280	4	2	10	17	44	8	5	300	480	—	—	0

FOOD	PORTION	CALS	FAT	SAT FAT	CHOL	PROT	CARB	SUGAR	FIBER	CALCI	SOD	POTAS	FOLIC	VIT C
JACK'S														
Great Combinations 12 inch Bacon Cheeseburger	¼ pie (4.7 oz)	360	18	9	45	20	31	4	2	250	770	350	—	0
Great Combinations 12 inch Double Cheese	¼ pie (4.9 oz)	380	19	11	50	21	32	5	2	450	670	290	—	0
Great Combinations 12 inch Pepperoni	¼ pie (5.2 oz)	410	19	9	40	19	42	5	3	300	830	280	—	0
Great Combinations 12 inch Pepperoni & Mushrooms	¼ pie (4.8 oz)	340	16	7	35	17	32	5	2	250	740	280	—	0
Great Combinations 12 inch Sausage	¼ pie (5.4 oz)	390	18	8	40	18	40	5	3	300	700	360	—	0
Great Combinations 12 inch Sausage & Mushroom	¼ pie (4.9 oz)	310	15	7	30	16	29	5	3	250	610	340	—	0
Great Combinations 12 inch Sausage & Pepperoni	¼ pie (4.8 oz)	350	19	8	40	17	29	4	2	250	770	300	—	0
Great Combinations 12 inch Supreme	¼ pie (5.2 oz)	350	18	8	40	17	30	3	5	250	750	320	—	1
Great Combinations 9 inch Double Cheese	½ pie (5.5 oz)	430	21	12	55	23	38	5	3	500	740	300	—	0
Great Combinations 9 inch Pepperoni & Sausage	½ pie (5.1 oz)	380	18	8	40	18	36	5	3	300	790	300	—	0
Naturally Rising 12 inch Bacon Cheeseburger	⅙ pie (5 oz)	350	15	7	40	18	35	7	2	250	680	310	—	0
Naturally Rising 12 inch Canadian Bacon	⅙ pie (4.9 oz)	280	9	5	30	16	34	7	2	250	590	280	—	0
Naturally Rising 12 inch Cheese	⅙ pie (4.5 oz)	290	10	6	25	15	35	7	2	250	500	260	—	0
Naturally Rising 12 inch Combination w/ Sausage & Pepperoni	⅙ pie (5.2 oz)	360	17	8	40	17	34	7	2	250	680	310	—	0

FOOD	PORTION	CALS	FAT	SAT FAT	CHOL	PROT	CARB	SUGAR	FIBER	CALCI	SOD	POTAS	FOLIC	VIT C
JACK'S (CONT.)														
Naturally Rising 12 inch Pepperoni	⅙ pie (4.9 oz)	350	16	8	40	17	35	7	2	250	710	260	—	0
Naturally Rising 12 inch Pepperoni Supreme	⅙ pie (5.1 oz)	340	16	8	35	16	34	11	2	250	670	300	—	0
Naturally Rising 12 inch Sausage	⅙ pie (5.1 oz)	340	15	7	35	17	34	7	2	250	600	330	—	0
Naturally Rising 12 inch Spicy Italian Sausage	⅙ pie (5.1 oz)	330	14	7	40	17	34	11	2	250	680	240	—	0
Naturally Rising 12 inch The Works	⅙ pie (5.3 oz)	330	14	7	35	16	34	7	2	250	580	340	—	0
Naturally Rising 9 inch Cheese	⅓ pie (4.7 oz)	300	10	6	25	15	38	7	2	250	500	270	—	0
Naturally Rising 9 inch Combination w/ Sausage & Pepperoni	¼ pie (4.2 oz)	300	14	7	35	14	29	5	2	200	560	260	—	0
Naturally Rising 9 inch Pepperoni	⅓ pie (5.2 oz)	360	16	8	40	17	38	7	2	250	720	300	—	0
Naturally Rising 9 inch Sausage	⅓ pie (5.4 oz)	360	16	7	35	17	38	7	2	250	620	340	—	0
Naturally Rising 9 inch The Works	¼ pie (4.5 oz)	280	12	6	30	13	29	6	2	250	480	280	—	0
Original 12 inch Canadian Bacon	¼ pie (4.4 oz)	280	10	5	30	16	31	5	2	250	620	270	—	0
Original 12 inch Cheese	⅓ pie (5 oz)	360	13	7	30	19	41	6	3	350	650	290	—	0
Original 12 inch Hamburger	¼ pie (4.4 oz)	300	14	7	35	16	28	4	2	250	580	270	—	0
Original 12 inch Pepperoni	¼ pie (4.3 oz)	330	15	7	35	16	31	4	2	250	720	240	—	0
Original 12 inch Sausage	¼ pie (4.3 oz)	300	14	7	30	15	28	4	2	250	580	290	—	0
Original 12 inch Spicy Italian Sausage	¼ pie (4.3 oz)	290	13	6	35	15	29	5	2	250	650	280	—	0
Original 9 inch Pepperoni	½ pie (5 oz)	380	18	8	40	18	37	5	3	300	820	270	—	0
Original 9 inch Sausage	½ pie (5.1 oz)	360	16	7	35	17	36	5	3	300	660	340	—	0
Pizza Bursts Combination Sausage & Pepperoni	6 pieces (3 oz)	250	12	4	20	8	26	3	2	60	500	230	—	0

FOOD	PORTION	CALS	FAT	SAT FAT	CHOL	PROT	CARB	SUGAR	FIBER	CALCI	SOD	POTAS	FOLIC	VIT C
JACK'S (CONT.)														
Pizza Bursts Pepperoni	6 pieces (3 oz)	260	14	5	20	9	25	3	2	100	560	200	—	0
Pizza Bursts Sausage	6 pieces (3 oz)	250	12	4	20	8	25	3	2	60	490	200	—	0
Pizza Bursts Supercheese	6 pieces (3 oz)	250	12	5	20	9	25	3	2	150	460	190	—	0
Pizza Bursts Supreme	6 pieces (3 oz)	250	13	4	20	8	26	3	2	60	520	200	—	0
JENO'S														
Crisp 'N Tasty Cheese	1 pie (6.8 oz)	460	19	6	20	19	52	6	2	350	860	—	—	0
KID CUISINE														
Backpacking Pizza Snack	6 pieces	230	11	5	20	8	23	4	1	60	480	—	—	1
Big League Hamburger	1 meal (8.3 oz)	400	11	4	35	14	61	32	5	100	550	—	—	1
Fire Chief Cheese	1 pie (5.2 oz)	340	10	5	20	19	44	7	2	200	760	—	—	0
Pirate Pizza w/ Cheese	1 meal (8 oz)	430	11	5	30	12	71	34	5	150	480	—	—	0
Poolside Pepperoni	1 (5.2 oz)	380	14	7	35	18	44	7	2	150	990	—	—	0
LEAN CUISINE														
Everyday Favorites French Bread Cheese	1 pkg (6 oz)	320	7	4	15	15	48	6	4	300	580	480	—	4
Everyday Favorites French Bread Deluxe	1 pkg (6.1 oz)	290	6	3	25	16	43	5	3	150	550	440	—	6
Everyday Favorites French Bread Pepperoni	1 pkg (5.25 oz)	300	8	4	25	15	43	6	3	100	590	410	—	1
Everyday Favorites French Bread Sun Dried Tomatoes	1 serv (6 oz)	340	8	5	20	19	48	8	3	350	580	500	—	1
MARIE CALLENDER'S														
French Bread Cheese	1 (7.2 oz)	530	24	14	60	28	50	5	4	500	980	—	—	0
French Bread Pepperoni	1 (7.5 oz)	570	28	14	65	29	50	5	4	450	1160	—	—	0
French Bread Supreme	1 (7.5 oz)	510	23	11	50	26	50	5	4	400	1200	—	—	0
PEPPERIDGE FARM														
Gourmet Crust Cheese	1 (4.4 oz)	390	20	7	90	12	39	11	6	200	770	—	—	2
Gourmet Crust Pepperoni	1 (4.5 oz)	420	23	9	90	15	39	8	5	150	810	—	—	4

FOOD	PORTION	CALS	FAT	SAT FAT	CHOL	PROT	CARB	SUGAR	FIBER	CALCI	SOD	POTAS	FOLIC	VIT C
RED BARON														
Deep Dish Single Pepperoni	1 pizza	460	25	9	35	17	41	3	2	200	910	—	—	1
STOUFFER'S														
French Bread Bacon Cheddar	1 piece (5.7 oz)	430	21	7	25	15	46	4	4	200	880	310	—	4
French Bread Cheese	1 piece (5.2 oz)	370	16	6	15	14	43	4	3	200	880	240	—	0
French Bread Cheeseburger	1 piece (6 oz)	420	20	6	30	17	44	3	3	200	800	320	—	2
French Bread Deluxe	1 piece (6.2 oz)	430	21	7	20	17	49	5	3	150	990	320	—	2
French Bread Double Cheese	1 piece (5.9 oz)	400	16	7	25	16	49	4	4	250	950	240	—	2
French Bread Pepperoni	1 piece (5.6 oz)	430	20	8	15	16	46	5	3	150	990	290	—	1
French Bread Pepperoni & Mushroom	1 piece (6.1 oz)	440	20	7	30	15	49	4	5	100	910	310	—	2
French Bread Sausage	1 piece (6 oz)	420	18	7	20	17	48	5	3	200	1260	330	—	2
French Bread Sausage & Pepperoni	1 piece (6.25 oz)	470	23	8	25	18	47	4	3	200	1340	350	—	5
French Bread Three Meat	1 piece (6.25 oz)	460	21	8	35	20	48	4	5	200	1200	370	—	4
French Bread Vegetable Deluxe	1 piece (6.4 oz)	380	16	6	20	14	46	4	4	300	780	230	—	0
French Bread White Pizza	1 piece (5.1 oz)	460	23	7	20	18	45	1	5	350	700	130	—	0
TOMBSTONE														
Double Top Pepperoni	⅙ pie (4.5 oz)	340	19	9	45	18	24	5	2	350	810	300	—	1
Double Top Sausage	⅙ pie (4.6 oz)	320	17	9	40	18	25	6	2	350	760	320	—	2
Double Top Sausage & Pepperoni	⅙ pie (4.6 oz)	340	19	9	45	19	25	5	2	350	820	320	—	1
Double Top Supreme	⅙ pie (4.7 oz)	330	18	9	40	18	25	5	2	300	780	310	—	2
Double Top Two Cheese	⅙ pie (5.2 oz)	380	19	11	50	22	29	6	2	500	760	320	—	2
For One ½ Less Fat Cheese	1 pie (6.5 oz)	460	10	5	20	23	43	8	3	400	940	450	—	2
For One ½ Less Fat Vegetable	1 pie (7.2 oz)	360	9	4	10	21	48	11	5	350	860	500	—	1

FOOD	PORTION	CALS	FAT	SAT FAT	CHOL	PROT	CARB	SUGAR	FIBER	CALCI	SOD	POTAS	FOLIC	VIT C
TOMBSTONE (CONT.)														
For One Extra Cheese	1 pie (6.9 oz)	520	28	13	50	26	47	8	3	500	940	450	—	1
For One Pepperoni	1 pie (6.9 oz)	550	32	14	55	25	41	8	3	400	1160	500	—	1
For One Supreme	1 pie (7.5 oz)	550	32	14	55	24	42	8	3	350	1090	500	—	4
Light Supreme	⅕ pie (4.8 oz)	270	9	4	20	17	30	6	3	200	720	370	—	1
Light Vegetable	⅕ pie (4.6 oz)	240	7	3	10	14	31	5	3	200	500	310	—	2
Original 12 inch Canadian Bacon	¼ pie (5.5 oz)	350	14	7	35	20	36	7	3	250	890	400	—	1
Original 12 inch Deluxe	⅕ pie (4.8 oz)	310	14	6	30	15	29	6	3	250	690	350	—	4
Original 12 inch Extra Cheese	¼ pie (5.1 oz)	350	15	8	30	18	35	7	3	350	680	350	—	1
Original 12 inch Hamburger	⅕ pie (4.4 oz)	310	15	7	30	15	29	5	2	200	670	320	—	2
Original 12 inch Pepperoni	¼ pie (5.3 oz)	400	21	9	40	19	35	7	3	300	930	400	—	1
Original 12 inch Sausage	⅕ pie (4.4 oz)	300	14	6	30	15	29	6	2	200	680	340	—	1
Original 12 inch Sausage & Mushroom	⅕ pie (4.6 oz)	300	14	6	30	15	29	6	3	200	680	350	—	1
Original 12 inch Sausage & Pepperoni	⅕ pie (4.4 oz)	320	16	7	30	15	29	6	2	250	740	330	—	1
Original 12 inch Supreme	⅕ pie (5.1 oz)	320	16	7	30	15	29	6	2	250	730	330	—	4
Original 9 inch Deluxe	⅓ pie (4.4 oz)	280	13	6	25	14	27	5	2	200	630	310	—	1
Original 9 inch Extra Cheese	½ pie (5.6 oz)	380	19	8	30	19	40	8	3	350	740	390	—	1
Original 9 inch Hamburger	⅓ pie (4 oz)	280	13	6	25	14	27	5	2	200	600	280	—	1
Original 9 inch Pepperoni	⅓ pie (4 oz)	300	15	7	30	14	27	5	2	200	680	290	—	1
Original 9 inch Pepperoni & Sausage	⅓ pie (4.1 oz)	300	15	7	30	14	27	5	2	200	710	320	—	1
Original 9 inch Sausage	⅓ pie (4 oz)	280	13	6	25	14	27	5	2	200	610	310	—	1
Original 9 inch Supreme	⅓ pie (4.4 oz)	310	16	7	30	15	27	5	2	200	720	300	—	2
Oven Rising Italian Sausage	⅙ pie (5.1 oz)	320	13	6	30	16	35	12	2	250	700	320	—	1
Oven Rising Pepperoni	⅙ pie (4.9 oz)	340	15	7	35	17	34	7	2	250	750	340	—	1
Oven Rising Supreme	⅙ pie (5.1 oz)	320	14	6	30	16	34	8	2	200	720	350	—	2

FOOD	PORTION	CALS	FAT	SAT FAT	CHOL	PROT	CARB	SUGAR	FIBER	CALCI	SOD	POTAS	FOLIC	VIT C
TOMBSTONE (CONT.)														
Oven Rising Three Cheese	⅙ pie (4.8 oz)	320	13	8	35	16	34	7	2	300	580	310	—	1
Oven Rising Three Meat	⅙ pie (5.1 oz)	340	15	7	35	17	34	7	2	250	750	350	—	1
Thin Crust Four Meat Combo	¼ pie (5 oz)	380	23	10	45	19	26	5	2	300	890	360	—	1
Thin Crust Italian Sausage	¼ pie (5 oz)	370	22	10	45	18	26	5	2	300	840	360	—	1
Thin Crust Pepperoni	¼ pie (4.8 oz)	400	25	11	50	18	25	5	2	300	920	350	—	1
Thin Crust Supreme	¼ pie (5 oz)	380	22	10	45	18	26	5	2	300	840	360	—	2
Thin Crust Supreme Taco	¼ pie (5.1 oz)	370	23	11	50	16	27	5	2	250	740	370	—	2
Thin Crust Three Cheese	¼ pie (4.7 oz)	360	21	11	45	19	25	5	2	400	690	290	—	1
TOTINO'S														
Crisp Crust Cheese	½ pie	320	14	5	20	15	34	4	2	300	620	—	—	0
WEIGHT WATCHERS														
Smart Ones Deluxe Combo	1 (6.57 oz)	380	11	6	40	23	47	3	6	350	550	—	—	5
Smart Ones Pepperoni	1 (5.56 oz)	390	12	4	45	23	46	3	4	450	650	—	—	5
TAKE-OUT														
cheese	12 in pie	1121	26	12	74	61	164	—	—	929	2680	875	470	10
cheese	⅛ of 12 in pie	140	3	2	9	8	21	—	—	116	336	110	59	1
cheese deep dish individual	1 (5.5 oz)	460	24	9	20	15	47	4	2	250	750	—	—	1
cheese meat & vegetables	12 in pie	1472	43	12	165	104	170	—	—	805	3054	1423	215	13
cheese meat & vegetables	⅛ of 12 in pie	184	5	2	21	13	21	—	—	101	382	178	27	2
pepperoni	12 in pie	1445	56	18	115	81	157	—	—	517	2133	1220	421	13
pepperoni	⅛ of 12 in pie	181	7	2	14	10	20	—	—	65	267	153	53	2
PIZZA DOUGH														
crust	1 slice (1.7 oz)	130	2	0	0	4	25	1	1	0	230	—	40	0
BETTY CROCKER														
Italian Herb Crust Mix	¼ crust (1.6 oz)	180	2	1	0	4	32	1	1	—	350	65	60	—
BOBOLI														
Thin Crust	⅕ crust (2 oz)	160	4	1	0	6	24	1	1	20	300	—	40	0
CARBSENSE														
Garlic & Herb as prep	1 slice	100	1	1	0	9	7	0	4	—	85	—	—	—
KETO														
Dough Mix as prep	1 slice	79	1	—	—	13	5	tr	3	—	95	—	—	—

FOOD	PORTION	CALS	FAT	SAT FAT	CHOL	PROT	CARB	SUGAR	FIBER	CALCI	SOD	POTAS	FOLIC	VIT C
MINICARB														
Parmesan Herb Mix as prep	1 slice	130	5	1	0	18	6	0	3	—	220	—	—	—
PILLSBURY														
Crust	⅕ crust (2 oz)	150	2	0	0	5	27	3	tr	0	380	—	—	0
ROBIN HOOD														
Crust	¼ crust	160	2	1	0	4	33	1	1	0	340	55	—	0

PIZZA SAUCE

FOOD	PORTION	CALS	FAT	SAT FAT	CHOL	PROT	CARB	SUGAR	FIBER	CALCI	SOD	POTAS	FOLIC	VIT C
HUNT'S														
Family Favorites	¼ cup	25	0	0	0	1	5	3	1	0	270	240	—	4
MUIR GLEN														
Organic	¼ cup (2.2 oz)	40	0	0	0	1	6	3	2	0	230	—	—	1
PROGRESSO														
Pizza Sauce	¼ cup (2.1 oz)	20	0	0	0	tr	4	2	1	0	170	—	—	5

PLANTAIN

FOOD	PORTION	CALS	FAT	SAT FAT	CHOL	PROT	CARB	SUGAR	FIBER	CALCI	SOD	POTAS	FOLIC	VIT C
fresh uncooked	1 (6.3 oz)	218	1	—	0	2	57	—	—	5	7	893	39	33
sliced cooked	½ cup	89	tr	—	0	1	24	—	—	2	4	358	20	8
TAKE-OUT														
ripe fried	2.8 oz	214	7	—	—	1	38	—	4	5	—	—	—	10

PLUM

FOOD	PORTION	CALS	FAT	SAT FAT	CHOL	PROT	CARB	SUGAR	FIBER	CALCI	SOD	POTAS	FOLIC	VIT C
CANNED														
purple in heavy syrup	1 cup	320	tr	tr	0	1	60	—	—	24	50	234	7	1
purple in heavy syrup	3	119	tr	tr	0	tr	31	—	—	12	26	121	3	1
purple in light syrup	1 cup	158	tr	tr	0	1	41	—	—	24	50	233	6	1
purple in light syrup	3	83	tr	tr	0	tr	22	—	—	13	26	123	3	1
purple juice pack	1 cup	146	tr	tr	0	1	38	—	—	25	3	389	—	7
purple juice pack	3	55	tr	tr	0	tr	14	—	—	9	1	147	—	3
purple water pack	1 cup	102	tr	tr	0	1	27	—	—	17	2	314	7	8
purple water pack	3	39	tr	tr	0	tr	10	—	—	6	1	120	3	3
EDEN														
Umeboshi Paste	1 tsp	5	0	0	0	0	1	0	0	0	600	15	—	0
Umeboshi Plums	1	5	0	0	0	0	1	0	0	0	710	20	—	0
FRESH														
plum	1	36	tr	tr	0	1	9	—	—	2	0	113	1	6
sliced	1 cup	91	1	tr	0	1	21	—	—	6	1	284	4	16
CHIQUITA														
Purple	2 med (4.6 oz)	80	1	0	0	1	19	10	2	0	0	—	—	12

POI

FOOD	PORTION	CALS	FAT	SAT FAT	CHOL	PROT	CARB	SUGAR	FIBER	CALCI	SOD	POTAS	FOLIC	VIT C
poi	½ cup	134	tr	tr	0	tr	33	—	—	19	14	220	—	5

FOOD	PORTION	CALS	FAT	SAT FAT	CHOL	PROT	CARB	SUGAR	FIBER	CALCI	SOD	POTAS	FOLIC	VIT C
POKEBERRY SHOOTS														
cooked	½ cup	16	tr	—	0	2	3	—	—	43	—	—	—	67
fresh	½ cup	18	tr	—	0	2	3	—	—	42	—	—	—	109
POLENTA														
FRIEDA'S														
Dried Tomato	4 oz	80	0	0	0	2	17	1	2	0	250	—	—	1
Italian Herb	4 oz	80	0	0	0	2	17	0	2	20	45	—	—	1
Mexicana	4 oz	80	0	0	0	2	17	0	2	0	200	—	—	9
Original	4 oz	80	0	0	0	2	16	0	2	0	198	—	—	0
Wild Mushroom	4 oz	80	0	0	0	2	17	0	2	0	200	—	—	0
MELISSA'S														
Original	4 oz	80	0	0	0	2	16	0	2	0	198	—	—	0
POLLACK														
atlantic fillet baked	5.3 oz	178	2	tr	137	38	0	—	—	116	166	689	—	—
atlantic baked	3 oz	100	1	tr	77	21	0	—	—	65	94	388	—	—
POMEGRANATE														
fresh	1	104	tr	—	0	1	26	—	—	5	5	399	—	9
POMEGRANATE JUICE														
CORTAS														
Concentrated Juice	1 tbsp (0.6 oz)	40	0	0	0	0	9	7	0	20	0	—	—	0
NAKED JUICE														
Pomegranaberry Blue	8 oz	130	1	—	—	1	33	31	2	20	10	400	—	9
Pomigranalicious	8 oz	150	0	0	0	1	38	37	0	0	10	340	—	48
POM WONDERFUL														
Pomegranate Blueberry	8 oz	140	0	0	0	1	34	28	0	40	45	—	—	0
Pomegranate Cherry	8 oz	140	0	0	0	1	33	28	0	60	35	—	—	0
Pomegranate Tangerine	8 oz	150	0	0	0	0	37	31	0	20	75	—	—	0
Pomegrante Juice	8 oz	140	0	0	0	1	35	34	0	40	30	—	—	0
POMPANO														
florida cooked	3 oz	179	10	4	54	20	0	—	—	36	65	541	—	—
florida raw	3 oz	140	8	3	43	16	0	—	—	19	55	324	—	—
POPCORN														
air-popped	1 cup (0.3 oz)	31	tr	tr	0	1	6	—	2	1	0	24	2	0
caramel coated	1 cup (1.2 oz)	152	5	1	—	1	28	14	2	15	72	38	—	0
caramel coated w/ peanuts	⅔ cup (1 oz)	114	2	tr	0	2	23	11	1	19	84	101	—	0
cheese	1 cup (0.4 oz)	58	4	1	1	1	6	—	1	12	98	29	—	tr
oil popped	1 cup (0.4 oz)	55	3	1	0	1	6	tr	1	1	97	25	2	0

FOOD	PORTION	CALS	FAT	SAT FAT	CHOL	PROT	CARB	SUGAR	FIBER	CALCI	SOD	POTAS	FOLIC	VIT C
CHESTER'S														
Butter	3 cups	160	12	2	0	2	15	0	2	—	330	—	—	—
Caramel Craze	¾ cup	130	2	0	0	1	27	18	1	—	220	—	—	—
Cheddar Cheese	3 cups	190	13	3	<5	3	17	2	3	—	300	—	—	—
Microwave Butter	5 cups	200	12	2	0	3	22	tr	4	—	300	—	—	—
CRACKER JACK														
Fat Free Butter Toffee	¾ cup	110	0	0	0	1	26	17	1	—	85	—	—	—
Fat Free Caramel	¾ cup	110	0	0	0	tr	26	17	1	—	70	—	—	—
Original	½ cup (1 oz)	120	2	0	0	2	23	15	1	0	70	—	—	0
ESTEE														
Caramel	1 cup	120	2	0	0	tr	26	1	1	—	90	0	—	—
HERR'S														
Regular	3 cups (1 oz)	140	11	2	0	2	11	1	3	0	250	—	—	0
HUSMAN'S														
Cheese Corn	2¼ cups (1 oz)	160	10	2	<5	2	15	0	1	10	220	—	—	0
JOLLY TIME														
America's Best 94% Fat Free	1 cup	20	0	0	0	tr	5	0	1	0	10	—	—	0
Blast O Butter	1 cup	45	3	1	0	1	5	0	1	0	85	—	—	0
Blast O Butter Light	1 cup	30	2	0	0	tr	4	0	1	0	75	—	—	0
Butter Licious	1 cup	35	2	0	0	tr	4	0	1	0	40	—	—	0
Butter Licious Light	1 cup	30	2	0	0	tr	4	0	tr	0	25	—	—	0
Crispy & White	1 cup	40	3	1	0	tr	4	0	1	0	40	—	—	0
Crispy & White Light	1 cup	25	1	0	0	tr	4	0	1	0	25	—	—	0
Healthy Pop 94% Fat Free	1 cup	20	0	0	0	tr	5	0	1	0	10	—	—	0
White Air Popped	5 cups	100	1	0	0	4	24	0	6	0	0	—	—	0
Yellow Air Popped	5 cups	100	1	0	0	4	24	tr	6	0	0	—	—	0
JUDY'S														
Sugar Free Popcorn Nut Brittle	¼ piece (1 oz)	100	5	1	0	1	3	0	tr	—	45	—	—	—
LANCE														
Cheese	1 pkg (0.6 oz)	90	5	2	0	2	9	0	2	0	210	55	—	0
Plain	1 pkg (0.5 oz)	70	3	1	0	1	10	0	1	0	135	5	—	0
White Cheddar	1 pkg (0.6 oz)	100	8	2	0	1	7	1	1	0	170	65	—	0
White Cheddar	1 pkg (0.9 oz)	150	11	3	0	2	10	1	1	20	240	90	—	0
MAUNA LOA														
Macadamia Nut Butter Corn Crunch	1 oz	150	8	4	1	1	18	11	1	—	140	—	—	—

FOOD	PORTION	CALS	FAT	SAT FAT	CHOL	PROT	CARB	SUGAR	FIBER	CALCI	SOD	POTAS	FOLIC	VIT C
NEWMAN'S OWN														
Microwave Butter Flavor	3½ cups	170	11	2	0	2	16	0	3	0	180	—	—	0
Microwave Light Butter	3½ cups	110	3	1	0	2	20	0	3	0	90	—	—	0
Microwave Light Natural	3½ cups	110	3	1	0	2	20	0	3	0	90	—	—	0
Microwave Natural	3½ cups	170	11	2	0	2	16	0	3	0	180	—	—	0
Popcorn unpopped	3 tbsp	110	2	0	0	4	27	0	7	0	0	—	—	0
ORVILLE REDENBACHER'S														
Gourmet Original	3 cups	92	1	tr	0	3	22	0	5	2	2	—	—	0
Hot Air	3 cups	92	1	tr	0	3	22	0	5	2	2	—	—	0
Microwave Butter	3 cups	168	13	3	0	2	15	0	4	1	388	—	—	0
Microwave Butter No Salt Added	3 cups	176	12	3	0	3	19	0	4	2	2	—	—	0
Microwave Butter Light	3 cups	122	6	1	0	3	20	0	5	2	357	—	—	0
Microwave Caramel	1 serv	179	10	2	0	1	23	12	3	18	47	—	—	0
Microwave Golden Cheddar	1 serv	169	13	3	0	2	15	0	3	2	373	—	—	0
Microwave Natural	3 cups	164	11	2	0	2	18	0	4	tr	512	—	—	0
Microwave Natural No Salt Added	3 cups	174	12	3	0	3	19	0	5	2	2	—	—	0
Microwave Natural Light	3 cups	118	5	1	0	3	19	0	5	2	382	—	—	0
Microwave Smartpop	1 serv	96	3	1	0	3	20	0	5	2	445	—	—	0
Microwave Smartpop Butter Snack Size	1 bag	155	4	1	0	5	34	6	0	3	477	—	—	0
Microwave Snack Size Butter	1 bag	287	22	5	0	3	25	0	6	2	647	—	—	0
Microwave Snack Size Butter Light	1 bag	183	8	2	0	4	30	0	7	2	539	—	—	0
Microwave White Cheddar	1 serv	169	13	3	0	2	15	0	3	2	373	—	—	0
Redenbudders Microwave Herb & Garlic	1 serv	176	13	3	0	2	16	0	4	1	499	—	—	0
Redenbudders Microwave Zesty Butter	1 serv	177	13	3	0	2	16	0	4	1	429	—	—	0
Redenbudders Movie Theater Butter Light	1 serv	113	5	1	0	3	20	0	5	2	321	—	—	0

FOOD	PORTION	CALS	FAT	SAT FAT	CHOL	PROT	CARB	SUGAR	FIBER	CALCI	SOD	POTAS	FOLIC	VIT C
ORVILLE REDENBACHER'S (CONT.)														
Redenbudders Movie Theater Microwave Butter	1 serv	176	13	3	0	2	16	0	4	1	499	—	—	0
Smart Pop Movie Theater Butter	1 serv	92	2	tr	0	3	20	0	5	16	307	—	—	0
White	3 cups	92	1	tr	0	3	22	0	5	2	2	—	—	0
PLANTERS														
Fiddle Faddle Caramel Fat Free	1 cup (1 oz)	110	0	0	0	tr	28	16	1	0	210	—	—	0
POP SECRET														
94% Fat Free Butter	1 cup (5 g)	20	0	0	0	tr	4	0	tr	0	40	10	—	0
94% Fat Free Natural	1 cup (5 g)	20	0	0	0	tr	4	0	tr	0	40	10	—	0
Butter	1 cup (7 g)	35	3	1	0	tr	4	0	tr	0	50	15	—	0
Cheddar Cheese	1 cup (6 g)	30	2	1	0	tr	3	0	tr	0	45	15	—	0
Jumbo Pop Butter	1 cup (7 g)	40	3	1	0	tr	4	0	tr	0	55	15	—	0
Jumbo Pop Movie Theater Butter	1 cup (7 g)	40	3	1	0	tr	4	0	tr	0	55	15	—	0
Light Butter	1 cup (5 g)	20	1	0	0	tr	4	0	tr	0	45	15	—	0
Light Movie Theater Butter	1 cup (5 g)	25	1	0	0	tr	4	0	tr	0	45	15	—	0
Light Natural	1 cup (5 g)	25	1	0	0	tr	4	0	tr	0	45	15	—	0
Movie Theater Butter	1 cup (7 g)	40	3	1	0	tr	3	0	tr	0	55	15	—	0
Nacho Cheese	1 cup (6 g)	30	2	1	0	tr	3	0	tr	0	50	15	—	0
Natural	1 cup (7 g)	35	3	1	0	tr	4	0	tr	0	65	15	—	0
Real Butter	1 cup (7 g)	35	3	1	0	tr	4	0	tr	0	60	10	—	0
POPPYCOCK														
The Original	½ cup	160	8	2	10	2	20	13	1	0	90	—	—	0
SMART BALANCE														
No Trans Fat Low Sodium Low Fat	1 cup	20	0	0	0	0	6	0	1	0	0	—	—	0
SMARTFOOD														
Butter	3 cups	150	9	2	5	2	15	2	1	—	240	—	—	—
Low Fat Toffee Crunch	¾ cup	110	1	0	0	1	25	19	1	—	220	—	—	—
Reduced Fat Golden Butter	3⅓ cups	130	4	1	0	3	21	0	4	—	410	—	—	—
Reduced Fat White Cheddar	3 cups	140	6	2	<5	4	19	1	3	—	280	—	—	—
White Cheddar	2 cups	190	12	3	5	3	17	5	2	—	310	—	—	—

FOOD	PORTION	CALS	FAT	SAT FAT	CHOL	PROT	CARB	SUGAR	FIBER	CALCI	SOD	POTAS	FOLIC	VIT C
SNYDER'S OF HANOVER														
Butter	⅝ oz	110	10	0	0	1	6	0	0	0	150	—	—	0
TOM'S														
Caramel Corn	1 pkg (1.6 oz)	180	3	1	0	1	39	23	2	—	110	—	—	—
UTZ														
Au Natural	3 cups (1 oz)	120	1	0	0	3	25	0	5	0	0	—	—	0
Butter	2 cups (1 oz)	170	12	2	0	2	13	tr	3	0	210	—	—	0
Cheese	2 cups (1 oz)	150	10	2	5	2	14	1	3	0	250	—	—	0
Hulless Puff'N Corn	2 cups (1 oz)	180	15	3	0	1	11	0	0	20	150	—	—	0
Hulless Puff'N Corn Hot Cheese	1 pkg (1.75 oz)	290	22	3	0	3	21	3	0	20	680	—	—	0
Hulless Puff'N Corn Cheese	2 cups (1 oz)	170	12	2	<5	2	13	0	0	20	210	—	—	0
White Cheddar	2 cups (1 oz)	150	9	2	<5	3	15	3	3	20	270	—	—	0
WEIGHT WATCHERS														
Butter	1 pkg (0.66 oz)	90	3	0	0	2	14	0	3	0	100	—	—	0
Butter Toffee	1 pkg (0.9 oz)	110	3	1	0	1	21	11	1	0	90	—	—	0
Caramel	1 pkg (0.9 oz)	100	1	0	0	1	22	11	1	0	45	—	—	0
Microwave	1 pkg (1 oz)	100	1	0	0	3	20	0	7	0	0	—	—	0
White Cheddar Cheese	1 pkg (0.66 oz)	90	4	1	0	2	12	0	2	0	125	—	—	0
POPCORN CAKES														
ORVILLE REDENBACHER'S														
BBQ Mini	8 (0.5 oz)	55	1	tr	0	0	12	1	1	5	124	—	—	tr
Butter	2 (0.6 oz)	134	1	tr	tr	2	13	1	2	6	79	—	—	tr
Butter Mini	8 (0.5 oz)	56	1	tr	1	2	11	tr	1	6	71	—	—	0
Caramel	1 (0.4 oz)	34	tr	0	0	1	8	2	1	2	16	—	—	0
Caramel Mini	7 (0.5 oz)	50	tr	tr	tr	1	12	3	1	3	24	—	—	0
Nacho Cheese Mini	8 (0.5 oz)	56	1	tr	1	2	11	tr	1	9	85	—	—	tr
Peanut Crunch Mini	7 (0.5 oz)	55	1	tr	tr	2	11	3	1	3	39			0
White Cheddar	2 (0.6 oz)	63	1	tr	tr	0	13	tr	2	0	83	—	—	6
White Cheddar Mini	8 (0.5 oz)	56	1	tr	tr	2	12	tr	1	5	67	—	—	0
POPOVER														
home recipe as prep w/ 2% milk	1 (1.4 oz)	87	3	1	46	4	11	—	—	38	82	65	7	tr
home recipe as prep w/ whole milk	1 (1.4 oz)	90	3	1	47	4	11	—	—	37	82	64	7	tr
mix as prep	1 (1.2 oz)	67	2	tr	—	3	10	—	—	9	143	25	—	—
POPPY SEEDS														
poppy seeds	1 tsp	15	1	tr	0	1	1	—	—	41	1	20	—	—

FOOD	PORTION	CALS	FAT	SAT FAT	CHOL	PROT	CARB	SUGAR	FIBER	CALCI	SOD	POTAS	FOLIC	VIT C
AMERICAN ALMOND														
Baker's Style Poppy Seed Filling	2 tbsp	120	5	0	0	2	18	16	tr	150	15	—	—	0
PORGY														
fresh	3 oz	77	tr	—	—	18	0	0	0	41	52	415	—	—
PORK														
(*see also* HAM, PORK DISHES)														
CANNED														
HORMEL														
Pickled Tidbits	2 oz	100	8	3	45	8	0	0	0	20	530	—	—	0
FRESH														
boston blade roast lean & fat cooked	3 oz	229	16	6	73	20	0	—	0	24	57	—	4	1
boston blade steak lean & fat cooked	3 oz	220	14	5	81	22	0	—	0	31	59	—	3	1
center loin roast lean bone in cooked	3 oz	169	8	3	67	23	0	—	0	21	56	—	3	1
center loin chop lean bone in cooked	3 oz	172	7	3	72	25	0	—	0	20	53	—	3	1
center rib chop lean & fat bone in cooked	3 oz	213	13	5	62	23	0	—	0	21	34	—	2	tr
center rib roast lean & fat bone in cooked	3 oz	217	13	5	62	23	0	—	0	24	39	—	3	tr
fresh ham rump lean roasted	3 oz	175	7	2	82	26	0	—	0	6	55	—	3	tr
fresh ham rump lean & fat roasted	3 oz	214	12	4	82	25	0	—	0	10	53	—	3	tr
fresh ham shank lean roasted	3 oz	183	9	3	78	24	0	—	0	6	54	—	5	tr
fresh ham shank lean & fat roasted	3 oz	246	17	6	78	22	0	—	0	13	50	—	4	tr
fresh ham whole lean roasted	3 oz	179	8	3	80	25	0	—	0	6	54	—	10	tr
fresh ham whole lean roasted diced	1 cup	285	13	4	127	40	0	—	0	9	86	—	16	tr
fresh ham whole lean & fat roasted	3 oz	232	15	6	80	23	0	—	0	12	51	—	9	tr
fresh ham whole lean & fat roasted diced	1 cup	369	24	9	127	36	0	—	0	19	81	—	14	tr
ground 97% fat free	4 oz	130	3	1	65	23	0	0	0	0	60	—	—	0
ground cooked	3 oz	252	18	7	80	22	0	—	0	19	62	—	5	1

FOOD	PORTION	CALS	FAT	SAT FAT	CHOL	PROT	CARB	SUGAR	FIBER	CALCI	SOD	POTAS	FOLIC	VIT C
leg loin & shoulder lean only roasted	3 oz	198	11	—	79	—	—	—	—	7	—	—	—	—
loin chop lean bone in braised	3 oz	191	11	4	71	21	0	—	0	20	53	—	3	1
loin chop lean bone in broiled	3 oz	199	12	4	71	22	0	—	0	20	68	—	3	1
loin roast lean bone in roasted	3 oz	210	13	5	79	23	0	—	0	25	25	—	4	tr
loin whole lean & fat braised	3 oz	203	12	4	68	23	0	—	0	18	41	—	3	1
loin whole lean & fat broiled	3 oz	206	12	4	68	23	0	—	0	16	53	—	4	1
loin whole lean & fat roasted	3 oz	211	12	5	70	23	0	—	0	16	50	—	5	1
lungs braised	3 oz	84	3	1	329	14	0	—	0	7	69	—	2	7
pancreas cooked	3 oz	186	9	3	268	24	0	—	0	14	36	—	4	5
ribs country style lean & fat braised	3 oz	252	18	7	74	20	0	—	0	25	50	—	3	1
shoulder arm picnic lean & fat roasted	3 oz	269	20	7	80	20	0	—	0	16	60	—	3	tr
shoulder whole lean & fat roasted	3 oz	248	18	7	77	20	0	—	0	20	58	—	4	tr
shoulder whole lean & fat roasted diced	1 cup	394	29	11	122	31	0	—	0	32	92	—	7	tr
shoulder whole lean roasted	3 oz	196	12	4	77	22	0	—	0	15	64	—	4	1
shoulder whole lean roasted diced	1 cup	311	18	6	122	34	0	—	0	24	101	—	7	1
sirloin chop lean & fat bone in braised	3 oz	208	13	5	70	22	0	—	0	15	43	—	3	1
sirloin roast lean & fat bone in cooked	3 oz	222	14	5	74	23	0	—	0	20	51	—	5	tr
spareribs braised	3 oz	338	26	10	103	25	0	—	0	40	79	—	3	0
spleen braised	3 oz	127	3	1	428	24	0	—	0	11	91	—	3	10
tail simmered	3 oz	336	30	11	110	15	0	—	0	11	21	—	3	0
tenderloin lean roasted	3 oz	139	4	1	67	24	0	—	0	5	48	—	5	tr
top loin chop boneless lean & fat cooked	3 oz	198	11	4	64	24	0	—	0	18	36	—	3	tr
top loin roast boneless lean & fat cooked	3 oz	192	10	4	66	24	0	—	0	4	37	—	7	tr
FREIRICH														
Porkette	4 oz	220	18	7	70	16	1	1	0	40	660	—	—	0

FOOD	PORTION	CALS	FAT	SAT FAT	CHOL	PROT	CARB	SUGAR	FIBER	CALCI	SOD	POTAS	FOLIC	VIT C
OSCAR MAYER														
Sweet Morsel Smoked Boneless Pork Shoulder Butt	3 oz	180	15	5	50	11	0	0	0	0	990	—	—	0
READY-TO-EAT														
TYSON														
Pork Pattie	1 (3.8 oz)	200	11	4	40	15	9	7	3	40	270	—	—	0
TAKE-OUT														
chicharrones pork cracklings fried	1 cup	844	72	—	—	27	22	—	tr	100	128	—	—	0

PORK DISHES

FOOD	PORTION	CALS	FAT	SAT FAT	CHOL	PROT	CARB	SUGAR	FIBER	CALCI	SOD	POTAS	FOLIC	VIT C
HORMEL														
Center Cut Loin Lemon Garlic	1 serv (4 oz)	130	5	2	45	19	1	0	0	0	690	—	—	1
Extra Lean Teriyaki	4 oz	140	4	2	50	20	5	4	0	0	400	—	—	0
Pork Roast Au Jus	1 serv (5 oz)	180	7	3	85	29	0	0	0	—	570	—	—	—
SMITHFIELD														
Pulled Pork w/ Barbecue Sauce	2 oz	90	4	2	20	9	7	6	—	20	220	—	—	2
Tenderloin Garlic & Herb	3 oz	100	3	1	60	17	2	0	tr	0	900	—	—	2
Tenderloin Hickory Sweet	4 oz	110	3	1	60	16	6	4	0	0	480	—	—	1
TYSON														
Lemon Pepper Pork Roast	1 serv (3 oz)	110	3	1	30	19	2	2	0	20	680	—	—	1
TAKE-OUT														
chinese spareribs	1 serv	776	166	21	54	—	—	—	—	—	716	—	—	—
pork roast	2 oz	70	3	1	40	10	0	—	—	—	390	—	—	1
tourtiere	1 piece (4.9 oz)	451	34	10	—	15	21	—	—	18	—	—	—	—

PORK RINDS

(*see* SNACKS)

POT PIE

FOOD	PORTION	CALS	FAT	SAT FAT	CHOL	PROT	CARB	SUGAR	FIBER	CALCI	SOD	POTAS	FOLIC	VIT C
AMY'S														
Broccoli	1 (7.5 oz)	430	22	10	45	11	46	3	4	—	630	—	—	—
Country Vegetable	1 (7.5 oz)	370	16	9	40	12	47	5	4	—	580	—	—	—
Shepherd's	1 (8 oz)	160	4	0	0	5	27	5	5	—	490	—	—	—
Vegetable	1 (7.5 oz)	420	19	12	50	9	54	3	4	—	590	—	—	—
Vegetable Non-Dairy	1 (7.5 oz)	320	9	1	0	7	50	3	4	—	590	—	—	—
BANQUET														
Beef	1 (7 oz)	400	23	11	30	9	38	8	1	20	1000	—	—	0
Cheesy Potato & Broccoli w/ Ham	1 (7 oz)	410	23	10	25	9	40	8	2	80	1220	—	—	0

FOOD	PORTION	CALS	FAT	SAT FAT	CHOL	PROT	CARB	SUGAR	FIBER	CALCI	SOD	POTAS	FOLIC	VIT C
BANQUET (CONT.)														
Chicken	1 (7 oz)	380	22	9	40	10	36	6	1	20	950	—	—	1
Chicken & Broccoli	1 (7 oz)	350	20	9	35	10	32	9	2	20	830	—	—	0
Family Size Hearty Chicken	1 cup	460	29	11	35	11	39	14	2	40	1010	—	—	0
Macaroni & Cheese	1 pkg (6.5 oz)	210	5	3	10	7	34	10	1	80	750	—	—	0
Turkey	1 (7 oz)	370	20	8	45	10	38	6	3	40	850	—	—	0
Vegetable Cheese	1 (7 oz)	340	17	7	10	6	39	19	1	80	920	—	—	0
HEALTHY CHOICE														
Colonial Chicken	1 (9.5 oz)	310	7	3	45	22	40	15	5	100	570	—	—	4
LEAN CUISINE														
Everyday Favorites Chicken Pie	1 pkg (9.5 oz)	300	8	3	30	19	38	14	—	100	580	830	—	15
Everyday Favorites Vegetable Eggroll	1 pkg (9 oz)	300	5	1	0	7	57	16	4	40	610	240	—	9
MARIE CALLENDER'S														
Beef	1 (9.5 oz)	680	42	21	20	16	53	7	1	40	1430	—	—	0
Chicken	1 (9.5 oz)	680	48	21	20	14	53	9	3	40	1100	—	—	0
Chicken & Broccoli	1 (9.5 oz)	670	43	12	25	16	54	11	4	60	1000	—	—	0
Chicken Au Gratin	1 (9.5 oz)	690	46	21	30	19	50	3	4	150	1300	—	—	0
Turkey	1 (9.5 oz)	680	46	19	15	13	56	10	5	40	1100	—	—	0
MORTON														
Macaroni & Cheese	1 (6.5 oz)	210	5	3	10	7	34	10	1	80	750	—	—	0
Vegetable w/ Beef	1 (7 oz)	340	21	9	20	5	33	8	2	20	1380	—	—	0
Vegetable w/ Chicken	1 (7 oz)	320	18	7	25	8	32	7	2	40	1040	—	—	0
Vegetable w/ Turkey	1 (7 oz)	310	18	9	25	8	29	8	2	40	1060	—	—	0
MRS. PATERSON'S														
Aussie Pie Chicken	1 (5.5 oz)	460	25	8	90	12	15	3	2	20	770	—	—	0
Aussie Pie Chicken Low Fat	1 (5.5 oz)	380	17	6	35	13	44	3	1	20	930	—	—	0
Aussie Pie Philly Steak	1 (5.5 oz)	420	24	8	40	11	39	3	2	20	860	—	—	0
STOUFFER'S														
Beef Pie	1 pkg (10 oz)	450	26	9	65	19	36	10	3	40	1140	260	—	1
Chicken Pie	1 pkg (10 oz)	540	33	10	25	23	38	11	4	80	1080	410	—	5
Turkey Pie	1 pkg (10 oz)	530	33	9	65	21	36	11	3	100	1040	320	—	2
SWANSON														
Beef	1 (7 oz)	376	19	8	22	12	39	4	5	26	739	236	—	1
Chicken	1 (7 oz)	416	22	8	19	9	45	5	2	50	814	192	—	2
Turkey	1 (7 oz)	440	24	9	18	12	44	5	2	40	748	236	—	2

FOOD	PORTION	CALS	FAT	SAT FAT	CHOL	PROT	CARB	SUGAR	FIBER	CALCI	SOD	POTAS	FOLIC	VIT C
TAKE-OUT														
beef	⅓ of 9 in pie (7.4 oz)	515	30	8	42	21	39	—	—	29	596	334	—	6
chicken	⅓ of 9 in pie (8.1 oz)	545	31	10	56	23	42	—	—	70	594	343	—	5

POTATO

(*see also* CHIPS, KNISH, PANCAKES)

FOOD	PORTION	CALS	FAT	SAT FAT	CHOL	PROT	CARB	SUGAR	FIBER	CALCI	SOD	POTAS	FOLIC	VIT C
CANNED														
potatoes	½ cup	54	tr	tr	0	1	12	—	—	5	—	206	6	5
DEL MONTE														
New Sliced	⅔ cup (5.4 oz)	60	0	0	0	1	13	0	2	20	360	—	—	9
New Whole	2 med (5.5 oz)	60	0	0	0	1	13	0	2	20	360	—	—	9
HORMEL														
Au Gratin & Bacon	1 can (7.5 oz)	250	14	5	25	8	23	1	2	100	840	—	—	0
S&W														
Whole Small	2 (5.5 oz)	60	0	0	0	1	13	0	2	20	360	—	—	9
FRESH														
baked skin only	1 skin (2 oz)	115	tr	tr	0	2	27	—	2	20	12	332	—	8
baked w/ skin	1 (6.5 oz)	220	tr	tr	0	5	51	—	—	20	16	844	22	26
baked w/o skin	½ cup	57	tr	tr	0	1	13	—	1	3	3	238	6	8
baked w/o skin	1 (5 oz)	145	tr	tr	0	3	34	—	2	8	8	610	14	20
boiled	½ cup	68	tr	tr	0	1	16	—	1	4	3	295	8	10
microwaved	1 (7 oz)	212	tr	tr	0	5	49	—	—	22	16	903	24	31
microwaved w/o skin	½ cup	78	tr	tr	0	2	18	—	—	4	5	321	10	12
raw w/o skin	1 (3.9 oz)	88	tr	tr	0	2	20	—	—	8	7	608	14	22
ARROWFARMS														
Yukon Gold	1 med (5 oz)	100	0	0	0	4	26	3	3	20	0	—	—	27
DOLE														
Idaho	1 (5.3 oz)	100	0	0	0	4	26	3	3	20	0	720	24	27
FROZEN														
french fries	10 strips	111	4	2	0	2	17	—	2	4	15	229	8	6
french fries thick cut	10 strips	109	4	2	0	2	17	—	—	5	23	240	9	5
hashed brown	½ cup	170	9	4	—	2	22	—	—	12	27	340	—	5
potato puffs	½ cup	138	7	3	0	2	19	—	—	19	462	236	10	4
potato puffs as prep	1	16	1	tr	0	tr	2	—	—	2	52	27	1	1
BIRDS EYE														
Baby Gourmet	7 (4 oz)	100	0	0	0	2	21	0	1	0	15	—	—	0
Whole	3	50	0	0	0	1	13	0	1	0	25	—	—	2
FILLO FACTORY														
Petite Fillo Puffs Potato & Herb	7 (4.6 oz)	280	8	4	15	8	44	0	1	—	250	—	—	—

FOOD	PORTION	CALS	FAT	SAT FAT	CHOL	PROT	CARB	SUGAR	FIBER	CALCI	SOD	POTAS	FOLIC	VIT C
HEALTHY CHOICE														
Cheddar Broccoli Potatoes	1 meal (10.5 oz)	330	7	3	25	13	53	8	6	200	550	—	—	27
LEAN CUISINE														
Everyday Favorites Deluxe Cheddar Potato	1 pkg (10.4 oz)	250	6	3	20	13	37	6	5	250	590	1080	—	18
Everyday Favorites Roasted Potatoes w/ Broccoli	1 pkg (10.25 oz)	260	6	4	15	12	39	7	7	250	590	920	—	12
OH BOY!														
Stuffed w/ Cheddar Cheese	1 (5 oz)	130	4	1	<5	3	22	0	2	60	270	—	—	1
STOUFFER'S														
Au Gratin	½ cup (5.75 oz)	130	6	3	15	4	15	3	1	100	590	250	—	4
Scalloped	½ cup (5.75 oz)	140	6	1	<5	4	17	3	2	100	450	230	—	5
TREE OF LIFE														
Organic French Fries	20 pieces (3 oz)	110	3	0	0	2	19	tr	1	20	75	—	—	0
WEIGHT WATCHERS														
Smart Ones Baked Broccoli & Cheese	1 pkg (10 oz)	250	6	4	20	11	39	9	6	250	570	—	—	12
MIX														
au gratin as prep	½ cup	160	9	6	29	6	14	—	—	146	528	483	10	12
instant mashed flakes as prep w/ whole milk & butter	½ cup	118	6	4	15	2	16	—	—	52	349	245	8	10
instant mashed flakes not prep	½ cup	78	tr	tr	0	2	18	—	—	5	24	239	9	18
instant mashed granules as prep w/ whole milk & butter	½ cup	114	5	3	15	2	15	—	—	37	270	152	8	6
instant mashed granules not prep	½ cup	372	1	tr	0	8	86	—	—	41	67	703	40	37
scalloped	½ cup	105	5	3	14	4	13	—	—	70	409	461	10	13
BETTY CROCKER														
Au Gratin as prep	½ cup	150	6	2	5	3	22	3	1	60	600	300	—	0
Au Gratin Low Fat Recipe	½ cup	110	1	1	<5	3	22	3	1	60	560	300	—	0
Cheddar & Bacon	½ cup	150	6	2	<5	3	21	2	1	40	650	280	—	0
Cheddar & Bacon Low Fat Recipe	½ cup	120	3	1	0	3	21	2	1	40	620	280	—	0
Cheddar & Sour Cream	½ cup	130	3	1	5	3	25	3	1	60	580	280	—	0

FOOD	PORTION	CALS	FAT	SAT FAT	CHOL	PROT	CARB	SUGAR	FIBER	CALCI	SOD	POTAS	FOLIC	VIT C
BETTY CROCKER (CONT.)														
Chicken & Vegetable	⅔ cup	140	4	1	<5	4	23	4	2	60	520	300	—	0
Chicken & Vegetable Low Fat Recipe	⅔ cup	120	3	1	<5	4	23	4	2	60	510	300	—	0
Hash Browns	½ cup	190	8	2	0	3	30	0	3	0	620	550	—	0
Homestyle Broccoli Au Gratin	½ cup	140	6	2	<5	3	21	6	2	40	530	300	—	0
Homestyle Broccoli Au Gratin Low Fat Recipe	½ cup	110	3	1	0	3	21	6	2	40	530	300	—	0
Homestyle Cheddar Cheese	½ cup	120	3	1	<5	3	21	2	1	60	600	310	—	0
Homestyle Cheddar Cheese Stove Top Recipe	½ cup	140	5	2	5	3	21	2	1	60	680	310	—	0
Homestyle Cheesy Scalloped	½ cup	140	6	2	<5	3	21	5	2	60	540	300	—	0
Homestyle Cheesy Scalloped Low Fat Recipe	½ cup	110	3	1	<5	3	21	5	3	60	540	300	—	0
Julienne	½ cup	150	6	2	<5	3	21	5	1	60	630	250	—	0
Mashed Butter & Herb	½ cup	160	7	2	3	2	21	1	1	60	400	310	—	—
Mashed Butter & Herb Reduced Fat Recipe	½ cup	130	5	2	<5	3	20	2	1	40	450	380	—	0
Mashed Chicken & Herb	½ cup	150	7	2	<5	3	21	2	1	40	520	360	—	0
Mashed Chicken & Herb Reduced Fat Recipe	½ cup	120	4	1	0	3	21	2	1	40	490	360	—	0
Mashed Four Cheese	½ cup	150	7	2	<5	3	20	3	2	60	570	360	—	0
Mashed Four Cheese Reduced Fat Recipe	½ cup	120	4	1	0	3	20	3	2	60	540	360	—	0
Mashed Potato Buds	⅔ cup	160	8	2	<5	3	19	2	1	20	460	370	—	0
Mashed Potato Buds Reduced Fat Recipe	⅔ cup	120	4	1	0	3	19	2	1	20	420	370	—	0

FOOD	PORTION	CALS	FAT	SAT FAT	CHOL	PROT	CARB	SUGAR	FIBER	CALCI	SOD	POTAS	FOLIC	VIT C
BETTY CROCKER (CONT.)														
Mashed Roasted Garlic	½ cup	150	8	2	<5	3	19	2	2	40	400	350	—	0
Mashed Roasted Garlic Reduced Fat Recipe	½ cup	130	5	1	0	3	19	2	2	40	380	350	—	0
Mashed Sour Cream & Chives	½ cup	150	7	2	5	3	21	3	1	60	440	390	—	0
Mashed Sour Cream & Chives Reduced Fat Recipe	½ cup	120	4	1	<5	3	21	3	1	60	420	390	—	0
Potato Shakers Original	⅔ cup	140	4	1	<5	3	23	2	2	20	580	550	—	0
Potato Shakers Original Low Fat Recipe	⅔ cup	120	2	0	<5	3	23	2	2	20	560	550	—	0
Ranch	½ cup	160	6	2	<5	3	25	4	2	60	610	300	—	0
Scalloped	½ cup	150	6	2	<5	3	23	3	1	60	620	320	—	0
Scalloped Low Fat Recipe	⅔ cup	110	1	0	0	3	23	3	1	60	580	320	—	0
Sour Cream'n Chive	½ cup	160	7	2	5	3	22	5	2	60	600	310	—	0
Three Cheese	½ cup	150	6	2	<5	3	23	3	1	60	600	300	—	0
Twice Baked Cheddar & Bacon as prep	⅔ cup	210	11	3	85	6	22	4	1	100	580	410	—	0
Twice Baked Cheddar & Bacon Low Fat Recipe	⅔ cup	130	3	1	<5	6	22	4	1	100	530	410	—	0
HUNGRY JACK														
Au Gratin as prep	½ cup	150	5	3	10	3	24	3	1	80	620	—	—	1
Cheddar & Bacon as prep	½ cup	150	5	3	10	4	24	3	2	80	540	—	—	1
Cheesy Scalloped as prep	½ cup	150	5	3	10	3	24	3	1	60	570	—	—	1
Creamy Scalloped as prep	½ cup	150	5	3	10	3	24	3	2	60	460	—	—	1
Mashed Butter Flavored as prep	½ cup	150	7	2	<5	3	19	2	1	60	350	—	—	0
Mashed Garlic Flavored as prep	½ cup	150	7	2	<5	3	19	2	1	60	360	—	—	0

FOOD	PORTION	CALS	FAT	SAT FAT	CHOL	PROT	CARB	SUGAR	FIBER	CALCI	SOD	POTAS	FOLIC	VIT C
HUNGRY JACK (CONT.)														
Mashed Parsley Butter as prep	½ cup	150	7	2	<5	3	19	2	1	60	380	—	—	0
Mashed Sour Cream 'n Chives as prep	½ cup	150	7	2	<5	3	19	2	1	60	380	—	—	0
Mashed Potato Flakes as prep	½ cup	160	7	2	3	2	21	0	1	60	240	—	—	0
Sour Cream & Chives as prep	½ cup	160	6	4	15	3	23	3	1	60	510	—	—	2
IDAHO														
Mashed Potato Granules as prep	½ cup	160	7	2	<5	3	22	2	2	60	300	—	—	0
IDAHOAN														
AuGratin as prep	½ cup	150	6	1	3	3	20	2	2	80	744	—	—	6
Hash Browns as prep	½ cup	160	8	1	0	2	18	0	1	40	110	—	—	1
Hash Browns Cheesy not prep	½ cup	120	2	1	0	2	23	1	2	20	450	—	—	6
Mashed Baked as prep	½ cup	110	3	1	0	3	19	2	2	40	450	—	—	9
Mashed Butter & Herb as prep	½ cup	110	3	1	0	2	20	2	1	20	560	—	—	9
Mashed Buttery Homestyle as prep	½ cup	110	3	1	0	2	20	2	1	20	450	—	—	6
Mashed Four Cheese as prep	½ cup	100	3	1	0	2	19	2	1	40	550	—	—	9
Mashed Southwest as prep	½ cup	110	3	1	0	2	20	2	2	20	520	—	—	5
Roasted Garlic as prep	½ cup	600	3	1	0	2	20	3	1	40	260	—	—	6
Scalloped as prep	½ cup	150	7	1	3	2	21	2	1	80	610	—	—	6
SHAKE 'N BAKE														
Perfect Potatoes Crispy Cheddar	⅙ pkg (7 g)	30	2	2	5	2	2	tr	0	40	380	45	—	0
Perfect Potatoes Herb & Garlic	⅙ pkg (7 g)	20	0	0	0	0	5	1	0	0	380	15	—	0
Perfect Potatoes Home Fries	⅙ pkg (7 g)	20	0	0	0	0	5	1	0	0	410	45	—	2
Perfect Potatoes Parmesan Peppercorn	⅙ pkg (7 g)	25	1	1	<5	1	3	1	0	40	300	40	—	0
Perfect Potatoes Savory Onion	⅙ pkg (7 g)	20	0	0	0	0	5	1	0	0	280	20	—	0
REFRIGERATED														

FOOD	PORTION	CALS	FAT	SAT FAT	CHOL	PROT	CARB	SUGAR	FIBER	CALCI	SOD	POTAS	FOLIC	VIT C
PURELYIDAHO														
Cheddar Crusted	¾ cup	120	1	0	3	2	26	tr	2	30	420	—	—	15
Oven Roasts	1 serv (3 oz)	70	0	0	0	2	17	1	2	0	0	—	—	12
SHELF-STABLE														
LUNCH BUCKET														
Scalloped w/ Ham Chunks	1 pkg (7.5 oz)	170	7	3	10	2	24	tr	3	20	660	—	—	0
MICRO CUP MEALS														
Microcup Meals Scalloped Potatoes w/ Ham	1 cup (7.5 oz)	240	14	6	35	7	20	1	2	20	920	—	—	0
TASTYBITE														
Bombay Potatoes	½ pkg (5 oz)	190	8	2	0	9	22	2	6	50	720	—	—	0
Mumbai Pav Bhaji	½ pkg (5 oz)	229	6	4	0	2	23	7	7	40	121	—	—	1
Simla Potatoes	½ pkg (5 oz)	180	8	2	0	5	23	2	1	20	650		—	0
TAKE-OUT														
au gratin w/ cheese	½ cup	178	10	4	18	7	17	—	—	156	548	375	—	12
baked topped w/ cheese sauce	1	475	29	11	19	15	47	—	—	310	381	1167	28	26
baked topped w/ cheese sauce & bacon	1	451	26	10	30	18	44	—	—	309	973	1179	28	29
baked topped w/ cheese sauce & broccoli	1	402	14	9	20	14	47	—	—	334	484	1440	61	49
baked topped w/ cheese sauce & chili	1	481	22	13	31	23	56	—	—	409	701	1570	50	32
baked topped w/ sour cream & chives	1	394	22	10	23	7	50	—	—	105	182	1383	32	34
cheese fries w/ ranch dressing	1 serv	3010	—	—	—	—	—	—	—	—	—	—	—	—
curry	1 serv (6 oz)	292	16	—	—	4	36	—	4	47	—	—	—	14
french fries	1 reg	235	12	4	0	3	29	—	—	12	124	541	25	4
hash brown	½ cup (2.5 oz)	151	9	4	9	2	16	—	—	7	290	267	8	6
indian yogurt potatoes	1 serv	315	9	4	18	7	52	—	0	—	216	—	—	—
mashed	½ cup	111	4	1	2	2	18	—	—	27	309	303	0	6
mustard potato salad	3.5 oz	120	6	0	0	1	16	—	—	—	393	—	—	12
o'brien	1 cup	157	3	2	7	5	30	—	—	70	421	516	16	32
potato dumpling	3.5 oz	334	1	—	—	7	74	—	3	—	1	—	—	—
potato pancakes	1 (1.3 oz)	101	7	1	35	2	11	—	—	9	188	291	9	8
potato salad	½ cup	179	10	2	86	3	14	—	—	24	661	317	8	13
potato salad w/ vegetables	3.5 oz	120	3	1	0	2	20	—	—	—	390	—	—	4

FOOD	PORTION	CALS	FAT	SAT FAT	CHOL	PROT	CARB	SUGAR	FIBER	CALCI	SOD	POTAS	FOLIC	VIT C
red new boiled	5 sm (5 oz)	120	0	0	0	3	27	3	2	20	5	680	—	24
scalloped	½ cup	127	5	—	7	4	18	—	—	66	435	401	—	13
twice baked w/ cheese	1 half (10 oz)	392	18	10	54	8	48	—	4	400	810	—	—	29

POTATO STARCH
potato starch	1 oz	96	tr	—	0	tr	24	—	—	10	1	4	—	0

POUT
ocean baked	3 oz	86	1	tr	57	18	0	—	—	11	66	—	—	—
ocean fillet baked	4.8 oz	139	2	1	91	29	0	—	—	18	107	—	—	—

PRETZELS
chocolate covered	1 oz	130	5	2	—	2	20	—	—	21	—	—	—	tr
dutch twist	4 (2.1 oz)	229	2	tr	0	6	48	—	2	21	1029	68	—	0
milk chocolate covered twists	4 (1 oz)	140	7	4	0	2	19	11	tr	40	125	—	—	0
pretzels	1 oz	108	1	tr	0	3	23	—	1	10	486	42	—	0
rods	4 (2 oz)	229	2	tr	0	6	48	—	2	21	1029	68	—	0
sticks	120 (2 oz)	229	2	tr	0	6	48	—	2	21	1029	68	—	0
sticks	10	10	tr	tr	tr	tr	2	—	—	1	48	3	—	0
twists	10 (2.1 oz)	229	2	tr	0	6	48	—	2	21	1029	68	—	0
whole wheat	2 med (2 oz)	205	2	tr	0	6	46	—	—	16	115	244	—	—
whole wheat	2 sm (1 oz)	103	1	tr	0	3	23	—	—	8	58	122	—	—
ARAMANA														
Soy Pretzels	15 (1 oz)	100	3	2	5	10	12	0	4	—	330	—	—	—
BACHMAN														
Thin'n Right	12 (1 oz)	120	1	0	0	3	23	tr	1	0	650	—	—	0
ESTEE														
Chocolate Covered	7	130	6	4	0	2	19	0	tr	—	270	0	—	—
Dutch	2 (1.1 oz)	130	1	0	0	3	26	tr	1	—	40	40	—	—
Unsalted	23 (1 oz)	120	1	0	0	3	25	tr	1	—	30	120	—	—
GARDETTO'S														
Mustard	1 pkg (0.5 oz)	50	1	0	0	1	10	0	tr	0	110	—	—	0
HERR'S														
Hard Sourdough	1 (1 oz)	100	0	0	0	3	23	0	2	0	450	—	—	0
LANCE														
Pretzels	1 pkg (1.25 oz)	140	1	0	0	4	28	1	tr	0	470	50	—	0
LANDIES CANDIES														
Sugar Free Chocolate	4 (1.5 oz)	220	12	7	<5	5	23	0	tr	20	390	—	—	0
LITTLE DEBBIE														
Mini Twists	1 pkg (1.2 oz)	140	1	0	0	4	28	tr	1	—	470	—	—	—
NABISCO														
Air Crisps Fat Free	23 pieces (1 oz)	110	0	0	0	2	23	2	tr	60	550	—	—	0

FOOD	PORTION	CALS	FAT	SAT FAT	CHOL	PROT	CARB	SUGAR	FIBER	CALCI	SOD	POTAS	FOLIC	VIT C
NESTLE														
Flipz Milk Chocolate Covered	9 pieces (1 oz)	130	5	4	<5	2	19	10	tr	0	135	—	—	0
Flipz White Fudge Covered	9 pieces (1 oz)	130	6	5	0	2	19	11	0	40	130	—	—	0
NEWMAN'S OWN														
Salted Rounds Organic	1 pkg (1.4 oz)	150	2	0	0	3	31	2	1	0	530	—	—	0
ROLD GOLD														
Crispy's Thins	4 (1 oz)	110	2	0	0	3	22	1	1	—	670	—	—	—
Fat Free Honey Mustard	17 (1 oz)	110	0	0	0	3	23	2	1	—	380	—	—	—
Fat Free Sticks	48 (1 oz)	110	0	0	0	3	23	1	1	—	530	—	—	—
Fat Free Thins	12 pieces (1 oz)	110	0	0	0	2	24	tr	1	—	520	—	—	—
Fat Free Tiny Twists	18 pieces (1 oz)	110	0	0	0	3	23	tr	1	—	420	—	—	—
Honey Mustard	16 (1 oz)	110	1	0	0	3	22	1	1	0	370	—	—	0
Rods	3 (1 oz)	110	1	0	0	3	22	1	1	—	610	—	—	—
Sharp Cheddar	22 (1 oz)	110	1	0	0	3	22	tr	1	0	370	—	—	0
Sour Dough Nuggets	11 (1 oz)	110	0	0	0	2	24	1	1	—	330	—	—	—
SNYDER'S OF HANOVER														
Dips White Fudge	1 oz	130	6	4	0	2	19	12	0	0	80	—	—	0
Hard Sourdough	1 oz	100	0	0	0	3	22	0	1	0	240	—	—	0
Hard Sourdough Unsalted	1 oz	100	0	0	0	3	22	0	1	0	90	—	—	0
Logs	1 oz	110	1	0	0	3	21	1	tr	0	360	—	—	0
Mini	1 oz	120	0	0	0	3	25	tr	tr	0	250	—	—	0
Mini Unsalted	1 oz	110	0	0	0	3	25	tr	tr	0	75	—	—	0
Nibblers	1 oz	120	0	0	0	3	25	tr	tr	0	200	—	—	0
Nibblers Honey Mustard & Onions	1 oz	130	3	0	0	3	23	tr	tr	0	95	—	—	0
Nibblers Oat Bran	1 oz	130	3	0	0	3	23	1	3	0	170	—	—	0
Nibblers Unsalted	1 oz	120	0	0	0	3	25	tr	tr	0	50	—	—	0
Oat Bran	1 oz	100	3	0	0	3	22	tr	2	0	260	—	—	0
Old Fashioned Dipping Stix	1 oz	100	0	0	0	3	22	tr	1	0	330	—	—	0
Olde Tyme Unsalted	1 oz	120	1	0	0	3	24	tr	1	0	75	—	—	0
Olde Tyme	1 oz	120	1	0	0	3	24	tr	1	0	120	—	—	0
Olde Tyme Stix	1 oz	120	1	0	0	3	23	tr	1	0	150	—	—	0
Pieces Buttermilk Ranch	1 oz	130	5	1	0	3	19	tr	tr	0	250	—	—	0
Pieces Cheddar Cheese	1 oz	190	6	1	0	2	18	tr	tr	0	260	—	—	0

FOOD	PORTION	CALS	FAT	SAT FAT	CHOL	PROT	CARB	SUGAR	FIBER	CALCI	SOD	POTAS	FOLIC	VIT C
SNYDER'S OF HANOVER (CONT.)														
Pieces Honey Mustard & Onions	1 oz	140	7	1	0	2	18	3	tr	0	240	—	—	0
Pieces Peppered Pizza	1 oz	150	8	2	0	2	16	1	tr	0	340	—	—	0
Rods	1 oz	120	2	0	0	4	24	tr	tr	0	400	—	—	0
Snaps	24 (1 oz)	110	1	0	0	3	24	0	tr	0	340	—	—	0
Thin	1 oz	130	0	0	0	3	23	1	tr	0	430	—	—	0
Whole Wheat Honey	1 oz	120	1	0	0	3	24	4	2	0	20	—	—	0
SPINZELS														
Braided	1 pkg (0.5 oz)	55	1	0	0	2	11	tr	tr	0	200	—	—	0
UTZ														
Country Store Stix	5 (1 oz)	110	1	0	0	3	22	tr	1	0	470	—	—	0
Fat Free Hard	1 (0.8 oz)	90	0	0	0	2	18	tr	tr	0	470	—	—	0
Fat Free Hard No Salt Added	1 (0.8 oz)	90	0	0	0	2	19	tr	tr	0	50	—	—	0
Fat Free Sour Dough Nuggets	10 (1 oz)	100	0	0	0	2	22	tr	1	0	470	—	—	0
Fat Free Stix	14 (1 oz)	100	0	0	0	3	23	1	1	0	280	—	—	0
Fat Free Thin	10 (1 oz)	100	0	0	0	2	22	1	1	0	480	—	—	0
Honey Mustard & Onion	⅓ cup (1 oz)	130	6	1	0	2	18	1	tr	0	270	—	—	0
Rods	3 (1 oz)	120	1	0	0	3	24	1	1	0	400	—	—	0
Specials	5 (1 oz)	110	1	0	0	3	21	tr	1	0	470	—	—	0
Specials Extra Dark	5 (1 oz)	110	1	0	0	3	21	tr	1	0	470	—	—	0
Specials Unsalted	5 (1 oz)	110	1	0	0	3	21	tr	1	0	80	—	—	0
Wheels	20 (1 oz)	100	0	0	0	2	22	1	1	0	480	—	—	0
WEGE														
Honey Wheat	1 (0.8 oz)	120	2	0	0	2	24	4	1	0	20	—	—	0
WEIGHT WATCHERS														
Oat Bran Nuggets	1 pkg (1.5 oz)	170	3	0	0	4	33	0	3	0	250	—	—	0
PRUNE JUICE														
canned	1 cup	181	tr	tr	0	2	45	—	3	30	11	706	1	11
OCEAN SPRAY														
100% Juice	8 oz	180	0	0	0	2	44	42	0	—	8	480	—	5
PRUNES														
canned in heavy syrup	1 cup	245	tr	tr	0	2	65	—	—	40	6	528	—	7
canned in heavy syrup	5	90	tr	tr	0	1	24	—	—	15	2	194	—	2
dried	1 cup	385	1	tr	0	4	101	—	12	82	6	1200	6	5
dried	10	201	tr	tr	0	2	53	—	6	43	3	626	3	3
dried cooked w/ sugar	½ cup	147	tr	tr	0	1	39	—	7	25	2	371	tr	3

FOOD	PORTION	CALS	FAT	SAT FAT	CHOL	PROT	CARB	SUGAR	FIBER	CALCI	SOD	POTAS	FOLIC	VIT C
dried cooked w/o sugar	½ cup	113	tr	tr	0	1	30	—	6	24	2	354	tr	3
AMERICAN ALMOND														
Baker's Style Ledvar	2 tbsp	90	0	0	0	0	21	17	1	0	120	—	—	1
ST DALFOUR														
French Prunes	3	100	0	0	0	1	22	9	3	20	5	—	—	0
SUNSWEET														
Dried Plums	5	100	0	0	0	1	24	12	3	20	5	290	—	0

PUDDING

MIX

FOOD	PORTION	CALS	FAT	SAT FAT	CHOL	PROT	CARB	SUGAR	FIBER	CALCI	SOD	POTAS	FOLIC	VIT C
banana as prep w/ 2% milk	½ cup (4.9 oz)	142	2	1	9	4	26	—	—	154	232	193	5	1
banana as prep w/ whole milk	½ cup (4.9 oz)	157	4	3	17	4	25	—	—	151	231	189	5	1
chocolate	½ cup (5 oz)	150	3	2	9	5	28	—	—	161	148	240	—	1
chocolate as prep w/ whole milk	½ cup (5 oz)	158	5	3	17	5	26	—	—	158	147	232	—	1
coconut cream	½ cup (4.9 oz)	148	4	3	9	4	25	—	—	154	226	223	—	1
instant banana as prep w/ 2% milk	½ cup (5.2 oz)	152	3	1	9	4	29	—	—	150	435	192	6	1
instant banana as prep w/ whole milk	½ cup (5.2 oz)	167	4	3	17	4	27	—	—	147	434	189	6	1
instant chocolate	½ cup (5.2 oz)	149	3	2	9	3	28	—	—	153	418	247	6	1
instant chocolate as prep w/ whole milk	½ cup (5.2 oz)	164	5	3	17	5	28	—	—	151	417	244	6	1
instant lemon	½ cup (5.2 oz)	155	4	1	9	4	30	—	—	149	394	190	6	1
instant vanilla	½ cup (5 oz)	147	2	1	9	2	28	—	—	146	407	185	6	1
lemon	½ cup (5.1 oz)	163	2	1	77	1	36	—	—	11	94	7	—	0
rice as prep w/ whole milk	½ cup (5.1 oz)	175	4	3	17	5	30	—	—	149	158	186	5	1
tapioca	½ cup (5 oz)	147	2	1	9	4	28	—	—	149	172	190	—	1
tapioca as prep w/ whole milk	½ cup (5 oz)	161	4	3	17	4	28	—	—	147	171	186	—	1
vanilla as prep w/ 2% milk	½ cup (4.9 oz)	141	2	1	9	4	26	—	—	153	224	194	—	1
vanilla as prep w/ whole milk	½ cup (4.9 oz)	155	4	3	17	2	26	—	—	150	223	190	—	1
BETTY CROCKER														
Rice as prep	1 serv	200	3	tr	9	1	33	21	—	150	70	5	24	—
JELL-O														
Americana Rice as prep w/ skim milk	½ cup (5.2 oz)	140	0	0	<5	5	29	19	0	150	160	210	—	0

FOOD	PORTION	CALS	FAT	SAT FAT	CHOL	PROT	CARB	SUGAR	FIBER	CALCI	SOD	POTAS	FOLIC	VIT C
JELL-O (CONT.)														
Americana Tapioca as prep w/ skim milk	½ cup (5.1 oz)	130	0	0	<5	4	28	21	0	150	180	200	—	0
Banana Cream as prep w/ 2% milk	½ cup (5.1 oz)	140	3	2	10	4	26	21	0	150	240	190	—	0
Butterscotch as prep w/ 2% milk	½ cup (5.2 oz)	160	3	2	10	4	30	25	0	150	190	190	—	0
Chocolate as prep w/ 2% milk	½ cup (5.2 oz)	150	3	2	10	5	28	21	tr	150	170	340	—	0
Chocolate Fudge as prep w/ 2% milk	½ cup (5.2 oz)	150	3	2	10	5	28	21	1	150	170	330	—	0
Coconut Cream as prep w/ 2% milk	½ cup (5.1 oz)	150	5	4	10	4	24	19	tr	150	210	220	—	0
Fat Free Chocolate as prep w/ skim milk	½ cup (5.2 oz)	130	0	0	<5	5	29	21	0	150	170	310	—	0
Fat Free Vanilla as prep w/ skim milk	½ cup (5.1 oz)	130	0	0	<5	4	28	22	0	150	200	210	—	0
Instant Banana Cream as prep w/ 2% milk	½ cup (5.2 oz)	150	3	2	10	4	29	24	0	150	410	190	—	0
Instant Butterscotch as prep w/ 2% milk	½ cup (5.2 oz)	150	3	2	10	4	29	24	0	150	450	190	—	0
Instant Chocolate as prep w/ 2% milk	½ cup (5.2 oz)	160	3	2	10	4	31	25	tr	150	470	270	—	0
Instant Chocolate Fudge as prep w/ 2% milk	½ cup (4.2 oz)	160	3	2	10	5	31	23	tr	150	440	330	—	0
Instant Coconut Cream as prep w/ 2% milk	½ cup (4.2 oz)	160	5	4	10	4	27	22	tr	150	320	220	—	0
Instant French Vanilla as prep w/ 2% milk	½ cup (4.2 oz)	150	3	2	10	4	29	24	0	150	410	190	—	0
Instant Lemon as prep w/ 2% milk	½ cup (4.2 oz)	150	3	2	10	4	29	25	0	150	370	190	—	0
Instant Pistachio as prep w/ 2% milk	½ cup (4.2 oz)	160	3	2	10	4	29	24	0	150	410	200	—	0
Instant Vanilla as prep w/ 2% milk	½ cup (4.2 oz)	150	3	2	10	4	29	25	0	150	410	190	—	0
Instant Fat Free Chocolate as prep w/ skim milk	½ cup (5.3 oz)	140	0	0	<5	5	31	25	tr	150	410	280	—	0
Instant Fat Free Devil's Food as prep w/ skim milk	½ cup (5.3 oz)	140	0	0	<5	5	31	25	tr	150	420	280	—	0

FOOD	PORTION	CALS	FAT	SAT FAT	CHOL	PROT	CARB	SUGAR	FIBER	CALCI	SOD	POTAS	FOLIC	VIT C
JELL-O (CONT.)														
Instant Fat Free Sugar Free Banana as prep w/ skim milk	½ cup (4.6 oz)	70	0	0	<5	4	12	6	0	150	410	210	—	0
Instant Fat Free Sugar Free Butterscotch as prep w/ skim milk	½ cup (4.6 oz)	70	0	0	<5	4	12	6	0	150	400	210	—	0
Instant Fat Free Sugar Free Chocolate as prep w/ skim milk	½ cup (4.6 oz)	80	0	0	<5	5	14	6	tr	150	390	320	—	0
Instant Fat Free Sugar Free Chocolate Fudge as prep w/ skim milk	½ cup (4.7 oz)	80	0	0	<5	5	14	6	tr	150	390	320	—	0
Instant Fat Free Sugar Free Vanilla as prep w/ skim milk	½ cup (4.6 oz)	70	0	0	<5	4	12	6	0	150	400	210	—	0
Instant Fat Free Sugar Free White Chocolate as prep w/ skim milk	½ cup (4.6 oz)	70	0	0	<5	4	12	6	0	150	400	210	—	0
Instant Fat Free Vanilla as prep w/ skim milk	½ cup (5.2 oz)	140	0	0	<5	4	29	25	0	150	410	200	—	0
Instant Fat Free White Chocolate as prep w/ skim milk	½ cup (5.2 oz)	140	0	0	<5	4	29	25	0	150	410	200	—	0
Lemon as prep	½ cup (4.4 oz)	140	2	1	75	tr	29	23	0	0	75	75	—	0
Milk Chocolate as prep w/ 2% milk	½ cup (5.2 oz)	150	3	2	10	4	28	22	tr	150	170	260	—	0
Sugar Free Chocolate as prep w/ 2% milk	½ cup (4.6 oz)	90	3	2	10	5	13	6	tr	150	170	330	—	0
Sugar Free Vanilla as prep w/ 2% milk	½ cup (4.5 oz)	80	3	2	10	4	11	6	0	150	170	190	—	0
Vanilla as prep w/ 2% milk	½ cup (5.1 oz)	150	3	2	9	0	30	19	0	150	408	—	—	0
KETO														
Banana not prep	½ scoop	62	3	—	10	7	3	0	2	—	105	—	—	—
Chocolate not prep	½ scoop	66	3	—	10	7	4	0	3	—	115	—	—	—
French Vanilla not prep	½ scoop	62	3	—	10	7	3	0	2	—	105	—	—	—

FOOD	PORTION	CALS	FAT	SAT FAT	CHOL	PROT	CARB	SUGAR	FIBER	CALCI	SOD	POTAS	FOLIC	VIT C
LOUISIANA PURCHASE														
Bread	1 serv (1.3 oz)	150	3	3	0	3	28	16	2	40	220	—	—	0
LUNDBERG														
Elegant Rice Cinnamon Raisin	½ cup (3.9 oz)	70	0	0	0	0	16	7	1	20	0	—	—	0
Elegant Rice Coconut	½ cup (3.9 oz)	70	2	2	0	0	13	5	1	0	0	—	—	0
Elegant Rice Honey Almond	½ cup (3.9 oz)	70	1	0	0	2	15	5	1	0	0	—	—	0
UNCLE BEN'S														
Rice Pudding Cinnamon & Raisins as prep	½ cup (1.5 oz)	160	1	0	0	2	37	16	1	20	150	—	32	0
READY-TO-EAT														
banana	1 pkg (5 oz)	180	5	1	—	3	30	23	—	120	278	156	—	—
chocolate	1 pkg (5 oz)	189	6	1	5	4	32	23	—	128	183	256	4	3
lemon	1 pkg (5 oz)	177	4	1	0	tr	36	—	—	3	199	1	—	—
rice	1 pkg (5 oz)	231	11	2	—	3	31	—	—	—	121	65	—	—
tapioca	1 pkg (5 oz)	169	5	1	—	3	28	—	—	119	168	148	—	—
vanilla	1 pkg (4 oz)	146	4	1	8	3	25	—	—	99	153	128	0	0
BOOST														
Vanilla	1 pkg (5 oz)	240	9	1	<5	7	33	20	0	250	125	250	84	36
HANDI-SNACKS														
Banana	1 serv (3.5 oz)	120	4	1	0	1	22	16	0	40	150	70	—	0
Butterscotch	1 serv (3.5 oz)	120	4	1	0	1	22	17	0	60	150	70	—	0
Chocolate	1 serv (3.5 oz)	130	4	1	0	2	23	18	tr	60	125	140	—	0
Chocolate Fudge	1 serv (3.5 oz)	130	4	1	0	2	23	18	tr	60	130	160	—	0
Fat Free Chocolate	1 serv (3.5 oz)	90	0	0	0	2	21	16	0	60	170	140	—	0
Fat Free Vanilla	1 serv (3.5 oz)	90	0	0	0	1	21	16	0	60	180	70	—	0
Tapioca	1 serv (3.5 oz)	120	4	1	0	2	21	14	0	60	120	75	—	0
Vanilla	1 serv (3.5 oz)	120	4	1	0	1	21	17	0	40	150	70	—	0
HEALTHY CHOICE														
Low Fat Chocolate Raspberry	½ cup (3.5 oz)	102	2	1	0	3	19	15	0	110	111	—	—	0
Low Fat Chocolate Almond	½ cup (3.5 oz)	109	2	1	0	3	21	15	0	113	109	—	—	0
Low Fat Double Chocolate Fudge	½ cup (3.5 oz)	101	1	tr	0	3	20	14	0	95	116	—	—	0
Low Fat French Vanilla	½ cup (3.5 oz)	98	1	1	0	2	20	16	0	122	122	—	—	0
Low Fat Tapioca	½ cup (3.5 oz)	101	1	1	1	2	21	14	0	81	115	—	—	0
HUNT'S														
Snack Pack Banana	1 serv (3.5 oz)	119	4	2	2	2	18	14	0	47	155	—	—	0
Snack Pack Butterscotch	1 serv (3.5 oz)	130	4	1	2	2	21	14	0	45	164	—	—	0

FOOD	PORTION	CALS	FAT	SAT FAT	CHOL	PROT	CARB	SUGAR	FIBER	CALCI	SOD	POTAS	FOLIC	VIT C
HUNT'S (CONT.)														
Snack Pack Chocolate	1 serv (3.5 oz)	143	5	1	1	2	22	17	0	58	139	—	—	0
Snack Pack Chocolate Fudge	1 serv (3.5 oz)	147	5	2	1	2	23	17	0	50	153	—	—	0
Snack Pack Chocolate Marshmallow	1 serv (3.5 oz)	134	5	1	1	2	21	16	0	36	212	—	—	0
Snack Pack Fat Free Chocolate	1 serv (3.5 oz)	86	tr	tr	1	2	19	14	0	42	134	—	—	0
Snack Pack Fat Free Tapioca	1 serv (3.5 oz)	82	tr	0	0	2	18	14	0	43	141	—	—	0
Snack Pack Fat Free Vanilla	1 serv (3.5 oz)	81	tr	0	0	2	18	13	0	43	146	—	—	0
Snack Pack Lemon	1 serv (3.5 oz)	124	3	1	0	tr	24	21	0	6	47	—	—	2
Snack Pack Milk Chocolate Variety	1 serv (3.5 oz)	143	5	1	2	2	22	18	0	53	136	—	—	0
Snack Pack Swirl Chocolate Caramel	1 serv (3.5 oz)	143	5	2	1	2	23	17	0	53	143	—	—	0
Snack Pack Swirl Chocolate Peanut Butter	1 serv (3.5 oz)	146	6	1	2	3	21	15	0	60	156	—	—	0
Snack Pack Swirl Smores	1 serv (3.5 oz)	136	5	1	1	2	21	18	0	36	94	—	—	0
Snack Pack Tapioca	1 serv (3.5 oz)	125	4	2	1	1	21	15	0	60	144	—	—	0
Snack Pack Toppers Chocolate Fudge w/ Rainbow Sprinkles	1 serv (4 oz)	164	6	2	tr	2	25	16	tr	48	145	—	—	1
Snack Pack Toppers Chocolate w/ Dinosaurs	1 serv (4 oz)	161	6	1	tr	2	25	18	tr	43	164	—	—	tr
Snack Pack Toppers Chocolate w/ Fun Chips	1 serv (4 oz)	176	6	2	1	2	28	21	tr	65	153	—	—	1
Snack Pack Toppers Vanilla w/ Chocolate Sprinkles	1 serv (4 oz)	164	6	2	tr	1	26	16	tr	43	129	—	—	0
Snack Pack Vanilla	1 serv (3.5 oz)	135	5	1	1	2	21	17	0	47	147	—	—	0
IMAGINE														
Banana	1 pkg (4 oz)	150	3	0	0	1	30	19	0	100	40	92	—	0
Butterscotch	1 pkg (4 oz)	150	3	0	0	1	31	17	0	100	45	69	—	0
Chocolate	1 pkg (4 oz)	170	3	0	0	1	38	22	1	100	65	149	—	0
Lemon	1 pkg (4 oz)	150	3	0	0	1	33	19	1	100	50	148	—	1

FOOD	PORTION	CALS	FAT	SAT FAT	CHOL	PROT	CARB	SUGAR	FIBER	CALCI	SOD	POTAS	FOLIC	VIT C
JELL-O														
Chocolate	1 serv (4 oz)	160	5	2	0	3	28	23	0	100	190	260	—	0
Chocolate Vanilla Swirls	1 serv (4 oz)	160	5	2	0	3	27	22	0	80	180	210	—	0
Fat Free Chocolate	1 serv (4 oz)	100	0	0	0	3	23	17	tr	80	190	240	—	0
Fat Free Chocolate Vanilla Swirl	1 serv (4 oz)	100	0	0	0	2	23	17	tr	60	200	—	—	0
Fat Free Chocolate Fudge & Caramel	1 serv (4 oz)	100	0	0	0	2	24	17	0	60	230	—	—	0
Fat Free Devil's Food	1 serv (4 oz)	100	0	0	0	3	23	18	tr	80	210	220	—	0
Fat Free Rocky Road	1 serv (4 oz)	100	0	0	0	3	23	17	tr	80	210	200	—	0
Fat Free Tapioca	1 serv (4 oz)	100	0	0	0	1	23	17	0	60	230	—	—	0
Fat Free Vanilla	1 serv (4 oz)	100	0	0	0	2	23	18	0	80	240	125	—	0
Fat Free Vanilla Caramel	1 serv (4 oz)	100	0	0	0	1	23	16	0	40	230	—	—	0
Vanilla	1 serv (4 oz)	160	5	2	0	2	25	21	0	80	170	125	—	0
NUTRABALANCE														
Low Lactose All Flavors	1 serv (4 oz)	225	8	—	0	7	31	—	—	—	220	204	—	—
SWISS MISS														
Butterscotch	1 pkg (4 oz)	156	6	1	1	2	24	19	0	62	182	—	—	0
Chocolate	1 pkg (4 oz)	166	6	2	1	3	26	23	0	83	177	—	—	0
Chocolate Fudge	1 pkg (4 oz)	175	6	2	1	3	28	22	0	79	207	—	—	0
Fat Free Chocolate	1 pkg (4 oz)	98	tr	0	0	2	22	16	0	54	141	—	—	0
Fat Free Chocolate Fudge	1 pkg (4 oz)	101	tr	0	0	2	23	17	0	50	147	—	—	0
Fat Free Vanilla	1 pkg (4 oz)	93	tr	0	0	2	21	14	0	52	168	—	—	0
Fat Free Parfait Vanilla Chocolate	1 pkg (4 oz)	96	tr	0	0	2	21	16	0	53	143	—	—	0
Lemon Meringue Pie	1 pkg (4 oz)	150	3	1	0	0	30	24	—	—	60	—	—	—
Low Fat Tapioca	1 pkg (4 oz)	130	3	1	0	3	25	20	—	20	200	—	—	—
Low Fat Vanilla	1 serv (4 oz)	120	2	1	0	2	24	18	—	200	190	—	—	—
Milk Chocolate	1 pkg (4 oz)	166	6	2	1	2	26	20	0	66	165	—	—	0
Parfait	1 pkg (4 oz)	164	6	2	1	3	25	22	0	88	196	—	—	0
Swirl Vanilla Chocolate Caramel	1 pkg (4 oz)	169	6	2	1	2	26	20	1	66	178	—	—	0
Swirl Chocolate Vanilla	1 pkg (4 oz)	169	6	1	1	2	26	21	0	61	159	—	—	0

FOOD	PORTION	CALS	FAT	SAT FAT	CHOL	PROT	CARB	SUGAR	FIBER	CALCI	SOD	POTAS	FOLIC	VIT C
SWISS MISS (CONT.)														
Swirl Chocolate Vanilla Chocolate	1 pkg (4 oz)	169	6	2	1	3	26	22	0	61	159	—	—	0
Tapioca	1 pkg (4 oz)	138	4	1	1	2	24	20	0	84	180	—	—	0
Vanilla	1 pkg (4 oz)	156	6	1	1	2	24	19	0	83	181	—	—	0
TAKE-OUT														
blancmange	1 serv (4.7 oz)	154	5	—	—	4	25	—	tr	149	—	—	—	tr
bread pudding	½ cup (4.4 oz)	212	7	3	83	7	31	—	—	143	291	282	16	1
bread w/ raisins	½ cup	180	5	2	77	5	31	—	—	124	185	266	13	1
chocolate	½ cup (5.5 oz)	221	6	3	17	5	40	—	—	152	137	252	7	1
corn	⅔ cup	181	9	4	122	7	21	—	—	67	92	268	42	5
queen of puddings	1 serv (4.4 oz)	266	10	—	—	6	41	—	tr	99	—	—	—	1
rice pudding	1 serv (6 oz)	220	8	—	—	6	34	—	tr	222	—	—	—	2
rice w/ raisins	½ cup	246	6	3	136	7	42	—	4	125	270	265	21	1
tapioca	½ cup (5.3 oz)	189	7	—	124	7	26	—	—	159	288	216	14	1
vanilla	½ cup (4.3 oz)	130	4	3	17	4	20	—	—	145	113	185	5	1
yorkshire	1 serv (3 oz)	177	8	—	57	6	22	—	tr	37	168	45	3	0
PUDDING POPS														
chocolate	1 (1.6 oz)	72	2	—	1	2	12	10	—	66	77	105	1	tr
vanilla	1 (1.6 oz)	75	2	—	1	2	13	11	—	61	50	65	2	tr
PUFFERFISH														
raw	3 oz	72	0	0	—	17	0	0	0	12	120	246	—	0
PUMMELO														
fresh	1	228	tr	—	0	5	59	—	—	23	7	1317	—	372
sections	1 cup	71	tr	—	0	1	18	—	—	7	2	411	—	116
PUMPKIN														
butter	1 tbsp	32	0	0	0	0	8	8	—	—	0	—	—	—
canned	½ cup	41	tr	tr	0	1	10	—	—	32	6	251	15	5
cooked mashed	½ cup	24	tr	tr	0	1	6	—	—	18	2	281	—	6
flowers cooked	½ cup	10	tr	tr	0	1	2	—	—	25	4	71	—	3
flowers raw	1	0	0	0	0	tr	tr	—	—	1	0	3	—	1
leaves cooked	½ cup	7	tr	tr	0	1	1	—	—	15	3	153	—	tr
leaves raw	½ cup	4	tr	tr	0	1	tr	—	—	8	2	87	—	2
raw cubed	½ cup	15	tr	tr	0	1	4	—	—	12	1	197	—	5
LIBBY'S														
Puree	½ cup	40	1	0	0	2	9	4	5	20	5	—	—	0
PUMPKIN SEEDS														
dried	1 oz	154	13	2	0	7	5	—	—	12	5	229	—	—
roasted	¼ cup	296	24	5	0	19	8	—	—	24	10	457	—	—
salted & roasted	¼ cup	296	24	5	0	19	8	—	—	24	324	457	—	—
whole roasted	¼ cup	71	3	1	0	3	9	—	—	9	3	147	—	—
whole roasted	1 oz	127	6	1	0	5	15	—	—	16	5	261	—	—
whole salted roasted	¼ cup	71	3	1	0	3	9	—	—	9	67	147	—	—

FOOD	PORTION	CALS	FAT	SAT FAT	CHOL	PROT	CARB	SUGAR	FIBER	CALCI	SOD	POTAS	FOLIC	VIT C
PURSLANE														
cooked	1 cup	21	tr	—	0	2	4	—	—	90	51	561	—	12
fresh	1 cup	7	tr	—	0	1	1	—	—	28	20	213	—	9
QUAIL														
breast w/o skin raw	1 (2 oz)	69	2	tr	—	13	0	—	—	5	31	146	—	3
w/ skin raw	1 quail (3.8 oz)	210	13	4	—	21	0	—	—	14	58	235	8	7
w/o skin raw	1 quail (3.2 oz)	123	4	1	—	20	0	—	—	12	47	218	—	—
QUICHE														
ATKINS														
Crustless Bacon & Onion	1 serv	320	27	14	175	18	2	2	0	350	540	—	—	0
Crustless Four Cheese	1 serv	290	24	15	45	22	2	1	0	350	270	—	—	2
Crustless Smoked Ham & Cheese	1 serv	290	24	13	170	18	2	2	0	350	470	—	—	0
TAKE-OUT														
cheese	1 slice (3 oz)	283	20	—	—	11	16	—	1	234	—	—	—	tr
lorraine	⅛ of 8 in pie	600	48	23	285	13	29	—	—	211	653	283	—	tr
mushroom	1 slice (3 oz)	256	18	—	—	9	17	—	1	180	—	—	—	tr
QUINCE														
fresh	1	53	tr	tr	0	tr	14	—	—	10	4	181	—	14
QUINOA														
quinoa not prep	1 cup (6 oz)	636	10	1	0	22	117	—	10	102	36	1258	83	0
RABBIT														
domestic w/o bone roasted	3 oz	167	7	2	70	25	0	—	—	16	40	325	9	0
wild w/o bone stewed	3 oz	147	3	1	104	28	0	—	—	15	38	292	—	—
RACCOON														
roasted	3 oz	217	12	—	—	25	0	—	—	—	—	—	—	—
RADICCHIO														
raw shredded	½ cup	5	tr	—	0	tr	1	—	—	4	4	60	12	2
RADISHES														
chinese dried	½ cup	157	tr	tr	0	5	37	—	—	165	161	2027	—	0
chinese raw	1 (12 oz)	62	tr	tr	0	2	14	—	—	91	71	767	—	74
chinese raw sliced	½ cup	8	tr	tr	0	tr	2	—	—	12	9	100	—	10
chinese sliced cooked	½ cup	13	tr	tr	0	tr	3	—	—	12	10	211	—	11
daikon dried	½ cup	157	tr	tr	0	5	37	—	—	365	161	2027	—	0
daikon raw	1 (12 oz)	62	tr	tr	0	2	14	—	—	91	71	767	—	74
daikon raw sliced	½ cup	8	tr	tr	0	tr	2	—	—	12	9	100	—	10
daikon sliced cooked	½ cup	13	tr	tr	0	tr	3	—	—	12	10	211	—	11
red raw	10	7	tr	tr	0	tr	2	—	—	9	11	104	12	10

FOOD	PORTION	CALS	FAT	SAT FAT	CHOL	PROT	CARB	SUGAR	FIBER	CALCI	SOD	POTAS	FOLIC	VIT C
red sliced	½ cup	10	tr	tr	0	tr	2	—	—	12	14	134	16	13
white icicle raw	1 (½ oz)	2	tr	tr	0	tr	tr	—	—	5	3	48	2	5
white icicle raw sliced	½ cup	7	tr	tr	0	1	1	—	—	14	8	140	7	15
EDEN														
Daikon Dried Shredded	2 tbsp	45	0	0	0	1	9	6	3	60	20	420	0	0
Daikon Pickled	2 slices	5	0	0	0	0	1	0	0	0	250	25	0	0
TAKE-OUT														
korean kimchee	½ cup	31	1	—	—	2	6	—	—	3	—	—	—	7
moo namul saengche korean salad	1 serv (3.7 oz)	34	tr	tr	0	1	8	6	2	19	547	247	15	13

RAISINS

FOOD	PORTION	CALS	FAT	SAT FAT	CHOL	PROT	CARB	SUGAR	FIBER	CALCI	SOD	POTAS	FOLIC	VIT C
chocolate coated	1 cup (6.7 oz)	741	28	17	5	8	130	—	—	163	68	976	—	tr
chocolate coated	10 (0.4 oz)	39	2	1	0	tr	7	—	—	9	4	51	—	0
golden seedless	1 cup	437	1	tr	0	5	115	—	8	76	17	1082	5	5
jumbo golden	¼ cup	130	0	0	0	1	31	29	2	20	10	—	—	0
seedless	1 cup	434	1	tr	0	5	115	—	8	71	17	1089	5	5
seedless	1 tbsp	27	tr	tr	0	tr	7	—	—	—	—	—	—	—
sultanas	1 oz	88	0	—	—	1	23	—	2	18	—	—	—	0
DOLE														
CinnaRaisins	1 pkg (1 oz)	95	0	0	0	1	22	20	2	20	5	220	—	0
ESTEE														
Chocolate Covered	¼ cup	180	6	5	<5	3	27	16	1	—	45	270	—	—
MARIANA														
Fruitn Yogurt Milk Chocolate Covered Raisins	32 pieces (1 oz)	130	5	3	0	1	20	17	2	20	40	—	—	0
NESTLÉ														
Chocolate Covered	1⅓ tbsp	70	3	2	0	tr	11	9	tr	0	0	—	—	0
SUN-MAID														
California Golden	¼ cup	130	0	0	0	1	31	29	2	20	10	310	—	—
California Seedless	1 box (1.5 oz)	130	0	0	0	1	33	30	2	20	10	—	—	—
TREE OF LIFE														
Organic	¼ cup (1.4 oz)	130	0	0	0	1	31	29	2	20	10	310	—	9

RASPBERRIES

FOOD	PORTION	CALS	FAT	SAT FAT	CHOL	PROT	CARB	SUGAR	FIBER	CALCI	SOD	POTAS	FOLIC	VIT C
canned in heavy syrup	½ cup	117	tr	tr	0	1	30	—	—	14	4	120	13	11
fresh	1 cup	61	1	tr	0	1	14	—	—	27	0	187	—	31
fresh	1 pint	154	2	tr	0	3	36	—	—	69	0	474	—	78
frozen sweetened	1 cup	256	tr	tr	0	2	65	—	—	38	1	285	65	41
frozen sweetened	1 pkg (10 oz)	291	tr	tr	0	2	74	—	—	43	1	324	74	47
frzn unsweetened	¾ cup	130	0	0	0	2	29	6	2	40	0	—	—	36

FOOD	PORTION	CALS	FAT	SAT FAT	CHOL	PROT	CARB	SUGAR	FIBER	CALCI	SOD	POTAS	FOLIC	VIT C
BIRDS EYE														
Red	5 oz	90	0	0	0	1	22	22	5	—	5	—	—	—
TREE OF LIFE														
Organic	⅔ cup (5 oz)	50	0	0	0	1	12	7	2	0	0	—	—	18

RASPBERRY JUICE

FOOD	PORTION	CALS	FAT	SAT FAT	CHOL	PROT	CARB	SUGAR	FIBER	CALCI	SOD	POTAS	FOLIC	VIT C
CRYSTAL LIGHT														
Raspberry Ice Drink	1 serv (8 oz)	5	0	0	0	0	0	0	0	0	20	60	—	0
Raspberry Ice Drink Mix as prep	1 serv (8 oz)	5	0	0	0	0	0	0	0	0	0	0	—	6
DOLE														
Country Raspberry	8 fl oz	140	0	0	0	0	35	—	—	—	35	200	—	60
FRESH SAMANTHA														
Raspberry Dream	1 cup (8 oz)	120	1	0	—	2	10	—	8	20	0	120	40	48
KOOL-AID														
Drink Mix as prep	1 serv (8 oz)	60	0	0	0	0	17	17	0	0	0	0	—	6
Raspberry Drink as prep w/ sugar	1 serv (8 oz)	100	0	0	0	0	25	25	0	0	30	0	—	6
Splash Blue Raspberry Drink	1 serv (8 oz)	120	0	0	0	0	30	30	0	0	35	15	—	0
NANTUCKET NECTARS														
Organic Very Raspberry	8 oz	120	0	0	0	0	30	29	—	—	30	—	—	—
SQUEEZIT														
Blue Raspberry	1 bottle (7 oz)	110	0	0	0	0	28	27	0	0	0	—	—	0

RED BEANS

FOOD	PORTION	CALS	FAT	SAT FAT	CHOL	PROT	CARB	SUGAR	FIBER	CALCI	SOD	POTAS	FOLIC	VIT C
CANNED														
GREEN GIANT														
Red Beans	½ cup (4.5 oz)	100	1	0	0	6	19	2	6	40	350	—	—	0
HUNT'S														
Small	½ cup (4.5 oz)	89	1	0	0	6	19	4	6	32	713	—	—	tr
VAN CAMP														
Red Beans	½ cup (4.6 oz)	90	0	0	0	6	20	3	5	20	560	—	—	0
DRIED														
HURST														
HamBeens w/ Ham	1 serv	120	1	0	0	8	20	1	10	40	63	—	—	1
MIX														
BEAN CUISINE														
Pasta & Beans Barcelona Red w/ Radiatore	1 serv	210	1	0	0	7	29	2	4	60	15	—	—	42

RELISH

FOOD	PORTION	CALS	FAT	SAT FAT	CHOL	PROT	CARB	SUGAR	FIBER	CALCI	SOD	POTAS	FOLIC	VIT C
cranberry orange	½ cup	246	tr	—	0	tr	64	—	—	15	44	53	—	25
hamburger	½ cup	158	1	tr	0	1	42	—	—	5	1338	93	—	3

FOOD	PORTION	CALS	FAT	SAT FAT	CHOL	PROT	CARB	SUGAR	FIBER	CALCI	SOD	POTAS	FOLIC	VIT C
hamburger	1 tbsp	19	tr	tr	0	tr	5	—	—	1	164	11	—	tr
hot dog	1 tbsp	14	tr	tr	0	tr	4	—	—	1	164	12	—	tr
hot dog	½ cup	111	1	tr	0	2	28	—	—	7	1332	95	—	1
piccalilli	1.4 oz	13	tr	—	—	tr	2	—	1	10	—	—	—	0
sweet	½ cup	159	1	tr	0	tr	43	—	—	4	990	30	—	1
sweet	1 tbsp	19	tr	tr	0	tr	5	—	—	0	122	4	—	tr
CLAUSSEN														
Sweet Pickle	1 tbsp (0.5 oz)	15	0	0	0	0	3	2	0	0	85	—	—	0
GREEN GIANT														
Corn	1 tbsp (0.6 oz)	20	0	0	0	0	5	2	0	0	40	—	—	0
MATOUK'S														
Hot Chow	2 tbsp	20	0	0	0	0	5	2	0	—	200	—	—	—
Kuchela	1 tsp	9	1	0	0	0	tr	0	0	—	80	—	—	—
VLASIC														
Fancy Sweet	1 tbsp	15	0	0	0	0	4	4		—	140	—	—	—

RENNIN

FOOD	PORTION	CALS	FAT	SAT FAT	CHOL	PROT	CARB	SUGAR	FIBER	CALCI	SOD	POTAS	FOLIC	VIT C
tablet	1 (0.9 g)	1	0	—	—	0	tr	—	—	34	234	3	—	0

RHUBARB

FOOD	PORTION	CALS	FAT	SAT FAT	CHOL	PROT	CARB	SUGAR	FIBER	CALCI	SOD	POTAS	FOLIC	VIT C
fresh	½ cup	13	tr	—	0	1	3	—	—	52	2	175	4	5
frozen	½ cup	60	tr	—	0	tr	3	—	—	132	1	73	6	3
frzn as prep w/ sugar	½ cup	139	tr	—	0	tr	37	—	—	174	2	115	6	4

RICE

(see also RICE CAKES, WILD RICE)

FOOD	PORTION	CALS	FAT	SAT FAT	CHOL	PROT	CARB	SUGAR	FIBER	CALCI	SOD	POTAS	FOLIC	VIT C
arborio	½ cup	100	0	—	0	2	22	—	—	—	5	—	—	—
brown long grain cooked	1 cup (6.8 oz)	216	2	tr	0	5	45	—	4	20	10	84	8	0
brown medium grain cooked	1 cup (6.8 oz)	218	2	tr	0	5	46	—	4	20	2	154	8	0
glutinous cooked	1 cup (6.1 oz)	169	tr	tr	0	4	37	—	2	3	9	17	2	0
starch	1 oz	98	0	0	0	tr	24	—	—	6	17	2	—	—
white long grain cooked	1 cup (5.5 oz)	205	tr	tr	0	4	45	—	1	16	2	55	92	0
white long grain instant cooked	1 cup (5.8 oz)	162	tr	tr	0	3	35	—	1	13	5	7	68	0
white medium grain cooked	1 cup (6.5 oz)	242	tr	tr	0	4	53	—	1	6	0	54	108	0
white short grain cooked	1 cup (6.5 oz)	242	tr	tr	0	4	53	—	—	2	0	48	110	0
AMY'S														
Bowls Brown Rice & Vegetables	1 pkg (10 oz)	240	8	1	0	9	36	7	5	—	510	—	—	—
BIRDS EYE														
Rice & Broccoli In Cheese Sauce	1 pkg	290	9	3	15	8	15	4	2	100	1110	—	—	21

FOOD	PORTION	CALS	FAT	SAT FAT	CHOL	PROT	CARB	SUGAR	FIBER	CALCI	SOD	POTAS	FOLIC	VIT C
BIRDS EYE (CONT.)														
White & Wild w/ Green Beans	1 cup (6.6 oz)	180	4	2	10	4	31	2	2	40	480	—	—	1
BUITONI														
Risotto Garden Vegetable	1 serv	210	1	0	0	4	47	1	0	20	930	—	—	0
Risotto Portobello Mushrooms	1 serv	210	0	0	0	5	48	0	0	0	930	—	—	0
Risotto Rosemary & Potatoes	1 serv	210	1	0	10	4	47	0	2	20	810	—	—	0
Risotto Tomato Basil	1 serv	210	1	0	0	4	46	1	0	0	870	—	—	0
CAROLINA														
Black Beans & Rice Mix as prep	1 serv	200	2	0	0	7	39	0	5	60	930	—	40	0
Gold as prep	1 cup	160	0	0	0	3	37	0	tr	0	0	—	80	0
Spanish Rice Mix as prep	1 serv	180	1	0	0	4	42	1	2	20	760	—	80	4
CHUN KING														
Fried Rice Mix	½ cup (1.4 oz)	126	tr	0	0	4	29	5	1	53	691	—	—	1
GOURMET HOUSE														
Brown & White not prep	¼ cup	160	10	0	0	7	34	1	1	0	0	113	—	0
GOYA														
Arroz Amarillo	¼ cup (1.6 oz)	170	0	0	0	4	37	0	1	0	546	—	—	0
GREEN GIANT														
Rice & Broccoli	1 pkg (10 oz)	320	12	4	15	8	44	1	2	150	1000	—	—	18
Rice Medley	1 pkg (10 oz)	240	3	2	5	6	46	3	2	40	880	—	—	6
Rice Pilaf	1 pkg (10 oz)	230	3	2	5	6	44	3	3	40	1020	—	—	5
White & Wild	1 pkg (10 oz)	250	5	1	0	6	45	3	3	60	1000	—	—	5
LA CHOY														
Fried Rice	1 cup (4.9 oz)	236	1	tr	0	5	53	6	2	17	1024	—	—	0
LIPTON														
Oriental Stir Fry as prep	1 cup	270	8	1	0	5	47	2	1	0	860	—	80	2
Rice & Sauce Alfredo Broccoli as prep	1 cup	320	12	5	15	9	46	4	1	150	990	—	100	6
Rice & Sauce Beef as prep	1 cup	270	8	1	0	6	47	1	1	0	1010	—	80	0
Rice & Sauce Cajun Style as prep	1 cup	270	7	1	0	7	46	1	1	0	910	—	80	4
Rice & Sauce Cajun Style w/ Beans as prep	1 cup	310	8	1	0	10	52	1	7	0	530	—	100	1

FOOD	PORTION	CALS	FAT	SAT FAT	CHOL	PROT	CARB	SUGAR	FIBER	CALCI	SOD	POTAS	FOLIC	VIT C
LIPTON (CONT.)														
Rice & Sauce Cheddar Broccoli as prep	1 cup	280	9	3	5	7	46	1	1	40	1010	—	100	5
Rice & Sauce Chicken & Parmesan Risotto as prep	1 cup	270	9	2	0	6	43	0	tr	0	830	—	100	0
Rice & Sauce Chicken Broccoli as prep	1 cup	280	9	2	0	7	46	1	2	20	910	—	100	6
Rice & Sauce Chicken Flavor as prep	1 cup	280	9	2	5	7	45	1	1	0	960	—	60	0
Rice & Sauce Creamy Chicken as prep	1 cup	290	11	3	0	6	45	2	1	0	830	—	80	0
Rice & Sauce Herb & Butter as prep	1 cup	280	11	4	10	6	43	0	tr	0	880	—	80	0
Rice & Sauce Medley as prep	1 cup	270	9	2	5	7	44	1	2	0	870	—	80	0
Rice & Sauce Mushroom as prep	1 cup	270	8	1	0	6	45	1	1	20	960	—	80	0
Rice & Sauce Mushroom & Herb as prep	1 cup	290	8	2	0	6	49	0	1	20	620	—	80	1
Rice & Sauce Oriental as prep	1 cup	280	8	1	0	7	48	2	2	20	940	—	60	2
Rice & Sauce Pilaf as prep	1 cup	260	11	1	0	6	44	1	1	20	930	—	80	0
Rice & Sauce Scampi Style as prep	1 cup	270	9	2	5	6	44	1	1	0	900	—	80	0
Rice & Sauce Spanish as prep	1 cup	270	8	1	0	6	47	2	2	0	900	—	80	5
Rice & Sauce Teriyaki as prep	1 cup	270	8	1	0	5	45	2	1	0	910	—	80	0
Roasted Chicken as prep	1 cup	260	8	1	0	4	46	1	1	0	880	—	80	0
Salsa Style as prep	1 cup	220	7	1	0	4	37	1	2	0	540	—	60	4
Southwestern Chicken Flavor as prep	1 cup	260	11	1	0	5	47	1	1	0	840	—	80	2
LUNDBERG														
One-Step Curry	1 cup (7.4 oz)	160	1	0	0	5	38	0	5	20	400	—	—	1
Quick Brown Rice Savory Vegetarian Chicken	1 cup (2.5 oz)	260	3	1	—	6	53	1	5	40	910	240	—	—

FOOD	PORTION	CALS	FAT	SAT FAT	CHOL	PROT	CARB	SUGAR	FIBER	CALCI	SOD	POTAS	FOLIC	VIT C
LUNDBERG (CONT.)														
Risotto Tomato Basil	1 serv	140	1	0	0	4	30	2	1	20	630	—	—	1
MAHATMA														
Jambalaya as prep	1 cup	190	1	0	0	5	42	1	1	20	1120	—	—	1
Nacho Cheese Mix as prep	1 serv	250	3	2	5	6	49	5	tr	60	1260	—	80	0
Thai Jasmine as prep	¾ cup	160	0	0	0	3	36	0	2	0	0	—	60	0
MELTING POT														
Risotto Milanese w/ Saffron	1 cup	210	0	0	0	4	48	1	0	0	70	—	—	5
Risotto Primavera	1 cup	200	1	0	0	5	44	3	1	0	85	—	—	1
Risotto Sun-Dried Tomatoes & Peas	1 cup	200	1	0	0	5	45	2	1	0	75	—	—	0
Risotto Three Cheese	1 cup	200	2	1	5	5	44	1	0	20	410	—	—	0
Risotto Wild Mushroom	1 cup	200	1	0	0	5	44	3	2	0	50	—	—	0
MINUTE														
Boil-In-Bag White as prep	1 cup (5.7 oz)	190	0	0	0	4	42	0	tr	0	10	15	80	0
Instant Brown as prep	⅔ cup	170	2	0	0	4	34	—	2	—	10	—	—	—
Instant White as prep	1 cup (5.7 oz)	160	0	0	0	3	36	0	tr	0	5	10	60	0
Long Grain & Wild Seasoned w/ Herbs as prep	1 cup (7.8 oz)	230	1	0	0	6	50	2	1	20	950	95	80	0
NEAR EAST														
Creative Grains Chicken & Herb as prep	1 cup	270	6	1	0	8	51	2	6	20	780	—	—	0
Creative Grains Creamy Parmesan as prep	1 cup	280	8	4	18	8	48	2	3	80	790	—	—	0
Creative Grains Roasted Garlic as prep	1 cup	220	5	1	0	6	41	1	5	20	570	—	—	0
Creative Grains Roasted Pecan as prep	1 cup	240	8	1	0	6	37	1	4	20	540	—	—	0
Long Grain & Wild Rice Roasted Vegetable & Chicken as prep	1 cup	220	5	2	9	5	43	1	2	20	730	—	—	6
Long Grain & Wild Rice Garlic & Herb as prep	1 cup	220	5	2	9	5	43	1	2	20	680	—	—	0

FOOD	PORTION	CALS	FAT	SAT FAT	CHOL	PROT	CARB	SUGAR	FIBER	CALCI	SOD	POTAS	FOLIC	VIT C
NEAR EAST (CONT.)														
Pilaf Brown Rice as prep	1 cup	210	5	2	9	5	41	1	3	20	670	—	—	0
Pilaf Chicken as prep	1 cup	220	5	2	9	5	43	1	2	20	800	—	—	9
Pilaf Mix Curry as prep	1 cup	220	5	2	9	4	44	0	2	20	600	—	—	4
Pilaf Mix Garlic & Herb as prep	1 cup	220	3	tr	0	5	44	0	1	0	680	—	—	0
Pilaf Mix Long Grain & Wild as prep	1 cup	220	5	2	9	5	43	0	2	20	800	—	—	2
Pilaf Mix Rice as prep	1 cup	220	5	2	9	5	44	0	1	0	780	—	—	0
Pilaf Mix Roasted Chicken & Garlic as prep	1 cup	220	4	1	6	5	44	1	2	20	570	—	—	0
Pilaf Mix Spanish Rice as prep	1 cup	310	8	5	21	5	54	2	2	20	1010	—	—	18
Pilaf Mix Toasted Almond as prep	1 cup	230	6	2	9	6	40	1	2	20	640	—	—	0
Pilaf Mix Wild Mushroom & Herb as prep	1 cup	220	5	2	9	5	44	1	2	20	530	—	—	0
RICE EXPRESSIONS														
Indian Basmati	1 cup	180	tr	0	0	4	40	0	tr	0	0	—	—	0
Organic Brown	1 cup	160	1	0	0	4	34	0	3	0	0	—	—	0
Organic Long Grain	1 cup	180	tr	0	0	4	40	0	tr	0	0	—	—	0
Organic Rice Pilaf	1 cup	170	3	0	0	4	32	1	2	20	470		—	5
Organic Tex Mex	1 cup	190	2	0	0	4	40	0	tr	0	540	—	—	0
RIVER RICE														
Brown Long Grain not prep	¼ cup	150	1	0	0	3	32	0	tr	0	0	—	—	0
S&W														
Arborio as prep	¾ cup	150	0	0	0	3	35	0	tr	0	0	—	60	0
Basmati Mix as prep	¾ cup	160	0	0	0	3	36	0	0	0	0	—	60	0
Brown Long Grain not prep	¼ cup	150	1	0	0	3	32	0	1	0	0	—	—	0
Long Grain Organic not prep	¼ cup	150	0	0	0	3	35	0	0	0	0	—	—	0
SUCCESS														
Beef Mix as prep	1 cup	240	7	1	0	5	42	2	2	40	984		80	1
Broccoli & Cheese	½ cup	130	4	2	0	2	21	4	tr	20	432	—	32	1
Brown	1 cup	150	1	0	0	4	33	0	2	20	5	—	—	0
Brown & Wild Mix	½ cup	120	3	1	0	3	21	1	2	20	432	—	—	0

FOOD	PORTION	CALS	FAT	SAT FAT	CHOL	PROT	CARB	SUGAR	FIBER	CALCI	SOD	POTAS	FOLIC	VIT C
SUCCESS (CONT.)														
Classic Chicken	½ cup	90	1	1	0	2	15	0	1	20	384	—	32	2
Grilled Chicken & Broccoli Mix as prep	1 cup	240	6	1	0	5	42	1	1	20	936	—	80	15
Long Grain & Wild	½ cup	120	3	1	0	3	21	2	tr	20	480	—	32	4
Pilaf	½ cup	120	3	1	0	3	21	3	1	20	336	—	40	0
Red Beans & Rice Mix as prep	1 cup	300	7	2	0	7	51	1	8	80	960	—	—	2
Spanish	½ cup	120	3	1	0	2	21	2	1	40	408	—	32	2
White as prep	1 cup	190	0	0	0	4	44	0	1	20	5	—	80	0
Yellow Mix as prep	1 cup	170	3	1	0	3	33	0	1	20	696	—	60	2
TASTYBITE														
Pilaf Curried Vegetable	½ pkg (4.5 oz)	180	6	3	0	5	26	3	9	50	440	—	—	1
Pilaf Green Peas	½ pkg (4.5 oz)	208	4	1	0	6	36	0	4	20	487	—	—	1
Pilaf Vegetable Kofta	½ pkg (4.5 oz)	229	5	2	0	7	39	0	7	30	531	—	—	8
UNCLE BEN'S														
White Converted as prep	1 cup	170	0	0	0	4	38	—	—	40	0	—	80	—
VAN CAMP														
Spanish	½ cup (4.5 oz)	90	2	tr	0	2	19	5	2	10	645	—	—	7
WATER MAID														
White Medium Grain not prep	¼ cup	160	0	0	0	2	37	0	tr	0	0	—	80	0
ZATARAIN'S														
Dirty Rice Mix as prep w/o meat and oil	½ cup	130	0	0	0	3	29	0	0	20	680	—	—	1
Red Beans & Rice as prep w/o oil	½ cup	100	0	0	0	4	21	1	4	40	490	—	—	0
TAKE-OUT														
coconut rice	1 serv	500	42	—	—	6	30	—	2	—	27	—	—	—
congee	½ cup (4.1 oz)	44	—	—	—	1	10	—	—	4	—	13	—	—
nasi goreng fried rice	1 serv	206	4	—	—	10	35	—	5	—	356	—	—	—
nasi goreng indonesian rice & vegetables	1 cup (4.9 oz)	130	0	0	0	4	28	1	1	20	530	—	—	5
paella	1 serv (7 oz)	308	16	3	92	23	17	—	3	52	580	386	—	10
pilaf	½ cup	84	3	1	22	4	11	—	3	21	362	206	24	15
risotto	1 serv (6.6 oz)	426	18	—	—	6	65	—	3	46	—	—	—	tr
spanish	¾ cup	363	27	10	35	11	19	—	—	22	1339	369	14	26

RICE CAKES

(*see also* POPCORN CAKES)

FOOD	PORTION	CALS	FAT	SAT FAT	CHOL	PROT	CARB	SUGAR	FIBER	CALCI	SOD	POTAS	FOLIC	VIT C
ESTEE														
Banana Nut	5	60	1	0	0	1	14	0	0	—	30	0	—	—
Cinnamon Spice	5	60	0	0	0	1	14	0	0	—	5	0	—	—
Granny Smith Apple	5	60	0	0	0	1	13	0	0	—	5	0	—	—
Mixed Berry	5	60	0	0	0	1	14	0	0	—	0	20	—	—
Peanut Butter Crunch	5	60	0	0	0	1	13	0	tr	—	80	0	—	—
LUNDBERG														
Nutra Farmed Brown Rice	1 (0.7 oz)	70	0	0	0	1	15	—	—	—	55	65	—	—
Nutra Farmed Sesame Tamari	1 (0.7 oz)	70	1	0	0	2	16	—	2	40	120	85	—	—
Organic Koku Sesame	1 (0.7 oz)	80	0	0	0	2	17	tr	2	60	35	—	—	—
TASTEMORR														
Rice Crisps Caramel	7	55	0	0	0	tr	12	3	0	—	46	—	—	—
WEIGHT WATCHERS														
Apple Cinnamon	1 oz	110	1	0	0	2	25	8	1	0	0	—	—	0
Butter	1 oz	110	2	0	0	2	21	0	1	0	280	—	—	0
Caramel	1 oz	110	1	0	0	2	24	8	1	0	30	—	—	0
White Cheddar	1 oz	100	1	0	0	3	22	0	1	20	280	—	—	0

ROCKFISH

FOOD	PORTION	CALS	FAT	SAT FAT	CHOL	PROT	CARB	SUGAR	FIBER	CALCI	SOD	POTAS	FOLIC	VIT C
pacific cooked	3 oz	103	2	tr	38	20	0	—	—	10	65	442	—	—
pacific cooked	1 fillet (5.2 oz)	180	3	1	66	36	0	—	—	18	114	774	—	—
pacific raw	3 oz	80	1	tr	29	16	0	—	—	8	51	344	—	—

ROE

(*see also individual fish names*)

FOOD	PORTION	CALS	FAT	SAT FAT	CHOL	PROT	CARB	SUGAR	FIBER	CALCI	SOD	POTAS	FOLIC	VIT C
fish	1 oz	11	tr	tr	30	2	tr	—	—	—	—	—	—	—
fresh baked	1 oz	58	2	1	136	8	1	—	—	—	—	—	—	—

ROLLS

FROZEN

FOOD	PORTION	CALS	FAT	SAT FAT	CHOL	PROT	CARB	SUGAR	FIBER	CALCI	SOD	POTAS	FOLIC	VIT C
NEW YORK														
Garlic	1 (2 oz)	210	10	2	0	3	26	1	1	0	370	—	—	0
PILLSBURY														
Dinner Rolls Crusty French	1	110	2	0	0	4	19	2	0	0	220	—	—	0
SARA LEE														
Deluxe Cinnamon Rolls w/o Icing	1 (2.7 oz)	370	15	9	40	5	41	21	1	20	300	—	—	0
READY-TO-EAT														
bialy	1 (2.2 oz)	138	0	0	0	14	32	—	1	—	167	—	—	—

FOOD	PORTION	CALS	FAT	SAT FAT	CHOL	PROT	CARB	SUGAR	FIBER	CALCI	SOD	POTAS	FOLIC	VIT C
brioche sweet roll	1 (3.5 oz)	410	23	14	190	10	41	5	3	43	495	201	—	tr
brown & serve	1 (1 oz)	85	2	tr	0	2	14	—	—	34	148	38	8	—
cheese	1 (2.3 oz)	238	12	4	—	5	29	—	—	78	236	—	—	—
cinnamon raisin	1 (2¾ in)	223	10	3	40	4	31	—	1	43	229	67	14	1
dinner	1 (1 oz)	85	2	tr	0	2	14	—	—	34	148	38	8	—
egg	1 (2½ in)	107	2	1	—	3	18	—	1	21	191	—	—	0
french	1 (1.3 oz)	105	2	tr	0	3	19	—	—	35	232	43	—	0
hamburger	1 (1½ oz)	123	2	1	—	4	22	—	—	60	241	60	—	—
hamburger multi-grain	1 (1½ oz)	113	2	1	0	4	19	—	2	41	197	—	—	0
hamburger reduced calorie	1 (1½ oz)	84	1	tr	0	4	18	—	3	26	190	34	—	—
hard	1 (3½ in)	167	2	tr	0	6	30	—	—	54	310	61	8	0
hot cross bun	1	202	4	—	—	5	38	—	1	72	—	—	—	0
hotdog	1 (1½ oz)	123	2	1	—	4	22	—	—	60	241	60	—	—
hotdog reduced calorie	1 (1½ oz)	84	1	tr	0	4	18	—	3	26	190	34	—	—
hotdog whole wheat	1 (1.5 oz)	110	2	0	0	5	19	2	2	20	220	—	—	0
kaiser	1 (3½ in)	167	2	tr	0	6	30	—	—	54	310	61	8	0
oat bran	1 (1.2 oz)	78	2	tr	0	3	13	—	1	28	136	—	—	0
rye	1 (1 oz)	81	1	tr	0	3	15	—	—	9	253	51	—	0
submarine	1 (4.7 oz)	155	2	tr	tr	5	30	—	—	24	313	49	—	0
wheat	1 (1 oz)	77	2	tr	0	2	13	—	—	50	96	—	—	0
whole wheat	1 (1 oz)	75	1	tr	0	3	15	—	—	30	135	77	8	0
BREAD DU JOUR														
Cracked Wheat	1 (1.2 oz)	100	1	0	0	3	17	2	1	40	200	—	16	0
Italian	1 (1.2 oz)	90	1	0	0	3	16	2	0	40	190	—	16	0
Sourdough	1 (1.2 oz)	90	1	0	0	3	17	1	0	100	190	—	24	0
COUNTRY KITCHEN														
Wheat Light	1	80	2	0	0	4	17	1	4	60	160	—	32	0
FREIHOFER'S														
Brown 'N Serve	1 (1 oz)	80	2	0	0	3	13	1	1	0	160	—	24	0
NATURAL OVENS														
Best Burger Bun	1	178	4	0	0	4	29	3	3	50	150	—	40	12
Better Wheat Buns	1	140	2	0	0	4	30	4	5	150	120	—	80	0
Gourmet Dinner	1	70	1	0	0	3	15	3	4	100	70	0	0	0
PEPPERIDGE FARM														
Brown & Serve Club	1 (1.6 oz)	120	1	0	0	5	22	1	2	40	240	—	—	0
Dinner Rolls Finger Poppy	1 (0.9 oz)	80	2	1	<5	3	12	2	tr	20	125	—	24	0
Parker House	1 (0.9 oz)	80	2	1	<5	2	13	2	tr	0	120	—	24	0

FOOD	PORTION	CALS	FAT	SAT FAT	CHOL	PROT	CARB	SUGAR	FIBER	CALCI	SOD	POTAS	FOLIC	VIT C
STROEHMANN														
Hamburger	1 (1.4 oz)	100	2	0	0	3	21	3	tr	20	210	—	40	0
Hamburger Potato	1 (1.9 oz)	140	2	0	0	4	28	5	tr	60	260	—	60	0
Hot Dog	1 (1.4 oz)	100	2	0	0	3	21	3	tr	20	210	—	40	0
Hot Dog Potato	1 (1.9 oz)	140	2	0	0	4	28	5	tr	60	260	—	60	0
WONDER														
Brown & Serve	1 (1 oz)	80	2	1	0	2	13	1	0	20	150	—	24	0
Brown & Serve Sourdough	1 (1 oz)	70	2	0	0	2	13	1	0	20	130	—	24	0
Brown & Serve Wheat	1 (1 oz)	80	2	0	0	2	13	1	0	40	140	—	16	0
Bun	1 (3 oz)	220	3	1	0	7	42	6	1	60	430	—	60	0
Club French	1 (1.6 oz)	120	2	0	0	4	23	2	0	20	230	—	—	0
Club Grain	1 (1.6 oz)	120	2	0	0	4	23	2	1	20	210	—	—	0
Club Sourdough	1 (1.6 oz)	120	2	0	0	4	23	1	0	20	230	—	—	0
Dinner	2 (1.6 oz)	130	1	0	0	4	25	3	1	60	240	—	32	0
Dinner Honey Rich	1 (1.3 oz)	100	2	0	0	3	17	3	0	20	160	—	32	0
Dinner Wheat	2 (1.6 oz)	140	3	0	0	3	24	4	1	60	240	—	16	0
Hamburger	1 (1.5 oz)	110	2	0	0	3	21	3	0	20	220	—	32	0
Hamburger	1 (2 oz)	150	2	0	0	4	28	4	1	40	290	—	40	0
Hamburger	1 (2.5 oz)	180	3	0	0	7	32	2	2	100	370	—	40	0
Hamburger Wheat	1 (1.5 oz)	120	2	1	0	4	21	1	1	60	210	—	—	0
Hamburger Wheat	1 (1.9 oz)	140	2	0	0	5	24	1	2	60	280	—	32	0
Hoagie French	1 (3 oz)	220	3	1	0	7	41	3	1	20	410	—	—	0
Hoagie Grain	1 (3 oz)	220	3	1	0	7	41	4	2	20	370	—	—	0
Hoagie Sourdough	1 (3 oz)	220	3	1	0	8	41	2	1	60	410	—	—	0
Hot Dog	1 (2 oz)	160	3	1	0	4	29	6	0	40	300	—	—	0
Kaiser	1 (2.2 oz)	180	3	1	0	5	33	2	1	60	270	—	—	0
Kaiser Hoagie	1 (3 oz)	220	3	1	0	7	41	3	1	20	410	—	—	0
Multigrain	1 (1.8 oz)	140	2	1	0	4	25	4	1	0	210	—	—	0
Potato Bun	1 (1.5 oz)	110	1	0	0	4	22	3	1	40	220	—	24	0
Steak	1 (2.5 oz)	190	3	1	0	6	36	1	1	60	360	—	60	0
REFRIGERATED														
cinnamon w/ frosting	1	109	4	1	—	2	17	—	—	10	250	19	—	—
crescent	1 (1 oz)	98	4	1	0	2	14	—	—	6	341	45	—	0
PILLSBURY														
Apple Cinnamon	1 (1.5 oz)	150	6	2	0	2	23	11	tr	0	320	—	—	0
Caramel	1 (1.7 oz)	170	7	2	0	2	24	10	tr	0	330	—	—	0
Cinnamon w/ Icing	1 (1.5 oz)	150	6	2	0	2	23	10	tr	0	340	—	—	0
Cinnamon w/ Icing Reduced Fat	1 (1.5 oz)	140	4	1	0	2	24	10	tr	0	340	—	—	0

FOOD	PORTION	CALS	FAT	SAT FAT	CHOL	PROT	CARB	SUGAR	FIBER	CALCI	SOD	POTAS	FOLIC	VIT C
PILLSBURY (CONT.)														
Cinnamon Raisin w/ Icing	1 (1.7 oz)	170	6	2	0	2	26	11	tr	0	320	—	—	0
Cornbread Twists	1 (1.4 oz)	140	6	2	0	3	18	4	0	0	330	—	—	0
Crecents Reduced Fat	1 (1 oz)	100	5	1	0	2	12	2	0	0	230	—	—	0
Crescent	1 (1 oz)	110	6	2	0	2	11	2	0	0	220	—	—	0
Dinner	1 (1.4 oz)	110	2	0	0	4	18	3	1	0	270	—	—	0
Dinner Wheat	1 (1.4 oz)	110	2	0	0	4	18	3	1	0	270	—	—	0
Orange Sweet Roll w/ Icing	1 (1.7 oz)	150	7	2	0	2	25	10	tr	0	340	—	—	0
ROSE APPLE														
fresh	3.5 oz	32	tr	—	0	1	7	—	—	20	—	—	—	22
ROSE HIP														
fresh	1 oz	26	0	0	0	1	5	—	—	73	42	83	—	tr
ROSELLE														
fresh	1 cup	28	tr	—	0	1	6	—	—	123	3	118	—	7
ROSEMARY														
dried	1 tsp	4	tr	—	0	tr	1	—	—	15	1	11	—	1
ROUGHY														
orange baked	3 oz	75	1	tr	22	16	0	—	—	—	69	—	—	—
RUTABAGA														
cooked mashed	½ cup	41	tr	tr	0	1	9	—	—	50	22	344	19	26
raw cubed	½ cup	25	tr	tr	0	1	6	—	—	33	14	236	14	18
SABLEFISH														
baked	3 oz	213	17	3	53	15	0	—	—	—	61	390	—	—
fillet baked	5.3 oz	378	30	6	95	26	0	—	—	—	108	693	—	—
smoked	3 oz	218	17	4	55	15	0	—	—	—	626	401	—	—
smoked	1 oz	72	6	1	18	5	0	—	—	—	206	132	—	—
SAFFLOWER														
seeds dried	1 oz	147	11	1	0	5	10	—	—	22	—	—	—	—
SAFFRON														
saffron	1 tsp	2	tr	—	0	tr	tr	—	—	1	1	12	—	—
SAGE														
ground	1 tsp	2	tr	tr	0	tr	tr	—	—	12	tr	7	—	tr
SALAD														
MIX														
DOLE														
All American Toss	2 cups (3.5 oz)	50	1	0	<5	4	7	4	2	40	160	—	—	12
American Blend	1½ cups (3 oz)	15	0	0	0	1	3	2	1	20	10	—	—	12
Classic	1½ cups (3 oz)	15	0	0	0	1	4	2	1	20	15	—	—	6
Classic Romaine Blend	1½ cups (3 oz)	15	0	0	0	1	3	2	1	20	10	—	—	9

FOOD	PORTION	CALS	FAT	SAT FAT	CHOL	PROT	CARB	SUGAR	FIBER	CALCI	SOD	POTAS	FOLIC	VIT C
DOLE (CONT.)														
Coleslaw	1½ cups (3 oz)	25	0	0	0	1	5	3	2	40	25	—	—	36
European Special Blend	2 cups (3 oz)	15	0	0	0	1	3	2	1	10	15	—	—	9
Garlic Caesar Complete w/ Dressing	1½ cups (3.5 oz)	180	15	3	5	3	8	7	1	60	420	—	—	18
Greek Marinade	1½ cups (3.5 oz)	100	8	2	<5	2	5	3	1	40	340	—	—	15
Greener Selection	1½ cups (3 oz)	15	0	0	0	1	3	2	1	20	10	—	—	12
Light Caesar Complete w/ Dressing	1½ cups (3.5 oz)	60	1	0	0	3	10	5	2	40	390	—	—	18
Light Herb Ranch Complete w/ Dressing	1½ cups (3.5 oz)	50	1	1	5	2	10	5	2	80	280	—	—	6
Light Roasted Garlic Caesar Complete w/ Dressing	1½ cups (3.5 oz)	60	1	0	0	3	11	4	1	40	400	—	—	15
Light Zesty Italian Complete w/ Dressing	1½ cups (3.5 oz)	50	1	0	0	2	11	5	1	40	290	—	—	9
Mediterranean Marinade	2 cups (3.5 oz)	90	8	1	0	1	5	3	1	40	180	—	—	18
Oriental Complete w/ Dressing	1½ cups (3.5 oz)	120	6	1	0	2	13	5	2	20	240	—	—	21
Romano Complete w/ Dressing	1½ cups (3.5 oz)	150	12	2	0	3	9	2	2	40	570	—	—	15
Sunflower Ranch Complete w/ Dressing	1½ cups (3.5 oz)	160	16	2	5	2	5	3	2	40	220	—	—	6
Tomato & Mozzarella Medley	2 cups (3.5 oz)	60	2	1	5	4	7	4	2	100	80	—	—	18
Triple Cheese Toss	2 cups (3.5 oz)	80	5	3	15	5	4	2	1	150	120	—	—	12
EARTHBOUND FARM														
Baby Caesar Mix	1 pkg (5 oz)	25	0	0	0	2	3	3	2	40	10	—	—	18
Baby Greens w/ Low Fat Honey Dijon Vinaigrette & Tomato Croutons	1 serv (3.5 oz)	90	3	0	0	3	15	6	2	60	380	—	—	5
Caesar w/ Garlic Croutons	1 serv (3.5 oz)	170	15	2	10	3	7	1	1	60	230	—	—	9
Italian Salad Organic	1⅔ cups (2.9 oz)	15	0	0	0	1	3	2	1	20	10	—	—	9
Mixed Baby Greens Organic	1 pkg (4 oz)	30	0	0	0	3	4	0	2	100	100	—	—	9

FOOD	PORTION	CALS	FAT	SAT FAT	CHOL	PROT	CARB	SUGAR	FIBER	CALCI	SOD	POTAS	FOLIC	VIT C
EARTHBOUND FARM (CONT.)														
Organic Baby Greens w/ Vinaigrette & Garlic Croutons	1 serv (3.5 oz)	230	20	3	0	3	11	0	1	60	290	—	—	5
Organic Baby Spinach w/ Sesame Soy Vinaigrette & Peanuts	1 serv (3.5 oz)	150	11	2	0	5	8	4	2	60	340	—	—	9
Organic Italian Salad w/ Blue Cheese Dressing & Walnuts	1 serv (3.5 oz)	190	17	3	15	4	4	2	1	60	210	—	—	6
Romaine Blend Organic	1⅔ cups (2.9 oz)	15	0	0	0	1	3	2	1	20	10	—	—	12
FRESH EXPRESS														
Baby Spinach Trio	4 cups (3 oz)	20	0	0	0	2	4	1	1	80	55	—	—	21
Fancy Field Greens	1½ cups (3 oz)	15	0	0	0	1	3	1	2	20	15	—	—	12
Original Iceberg Garden w/ Zip	1½ cups (3 oz)	15	0	0	0	1	3	2	1	20	10	—	—	6
Veggie Lover's	1½ cups (3 oz)	20	0	0	0	1	4	2	1	20	15	—	—	15
KRAKUS														
Bordeaux	1 pkg (5 oz)	35	0	0	0	2	5	1	2	80	20	—	—	6
READY PAC														
All American	2.5 cups	15	0	0	0	1	3	1	1	20	10	—	—	4
Bowl Salad Chef	1 pkg	350	25	8	70	21	9	5	2	350	1060	—	—	6
Bowl Salad Chicken Caesar	1 pkg	380	27	7	75	26	8	3	2	350	1050	—	—	24
Bowl Salad Greek	1 pkg	400	35	8	20	6	5	2	3	150	910	—	—	21
Bowl Salad Spinach Bacon	1 pkg	300	17	6	155	17	22	13	1	150	980	—	—	4
Bowl Salad Spring Mix Veggie	1 pkg	330	23	5	15	12	18	6	3	300	1120	—	—	48
Caesar Romaine	1½ cups	15	0	0	0	1	2	1	1	20	5	—	—	5
Classic Crisp Salad	2¼ cups	10	0	0	0	tr	2	tr	tr	20	5	—	—	9
Continental	3 cups	20	0	0	0	1	4	2	2	40	15	—	—	15
Costa Brava	3 cups	15	0	0	0	1	3	2	2	40	20	—	—	15
Hearty Green Salad	2½ cups	10	0	0	0	tr	2	tr	tr	20	5	—	—	9
Lafayette	3 cups	10	0	0	0	0	3	1	1	20	5	—	—	5
Milano	3 cups	15	0	0	0	1	3	0	2	40	15	—	—	9
Organic Caesar Romaine	2¼ cups	15	0	0	0	tr	2	tr	tr	20	20	—	—	9
Organic Mesclun Blend	1 pkg (4.5 oz)	35	0	0	0	3	7	0	3	40	40	—	—	6

FOOD	PORTION	CALS	FAT	SAT FAT	CHOL	PROT	CARB	SUGAR	FIBER	CALCI	SOD	POTAS	FOLIC	VIT C
READY PAC (CONT.)														
Organic Monterey	3 cups	15	0	0	0	1	3	1	2	40	10	—	—	18
Parisian	2 cups	20	0	0	0	1	4	1	1	40	20	—	—	12
Portofino	1 pkg (5 oz)	25	0	0	0	3	4	0	2	150	125	—	—	0
Santa Barbara	3½ cups	15	0	0	0	1	3	1	tr	20	20	—	—	0
Spring Mix	1 pkg (5 oz)	35	0	0	0	3	7	0	3	40	40	—	—	6
SUDDENLY SALAD														
Caesar	¾ cup	220	9	2	0	5	30	3	1	20	580	130	—	0
Caesar Low Fat Recipe	¾ cup	170	3	0	0	5	30	3	1	20	580	130	—	0
Italian Pepperoni	1 cup	190	4	1	0	6	35	7	2	20	680	200	—	0
Italian Pepperoni Low Fat Recipe	1 cup	180	2	0	0	6	35	7	2	20	680	200	—	0
Ranch & Bacon	¾ cup	330	20	3	15	7	30	3	1	20	480	200	—	0
Ranch & Bacon Low Fat Recipe	¾ cup	180	2	0	<5	7	30	3	1	20	530	200	—	0
WEIGHT WATCHERS														
Caesar Salad	1 serv (3.5 oz)	60	0	0	0	2	11	1	1	40	600	—	—	9
Caesar Salad w/ Cookies	1 pkg (4.3 oz)	160	3	1	0	4	29	12	3	40	670	—	—	9
European Salad	1 serv (3.5 oz)	60	0	0	0	2	13	9	2	40	530	—	—	9
European Salad w/ Cookies	1 pkg (4.3 oz)	160	3	1	0	3	31	11	2	40	620	—	—	9
Garden Salad	1 serv (3.5 oz)	60	0	0	0	2	12	4	1	20	270	—	—	9
Garden Salad w/ Cookies	1 pkg (4 oz)	120	2	1	0	3	24	10	2	20	340	—	—	9
TAKE-OUT														
caesar	2 cups (5 oz)	235	20	2	10	5	11	3	1	40	440	—	—	24
chef w/o dressing	1½ cups	386	28	13	244	24	9	—	—	317	279	330	56	15
tossed w/o dressing	1½ cups	32	tr	0	0	3	7	—	—	26	53	356	77	48
tossed w/o dressing	¾ cup	16	0	0	0	1	3	—	—	13	27	179	39	24
tossed w/o dressing w/ cheese & egg	1½ cups	102	6	3	98	9	5	—	—	100	119	371	85	10
tossed w/o dressing w/ chicken	1½ cups	105	2	tr	72	17	4	—	—	37	209	447	67	17
tossed w/o dressing w/ pasta & seafood	1½ cups (14.6 oz)	380	21	3	50	16	32	—	—	73	1572	600	100	38
tossed w/o dressing w/ shrimp	1½ cups	107	2	tr	180	15	7	—	—	60	487	404	87	9
waldorf	½ cup	79	6	2	8	1	6	—	1	12	49	78	6	2

SALAD DRESSING

FOOD	PORTION	CALS	FAT	SAT FAT	CHOL	PROT	CARB	SUGAR	FIBER	CALCI	SOD	POTAS	FOLIC	VIT C
MIX														
ET TU														
Caesar Salad Kit	1 serv	140	12	1	5	2	6	0	0	0	115	—	—	0
GOOD SEASONS														
Cheese Garlic as prep	2 tbsp (1 oz)	140	16	3	0	0	1	1	0	0	330	15	—	0
Fat Free Honey Mustard as prep	2 tbsp (1.2 oz)	20	0	0	0	0	5	4	0	0	280	30	—	0
Fat Free Italian as prep	2 tbsp (1.1 oz)	10	0	0	0	0	2	3	0	0	290	110	—	0
Fat Free Ranch as prep	2 tbsp (1.2 oz)	20	0	0	0	0	5	4	0	0	250	30	—	0
Fat Free Zesty Herb as prep	2 tbsp (1.1 oz)	10	0	0	0	0	2	1	0	0	260	70	—	0
Garlic & Herbs as prep	2 tbsp (1 oz)	140	15	2	0	0	1	1	0	0	340	10	—	0
Gourmet Parmesan Italian as prep	2 tbsp (1.1 oz)	150	16	3	0	0	2	1	0	0	330	25	—	0
Honey French as prep	2 tbsp (1.2 oz)	160	15	2	0	0	5	4	0	0	250	30	—	0
Honey Mustard as prep	2 tbsp (1.1 oz)	150	15	2	0	0	3	2	0	0	240	15	—	0
Italian as prep	2 tbsp	130	14	2	0	0	3	1	—	—	340	—	—	—
Italian not prep	⅛ pkg (3 g)	5	0	0	0	0	1	tr	—	—	320	—	—	—
Mexican Spice as prep	2 tbsp (1.1 oz)	140	15	3	0	0	2	1	0	0	310	65	—	0
Mild Italian as prep	2 tbsp (1.1 oz)	150	15	3	0	0	2	2	0	0	370	10	—	0
Oriental Sesame as prep	2 tbsp (1.1 oz)	150	16	3	0	0	3	2	0	0	360	15	—	0
Reduced Calorie Italian as prep	2 tbsp (1 oz)	50	5	1	0	0	2	1	0	0	280	15	0	—
Reduced Calorie Zesty Italian as prep	2 tbsp (1 oz)	50	5	1	0	0	2	1	0	0	260	30	—	0
Roasted Garlic as prep	2 tbsp (1.1 oz)	150	15	2	0	0	2	1	0	0	340	15	—	0
Zesty Italian as prep	2 tbsp (1 oz)	140	15	2	0	0	1	1	0	0	220	15	—	0
MCCORMICK														
Mediterrenean Potato Salad	1 tbsp	25	0	0	—	tr	4	3	1	—	460	—	—	—
Pasta Salad Vinaigrette	1 tsp (5 g)	15	0	0	—	0	2	1	—	—	590	—	—	—

FOOD	PORTION	CALS	FAT	SAT FAT	CHOL	PROT	CARB	SUGAR	FIBER	CALCI	SOD	POTAS	FOLIC	VIT C
READY-TO-EAT														
blue cheese	1 tbsp	77	8	2	—	1	1	—	—	12	—	—	—	tr
french	1 tbsp	67	6	2	—	tr	3	—	—	2	214	12	—	—
french reduced calorie	1 tbsp	22	1	tr	1	0	4	—	—	2	128	13	—	—
italian	1 tbsp	69	7	1	—	tr	2	—	—	1	116	2	—	—
italian reduced calorie	1 tbsp	16	2	tr	1	tr	1	—	—	0	118	2	—	—
russian	1 tbsp	76	8	1	—	tr	2	—	—	3	133	24	—	1
russian reduced calorie	1 tbsp	23	1	tr	1	tr	5	—	—	3	141	26	—	—
sesame seed	1 tbsp	68	7	1	0	1	1	—	—	—	153	—	—	—
thousand island	1 tbsp	59	6	1	—	tr	2	—	—	2	109	18	—	—
thousand island reduced calorie	1 tbsp	24	2	tr	2	tr	3	—	—	2	153	17	—	—
ANNIE CHUN'S														
Lemongrass	2 tbsp	60	3	0	0	0	6	5	0	0	75	—	—	0
Sesame Cilantro	1 tbsp	4	0	—	0	0	4	4	0	0	400	—	—	0
CARB OPTIONS														
Italian	2 tbsp	70	8	1	0	0	0	0	0	0	350	—	—	0
Ranch	2 tbsp	150	17	3	10	0	0	0	0	0	210	—	—	0
DREW'S														
Low Carb Garlic Italian	1 tbsp	80	9	1	0	0	0	0	0	—	90	—	—	—
Low Carb Lemon Tahini Goddess	1 tbsp	80	9	1	0	0	1	0	0	—	90	—	—	—
Low Carb Sesame Orange	1 tbsp	80	9	1	0	0	2	0	0	—	90	—	—	—
ESTEE														
Creamy French	2 tbsp (1 oz)	10	0	0	0	0	2	2	—	—	80	0	—	—
Italian	2 tbsp	5	0	0	0	0	1	1	0	—	80	0	—	—
HELLMANN'S														
Citrus Splash Ruby Red Ginger	2 tbsp (1 oz)	90	7	1	—	0	8	7	—	—	400	—	—	6
KRAFT														
⅓ Less Fat Catalina	2 tbsp (1.2 oz)	80	5	1	0	0	9	8	0	0	400	70	—	0
⅓ Less Fat Cucumber Ranch	2 tbsp (1.1 oz)	60	5	1	0	0	2	2	0	0	480	20	—	0
⅓ Less Fat Italian	2 tbsp (1.1 oz)	70	7	1	0	0	3	2	0	20	240	25	—	0
⅓ Less Fat Ranch	2 tbsp (1.1 oz)	110	11	2	10	0	1	1	0	0	310	40	—	0
⅓ Less Fat Thousand Island	2 tbsp (1.2 oz)	70	5	1	10	0	7	5	0	0	340	60	—	0
Bacon & Tomato	2 tbsp (1.1 oz)	140	14	3	<5	tr	2	2	0	0	280	35	—	0
Buttermilk Ranch	2 tbsp (1.1 oz)	150	16	3	<5	0	1	tr	0	0	240	20	—	0

FOOD	PORTION	CALS	FAT	SAT FAT	CHOL	PROT	CARB	SUGAR	FIBER	CALCI	SOD	POTAS	FOLIC	VIT C
KRAFT (CONT.)														
Caesar Italian	2 tbsp (1.1 oz)	100	10	2	0	tr	2	1	0	20	480	25	—	0
Caesar Ranch	2 tbsp (1.1 oz)	110	11	2	10	1	1	0	0	20	290	30	—	0
Catalina	2 tbsp (1.1 oz)	120	10	2	0	0	7	7	0	0	390	35	—	0
Catalina w/ Honey	2 tbsp (1.1 oz)	130	11	2	0	0	7	6	0	0	320	70	—	0
Classic Caesar	2 tbsp (1.1 oz)	110	11	2	10	1	1	0	0	20	290	30	—	0
Coleslaw	2 tbsp (1.1 oz)	130	11	2	15	0	7	7	0	0	410	5	—	0
Creamy French	2 tbsp (1.1 oz)	160	15	3	0	0	5	5	0	0	270	20	—	0
Creamy Garlic	2 tbsp (1.1 oz)	110	11	2	0	0	2	2	0	0	360	25	—	0
Creamy Italian	2 tbsp (1.1 oz)	110	11	2	0	0	2	2	0	0	250	15	—	0
Cucumber Ranch	2 tbsp (1.1 oz)	140	15	2	0	0	2	2	0	0	220	20	—	0
Free Blue Cheese	2 tbsp (1.2 oz)	45	0	0	0	0	11	2	1	0	360	30	—	0
Free Caesar Italian	2 tbsp (1.2 oz)	25	0	0	0	tr	4	3	0	20	480	50	—	0
Free Catalina	2 tbsp (1.2 oz)	35	0	0	0	0	8	7	tr	0	320	40	—	0
Free Classic Caesar	2 tbsp (1.2 oz)	45	0	0	0	tr	11	2	tr	0	360	50	—	0
Free Creamy Italian	2 tbsp (1.2 oz)	50	0	0	0	0	12	4	tr	0	330	25	—	0
Free French	2 tbsp (1.2 oz)	45	0	0	0	0	11	5	tr	0	300	25	—	0
Free Garlic Ranch	2 tbsp (1.2 oz)	45	0	0	0	0	11	2	1	0	320	30	—	0
Free Honey Dijon	2 tbsp (1.2 oz)	45	0	0	0	0	10	4	1	0	330	35	—	0
Free Italian	2 tbsp (1.2 oz)	20	0	0	0	0	4	2	0	0	430	40	—	0
Free Peppercorn Ranch	2 tbsp (1.2 oz)	45	0	0	0	0	11	2	tr	0	330	35	—	0
Free Ranch	1 tbsp (1.2 oz)	50	0	0	0	0	11	2	1	0	350	30	—	0
Free Red Wine Vinegar	2 tbsp (1.1 oz)	15	0	0	0	0	3	3	0	0	410	10	—	0
Free Thousand Island	2 tbsp (1.2 oz)	40	0	0	0	0	9	5	1	0	280	40	—	0
Garlic Ranch	2 tbsp (1.1 oz)	180	19	3	10	0	1	tr	0	0	270	15	—	0
Herb Vinaigrette	2 tbsp (1.1 oz)	140	15	2	0	0	tr	0	0	0	250	10	—	0
Honey Dijon	2 tbsp (1.1 oz)	110	10	2	0	0	6	4	0	0	210	35	—	0
Honey Mustard	2 tbsp (1.1 oz)	110	10	2	0	0	6	4	0	0	210	35	—	0
House Italian w/ Olive Oil Blend	2 tbsp (1.1 oz)	120	12	2	<5	0	2	2	0	0	240	20	—	0
Peppercorn Ranch	2 tbsp (1 oz)	170	18	3	10	tr	1	1	0	20	270	15	—	0
Pesto Italian	2 tbsp (1.1 oz)	90	9	2	0	0	2	1	0	0	310	15	—	0
Ranch	2 tbsp (1 oz)	170	18	3	10	0	1	1	0	0	280	10	—	0
Roka Blue Cheese	2 tbsp (1.1 oz)	130	13	3	<5	tr	2	tr	tr	0	310	35	—	0
Russian	2 tbsp (1.2 oz)	130	10	2	0	0	10	10	0	0	310	40	—	0
Sour Cream & Onion Ranch	2 tbsp (1 oz)	170	18	3	10	0	1	1	0	0	250	45	—	0
Thousand Island	2 tbsp (1.1 oz)	110	10	2	10	0	5	4	0	0	310	40	—	0

FOOD	PORTION	CALS	FAT	SAT FAT	CHOL	PROT	CARB	SUGAR	FIBER	CALCI	SOD	POTAS	FOLIC	VIT C
KRAFT (CONT.)														
Thousand Island w/ Bacon	2 tbsp (1.1 oz)	130	12	2	0	0	5	5	0	0	200	35	—	0
Tomato & Herb Italian	2 tbsp (1.1 oz)	100	9	1	0	0	3	3	0	0	340	80	—	0
Zesty Italian	2 tbsp (1.1 oz)	110	11	1	0	0	2	1	0	0	540	10	—	0
LAMARTINIQUE														
Blue Cheese Vinaigrette	2 tbsp	160	17	6	5	2	0	0	0	40	450	—	—	0
Poppy Seed	2 tbsp	170	15	4	0	0	8	7	0	0	330	—	—	0
NASOYA														
Creamy Dill	2 tbsp	70	7	1	0	0	2	1	0	—	135	—	—	—
Creamy Italian	2 tbsp	60	6	1	0	0	2	1	0	—	180	—	—	—
Garden Herb	2 tbsp	70	7	1	0	0	2	1	0	—	140	—	—	—
Sesame Garlic	2 tbsp	60	6	1	0	0	2	1	0	—	130	—	—	—
Thousand Island	2 tbsp	70	6	1	0	0	3	2	0	—	115	—	—	—
NEWMAN'S OWN														
Balsamic Vinaigrette	2 tbsp (1.1 oz)	90	9	1	0	0	3	1	0	0	350	—	—	0
Caesar	2 tbsp (1.1 oz)	150	16	2	<5	1	1	1	0	0	450	—	—	0
Light Italian	2 tbsp (1.1 oz)	20	1	0	0	0	3	2	0	0	380	—	—	0
Olive Oil & Vinegar	2 tbsp (1 oz)	150	16	3	0	0	1	1	0	0	150	—	—	0
Ranch	2 tbsp (1 oz)	180	19	3	<5	1	2	1	0	0	170	—	—	0
OLD DUTCH														
Sweet & Sour	2 tbsp	50	0	0	0	0	13	13	0	0	480	—	—	0
PAUL'S														
No-Fat Raspberry & Balsamic	2 tbsp	20	0	0	0	0	5	5	—	—	45	—	—	—
No-Oil Orange & Basil	2 tbsp	15	0	0	0	0	4	4	0	—	64	—	—	—
SEVEN SEAS														
⅓ Less Fat Creamy Italian	2 tbsp (1.1 oz)	60	5	1	0	0	2	2	0	0	500	0	—	0
⅓ Less Fat Italian w/ Olive Oil Blend	2 tbsp (1.1 oz)	45	4	0	0	0	2	2	0	0	460	10	—	0
⅓ Less Fat Ranch	2 tbsp (1.1 oz)	100	9	2	0	0	5	2	0	0	320	10	—	0
⅓ Less Fat Red Wine Vinegar & Oil	2 tbsp (1.1 oz)	45	4	0	0	0	3	2	0	0	320	10	—	0
⅓ Less Fat Viva Italian	2 tbsp (1.1 oz)	45	4	0	0	0	2	1	0	0	320	10	—	0
2 Cheese Italian	2 tbsp (1.1 oz)	70	7	1	0	0	3	2	0	0	240	25	—	0
Chunky Blue Cheese	2 tbsp (1.1 oz)	130	13	3	<5	tr	2	tr	tr	0	310	35	—	0
Classic Caesar	2 tbsp (1.1 oz)	100	10	2	0	tr	2	1	0	20	480	25	—	0

FOOD	PORTION	CALS	FAT	SAT FAT	CHOL	PROT	CARB	SUGAR	FIBER	CALCI	SOD	POTAS	FOLIC	VIT C
SEVEN SEAS (CONT.)														
Creamy Italian	2 tbsp (1.1 oz)	120	12	2	0	0	1	1	0	0	510	10	—	0
Free Ranch	2 tbsp (1.2 oz)	45	0	0	0	0	11	2	1	0	330	35	—	0
Free Red Wine Vinegar	2 tbsp (1.1 oz)	15	0	0	0	0	3	3	0	0	410	10	—	0
Free Sour Cream & Onion Ranch	2 tbsp (1.2 oz)	50	0	0	0	0	11	3	1	0	300	35	—	0
Free Viva Italian	2 tbsp (1.1 oz)	10	0	0	0	0	2	1	1	0	480	30	—	0
Green Goddess	2 tbsp (1.1 oz)	130	13	2	0	0	1	tr	0	0	260	15	—	0
Herbs & Spices	2 tbsp (1.1 oz)	90	9	1	0	0	1	1	0	0	290	5	—	0
Ranch	2 tbsp (1.1 oz)	160	17	3	<5	0	2	1	0	0	260	20	—	0
Red Wine Vinegar & Oil	2 tbsp (1.1 oz)	90	9	1	0	0	2	2	0	0	500	10	—	0
Viva Italian	2 tbsp (1.1 oz)	90	9	1	0	0	2	1	0	0	370	10	—	0
Viva Russian	2 tbsp (1.1 oz)	150	16	3	0	0	3	2	0	0	210	50	—	0
STEEL'S														
Honey Mustard	1 tbsp	90	7	1	0	0	0	0	0	—	125	—	—	—
Sweet Ginger Lime	1 tbsp	68	7	0	0	0	1	0	1	—	0	—	—	—
WEIGHT WATCHERS														
Fat Free Caesar	1 pkg (0.75 oz)	5	0	0	0	0	1	1	0	0	290	—	—	0
Fat Free Caesar	2 tbsp	10	0	0	0	0	1	1	0	0	390	—	—	0
Fat Free Creamy Italian	2 tbsp	30	0	0	0	0	7	2	0	0	360	—	—	0
Fat Free French Style	2 tbsp	40	0	0	0	0	9	6	0	0	200	—	—	0
Fat Free Honey Dijon	2 tbsp	45	0	0	0	0	11	5	0	0	150	—	—	0
Fat Free Italian	2 tbsp	10	0	0	0	0	2	1	0	0	360	—	—	0
Fat Free Ranch	2 tbsp	35	0	0	0	0	7	3	0	0	270	—	—	0
Fat Free Ranch	1 pkg (0.75 oz)	25	0	0	0	0	6	2	0	0	200	—	—	0
WISHBONE														
Caesar	2 tbsp (1 oz)	90	10	2	5	1	2	2	0	0	300	—	—	0
Chunky Blue Cheese	2 tbsp (1 oz)	150	17	3	0	1	3	1	0	20	290	—	—	0
Classic House Italian	2 tbsp (1 oz)	140	14	2	5	0	2	1	0	0	360	—	—	0
Classic Olive Oil Italian	2 tbsp (1 oz)	60	5	1	0	0	4	3	0	0	350	—	—	0
Creamy Caesar	2 tbsp (1 oz)	180	18	3	10	1	1	1	0	20	290	—	—	0
Creamy Italian	2 tbsp (1 oz)	110	10	2	0	1	4	1	0	20	240	—	—	0
Creamy Roasted Garlic	2 tbsp (1 oz)	110	10	2	0	1	3	3	0	0	240	—	—	0
Deluxe French	2 tbsp (1 oz)	120	11	2	0	0	5	4	0	0	170	—	—	0
Fat Free Chunky Blue Cheese	2 tbsp (1 oz)	35	0	0	0	0	7	1	tr	20	290	—	—	0

FOOD	PORTION	CALS	FAT	SAT FAT	CHOL	PROT	CARB	SUGAR	FIBER	CALCI	SOD	POTAS	FOLIC	VIT C
WISHBONE (CONT.)														
Fat Free Creamy Italian	2 tbsp (1 oz)	35	0	0	0	0	9	3	tr	0	250	—	—	0
Fat Free Creamy Roasted Garlic	2 tbsp (1 oz)	40	0	0	0	0	9	3	0	20	280	—	—	0
Fat Free Deluxe French	2 tbsp (1 oz)	30	0	0	0	0	7	6	tr	0	230	—	—	0
Fat Free Honey Dijon	2 tbsp (1 oz)	45	0	0	0	1	10	9	0	20	270	—	—	0
Fat Free Italian	2 tbsp (1 oz)	10	0	0	0	0	2	1	0	0	280	—	—	0
Fat Free Parmesan & Onion	2 tbsp (1 oz)	45	0	0	0	1	9	2	tr	20	320	—	—	0
Fat Free Ranch	2 tbsp (1 oz)	40	0	0	0	0	9	2	tr	20	280	—	—	0
Fat Free Red Wine Vinaigrette	2 tbsp (1 oz)	35	0	0	0	0	7	6	0	0	230	—	—	0
Fat Free Sweet N' Spicy French	2 tbsp (1 oz)	30	0	0	0	0	7	6	0	0	220	—	—	0
Fat Free Thousand Island	2 tbsp (1 oz)	35	0	0	0	0	9	6	tr	0	290	—	—	0
Italian	2 tbsp	80	8	1	0	0	3	2	0	0	490	—	—	0
Lite French	2 tbsp (1 oz)	50	2	1	5	0	8	7	0	0	240	—	—	0
Lite Italian	2 tbsp (1 oz)	15	1	0	0	0	2	1	0	0	500	—	—	0
Lite Ranch	2 tbsp (1 oz)	100	8	1	5	0	5	1	0	0	300	—	—	0
Olive Oil Vinaigrette	2 tbsp (1 oz)	60	5	1	0	0	4	3	0	0	250	—	—	0
Oriental	2 tbsp (1 oz)	70	5	1	0	0	5	3	0	0	440	—	—	0
Parmesan & Onion	2 tbsp (1 oz)	110	10	2	5	1	5	1	0	20	260	—	—	0
Ranch	2 tbsp (1 oz)	160	17	3	10	0	1	1	0	20	200	—	—	0
Red Wine Vinaigrette	2 tbsp (1 oz)	80	5	1	0	0	9	8	0	0	230	—	—	0
Robusto Italian	2 tbsp (1 oz)	90	8	1	0	0	4	3	0	0	550	—	—	2
Russian	2 tbsp (1 oz)	110	6	1	0	0	15	7	0	0	350	—	—	0
Sweet N' Spicy French	2 tbsp (1 oz)	140	12	2	0	0	6	5	0	0	330	—	—	0
TAKE-OUT														
vinegar & oil	1 tbsp	72	8	2	0	0	tr	—	—	—	tr	1	—	—
SALMON														
CANNED														
chum w/ bone	1 can (13.9 oz)	521	20	5	144	79	0	—	—	920	1797	—	—	—
chum w/ bone	3 oz	120	5	1	33	18	0	—	—	212	414	—	—	—
pink w/ bone	1 can (15.9 oz)	631	27	7	—	90	0	—	—	969	2514	1982	70	0
pink w/ bone	3 oz	118	5	1	—	17	0	—	—	181	471	277	13	0
sockeye w/ bone	3 oz	130	6	1	37	17	0	—	—	203	458	321	8	0
sockeye w/ bone	1 can (12.9 oz)	566	27	6	161	76	0	—	—	883	1987	1392	36	0

FOOD	PORTION	CALS	FAT	SAT FAT	CHOL	PROT	CARB	SUGAR	FIBER	CALCI	SOD	POTAS	FOLIC	VIT C
BUMBLE BEE														
Keta	½ cup (3.5 oz)	160	8	—	—	20	0	—	—	150	490	290	—	0
Red	½ cup (3.5 oz)	180	10	—	—	20	0	—	—	150	490	290	—	0
CHICKEN OF THE SEA														
Pink Chunk In Water	¼ cup	60	2	1	20	10	0	0	0	0	280	—	—	0
Pink Skinless Boneless	¼ cup	60	2	1	20	10	0	0	0	0	280	—	—	0
LIBBY'S														
Alaskan Sockeye Red	¼ cup	110	7	2	40	13	0	0	0	100	270	—	—	—
Pink Skinless Boneless	¼ cup	50	1	0	20	11	0	0	0	0	150	—	—	0
FRESH														
atlantic baked	3 oz	155	7	1	60	22	0	—	—	13	48	534	—	—
chinook baked	3 oz	196	11	3	72	22	0	—	—	24	51	429	—	4
chum baked	3 oz	131	4	1	81	22	0	—	—	12	54	467	—	—
coho cooked	½ fillet (5.4 oz)	286	12	2	76	42	0	—	—	—	91	828	—	2
coho cooked	3 oz	157	6	1	42	23	0	—	—	—	50	454	—	1
coho raw	3 oz	124	5	1	33	18	0	—	—	—	39	359	—	1
pink baked	3 oz	127	4	1	57	22	0	—	—	—	73	352	—	—
roe raw	1 oz	59	3	—	—	7	tr	—	—	—	—	—	—	5
sockeye cooked	3 oz	183	9	2	74	23	0	—	—	6	102	582	—	—
sockeye cooked	½ fillet (5.4 oz)	334	17	3	135	42	0	—	—	11	102	582	—	—
sockeye raw	3 oz	143	7	1	53	18	0	—	—	5	40	332	—	—
SMOKED														
chinook	1 oz	33	1	tr	7	5	0	—	—	3	220	49	1	—
LASCCO														
Nova Sliced	2 oz	60	1	0	20	10	3	0	0	—	960	—	—	—
TAKE-OUT														
roulette w/ spinach stuffing	1 serv (4 oz)	160	6	2	45	13	10	0	tr	40	400	—	—	6
salmon cake	1 (3 oz)	241	15	7	104	18	6	—	—	203	602	290	7	tr
SALSA														
black bean & corn	2 tbsp (1 oz)	15	0	0	0	1	3	1	tr	20	45	—	—	5
citrus	2 tbsp (1 oz)	10	0	0	0	0	2	2	0	0	7	—	—	1
peach	2 tbsp	15	0	0	0	0	4	4	0	0	90	—	—	5
CHI-CHI'S														
Con Queso	2 tbsp (1.1 oz)	90	7	3	15	3	4	3	0	80	480	—	—	0
Hot	2 tbsp (1 oz)	10	0	0	0	0	2	1	0	0	160	—	—	0
Medium	2 tbsp (1 oz)	10	0	0	0	0	2	1	0	0	140	—	—	0
Mild	2 tbsp (1 oz)	10	0	0	0	0	1	1	0	0	140	—	—	0
Picante Hot	2 tbsp (1 oz)	10	0	0	0	0	2	2	0	0	270	—	—	0
Picante Medium	2 tbsp (1 oz)	10	0	0	0	0	2	2	0	0	200	—	—	0

FOOD	PORTION	CALS	FAT	SAT FAT	CHOL	PROT	CARB	SUGAR	FIBER	CALCI	SOD	POTAS	FOLIC	VIT C
CHI-CHI'S (CONT.)														
Picante Mild	2 tbsp (1 oz)	10	0	0	0	0	2	2	0	0	210	—	—	0
Verde Medium	2 tbsp (1.2 oz)	15	0	0	0	0	3	2	0	0	180	—	—	2
Verde Mild	2 tbsp (1.2 oz)	15	0	0	0	0	3	2	0	0	180	—	—	2
DEL SALSA														
Fire Roasted All Flavors	2 tbsp	8	0	0	0	0	2	0	0	—	70	—	—	—
GRINGO BILLY'S														
Salsa Mix	1 tsp	5	1	0	0	0	1	0	1	—	233	—	—	—
GUILTLESS GOURMET														
Roasted Red Pepper	2 tbsp	10	0	0	0	0	2	1	0	20	130	—	—	0
Southwestern Grill	2 tbsp	15	0	0	0	0	2	0	0	20	115	—	—	0
HUNT'S														
Alfresco All Varieties	2 tbsp (1.1 oz)	10	tr	tr	0	tr	2	2	tr	15	161	—		tr
Hot	2 tbsp (1.1 oz)	27	tr	0	0	1	6	1	1	10	236	—	—	5
Medium	2 tbsp (1.1 oz)	27	tr	0	0	1	6	1	1	10	236	—	—	5
Mild	2 tbsp (1.1 oz)	27	tr	0	0	1	6	1	1	10	236	—	—	5
Picante All Varieties	2 tbsp (1.1 oz)	11	tr	0	0	1	2	1	tr	5	256	—	—	2
Squeeze Mild & Medium	2 tbsp (1.1 oz)	27	tr	0	0	1	6	2	1	10	236	—	—	5
MUIR GLEN														
Black Bean & Corn Medium	2 tbsp (1.1 oz)	15	0	0	0	1	3	1	tr	0	125	—	—	4
Chipotle Medium	2 tbsp (1.1 oz)	10	0	0	0	0	2	1	0	0	125	—	—	5
Fire Roasted Tomato Medium	2 tbsp (1.1 oz)	10	0	0	0	0	2	1	0	0	125	—	—	4
Garlic Cilantro Medium	2 tbsp (1.1 oz)	10	0	0	0	0	2	1	0	0	125	—	—	5
Habanero Hot	2 tbsp (1.1 oz)	10	0	0	0	0	2	1	0	0	125	—	—	4
Organic Medium	2 tbsp (1.1 oz)	10	0	0	0	0	2	1	0	0	125	—	—	5
Organic Mild	2 tbsp (1.1 oz)	10	0	0	0	0	2	1	0	0	125	—	—	1
Roasted Garlic Medium	2 tbsp (1.1 oz)	10	0	0	0	0	2	1	0	0	125	—	—	4
NEWMAN'S OWN														
Bandito Hot	2 tbsp (1.1 oz)	10	0	0	0	0	2	1	tr	0	150	—	—	0
Bandito Medium	2 tbsp (1.1 oz)	10	0	0	0	0	2	1	tr	0	105	—	—	0
Bandito Mild	2 tbsp (1.1 oz)	10	0	0	0	0	2	1	tr	0	105	—	—	0
Peach	2 tbsp (1.1 oz)	25	0	0	0	0	6	5	1	0	90	—	—	0
Pineapple	2 tbsp (1.1 oz)	15	0	0	0	0	3	3	1	0	90	—	—	0
Roasted Garlic	2 tbsp (1.1 oz)	10	0	0	0	1	2	1	1	0	150	—	—	0
PACE														
Picante Mild or Medium	2 tbsp	10	0	0	0	0	2	1	0	0	220	—	—	2

FOOD	PORTION	CALS	FAT	SAT FAT	CHOL	PROT	CARB	SUGAR	FIBER	CALCI	SOD	POTAS	FOLIC	VIT C
PACE (CONT.)														
Thick & Chunky Mild or Medium	2 tbsp	10	0	0	0	0	2	1	0	0	220	—	—	6
ROSARITA														
Extra Chunky Medium	2 tbsp (1 oz)	7	tr	0	0	tr	1	1	tr	10	229	—	—	3
Green Tomatillo Medium	2 tbsp (1 oz)	8	tr	0	0	tr	2	2	1	5	188	—	—	1
Picante Zesty Jalapeño Hot	2 tbsp (1 oz)	8	tr	0	0	tr	2	1	1	8	246	—	—	2
Picante Zesty Jalapeño Medium	2 tbsp (1 oz)	9	tr	0	0	tr	2	1	1	7	254	—	—	1
Picante Zesty Jalapeño Mild	2 tbsp (1 oz)	8	tr	0	0	tr	2	1	tr	7	239	—	—	1
Roasted Mild	2 tbsp (1 oz)	10	tr	0	0	tr	2	1	1	12	233	—	—	3
Traditional Medium	2 tbsp (1 oz)	7	tr	0	0	tr	2	1	1	11	234	—	—	4
Traditional Mild	2 tbsp (1 oz)	7	tr	0	0	1	1	1	1	13	247	—	—	3
SNYDER'S OF HANOVER														
Mild	2 tbsp	10	0	0	0	0	2	2	0	0	220	—	—	0
TACO BELL														
Smooth 'N Zesty Picante Medium	2 tbsp (1.1 oz)	15	0	0	0	0	3	2	tr	0	190	—	—	0
Smooth 'N Zesty Picante Mild	2 tbsp (1.1 oz)	15	0	0	0	0	3	2	tr	0	190	—	—	0
Thick 'N Chunky Salsa Hot	2 tbsp (1.1 oz)	15	0	0	0	0	2	2	tr	0	240	—	—	0
Thick 'N Chunky Salsa Medium	2 tbsp (1.1 oz)	15	0	0	0	0	2	2	tr	0	240	—	—	0
Thick 'N Chunky Salsa Mild	2 tbsp (1.1 oz)	15	0	0	0	tr	3	2	tr	0	240	—	—	0
TOSTITOS														
Con Queso	2.3 oz	80	5	2	<10	2	10	tr	<2	—	560	—	—	—
Hot	2.3 oz	30	0	0	0	2	6	2	2	—	520	—	—	—
Low Fat Con Queso	2.5 oz	80	3	2	<10	2	8	tr	tr	—	560	—	—	—
Medium	2.3 oz	30	0	0	0	2	6	2	2	—	520	—	—	—
Mild	2.3 oz	30	0	0	0	2	6	2	2	—	520	—	—	—
Restaurant Style	2.2 oz	30	0	0	0	<2	6	2	<2	—	420	—	—	—
Ultimate Garden	2.4 oz	30	0	0	0	2	6	2	2	—	460	—	—	—
TREE OF LIFE														
Medium	2 tbsp (1 oz)	10	0	0	0	0	2	1	—	20	30	—	—	4
Mild	2 tbsp (1 oz)	10	0	0	0	0	2	1	—	20	30	—	—	4
UTZ														
Chunky	2 tbsp (1 fl oz)	60	0	0	0	2	14	4	4	0	190	—	—	0

FOOD	PORTION	CALS	FAT	SAT FAT	CHOL	PROT	CARB	SUGAR	FIBER	CALCI	SOD	POTAS	FOLIC	VIT C
SALSIFY														
fresh sliced cooked	½ cup	46	tr	—	0	2	10	—	—	32	11	192	—	3
raw sliced	½ cup	55	tr	—	0	2	12	—	—	40	13	255	—	5
SALT SUBSTITUTES														
EDEN														
Shiso Leaf Powder	1 tsp	0	0	0	0	0	0	0	2	0	200	—	—	0
ESTEE														
Salt-It	¼ tsp	0	0	0	0	0	0	0	0	—	560	0	—	—
HALSOSALT														
All Flavors	¼ tsp (7 g)	1	0	0	0	0	0	—	—	—	0	358	—	—
MOLLY MCBUTTER														
Lite Sodium	1 tsp	5	0	0	0	0	2	—	—	—	90	0	—	—
MORTON														
Salt Substitute	¼ tsp (1.2 g)	tr	0	0	0	0	tr	—	—	7	tr	610	—	—
MRS. DASH														
Onion & Herb	¼ tsp	0	0	0	0	0	0	0	0	—	0	10	—	—
NOSALT														
Salt Alternative	1 pkg (0.75 g)	0	0	0	0	2	0	—	—	—	0	375	—	—
SALT/SEASONED SALT														
salt	1 tbsp (18 g)	0	0	0	0	0	0	—	—	4	6976	1	—	—
salt	1 tsp (6 g)	0	0	0	0	0	0	—	—	1	2325	0	—	—
EDEN														
Atlantic Sea Salt	¼ tsp	0	0	0	0	0	0	0	0	tr	467	tr	0	0
Brittany Sea Salt	¼ tsp	0	0	0	0	0	0	0	0	tr	552	tr	0	0
MCCORMICK														
Celery Salt	¼ tsp	0	0	0	0	0	0	0	0	—	250	—	—	—
MORTON														
Garlic	1 tsp	3	tr	—	0	—	—	—	—	10	—	—	—	—
Iodized	1 tsp	tr	0	—	0	—	—	—	—	2	—	—	—	—
Kosher	1 tsp	0	0	—	0	—	—	—	—	0	—	—	—	—
Lite	¼ tsp (1.4 g)	tr	0	0	0	0	tr	—	—	1	280	350	—	—
Nature's Season Seasoning Blend	1 tsp	3	tr	—	0	—	—	—	—	5	—	—	—	—
Non-Iodized	1 tsp	0	0	—	0	—	—	—	—	2	—	—	—	—
Seasoned	1 tsp	4	tr	—	0	—	—	—	—	12	—	—	—	—
SANDWICHES														
AMY'S														
Pocket Sandwich Broccoli & Cheese	1 (4.5 oz)	270	10	4	15	8	37	4	3	—	560	—	—	—
Pocket Sandwich Roasted Vegetables	1 (4.5 oz)	220	8	2	0	6	35	5	4	—	480	—	—	—
Pocket Sandwich Spinach Feta	1 (4.5 oz)	250	9	5	20	11	34	4	3	—	590	—	—	—

FOOD	PORTION	CALS	FAT	SAT FAT	CHOL	PROT	CARB	SUGAR	FIBER	CALCI	SOD	POTAS	FOLIC	VIT C
AMY'S (CONT.)														
Pocket Sandwich Tofu Scramble	1 (4 oz)	160	6	0	0	11	23	2	tr	—	520	—	—	—
Pocket Sandwich Vegetable Pie	1 (5 oz)	300	9	2	0	5	45	5	3	—	490	—	—	—
Toaster Pops Grilled Cheese	1	180	8	4	20	8	19	3	0	—	220	—	—	—
CROISSANT POCKETS														
Chicken Parmesan	1 piece	370	20	7	15	11	36	10	4	—	760	—	—	—
HEALTHY CHOICE														
Bread Stuffs Chicken & Broccoli	1 (6.1 oz)	310	4	2	25	17	50	11	2	100	600	—	—	6
Bread Stuffs Ham & Cheese w/ Broccoli	1 (6.1 oz)	320	5	2	20	21	46	10	1	250	590	—	—	9
Bread Stuffs Italian Style Meatball	1 (6.1 oz)	330	5	2	20	16	52	12	4	200	600	—	—	0
Bread Stuffs Philly Beef Steak	1 (6.1 oz)	310	5	2	20	17	50	10	3	200	600	—	—	0
HOT POCKETS														
Four Cheese Pizza	1 (4.5 oz)	380	17	8	45	11	45	10	3	250	680	—	—	—
LEAN POCKETS														
Chicken Fajita	1 (4.5 oz)	260	7	3	25	11	38	7	3	200	730	—	—	—
SMUCKER'S														
Uncrustables Grape	1 (2 oz)	200	8	2	0	7	27	12	2	60	260	—	—	1
TAKE-OUT														
chicken fillet plain	1	515	29	9	60	24	39	—	—	60	957	358	28	9
chicken fillet w/ cheese lettuce mayonnaise & tomato	1	632	39	12	76	29	42	—	—	258	1238	334	46	3
croque monsieur	1 (12.4 oz)	765	46	26	152	41	43	9	2	1089	1018	437	41	9
fish fillet w/ tartar sauce	1	431	55	5	—	17	41	—	—	84	615	339	44	3
fish fillet w/ tartar sauce & cheese	1	524	29	8	68	21	48	—	—	185	939	353	32	3
fried egg w/ cheese	1	340	19	7	291	16	26	—	—	225	804	188	36	2
fried egg w/ cheese & ham	1	348	16	7	245	19	31	—	—	212	1005	209	43	3
ham w/ cheese	1	353	15	6	58	21	33	—	—	130	772	290	71	3
roast beef submarine sandwich w/ tomato lettuce & mayonnaise	1	411	13	7	73	29	44	—	—	41	845	330	45	6

FOOD	PORTION	CALS	FAT	SAT FAT	CHOL	PROT	CARB	SUGAR	FIBER	CALCI	SOD	POTAS	FOLIC	VIT C
roast beef w/ cheese	1	402	18	9	77	32	27	—	—	183	1634	345	41	0
roast beef plain	1	346	14	4	52	22	33	—	—	54	792	316	40	2
steak w/ tomato lettuce salt & mayonnaise	1	459	14	4	73	30	52	—	—	91	798	525	89	6
submarine w/ salami ham cheese lettuce tomato onion & oil	1	456	19	7	35	22	51	—	—	189	1650	394	—	12
tuna salad submarine sandwich w/ lettuce & oil	1	584	28	5	47	30	55	—	—	74	1294	335	58	4

SAPODILLA

FOOD	PORTION	CALS	FAT	SAT FAT	CHOL	PROT	CARB	SUGAR	FIBER	CALCI	SOD	POTAS	FOLIC	VIT C
fresh	1	140	2	—	0	1	34	—	—	36	20	328	—	25
fresh cut up	1 cup	199	3	—	0	1	48	—	—	51	29	465	—	35

SAPOTES

FOOD	PORTION	CALS	FAT	SAT FAT	CHOL	PROT	CARB	SUGAR	FIBER	CALCI	SOD	POTAS	FOLIC	VIT C
fresh	1	301	1	—	0	5	76	—	—	88	21	773	—	45

SARDINES

FOOD	PORTION	CALS	FAT	SAT FAT	CHOL	PROT	CARB	SUGAR	FIBER	CALCI	SOD	POTAS	FOLIC	VIT C
CANNED														
atlantic in oil w/ bone	1 can (3.2 oz)	192	11	1	131	23	0	—	—	351	465	365	11	—
atlantic in oil w/ bone	2	50	3	tr	34	6	0	—	—	92	121	95	3	—
pacific in tomato sauce w/ bone	1 can (13 oz)	658	44	11	225	61	0	—	—	887	1532	1262	89	4
pacific in tomato sauce w/ bone	1	68	5	1	23	6	0	—	—	91	157	130	9	tr
BUMBLE BEE														
In Hot Sauce	½ can (2 oz)	109	8	2	30	9	tr	tr	0	200	230	—	—	0
In Mustard	½ can (2 oz)	88	5	2	35	10	1	tr	0	300	260	—	—	0
In Oil	½ can (2 oz)	125	7	2	39	15	0	0	0	300	240	—	—	0
In Water	½ can (2 oz)	83	3	1	60	15	0	0	0	300	190	—	—	—
GOYA														
In Tomato Sauce	2 pieces (2.2 oz)	50	1	0	45	8	20	1	2	250	15	—	—	1
KING OSCAR														
In Olive Oil	1 can (3.75 oz)	150	11	3	120	14	0	0	0	220	340	—	—	0
Skinless Boneless In Soya Oil	3 pieces (1.9 oz)	120	7	2	20	13	0	0	0	80	350	—	—	1
SEASON														
Brisling In Water	1 can (3.75 oz)	145	10	4	120	14	0	0	0	210	340	—	—	0
FRESH														
raw	3.5 oz	135	5	—	—	19	0	—	—	85	100	—	—	—

SAUCE

(see also BARBECUE SAUCE, GRAVY, PIZZA SAUCE, SPAGHETTI SAUCE)

FOOD	PORTION	CALS	FAT	SAT FAT	CHOL	PROT	CARB	SUGAR	FIBER	CALCI	SOD	POTAS	FOLIC	VIT C
JARRED														
fish sauce chinese	1 tbsp	9	0	0	—	2	tr	—	0	2	1224	52	—	0
fish sauce vietnamese nuoc mam	1 tbsp	6	0	0	0	1	1	—	0	8	1390	52	9	0
hoisin	1 tbsp	35	1	—	0	1	7	—	tr	5	258	19	4	0
morroccan tagine	½ cup (4 oz)	70	3	0	0	2	10	10	1	20	1140	—	—	30
oyster	1 tbsp	8	0	0	0	tr	2	—	0	5	437	9	2	0
teriyaki	1 tbsp	15	0	0	0	1	3	—	—	4	690	41	4	0
A1														
Bold Steak Sauce	1 tbsp	20	0	0	0	0	5	4	—	—	190	—	—	—
ANNIE CHUN'S														
Shiitake Mushroom	1 tbsp	15	0	0	0	1	3	2	0	0	190	—	—	0
Thai Peanut	2 tbsp	120	7	1	0	4	10	8	1	0	230	—	—	—
ARMOUR														
Chili Hot Dog	¼ cup (2.2 oz)	120	9	4	20	4	5	2	0	0	310	—	—	0
Meatless Sloppy Joe Sauce	¼ cup (2.2 oz)	30	0	0	0	0	7	6	0	0	430	—	—	1
ATKINS														
Steak Sauce	1 tbsp	5	0	0	0	0	1	0	0	0	180	—	—	0
Teriyaki	1 tbsp	10	1	0	0	0	1	0	0	0	300	—	—	0
BOAR'S HEAD														
Ham Glaze Brown Sugar & Spice	2 tbsp (1.4 oz)	120	0	0	0	0	30	29	0	40	95	—	—	0
CARB OPTIONS														
Alfredo	¼ cup	110	10	4	30	1	2	0	0	40	390	—	—	0
Asian Teriyaki Marinade	1 tbsp	5	1	—	—	0	1	0	0	—	500	—	—	—
Cheese	¼ cup	90	8	3	25	2	2	0	0	60	480	—	—	0
Garden Style	½ cup	80	5	1	0	2	7	4	2	40	540	—	—	5
Steak Sauce	1 tbsp	5	0	0	0	0	1	0	0	—	200	—	—	—
CHEEZ WHIZ														
Cheese	2 tbsp (1.2 oz)	90	7	5	20	4	3	tr	0	100	540	105	—	0
Cheese Jalapeño Pepper	2 tbsp (1.2 oz)	90	7	5	25	4	3	2	0	100	510	90	—	0
Cheese Mild Salsa	2 tbsp (1.2 oz)	100	7	5	25	4	3	2	0	100	530	85	—	0
CHI-CHI'S														
Enchilada	¼ cup (2.1 oz)	30	2	1	0	0	3	0	0	0	210	—	—	0
Taco	1 tbsp (0.5 oz)	10	0	0	0	0	1	1	0	0	75	—	—	0
CHUN KING														
Sweet And Sour	2 tbsp (1.2 oz)	58	tr	0	0	tr	14	14	0	1	104	—	—	0
Teriyaki	1 tbsp (0.6 oz)	17	tr	0	0	1	3	2	0	2	917	—	—	0
Teriyaki Hot	1 tbsp (0.6 oz)	17	tr	0	0	2	3	2	0	4	995	—	—	0

FOOD	PORTION	CALS	FAT	SAT FAT	CHOL	PROT	CARB	SUGAR	FIBER	CALCI	SOD	POTAS	FOLIC	VIT C
CONSORZIO														
Marinade Baja Lime	1 tbsp	60	6	—	0	0	3	0	—	—	140	—	—	—
DEL MONTE														
Seafood Cocktail	¼ cup (2.7 oz)	100	0	0	0	1	24	22	0	0	910	—	—	2
Sloppy Joe Hickory Flavor	¼ cup (2.4 oz)	70	0	0	0	1	18	15	0	0	700	—	—	1
Sloppy Joe Original	¼ cup (2.4 oz)	70	0	0	0	1	16	13	0	0	680	—	—	1
FRITOS														
Texas-Style Chili Hearty Topping	2.3 oz	50	2	1	10	2	8	2	1	—	330	—	—	—
Utimate Taco Hearty Topping	2.3 oz	50	2	1	10	2	8	2	1	—	330	—	—	—
GEBHARDT														
Enchilada Sauce	¼ cup (2.2 oz)	35	2	1	0	1	4	0	1	1	218	—	—	1
Hot Dog Chili Sauce	¼ cup (2.2 oz)	60	3	1	1	3	6	0	2	30	274	—	—	1
Hot Sauce	1 tsp (5 g)	1	tr	0	0	tr	tr	0	0	tr	89	—	—	tr
GREEN GIANT														
Sloppy Joe	¼ cup (2.6 oz)	50	0	0	0	2	11	8	2	0	420	—	—	0
Sloppy Joe as prep w/ meat	1 serv (4.4 oz)	200	11	4	45	14	11	8	2	20	470	—	—	0
GRINGO BILLY'S														
Chipotle Dipping & Grilling Sauce	1 tsp	5	0	0	0	0	1	0	0	—	35	—	—	—
HORMEL														
Not-So-Sloppy-Joe Sauce	¼ cup (2.2 oz)	70	0	0	0	1	15	3	1	20	720	—	—	1
HOUSE OF TSANG														
Bangkok Padang	1 tbsp (0.6 oz)	45	3	1	0	1	4	3	0	0	240	—	—	0
Hoisin	1 tsp (6 g)	15	0	0	0	0	4	3	0	0	120	—	—	0
Mandarin Marinade	1 tbsp (0.6 oz)	25	0	0	0	0	6	5	0	0	680	—	—	0
Saigon Sizzle	1 tbsp (0.6 oz)	40	1	0	0	0	8	6	0	0	350	—	—	0
Spicy Brown Bean	1 tsp (6 g)	15	0	0	0	0	3	3	0	0	130	—	—	0
Stir Fry Classic	1 tbsp (0.6 oz)	25	1	0	0	0	4	3	0	0	570	—	—	0
Stir Fry Sweet & Sour	1 tbsp (0.6 oz)	30	0	0	0	0	7	6	0	0	45	—	—	0
Stir Fry Szechuan Spicy	1 tbsp (0.6 oz)	20	1	0	0	0	4	3	0	0	490	—	—	0
Sweet & Sour Concentrate	1 tsp (6 g)	10	0	0	0	0	3	2	0	0	15	—	—	0
Teriyaki Korean	1 tbsp (0.6 oz)	30	1	0	0	0	6	4	0	0	430	—	—	0
JOK'N'AL														
Cocktail	¼ cup	29	0	0	0	0	6	2	—	—	400	—	—	—
Plum	1 tbsp	10	0	0	0	0	2	1	—	—	40	—	—	—

FOOD	PORTION	CALS	FAT	SAT FAT	CHOL	PROT	CARB	SUGAR	FIBER	CALCI	SOD	POTAS	FOLIC	VIT C
JUST RITE														
Hot Dog	¼ cup (2.2 oz)	50	3	1	2	2	5	0	2	16	265	—	—	1
KIKKOMAN														
Teriyaki	1 tbsp	15	0	0	0	1	3	2	0	—	610	—	—	—
KRAFT														
Cocktail	¼ cup (2.3 oz)	60	1	0	0	1	13	9	1	0	800	270	—	6
Fat Free Tartar Sauce	2 tbsp (1.1 oz)	25	0	0	0	0	5	4	0	0	200	20	—	0
Lemon & Herb Tartar Sauce	2 tbsp (1 oz)	150	16	3	15	0	tr	tr	0	0	170	10	—	0
Reduced Fat Sandwich Spread	1 tbsp (0.5 oz)	35	3	0	0	0	3	3	0	0	130	5	—	0
Sandwich Spread	1 tbsp (0.5 oz)	50	4	1	<5	0	3	2	0	0	105	0	—	0
Sweet'n Sour	2 tbsp (1.2 oz)	60	0	0	0	0	14	12	0	0	125	20	—	0
Tartar	2 tbsp (1.1 oz)	90	9	2	10	0	4	0	2	0	170	15	—	0
LA CHOY														
Duck Sauce Sweet & Sour	2 tbsp (1.3 oz)	61	tr	0	0	tr	15	15	0	1	128	—	—	1
Sweet & Sour	2 tbsp (1.2 oz)	58	tr	0	0	tr	14	14	0	1	104	—	—	0
Teriyaki	1 tbsp (0.6 oz)	17	tr	0	0	1	3	2	0	2	917	—	—	0
LEA & PERRINS														
Worcestershire	1 tsp	5	0	0	0	0	1	1	—	—	65	—	—	—
MANWICH														
Bold	¼ cup (2.2 oz)	62	1	0	0	1	13	11	1	28	802	—	—	5
Mexican	¼ cup (2.2 oz)	27	tr	0	0	1	5	5	1	18	552	—	—	4
Original	¼ cup (2.2 oz)	32	tr	0	0	1	6	5	1	13	365	—	—	4
Taco Season	¼ cup (2.2 oz)	27	tr	tr	0	1	6	4	1	22	552	—	—	2
Thick & Chunky	¼ cup (2.3 oz)	44	tr	0	0	1	9	7	1	19	737	—	—	4
MATOUK'S														
Flambeau Sauce	1 tsp	0	0	0	0	0	0	0	0	—	140	—	—	—
MCCORMICK														
Flavor Medleys Garlic & Herb	2 tbsp	50	5	—	—	0	5	4	—	—	390	—	—	—
Flavor Medleys Italian Herb	2 tbsp	50	4	—	—	0	4	3	—	—	370	—	—	—
Flavor Medleys Lemon Pepper	2 tbsp	50	4	—	—	0	4	3	—	—	450	—	—	—
Flavor Medleys Tomato & Basil	2 tbsp	50	3	—	—	0	4	3	—	—	400	—	—	—
NEWMAN'S OWN														
Spicy Simmer Sauce Diavolo	½ cup (4.4 oz)	70	3	0	0	0	10	4	3	60	510	—	—	0
OLD EL PASO														
Enchilada Mild	¼ cup	20	1	0	0	0	3	tr	0	0	220	—	—	1
OPEN RANGE														
Hot Dog Chili	¼ cup (2.2 oz)	61	3	2	3	3	6	1	2	16	255	—	—	1

FOOD	PORTION	CALS	FAT	SAT FAT	CHOL	PROT	CARB	SUGAR	FIBER	CALCI	SOD	POTAS	FOLIC	VIT C
PACE														
Enchilada Sauce	¼ cup	36	0	0	0	0	6	4	0	0	290	—	—	0
Taco Sauce	¼ cup	32	2	0	0	0	4	2	0	0	150	—	—	0
PROGRESSO														
Alfredo	½ cup (4.4 oz)	200	15	10	50	8	7	2	1	250	850	—	—	0
SAUCE ARTURO														
Original	¼ cup (2.2 fl oz)	50	1	0	0	1	8	4	0	0	680	—	—	6
STEEL'S														
Sugar Free Cocktail w/ Dill & Lemon	¼ cup	36	0	0	0	1	1	1	1	—	160	—	—	—
Sugar Free Hoisin	2 tbsp	15	0	0	0	1	2	1	1	—	440	—	—	—
Sugar Free Peanut Sauce	1 tbsp	34	2	—	—	2	7	0	5	—	150	—	—	—
Sugar Free Sweet & Sour	2 tbsp	10	0	0	0	0	2	0	0	—	155	—	—	—
TABASCO														
Caribbean Steak Sauce	1 tbsp (0.6 oz)	15	0	0	0	0	4	3	0	0	160	—	—	0
Garlic Basting Sauce	1 tbsp (0.6 oz)	20	0	0	0	0	4	4	0	0	250	—	—	0
Habanero Sauce	1 tsp (0.2 oz)	5	0	0	0	0	1	tr	0	0	140	—	—	0
Hot Sauce w/ Garlic	1 tsp (0.2 oz)	0	0	0	0	0	0	0	0	0	95	—	—	0
Jalapeño Pepper Sauce	1 tbsp	15	0	0	0	tr	3	0	tr	0	3200	—	—	0
New Orleans Steak Sauce	1 tbsp (0.6 oz)	15	0	0	0	0	4	3	0	0	270	—	—	0
Pepper Sauce	1 tsp (0.2 oz)	0	0	0	0	0	0	0	0	0	30	—	—	0
TACO BELL														
Taco Sauce Medium	2 tbsp (1.1 oz)	15	0	0	0	0	3	1	tr	0	160	—	—	0
Taco Sauce Mild	2 tbsp (1.1 oz)	15	0	0	0	0	3	1	tr	0	160	—	—	0
The Restaurant Hot Sauce	1 tsp (5 g)	0	0	0	0	0	0	0	0	0	50	—	—	0
TOSTITOS														
Beef Fiesta Nacho	2.4 oz	120	8	3	10	4	6	2	tr	—	500	—	—	—
Chicken Quesadilla Topping	2.5 oz	90	6	2	10	4	6	2	tr	—	600	—	—	—
WALDEN FARMS														
Calorie Free Seafood Sauce	1 tbsp	0	0	0	0	0	0	0	0	—	290	—	—	—
Scampi Sauce Calorie Free	2 tbsp	0	0	0	0	0	0	0	0	—	130	—	—	—

FOOD	PORTION	CALS	FAT	SAT FAT	CHOL	PROT	CARB	SUGAR	FIBER	CALCI	SOD	POTAS	FOLIC	VIT C
WILD THYME FARMS														
Chili Ginger Honey	1 tbsp	30	0	0	0	0	8	8	—	—	0	—	—	1
MIX														
cheese as prep w/ milk	1 cup	307	17	9	53	16	23	—	—	570	1566	554	—	2
curry as prep w/ milk	1 cup	270	15	6	35	11	26	—	—	485	1276	—	—	—
mushroom as prep w/ milk	1 cup	228	10	5	34	11	24	—	—	—	1533	—	—	—
sour cream as prep w/ milk	1 cup	509	30	16	91	19	45	—	—	546	1007	733	—	—
stroganoff as prep	1 cup	271	11	7	38	12	34	—	—	521	1829	672	—	—
sweet & sour as prep	1 cup	294	tr	tr	0	1	73	—	—	41	779	66	—	—
teriyaki as prep	1 cup	131	1	tr	0	4	28	—	—	112	4791	216	—	—
white as prep w/ milk	1 cup	241	13	6	34	10	21	—	—	424	796	443	—	—
DURKEE														
A La King as prep	1 cup	60	4	1	0	1	8	2	0	80	800	—	—	9
Cheese as prep	¼ cup	25	2	1	2	1	4	0	0	40	260	—	—	0
Hollandaise as prep	2 tbsp	10	0	0	0	0	2	0	0	0	70	—	—	0
White as prep	¼ cup	20	1	0	0	0	5	0	0	0	330	—	—	0
FRENCH'S														
Cheese as prep	¼ cup	25	1	0	0	1	4	0	0	0	250	—	—	0
Hollandaise as prep	2 tbsp	10	0	0	0	0	2	0	0	0	75	—	—	0
MANWICH														
Mix	¼ oz	22	tr	0	0	tr	5	0	tr	8	355	—	—	0
MCCORMICK														
Bernaise Blend	1 tsp (3 g)	10	0	0	—	0	1	—	—	—	130	—	—	—
Chicken Dijon Blend	1⅔ tbsp (10 g)	40	2	—	<5	tr	5	1	—	0	420	—	—	0
Green Peppercorn Blend as prep	¼ cup	20	0	0	—	tr	3	1	—	—	360	—	—	—
Grill Mates Mesquite Marinade as prep	1 tbsp	15	0	0	—	0	2	2	—	—	610	—	—	—
Grill Mates Southwest Marinade	2 tsp (5 g)	15	0	0	—	0	2	—	tr	—	440	—	—	—
Hollandaise Blend	2 tsp (4 g)	15	0	—	15	0	1	—	—	—	110	—	—	—
Hunter Blend as prep	¼ cup	25	0	0	—	tr	4	1	—	—	270	—	—	—
Meat Marinade	1 tsp (4 g)	15	0	0	—	0	2	tr	—	—	240	—	—	—

FOOD	PORTION	CALS	FAT	SAT FAT	CHOL	PROT	CARB	SUGAR	FIBER	CALCI	SOD	POTAS	FOLIC	VIT C
MCCORMICK (CONT.)														
Pepper Medley Blend as prep	¼ cup	30	2	—	—	1	3	tr	—	—	310	—	—	—
White Blend	2 tsp (6 g)	20	1	—	—	tr	3	—	—	—	300	—	—	—
SHELF-STABLE														
CHEEZ WHIZ														
Cheese Sqeezable	2 tbsp (1.2 oz)	100	8	4	15	2	4	1	0	60	470	30	—	0
TAKE-OUT														
bearnaise	1 oz	177	19	12	21	1	1	—	tr	49	257	63	1	tr
cucumber yogurt sauce	1.5 tbsp	20	0	0	2	2	3	—	0	60	20	—	—	4

SAUERKRAUT

FOOD	PORTION	CALS	FAT	SAT FAT	CHOL	PROT	CARB	SUGAR	FIBER	CALCI	SOD	POTAS	FOLIC	VIT C
canned	½ cup	22	tr	tr	0	1	5	—	—	36	780	201	—	17
B&G														
Sauerkraut	2 tbsp (1 oz)	6	0	0	0	0	1	0	1	0	180	—	—	2
BOAR'S HEAD														
Sauerkraut	2 tbsp (1 oz)	5	0	0	0	0	1	0	tr	0	180	—	—	2
CLAUSSEN														
Sauerkraut	¼ cup (1.1 oz)	5	0	0	0	0	1	0	1	0	210	—	—	4
DEL MONTE														
Bavarian Style	2 tbsp (1 oz)	15	0	0	0	0	4	3	0	0	180	—	—	1
Sauerkraut	2 tbsp (1 oz)	0	0	0	0	0	1	0	1	0	180	—	—	1
EDEN														
Organic	½ cup	25	0	0	0	2	4	1	3	40	580	160	0	12
S&W														
Canned	2 tbsp (1 oz)	5	0	0	0	0	1	0	0	0	220	—	—	2
Red Cabbage	2 tbsp (1 oz)	15	0	0	0	0	3	2	0	0	160	—	—	1
SILVER FLOSS														
Sauerkraut	½ cup	20	0	0	0	0	5	1	4	0	740	—	—	9

SAUSAGE

FOOD	PORTION	CALS	FAT	SAT FAT	CHOL	PROT	CARB	SUGAR	FIBER	CALCI	SOD	POTAS	FOLIC	VIT C
bierschinken	3.5 oz	174	11	—	—	18	tr	—	—	15	753	261	—	—
bierwurst	3.5 oz	258	21	—	—	16	0	—	—	—	—	—	—	—
blutwurst uncooked	3.5 oz	424	39	—	—	13	0	—	—	7	680	38	—	—
bockwurst	3.5 oz	276	25	—	—	12	0	—	—	—	700	—	—	—
bratwurst pork cooked	1 link (3 oz)	256	22	8	51	12	2	—	—	38	473	180	—	1
bratwurst pork & beef	1 link (2.5 oz)	226	19	7	44	10	2	—	—	34	778	197	—	20
chipolata	3.5 oz	342	32	12	66	14	1	1	0	16	747	160	3	1
chorizo	3.5 oz	499	45	17	70	20	4	4	tr	12	2300	180	3	0
fleischwurst	3.5 oz	305	29	—	—	12	0	—	—	14	829	199	—	—
free range chicken breakfast	2 links (2.7 oz)	110	6	1	45	14	1	1	0	0	570	—	—	0

FOOD	PORTION	CALS	FAT	SAT FAT	CHOL	PROT	CARB	SUGAR	FIBER	CALCI	SOD	POTAS	FOLIC	VIT C
gelbwurst uncooked	3.5 oz	363	33	—	—	12	0	—	—	—	640	285	—	—
italian pork cooked	1 (3 oz)	268	21	8	65	17	1	—	—	20	765	253	—	1
jagdwurst	3.5 oz	211	16	—	—	16	0	—	—	14	818	260	—	—
kielbasa pork	1 oz	88	8	3	19	8	1	—	—	12	305	77	—	6
knockwurst pork & beef	1 (2.4 oz)	209	19	7	39	8	1	—	—	7	687	136	—	18
mettwurst uncooked	3.5 oz	483	45	—	—	13	0	—	—	13	1090	213	—	—
plockwurst uncooked	3.5 oz	312	45	—	—	19	0	—	—	—	—	—	—	—
polish pork	1 (8 oz)	739	65	23	158	32	4	—	—	26	1989	538	—	2
pork cooked	1 link (½ oz)	48	4	1	11	3	tr	—	—	4	168	47	—	0
regensburger uncooked	3.5 oz	354	31	—	—	13	0	—	—	—	—	—	—	—
vienna canned	1 (½ oz)	45	4	1	8	2	tr	—	—	2	152	16	—	0
vienna canned	7 (4 oz)	315	28	10	59	12	2	—	—	12	1077	114	—	0
weisswurst uncooked	3.5 oz	305	27	—	—	11	0	—	—	25	620	122	—	—
zungenwurst (tongue)	3.5 oz	285	24	—	—	17	0	—	—	—	—	—	—	—
ARMOUR														
Vienna Sausage 25% Less Fat	3 (1.9 oz)	130	11	4	50	6	1	0	0	40	420	—	—	0
Vienna Sausage 50% Less Fat	3 (1.9 oz)	90	7	3	40	5	1	1	0	40	420	—	—	0
Vienna Sausage Chicken & Beef	3 (1.9 oz)	120	10	4	65	6	1	1	0	40	620	—	—	0
Vienna Sausage Hot'n Spicy	3 (2.1 oz)	150	13	5	50	5	2	0	0	60	660	—	—	0
Vienna Sausage In BBQ Sauce	3 (2.1 oz)	150	13	5	50	5	3	3	0	40	580	—	—	0
Vienna Sausage In Beef Stock	3 (1.9 oz)	150	14	6	50	5	0	0	0	40	430	—	—	0
Vienna Sausage Jalapeño In Beef Stock	3 (1.9 oz)	170	16	6	50	5	1	0	0	40	420	—	—	0
BANNER														
Sausage Stomachs	2 oz	90	5	3	95	0	0	0	0	0	430	—	—	0
Sausage Tripe	2 oz	90	5	3	85	9	2	0	0	0	430	—	—	0
BILINSKI'S														
Chicken Bratworst With Wild Rice	1 (2 oz)	70	2	1	25	11	2	—	0	0	280	—	—	1
Chicken Cajun-Style Andouille	2 oz	80	4	2	60	9	1	—	0	60	300	—	—	0

FOOD	PORTION	CALS	FAT	SAT FAT	CHOL	PROT	CARB	SUGAR	FIBER	CALCI	SOD	POTAS	FOLIC	VIT C
BILINSKI'S (CONT.)														
Chicken Italian With Peppers	1 (2 oz)	70	4	1	60	9	1	—	0	60	270	—	—	0
Chicken With Apples & Chardonnay	2 oz	70	6	2	60	10	3	—	0	60	350	—	—	0
Chicken With Cilantro	2 oz	70	4	1	40	9	1	—	1	—	270	—	—	0
Chicken With Jalapeños	2 oz	70	4	2	55	9	0	0	0	—	270	—	—	5
Chicken With Pesto	2 oz	90	5	2	40	10	0	0	0	60	320	—	—	5
Chicken With Spinach	2 oz	70	4	1	40	9	1	—	1	0	270	—	—	0
Chicken With Sun-Dried Tomato	2 oz	70	4	2	40	10	2	—	0	40	280	—	—	5
BOAR'S HEAD														
Bratwurst	1 (4 oz)	300	25	11	75	19	0	0	0	20	650	—	—	0
Hot Smoked	1 (3.2 oz)	280	25	10	55	12	1	0	0	0	740	—	—	0
Kielbasa	2 oz	120	10	4	50	9	0	0	0	0	440	—	—	0
Knockwurst	1 (4 oz)	310	27	11	50	15	1	0	0	20	950	—	—	0
BROWN'N SERVE														
Turkey	3 (2.1 oz)	120	8	3	35	10	2	1	0	40	370	—	—	0
HORMEL														
Kielbasa	2 oz	150	13	5	40	8	—	—	—	0	530	—	—	0
Light & Lean 97 Dinner Smoked	2 oz	60	2	1	20	8	2	2	0	0	640	—	—	6
Pickled Hot	6 (2 oz)	140	11	5	40	8	1	1	0	0	380	—	—	9
Pickled Smoked	6 (2 oz)	140	11	5	40	8	1	1	0	0	380	—	—	9
Smoked Summer	2 oz	200	18	8	55	8	2	2	0	—	970	—	—	—
Vienna	2 oz	140	14	5	45	5	0	0	0	40	420	—	—	0
Vienna Chicken	2 oz	110	9	3	55	6	1	0	0	40	400	—	—	0
JENNIE-O														
Italian Hot	1 (3.9 oz)	160	10	3	60	17	2	—	—	20	850	—	—	—
JONES														
Light 50% Less Fat	2 (1.6 oz)	100	8	3	25	7	1	—	—	—	230	—	—	—
Little Pork	3	190	17	7	45	8	1	—	—	—	420	—	—	—
LITTLE SIZZLERS														
Brown & Serve	2 patties (1.8 oz)	190	18	6	40	7	1	1	0	0	560	—	—	0
Brown & Serve	3 links (2.1 oz)	190	22	8	45	8	1	1	0	0	670	—	—	0
Cooked	2 patties (1.8 oz)	230	22	8	45	8	0	0	0	0	610	—	—	0
Cooked	3 links (1.8 oz)	230	22	8	45	8	0	0	0	0	610	—	—	0
Heat & Serve Pork cooked	3 links (1.8 oz)	230	22	8	45	8	0	0	0	0	610	—	—	0

FOOD	PORTION	CALS	FAT	SAT FAT	CHOL	PROT	CARB	SUGAR	FIBER	CALCI	SOD	POTAS	FOLIC	VIT C
LOUIS RICH														
Polska Kielbasa	2 oz	90	5	2	35	8	2	tr	0	0	490	—	—	0
Turkey Hot	2.5 oz	120	8	3	55	12	1	0	0	40	430	—	—	0
Turkey Original	2.5 oz	120	8	3	55	12	1	0	0	40	430	—	—	0
Turkey Smoked	2 oz	90	5	2	30	8	2	1	0	0	490	—	—	0
MURRAY'S														
Chicken Hot Italian	3 oz	130	7	2	85	16	1	—	—	20	670	—	—	0
Chicken Spinach & Garlic	3 oz	100	5	2	50	12	1	—	—	20	640	—	—	5
Chicken Sun Dried Tomato	3 oz	110	5	2	55	18	2	—	—	20	420	—	—	1
Chicken Sweet Italian	3 oz	130	7	2	85	16	1	—	—	20	670	—	—	0
OLD SMOKEHOUSE														
Summer Sausage	2 oz	200	18	8	55	8	2	2	0	0	970	—	—	6
OSCAR MAYER														
Pork cooked	2 links (1.7 oz)	170	15	5	40	9	1	0	0	0	410	—	—	0
Smokies Beef	1 (1.5 oz)	120	11	5	30	5	1	tr	0	0	420	—	—	0
Smokies Cheese	1 (1.5 oz)	130	12	5	30	6	1	tr	0	0	450	—	—	0
Smokies Link	1 (1.5 oz)	130	12	4	25	5	1	tr	0	0	430	—	—	0
Smokies Little	6 (2 oz)	170	15	6	35	7	1	tr	0	40	570	—	—	0
Smokies Little Cheese	6 (2 oz)	180	16	6	40	7	1	0	0	40	590	—	—	0
PERDUE														
Hot Italian Turkey Cooked	1 link (2.4 oz)	150	9	3	60	16	1	—	—	—	470	—	—	—
Sweet Italian Turkey Cooked	1 link (2.4 oz)	150	9	3	60	16	1	—	—	—	490	—	—	—
SHADY BROOK														
Turkey Breakfast	2 oz	80	4	2	35	10	—	—	—	—	480	—	—	—
Turkey Hot Italian	2 oz	100	5	2	40	12	—	—	—	—	460	—	—	—
Turkey Old World Style	4 oz	190	11	3	65	20	—	—	—	—	850	—	—	—
Turkey Sweet Italian	1 (2.5 oz)	110	7	2	50	13	1	1	—	20	570	—	—	—
TURKEY STORE														
Breakfast	2 links (2 oz)	140	11	3	45	8	1	—	—	20	360	—	—	—
Breakfast Sausage Patties Mild	2 patties (2.3 oz)	160	13	4	50	10	1	—	—	—	420	—	—	—
WAMPLER														
Breakfast Turkey	2 (2.4 oz)	110	6	2	45	13	1	1	—	20	440	—	—	—
Italian Turkey	1 (2.7 oz)	120	6	2	50	14	1	1	—	20	480	—	—	—

FOOD	PORTION	CALS	FAT	SAT FAT	CHOL	PROT	CARB	SUGAR	FIBER	CALCI	SOD	POTAS	FOLIC	VITC
TAKE-OUT														
pork	1 link (0.5 oz)	48	4	1	11	3	tr	—	—	4	168	47	—	0
pork	1 patty (1 oz)	100	8	3	22	5	tr	—	—	9	349	97	—	0

SAUSAGE DISHES

FOOD	PORTION	CALS	FAT	SAT FAT	CHOL	PROT	CARB	SUGAR	FIBER	CALCI	SOD	POTAS	FOLIC	VITC
TAKE-OUT														
italian sausage w/ peppers & onions	1 cup	210	11	—	70	17	14	—	—	—	1120	—	—	—
sausage roll	1 (2.3 oz)	311	24	—	—	5	22	—	1	46	—	—	—	0

SAUSAGE SUBSTITUTES

FOOD	PORTION	CALS	FAT	SAT FAT	CHOL	PROT	CARB	SUGAR	FIBER	CALCI	SOD	POTAS	FOLIC	VITC
nonmeat sausage	1 link (25 g)	64	5	1	0	5	2	—	—	16	222	58	7	0
nonmeat sausage	1 patty (38 g)	97	7	1	0	7	4	—	—	24	137	88	10	0
BOCA BURGERS														
Breakfast Patties	1 (1.3 oz)	70	3	0	0	9	4	1	2	40	300	210	—	0
GARDENSAUSAGE														
Patty	1 (2.5 oz)	140	3	2	5	7	20	2	5	350	460	—	—	0
LIGHTLIFE														
Gimme Lean	2 oz	70	0	0	0	9	8	1	1	—	290	—	—	—
Lean Links Breakfast	1 (1.2 oz)	60	3	1	0	4	4	1	0	—	130	—	—	—
Lean Links Italian	1 (1.4 oz)	60	2	1	0	5	5	1	0	—	160	—	—	—
Light	2 patties (2.3 oz)	80	0	0	0	11	10	1	1	—	340	—	—	—
LOMA LINDA														
Linketts	1 (1.2 oz)	70	5	1	0	7	1	0	1	0	160	15	—	0
Little Links	2 (1.6 oz)	90	6	1	0	8	2	0	2	0	230	25	—	0
MORNINGSTAR FARMS														
Breakfast Links	2	60	2	1	0	8	2	0	2	0	340	60	—	0
Breakfast Patties	1 (1.3 oz)	80	3	1	0	10	3	tr	2	0	270	110	—	0
Grillers	1 patty (2.2 oz)	140	7	2	0	14	5	u	3	40	260	130	—	0
Sausage Style Recipe Crumbles	⅔ cup (1.9 oz)	90	3	0	0	11	5	tr	2	20	370	80	—	0
NATURAL TOUCH														
Vegan Sausage Crumbles	½ cup (1.9 oz)	60	0	0	0	10	4	0	2	40	300	80	—	0
QURON														
Meat-Free Links	2 (1.6 oz)	70	3	0	0	8	2	0	1	30	210	—	—	0
WORTHINGTON														
Leanies	1 link (1.4 oz)	100	7	1	0	7	2	tr	1	20	430	40	—	0
Prosage Links	2 (1.6 oz)	60	3	1	0	8	2	0	2	0	340	60	—	0
Saucettes	1 link (1.3 oz)	90	6	1	0	6	1	0	1	0	200	25	—	0
Super Links	1 (1.7 oz)	110	8	1	0	7	2	0	1	0	350	30	—	0
Veja Links	1 (1.1 oz)	50	3	1	0	5	1	0	0	0	190	20	—	0
YVES														
Veggie Breakfast Links	1 (1.6 oz)	60	0	0	0	11	3	1	2	40	390	110	—	0

FOOD	PORTION	CALS	FAT	SAT FAT	CHOL	PROT	CARB	SUGAR	FIBER	CALCI	SOD	POTAS	FOLIC	VIT C
YVES (CONT.)														
Veggie Breakfast Patties	1 (2 oz)	70	2	0	0	11	4	1	2	60	350	290	—	0
SAVORY														
ground	1 tsp	4	tr	—	0	tr	1	—	—	30	tr	15	—	—
SCALLOPS														
raw	3 oz	75	1	tr	28	14	2	—	—	21	137	274	—	—
TAKE-OUT														
breaded & fried	2 lg	67	3	1	19	6	3	—	—	13	144	103	—	—
SCONES														
FINNEGAN'S														
Cranberry	1 (2.7 oz)	90	2	0	0	2	20	1	1	60	176	—	—	0
Irish Raisin	1 (2 oz)	170	4	1	0	4	31	5	1	10	290	—	—	0
HEALTH VALLEY														
Apple Kiwi	1	180	0	0	0	4	43	18	5	0	190	—	—	5
Cinnamon Raisin	1	180	0	0	0	4	43	18	5	0	190	—	—	5
Cranberry Orange	1	180	0	0	0	4	43	18	5	0	190	—	—	5
Mountain Blueberry	1	180	0	0	0	4	43	18	5	0	190	—	—	5
Pineapple Banana	1	180	0	0	0	4	43	18	5	0	190	—	—	5
KING ARTHUR														
Cranberry Orange as prep	1	248	8	5	47	5	39	14	0	116	174	—	—	2
TAKE-OUT														
apricot	1	232	7	—	34	5	39	—	—	—	201	—	—	—
blueberry	1 (3 oz)	270	9	4	10	7	41	7	2	40	600	—	—	0
cheese	1 (3.5 oz)	364	18	—	—	10	44	—	2	250	—	—	—	tr
orange poppy	1 (3 oz)	260	6	4	30	6	47	12	2	80	400	—	—	0
plain	1 (3.5 oz)	362	14	—	—	8	54	—	2	180	—	—	—	tr
raisin	1 (3 oz)	270	8	3	10	6	43	12	2	40	490	—	—	0
SCUP														
fresh baked	3 oz	115	3	—	—	21	0	—	—	44	46	313	—	—
SEA BASS														
(*see* BASS)														
SEA CUCUMBER														
dried	1 oz	74	1	—	17	14	1	—	0	87	1411	101	—	0
fresh	1 oz	20	tr	—	14	5	tr	—	0	81	143	12	—	0
SEA TROUT														
(*see* TROUT)														
SEA URCHIN														
canned	1 oz	39	1	—	—	4	3	—	0	—	—	—	—	0
fresh	1 oz	36	1	—	—	4	3	—	tr	2	32	51	—	3
roe paste	1 tbsp	19	tr	—	—	2	3	—	0	6	658	31	—	0

FOOD	PORTION	CALS	FAT	SAT FAT	CHOL	PROT	CARB	SUGAR	FIBER	CALCI	SOD	POTAS	FOLIC	VIT C
SEAWEED														
agar dried	1 oz	87	tr	tr	0	2	23	—	—	78	29	321	—	0
agar fresh	1 oz	tr	tr	tr	0	tr	2	—	—	15	3	64	—	0
hijiki dried	1 tbsp	9	0	0	0	1	2	—	1	70	—	—	—	0
irishmoss fresh	1 oz	14	tr	tr	0	tr	4	—	—	21	19	18	—	—
kelp fresh	1 oz	12	tr	tr	0	tr	3	—	—	48	66	25	51	—
kombu fresh	1 oz	12	tr	tr	0	tr	3	—	—	48	66	25	51	—
laver fresh	1 oz	10	tr	tr	0	2	1	—	—	20	14	101	—	11
nori fresh	1 oz	10	tr	tr	0	2	1	—	—	20	14	101	—	11
nori sheet dried	1 (8 × 8 in)	5	0	0	0	1	1	—	1	7	18	45	—	0
seahair dried	1 tbsp	13	0	0	0	1	3	—	tr	38	—	—	—	—
spirulina dried	1 oz	83	2	1	0	16	7	—	—	—	309	388	—	13
spirulina fresh	1 oz	7	tr	tr	0	2	1	—	—	—	28	36	—	tr
tangle fresh	1 oz	12	tr	tr	0	tr	3	—	—	48	66	25	51	—
wakame fresh	1 oz	13	tr	tr	0	1	3	—	—	43	249	14	—	1
SEITAN														
(*see* WHEAT)														
SEMOLINA														
dry	1 cup (5.9 oz)	601	2	tr	0	21	122	—	7	28	2	311	129	0
SESAME														
seeds	1 tsp	16	2	—	0	1	tr	—	—	4	1	11	—	—
sesame butter	1 tbsp	95	8	1	0	3	4	—	1	154	2	93	—	0
sesame crunch candy	20 pieces (1.2 oz)	181	12	2	0	4	18	—	—	—	—	—	—	—
sesame crunch candy	1 oz	146	9	1	0	3	14	—	—	—	—	—	—	—
tahini from roasted & toasted kernels	1 tbsp	89	8	1	0	3	3	—	—	64	17	62	—	0
tahini from stone ground kernels	1 tbsp	86	7	1	0	3	4	—	—	63	11	62	—	0
tahini from unroasted kernels	1 tbsp	85	8	1	0	3	3	—	—	20	0	64	—	—
EDEN														
Organic Seaweed Gomasio	1 serv (1.5 oz)	10	1	0	0	0	0	0	0	0	35	0	0	0
Organic Gomasio	½ tsp	10	1	0	0	0	0	0	tr	0	40	0	0	0
Organic Gomasio Garlic	½ tsp	10	1	0	0	0	0	0	tr	0	35	0	0	0
MARANATHA														
Raw Tahini	2 tbsp	190	16	2	0	6	9	0	3	20	80	—	—	0
Roasted Tahini	2 tbsp	210	16	2	0	6	10	0	2	20	80	—	—	0

FOOD	PORTION	CALS	FAT	SAT FAT	CHOL	PROT	CARB	SUGAR	FIBER	CALCI	SOD	POTAS	FOLIC	VIT C
SESBANIA														
flower	1	1	0	0	0	tr	tr	—	—	1	0	5	—	2
flowers	1 cup	5	tr	—	0	tr	1	—	—	4	3	37	—	15
flowers cooked	1 cup	23	tr	—	0	1	5	—	—	23	11	111	—	39
SHAD														
american baked	3 oz	214	15	—	—	18	0	—	—	51	56	418	—	—
roe baked w/ butter & lemon	1 oz	36	1	—	—	6	tr	—	—	4	21	38	—	—
roe raw	1 oz	37	tr	—	103	7	tr	—	—	—	—	—	—	4
SHARK														
fin dried	1 oz	32	tr	—	—	7	—	—	—	48	5	16	—	0
raw	3 oz	111	4	1	43	18	0	—	—	29	67	136	—	—
TAKE-OUT														
batter-dipped & fried	3 oz	194	12	3	50	16	5	—	—	52	103	132	—	—
SHEEPSHEAD FISH														
cooked	3 oz	107	1	tr	—	22	0	—	—	32	62	435	—	—
cooked	1 fillet (6.5 oz)	234	3	1	—	48	0	—	—	70	136	952	—	—
raw	3 oz	92	2	1	—	17	0	—	—	18	61	344	—	—
SHELLFISH														
(*see individual names,* SHELLFISH SUBSTITUTES)														
SHELLFISH SUBSTITUTES														
crab imitation	3 oz	87	1	—	17	10	1	—	—	11	715	77	—	—
scallop imitation	3 oz	84	tr	—	18	11	9	—	—	7	676	88	—	—
shrimp imitation	3 oz	86	1	—	31	11	8	—	—	16	599	76	—	—
surimi	1 oz	28	tr	—	8	4	2	—	—	2	40	31	—	—
surimi	3 oz	84	1	—	25	13	6	—	—	7	122	95	—	—
LOUIS KEMP														
Crab Delights	½ cup (3 oz)	90	0	0	10	10	12	8	2	0	410	—	—	0
Lobster Delights	½ cup (3 oz)	80	0	0	10	8	12	4	0	0	420	—	—	0
Scallop Delights	13 pieces (3 oz)	80	0	0	10	9	12	3	0	0	550	—	—	0
SHELLIE BEANS														
canned	½ cup	37	tr	tr	0	2	8	—	—	36	408	133	—	4
SHERBET														
orange	½ cup (4 fl oz)	132	2	1	5	1	29	—	—	52	44	92	4	4
orange	1 bar (2.75 fl oz)	91	1	1	3	1	20	—	—	36	30	63	3	3
orange	½ gal	2158	31	19	113	17	469	—	—	827	706	1585	111	31
BREYERS														
Orange	½ cup	120	2	1	5	1	26	19	0	40	35	—	—	4
Rainbow	½ cup	120	2	1	5	1	26	20	0	40	35	—	—	1
TURKEY HILL														
Fruit Rainbow	½ cup	120	1	—	5	—	26	—	—	—	20	—	—	—
Orange Grove	½ cup	120	1	—	5	—	26	—	—	—	20	—	—	—

FOOD	PORTION	CALS	FAT	SAT FAT	CHOL	PROT	CARB	SUGAR	FIBER	CALCI	SOD	POTAS	FOLIC	VIT C
SHRIMP														
canned	3 oz	102	2	tr	147	20	1	—	—	50	143	179	2	—
canned	1 cup	154	3	tr	222	30	1	—	—	75	216	269	2	—
chinese shrimp paste	1 tbsp	15	tr	—	45	3	1	—	—	125	2000	—	—	0
cooked	4 large	22	tr	tr	43	5	0	—	—	9	49	40	1	—
raw	4 large	30	tr	tr	43	6	tr	—	—	15	42	52	1	—
BUMBLE BEE														
Medium	⅓ can (2 oz)	45	tr	0	115	10	0	1	0	—	650	—	—	—
Orleans Tiny Cocktail	½ can (3 oz)	44	0	—	114	—	0	1	0	—	650	—	—	—
GORTON'S														
Popcorn Garlic & Herb	22 pieces (3.6 oz)	270	14	3	90	11	24	3	—	40	600	—	—	—
Popcorn Original	20 pieces (3.2 oz)	240	13	3	65	9	22	1	—	40	780	—	—	—
TAKE-OUT														
breaded & fried	3 oz	206	10	2	150	18	10	—	—	57	292	191	7	—
gingered	4	80	tr	tr	140	—	—	—	—	—	920	—	—	—
jambalaya	¾ cup	188	5	2	50	11	26	—	8	67	83	422	15	19
scampi	2 cups	438	480	10	20	—	—	—	—	—	584	—	—	—
SMELT														
rainbow cooked	3 oz	106	3	tr	76	19	0	—	—	65	65	316	—	—
rainbow raw	3 oz	83	2	tr	60	15	0	—	—	51	51	247	—	—
SMOOTHIE														
(*see* FRUIT DRINKS)														
SNACKS														
cheese puffs	1 oz	157	10	2	1	2	15	—	tr	16	298	47	34	0
corn puffs cheese	1 bag (8 oz)	1256	78	15	9	17	122	—	2	131	2383	376	272	tr
corn twists cheese	1 oz	157	10	2	1	2	15	—	tr	16	298	47	34	0
corn twists cheese	1 bag (8 oz)	1256	78	15	9	17	122	—	2	131	2383	376	272	tr
oriental mix	1 oz	155	12	—	0	6	9	—	—	22	235	147	25	tr
pork skins	1 oz	154	9	3	27	17	0	—	—	8	521	36	—	tr
pork skins barbecue	1 oz	152	9	3	33	16	1	—	—	12	756	51	—	tr
trail mix	1 oz	131	8	2	0	4	13	—	—	22	65	194	20	tr
trail mix	1 cup (5.3 oz)	693	44	8	0	21	67	—	—	117	343	1028	107	2
trail mix tropical	1 oz	115	5	2	0	2	19	—	—	16	3	201	12	2
trail mix w/ chocolate chips	1 oz	137	9	2	—	4	13	—	—	31	34	184	18	tr
trail mix w/ chocolate chips	1 cup (5.1 oz)	707	47	9	—	21	66	—	—	159	177	946	95	2
BAKEN-ETS														
BBQ	9 (0.5 oz)	70	5	2	10	7	tr	0	tr	—	400	—	—	—
Hot N'Spicy	7 (0.5 oz)	70	5	2	20	8	tr	0	tr	—	440	—	—	—

FOOD	PORTION	CALS	FAT	SAT FAT	CHOL	PROT	CARB	SUGAR	FIBER	CALCI	SOD	POTAS	FOLIC	VIT C
BAKEN-ETS (CONT.)														
Hot N'Spicy Cracklins	8 (0.5 oz)	80	5	2	20	7	tr	0	tr	—	320	—	—	—
Regular	9 (0.5 oz)	80	5	3	20	8	tr	0	tr	—	330	—	—	—
Regular Cracklins	8 (0.5 oz)	40	6	2	15	7	tr	0	tr	—	550	—	—	—
BARBARA'S BAKERY														
Cheese Puffs Bakes	1½ cups (1 oz)	160	11	2	0	2	13	1	0	—	190	—	—	—
Cheese Puffs Jalapeño	¾ cup (1 oz)	150	10	2	0	2	16	0	0	—	130	—	—	—
Cheese Puffs Original	¾ cup (1 oz)	150	10	2	0	2	16	0	0	—	130	—	—	—
BOWLBY'S														
Bits Almond	½ cup	100	19	3	0	4	5	1	1	0	95	—	—	0
Bits Pecan	½ cup	200	19	3	0	4	5	1	1	0	95	—	—	0
Bits Ranch	½ cup	170	16	2	0	4	7	2	0	0	170	—	—	0
Bits Salsa	½ cup	170	16	2	0	2	7	2	0	0	230	—	—	0
Bits Sour Cream Cream Onion & Dill	½ cup	170	16	2	0	4	7	2	0	0	190	—	—	0
Bits'N'Pops	¾ cup	130	7	3	13	1	16	13	1	10	90	—	—	1
Mix-Ups Country Mix	½ cup	170	14	2	0	5	8	1	1	0	150	—	—	0
Mix-Ups Nuttyest-Of-All	½ cup	160	13	2	0	5	8	2	1	20	130	—	—	0
Mix-Ups Trail Mix	½ cup	165	12	2	0	4	11	6	1	0	135	—	—	0
BUGLES														
Baked Original	1⅓ cups	130	4	1	0	2	23	2	—	—	380	—	—	—
Chile Con Queso	1⅓ cups	160	9	7	0	2	18	1	—	—	310	—	—	—
Nacho	1½ cups	160	9	7	0	1	18	1	—	—	300	—	—	—
Original	1½ cups	160	9	8	0	1	18	1	tr	—	310	—	—	—
Smokin' BBQ	1⅓ cups	150	8	7	0	1	19	2	—	—	330	—	—	—
CHEETOS														
Crunchy	21 pieces (1 oz)	160	10	3	0	2	15	1	tr	—	290	—	—	—
Curls	15 pieces (1 oz)	150	10	3	0	2	15	1	1	—	290	—	—	—
Flamin' Hot	21 pieces (1 oz)	160	10	2	0	2	15	1	tr	—	280	—	—	—
Nacho Cheese	23 pieces (1 oz)	160	10	3	0	2	15	0	tr	—	260	—	—	—
Puffed Balls	38 pieces (1 oz)	150	10	3	0	2	15	1	tr	—	300	—	—	—
Puffs	29 pieces (1 oz)	160	10	3	0	2	15	tr	tr	—	370	—	—	—
Zig Zags	17 pieces (1 oz)	170	11	3	<5	2	17	tr	tr	—	370	—	—	—

FOOD	PORTION	CALS	FAT	SAT FAT	CHOL	PROT	CARB	SUGAR	FIBER	CALCI	SOD	POTAS	FOLIC	VIT C
CHEX MIX														
Cheddar	⅔ cup	140	5	1	0	3	21	2	2	—	330	—	—	—
Hot'N Spicy	⅔ cup	130	5	1	0	3	21	2	2	—	390	—	—	—
Nacho Fiesta	⅔ cup	120	4	1	0	2	22	2	1	—	350	60	—	—
Party Blend Bold	⅔ cup	140	6	1	0	3	20	2	2	—	290	60	8	—
Peanut Lovers	⅔ cup	140	6	1	0	3	19	2	1	—	370	80	—	—
Traditional	⅔ cup	130	4	1	0	2	22	2	1	—	50	—	8	—
DAKOTA GOURMET														
Amazing Corn Classic	1 pkg (1 oz)	360	7	1	0	10	78	—	5	6	813	768	—	3
Amazing Corn Cool Ranch	1 pkg (1 oz)	367	9	1	2	10	74	—	5	31	1073	754	—	4
Amazing Corn Mesquite BBQ	1 pkg (1 oz)	369	8	1	0	11	76	—	5	11	725	764	—	4
Heart Smart Toasted Corn	⅓ cup (1 oz)	110	2	0	0	3	22	0	3	0	280	—	—	0
Toasted Corn Heart Smart	1 pkg (1.75 oz)	177	3	tr	0	5	39	0	2	7	470	388	72	2
Trail Mix Heart Smart	1 pkg (1.75 oz)	172	0	0	0	4	39	25	3	32	156	271	45	1
EDEN														
Rice Puffs Five Flavor Arare	1 oz	110	0	0	0	3	24	0	2	40	160	25	—	0
FRITO LAY														
Funyuns	13 (1 oz)	140	7	2	0	2	18	tr	tr	—	270	—	—	—
Munchos	16 (1 oz)	160	10	2	0	1	16	0	1	—	230	—	—	—
Munchos BBQ	14 (1 oz)	160	10	2	0	1	15	2	1	—	250	—	—	—
GLENNY'S														
Soy Crisps All Flavors	5	60	4	3	0	2	8	0	1	—	30	—	—	—
GRAM'S GOURMET														
Crunchies Pork Rinds	⅛ pkg (0.5 oz)	70	5	2	—	8	0	0	0	—	190	—	—	—
HEALTH VALLEY														
Cheddar Lites Green Onion	1¾ cups	120	3	—	5	3	21	1	1	40	170	—	—	0
Cheddar Lites Original	1¾ cups	120	3	—	5	3	21	1	1	40	170	—	—	0
Corn Puffs Caramel	2 cups	120	2	—	0	2	25	7	1	0	80	—	—	0
Low Fat Potato Puffs Cheddar Cheese	1½ cups	110	3	—	5	2	21	1	1	40	260	—	—	6
Low Fat Potato Puffs Garlic w/ Cheese	1½ cups	260	3	—	0	2	21	1	1	40	260	—	—	6

FOOD	PORTION	CALS	FAT	SAT FAT	CHOL	PROT	CARB	SUGAR	FIBER	CALCI	SOD	POTAS	FOLIC	VIT C
HEALTH VALLEY (CONT.)														
Low Fat Potato Puffs Zesty Ranch	1½ cups	110	3	—	0	2	21	1	1	40	260	—	—	6
J&J														
Microwave Pork Rinds All Flavors	1 oz	130	4	2	0	23	tr	—	0	—	160	—	—	—
LANCE														
Cheese Balls	1 pkg (1 oz)	150	8	2	0	2	16	1	0	20	300	50	—	0
Crunchy Cheese Twists	1 pkg (1.25 oz)	190	4	—	0	2	15	0	0	20	280	50	—	0
Gold-N-Chees	1 pkg (1 oz)	130	5	2	0	3	18	0	1	20	290	40	—	0
Onion Rings	1 pkg (0.9 oz)	100	8	2	0	1	7	1	1	0	170	65	—	0
Pork Skins	1 pkg (0.4 oz)	65	4	2	10	6	1	0	0	0	230	15	—	0
Pork Skins BBQ	1 pkg (0.4 oz)	60	4	2	10	6	1	0	0	0	330	10	—	0
MARANATHA														
High Energy Mix	¼ cup	120	7	1	0	3	15	12	2	20	0	—	—	0
Organic Harvest Mix	¼ cup	150	9	1	0	4	15	2	2	20	0	—	—	0
Organic Nature Mix	¼ cup	150	9	2	0	4	15	2	2	20	0	—	—	0
Snack Attack Mix	¼ cup	140	8	3	0	2	16	12	2	20	0	—	—	2
Trail Mix Organic Raw	¼ cup	140	9	2	0	5	13	10	2	20	4	—	—	0
Trail Mix Deluxe	¼ cup	150	11	1	0	5	11	8	2	20	0	—	—	0
Trail Mix Navajo	¼ cup	140	9	1	0	4	13	8	4	20	3	—	—	1
Trail Mix Olympic w/ Chocolate	¼ cup	140	8	2	0	4	16	13	2	20	13	—	—	0
Trail Mix Organic Delight	¼ cup	150	10	2	0	4	12	8	2	20	3	—	—	0
MAUNA LOA														
Tropical Nut & Fruit	¼ cup	180	8	2	0	3	23	14	2	—	50	—	—	—
OLD DUTCH FOODS														
Baked Cheese Curls	2 cups (1.1 oz)	180	12	3	0	2	15	1	tr	20	340	—	—	4
Cheese Puffcorn Curls	2 cups (1.1 oz)	170	12	1	0	2	15	1	0	0	310	55	—	0
PLANTERS														
Cheez Mania Original	42 pieces (1 oz)	150	10	2	<5	2	15	tr	1	0	300	—	—	0
PUMPKORN														
Caramel	⅓ cup	150	11	2	0	9	4	—	2	20	85	—	16	0
Chili	⅓ cup	150	11	2	0	9	4	—	2	20	100	—	16	0
Curry	⅓ cup	150	11	2	0	9	4	—	2	20	100	—	16	0
Maple Vanilla	⅓ cup	150	11	2	0	9	4	—	2	20	100	—	16	0

FOOD	PORTION	CALS	FAT	SAT FAT	CHOL	PROT	CARB	SUGAR	FIBER	CALCI	SOD	POTAS	FOLIC	VIT C
PUMPKORN (CONT.)														
Mesquite	⅓ cup	150	11	2	0	9	4	—	2	20	110	—	16	0
Original	⅓ cup	150	11	2	0	10	4	—	2	20	110	—	16	0
ROBERT'S AMERICAN GOURMET														
Pirate's Booty Puffed Rice & Corn w/ Cheddar	1 oz	120	3	0	0	3	22	0	4	40	137	—	—	0
ROLD GOLD														
Snack Mix Colossal Cheddar	1 pkg (1 oz)	140	7	2	0	3	17	2	1	20	230	—	—	0
SNYDER'S OF HANOVER														
Cheese Twists	1 oz	230	14	2	0	1	10	0	0	20	280	—	—	0
Fried Pork Skins	1 oz	80	4	2	30	8	1	0	0	0	115	—	—	0
Fried Pork Skins Barbecue	1 oz	80	4	2	20	8	1	0	0	0	106	—	—	0
Kruncheez	1.25 oz	200	10	1	0	2	19	tr	tr	20	210	—	—	0
Onion Toasters	1 oz	188	10	1	0	2	21	tr	tr	80	350	—	—	0
UTZ														
Caramel Corn Clusters	1⅛ cups (1 oz)	120	2	0	0	tr	24	13	tr	0	140	—	—	0
Cheese Balls	50 (1 oz)	150	9	3	0	2	16	tr	tr	0	260	—	—	0
Cheese Curls	18 (1 oz)	150	9	3	0	2	16	tr	tr	0	260	—	—	0
Cheese Curls Crunchy	30 (1 oz)	160	10	2	0	2	16	tr	0	0	200	—	—	0
Cheese Curls Reduced Fat	32 (1 oz)	140	6	1	<5	3	18	tr	2	20	300	—	—	0
Onion Rings	41 (1 oz)	140	7	1	0	1	18	2	0	0	340	—	—	0
Party Mix	¾ cup (1 oz)	140	6	1	0	2	19	tr	1	20	250	—	—	0
Pork Cracklins	0.5 oz	90	7	3	15	6	0	—	—	—	300	—	—	—
Pork Cracklins Hot & Spicy	0.5 oz	80	5	2	15	8	0	—	—	—	340	—	—	—
Pork Rinds	0.5 oz	80	5	2	15	8	0	—	—	—	230	—	—	—
Pork Rinds BBQ	0.5 oz	80	5	2	15	8	0	—	—	—	280	—	—	—
WEIGHT WATCHERS														
Cheese Curls	1 pkg (0.5 oz)	70	3	1	0	1	10	0	0	0	85	—	—	0
SNAIL														
cooked	3 oz	233	1	tr	110	41	13	—	—	96	350	590	10	—
raw	3 oz	117	tr	tr	55	20	7	—	—	48	175	295	5	—
TAKE-OUT														
escargot cooked	5	25	0	0	15	4	1	—	0	5	25	95	0	0
SNAKE														
fresh	3 oz	78	tr	—	—	17	3	—	0	15	57	303	—	3
SNAPPER														
cooked	1 fillet (6 oz)	217	3	1	80	45	0	—	—	69	96	887	—	—
cooked	3 oz	109	1	tr	40	22	0	—	—	34	48	444	—	—
raw	3 oz	85	1	tr	31	17	0	—	—	27	54	355	—	—

SODA

FOOD	PORTION	CALS	FAT	SAT FAT	CHOL	PROT	CARB	SUGAR	FIBER	CALCI	SOD	POTAS	FOLIC	VIT C
club	12 oz	0	0	0	0	0	0	—	—	17	75	6	0	0
cola	12 oz	151	tr	—	0	tr	39	—	—	9	14	4	0	0
cream	12 oz	191	0	0	0	0	49	—	—	19	43	4	0	0
diet cola	12 oz	2	0	0	0	tr	tr	—	—	12	21	0	0	0
diet cola w/ equal	12 oz	2	0	0	0	tr	tr	—	—	12	21	0	0	0
diet cola w/ saccharin	12 oz	2	0	0	0	tr	tr	—	—	14	57	7	0	0
ginger ale	12 oz can	124	0	—	0	tr	32	—	—	12	25	5	0	0
grape	12 oz	161	0	0	0	0	42	—	—	12	57	3	0	0
lemon lime	12 oz	149	0	0	0	0	38	—	—	9	41	4	0	0
orange	12 oz	177	0	0	0	0	46	—	—	19	49	9	0	0
pepper type	12 oz	151	tr	—	0	0	38	—	—	12	38	2	0	0
quinine	12 oz	125	0	0	0	0	32	—	—	5	15	1	0	0
root beer	12 oz	152	0	0	0	tr	39	—	—	19	49	3	0	0
shirley temple	1 serv	159	0	0	0	0	41	—	0	11	34	23	—	—
tonic water	12 oz	125	0	0	0	0	32	—	—	5	15	1	0	0
7 UP														
Diet	8 oz	0	0	0	0	0	0	0	—	—	30	—	—	—
Original	1 can	140	0	0	0	0	39	39	—	—	75	—	—	—
Plus Mixed Berry	8 oz	10	0	0	0	0	2	1	—	100	130	—	—	6
A & W														
Root Beer	1 can (12 oz)	170	0	0	0	0	46	46	—	—	45	—	—	—
BARQ'S														
Root Beer	1 can (12 oz)	160	0	0	0	0	45	45	—	—	70	—	—	—
BARRITTS														
Ginger Beer	1 bottle (12 oz)	200	0	0	0	0	49	49	—	—	40	—	—	—
BEST HEALTH														
Root Beer	1 bottle (12 oz)	165	0	0	0	0	42	42	—	—	35	—	—	—
Vanilla Cream	1 bottle (12 oz)	170	0	0	0	0	43	43	—	—	30	—	—	—
BONG WATER														
Chronic Tonic	12 oz	144	0	0	0	0	36	36	—	—	32	—	—	—
Cottonmouth Quencher	12 oz	165	0	0	0	0	42	42	—	—	29	—	—	—
Green Dreams	12 oz	165	0	0	0	0	42	42	—	—	30	—	—	—
Purple Haze	12 oz	165	0	0	0	0	42	42	—	—	30	—	—	—
BRIAR'S														
Black Cherry	1 bottle (12 oz)	180	0	0	0	0	45	45	—	—	35	—	—	—
Cream	1 bottle (12 oz)	180	0	0	0	0	45	45	—	—	50	—	—	—
Diet Root Beer	8 oz	4	0	0	0	0	1	0	—	—	10	—	—	—
Orange Cream	8 oz	120	0	0	0	0	31	31	—	—	30	—	—	—
Red Birch	8 oz	104	0	0	0	0	26	26	—	—	7	—	—	—
Root Beer	1 bottle (12 oz)	168	0	0	0	0	42	42	—	—	15	—	—	—

FOOD	PORTION	CALS	FAT	SAT FAT	CHOL	PROT	CARB	SUGAR	FIBER	CALCI	SOD	POTAS	FOLIC	VIT C
CANADA DRY														
Ginger Ale	1 can (12 oz)	140	0	0	0	0	35	35	0	—	50	—	—	—
Tonic Water	8 fl oz	90	0	0	0	0	24	24	0	—	15	—	—	—
CAPT'N ELI'S														
Root Beer	8 oz	165	0	0	0	0	49	40	—	—	35	—	—	—
CHRONIC 187														
Orange	1 bottle (12 oz)	300	0	0	0	0	77	75	—	—	53	—	—	—
COCA-COLA														
C2	8 oz	48	0	0	0	0	12	12	—	—	30	—	—	—
Classic	1 can (12 oz)	140	0	0	0	0	39	39	—	—	50	—	—	—
Diet	1 can (12 oz)	0	0	0	0	0	0	0	—	—	40	—	—	—
DR PEPPER														
Diet	1 can (12 oz)	tr	0	—	0	—	—	—	—	0	—	—	—	—
Original	1 can (12 oz)	150	0	0	0	0	40	40	—	—	55	—	—	—
FANTA														
Orange	1 can (12 oz)	160	0	0	0	0	44	44	—	—	50	—	—	—
FIREFIGHTER														
Backdraft Root Beer	8 oz	90	0	0	0	0	22	22	—	—	10	—	—	—
Courageous Cola	8 oz	90	0	0	0	0	20	20	—	—	10	—	—	—
Flashover Orange	8 oz	20	0	0	0	0	24	24	—	—	10	—	—	—
Incendiary Citrus	8 oz	90	0	0	0	0	23	23	—	—	10	—	—	—
Rolling Code Black Cherry	8 oz	90	0	0	0	0	23	23	—	—	10	—	—	—
HANSEN'S														
Black Cherry	8 fl oz	110	0	0	0	0	30	29	—	—	0	—	—	—
Diet All Flavors	1 can	0	0	0	0	0	0	0	—	—	0	—	—	—
Ginger Beer	8 fl oz	100	0	0	0	0	28	28	—	—	0	—	—	—
Natural Black Cherry	1 can	160	0	0	0	0	44	43	—	—	0	—	—	—
Natural Cherry Vanilla	1 can	140	0	0	0	0	39	39	—	—	0	—	—	—
Natural Creamy Rootbeer	1 can	160	0	0	0	0	44	44	—	—	0	—	—	—
Natural Ginger Ale	1 can	140	0	0	0	0	37	37	—	—	0	—	—	—
Natural Grapefruit	1 can	130	0	0	0	0	38	36	—	—	0	—	—	—
Natural Key Lime	1 can	130	0	0	0	0	37	36	—	—	0	—	—	—
Natural Kiwi Strawberry	1 can	130	0	0	0	0	38	36	—	—	0	—	—	—
Natural Mandarin Lime	1 can	130	0	0	0	0	37	35	—	—	0	—	—	—
Natural Orange Mango	1 can	170	0	0	0	0	46	46	—	—	0	—	—	—
Natural Raspberry	1 can	130	0	0	0	0	36	37	—	—	0	—	—	—
Natural Tangerine	1 can	160	0	0	0	0	43	35	—	—	0	—	—	—

FOOD	PORTION	CALS	FAT	SAT FAT	CHOL	PROT	CARB	SUGAR	FIBER	CALCI	SOD	POTAS	FOLIC	VIT C
HANSEN'S (CONT.)														
Natural Tropical Passion	1 can	160	0	0	0	0	43	42	—	—	0	—	—	—
Natural Vanilla Cola	1 can	140	0	0	0	0	39	37	—	—	0	—	—	—
Orange Creme	8 fl oz	110	0	0	0	0	31	31	—	—	0	—	—	—
Sangria	8 fl oz	110	0	0	0	0	30	30	—	—	0	—	—	—
Sarsaparilla	8 fl oz	110	0	0	0	0	30	30	—	—	0	—	—	—
Sparkling Orangeade	8 fl oz	100	0	0	0	0	25	25	—	—	10	20	—	—
Vanilla Creme	8 fl oz	110	0	0	0	0	30	30	—	—	0	—	—	—
HEALTH VALLEY														
Ginger Ale	1 bottle	160	0	0	0	0	40	40	0	0	0	—	—	0
Rootbeer Old Fashioned	1 bottle	160	0	0	0	0	40	40	0	0	0	—	—	0
Sarsaparilla Rootbeer	1 bottle	160	0	0	0	0	40	40	0	0	0	—	—	0
HIBALL														
Club	1 bottle	5	0	0	0	1	0	0	0	—	20	—	—	—
Tonic Water	1 bottle	120	0	0	0	1	31	29	—	—	15	—	—	—
IBC														
Cream	1 bottle (12 oz)	180	0	0	0	0	48	48	—	—	75	—	—	—
Root Beer	1 can	160	0	0	0	0	43	43	—	—	55	—	—	—
JOLT														
Blue	8 oz	120	0	0	0	0	32	32	—	—	50	—	—	—
Cherry Bomb	8 oz	90	0	0	0	0	25	25	—	—	25	—	—	—
Cola	8 oz	100	0	0	0	0	27	27	—	—	10	—	—	—
Red	8 oz	120	0	0	0	0	33	33	—	—	40	—	—	—
Ultra	8 oz	0	0	0	0	0	0	0	0	—	30	—	—	—
JONES SODA														
Sugar Free All Flavors	1 bottle (12 oz)	0	0	0	0	0	0	0	—	—	10	—	—	—
KUTZTOWN														
Birch Beer	1 bottle (12 oz)	160	0	0	0	0	39	39	—	—	20	—	—	—
Red Cream	1 bottle (12 oz)	150	0	0	0	0	39	39	—	—	25	—	—	—
Sarsaparilla	1 bottle (12 oz)	150	0	0	0	0	38	28	—	—	25	—	—	—
LIKE														
Cola	1 oz	13	0	—	0	—	—	—	—	0	—	—	—	—
LUCOZADE														
Soda	7 oz	136	0	0	0	0	36	—	0	10	—	—	—	0
MINUTE MAID														
Valencia Orange	1 can (12 oz)	180	0	0	0	0	47	47	—	—	30	—	—	—
MOUNTAIN DEW														
Pitch Black	8 oz	110	0	0	0	0	31	—	—	—	35	—	—	—

FOOD	PORTION	CALS	FAT	SAT FAT	CHOL	PROT	CARB	SUGAR	FIBER	CALCI	SOD	POTAS	FOLIC	VIT C
OLDE BROOKLYN														
Flatbush Orange	8 oz	130	0	0	0	0	33	33	—	—	25	—	—	—
Williamsburg Root Beer	8 oz	120	0	0	0	0	32	32	—	—	25	—	—	—
OLDE PHILADELPHIA														
Black Cherry	1 bottle (12 oz)	180	0	0	0	0	45	45	—	—	40	—	—	—
Cream	1 bottle (12 oz)	190	0	0	0	0	47	47	—	—	40	—	—	—
Cream Diet	1 bottle (12 oz)	0	0	0	0	0	0	0	—	—	0	—	—	—
Grape	1 bottle (12 oz)	180	0	0	0	0	45	45	—	—	40	—	—	—
Orange Cream	1 bottle (12 oz)	190	0	0	0	0	49	49	—	—	40	—	—	—
Pineapple	1 bottle	190	0	0	0	0	48	48	—	—	40	—	—	—
Root Beer	1 bottle (12 oz)	180	0	0	0	0	44	44	—	—	35	—	—	—
ORANGINA														
Sparkling Citrus	8 oz	90	0	0	0	0	23	21	—	40	0	—	—	9
PENNSYLVANIA DUTCH														
Birch Beer	8 fl oz	110	0	0	0	0	28	28	—	—	30	—	—	—
PEPSI														
Blue Berry Cola Fusion	8 fl oz	100	0	0	0	0	28	27	—	—	25	—	—	—
Diet	1 can (12 oz)	0	0	0	0	0	0	0	—	—	35	—	—	—
Edge	1 can (12 oz)	70	0	0	0	0	20	20	—	—	40	—	—	—
Regular	1 can (12 oz)	150	0	0	0	0	41	41	—	—	35	—	—	—
Vanilla	1 can	160	0	0	0	0	43	42	—	—	40	—	—	—
Vanilla Diet	1 can	0	0	0	0	0	0	0	0	—	25	—	—	—
PRISM														
Green Tea Soda Cola	8 oz	105	0	0	0	0	26	26	—	—	7	—	—	—
Lemon Lime	8 oz	117	0	0	0	0	29	29	—	—	2	—	—	—
QIBLA														
Cola	1 bottle (18 oz)	185	tr	—	—	tr	11	—	—	—	—	—	—	—
Diet Cola	1 bottle (18 oz)	1	0	0	0	0	0	0	0	—	—	—	—	—
SARANAC														
Diet Root Beer	1 bottle (12 oz)	35	0	0	0	0	9	9	—	—	55	—	—	—
Ginger Beer	1 bottle (12 oz)	160	0	0	0	0	42	42	—	—	55	—	—	—
Root Beer	1 bottle (12 oz)	180	0	0	0	0	46	46	—	—	55	—	—	—
SCHWEPPES														
Ginger Ale	8 oz	120	0	0	0	0	34	32	0	—	60	—	—	—
SEAGRAM'S														
Ginger Ale	1 can (12 oz)	130	0	0	0	0	35	35	—	—	45	—	—	—
SEX COLA														
All Flavors	1 bottle (12 oz)	0	0	0	0	0	0	0	0	—	0	—	—	—
SHASTA														
Black Cherry	1 can (12 oz)	170	0	0	0	0	41	41	0	—	54	—	—	—
Caffeine Free Cola	1 can (12 oz)	160	0	0	0	0	41	41	—	—	45	—	—	—
Cherry Cola	1 can (12 oz)	160	0	0	0	0	39	39	—	—	45	—	—	—

FOOD	PORTION	CALS	FAT	SAT FAT	CHOL	PROT	CARB	SUGAR	FIBER	CALCI	SOD	POTAS	FOLIC	VIT C
SHASTA (CONT.)														
Club Soda	1 can (12 oz)	0	0	0	0	0	0	0	—	—	90	—	—	—
Cola	1 can (12 oz)	170	0	0	0	0	42	42	0	—	45	—	—	—
Creme	1 can (12 oz)	190	0	0	0	0	47	47	0	—	45	—	—	—
Diet Black Cherry	1 can (12 oz)	0	0	0	0	0	0	0	0	—	55	—	—	—
Diet Caffeine Free Cola	1 can (12 oz)	0	0	0	0	0	0	0	0	—	55	—	—	—
Diet Cherry Cola	1 can (12 oz)	0	0	0	0	0	0	0	0	—	55	—	—	—
Diet Cola	1 can (12 oz)	0	0	0	0	0	0	0	0	—	45	—	—	—
Diet Creme	1 can (12 oz)	0	0	0	0	0	0	0	0	—	55	—	—	—
Diet Doc Shasta	1 can (12 oz)	0	0	0	0	0	0	0	0	—	45	—	—	—
Diet Ginger Ale	1 can (12 oz)	0	0	0	0	0	0	0	0	—	55	—	—	—
Diet Grape	1 can (12 oz)	0	0	0	0	0	0	0	0	—	55	—	—	—
Diet Grapefruit	1 can (12 oz)	0	0	0	0	0	0	0	0	—	55	—	—	—
Diet Grapefruit	1 can (12 oz)	0	0	0	0	0	0	0	0	—	45	—	—	—
Diet Kiwi-Strawberry	1 can (12 oz)	0	0	0	0	0	0	0	0	—	45	—	—	—
Diet Lemon-Lime Twist	1 can (12 oz)	0	0	0	0	0	0	0	0	—	55	—	—	—
Diet Orange	1 can (12 oz)	0	0	0	0	0	0	0	0	—	55	—	—	—
Diet Pineapple-Orange	1 can (12 oz)	0	0	0	0	0	0	0	0	—	55	—	—	—
Diet Raspberry Creme	1 can (12 oz)	0	0	0	0	0	0	0	0	—	45	—	—	—
Diet Red Pop	1 can (12 oz)	0	0	0	0	0	0	0	0	—	55	—	—	—
Diet Root Beer	1 can (12 oz)	0	0	0	0	0	0	0	0	—	55	—	—	—
Diet Strawberry	1 can (12 oz)	0	0	0	0	0	0	0	0	—	55	—	—	—
Diet Strawberry-Peach	1 can (12 oz)	0	0	0	0	0	0	0	0	—	55	—	—	—
Doc Shasta	1 can (12 oz)	160	0	0	0	0	39	39	0	—	45	—	—	—
Fruit Punch	1 can (12 oz)	200	0	0	0	0	50	50	0	—	45	—	—	—
Ginger Ale	1 can (12 oz)	130	0	0	0	0	32	32	0	—	45	—	—	—
Grape	1 can (12 oz)	190	0	0	0	0	48	48	0	—	45	—	—	—
Kiwi-Strawberry	1 can (12 oz)	170	0	0	0	0	43	43	0	—	45	—	—	—
Lemon-Lime Twist	1 can (12 oz)	150	0	0	0	0	38	38	0	—	45	—	—	—
Moon Mist	1 can (12 oz)	180	0	0	0	0	46	46	0	—	45	—	—	—
Orange	1 can (12 oz)	200	0	0	0	0	49	49	0	—	45	—	—	—
Peach	1 can (12 oz)	170	0	0	0	0	43	43	0	—	45	—	—	—
Pineapple	1 can (12 oz)	200	0	0	0	0	51	51	0	—	45	—	—	—
Pineapple-Orange	1 can (12 oz)	180	0	0	0	0	46	46	0	—	45	—	—	—
Quinine/Tonic	1 can (12 oz)	130	0	0	0	0	32	32	0	—	45	—	—	—
Raspberry Creme	1 can (12 oz)	170	0	0	0	0	44	44	0	—	45	—	—	—
Red Pop	1 can (12 oz)	170	0	0	0	0	43	43	0	—	45	—	—	—
Root Beer	1 can (12 oz)	170	0	0	0	0	42	42	0	—	45	—	—	—

FOOD	PORTION	CALS	FAT	SAT FAT	CHOL	PROT	CARB	SUGAR	FIBER	CALCI	SOD	POTAS	FOLIC	VIT C
SHASTA (CONT.)														
Strawberry	1 can (12 oz)	190	0	0	0	0	46	46	0	—	45	—	—	—
Strawberry-Peach	1 can (12 oz)	170	0	0	0	0	42	42	0	—	45	—	—	—
SKI														
Citrus	1 bottle (10 oz)	150	0	0	0	0	40	40	—	—	40	—	—	—
STEAP														
Green Tea Soda Root Beer	8 oz	90	0	0	0	0	23	23	—	—	35	—	—	36
Organic Green Tea Soda Raspberry	8 oz	90	0	0	0	0	23	23	—	—	35	—	—	12
STEWART'S														
Cream	1 bottle (12 oz)	180	0	0	0	0	45	45	—	—	50	—	—	—
Diet Cream	1 bottle (12 oz)	0	0	0	0	0	0	0	0	—	25	—	—	—
Root Beer	1 bottle (12 oz)	160	0	0	0	0	41	41	—	—	51	—	—	—
Strawberries N' Cream	1 bottle	200	—	—	—	0	50	50	—	—	65	—	—	—
Wishniak Black Cherry	1 bottle	180	—	—	—	0	47	47	—	—	65	—	—	—
SUNKIST														
Orange	1 can	190	0	0	0	0	52	52	0	—	45	—	—	—
THOMAS KEMPER														
Black Cherry	1 bottle	177	0	0	0	0	40	27	—	—	40	—	—	—
Old Fashion Birch	1 bottle	170	0	0	0	0	43	29	—	—	70	—	—	—
Orange Cream	1 bottle	180	0	0	0	0	37	30	—	—	64	—	—	—
Pure Draft Honey Cola	1 bottle	140	0	0	0	0	35	27	—	—	15	—	—	—
Pure Draft Root Beer	1 bottle	160	0	0	0	0	41	36	—	—	80	—	—	—
Vanilla Cream	1 bottle	170	0	0	0	0	43	29	—	—	70	—	—	—
THREE DRINKS														
Citrus	12 oz	12	0	0	0	0	3	2	—	—	20	—	—	—
TOMMYKNOCKER														
Almond Creme	1 bottle (12 oz)	150	0	0	0	0	40	40	—	—	19	—	—	—
Key Lime Creme	1 bottle (12 oz)	180	0	0	0	0	45	45	—	—	29	—	—	—
Orange Creme	1 bottle (12 oz)	180	0	0	0	0	45	45	—	—	29	—	—	—
Root Beer	1 bottle (12 oz)	150	0	0	0	0	40	40	—	—	19	—	—	—
Root Beer Float	1 bottle (12 oz)	110	0	0	0	0	29	28	—	—	20	—	—	—
Strawberry Creme	1 bottle (12 oz)	150	0	0	0	0	40	40	—	—	19	—	—	—
VERMONT SWEETWATER														
Coutry Apple Jack	1 bottle	180	0	0	0	0	42	42	0	—	8	—	—	—
Kickin' Cow Cola	1 bottle	129	0	0	0	0	33	33	0	—	8	—	—	—
Mango Moonshine	1 bottle	180	0	0	0	0	42	42	0	—	8	—	—	—
Maple	1 bottle	101	0	0	0	0	27	27	0	—	2	—	—	—
Raspberry Rhubarb Ramble	1 bottle	180	0	0	0	0	42	42	0	—	8	—	—	—

FOOD	PORTION	CALS	FAT	SAT FAT	CHOL	PROT	CARB	SUGAR	FIBER	CALCI	SOD	POTAS	FOLIC	VIT C
VERMONT SWEETWATER (CONT.)														
Tangerine Cream Twister	1 bottle	180	0	0	0	0	42	42	0	—	8	—	—	—
Vermont Maple Seltzer	1 bottle	53	0	0	0	0	12	12	0	—	0	—	—	—
VIRGIL'S														
Micro Brewed Root Beer	1 bottle (12 oz)	160	0	0	0	0	42	42	—	—	0	—	—	—
WHITE T														
All Flavors	1 bottle (12 oz)	128	0	0	0	0	33	33	0	—	15	—	—	—
Diet All Flavors	1 bottle (12 oz)	0	0	0	0	0	0	0	0	—	15	—	—	—
YOO-HOO														
Original	9 fl oz	150	tr	tr	0	3	31	—	tr	100	200	250	8	6
Z COLA														
No Artifical Sweeteners	8 oz	0	0	0	0	0	1	0	0	—	35	—	—	—
SOLE														
cooked	3 oz	99	1	tr	58	21	0	—	—	16	89	292	—	—
cooked	1 fillet (4.5 oz)	148	2	tr	86	31	0	—	—	23	133	436	—	—
lemon raw	3.5 oz	85	1	—	—	17	0	—	—	—	80	298	—	—
raw	3.5 oz	90	1	—	50	18	0	—	—	29	100	309	—	0
TAKE-OUT														
breaded & fried	3.2 oz	211	11	3	31	13	15	—	—	17	484	292	51	0
SORGHUM														
sorghum	1 cup (6.7 oz)	651	6	1	0	22	143	—	—	54	12	672	—	0
SOUFFLÉ														
lemon chilled	1 cup	176	tr	—	2	9	34	—	—	175	108	—	—	—
raspberry chilled	1 cup	173	tr	—	3	10	34	—	—	190	108	—	—	—
spinach	1 cup	218	18	7	184	11	3	—	—	230	763	202	62	3
ATKINS														
Broccoli Cheddar & Bacon	1 serv	200	15	8	205	12	3	2	1	200	520	—	—	24
SOUP														
CANNED														
asparagus cream of as prep w/ milk	1 cup	161	8	3	22	6	16	—	—	175	1041	359	—	4
asparagus cream of as prep w/ water	1 cup	87	4	1	5	1	11	—	—	29	981	173	—	3
beef broth ready-to-serve	1 cup	16	1	tr	tr	3	tr	—	—	15	782	130	—	0
beef broth ready-to-serve	1 can (14 oz)	27	1	tr	1	5	tr	—	—	25	1294	214	—	0
beef noodle as prep w/water	1 cup	84	3	1	5	5	9	—	—	15	952	99	4	tr
black bean turtle soup	1 cup	218	1	tr	0	14	40	—	17	84	922	739	146	6

FOOD	PORTION	CALS	FAT	SAT FAT	CHOL	PROT	CARB	SUGAR	FIBER	CALCI	SOD	POTAS	FOLIC	VIT C
black bean as prep w/water	1 cup	116	2	tr	0	6	20	—	—	45	1198	273	25	1
celery cream of as prep w/ milk	1 cup	165	10	4	32	6	15	—	—	186	1010	309	9	1
celery cream of as prep w/ water	1 cup	90	6	1	15	2	9	—	—	40	949	123	2	tr
celery cream of not prep	1 can (10¾ oz)	219	14	3	34	4	21	—	—	98	2308	299	6	1
cheese as prep w/ milk	1 cup	230	15	9	48	9	16	—	—	288	1020	340	—	1
cheese as prep w/ water	1 cup	155	10	7	30	5	11	—	—	142	959	154	—	0
cheese not prep	1 can (11 oz)	377	25	16	72	13	26	—	—	345	2331	374	—	0
chicken broth as prep w/ water	1 cup	39	1	tr	1	5	1	—	—	9	776	210	—	0
chicken cream of as prep w/ milk	1 cup	191	11	5	27	7	15	—	—	180	1046	273	8	1
chicken cream of as prep w/ water	1 cup	116	7	2	10	3	9	—	—	34	986	87	2	tr
chicken gumbo as prep w/ water	1 cup	56	1	tr	5	3	8	—	—	24	955	75	—	5
chicken noodle as prep w/ water	1 cup	75	2	1	7	4	9	—	—	17	1107	55	2	tr
chicken rice as prep w/ water	1 cup	251	2	tr	7	4	7	—	—	17	814	100	1	tr
clam chowder manhattan as prep w/ water	1 cup	77	2	tr	3	2	12	—	—	26	1029	188	10	4
clam chowder new england as prep w/ water	1 cup	95	3	tr	5	5	12	—	—	43	914	146	4	2
clam chowder new england as prep w/ milk	1 cup	163	7	3	22	9	17	—	—	187	992	300	10	4
consommé w/ gelatin not prep	1 can (10½ oz)	71	0	0	0	13	4	—	—	21	1550	373	7	2
consommé w/ gelatin as prep w/ water	1 cup	29	0	0	0	5	2	—	—	8	637	153	3	1
escarole ready-to-serve	1 cup	27	2	1	2	2	2	—	—	32	3865	—	—	—
french onion as prep w/ water	1 cup	57	2	tr	0	4	8	—	—	26	1053	69	15	1
gazpacho ready-to-serve	1 cup	57	2	tr	0	9	1	—	—	24	1183	224	—	3
minestrone as prep w/water	1 cup	83	3	1	2	4	11	—	—	34	911	312	16	1
mushroom cream of as prep w/ milk	1 cup	203	14	5	20	6	15	—	—	178	1076	270	—	2

FOOD	PORTION	CALS	FAT	SAT FAT	CHOL	PROT	CARB	SUGAR	FIBER	CALCI	SOD	POTAS	FOLIC	VIT C
mushroom cream of as prep w/ water	1 cup	129	9	2	2	2	9	—	—	46	1031	101	—	1
oyster stew as prep w/ milk	1 cup	134	8	5	32	6	10	—	—	167	1040	235	—	4
oyster stew as prep w/ water	1 cup	59	4	3	14	2	4	—	—	22	980	49	—	3
pepperpot as prep w/ water	1 cup	103	5	2	10	6	9	—	—	23	970	152	tr	1
potato cream of as prep w/ milk	1 cup	148	6	4	22	6	17	—	—	166	1060	323	9	1
potato cream of as prep w/ water	1 cup	73	2	1	5	2	11	—	—	20	1000	137	3	0
scotch broth as prep w/ water	1 cup	80	3	1	5	5	9	—	—	15	1012	159	—	1
split pea w/ ham as prep w/ water	1 cup	189	4	2	8	10	28	—	—	22	1008	399	3	1
tomato as prep w/ milk	1 cup	160	6	3	17	6	22	—	—	159	932	450	21	68
tomato as prep w/ water	1 cup	86	2	tr	0	2	17	—	—	13	872	263	15	67
vegetarian vegetable as prep w/ water	1 cup	72	2	tr	0	2	12	—	—	21	823	209	11	1
vichyssoise	1 cup	148	6	4	22	6	17	—	—	166	1060	323	9	1
AMY'S														
Organic Barley	1 cup	50	1	0	0	1	10	4	2	—	580	—	—	—
Organic Black Bean Vegetable	1 cup	110	1	0	0	6	22	6	5	—	580	—	—	—
Organic Cream Of Mushroom	1 cup	120	9	2	5	2	10	2	2	—	590	—	—	—
Organic Cream Of Tomato	1 cup	100	2	2	10	2	17	11	4	—	590	—	—	—
Organic Lentil	1 cup	130	4	1	0	8	19	3	9	—	590	—	—	—
Organic Minestrone	1 cup	90	2	0	0	3	17	5	3	—	540	—	—	—
Organic No Chicken Noodle Soup	1 cup	90	3	0	0	5	12	4	2	—	480	—	—	—
Organic Vegetable	1 cup	35	0	0	0	1	8	4	1	—	680	—	—	—
BOSTON MARKET														
Chicken Broth Reduced Sodium	1 cup	15	1	0	0	1	1	0	0	0	760	—	—	0
BUTTERBALL														
Chicken Broth Reduced Sodium 99% Fat Free	1 cup	10	0	0	0	1	2	0	0	—	620	—	—	—

FOOD	PORTION	CALS	FAT	SAT FAT	CHOL	PROT	CARB	SUGAR	FIBER	CALCI	SOD	POTAS	FOLIC	VIT C
CAMPBELL'S														
98% Fat Free Cream Of Chicken as prep	1 cup	70	2	1	10	3	10	1	tr	20	890	—	—	0
Cheddar Cheese	1 cup	110	5	3	10	3	12	2	1	80	950	—	—	0
Cheddar Cheese as prep	1 cup	134	8	4	19	4	11	1	1	122	1083	30	—	tr
Chicken Vegetable as prep	1 cup	74	3	1	9	3	9	1	1	16	985	125	—	1
Chicken Broth	½ cup	20	1	0	<5	1	1	1	0	0	770	—	—	0
Chicken Gumbo as prep	1 cup	55	1	1	5	2	9	2	1	23	985	87	—	0
Chunky Beef Barley	1 cup	160	3	1	25	10	22	4	2	20	920	—	—	1
Chunky Chicken Corn Chowder	1 cup	230	13	4	20	8	21	4	3	20	800	—	—	0
Chunky New England Clam Chowder	1 cup	240	13	2	15	7	23	1	2	20	890	—	—	2
Chunky Old Fashioned Vegetable Beef	1 cup	130	3	2	15	9	18	2	6	40	910	—	—	0
Chunky Sirloin Burger w/ Country Vegetables	1 cup	180	8	5	20	10	17	4	3	20	890	—	—	1
Chunky Classic Chicken Noodle	1 cup	100	3	1	20	9	16	3	2	20	860	—	—	0
Chunky Vegetable	1 cup	130	4	1	0	3	22	5	4	40	870	—	—	1
Clam Chowder New England as prep	1 cup	89	3	1	3	4	13	tr	1	29	979	127	—	2
Classics Chicken Rice	1 cup (8.1 oz)	80	2	1	5	2	14	0	1	0	850	—	—	0
Classics Beef Noodle	1 cup	70	3	1	15	5	8	1	1	300	920	—	—	0
Classics Minestrone	1 cup	90	1	1	<5	4	17	3	3	20	960	—	—	0
Classics Old Fashioned Vegetable	1 cup	90	2	1	<5	3	16	3	2	20	940	—	—	0
Classics Vegetarian Vegetable as prep	1 cup	90	1	0	0	3	18	6	2	20	790	—	—	0
Consommé as prep	1 cup	24	tr	0	tr	5	1	1	tr	7	817	56	—	0
Cream Of Asparagus as prep	1 cup	72	4	1	2	2	9	3	1	25	749	68	—	1
Cream Of Mushroom as prep	1 cup	108	7	2	2	2	9	1	2	21	872	78	—	tr

FOOD	PORTION	CALS	FAT	SAT FAT	CHOL	PROT	CARB	SUGAR	FIBER	CALCI	SOD	POTAS	FOLIC	VIT C
CAMPBELL'S (CONT.)														
Cream Of Celery as prep	1 cup	107	7	2	2	2	9	1	1	30	903	110	—	tr
Cream Of Chicken as prep	1 cup	120	8	3	10	3	10	1	1	20	880	—	—	0
Cream of Chicken w/ Herbs	1 cup	90	4	2	10	3	10	2	1	20	890	—	—	0
Fiesta Tomato as prep	1 cup	72	tr	tr	1	1	16	8	1	33	856	302	—	7
Garden Vegetable as prep	1 cup	69	2	1	3	3	11	2	1	21	857	186	—	3
Green Pea as prep	1 cup	173	3	1	1	9	29	4	4	20	888	337	—	0
Healthy Request Chicken Noodle as prep	1 cup	70	2	1	15	3	9	1	0	300	480	—	—	0
Healthy Request Chicken Rice as prep	1 cup	60	2	1	10	2	8	1	tr	0	420	—	—	12
Healthy Request Cream Of Mushroom as prep	1 cup	66	2	1	4	2	10	2	1	122	475	464	—	0
Healthy Request Cream Of Chicken & Broccoli as prep	1 cup	78	3	1	6	3	10	2	1	21	460	402	—	3
Healthy Request Cream Of Chicken as prep	1 cup	70	3	1	10	2	12	2	tr	0	430	330	—	0
Healthy Request Hearty Pasta w/ Vegetables	1 cup	87	1	tr	1	3	17	7	2	30	474	614	—	2
Healthy Request Tomato as prep	1 cup	91	2	tr	1	2	18	9	2	15	456	252	—	31
Healthy Request Vegetable as prep	1 cup	84	1	tr	1	3	17	5	2	25	473	542	—	1
Home Cookin' Chicken Vegetable	1 cup (8.4 oz)	130	4	1	10	6	20	6	3	40	820	—	—	1
Italian Tomato as prep	1 cup	105	tr	tr	1	2	23	16	4	40	820	394	—	23
Kitchen Classics Bean w/ Bacon	1 cup	180	4	2	5	9	28	4	8	60	820	—	—	0
Kitchen Classics Chicken Noodle	1 cup	980	1	1	10	6	13	1	1	20	870	—	—	0
Kitchen Classics Chicken w/ White & Wild Rice	1 cup	100	1	1	10	5	18	1	2	20	800	—	—	0
Kitchen Classics Lentil	1 cup	120	1	1	5	7	23	1	5	50	750	—	—	0

FOOD	PORTION	CALS	FAT	SAT FAT	CHOL	PROT	CARB	SUGAR	FIBER	CALCI	SOD	POTAS	FOLIC	VIT C
CAMPBELL'S (CONT.)														
Low Sodium Chicken w/ Noodles	1 can (10.75 oz)	162	5	2	40	14	16	3	2	34	85	296	—	3
Low Sodium Chunky Vegetable Beef	1 can (10.75 oz)	159	4	1	39	13	17	5	3	49	64	400	—	10
Low Sodium Cream of Mushroom	1 can (10.75 oz)	200	13	4	12	3	18	5	2	69	48	122	—	1
Low Sodium Green Pea	1 can (10.75 oz)	235	4	2	4	12	38	4	6	43	27	451	—	4
Low Sodium Tomato w/ Pieces	1 can (10.75 oz)	170	5	2	6	4	28	17	3	48	36	593	—	37
Ready To Serve Bean w/ Bacon 'N Ham	1 can (10.5 oz)	274	7	2	13	14	41	8	11	101	1299	653	—	7
Ready To Serve Chicken Noodle	1 cup	80	2	1	15	3	11	1	1	0	890	—	—	0
Ready To Serve Chicken w/ Rice	1 can (10.5 oz)	122	2	1	11	5	20	4	2	48	1132	298	—	0
Ready-To-Serve Vegetable Beef	1 can (10.5 oz)	143	1	tr	10	9	26	5	5	77	1243	474	—	1
Savory Tomato & Dill as prep	1 cup	99	2	tr	tr	2	20	11	2	28	811	0	—	25
Select Chicken & Pasta w/ Roasted Garlic	1 cup (8.4 oz)	100	1	1	10	7	16	4	2	20	840	—	—	0
Select Chicken Rice	1 cup	100	1	1	5	6	17	2	2	20	990	—	—	1
Select Chicken w/ Egg Noodles	1 cup	110	2	1	15	9	14	1	1	20	990	—	—	0
Select Creamy Potato w/ Roasted Garlic	1 cup	180	10	3	10	3	20	3	2	20	770	—	—	0
Select Fiesta Vegetable	1 cup (8.4 oz)	120	1	0	0	4	24	7	3	40	810	—	—	4
Select Herbed Chicken w/ Roasted Vegetables	1 cup	90	1	1	15	7	14	2	1	20	890	—	—	0
Select Italian Style Wedding	1 cup	110	3	2	10	8	16	3	2	60	840	—	—	0
Select Mexican Chicken Tortilla	1 cup	150	3	2	10	8	22	1	4	60	890	—	—	1

FOOD	PORTION	CALS	FAT	SAT FAT	CHOL	PROT	CARB	SUGAR	FIBER	CALCI	SOD	POTAS	FOLIC	VIT C
CAMPBELL'S (CONT.)														
Select Roasted Chicken w/ Long Grain & Wild Rice	1 cup	130	1	1	10	6	17	2	1	20	890	—	—	0
Select Roasted Chicken w/ Rotini & Penne Pasta	1 cup	90	1	1	10	6	16	4	2	20	840	—	—	0
Select Rosemary Chicken w/ Roasted Potatoes	1 cup	110	1	0	10	8	18	2	2	20	820	—	—	0
Select Split Pea w/ Ham	1 cup (8.4 oz)	170	2	1	10	10	30	6	6	40	860	—	—	2
Select Tuscany-Style Minestrone	1 cup (8.4 oz)	190	9	2	5	5	21	5	5	80	870	—	—	2
Soup At Hand Blended Vegetable Medley	1 pkg (10.75 oz)	110	2	2	10	3	21	10	4	20	950	—	—	36
Vegetable Beef as prep	1 cup	68	2	1	8	5	9	1	2	18	897	121	—	4
COLLEGE INN														
Beef Broth 99% Fat Free	1 cup	20	1	0	0	4	0	0	0	0	910	—	—	0
Beef Broth Fat Free Lower Sodium	1 cup	15	0	0	0	4	0	0	0	0	450	—	—	0
Chicken Broth Light & Fat Free	1 cup	5	0	0	0	1	0	0	0	0	450	—	—	0
GOLD'S														
Borscht Unsalted	1 cup	70	0	0	0	1	17	16	1	20	45	—	—	2
HEALTH VALLEY														
5 Bean Vegetable	1 cup	250	0	0	0	10	32	9	10	80	250	—	—	12
Beef Broth Fat Free	1 cup	20	0	0	0	5	0	2	0	0	160	—	—	0
Beef Broth Fat Free No Salt	1 cup	20	0	0	0	5	0	2	0	0	160	—	—	0
Black Bean & Vegetable	1 cup	110	0	0	0	11	24	8	9	40	280	—	—	9
Chicken Broth	1 cup	45	2	—	25	7	0	0	0	0	250	—	—	0
Chicken Broth Fat Free	1 cup	30	0	0	0	7	0	0	0	0	170	—	—	0
Chicken Broth No Salt	1 cup	45	2	—	25	7	0	0	0	0	25	—	—	0
Country Corn & Vegetable	1 cup	70	0	0	0	5	17	8	7	40	135	—	—	6
Garden Vegetable	1 cup	80	0	0	0	6	17	8	4	40	250	—	—	15

FOOD	PORTION	CALS	FAT	SAT FAT	CHOL	PROT	CARB	SUGAR	FIBER	CALCI	SOD	POTAS	FOLIC	VIT C
HEALTH VALLEY (CONT.)														
Italian Plus Carotene	1 cup	80	0	0	0	7	19	5	6	40	240	—	—	6
Lentil & Carrot	1 cup	100	0	0	0	10	25	7	10	60	220	—	—	2
Organic Black Bean	1 cup	110	0	0	0	8	28	14	10	40	45	—	—	24
Organic Lentil No Salt	1 cup	90	0	0	0	9	20	7	9	40	40	—	—	4
Organic Minestrone	1 cup	100	0	0	0	8	23	6	8	40	190	—	—	9
Organic Mushroom Barley No Salt	1 cup	60	0	0	0	5	15	5	5	20	95	—	—	7
Organic Potato Leek	1 cup	70	0	0	0	4	15	5	3	20	230	—	—	0
Organic Potato Leek No Salt	1 cup	70	0	0	0	4	15	5	3	20	35	—	—	0
Organic Split Pea	1 cup	110	0	0	0	10	23	5	8	20	160	—	—	1
Organic Split Pea No Salt	1 cup	110	0	0	0	10	23	5	8	20	115	—	—	1
Organic Tomato	1 cup	90	0	0	0	4	22	20	4	20	250	—	—	12
Organic Vegetable No Salt	1 cup	80	0	0	0	5	18	10	6	40	80	—	—	5
Pasta Bolognese	1 cup	100	0	0	0	4	20	4	4	60	290	—	—	12
Pasta Cacciatore	1 cup	100	0	0	0	4	20	6	4	60	290	—	—	12
Pasta Romano	1 cup	100	0	0	0	4	20	6	4	60	290	—	—	12
Real Italian Minestrone	1 cup	90	0	0	0	8	21	6	8	40	210	—	—	5
Rotini & Vegetable	1 cup	100	0	0	0	4	20	4	4	60	290	—	—	12
Split Pea & Carrots	1 cup	110	0	0	0	8	17	7	4	40	230	—	—	9
Super Broccoli Carotene	1 cup	70	0	0	0	6	16	12	7	40	240	—	—	9
Tomato Vegetable	1 cup	80	0	0	0	6	17	9	5	40	240	—	—	9
Vegetable Barley	1 cup	90	0	0	0	6	19	4	4	40	210	—	—	15
Vegetable Power Carotene	1 cup	70	0	0	0	5	17	7	6	40	240	—	—	6
HEALTHY CHOICE														
Bean & Ham	1 cup (8.7 oz)	166	1	tr	4	9	31	3	7	74	570	979	—	6
Beef & Potato	1 cup (8.5 oz)	116	1	1	5	11	16	3	tr	21	452	919	—	5
Broccoli Cheddar	1 cup (8.4 oz)	116	2	1	4	4	22	1	2	55	304	130	—	1
Chicken Corn Chowder	1 cup (8.8 oz)	176	3	1	8	8	30	2	2	23	466	1101	—	9
Chicken Pasta	1 cup (8.6 oz)	119	3	1	6	7	18	0	1	37	493	758	—	3
Chicken Rice	1 cup (8.4 oz)	119	2	1	6	9	19	3	3	18	324	672	—	5
Chili Beef	1 cup (9.1 oz)	189	2	1	12	15	32	5	5	88	441	1899	—	1

FOOD	PORTION	CALS	FAT	SAT FAT	CHOL	PROT	CARB	SUGAR	FIBER	CALCI	SOD	POTAS	FOLIC	VIT C
HEALTHY CHOICE (CONT.)														
Clam Chowder	1 cup (8.8 oz)	123	1	1	12	6	23	3	2	32	481	562	—	2
Classic Italian Bean and Pasta	1 cup (8 oz)	100	2	1	0	6	17	0	3	60	480	—	—	0
Country Vegetable	1 cup	100	1	0	0	4	21	4	5	40	480	—	—	2
Cream Of Mushroom	1 cup (8.8 oz)	77	1	tr	tr	4	14	0	1	112	450	360	—	1
Cream Of Celery as prep	1 cup	73	2	1	3	1	14	2	3	16	366	470	—	1
Cream Of Chicken Vegetable	1 cup (8.9 oz)	127	2	1	10	7	21	0	1	36	384	945	—	1
Cream Of Roasted Chicken as prep	1 cup	80	3	1	4	2	13	1	3	11	349	318	—	tr
Cream Of Roasted Garlic as prep	1 cup	57	1	tr	2	1	13	0	3	8	489	67	—	tr
Garden Vegetable	1 cup (8.6 oz)	108	1	1	tr	5	22	0	6	55	454	—	—	1
Lentil	1 cup (8.7 oz)	135	1	tr	tr	10	28	2	5	67	472	1455	—	1
Minestrone	1 cup (8.6 oz)	107	1	tr	1	5	24	4	5	60	370	1073	—	1
Old Fashioned Chicken Noodle	1 cup	110	2	1	10	8	17	0	3	20	480	—	—	1
Roasted Italian Style Chicken	1 cup	120	2	1	15	9	18	4	4	60	480	—	—	4
Split Pea & Ham	1 cup (8.8 oz)	164	2	1	7	11	26	6	5	50	468	1460	—	13
Tomato Garden	1 cup (8.6 oz)	101	1	1	1	4	19	8	5	70	468	961	—	1
Turkey Wild Rice	1 cup (8.4 oz)	72	1	tr	3	10	9	5	3	27	407	727	—	1
Vegetable Beef	1 cup (8.8 oz)	96	1	tr	2	11	14	3	2	31	433	1434	—	2
Zesty Gumbo	1 cup	100	2	1	20	6	16	2	3	40	480	—	—	5
HERB-OX														
Beef Liquid	2 tsp (0.4 oz)	20	0	0	0	2	2	1	0	0	570	—	—	0
Chicken Liquid	2 tsp (0.4 oz)	15	0	0	0	1	1	0	0	0	620	—	—	0
IMAGINE														
Creamy Broccoli	1 serv (8 oz)	70	2	0	0	3	10	4	2	40	370	—	—	5
Creamy Butternut Squash	1 serv (8 oz)	120	2	2	0	2	23	14	2	40	370	—	—	0
Creamy Mushroom	1 serv (8 oz)	80	3	1	0	4	10	1	2	20	310	—	—	0
Creamy Potato Leek	1 serv (8 oz)	90	3	0	0	2	14	tr	2	20	380	—	—	0
Creamy Sweet Corn	1 serv (8 oz)	100	3	1	0	4	15	6	1	0	540	—	—	0
Creamy Tomato	1 serv (8 oz)	90	2	0	0	8	17	10	2	40	520	—	—	0
Vegetable Broth	1 serv (8 oz)	45	1	0	0	0	7	5	1	20	500	—	—	0
Zesty Gazpacho	1 serv (8 oz)	80	0	0	0	tr	8	5	tr	90	720	—	—	11
MANISCHEWITZ														
Clear Chicken Condensed	½ cup	15	1	0	0	tr	2	0	2	0	740	—	—	1

FOOD	PORTION	CALS	FAT	SAT FAT	CHOL	PROT	CARB	SUGAR	FIBER	CALCI	SOD	POTAS	FOLIC	VIT C
NATURAL CHOICE														
Orangic Vegan Classic Tomato	1 cup	100	1	0	0	2	22	8	2	20	317	—	—	15
Organic Vegan Classic Mushroom	1 cup	50	2	0	0	2	9	3	2	20	435	—	—	4
Organic Vegan Country Corn	1 cup	100	1	0	0	3	24	6	3	20	377	—	—	6
Organic Vegan Kabocha Squash	1 cup	60	1	0	0	2	14	8	1	40	370	—	—	12
Organic Vegan Southern Greens	1 cup	80	3	0	0	2	13	5	2	40	399	—	—	12
Organic Vegan Split Pea	1 cup	120	1	0	0	7	21	4	7	20	420	—	—	2
Organic Vegan Vegetable Curry	1 cup	110	4	1	0	4	17	4	2	40	392	—	—	9
PACIFIC														
Free Range Organic Chicken Broth	1 cup	5	0	0	0	1	1	—	—	—	570	—	—	—
PROGRESSO														
99% Fat Free Beef Barley	1 cup (8.5 oz)	140	2	1	20	11	20	4	3	20	470	—	—	4
99% Fat Free Beef Vegetable	1 cup (8.5 oz)	160	2	1	10	11	24	4	3	0	870	—	—	5
99% Fat Free Chicken Rice w/ Vegetables	1 cup (8.4 oz)	110	2	0	10	7	16	2	1	20	780	—	—	0
99% Fat Free Lentil	1 cup (8.5 oz)	130	2	0	0	8	20	1	6	40	440	—	—	0
99% Fat Free Minestrone	1 cup (8.5 oz)	130	2	0	0	7	23	3	4	40	710	—	—	0
99% Fat Free Split Pea	1 cup (8.9 oz)	170	2	0	0	10	29	5	5	0	620	—	—	0
99% Fat Free Tomato Garden Vegetable	1 cup (8.6 oz)	100	2	0	0	3	19	7	2	20	660	—	—	5
99% Fat Free Vegetable	1 cup (8.4 oz)	70	1	0	0	2	13	3	2	0	870	—	—	0
99% Fat Free White Cheddar Potato	1 cup (8.6 oz)	140	3	2	5	4	26	2	2	40	930	—	—	6
Bean & Ham	1 cup (8.4 oz)	160	2	1	10	10	25	3	8	80	870	—	—	0
Beef & Vegetable	1 cup	130	3	2	20	10	16	4	2	20	850	—	—	6
Beef Barley	1 cup (8.5 oz)	130	4	2	25	10	13	4	3	40	780	—	—	0
Beef Minestrone	1 cup (8.5 oz)	140	3	1	10	10	18	3	3	20	970	—	—	2
Beef Noodle	1 cup (8.5 oz)	140	4	2	30	13	15	2	1	20	950	—	—	0
Cheese & Herb Tortellini Tomato	1 cup (8.6 oz)	140	3	1	<5	4	23	9	2	60	700	—	—	1

FOOD	PORTION	CALS	FAT	SAT FAT	CHOL	PROT	CARB	SUGAR	FIBER	CALCI	SOD	POTAS	FOLIC	VIT C
PROGRESSO (CONT.)														
Chickarina	1 cup (8.3 oz)	130	5	2	20	8	12	tr	tr	20	1010	—	—	0
Chicken Minestrone	1 cup (8.4 oz)	110	2	0	15	9	15	2	2	20	890	—	—	0
Chicken Vegetable	1 cup (8.4 oz)	90	2	0	15	7	13	2	2	0	820	—	—	0
Chicken & Wild Rice	1 cup (8.4 oz)	100	2	1	15	7	15	1	1	0	850	—	—	0
Chicken Barley	1 cup (8.5 oz)	110	2	0	15	8	16	2	3	0	850	—	—	0
Chicken Broth	1 cup (8.2 oz)	20	2	0	0	1	1	0	0	0	920	—	—	0
Chicken Rice w/ Vegetable	1 cup	100	2	0	10	6	15	1	1	20	820	—	—	0
Clam & Rotini Chowder	1 cup (8.8 oz)	190	9	2	10	7	21	3	0	80	800	—	—	0
Escarole In Chicken Broth	1 cup (8.1 oz)	25	1	0	<5	1	3	tr	1	20	930	—	—	0
Hearty Black Bean	1 cup (8.5 oz)	170	2	0	<5	8	30	2	10	60	730	—	—	0
Hearty Penne In Chicken Broth	1 cup (8.4 oz)	80	1	0	0	4	14	1	tr	0	1020	—	—	0
Hearty Tomato	1 cup (8.7 oz)	100	2	0	0	2	19	11	1	0	800	—	—	12
Herb Rotini Vegetable	1 cup (9.1 oz)	120	2	0	0	5	21	5	4	40	990	—	—	0
Homestyle Chicken w/ Vegetable	1 cup (8.4 oz)	90	2	0	15	7	11	1	tr	0	900	—	—	0
Italian Herb Shells Minestrone	1 cup (9.1 oz)	120	2	0	0	5	22	4	4	40	1050	—	—	0
Macaroni & Bean	1 cup (8.6 oz)	160	4	1	<5	7	23	1	6	40	800	—	—	0
Manhattan Clam Chowder	1 cup (8.4 oz)	110	2	0	10	12	11	3	3	40	710	—	—	4
Meatballs & Pasta Pearls	1 cup (8.3 oz)	140	7	3	15	7	13	0	0	40	700	—	—	0
Minestrone Parmesan	1 cup (8.3 oz)	100	3	1	0	3	16	3	3	40	700	—	—	1
New England Clam Chowder	1 cup (8.4 oz)	190	10	3	15	6	20	3	1	40	920	—	—	4
Oregano Penne Italian Style Vegetable	1 cup (8.7 oz)	90	2	0	0	3	15	2	1	20	960	—	—	0
Peppercorn Penne Vegetable	1 cup (9.1 oz)	100	1	0	0	3	20	3	2	0	920	—	—	0
Potato Broccoli & Cheese	1 cup (8.8 oz)	160	6	2	<5	5	21	4	1	80	960	—	—	6
Potato Ham & Cheese	1 cup (8.6 oz)	170	7	2	10	6	21	3	1	60	860	—	—	2
Rich & Hearty Beef Pot Roast	1 cup	130	2	1	20	10	17	4	2	40	990	—	—	0

FOOD	PORTION	CALS	FAT	SAT FAT	CHOL	PROT	CARB	SUGAR	FIBER	CALCI	SOD	POTAS	FOLIC	VIT C
PROGRESSO (CONT.)														
Rich & Hearty Chicken & Homestyle Noodles	1 cup	110	3	1	30	8	14	2	1	20	990	—	—	0
Roasted Garlic Pasta Lentil	1 cup (9.3 oz)	120	2	0	0	7	20	2	5	20	960	—	—	0
Rotisserie Seasoned Chicken	1 cup (8.5 oz)	100	2	0	15	7	15	2	2	0	920	—	—	0
Spicy Chicken & Penne	1 cup (8.5 oz)	110	2	0	15	9	14	2	1	0	950	—	—	0
Split Pea w/ Ham	1 cup (8.4 oz)	150	4	2	15	9	20	3	5	40	830	—	—	2
Tomato	1 cup (8.5 oz)	100	2	0	0	2	19	10	1	0	790	—	—	12
Tomato Basil	1 cup (8.8 oz)	100	2	0	0	2	19	10	1	0	790	—	—	12
Tomato Vegetable	1 cup (8.5 oz)	90	2	0	0	3	15	8	4	20	990	—	—	1
Tortellini In Chicken Broth	1 cup (8.3 oz)	70	2	1	10	3	10	1	2	20	970	—	—	0
Traditional Chicken & Herb Dumplings	1 cup	110	3	1	30	7	15	1	1	20	750	—	—	0
Traditional Chicken Noodle	1 cup	100	2	1	25	9	13	2	1	20	980	—	—	0
Traditional Hearty Chicken & Rotini	1 cup	100	2	1	15	8	12	1	1	20	940	—	—	0
Turkey Noodle	1 cup	90	2	0	20	7	11	1	1	0	1060	—	—	0
Turkey Rice w/ Vegetables	1 cup (8.5 oz)	110	1	0	15	7	18	2	1	20	1040	—	—	1
Vegetable Classics Green Split Pea	1 cup	170	3	1	5	10	28	6	4	0	870	—	—	0
Vegetable Classics Lentil	1 cup	180	2	0	0	10	30	1	5	40	880	—	—	0
Vegetable Classics Tomato Rotini	1 cup	140	1	0	0	4	30	12	2	20	1000	—	—	18
Vegetable Classics Vegetable	1 cup	80	1	0	0	3	16	6	2	20	940	—	—	0
Vegetables Classics Minestrone	1 cup	110	2	0	0	4	19	2	5	40	980	—	—	0
Vegetable Classics French Onion	1 cup	50	2	1	<5	tr	9	3	1	20	900	—	—	0
SNOW'S														
Clam Chowder	1 cup	200	15	4	15	5	13	3	1	40	900	—	—	4
STREIT'S														
Hearty Vegetarian Vegetable	1 cup	90	0	0	0	3	19	7	3	20	520	—	—	0
Mushroom Barley	1 cup	100	2	0	0	3	17	4	3	20	890	—	—	2

FOOD	PORTION	CALS	FAT	SAT FAT	CHOL	PROT	CARB	SUGAR	FIBER	CALCI	SOD	POTAS	FOLIC	VIT C
SWANSON														
Beef Broth 100% Fat Free Lower Sodium	1 cup	15	0	—	<5	2	1	1	—	—	440	—	—	—
Beef Broth 99% Fat Free	1 cup	10	1	—	—	2	0	0	0	—	890	—	—	—
Beef Broth Onion Seasoned	1 cup (8.4 oz)	20	0	0	0	2	2	1	tr	—	890	—	—	—
Chicken Broth 100% Fat Free 33% Less Sodium	1 cup	15	0	0	0	3	1	1	—	—	570	—	—	—
Chicken Broth 99% Fat Free	1 cup	15	1	0	<5	1	1	1	—	—	960	—	—	—
Vegetable Broth	1 cup	19	1	0	1	1	3	3	0	14	996	42	—	0
WALNUT ACRES														
Organic Country Corn Chowder	1 cup (8.8 oz)	150	3	2	10	4	28	8	2	80	690	—	—	15
WEIGHT WATCHERS														
Chicken & Rice	1 can (10.5 oz)	110	2	0	10	6	17	11	4	60	720	—	—	0
Chicken Noodle	1 can (10.5 oz)	150	2	1	30	9	25	15	4	60	740	—	—	0
Minestrone	1 can (10.5 oz)	130	2	1	5	5	23	7	6	100	760	—	—	1
Vegetable	1 can (10.5 oz)	130	1	0	0	4	27	11	6	80	680	—	—	2
FROZEN														
BIRDS EYE														
Hearty Spoonfuls Pasta & Chicken	1 bowl (11.2 oz)	140	2	0	20	11	19	3	2	40	1000	—	—	1
NATURE'S ENTREE														
Chowder	1 pkg (12 oz)	230	6	3	15	16	26	5	5	150	960	—	—	9
Tortellini Minestrone	1 pkg (12 oz)	360	9	1	10	22	48	6	5	80	960	—	—	9
MIX														
asparagus cream of as prep w/ water	1 cup	59	2	tr	tr	2	9	—	—	—	801	—	—	—
beef broth	1 pkg (0.2 oz)	14	1	tr	1	1	1	—	—	4	1019	27	—	—
beef broth as prep w/ water	1 cup	19	1	tr	1	1	2	—	—	10	1368	36	—	—
beef broth cube	1 cube (3.6 g)	6	tr	tr	tr	1	1	—	—	—	864	15	—	—
beef broth cube as prep w/ water	1 cup	8	tr	tr	tr	1	1	—	—	—	1152	20	—	—
celery cream of as prep w/ water	1 cup	63	2	tr	1	3	10	—	—	—	839	—	—	—
chicken broth	1 pkg (0.2 oz)	16	1	tr	1	1	1	—	—	11	1116	19	—	tr
chicken broth as prep w/ water	1 cup	21	1	tr	1	1	1	—	—	15	1484	25	—	tr
chicken broth cube	1 cube (4.8 g)	9	tr	tr	1	1	1	—	—	—	1152	18	—	—

FOOD	PORTION	CALS	FAT	SAT FAT	CHOL	PROT	CARB	SUGAR	FIBER	CALCI	SOD	POTAS	FOLIC	VIT C
chicken broth cube as prep w/ water	1 cup	13	tr	tr	1	1	2	—	—	—	792	24	—	—
chicken cream of as prep w/ water	1 cup	107	5	3	3	2	13	—	—	76	1184	215	—	—
chicken noodle as prep w/ water	1 cup	53	1	tr	3	3	7	—	—	32	1284	31	1	tr
french onion not prep	1 pkg (1.4 oz)	115	2	1	2	5	21	—	—	55	3493	260	6	1
leek as prep w/ water	1 cup	71	2	1	3	2	11	—	—	—	966	—	—	—
onion as prep w/ water	1 cup	28	1	tr	0	1	5	—	—	13	848	63	2	tr
tomato as prep w/ water	1 cup	102	2	1	1	2	19	—	—	54	943	295	7	5
ALPINE AIRE														
Low Carb Bay Shrimp Bisque	1 pkg	150	11	6	35	6	6	1	1	—	500	—	—	—
Low Carb Beefy Vegetable	1 pkg	100	4	2	30	9	7	1	1	—	1260	—	—	—
Low Carb Broccoli Cheddar	1 pkg	140	10	6	35	6	6	1	2	—	640	—	—	—
Low Carb Mushroom & Chicken w/ Roasted Garlic	1 pkg	130	8	5	35	7	7	2	1	—	650	—	—	—
ARMOUR														
Bouillon Cubes Beef	1 (4 g)	5	0	0	0	0	1	0	0	0	920	—	—	0
Bouillon Cubes Chicken	1 (4 g)	5	0	0	0	0	1	0	0	0	910	—	—	0
AZUMAYA														
Thin Cut Noodle	1 cup	120	0	0	0	5	24	2	tr	20	820	—	—	0
Wide Cut Noodle	1 cup	120	0	0	0	5	24	2	tr	20	800	—	—	0
BEAN CUISINE														
13 Bean Bouillabasse	1 cup	220	0	0	0	6	17	1	5	80	0	—	—	9
Island Black Bean	1 cup	210	0	0	0	6	17	1	7	150	0	—	—	27
Lots of Lentil	1 cup	230	0	0	0	6	17	1	5	60	5	—	—	18
Mesa Maize	1 cup	160	0	0	0	6	18	2	6	40	10	—	—	5
White Bean Provençal	1 cup	250	1	0	0	10	32	4	11	150	15	—	—	21
CUP-A-SOUP														
Broccoli & Cheese as prep	1 serv (6 oz)	70	3	1	5	2	9	2	tr	40	550	—	—	4
Chicken Vegetable as prep	1 serv (6 oz)	50	1	0	10	1	10	1	0	0	520	—	16	0

FOOD	PORTION	CALS	FAT	SAT FAT	CHOL	PROT	CARB	SUGAR	FIBER	CALCI	SOD	POTAS	FOLIC	VIT C
CUP-A-SOUP (CONT.)														
Chicken Broth as prep	1 serv (6 oz)	20	0	0	0	1	3	0	0	0	440	—	—	0
Chicken Broth w/ Pasta Fat Free as prep	1 serv (6 oz)	45	0	0	0	2	8	0	0	0	450	—	16	0
Chicken Noodle as prep	1 serv (6 oz)	50	1	0	10	2	8	0	0	0	540	—	16	0
Cream Of Chicken as prep	1 serv (6 oz)	70	2	0	0	1	12	2	tr	0	640	—	—	0
Creamy Chicken Vegetable as prep	1 serv (6 oz)	80	5	2	0	2	10	2	tr	20	590	—	—	0
Creamy Mushroom as prep	1 serv (6 oz)	60	2	0	0	1	10	1	0	0	610	—	—	0
Green Pea as prep	1 serv (6 oz)	80	1	0	0	4	12	1	3	0	520	—	—	0
Hearty Chicken Noodle as prep	1 serv (6 oz)	60	1	0	15	3	10	0	0	0	590	—	16	0
Ring Noodle as prep	1 serv (6 oz)	50	1	0	10	2	9	0	0	0	560	—	16	0
Spring Vegetable as prep	1 serv (6 oz)	45	1	0	10	2	21	1	tr	0	500	—	16	0
Tomato as prep	1 serv (6 oz)	100	1	0	5	2	20	14	tr	100	510	—	—	4
FANTASTIC														
Noodle Bowls Mandarin Broccoli	1 pkg (2.2 oz)	220	0	0	0	10	40	2	4	40	1260	—	—	24
HEALTH VALLEY														
Chicken Noodles w/ Vegetables	1 serv	110	0	0	0	3	24	1	3	20	190	—	—	6
Corn Chowder w/ Tomatoes	1 serv	100	0	0	0	4	21	1	3	20	190	—	—	9
Creamy Potato w/ Broccoli	1 serv	70	0	0	0	4	17	2	3	60	190	—	—	12
Garden Split Pea w/ Carrots	1 serv	130	0	0	0	8	22	2	2	40	190	—	—	6
Lentil w/ Couscous	1 serv	130	0	0	0	7	28	1	5	40	190	—	—	5
Pasta Italiano	1 serv	140	0	0	0	5	31	1	3	20	190	—	—	12
Pasta Marinara	1 serv	100	0	0	0	5	20	1	1	40	190	—	—	6
Pasta Parmesan	1 serv	100	0	0	0	5	20	1	1	40	190	—	—	6
Spicy Black Bean w/ Couscous	1 serv	130	0	0	0	6	29	3	5	40	190	—	—	4
Zesty Black Bean w/ Rice	1 serv	100	0	0	0	5	22	2	4	40	190	—	—	4
HERB-OX														
Beef Bouillon	1 cube (3.5 g)	5	0	0	0	0	tr	0	0	0	900	—	—	0
Beef Instant Bouillon Powder	1 tsp (4 g)	5	0	0	0	0	tr	0	0	0	1020	—	—	0

FOOD	PORTION	CALS	FAT	SAT FAT	CHOL	PROT	CARB	SUGAR	FIBER	CALCI	SOD	POTAS	FOLIC	VIT C
HERB-OX (CONT.)														
Beef Instant Broth & Seasoning Pack	1 pkg (4.5 g)	5	0	0	0	0	tr	0	0	0	1020	—	—	0
Beef Instant Broth & Seasoning Pack Low Sodium	1 pkg (4 g)	10	0	0	0	0	2	1	0	0	5	—	—	0
Chicken Bouillon	1 cube (4 g)	5	0	0	0	0	tr	0	0	0	1100	—	—	0
Chicken Instant Bouillon Powder	1 tsp (4 g)	5	0	0	0	0	tr	0	0	0	1100	—	—	0
Chicken Instant Broth & Seasoning Pack	1 pkg (4 g)	5	0	0	0	0	tr	0	0	0	1100	—	—	0
Chicken Instant Broth & Seasoning Pack Low Sodium	1 pkg (4 g)	10	0	0	0	0	2	1	0	0	5	—	—	0
Vegetable Bouillon	1 cube (4 g)	5	0	0	0	0	tr	0	0	0	980	—	—	0
HODGSON MILL														
Choice Bean not prep	¼ cup (1.5 oz)	150	0	0	0	9	27	2	11	60	5	—	—	9
HURST														
15 Bean Soup Beef	1 serv (6 oz)	120	1	0	0	8	20	1	9	40	310	—	—	0
15 Bean Soup Cajun	1 serv	120	1	0	0	8	20	1	9	40	100	—	—	0
15 Bean Soup Chicken	1 serv (6 oz)	120	1	0	0	8	20	1	9	40	250	—	—	0
15 Bean Soup Chili	1 serv (6 oz)	120	1	0	0	8	20	1	9	40	170	—	—	0
15 Bean Soup Ham	1 serv	120	1	0	0	8	20	1	9	40	70	—	—	0
HamBeens Great Northern Bean	1 serv	120	1	0	0	7	22	1	11	60	470	—	—	1
HamBeens Navy Bean	1 serv	120	1	0	0	8	21	1	11	40	470	—	—	0
Pasta Fagioli	1 serv	120	1	0	0	8	23	1	9	40	540	—	—	0
Spanish American Pinto Bean	1 serv	120	1	0	0	7	22	1	6	40	350	—	—	2
Spanish-American Black Bean	1 serv	120	1	0	0	7	22	1	8	40	280	—	—	0
LIPTON														
Chicken Noodle w/ White Chicken Meat as prep	1 cup	80	2	1	15	3	11	0	0	0	690	—	24	0
Extra Noodle w/ Chicken Broth as prep	1 cup	90	2	1	25	3	15	1	tr	0	680	—	32	0
Giggle Noodle w/ Chicken Broth as prep	1 cup	70	2	1	20	2	11	1	0	0	750	—	16	0

FOOD	PORTION	CALS	FAT	SAT FAT	CHOL	PROT	CARB	SUGAR	FIBER	CALCI	SOD	POTAS	FOLIC	VIT C
LIPTON (CONT.)														
Recipe Secrets Beefy Mushroom	1½ tbsp (0.4 oz)	35	0	0	0	1	7	2	0	0	640	—	—	0
Recipe Secrets Beefy Onion	1 tbsp (0.3 oz)	25	1	0	0	1	5	0	0	0	610	—	—	0
Recipe Secrets Fiesta Herb w/ Red Pepper as prep	1 cup	30	0	0	0	1	6	tr	0	0	560	—	—	0
Recipe Secrets Golden Herb w/ Lemon as prep	1 cup	35	1	0	0	tr	7	0	0	0	510	—	—	0
Recipe Secrets Golden Onion	1⅔ tbsp (0.5 oz)	50	1	0	0	1	9	2	0	0	700	—	—	0
Recipe Secrets Italian Herb w/ Tomato as prep	1 cup	40	1	0	0	tr	9	3	0	0	510	—	—	2
Recipe Secrets Onion as prep	1 cup	20	0	0	0	0	4	0	tr	0	610	—	—	0
Recipe Secrets Onion Mushroom as prep	1 cup	30	1	0	0	1	5	0	0	0	640	—	—	0
Recipe Secrets Savory Herb w/ Garlic as prep	1 cup	30	0	0	0	1	6	0	0	0	480	—	—	0
Recipe Secrets Vegetable as prep	1 cup	30	0	0	0	tr	7	2	1	0	600	—	—	2
Ring-O-Noodle w/ Chicken Broth as prep	1 cup	70	2	1	15	2	10	1	0	0	720	—	24	0
Soup Secrets Chicken 'N Onion as prep	1 cup	120	2	0	5	4	24	1	1	40	740	—	24	1
Soup Secrets Chicken w/ Pasta & Beans as prep	1 cup	110	2	0	5	5	19	1	3	40	700	—	32	1
Soup Secrets Country Chicken w/ Pasta & Herbs as prep	1 cup	100	2	0	5	4	18	1	1	20	740	—	32	0
Soup Secrets Homestyle Lentil w/ Bow Tie Pasta as prep	1 cup	130	1	0	0	7	22	1	5	0	750	—	32	0
Soup Secrets Minestrone as prep	1 cup	110	1	0	0	4	21	4	4	40	750	—	49	4
Spiral Pasta w/ Chicken Broth as prep	1 cup	60	1	0	0	2	11	1	0	0	660	—	24	0

FOOD	PORTION	CALS	FAT	SAT FAT	CHOL	PROT	CARB	SUGAR	FIBER	CALCI	SOD	POTAS	FOLIC	VIT C
MINICARB														
Miso w/ Tofu & Shiitake	1 pkg	33	1	0	0	1	5	2	1	—	420	—	—	—
Szechuan Beef	1 pkg	24	1	0	0	1	4	0	0	—	1325	—	—	—
Thai Coconut Cream	1 pkg	100	6	4	3	3	9	0	1	—	770	—	—	—
MISO-CUP														
Golden Vegetable as prep	1 cup	30	1	—	0	2	3	1	tr	—	780	—	—	—
Miso Reduced Sodium as prep	1 cup	25	1	—	0	2	3	tr	tr	—	270	—	—	—
Organic Miso as prep	1 cup	35	1	—	0	2	4	tr	tr	—	480	—	—	—
Savory Seaweed as prep	1 cup	30	1	—	0	3	3	1	tr	—	690	—	—	—
RAMEN NOODLE														
Beef as prep	1 pkg (2.2 oz)	280	11	6	tr	6	40	3	3	31	1236	—	—	0
Beef Low Fat as prep	1 pkg (2.2 oz)	216	1	tr	1	6	45	3	2	39	1361	—	—	1
Chicken as prep	1 pkg (2.2 oz)	279	11	5	1	6	40	3	6	27	1360	—	—	2
Chicken Low Fat as prep	1 pkg (2.2 oz)	216	1	tr	tr	7	44	3	2	35	1335	—	—	1
Oriental Low Fat as prep	1 pkg (2.2 oz)	217	1	tr	0	7	45	3	2	49	1359	—	—	1
Shrimp as prep	1 pkg (2.2 oz)	294	13	4	1	6	39	3	3	35	972	—	—	1
Shrimp Low Fat as prep	1 pkg (2.2 oz)	218	1	tr	5	7	45	3	3	27	1111	—	—	1
Tomato as prep	1 pkg (2.2 oz)	295	13	5	tr	6	39	4	2	37	822	—	—	6
RAPUNZEL														
Cubes Vegetable Bouillon No Salt Added	½ cube	25	2	—	—	2	0	0	0		130	—	—	—
Cubes Vegetable Bouillon w/ Sea Salt	½ cube	15	1	—	—	tr	0	0	0		1000	—	—	—
Cubes Vegetable Bouillon w/ Sea Salt & Herbs	½ cube	15	2	—	—	tr	0	0	0	—	950	—	—	—
SLIM-FAST														
Creamy Broccoli	1 pkg	210	5	2	20	10	30	13	5	400	890	400	120	60
Creamy Chicken	1 pkg	220	5	2	20	10	33	15	5	400	890	400	120	60
Creamy Potato Cheddar & Chive	1 pkg	220	5	2	15	10	35	15	5	400	890	400	120	60
STEERO														
Beef Bouillon Cube	1 (3.5 g)	5	0	0	—	0	1	—	—	—	900	—	—	—

FOOD	PORTION	CALS	FAT	SAT FAT	CHOL	PROT	CARB	SUGAR	FIBER	CALCI	SOD	POTAS	FOLIC	VIT C
STEERO (CONT.)														
Beef Bouillon Cube Reduced Sodium	1 cube (3.5 oz)	5	0	0	—	0	1	—	—	—	600	300	—	—
Beef Bouillon Instant	1 tsp (3.5 oz)	5	0	0	—	0	1	—	—	—	900	—	—	—
Beef Bouillon Instant Reduced Sodium	1 tsp (3.5 oz)	5	0	0	—	0	1	—	—	—	600	300	—	—
Chicken Bouillon Cube	1 (3.5 g)	5	0	0	—	0	1	—	—	—	900	—	—	—
Chicken Bouillon Cube Reduced Sodium	1 (3.5 g)	5	0	0	—	0	1	—	—	—	600	135	—	—
Chicken Bouillon Instant	1 tsp (3.5 g)	5	0	0	—	0	1	—	—	—	900	—	—	—
Chicken Bouillon Instant Reduced Sodium	1 tsp (3.5 g)	5	0	0	—	0	1	—	—	—	600	135	—	—
THAI KITCHEN														
Instant Rice Noodle Bangkok Curry	1 pkg	192	5	0	0	3	35	2	0	0	400	—	—	0
Rice Noodle Bowl Roasted Garlic	1 bowl	170	2	0	0	3	35	2	0	0	390	—	—	0
Rice Noodle Bowl Spring Onion	1 bowl	170	2	0	0	3	35	2	0	0	400	—	—	0
WEIGHT WATCHERS														
Instant Beef Broth	1 pkg (0.16 oz)	10	0	0	0	0	2	2	0	0	800	—	—	0
Instant Chicken Broth	1 pkg (0.16 oz)	10	0	0	0	0	2	2	0	0	830	—	—	0
WYLER'S														
Beef Bouillon Cube	1 (3.5 g)	5	0	0	—	0	1	—	—	—	900	—	—	—
Beef Bouillon Cube Reduced Sodium	1 (3.5 g)	5	0	0	—	0	1	—	—	—	600	300	—	—
Beef Bouillon Instant	1 tsp (3.5 g)	5	0	0	—	0	1	—	—	—	900	—	—	—
Beef Bouillon Instant Reduced Sodium	1 tsp (3.5 g)	5	0	0	—	0	1	—	—	—	600	300	—	—
Chicken Bouillon Cube	1 (3.5 g)	5	0	0	—	0	1	—	—	—	900	—	—	—

FOOD	PORTION	CALS	FAT	SAT FAT	CHOL	PROT	CARB	SUGAR	FIBER	CALCI	SOD	POTAS	FOLIC	VIT C
WYLER'S (CONT.)														
Chicken Bouillon Cube Reduced Sodium	1 (3.5 g)	5	0	0	—	0	1	—	—	—	900	—	—	—
Chicken Bouillon Instant	1 tsp (3.5)	5	0	0	—	0	1	—	—	—	900	—	—	—
Chicken Bouillon Instant Reduced Sodium	1 tsp (3.5 g)	5	0	0	—	0	1	—	—	—	600	135	—	—
SHELF-STABLE														
ANNIE CHUN'S														
Ginger Chicken	1 cup	30	0	0	0	4	3	3	0	0	730	—	—	1
Shiitake Mushroom	1 cup	25	0	0	0	2	3	2	0	0	90	—	—	0
Traditional Miso	1 cup	35	1	0	0	2	5	2	1	20	870	—	—	0
HORMEL														
Micro Cup Bean & Ham	1 cup (7.5 oz)	190	4	1	15	9	29	2	7	20	680	—	—	1
Micro Cup Beef Vegetable	1 cup (7.5 oz)	90	1	0	10	6	15	3	1	20	790	—	—	0
Micro Cup Broccoli Cheese w/ Ham	1 cup (7.5 oz)	170	13	5	40	4	10	3	1	60	710	—	—	6
Micro Cup Chicken & Rice	1 cup (7.5 oz)	110	3	1	15	5	17	3	1	20	950	—	—	1
Micro Cup Chicken Noodle	1 cup (7.5 oz)	110	3	2	35	8	13	0	0	20	790	—	—	0
Micro Cup New England Clam Chowder	1 cup (7.5 oz)	130	5	3	25	5	17	0	1	20	820	—	—	0
Micro Cup Potato Cheese w/ Ham	1 cup (7.5 oz)	190	13	5	50	4	15	2	1	60	750	—	—	0
LUNCH BUCKET														
Chicken Noodle	1 pkg (7.25 oz)	80	2	1	10	2	13	0	0	20	830	—	—	0
Country Vegetable	1 pkg (7.25 oz)	60	1	0	0	1	14	1	3	20	750	—	—	1
TASTYBITE														
Tom Yum	½ pkg (5.3 oz)	92	7	5	0	2	6	0	1	20	740	—	—	0
TAKE-OUT														
albondigas meatball soup	1 bowl	318	17	7	71	—	—	—	—	—	1385	—	—	—
beef stew soup	1 cup (8.8 oz)	221	5	2	60	23	20	—	—	32	461	527	25	14
black bean turtle soup	1 cup	241	1	tr	0	15	45	—	10	103	6	801	158	0

FOOD	PORTION	CALS	FAT	SAT FAT	CHOL	PROT	CARB	SUGAR	FIBER	CALCI	SOD	POTAS	FOLIC	VIT C
brunswick stew soup	1 cup (8.5 oz)	232	6	2	71	27	17	—	—	39	438	509	21	14
caldo de res beef soup	1 bowl	327	12	4	50	—	—	—	—	—	1861	—	—	—
chinese velvet corn	1¼ cups	135	0	0	1	—	—	—	—	—	708	—	—	—
corn & cheese chowder	¾ cup	215	12	7	66	9	21	—	3	220	386	337	12	7
egg drop	1 cup	73	4	1	103	—	—	—	—	—	729	—	—	—
gazpacho	1 cup	46	tr	—	0	1	5	—	—	28	63	—	—	—
greek lemon	¾ cup	63	2	1	83	4	7	—	2	22	386	45	8	4
hot & sour	1 serv (14 oz)	173	8	2	87	15	8	1	1	50	475	197	9	1
middle eastern chilled fruit	1 cup	99	0	0	0	—	—	—	—	—	12	—	—	—
middle eastern chilled yogurt & cucumber	1 bowl	85	3	—	6	—	—	—	—	—	66	—	—	—
minestrone	1 cup	154	0	tr	5	—	—	—	—	—	790	—	—	—
miso w/ tofu	1 bowl	36	0	0	1	—	—	—	—	—	309	—	—	—
onion soup gratinee	1 serv	492	27	16	77	25	38	6	4	637	1325	528	57	11
oxtail	5 oz	64	3	—	—	4	7	—	—	58	—	—	—	0
pasta e fagioll	1 cup (8.8 oz)	194	5	1	3	9	30	—	—	62	790	522	49	12
ratatouille	1 cup (7.5 oz)	266	25	3	0	2	12	—	—	56	329	485	34	41
thai lemon grass	1 bowl	100	4	—	65	10	5	—	—	—	553	—	—	—
vietnamese pho beef noodle	1 serv (7.8 oz)	480	12	5	46	15	78	2	1	44	43	334	33	50
wonton soup	1 cup	205	3	1	89	16	26	—	1	32	322	226	15	5
zupa koprowa polish dill soup	1 bowl	54	2	—	55	11	6	—	—	—	524	—	—	—
zuppa toscana	1 bowl	543	123	18	45	—	—	—	—	—	1673	—	—	—

SOUR CREAM

FOOD	PORTION	CALS	FAT	SAT FAT	CHOL	PROT	CARB	SUGAR	FIBER	CALCI	SOD	POTAS	FOLIC	VIT C
sour cream	1 tbsp (0.4 oz)	26	3	2	5	tr	1	—	—	14	6	17	1	tr
sour cream	1 cup (8 oz)	493	48	30	102	7	10	—	—	268	123	331	25	2
BREAKSTONE'S														
Free	2 tbsp (1.1 oz)	35	0	0	<5	2	6	2	0	40	25	70	—	0
Reduced Fat	2 tbsp (1.1 oz)	45	4	3	15	1	2	2	0	40	20	65	—	0
Sour Cream	2 tbsp (1 oz)	60	5	4	20	tr	1	1	0	20	10	—	—	0
CABOT														
Light	2 tbsp	35	3	2	10	1	2	0	0	40	25	—	—	0
No Fat	2 tbsp	20	0	0	0	1	3	2	0	40	40	—	—	0
Sour Cream	2 tbsp	50	5	3	15	1	1	0	0	20	35	—	—	0
CROWLEY														
Sour Cream	2 tbsp	60	5	4	20	tr	1	1	0	40	15	—	—	0

FOOD	PORTION	CALS	FAT	SAT FAT	CHOL	PROT	CARB	SUGAR	FIBER	CALCI	SOD	POTAS	FOLIC	VIT C
KNUDSEN														
Free	2 tbsp (1.1 oz)	35	0	0	<5	2	6	2	0	40	25	70	—	0
Hampshire	2 tbsp (1 oz)	60	6	4	25	tr	1	1	0	20	15	45	—	0
Light	2 tbsp (1.1 oz)	50	3	2	10	2	2	2	0	60	10	70	—	0
LAND O LAKES														
Fat Free	2 tbsp (1.1 oz)	25	0	0	<5	2	4	2	0	60	40	—	—	0
Light	2 tbsp (1 oz)	40	3	2	10	1	3	2	0	40	35	—	—	0
Sour Cream	2 tbsp (1 oz)	60	6	4	15	tr	1	1	0	20	30	—	—	0

SOUR CREAM SUBSTITUTES

FOOD	PORTION	CALS	FAT	SAT FAT	CHOL	PROT	CARB	SUGAR	FIBER	CALCI	SOD	POTAS	FOLIC	VIT C
nondairy	1 cup	479	45	41	0	6	15	—	—	6	235	369	0	0
nondairy	1 oz	59	6	5	0	1	2	—	—	1	29	46	0	0

SOURSOP

FOOD	PORTION	CALS	FAT	SAT FAT	CHOL	PROT	CARB	SUGAR	FIBER	CALCI	SOD	POTAS	FOLIC	VIT C
fresh	1	416	2	—	0	6	105	—	—	88	87	1739	—	129
fresh cut up	1 cup	150	1	—	0	2	38	—	—	32	31	626		46

SOY

(*see also* CHEESE SUBSTITUTES, ICE CREAM AND FROZEN DESSERTS, MILK SUBSTITUTES, MISO, SOY SAUCE, SOYBEANS, TEMPEH, TOFU, YOGURT FROZEN)

FOOD	PORTION	CALS	FAT	SAT FAT	CHOL	PROT	CARB	SUGAR	FIBER	CALCI	SOD	POTAS	FOLIC	VIT C
lecithin	1 tbsp	104	14	2	0	0	0	0	0	—	—	—	—	—
soy milk	1 cup	79	5	1	0	7	4	—	—	10	30	338	4	0
soya cheese	1.4 oz	128	11	—	—	7	tr	—	0	180	—	—	—	0
BOB'S RED MILL														
Flour	⅓ cup	130	6	—	0	11	11	0	5	—	0	—	—	—
DAKOTA GOURMET														
Soy Nuts	1 oz	129	7	1	0	11	9	—	1	72	217	367	55	1
FEARN														
Granules	¼ cup	110	1	—	0	22	13	5	8	—	5	—	—	—
Powder	¼ cup	100	5	—	0	10	7	0	4	—	1	—	—	—
GENISOY														
Soy Nuts Deep Sea Salted	1 oz	120	4	1	0	12	9	3	5	60	150	—	—	0
Soy Nuts Old Hickory Smoked	1 oz	120	4	1	0	12	9	5	5	60	490	—	—	0
Soy Nuts Praline	55 pieces (1 oz)	120	3	0	0	6	18	16	2	30	110	—	—	0
Soy Nuts Unsalted	1 oz	120	4	0	0	12	9	3	5	60	10	—	—	0
Soy Nuts Zesty Barbeque	1 oz	120	4	1	0	12	9	5	5	60	420	—	—	0
HEALTH TRIP														
Soynut Butter Honey Sweet	2 tbsp	170	13	2	0	8	9	3	1	40	70	—	—	0
Soynut Butter Original	2 tbsp	180	13	2	0	9	8	1	1	40	70	—	—	0
Soynut Butter Unsalted	2 tbsp	180	13	2	0	9	8	1	1	40	0	—	—	0
I.M. HEALTHY														
SoyNut Butter Chocolate	2 tbsp (1.1 oz)	190	14	2	0	5	12	7	4	20	50	—	—	0

FOOD	PORTION	CALS	FAT	SAT FAT	CHOL	PROT	CARB	SUGAR	FIBER	CALCI	SOD	POTAS	FOLIC	VIT C
I.M. HEALTHY (CONT.)														
SoyNut Butter Honey Creamy	2 tbsp (1.1 oz)	170	11	2	0	7	12	2	2	30	150	—	—	0
SoyNut Butter Original Creamy	2 tbsp (1.1 oz)	170	11	2	0	8	10	3	1	50	170	—	—	0
SoyNut Butter Unsweetened Chunky	2 tbsp (1.1 oz)	160	13	2	0	7	5	1	5	60	160	—	—	0
SoyNut Butter Unsweetened Creamy	2 tbsp (1.1 oz)	160	13	2	0	7	5	1	5	60	160	—	—	0
LOMA LINDA														
Soyagen All Purpose	¼ cup (1 oz)	130	6	1	0	6	12	7	3	100	150	270	—	5
Soyagen Carob	¼ cup (1 oz)	130	6	1	0	6	13	7	2	100	170	270	—	5
Soyagen No Sucrose	¼ cup (1 oz)	130	6	1	0	6	12	7	3	100	160	270	—	2
NATURAL TOUCH														
Roasted Soy Butter	2 tbsp (1.1 oz)	170	11	2	0	6	10	3	1	0	170	150	—	0
REVIVAL														
Shake Chocolate Daydream Fructose	1 pkg	240	3	1	0	20	36	32	2	500	290	410	—	—
Shake Strawberry Smile Unsweetened	1 pkg	130	2	1	0	20	4	0	0	500	200	400	—	—
Shake Strawberry Smile Fructose	1 pkg	225	2	1	0	20	33	29	0	500	250	400	—	—
Shake Strawberry Smile Splenda	1 pkg	130	2	1	0	20	4	1	0	500	200	400	—	—
Soy Shake Plain	1 pkg	110	2	1	0	20	2	1	0	20	360	20	—	—
Soy Shake Vanilla Pleasure	1 pkg	220	2	1	0	20	31	28	0	500	290	230	—	—
Soy Shake Vanilla Pleasure Splenda	1 pkg	120	2	1	0	20	6	1	0	500	290	250	—	—
Soy Shake Vanilla Pleasure Unsweetened	1 pkg	120	2	1	0	20	6	1	0	500	290	230	—	—
Soynuts Chocolate Covered	⅙ cup	70	4	2	2	2	7	6	tr	27	8	—	—	—
Soynuts Hot Jalapeño & Cheddar	⅙ cup	78	4	1	0	5	5	tr	2	20	68	—	—	—
Soynuts Unsalted	⅙ cup	78	4	1	0	5	5	tr	2	29	2	—	—	—
Soynuts Yogurt Covered	⅙ cup	720	4	3	0	2	8	7	tr	20	12	—	—	—

FOOD	PORTION	CALS	FAT	SAT FAT	CHOL	PROT	CARB	SUGAR	FIBER	CALCI	SOD	POTAS	FOLIC	VIT C
SOY JUICY														
All Flavors	8 oz	160	3	1	0	7	25	24	1	200	30	20	—	60
SOY WONDER														
Creamy	2 tbsp	170	11	2	0	8	10	3	1	50	170	—	—	0
Crunchy	2 tbsp	170	11	2	0	8	10	3	1	50	170	—	—	0
SOY SAUCE														
shoyu	1 tbsp	9	tr	tr	0	1	2	—	—	3	1029	32	3	0
soy sauce	1 tbsp	7	tr	tr	0	tr	1	—	—	1	1024	27	2	0
tamari	1 tbsp	11	tr	tr	0	2	1	—	—	4	1005	38	3	0
CHUN KING														
Lite	1 tbsp (0.5 oz)	15	tr	0	0	2	2	2	0	3	542	—	—	0
Soy Sauce	1 tbsp (0.6 oz)	11	tr	0	0	2	1	1	0	6	1227	—	—	0
EDEN														
Organic Shoyu Reduced Sodium	1 tbsp	10	0	0	0	2	2	0	0	0	500	60	—	0
Organic Tamari	1 tbsp	15	0	0	0	2	2	0	0	0	860	80	—	0
Ponzu Sauce	1 tbsp	5	0	0	0	0	1	0	0	0	340	15	—	0
Shoyu	1 tbsp	15	0	0	0	2	2	0	0	0	1010	85	0	0
HOUSE OF TSANG														
Ginger Flavored	1 tbsp (0.6 oz)	20	0	0	0	1	4	3	0	0	730	—	—	0
Light	1 tbsp (0.6 oz)	5	0	0	0	1	0	0	0	0	900	—	—	0
Low Sodium	1 tbsp (0.6 oz)	5	0	0	0	0	0	0	0	0	280	—	—	0
Low Sodium Ginger	1 tbsp (0.6 oz)	10	0	0	0	0	2	1	0	0	280	—	—	0
Low Sodium Mushroom	1 tbsp (0.6 oz)	10	0	0	0	0	2	1	0	0	280	—	—	0
JUST RITE														
Soy Sauce	1 tbsp (0.5 oz)	11	tr	0	0	2	1	1	0	6	1227	—	—	0
KIKKOMAN														
Lite	1 tbsp (0.5 oz)	10	0	0	0	1	1	—	—	—	575	—	—	—
Soy Sauce	1 tbsp (0.5 oz)	10	0	0	0	2	0	0	0	—	920	—	—	—
LA CHOY														
Lite	1 tbsp (0.5 oz)	15	tr	0	0	2	2	2	0	3	542	—	—	0
Soy Sauce	1 tbsp (0.6 oz)	11	tr	0	0	2	1	1	0	6	1227	—	—	0
TREE OF LIFE														
Shoyu	1 tbsp (0.5 oz)	15	0	0	0	2	1	1	—	—	960	—	—	—
Tamari Wheat Free	1 tbsp (0.5 oz)	15	0	0	0	2	1	1	—	—	940	—	—	—
SOYBEANS														
dried cooked	1 cup	298	15	2	0	29	17	—	—	175	1	886	93	3
dry roasted	½ cup	387	19	3	0	34	28	—	—	232	2	1173	176	4
green cooked	½ cup	127	6	1	0	11	10	—	4	—	13	485	100	—
roasted	½ cup	405	22	3	0	30	29	—	—	119	140	1264	182	2
roasted & toasted	1 cup	490	26	3	0	40	33	—	—	149	4	1588	244	2
roasted & toasted salted	1 cup	490	26	3	0	40	33	—	—	149	176	1588	244	2

FOOD	PORTION	CALS	FAT	SAT FAT	CHOL	PROT	CARB	SUGAR	FIBER	CALCI	SOD	POTAS	FOLIC	VIT C
sprouts raw	½ cup	43	2	tr	0	5	3	—	—	23	5	169	60	5
sprouts steamed	½ cup	38	2	tr	0	4	3	—	—	28	5	167	—	4
sprouts stir fried	1 cup	125	7	1	0	13	9	—	—	82	14	567	—	12
ARROWHEAD														
Organic not prep	¼ cup	180	8	—	0	15	14	3	10	—	0	—	—	—
EDEN														
Organic Black	½ cup (4.6 oz)	120	6	1	0	11	8	1	7	80	30	310	24	0
SEAPOINT FARMS														
Edamame Organic	½ cup (2.6 oz)	100	3	0	0	8	9	1	4	50	30	—	—	5
Edamame In Pods frzn	½ cup (2.6 oz)	100	3	0	0	8	9	1	4	50	30	—	—	5
Edamame Rice Bowl Kung Pao Vegetable	1 pkg (12 oz)	420	6	1	0	15	72	14	6	60	960	—	—	24
Edamame Rice Bowl Szechwan Vegetables	1 pkg (12 oz)	420	4	1	0	13	80	22	6	50	510	—	—	30
Edamame Rice Bowl Teriyaki Vegetable	1 pkg (12 oz)	430	5	1	0	14	83	21	5	80	1130	—	—	12
Edamame Rice Bowl Vegetable Fried Rice	1 pkg (11 oz)	220	6	1	40	11	31	6	1	80	950	—	—	6
Edamame Shelled	½ cup (2.6 oz)	100	3	0	0	8	9	1	4	50	30	—	—	5

SPAGHETTI

(*see* PASTA, PASTA DINNERS, PASTA SALAD, SPAGHETTI SAUCE)

SPAGHETTI SAUCE

FOOD	PORTION	CALS	FAT	SAT FAT	CHOL	PROT	CARB	SUGAR	FIBER	CALCI	SOD	POTAS	FOLIC	VIT C
JARRED														
marinara sauce	1 cup	171	8	tr	0	4	25	—	—	44	1572	1061	—	32
spaghetti sauce	1 cup	272	12	2	0	12	40	—	—	70	1236	957	—	28
AMY'S														
Family Marinara	½ cup	50	1	0	0	1	8	5	3	—	590	—	—	—
Garlic Mushroom	½ cup	120	7	3	5	3	10	5	3	—	680	—	—	—
Puttanesca	½ cup	40	2	0	0	1	5	2	1	—	680	—	—	—
Tomato Basil	½ cup	80	3	0	0	2	11	6	3	—	580	—	—	—
Wild Mushroom	½ cup	60	3	0	0	2	7	4	2	—	580	—	—	—
BARILLA														
Restaurant Creations Cheese & Tomatoes	¼ cup	110	8	1	3	1	5	1	1	40	400	—	—	2
Restaurant Creations Garlic Herbs & Tomatoes	¼ cup	100	8	1	3	1	6	3	2	20	460	—	—	2

FOOD	PORTION	CALS	FAT	SAT FAT	CHOL	PROT	CARB	SUGAR	FIBER	CALCI	SOD	POTAS	FOLIC	VIT C
BARILLA (CONT.)														
Restaurant Creations Pesto & Tomatoes	¼ cup	150	12	2	3	2	7	2	2	40	400	—	—	2
CLASSICO														
Italian Sausage	½ cup	90	2	1	5	5	13	8	2	60	470	—	—	6
COLAVITA														
Garden Style	½ cup (4.4 oz)	60	3	0	0	3	12	0	3	40	290	—	—	4
DEL MONTE														
Chunky Garlic & Herb	½ cup (4.4 oz)	60	2	0	0	2	11	9	1	40	490	—	—	2
Chunky Italian Herb	½ cup (4.4 oz)	60	1	0	0	2	12	8	1	40	520	—	—	2
Tomato & Basil	½ cup (4.4 oz)	70	1	0	0	2	16	11	3	40	600	—	—	9
Traditional	½ cup (4.4 oz)	60	1	0	0	2	15	10	3	40	590	—	—	9
With Garlic & Onion	½ cup (4.4 oz)	80	1	0	0	2	16	10	2	40	490	—	—	6
With Green Peppers & Mushrooms	½ cup (4.4 oz)	80	1	0	0	2	16	10	3	40	490	—	—	6
With Meat	½ cup (4.4 oz)	60	1	0	4	3	14	9	3	40	720	—	—	9
With Mushrooms	½ cup (4.4 oz)	60	1	0	0	2	14	9	2	40	630	—	—	9
EDEN														
Organic Lightly Seasoned	½ cup (4.4 oz)	80	3	0	0	3	12	6	3	80	320	530	0	2
FRANCESCO RINALDI														
Alfredo	¼ cup (2.1 oz)	70	5	3	15	2	4	1	0	80	410	—	—	0
Chunky Garden Mushroom & Onion	½ cup (4.4 oz)	80	2	0	0	3	12	6	3	40	690	—	—	0
Chunky Garden Tomato Garlic & Onion	½ cup (4.4 oz)	80	2	0	0	3	12	6	3	40	690	—	—	0
Dolce Sweet & Tasty Tomato	½ cup (4.4 oz)	110	5	1	0	2	15	11	3	40	610	—	—	0
Dolce Three Cheese	½ cup (4.4 oz)	90	2	1	0	3	15	11	3	40	490	—	—	0
Dulce Super Mushroom	½ cup (4.4 oz)	110	5	1	0	3	15	11	3	40	490	—	—	0
Hearty Diavolo	½ cup (4.4 oz)	70	4	1	0	2	7	4	3	40	550	—	—	0
Hearty Mushroom Pepper & Onion	½ cup (4.4 oz)	80	3	1	0	3	10	7	3	40	690	—	—	0
Hearty Tomato & Basil	½ cup (4.4 oz)	80	3	0	0	2	11	7	4	60	730	—	—	0
Puttanesca	½ cup (4.3 oz)	70	4	1	0	2	8	7	tr	0	720	—	—	0
Tomato Alfredo	¼ cup (2.1 oz)	60	4	2	10	2	4	4	0	40	290	—	—	0

FOOD	PORTION	CALS	FAT	SAT FAT	CHOL	PROT	CARB	SUGAR	FIBER	CALCI	SOD	POTAS	FOLIC	VIT C
FRANCESCO RINALDI (CONT.)														
Traditional Meat Flavored	½ cup (4.4 oz)	90	4	1	4	2	11	7	3	0	700	—	—	0
Traditional Mushroom	½ cup (4.4 oz)	90	4	1	0	2	11	7	3	0	700	—	—	0
Traditional No Salt Added	½ cup (4.4 oz)	70	3	0	0	2	10	9	tr	40	25	—	—	6
Traditional Original	½ cup (4.4 oz)	90	4	1	0	2	11	2	3	0	700	—	—	0
Traditional Original	½ cup (4.4 oz)	90	4	1	0	2	11	7	3	0	700	—	—	0
Vodka Sauce	¼ cup (2.1 oz)	60	4	2	10	2	4	4	0	0	290	—	—	0
HEALTHY CHOICE														
Chunky Italian Vegetable	½ cup (4.4 oz)	40	tr	0	0	2	9	7	2	40	299	315	—	6
Chunky Mushroom	½ cup (4.4 oz)	42	tr	0	0	2	9	8	2	50	297	—	—	6
Garlic & Herbs	½ cup (4.4 oz)	49	tr	0	0	2	10	7	2	33	337	489	—	8
Garlic Lovers Garlic & Mushroom	½ cup (4.4 oz)	44	tr	0	0	2	10	8	2	35	362	398	—	10
Garlic Lovers Roasted Garlic	½ cup (4.4 oz)	52	tr	0	0	2	12	8	3	25	293	409	—	7
Garlic Lovers Roasted Garlic & Sun Dried Tomato	½ cup (4.4 oz)	52	tr	0	0	2	11	8	3	29	357	893	—	14
Super Chunky Mushroom & Sweet Peppers	½ cup (4.4 oz)	43	tr	0	0	2	9	6	2	37	308	—	—	7
Super Chunky Tomato Mushroom & Garlic	½ cup (4.4 oz)	45	tr	0	0	2	10	8	2	40	372	409	—	6
Super Chunky Vegetable Primavera	½ cup (4.4 oz)	43	tr	0	0	2	9	7	2	35	327	384	—	4
Traditional	½ cup (4.4 oz)	48	tr	0	0	2	11	8	2	33	378	485	—	10
With Mushrooms	½ cup (4.4 oz)	48	tr	0	0	2	11	8	2	33	378	485	—	6
HUNT'S														
Basil Garlic & Oregano	½ cup	15	0	0	0	tr	3	2	tr	0	350	180	—	4
Cheese & Garlic	½ cup	50	1	0	0	3	9	7	2	40	600	430	—	6
Chunky Vegetable	½ cup	50	1	0	0	2	11	8	3	20	560	340	—	6
Diced In Tomato Sauce	½ cup	30	0	0	0	tr	7	4	1	60	430	—	—	12
Family Favorites Lasagna	¼ cup	30	0	0	0	1	6	5	1	0	330	180	—	9

FOOD	PORTION	CALS	FAT	SAT FAT	CHOL	PROT	CARB	SUGAR	FIBER	CALCI	SOD	POTAS	FOLIC	VIT C
HUNT'S (CONT.)														
Four Cheese	½ cup	50	1	0	0	3	10	7	3	40	600	370	—	9
Italian Sausage	½ cup	60	2	0	0	2	10	7	3	20	590	400	—	12
Light	½ cup	45	0	0	0	2	9	6	3	20	430	400	—	9
Meat	½ cup	68	1	0	0	3	11	7	3	20	610	380	—	9
No Added Sugar	½ cup	45	1	0	0	2	9	6	3	20	610	—	—	12
Roasted Garlic & Onion	½ cup	50	1	0	0	2	10	7	3	20	540	400	—	9
Traditional	½ cup	50	1	0	0	2	10	7	3	20	580	390	—	9
With Mushrooms	½ cup	50	1	0	0	2	10	7	3	20	600	410	—	9
MUIR GLEN														
Organic Balsamic Roasted Onion	½ cup (4.4 oz)	50	1	0	0	2	10	5	0	40	320	—	—	9
Organic Cabernet Marinara	½ cup (4.4 oz)	50	1	0	0	2	10	4	0	40	330	—	—	9
Organic Chunky Herb	½ cup (4.4 oz)	50	1	0	0	2	10	5	0	40	320	—	—	9
Organic Garden Vegetable	½ cup (4.4 oz)	50	1	0	0	2	10	4	0	40	120	—	—	9
Organic Garlic & Onion	½ cup (4.4 oz)	55	1	0	0	2	10	5	0	40	320	—	—	9
Organic Garlic Roasted Garlic	½ cup (4.4 oz)	50	1	0	0	2	10	4	0	40	320	—	—	9
Organic Green Olive	½ cup (4.4 oz)	60	2	0	0	2	10	4	0	40	350	—	—	9
Organic Italian Herb	½ cup (4.4 oz)	55	1	0	0	2	10	5	0	40	320	—	—	9
Organic Mushroom Marinara	½ cup (4.4 oz)	45	0	0	0	2	10	4	0	40	120	—	—	6
Organic Portabello Mushroom	½ cup (4.4 oz)	50	0	0	0	2	10	4	0	40	330	—	—	6
Organic Sun Dried Tomato	½ cup (4.4 oz)	55	1	1	0	2	10	4	1	40	170	—	—	6
Organic Tomato Basil	½ cup (4.4 oz)	50	1	1	0	2	12	4	0	40	370	—	—	6
NEWMAN'S OWN														
Marinara Venetian	½ cup (4.4 oz)	60	2	0	0	2	9	7	3	60	590	—	—	0
Marinara Venetian w/ Mushrooms	½ cup (4.4 oz)	60	2	0	0	2	9	7	3	60	590	—	—	0
Pasta Sauce Bambolina	½ cup (4.5 oz)	100	5	1	0	1	15	9	5	40	590	—	—	0
Pasta Sauce Roasted Garlic & Red & Green Peppers	½ cup (4.7 oz)	70	3	0	0	2	11	6	4	0	460	—	—	0

FOOD	PORTION	CALS	FAT	SAT FAT	CHOL	PROT	CARB	SUGAR	FIBER	CALCI	SOD	POTAS	FOLIC	VIT C
NEWMAN'S OWN (CONT.)														
Pasta Sauce Say Cheese	½ cup (4.4 oz)	90	3	2	<5	3	14	8	3	60	510	—	—	0
Sockarooni	½ cup	60	2	0	0	2	9	7	3	60	590	—	—	0
PREGO														
Pasta Bake Sauce Tomato Garlic & Basil	1 serv (3.4 oz)	80	4	1	0	1	11	10	2	20	530	—	—	6
Traditional	½ cup (4.2 oz)	140	5	2	0	2	23	15	2	40	610	—	—	9
PROGRESSO														
Marinara	½ cup (4.3 oz)	80	5	1	<5	2	8	5	2	20	480	—	—	0
Meat Flavored	½ cup (4.4 oz)	100	5	1	5	4	12	9	3	40	610	—	—	0
Sauce	½ cup (4.4 oz)	100	5	1	<5	3	12	8	2	20	620	—	—	2
RAGU														
Chunky Garden Style Tomato Garlic & Onion	½ cup (4.5 oz)	110	3	0	0	2	18	13	2	40	520	—	—	5
SARA LEE														
Chunky Garden Mushroom & Peppers	½ cup (4.4 oz)	80	2	0	0	3	12	6	3	40	690	—	—	0
TREE OF LIFE														
Pasta Sauce	½ cup (4 oz)	50	2	—	0	2	9	8	—	20	290	—	—	15
Pasta Sauce Fat Free Classic	½ cup (3.9 oz)	40	0	0	0	2	8	6	0	20	250	—	—	18
Pasta Sauce Fat Free Mushroom & Basil	½ cup (3.9 oz)	30	0	0	0	1	7	6	0	0	300	—	—	12
Pasta Sauce Fat Free Onion & Garlic	½ cup (3.9 oz)	30	0	0	0	1	7	6	0	0	240	—	—	12
Pasta Sauce Fat Free Sweet Pepper	½ cup (3.9 oz)	30	0	0	0	1	7	6	0	0	280	—	—	18
Pasta Sauce No Salt Added	½ cup (3.9 oz)	50	2	—	0	2	9	8	—	20	0	—	—	15
WALDEN FARMS														
Alfredo Sauce Calorie Free	¼ cup	0	0	0	0	0	0	0	0	—	20	—	—	—
Marinara Calorie Free	⅓ cup	0	0	0	0	1	0	0	0	—	350	—	—	—
MIX														
DURKEE														
Spaghetti Sauce as prep	½ cup	15	0	0	0	0	5	1	0	0	390	—	—	1
With Mushrooms as prep	½ cup	15	0	0	0	1	4	2	0	0	520	—	—	0

FOOD	PORTION	CALS	FAT	SAT FAT	CHOL	PROT	CARB	SUGAR	FIBER	CALCI	SOD	POTAS	FOLIC	VIT C
FRENCH'S														
Italian as prep	½ cup	16	0	0	0	0	5	1	0	0	390	—	—	1
Mushroom as prep	½ cup	20	1	0	2	1	4	1	0	40	760	—	—	2
Thick as prep	½ cup	10	0	0	0	0	4	1	0	0	630	—	—	0
MCCORMICK														
Alfredo Pasta Blend as prep	½ cup	60	2	—	10	—	4	2	0	40	680	—	—	0
Pasta Rosa Blend	1 tbsp (10 g)	40	2	1	<5	1	4	2	0	0	540	—	—	0
Pesto Pasta Sauce as prep	2 tsp (4 g)	10	0	0	—	tr	tr	—	—	20	480	—	—	—
Primavera Pasta Blend	1 tbsp (7 g)	30	1	—	—	0	4	tr	—	—	490	—	—	—
Spaghetti Sauce	1 tbsp (8 g)	25	0	0	—	0	5	3	—	—	490	—	—	—
REFRIGERATED														
BUITONI														
Alfredo Portabello Mushroom	¼ cup	100	8	5	20	2	5	2	0	40	340	—	—	0
Alfredo Light	¼ cup	80	5	4	20	4	5	2	0	100	370	—	—	0
Marinara	½ cup	80	3	1	0	2	11	7	2	60	580	—	—	1
Marinara Portabello Mushroom	½ cup	80	3	1	0	2	11	7	2	60	520	—	—	1
Marinara Roasted Garlic	½ cup	60	2	1	0	2	9	6	1	60	580	—	—	1
Pesto w/ Basil	¼ cup	300	26	6	20	7	9	4	2	200	560	—	—	0
Pesto w/ Basil Reduced Fat	¼ cup	230	18	4	15	7	9	5	2	200	560	—	—	0
Pesto w/ Sun Dried Tomatoes	¼ cup	210	18	3	5	4	8	4	2	100	400	—	—	0
Tomato Herb Parmesan	½ cup	120	8	3	10	0	9	7	2	100	790	—	—	0
DI GIORNO														
Alfredo	¼ cup (2.2 oz)	180	18	7	25	3	3	2	0	80	600	65	0	0
Basil Pesto	¼ cup (2.2 oz)	320	31	6	15	7	2	tr	tr	250	530	100	8	0
Four Cheese	¼ cup (2.2 oz)	160	15	7	30	5	3	2	0	150	410	75	0	0
Garlic Pesto	¼ cup (2.1 oz)	340	33	7	15	7	3	tr	tr	250	540	65	0	0
Light Alfredo Sauce	¼ cup (2.4 oz)	140	9	6	30	5	9	3	0	100	600	90	0	0
Marinara	½ cup (4.5 oz)	70	0	0	0	2	15	10	2	40	220	400	0	0
Plum Tomato Cream Sauce	½ cup (4.4 oz)	160	13	7	40	3	8	6	2	100	370	360	0	1
Plum Tomato & Mushroom	½ cup (4.4 oz)	60	0	0	0	2	13	10	2	40	260	400	0	0
Roasted Red Bell Pepper Cream Sauce	¼ cup (2.3 oz)	140	10	6	35	4	8	3	0	80	510	70	0	0

FOOD	PORTION	CALS	FAT	SAT FAT	CHOL	PROT	CARB	SUGAR	FIBER	CALCI	SOD	POTAS	FOLIC	VIT C
TAKE-OUT														
bolognese	5 oz	195	15	—	—	11	4	—	tr	36	—	—	—	7

SPANISH FOOD

CANNED

CHI-CHI'S

FOOD	PORTION	CALS	FAT	SAT FAT	CHOL	PROT	CARB	SUGAR	FIBER	CALCI	SOD	POTAS	FOLIC	VIT C
Pico De Gallo	2 tbsp (1.2 oz)	10	0	0	0	0	2	2	0	0	170	—	—	2
DERBY														
Tamales	3 (6.5 oz)	253	17	8	23	7	21	0	4	30	1034	—	—	7
GEBHARDT														
Enchiladas	2 (5.7 oz)	258	19	9	25	4	20	0	3	28	687	—	—	2
Tamales	2 (5.7 oz)	268	21	10	28	5	19	1	3	27	770	—	—	2
Tamales Jumbo	2 (6.9 oz)	332	25	12	34	6	24	0	3	36	930	—	—	2
HORMEL														
Tamales Beef	3 (7.5 oz)	280	21	8	35	6	20	1	3	20	1010	—	—	0
Tamales Chicken	3 (7.5 oz)	210	11	4	50	6	22	2	2	40	1020	—	—	1
Tamales Hot Spicy Beef	3 (7.5 oz)	280	21	8	35	6	20	1	3	20	1010	—	—	0
Tamales Jumbo Beef	2 (6.9 oz)	270	20	8	35	5	18	1	3	20	940	—	—	0
ROSARITA														
Enchilada Sauce Mild	¼ cup (2.1 oz)	23	1	tr	0	1	3	3	0	11	409	—	—	1
VAN CAMP														
Tamales	2 (5 oz)	210	13	5	20	5	20	1	3	20	610	—	—	1
FROZEN														
AMY'S														
Black Bean Vegetable Enchilada	1 (4.75 oz)	130	4	0	0	4	20	1	2	—	390	—	—	—
Bowls Santa Fe Enchilada	1 pkg (10 oz)	340	9	2	5	17	47	5	10	—	780	—	—	—
Burrito Bean & Cheese	1 (6 oz)	280	8	3	10	10	43	1	6	—	540	—	—	—
Burrito Bean & Rice Non-Dairy	1 (6 oz)	270	6	1	0	9	48	2	5	—	550	—	—	—
Burrito Black Bean Vegetable	1 (6 oz)	320	8	1	0	9	54	4	4	—	540	—	—	—
Burrito Breakfast	1 (6 oz)	210	6	tr	0	9	38	4	5	—	540	—	—	—
Burrito Especial	1 (6 oz)	260	6	2	5	8	45	4	3	—	620	—	—	—
Cheese Enchilada	1 (4.75 oz)	210	12	6	35	10	13	2	2	—	440	—	—	—
Mexican Tamale Pie	1 (8 oz)	150	3	0	0	5	27	2	4	—	590	—	—	—

FOOD	PORTION	CALS	FAT	SAT FAT	CHOL	PROT	CARB	SUGAR	FIBER	CALCI	SOD	POTAS	FOLIC	VIT C
BANQUET														
Chimichanga Meal	1 meal (9.5 oz)	500	24	8	20	13	56	9	9	60	1180	—	—	6
Enchilada Beef	1 pkg (11 oz)	370	12	5	20	10	54	7	6	150	1330	—	—	0
Enchilada Cheese	1 pkg (11 oz)	360	10	4	20	12	56	7	6	200	1500	—	—	2
Enchilada Chicken	1 pkg (11 oz)	350	10	3	25	12	54	7	9	150	1580	—	—	0
Enchilada Beef & Tamale Combo	1 pkg (11 oz)	450	20	6	30	10	50	7	9	150	1530	—	—	0
Mexican Style Enchilada Combo	1 meal (11 oz)	360	11	5	20	10	55	7	9	150	1390	—	—	3
CHI-CHI'S														
Burro Beef	1 pkg (15.9 oz)	590	19	8	55	27	76	7	11	250	2060	—	—	3
Burro Chicken	1 pkg (15.9 oz)	540	14	5	55	26	77	8	10	200	2110	—	—	9
Chimichanga Beef	1 pkg (15.9 oz)	630	24	9	55	28	75	8	10	200	2050	—	—	9
Chimichanga Chicken	1 pkg (15.9 oz)	580	19	6	50	25	78	8	10	200	2100	—	—	12
Enchilada Chicken Suprema	1 pkg (15.9 oz)	600	20	9	70	26	80	9	11	200	2310	—	—	4
Enchilada Baja	1 pkg (15.9 oz)	590	20	9	50	27	75	7	15	200	1920	—	—	5
HEALTH IS WEALTH														
Burrito Munchees	10 (5 oz)	310	7	2	5	11	53	2	6	60	610	—	—	5
Mexican Munchees	2 (1 oz)	49	1	0	0	2	8	0	1	20	110	—	—	1
HEALTHY CHOICE														
Chicken Enchilada Suprema	1 meal (11.3 oz)	300	7	3	40	13	46	8	4	100	560	—	—	18
Chicken Enchiladas Suiza	1 meal (10 oz)	280	6	3	40	14	43	4	5	100	410	—	—	2
Chicken Breast Con Queso Burrito	1 meal (10.55 oz)	350	6	3	35	14	60	11	6	100	590	—	—	6
LEAN CUISINE														
Everyday Favorites Chicken Enchilada Suiza	1 pkg (9 oz)	280	5	2	25	11	48	7	3	150	520	340	—	2
PATIO														
Beef & Cheese Enchiladas Chili 'N Beans	1 meal (15.5 oz)	670	30	14	60	19	80	6	12	250	2400	—	—	0
Beef Enchiladas Chili 'N Beans	1 meal (15.5 oz)	540	27	10	50	12	73	6	12	250	2690	—	—	0
Burrito Bean & Cheese	1 (5 oz)	300	9	5	15	9	45	1	4	40	690	—	—	0
Burrito Beef & Bean Hot	1 (5 oz)	320	12	5	25	10	43	4	4	20	840	—	—	1

FOOD	PORTION	CALS	FAT	SAT FAT	CHOL	PROT	CARB	SUGAR	FIBER	CALCI	SOD	POTAS	FOLIC	VIT C
PATIO (CONT.)														
Burrito Beef & Bean Mild	1 (5 oz)	330	12	4	20	10	45	3	4	20	890	—	—	1
Burrito Chicken	1 (5 oz)	290	6	3	20	11	44	6	2	60	740	—	—	0
Burritos Beef & Bean Medium	1 (5 oz)	310	10	5	20	10	45	5	4	0	660	—	—	1
Burritos Beef & Bean Red Chili Pepper Red Hot	1 (5 oz)	320	12	5	20	10	42	4	4	20	850	—	—	0
Enchilada Beef	1 meal (12 oz)	320	12	5	25	12	52	4	9	150	1700	—	—	4
Enchilada Cheese	1 meal (12 oz)	370	12	5	25	11	54	7	7	150	1570	—	—	0
Enchilada Chicken	1 meal (12 oz)	400	12	4	35	13	60	6	8	200	1470	—	—	0
Fiesta	1 meal (12 oz)	350	11	5	25	11	53	5	7	150	1760	—	—	0
Mexican Style	1 meal (13.25 oz)	470	19	6	20	15	59	5	10	100	2210	—	—	2
STOUFFER'S														
Chicken Enchilada	1 serv (4.8 oz)	230	11	5	30	7	25	4	3	150	530	220	—	0
TYSON														
Beef Fajita	3½ pieces (12.5 oz)	550	16	4	20	28	75	8	6	100	1130	—	—	30
Chicken Fajita	3½ pieces (13.1 oz)	460	11	3	45	28	61	10	6	80	1220	—	—	36
WEIGHT WATCHERS														
Smart Ones Chicken Enchiladas Suiza	1 pkg (9 oz)	270	9	5	50	15	33	8	2	250	660	—	—	4
Smart Ones Santa Fe Style Rice & Beans	1 pkg (10 oz)	290	8	4	20	12	43	6	6	200	590	—	—	2
MIX														
GEBHARDT														
Menudo Mix	¼ tsp (0.4 g)	1	tr	0	0	tr	tr	tr	tr	1	52	—	—	tr
MCCORMICK														
Burrito Seasoning	1 tbsp (8 g)	25	1	—	—	tr	5	1	tr	—	500	—	—	—
Fajitas Marinade Mix	2 tsp (4 g)	15	0	0	—	0	2	—	—	—	250	—	—	—
Taco Seasoning Hot	2 tsp (6 g)	20	0	0	—	tr	3	1	tr	—	430	—	—	—
Taco Seasoning Mild	2 tsp (7 g)	20	0	0	—	tr	4	1	tr	—	460	—	—	—
TACO BELL														
Home Originals Chicken Fajita Dinner as prep	2 (6.9 oz)	340	9	2	40	21	45	7	3	60	1120	—	—	27

FOOD	PORTION	CALS	FAT	SAT FAT	CHOL	PROT	CARB	SUGAR	FIBER	CALCI	SOD	POTAS	FOLIC	VIT C
TACO BELL (CONT.)														
Home Originals Chicken Fajita Seasoning Mix	1 tbsp (8 g)	25	0	0	0	tr	5	1	2	0	540	—	—	1
Home Originals Soft Taco Dinner as prep	2 (6.3 oz)	410	18	4	60	21	41	5	2	40	1090	—	—	0
Home Originals Taco Dinner as prep	2 (4.4 oz)	280	15	5	50	16	19	2	2	40	580	—	—	0
Home Originals Taco Seasoning Mix	2 tsp (6 g)	20	0	0	0	tr	3	0	tr	0	450	—	—	0
Home Originals Ultimate Bean Burrito Dinner as prep	1 (4.4 oz)	200	5	2	0	6	34	4	3	40	710	—	—	0
Home Originals Ultimate Nachos as prep	12 pieces (4.6 oz)	240	11	3	0	6	31	2	4	100	680	—	—	0
READY-TO-EAT														
taco shell baked	1 med (0.5 oz)	61	3	tr	0	1	8	—	tr	21	48	23	1	0
taco shell baked w/o salt	1 med (½ oz)	61	3	tr	0	1	8	—	tr	21	2	23	1	0
CHI-CHI'S														
Taco Shells White Corn	2 (1.2 oz)	170	8	2	0	3	22	0	2	0	0	—	—	0
Taco Shells Yellow Corn	2 shells (1.2 oz)	170	8	0	0	2	22	0	2	0	0	—	—	0
GEBHARDT														
Taco Shells	3 (1.1 oz)	155	8	2	0	2	19	0	3	tr	1		—	0
LA MEXICANA														
Flour Burritos	1 (1.6 oz)	160	5	1	0	4	26	2	2	80	580	—	—	0
ROSARITA														
Taco Shells	3 (1.1 oz)	155	8	2	0	2	19	0	3	tr	1	—	—	0
Tostada Shells	2 (1 oz)	125	5	1	37	2	17	tr	0	27	20	—	—	0
TACO BELL														
Home Originals Taco Shells	3 (1.1 oz)	150	6	1	0	2	21	0	2	0	5	—	—	0
TAKE-OUT														
burrito w/ apple	1 lg (5.4 oz)	484	20	7	7	5	73	—	—	32	443	218	4	2
burrito w/ apple	1 sm (2.6 oz)	231	10	5	3	3	35	—	—	15	211	104	4	tr
burrito w/ beans	2 (7.6 oz)	448	14	7	5	14	71	—	—	113	986	653	118	2
burrito w/ beans & cheese	2 (6.5 oz)	377	12	7	27	15	55	—	—	214	1166	496	81	2
burrito w/ beans & chili peppers	2 (7.2 oz)	413	15	8	33	16	58	—	—	100	1043	580	118	1

FOOD	PORTION	CALS	FAT	SAT FAT	CHOL	PROT	CARB	SUGAR	FIBER	CALCI	SOD	POTAS	FOLIC	VIT C
burrito w/ beans & meat	2 (8.1 oz)	508	18	8	48	22	66	—	—	105	1335	656	73	2
burrito w/ beans cheese & beef	2 (7.1 oz)	331	13	7	125	15	40	—	—	131	990	410	61	5
burrito w/ beans cheese & chili peppers	2 (11.8 oz)	663	23	11	158	33	85	—	—	288	2060	810	146	7
burrito w/ beef	2 (7.7 oz)	523	21	10	65	27	59	—	—	84	1492	739	39	1
burrito w/ beef & chili peppers	2 (7.1 oz)	426	17	8	54	22	49	—	—	87	1116	499	37	2
burrito w/ beef cheese & chili peppers	2 (10.7 oz)	634	25	10	170	41	64	—	—	223	2091	667	58	4
burrito w/ cherry	1 lg (5.4 oz)	484	20	7	7	5	73	—	—	32	443	218	4	2
burrito w/ cherry	1 sm (2.6 oz)	231	10	5	3	3	35	—	—	15	211	104	4	tr
chimichanga w/ beef	1 (6.1 oz)	425	20	9	9	20	43	—	—	63	910	587	31	5
chimichanga w/ beef & cheese	1 (6.4 oz)	443	23	11	51	20	39	—	—	238	956	203	34	3
chimichanga w/ beef & red chili peppers	1 (6.7 oz)	424	19	8	9	18	46	—	—	71	1169	613	34	tr
chimichanga w/ beef cheese & red chili peppers	1 (6.3 oz)	364	18	8	50	15	38	—	—	218	895	330	33	2
enchilada eggplant	1	142	5	—	7	—	—	—	—	124	—	—	—	—
enchilada w/ cheese	1 (5.7 oz)	320	19	11	44	10	29	—	—	324	784	240	34	tr
enchilada w/ cheese & beef	1 (6.7 oz)	324	18	9	40	12	30	—	—	228	1320	574	192	1
enchirito w/ cheese beef & beans	1 (6.8 oz)	344	16	8	49	18	34	—	—	217	1251	560	254	5
frijoles w/ cheese	1 cup (5.9 oz)	226	8	4	36	11	29	—	—	188	882	605	111	2
nachos w/ cheese	6 to 8 (4 oz)	345	19	8	18	9	36	—	—	272	816	172	10	1
nachos w/ cheese & jalapeño peppers	6 to 8 (7.2 oz)	607	34	14	83	17	60	—	—	620	1736	292	19	tr
nachos w/ cheese beans ground beef & peppers	6 to 8 (8.9 oz)	568	31	12	21	20	56	—	—	384	1800	451	39	5
nachos w/ cinnamon & sugar	6 to 8 (3.8 oz)	592	36	18	39	7	63	—	—	85	439	75	7	8
quesadilla	1	290	16	8	40	—	—	—	—	—	470	—	—	—
taco	1 sm (6 oz)	370	21	11	57	21	27	—	—	221	802	473	23	2
taco salad	1½ cups	279	15	7	44	13	24	—	—	192	763	416	40	4
taco salad w/ chili con carne	1½ cups	288	13	6	4	17	27	—	—	246	886	393	64	3

FOOD	PORTION	CALS	FAT	SAT FAT	CHOL	PROT	CARB	SUGAR	FIBER	CALCI	SOD	POTAS	FOLIC	VIT C
tostada w/ beans & cheese	1 (5.1 oz)	223	10	5	30	10	27	—	—	211	543	403	75	1
tostada w/ beans beef & cheese	1 (7.9 oz)	334	17	11	75	16	30	—	—	190	870	490	97	4
tostada w/ beef & cheese	1 (5.7 oz)	315	16	10	41	19	23	—	—	217	896	572	15	3
tostada w/ guacamole	2 (9.2 oz)	360	23	10	39	12	32	—	—	424	789	649	110	4

SPICES

(*see individual names*, HERBS/SPICES)

SPINACH

CANNED

FOOD	PORTION	CALS	FAT	SAT FAT	CHOL	PROT	CARB	SUGAR	FIBER	CALCI	SOD	POTAS	FOLIC	VIT C
spinach	½ cup	25	1	tr	0	3	4	—	—	135	29	370	105	15
DEL MONTE														
Chopped	½ cup (4 oz)	30	0	0	0	2	4	0	2	100	360	—	—	15
No Salt Added	½ cup (4 oz)	30	0	0	0	2	4	0	2	100	85	—	—	15
Whole Leaf	½ cup (4 oz)	30	0	0	0	2	4	0	2	100	360	—	—	15
S&W														
Spinach	½ cup (4.5 oz)	30	0	0	0	3	4	1	2	80	440	410	—	12
FRESH														
baby raw	2 cups	20	0	0	0	1	5	0	3	30	80	—	—	8
cooked	½ cup	21	tr	tr	0	3	3	—	2	122	63	419	131	9
malabar cooked	1 cup (1.5 oz)	10	tr	—	0	1	1	—	1	55	24	113	50	1
mustard chopped cooked	½ cup	14	tr	—	0	2	3	—	—	142	—	—	—	59
mustard raw chopped	½ cup	17	tr	—	0	2	3	—	—	158	—	—	—	98
new zealand chopped cooked	½ cup	11	tr	tr	0	1	2	—	—	43	97	92	—	14
new zealand raw	½ cup	4	tr	tr	0	tr	1	—	—	16	36	36	—	8
raw chopped	¼ cup	6	tr	tr	0	1	1	—	1	28	22	156	54	8
raw chopped	1 pkg (10 oz)	46	1	tr	0	6	7	—	—	202	160	1139	397	57
DOLE														
Baby Spinach	3½ cups (3 oz)	35	0	0	0	2	9	0	4	60	135	—	—	12
FRESH EXPRESS														
Baby Spinach	3 cups	20	0	0	0	2	3	0	2	80	65	—	—	24
READY PAC														
Baby	2 cups	20	0	0	0	1	5	0	3	30	80	—	—	8
Microwave Spinach as prep	½ cup	20	0	0	0	2	3	0	tr	80	60	—	—	6
FROZEN														
cooked	½ cup	27	tr	tr	0	3	5	—	—	139	82	283	102	12
AMY'S ORGANIC														
Snacks Spinach Feta	5–6 pieces	170	6	3	15	7	24	3	2	—	430	—	—	—

FOOD	PORTION	CALS	FAT	SAT FAT	CHOL	PROT	CARB	SUGAR	FIBER	CALCI	SOD	POTAS	FOLIC	VIT C
BIRDS EYE														
Chopped	⅓ cup	20	0	0	0	—	—	—	2	80	80	—	—	15
Creamed	½ cup	100	7	3	35	3	7	3	1	80	660	—	—	5
Cut Leaf	1 cup	20	0	0	0	2	2	1	2	60	110	—	—	6
FRESH LIKE														
Cut Leaf	3.5 oz	21	tr	—	—	3	4	—	1	108	81	344	—	26
GREEN GIANT														
Butter Sauce	½ cup (3.4 oz)	40	2	1	<5	2	5	tr	2	100	280	—	—	18
Creamed Low Fat Sauce	½ cup	80	3	1	0	3	9	5	1	100	510	—	—	5
Cut Leaf	¾ cup (2.6 oz)	25	0	0	0	3	3	0	3	100	65	—	—	12
Harvest Fresh	½ cup (3.5 oz)	25	0	0	0	3	3	0	2	100	240	—	—	21
HEALTH IS WEALTH														
Spinach Munchees	2 (1 oz)	60	3	0	0	2	9	0	1	40	105	—	—	2
Spinach Feta Munchees	2 (1 oz)	70	3	1	5	2	9	0	1	40	115	—	—	2
STOUFFER'S														
Creamed	1 serv (4.5 oz)	160	12	4	15	4	8	2	2	100	380	410	—	5
Soufflé	1 serv (4 oz)	150	10	2	120	6	9	4	0	100	480	430	—	1
TREE OF LIFE														
Organic	1 cup (3 oz)	20	0	0	0	2	2	1	2	60	110	—	—	6
SHELF-STABLE														
TASTYBITE														
Kashmir Spinach	½ pkg (5 oz)	170	10	4	35	10	8	1	3	220	960	—	—	0
TAKE-OUT														
indian saag	1 serv	28	2	tr	0	2	2	—	1	—	44	—	—	—
spanakopita spinach pie	1 cup (6 oz)	196	3	2	30	14	35	4	4	250	590	—	—	9

SPINACH JUICE
juice	7 oz	14	0	0	0	2	2	—	—	2	146	824	—	58

SPORTS DRINKS
(*see* ENERGY DRINKS)

SPOT
baked	3 oz	134	5	2	—	20	0	—	—	15	32	541	—	—

SPROUTS
kidney bean	½ cup	27	tr	tr	0	4	4	—	—	16	—	172	—	36
lentil sprouts	½ cup	40	tr	tr	0	3	8	—	—	9	4	122	38	6
mung bean	½ cup	16	tr	tr	0	2	3	—	—	7	3	77	32	7
mung bean canned	½ cup	8	tr	tr	0	1	1	—	—	9	—	17	6	tr
mung bean cooked	½ cup	13	tr	tr	0	1	3	—	—	7	6	63	—	7
pea	½ cup	77	tr	tr	0	5	17	—	—	21	12	229	87	6
radish	½ cup	8	tr	tr	0	1	1	—	—	10	1	16	18	6
CHUN KING														
Bean Sprouts	1 cup (3 oz)	11	tr	0	0	1	1	0	1	36	17	—	—	20

FOOD	PORTION	CALS	FAT	SAT FAT	CHOL	PROT	CARB	SUGAR	FIBER	CALCI	SOD	POTAS	FOLIC	VIT C
FRESH ALTERNATIVES														
BroccoSprouts	½ cup (1 oz)	10	0	0	0	1	1	0	1	20	0	—	—	9
Deli Blend	½ cup (1 oz)	10	0	0	0	1	1	0	tr	0	0	—	—	9
Salad Blend	½ cup (1 oz)	10	0	0	0	1	2	0	tr	0	0	—	—	12
Sandwich Blend	½ cup (1 oz)	5	0	0	0	1	1	0	tr	0	0	—	—	12
LA CHOY														
Bean Sprouts	1 cup (2.9 oz)	11	tr	0	0	1	1	0	1	36	17	—	—	20
TAKE-OUT														
mung bean stir fried	½ cup	31	tr	tr	0	3	7	—	—	8	—	—	—	—
SQUAB														
boneless baked	3.5 oz	175	3	1	75	37	0	0	0	15	100	400	8	0
breast w/o skin raw	1 (3.5 oz)	135	5	1	91	22	0	—	—	—	—	—	—	—
w/o skin raw	1 squab (5.9 oz)	239	13	3	—	29	0	—	—	—	—	—	—	—
SQUASH														
CANNED														
crookneck sliced	½ cup	14	tr	tr	0	1	3	—	—	13	5	104	11	3
FRESH														
acorn cooked mashed	½ cup	41	tr	tr	0	1	11	—	3	32	3	321	14	8
acorn cubed baked	½ cup	57	tr	tr	0	1	15	—	2	45	4	446	19	11
butternut baked	½ cup	41	tr	tr	0	1	11	—	2	42	4	290	20	15
crookneck sliced cooked	½ cup	18	tr	tr	0	1	4	—	1	24	1	173	18	5
hubbard baked	½ cup	51	tr	tr	0	3	11	—	3	17	8	365	17	10
hubbard cooked mashed	½ cup	35	tr	tr	0	2	8	—	3	12	6	252	12	8
scallop sliced cooked	½ cup	14	tr	tr	0	1	3	—	1	14	1	126	19	10
spaghetti cooked	½ cup	23	tr	tr	0	1	5	—	2	17	14	91	6	3
MARTIN FARMS														
Butternut Fresh Cut	½ cup	40	0	0	0	1	10	5	1	40	3	300	20	18
FROZEN														
butternut cooked mashed	½ cup	47	tr	tr	0	1	12	—	3	23	2	160	—	4
crookneck sliced cooked	½ cup	24	tr	tr	0	1	5	—	—	19	6	243	12	7
BIRDS EYE														
Cooked Squash	½ cup	50	0	0	0	—	—	—	4	20	0	—	—	12
Sliced Yellow	⅔ cup	15	0	0	0	tr	2	1	1	0	15	—	—	0
SQUASH SEEDS														
roasted	1 oz	148	12	2	0	9	4	—	—	12	5	229	—	—
salted & roasted	1 oz	148	12	2	0	9	4	—	—	12	5	229	—	—

FOOD	PORTION	CALS	FAT	SAT FAT	CHOL	PROT	CARB	SUGAR	FIBER	CALCI	SOD	POTAS	FOLIC	VIT C
seeds dried	1 oz	154	13	2	0	7	5	—	—	12	5	229	—	—
seeds whole roasted	1 oz	127	6	1	0	5	15	—	—	16	5	261	—	—

SQUID
fried	3 oz	149	6	2	221	15	7	—	—	33	260	237	—	4
raw	3 oz	78	1	tr	198	13	3	—	—	27	37	209	—	4
TAKE-OUT														
calamari deep fried	1 serv	451	423	3	25	—	—	—	—	—	546	—	—	—

SQUIRREL
roasted	3 oz	147	4	tr	103	26	0	—	—	2	102	300	—	—

STARFRUIT
fresh	1	42	tr	—	0	1	10	—	—	6	2	207	—	27

STRAWBERRIES
CANNED														
in heavy syrup	½ cup	117	tr	tr	0	1	30	—	—	16	5	109	36	40
FRESH														
strawberries	1 cup	45	1	tr	0	1	10	—	4	21	2	247	26	85
strawberries	1 pint	97	1	tr	0	2	22	—	—	45	4	530	57	182
FROZEN														
sweetened sliced	1 cup	245	tr	tr	0	1	66	—	—	29	8	249	38	106
sweetened sliced	1 pkg (10 oz)	273	tr	tr	0	2	74	—	—	31	9	277	42	118
unsweetened	1 cup	52	tr	tr	0	1	14	—	—	23	3	220	25	61
whole sweetened	1 cup	200	tr	tr	0	1	54	—	—	29	3	249	10	101
whole sweetened	1 pkg (10 oz)	223	tr	tr	0	1	60	—	—	32	3	277	11	112
BIRDS EYE														
In Syrup	½ cup	120	0	0	0	1	31	28	1	—	0	—	—	—
Lite Syrup	1 pkg (10 oz)	120	0	0	0	1	31	28	1	—	0	—	—	—
Whole	½ cup	100	0	0	0	tr	25	23	1	—	0	—	—	36
TREE OF LIFE														
Organic	¾ cup (5 oz)	50	0	0	0	1	13	8	2	0	0	—	—	36

STRAWBERRY JUICE
CAPRI SUN														
Strawberry Cooler Drink	1 pkg (7 oz)	90	0	0	0	0	25	25	0	0	20	20	—	0
CERES														
Strawberry	8 oz	115	0	0	0	0	28	24	1	20	35	216	—	60
KOOL-AID														
Drink as prep w/ sugar	1 serv (8 oz)	100	0	0	0	0	25	25	0	0	30	0	—	6
Drink Mix as prep	1 serv (8 oz)	60	0	0	0	0	16	16	0	0	0	0	—	6
SQUEEZIT														
Strawberry	1 bottle (7 oz)	110	0	0	0	0	29	27	0	0	0	—	—	0
VERYFINE														
Juice-Ups	8 fl oz	140	0	0	0	0	36	36	0	0	15	—	—	60

STUFFING/DRESSING

FOOD	PORTION	CALS	FAT	SAT FAT	CHOL	PROT	CARB	SUGAR	FIBER	CALCI	SOD	POTAS	FOLIC	VIT C
bread as prep w/ water & fat	½ cup	251	15	6	tr	5	25	—	—	46	627	63	20	tr
bread as prep w/ water egg & fat	½ cup	107	7	4	75	3	9	—	—	31	319	80	12	3
bread dry as prep	½ cup	178	9	2	—	3	22	—	3	32	543	74	17	—
cornbread as prep	½ cup	179	9	2	0	3	22	—	—	26	455	62	8	1
KELLOGG'S														
Croutettes Mix	1 cup (1.2 oz)	120	0	0	0	5	25	0	0	40	460	50	—	0
PEPPERIDGE FARM														
Corn Bread	¾ cup (1.5 oz)	170	2	0	0	4	33	2	2	40	480	—	—	0
Herb Seasoned	¾ cup (1.5 oz)	170	2	0	0	5	33	2	3	40	600	—	—	0
Herb Seasoned Cubed	¾ cup (1.3 oz)	140	2	0	0	4	28	2	2	40	530	—	—	0
One Step Chicken	½ cup (1.2 oz)	140	4	1	<5	4	23	tr	tr	0	440	—	—	0
One Step Southwestern Corn Bread	½ cup (1.2 oz)	150	5	1	0	4	23	2	tr	0	440	—	—	0
One Step Turkey	½ cup (1.2 oz)	150	5	1	<5	4	22	3	tr	0	500	—	—	0
STOVE TOP														
Chicken as prep w/ margarine	½ cup (3.6 oz)	170	9	2	0	4	20	3	tr	20	510	90	16	0
Cornbread as prep w/ margarine	½ cup (3.6 oz)	170	8	2	0	3	21	3	1	20	580	85	16	0
Flexible Serve Chicken as prep w/ margarine	½ cup (3.3 oz)	170	8	2	0	3	19	3	tr	20	520	70	16	0
Flexible Serve Cornbread as prep w/ margarine	½ cup (3.3 oz)	160	8	2	0	3	19	3	1	0	560	70	16	0
Flexible Serve Homestyle Herb as prep w/ margarine	½ cup (3.3 oz)	170	8	2	0	3	19	3	1	20	500	75	16	0
For Beef as prep w/ margarine	½ cup (3.7 oz)	180	9	2	0	4	22	4	1	20	540	100	16	0
For Pork as prep w/ margarine	½ cup (3.6 oz)	170	9	2	0	4	20	3	1	20	530	95	24	0
For Turkey as prep w/ margarine	½ cup (3.6 oz)	170	9	2	0	4	20	3	tr	20	530	90	16	0
Long Grain & Wild Rice as prep w/ margarine	½ cup (3.7 oz)	180	9	2	0	4	22	3	tr	20	500	75	16	0
Lower Sodium Chicken as prep w/ margarine	½ cup (3.6 oz)	180	9	2	0	4	21	3	tr	20	340	90	16	0
Microwave Chicken as prep w/ margarine	½ cup (3.5 oz)	160	7	2	0	4	20	3	tr	20	480	70	16	0

FOOD	PORTION	CALS	FAT	SAT FAT	CHOL	PROT	CARB	SUGAR	FIBER	CALCI	SOD	POTAS	FOLIC	VIT C
STOVETOP (CONT.)														
Microwave Homestyle Cornbread as prep w/ margarine	½ cup (3 oz)	160	7	2	0	3	20	3	tr	0	480	70	16	0
Mushroom & Onion as prep w/ margarine	½ cup (3.6 oz)	180	9	2	0	4	20	3	tr	20	480	85	16	0
San Francisco Style as prep w/ margarine	½ cup (3.6 oz)	170	9	2	0	4	20	3	1	20	530	100	24	0
Savory Herb as prep w/ margarine	½ cup (3.6 oz)	170	9	2	0	4	20	3	1	40	530	95	16	0
Traditional Sage as prep w/ margarine	½ cup (3.6 oz)	180	9	2	0	4	21	3	1	20	530	110	16	0
TAKE-OUT														
bread	½ cup (3½ oz)	195	8	2	0	4	26	—	3	74	534	152	19	2
sausage	½ cup	292	11	2	12	8	40	—	1	17	258	96	3	2
STURGEON														
cooked	3 oz	115	4	1	—	18	0	—	—	—	—	309	—	—
raw	3 oz	90	3	1	—	14	0	—	—	—	—	241	—	—
roe raw	1 oz	59	3	—	—	7	tr	—	—	—	—	—	—	5
smoked	3 oz	147	4	1	—	27	0	—	—	—	—	—	—	—
smoked	1 oz	48	1	tr	—	9	0	—	—	—	—	—	—	—
SUCKER														
white baked	3 oz	101	3	tr	45	18	0	—	—	76	44	414	—	—
SUGAR														
brown packed	1 cup (7.7 oz)	828	0	0	0	0	214	214	—	167	86	762	1	0
brown unpacked	1 cup (5.1 oz)	546	0	0	0	0	141	—	—	123	57	502	1	0
maple	1 piece (1 oz)	100	tr	—	0	0	26	—	—	26	3	78	0	0
powdered	1 tbsp (0.3 oz)	31	0	0	0	0	8	8	—	0	0	0	0	0
powdered unsifted	1 cup (4.2 oz)	467	tr	—	0	tr	119	115	—	1	2	3	0	0
sugarcane stem	3 oz	54	0	0	0	1	14	—	3	2	—	—	—	1
white	1 tsp (4 g)	15	0	0	0	0	4	4	—	0	0	0	0	0
white	1 packet (6 g)	25	0	0	0	0	6	—	—	tr	tr	tr	—	0
white	1 cup (7 oz)	773	0	0	0	0	200	200	—	2	3	4	0	0
white	1 tbsp	45	0	0	0	0	12	—	—	tr	tr	tr	—	0
BILLINGTON'S														
Muscovado Light Brown	1 tsp	15	0	0	0	0	4	4	—	—	0	—	—	—
DOMINO														
Dark Brown	1 tsp	15	0	0	0	0	4	4	—	—	0	—	—	—
Light Brown	1 tsp	15	0	0	0	0	4	4	—	—	0	—	—	—
White	1 tsp	15	0	0	0	0	4	—	—	—	0	—	—	—
MAUI BRAND														
Raw Sugar	1 tsp	15	0	0	0	0	4	4	—	—	0	—	—	—

FOOD	PORTION	CALS	FAT	SAT FAT	CHOL	PROT	CARB	SUGAR	FIBER	CALCI	SOD	POTAS	FOLIC	VIT C
PRINCESS OF YUM														
Citrus Lemon	2.5 tsp	40	0	0	0	0	10	10	—	—	0	—	—	—
French Vanilla	2.5 tsp	40	0	0	0	0	10	10	—	—	0	—	—	—

SUGAR SUBSTITUTES

FOOD	PORTION	CALS	FAT	SAT FAT	CHOL	PROT	CARB	SUGAR	FIBER	CALCI	SOD	POTAS	FOLIC	VIT C
EQUAL														
Packet	1 pkg	0	0	0	0	0	tr	tr	—	—	0	—	—	—
FRAN GARE'S														
Miracle Sweet	1 tsp	10	0	0	0	0	5	0	0	—	0	—	—	—
KETO														
Sweet	½ tsp	0	0	0	0	0	0	0	0	—	0	—	—	—
LO HAN														
Sweet	2 scoops	2	0	0	0	0	2	0	tr	—	0	—	—	—
SOMERSWEET														
Sweetener	¼ tsp	0	0	0	0	0	tr	0	tr	—	0	—	—	—
SPLENDA														
Sugar Blend For Baking	½ tsp	10	0	0	0	0	2	2	—	—	0	—	—	—
Sweetener	1 pkg	0	0	0	0	0	tr	tr	0	0	0	—	—	0
STEEL'S														
Brown	1 tsp	10	0	0	0	0	1	0	0	—	0	—	—	—
Sugar Substitute	1 tsp	10	0	0	0	0	1	0	0	—	0	—	—	—
STEVITA														
Spoonable	⅓ tsp	0	0	0	0	0	0	0	0	—	0	0	—	—
SUGAR TWIN														
Packets	1	0	0	0	0	0	tr	—	—	—	0	0	—	—
Spoonable Brown	1 tsp	0	0	0	0	0	0	0	0	—	0	—	—	—
Spoonable White	1 tsp	0	0	0	0	0	0	0	0	—	0	—	—	—
WEIGHT WATCHERS														
Sweetener	1 serv (1 g)	5	0	0	0	0	1	1	0	0	30	—	—	0

SUGAR-APPLE

FOOD	PORTION	CALS	FAT	SAT FAT	CHOL	PROT	CARB	SUGAR	FIBER	CALCI	SOD	POTAS	FOLIC	VIT C
fresh	1	146	tr	—	0	3	37	—	—	37	15	384	—	66
fresh cut up	1 cup	236	1	—	0	5	59	—	—	59	24	619	—	91

SUNCHOKE

FOOD	PORTION	CALS	FAT	SAT FAT	CHOL	PROT	CARB	SUGAR	FIBER	CALCI	SOD	POTAS	FOLIC	VIT C
fresh raw sliced	½ cup	57	tr	0	0	2	13	—	—	10	—	—	—	3

SUNFISH

FOOD	PORTION	CALS	FAT	SAT FAT	CHOL	PROT	CARB	SUGAR	FIBER	CALCI	SOD	POTAS	FOLIC	VIT C
pumpkinseed baked	3 oz	97	1	tr	73	21	0	—	—	87	87	381	—	—

SUNFLOWER

FOOD	PORTION	CALS	FAT	SAT FAT	CHOL	PROT	CARB	SUGAR	FIBER	CALCI	SOD	POTAS	FOLIC	VIT C
seeds dried	1 cup	821	71	7	0	33	27	—	—	168	4	992	—	—
seeds dried	1 oz	162	14	7	0	33	5	—	—	33	1	196	—	—
seeds dry roasted	1 cup	745	64	7	0	25	31	—	—	90	4	1088	—	—
seeds dry roasted	1 oz	165	14	1	0	5	7	—	—	20	1	241	—	—

FOOD	PORTION	CALS	FAT	SAT FAT	CHOL	PROT	CARB	SUGAR	FIBER	CALCI	SOD	POTAS	FOLIC	VIT C
seeds dry roasted salted	1 oz	165	14	1	0	5	7	—	—	20	195	241	—	—
seeds dry roasted salted	1 cup	745	64	7	0	25	31	—	—	90	975	1088	—	—
seeds oil roasted	1 cup	830	78	8	0	29	20	—	—	76	4	652	316	2
seeds oil roasted salted	1 oz	175	16	2	0	6	4	—	—	16	201	137	67	tr
seeds oil roasted salted	1 cup	830	78	8	0	29	20	—	—	76	804	6528	316	2
seeds toasted	1 cup	826	76	8	0	23	28	—	—	76	4	658	—	—
seeds toasted	1 oz	176	16	2	0	5	6	—	—	16	1	139	—	—
seeds toasted salted	1 oz	176	16	2	0	5	6	—	—	16	204	139	—	—
seeds toasted salted	1 cup	826	76	8	0	23	28	—	—	76	817	658	—	—
sunflower butter	1 tbsp	93	8	1	0	3	4	—	—	19	82	12	—	tr
sunflower butter w/o salt	1 tbsp	93	8	1	0	3	4	—	—	19	1	12	—	tr
DAKOTA GOURMET														
Honey Roasted Kernels	1 pkg (1 oz)	158	12	1	0	6	8	4	1	28	56	164	0	—
Lightly Salted Kernels	1 pkg (1 oz)	168	14	1	0	6	5	1	2	28	85	164	0	0
FRITO LAY														
Seeds	1 oz	180	15	2	0	7	5	tr	2	—	25	—	—	—
LANCE														
Seeds In Shell	⅔ cup (1.8 oz)	160	13	3	0	6	5	1	2	20	30	200	—	0
Seeds Roasted & Shelled	1 pkg (1⅛ oz)	190	16	3	0	7	6	1	2	20	100	150	—	0
MARANATHA														
Tamari Seeds	¼ cup	160	14	2	0	6	7	1	2	20	140	—	—	0
SUNGOLD														
SunButter	2 tbsp	200	16	2	0	7	7	3	4	20	120	—	—	0

SUSHI

TAKE-OUT

FOOD	PORTION	CALS	FAT	SAT FAT	CHOL	PROT	CARB	SUGAR	FIBER	CALCI	SOD	POTAS	FOLIC	VIT C
california roll	1 piece (0.8 oz)	28	1	tr	1	1	4	tr	—	13	37	37	5	1
fresh salmon rolls	4 pieces	250	7	1	20	11	37	5	3	20	590	—	—	9
sashimi	1 serv (6 oz)	198	7	1	63	24	4	1	—	25	718	668	8	4
tuna roll	1 piece (0.7 oz)	23	tr	tr	3	2	3	tr	—	2	33	24	1	tr
vegetable roll	1 piece (1.2 oz)	27	1	tr	0	1	5	tr	—	20	47	60	16	3
vinegared ginger	⅓ cup (1.6 oz)	48	tr	tr	0	1	12	4	—	8	6	189	5	2
wasabi	2 tsp (0.3 oz)	5	tr	0	0	tr	1	—	—	6	124	28	0	0
yellowtail roll	1 piece (0.6 oz)	25	1	tr	0	1	3	tr	—	12	32	14	3	1

SWAMP CABBAGE

FOOD	PORTION	CALS	FAT	SAT FAT	CHOL	PROT	CARB	SUGAR	FIBER	CALCI	SOD	POTAS	FOLIC	VIT C
chopped cooked	½ cup	10	tr	—	0	1	2	—	—	26	60	139	—	8
raw chopped	1 cup	11	tr	—	0	1	2	—	—	43	63	174	—	31

FOOD	PORTION	CALS	FAT	SAT FAT	CHOL	PROT	CARB	SUGAR	FIBER	CALCI	SOD	POTAS	FOLIC	VIT C
SWEET POTATO														
(*see also* YAM)														
baked w/ skin	1 (3½ oz)	118	tr	tr	0	2	28	—	3	32	12	397	26	28
canned in syrup	½ cup	106	tr	tr	0	1	25	—	—	16	38	189	—	11
canned pieces	1 cup	183	tr	tr	0	3	42	—	—	44	107	625	33	53
frzn cooked	½ cup	88	tr	tr	0	2	21	—	—	31	7	332	20	8
leaves cooked	½ cup	11	tr	tr	0	1	2	—	—	8	4	153	—	1
mashed	½ cup	172	tr	tr	0	3	40	—	3	35	21	301	18	28
TAKE-OUT														
candied	3½ oz	144	3	1	0	1	29	—	—	27	73	198	12	7
SWEETBREADS														
beef braised	3 oz	230	15	—	—	23	0	—	—	14	51	209	—	17
lamb braised	3 oz	199	13	6	340	19	0	—	—	10	44	247	11	17
veal braised	3 oz	218	12	—	—	25	0	—	—	—	—	—	—	5
SWISS CHARD														
cooked	½ cup	18	tr	—	0	2	4	—	3	51	158	483	—	16
raw chopped	½ cup	3	tr	—	0	tr	1	—	—	9	38	68	—	5
SWORDFISH														
cooked	3 oz	132	4	1	43	22	0	—	—	5	98	314	—	1
raw	3 oz	103	3	1	33	17	0	—	—	4	76	245	—	1
SYRUP														
corn dark	1 cup (11.5 oz)	925	tr	—	0	0	251	—	—	58	608	144	0	0
corn dark	1 tbsp (0.7 oz)	56	0	—	0	0	15	—	—	4	31	9	0	0
corn light	1 cup (11.5 oz)	925	tr	—	0	0	251	168	—	10	395	13	0	0
corn light	1 tbsp (0.7 oz)	56	0	—	0	0	15	10	—	1	24	1	0	0
date syrup	1 tbsp	63	tr	—	—	tr	15	—	0	12	—	—	—	—
malt	1 tbsp (0.8 oz)	76	0	—	0	2	17	—	—	15	8	77	3	0
malt	1 cup (13 oz)	1222	tr	—	0	24	274	—	—	234	134	1229	46	0
maple	1 cup (11.1 oz)	824	1	—	0	tr	212	191	—	211	27	643	1	0
maple	1 tbsp (0.8 oz)	52	0	—	0	0	13	12	—	13	2	41	0	0
raspberry	1 oz	76	0	0	0	tr	19	—	—	8	1	45	—	8
rose hip	1 oz	9	0	0	—	0	2	2	0	—	—	—	—	—
sorghum	1 tbsp (0.7 oz)	61	0	0	0	0	16	16	—	31	2	210	—	—
sorghum	1 cup (11.6 oz)	957	0	0	0	0	247	247	—	495	28	3300	—	—
DAVINCI GOURMET														
Sugar Free All Flavors	1 tbsp	0	0	0	0	0	0	0	0	—	5	—	—	—
EDEN														
Organic Barley Malt	1 tbsp	60	0	0	0	1	14	8	0	0	0	65	0	0
ESTEE														
Blueberry	¼ cup	80	0	0	0	0	20	20	0	—	70	0	—	—
HERSHEY'S														
Strawberry	2 tbsp	100	0	0	0	0	26	—	—	—	10	—	—	—

FOOD	PORTION	CALS	FAT	SAT FAT	CHOL	PROT	CARB	SUGAR	FIBER	CALCI	SOD	POTAS	FOLIC	VIT C
KARO														
Corn Syrup Light	2 tbsp (1 oz)	120	0	0	0	0	31	12	—	—	35	—	—	—
QUIK														
Strawberry	2 tbsp (1.5 oz)	110	0	0	0	0	27	26	0	0	0	5	—	0
SMUCKER'S														
Apricot	¼ cup	210	0	0	0	0	52	52	—	—	0	—	—	—
Blackberry	¼ cup	210	0	0	0	0	52	52	—	—	0	—	—	—
Plate Scapers Kiwi Lime	2 tbsp (1.3 oz)	100	0	0	0	0	25	13	—	—	10	—	—	—
Plate Scapers Mango Orange	2 tbsp	100	0	0	0	0	24	13	—	—	0	—	—	1
Plate Scapers Raspberry	2 tbsp (1.3 oz)	100	0	0	0	0	25	13	—	—	5	—	—	—
TAHINI														
(*see* SESAME)														
TAMARIND														
fresh	1	5	tr	tr	0	tr	1	—	—	1	1	13	—	tr
fresh cut up	1 cup	287	1	tr	0	3	75	—	—	89	33	753	—	4
TANGERINE														
CANNED														
in light syrup	½ cup	76	tr	tr	0	1	20	—	—	9	8	99	—	25
juice pack	½ cup	46	tr	tr	0	1	12	—	—	14	7	165	—	43
FRESH														
sections	1 cup	86	tr	tr	0	1	22	—	—	27	3	305	40	60
tangerine	1	37	tr	tr	0	1	9	—	—	12	1	132	17	26
CHIQUITA														
Tangerine	1 med (3.5 oz)	50	1	0	0	1	15	12	2	40	0	—	—	30
TANGERINE JUICE														
canned sweetened	1 cup	125	1	tr	0	1	30	—	—	45	2	443	—	55
fresh	1 cup	106	tr	tr	0	1	25	—	—	44	2	440	—	77
frzn sweetened as prep	1 cup	110	tr	tr	0	1	27	—	—	18	2	273	11	58
frzn sweetened not prep	6 oz	344	1	tr	0	3	83	—	—	57	7	850	35	182
FRESH SAMANTHA														
Fresh Juice	1 cup (8 oz)	110	0	0	0	2	8	—	0	40	0	130	8	66
NAKED JUICE														
Tangerine Scream	8 oz	110	0	0	0	1	25	25	0	40	0	440	—	78
ODWALLA														
Juice	8 fl oz	110	0	0	0	1	25	24	0	40	25	440	—	78
TAPIOCA														
pearl dry	½ cup (2.7 oz)	272	tr	tr	0	tr	67	—	1	15	1	9	3	0
starch	1 oz	98	tr	—	—	17	24	—	—	3	1	6	—	0

FOOD	PORTION	CALS	FAT	SAT FAT	CHOL	PROT	CARB	SUGAR	FIBER	CALCI	SOD	POTAS	FOLIC	VIT C
MINUTE														
Minute Tapioca	1½ tsp (6 g)	20	0	0	0	0	5	0	0	0	0	0	—	0
TARO														
chips	1 oz	141	7	2	0	1	19	—	—	17	97	214	—	1
chips	10 (0.8 oz)	115	6	1	0	1	16	—	—	14	79	174	—	1
leaves cooked	½ cup	18	tr	tr	0	2	3	—	—	63	2	341	—	26
raw sliced	½ cup	56	tr	tr	0	1	14	—	—	22	6	307	—	2
shoots sliced cooked	½ cup	10	tr	tr	0	1	2	—	—	9	1	240	—	—
sliced cooked	½ cup (2.3 oz)	94	tr	tr	0	tr	23	—	—	12	10	319	—	3
tahitian sliced cooked	½ cup	30	tr	tr	0	3	5	—	—	101	37	423	—	26
TARPON														
fresh	3 oz	87	2	—	—	17	0	0	0	46	70	306	—	—
TARRAGON														
ground	1 tsp	5	tr	—	0	tr	1	—	—	18	1	48	—	—
TEA/HERBAL TEA														
(see also ICED TEA)														
HERBAL														
chamomile brewed	1 cup	2	tr	tr	0	0	tr	0	0	5	2	21	1	0
CELESTIAL SEASONINGS														
Mandarin Orange Spice	1 tea bag	0	0	0	0	0	tr	0	—	—	0	—	—	—
EDEN														
Organic Genmaicha Tea	1 cup	0	0	0	0	0	0	0	0	0	0	0	0	0
Organic Kukicha Tea	1 cup	0	0	0	0	0	0	0	0	0	0	0	0	0
GUAYAKI														
Yerba Mate Magical Mint	1 tea bag	5	0	0	0	—	1	—	—	—	—	—	—	—
Yerba Mate Organic Chai Spice	1 tea bag	5	0	0	0	—	1	—	—	—	—	—	—	—
Yerba Mate Organic Chocolate	1 tea bag	5	0	0	0	—	1	—	—	—	—	—	—	—
Yerba Mate Organic Orange Blossom	1 tea bag	5	0	0	0	—	1	—	—	—	—	—	—	—
Yerba Mate Organic Rooiboost	1 tea bag	5	0	0	0	0	1	0	—	—	3	40	—	—
Yerba Mate Organic Traditional	1 tea bag	5	0	0	0	0	1	0	—	—	3	40	—	—

FOOD	PORTION	CALS	FAT	SAT FAT	CHOL	PROT	CARB	SUGAR	FIBER	CALCI	SOD	POTAS	FOLIC	VIT C
LIPTON														
Bedtime Story	1 tea bag	0	0	0	0	0	1	0	—	—	0	—	—	0
Cinnamon Apple	1 tea bag	0	0	0	0	0	1	0	—	—	0	—	—	0
Ginger Twist	1 tea bag	0	0	0	0	0	0	0	0	—	0	—	—	—
Lemon	1 tea bag	0	0	0	0	0	1	0	—	—	0	—	—	0
Orange	1 tea bag	0	0	0	0	0	1	0	—	—	0	—	—	0
Peppermint	1 tea bag	0	0	0	0	0	1	0	—	—	0	—	—	0
Quietly Chamomile	1 tea bag	0	0	0	0	0	1	0	—	—	0	—	—	0
SILK														
Chai	1 cup	140	4	0	0	6	19	14	0	300	50	—	—	0
REGULAR														
brewed tea	6 oz	2	0	0	0	0	1	—	0	0	5	66	9	0
instant unsweetened as prep w/ water	8 oz	2	0	0	0	tr	tr	—	—	5	8	47	1	0
ACTIVITEA														
Green Tea	1 cup	36	0	0	0	0	3	tr	—	—	3	—	—	—
CELESTIAL SEASONINGS														
Green Tea Raspberry Garden as prep	1 cup	0	0	0	0	0	0	0	0	—	0	—	—	—
Green Tea Honey Lemon Ginseng	1 cup	0	0	0	0	0	0	0	0	—	0	—	—	—
Honey Darjeeling as prep	1 cup	0	0	0	0	0	0	0	0	—	0	—	—	—
DAVINCI GOURMET														
Sugar Free Tea Concentrate Green	2 tbsp	0	0	0	0	0	0	0	0	—	5	—	—	—
Sugar Free Tea Concentrate Lemon	2 tbsp	0	0	0	0	0	0	0	0	—	5	—	—	—
Sugar Free Tea Concentrate Spiced Chai	1.5 tbsp	0	0	0	0	0	0	0	0	—	15	—	—	—
GENERAL FOODS														
International Instant Tea Decaffeinated English Breakfast Creme	1 serv (8 oz)	70	2	1	0	0	13	10	0	0	105	220	—	0
International Instant Tea Decaffeinated Viennese Cinnamon Creme	1 serv (8 oz)	70	2	1	0	0	13	10	0	0	105	220	—	0

FOOD	PORTION	CALS	FAT	SAT FAT	CHOL	PROT	CARB	SUGAR	FIBER	CALCI	SOD	POTAS	FOLIC	VIT C
International Instant Tea English Breakfast Creme as prep	1 serv (8 oz)	70	2	1	0	0	13	10	0	0	65	70	—	0
International Instant Tea English Raspberry Creme as prep	1 serv (8 oz)	70	2	1	0	0	13	11	0	0	65	80	—	0
International Instant Tea Island Orange Creme as prep	1 serv (8 oz)	70	2	1	0	0	13	11	0	0	65	80	—	0
International Instant Tea Viennese Cinnamon Creme as prep	1 serv (8 oz)	70	2	1	0	0	13	11	0	0	65	80	—	0
GUAYAKI														
Yerba Mate Organic Greener Green Tea	1 tea bag	5	0	0	0	0	1	0	—	—	3	40	—	—
LIPTON														
Brisk Tea as prep	1 serv	0	0	0	0	0	0	0	0	0	0	—	—	0
Decaffeinated Brisk Tea as prep	1 serv	0	0	0	0	0	0	0	0	0	0	—	—	0
English Blend as prep	1 cup	0	0	0	0	0	0	0	0	0	0	—	—	0
Flavored Decaffeinated Orange & Spice	1 tea bag	0	0	0	0	0	0	0	—	—	0	—	—	0
Green Tea	1 tea bag	0	0	0	0	0	0	0	—	—	0	25	—	—
Loose Tea	1 tsp (2 g)	0	0	0	0	0	0	0	0	—	0	—	—	0
LOW CARB CREATIONS														
Chai as prep	1 cup	25	2	0	0	0	3	tr	0	0	50	—	—	0
PACIFIC CHAI														
All Flavors as prep	1 serv	93	1	1	0	2	18	11	0	80	30	—	—	0
PARADISE														
Tropical Tea	8 fl oz	1	0	0	0	0	tr	0	0	—	7	—	—	—
Tropical Tea Decafe	8 fl oz	1	0	0	0	0	tr	0	0	—	7	—	—	—
Tropical Tea Passion Fruit	8 fl oz	1	0	0	0	0	tr	0	0	—	7	—	—	—
SALADA														
Green Tea	1 cup	0	0	0	0	0	0	0	0	0	0	—	—	0
Green Tea Decaffeinated	1 tea bag	0	0	0	0	0	0	0	—	—	0	—	—	—

FOOD	PORTION	CALS	FAT	SAT FAT	CHOL	PROT	CARB	SUGAR	FIBER	CALCI	SOD	POTAS	FOLIC	VIT C
TETLEY														
British Blend Round Teabags	1 cup	0	0	0	0	0	0	0	0	—	0	31	—	—
Decaffeinated Tea Bag as prep	1	0	0	0	0	0	0	0	0	—	0	25	—	—
Tea Bag as prep	1	0	0	0	0	0	0	0	0	—	0	28	—	—
TAKE-OUT														
chai spiced latte decaf	1 cup	130	3	1	0	2	23	18	0	80	45	—	—	0
TEMPEH														
tempeh	½ cup	165	6	1	0	16	14	—	—	77	5	305	43	0
LIGHTLIFE														
Garden Vege	4 oz	200	8	1	0	21	12	3	6	—	399	—	—	—
Quinoa Sesame	4 oz	220	8	1	0	21	15	3	7	—	0	—	—	—
Smokey Strips	3 slices (2 oz)	80	3	1	0	8	6	0	1	—	230	—	—	—
Soy	4 oz	210	8	1	0	24	11	3	7	—	0	—	—	—
Three Grain	4 oz	200	7	1	0	20	13	3	6	—	0	—	—	—
Wild Rice	4 oz	190	7	1	0	19	13	3	6	—	0	—	—	—
TURTLE ISLAND														
Five Grain	3 oz	190	6	1	0	11	20	0	6	80	10	—	—	0
Low Fat Millet	3 oz	130	2	1	0	8	20	0	3	20	10	—	—	0
Soy	3 oz	160	4	1	0	13	20	0	7	60	15	—	—	0
Wild Rice Rhapsody	3 oz	160	4	1	0	13	20	0	7	40	15	—	—	0
WHITE WAVE														
Five Grain	⅓ block	140	4	1	0	12	15	2	4	20	0	—	—	0
Organic Original Soy	⅓ block	150	6	1	0	16	10	0	6	20	0	—	—	0
Organic Sea Veggie	⅓ block	120	3	0	0	12	11	0	8	100	25	—	—	0
Soy Rice	⅓ block	140	5	1	0	12	13	2	5	20	0	—	—	0
THYME														
ground	1 tsp	4	tr	tr	0	tr	1	—	—	26	1	11	—	—
TILEFISH														
cooked	3 oz	125	4	1	—	21	0	—	—	22	50	435	—	—
cooked	½ fillet (5.3 oz)	220	7	1	—	37	0	—	—	39	88	768	—	—
raw	3 oz	81	2	tr	—	15	0	—	—	22	45	368	—	—
TOFU														
firm	¼ block (3 oz)	118	7	1	0	13	3	—	1	166	11	192	24	tr
firm	½ cup	183	11	2	0	20	5	—	2	258	17	298	37	tr
fresh fried	1 piece (0.5 oz)	35	3	tr	0	2	1	—	tr	48	2	19	4	0
fuyu salted & fermented	1 block (⅓ oz)	13	1	tr	0	1	1	—	tr	5	316	8	—	—
koyadofu dried frozen	1 piece (½ oz)	82	5	1	0	8	2	—	tr	62	1	3	16	tr
okara	½ cup	47	1	tr	0	2	8	—	1	49	6	130	—	0

FOOD	PORTION	CALS	FAT	SAT FAT	CHOL	PROT	CARB	SUGAR	FIBER	CALCI	SOD	POTAS	FOLIC	VIT C
regular	¼ block (4 oz)	88	6	1	0	9	2	—	1	122	8	141	17	tr
regular	½ cup	94	6	1	0	6	2	—	1	130	9	150	19	tr
AZUMAYA														
Baked Chili Picante	2 pieces	200	10	2	0	20	9	3	2	100	320	—	—	0
Baked Mesquite	2 pieces	100	10	2	0	20	6	tr	2	100	480	—	—	0
Baked Spicy Thai Peanut	2 pieces	190	10	2	0	20	6	2	2	100	500	—	—	0
Baked Teriyaki	2 pieces	200	10	2	0	20	9	3	2	100	730	—	—	0
Extra Firm	1 serv (2.8 oz)	70	4	1	0	8	2	0	1	150	0	—	—	0
Firm	1 serv (2.8 oz)	70	4	1	0	7	2	0	0	150	0	—	—	0
Lite Extra Firm	1 serv (2.8 oz)	60	2	0	0	8	3	0	1	300	30	—	—	0
Lite Silken	1 serv (3.2 oz)	40	1	0	0	5	3	0	0	300	45	—	—	0
Silken	1 serv (3.2 oz)	40	2	0	0	4	1	tr	—	60	0	—	—	0
GALAXY														
Slices Hickory Smoked	1 slice (1 oz)	50	2	0	0	2	5	2	0	250	340	—	—	0
Slices Italian Garlic Herb	1 slice (1 oz)	50	2	0	0	2	5	2	0	250	390	—	—	0
Slices Original	1 slice (1 oz)	50	2	0	0	2	5	2	0	250	340	—	—	0
Slices Savory	1 slice (1 oz)	50	2	0	0	2	5	2	0	250	390	—	—	0
HINOICHI														
Firm	1 inch slice (3 oz)	60	3	0	0	6	2	0	1	100	10	—	—	0
LONG LIFE														
Tofu	3 oz	60	3	0	0	6	2	0	1	100	10	—	—	0
NASOYA														
5 Spice	1 serv (3 oz)	70	4	1	0	7	0	1	0	40	220	—	—	0
Baked Mesquite Smoke	2 pieces	220	9	2	0	21	17	tr	3	100	560	—	—	0
Baked Teriyaki	2 pieces	230	9	2	0	20	21	3	3	100	700	—	—	0
Baked TexMex	2 pieces	230	9	2	0	21	21	3	4	100	360	—	—	0
Baked Thai Peanut	2 pieces	240	10	2	0	21	19	2	3	100	540	—	—	0
Extra Firm	1 serv (3 oz)	90	5	1	0	8	3	0	0	60	0	—	—	0
Firm	1 serv (3 oz)	70	4	1	0	7	2	0	tr	100	0	—	—	0
Firm Enriched	1 serv (3 oz)	45	1	0	0	7	0	0	0	300	30	—	—	0
Garlic & Onion	1 serv (3 oz)	70	4	1	0	7	1	1	0	40	250	—	—	0
Silken	1 serv (3.2 oz)	45	3	1	0	4	2	tr	0	60	5	—	—	0
Soft	1 serv (3 oz)	60	4	1	0	7	1	0	0	100	0	—	—	0
TofuMate Breakfast Scramble	¼ pkg	15	0	0	0	1	3	0	—	20	330	—	—	1

FOOD	PORTION	CALS	FAT	SAT FAT	CHOL	PROT	CARB	SUGAR	FIBER	CALCI	SOD	POTAS	FOLIC	VIT C
NASOYA (CONT.)														
TofuMate Eggless Salad	¼ pkg	15	0	0	0	0	4	0	—	20	310	—	—	0
TofuMate Mandarin Stirfry	¼ pkg	30	0	0	0	1	6	3	—	40	310	—	—	1
TofuMate Mediterranean Herb	¼ pkg	15	0	0	0	1	3	1	—	20	330	—	—	4
TofuMate Szechwan Stirfry	¼ pkg	25	0	0	0	1	4	0	—	40	280	—	—	1
TofuMate Texas Taco	¼ pkg	15	0	0	0	1	3	0	0	20	360	—	—	0
PETE'S TOFU														
Dessert Peach Mango	1 serv (6 oz)	120	3	0	0	4	20	17	0	40	5			—
Dessert Very Berry	1 serv (6 oz)	120	3	1	0	6	17	14	0	50	25			—
Medium Firm	3 oz	70	4	1	0	6	2	0	0	100	0			—
Soft	3 oz	56	3	1	0	5	2	0	0	20	1			—
Super Firm Italian Herb	3 oz	120	7	1	0	13	1	0	tr	100	10			—
Super Firm	3 oz	130	8	2	0	12	2	0	0	100	5			—
Tofu 2 Go Lemon Pepper	2 pieces + sauce	160	9	1	0	13	9	7	2	300	400			—
Tofu 2 Go Santa Fe	2 pieces + sauce	150	9	1	0	14	6	4	2	300	340			—
Tofu 2 Go Sesame Ginger	2 pieces + sauce	160	10	2	0	13	7	4	2	300	390			—
Tofu 2 Go Thai Tango	2 pieces + sauce	165	10	2	0	12	9	7	2	250	380			—
TREE OF LIFE														
30% Reduced Fat Firm	⅕ block (3.2 oz)	90	4	0	0	10	4	0	2	40	5	—	—	0
Easymeal Pasta Primavera as prep	1 serv	460	16	3	10	20	54	4	3	200	790	—	—	24
Easymeal Southwest Medley as prep	1 serv	380	14	2	0	15	44	4	3	200	790	—	—	12
Easymeal Teriyaki Stir Fry as prep	1 serv	270	14	2	0	13	24	8	6	200	560	—	—	42
Easymeal Thai Stir Fry as prep	1 serv	270	14	2	0	14	21	8	6	200	230	—	—	6
Organic Baked	⅓ block (2.7 oz)	150	8	1	0	16	5	0	0	250	310	—	—	0
Organic Baked Island Spice	⅓ pkg (2.7 oz)	130	7	1	0	15	3	0	0	150	320	—	—	0
Organic Baked Oriental	⅓ pkg (2.7 oz)	130	7	1	0	15	5	2	0	150	330	—	—	0

FOOD	PORTION	CALS	FAT	SAT FAT	CHOL	PROT	CARB	SUGAR	FIBER	CALCI	SOD	POTAS	FOLIC	VIT C
TREE OF LIFE (CONT.)														
Organic Baked Savory	⅓ block (2.7 oz)	140	7	1	0	15	4	0	0	250	310	—	—	0
Organic Firm	⅕ block (3.2 oz)	100	5	0	0	9	2	0	0	150	5	—	—	0
Raw Firm	⅕ block (3.2 oz)	100	5	0	0	9	2	0	0	150	5	—	—	0
WHITE WAVE														
Baked Garlic Herb Italian	1 piece	120	6	1	0	13	3	0	1	40	240	—	—	1
Baked Hickory Smoke BBQ	1 piece	75	3	1	0	8	4	3	1	60	140	—	—	0
Baked Roma Italian Basil	1 piece	100	6	1	0	8	3	1	2	60	220	—	—	0
Baked Teriyaki Oriental	1 piece	120	6	1	0	13	3	0	1	40	240	—	—	1
Baked Thai Style	1 piece	120	6	1	0	13	3	0	1	40	240	—	—	1
Baked Zesty Lemon Pepper	1 piece	120	8	1	0	8	3	1	1	60	100	—	—	0
Extra Firm	¼ block	80	5	1	0	10	1	0	1	100	10	—	—	0
Organic Extra Firm	⅕ block	90	6	1	0	10	1	0	1	100	10	—	—	0
Organic Soft	⅕ block	90	6	1	0	10	1	0	1	100	10	—	—	0
Reduced Fat	⅕ block	90	4	0	0	10	4	0	2	40	5	—	—	0
TOMATILLO														
fresh	1 (1.2 oz)	11	tr	—	0	tr	2	—	—	2	0	91	2	4
fresh chopped	½ cup	21	1	—	0	1	4	—	—	4	1	177	4	8
TOMATO														
CANNED														
paste	½ cup	110	1	tr	0	5	25	—	6	46	86	1221	—	55
puree	1 cup	102	tr	tr	0	4	25		6	37	532	1051	—	88
puree w/o salt	1 cup	102	tr	tr	0	4	25	—	6	37	49	1051	—	88
red whole	½ cup	24	tr	tr	0	1	5	—	—	32	195	265	—	18
sauce	½ cup	37	tr	tr	0	2	9	—	2	17	738	452	—	16
sauce spanish style	½ cup	40	tr	tr	0	2	9	—	2	20	—	576	—	11
sauce w/ mushrooms	½ cup	42	tr	tr	0	2	10	—	—	16	552	464	—	15
sauce w/ onion	½ cup	52	tr	tr	0	1	12	—	—	20	672	504	—	16
stewed	½ cup	34	tr	tr	0	1	8	—	—	47	325	307	—	17
w/ green chiles	½ cup	18	tr	tr	0	1	4	—	—	24	481	129	—	8
wedges in tomato juice	½ cup	34	tr	tr	0	1	8	—	—	34	285	329	—	19

FOOD	PORTION	CALS	FAT	SAT FAT	CHOL	PROT	CARB	SUGAR	FIBER	CALCI	SOD	POTAS	FOLIC	VIT C
AMORE														
Sun-Dried Tomato Paste	1 tsp (6 g)	15	1	0	0	0	tr	0	0	0	115	—	—	0
BIG R														
Cajun Stewed	½ cup (4.2 oz)	25	0	0	0	1	4	4	1	—	150	—	—	0
Diced w/ Chilies	½ cup (4.2 oz)	25	0	0	0	1	4	3	1	—	340	—	—	6
Mexican Stewed	½ cups (4.2 oz)	25	0	0	0	1	5	3	1	—	190	—	—	6
Stewed	½ cup (4.2 oz)	25	0	0	0	1	5	3	1	40	190	—	—	6
Whole	½ cup (4.2 oz)	25	0	0	0	1	5	3	1	—	190	—	—	6
CENTO														
Puree	¼ cup	25	0	0	0	1	5	3	1	0	15	—	—	9
CLAUSSEN														
Halves	1 serv (1 oz)	5	0	0	0	0	1	0	tr	0	320	—	—	0
CONTADINA														
Italian Paste	2 tbsp	35	1	—	0	1	7	4	1	0	290	—	—	6
Italian Paste Roasted Garlic	2 tbsp	35	1	—	0	1	6	1	1	20	300	—	—	5
Paste	2 tbsp (1.2 oz)	30	0	0	0	2	6	3	1	0	20	—	—	6
Puree	¼ cup (2.2 oz)	20	0	0	0	tr	4	1	tr	0	15	—	—	9
Recipe Ready Diced Roasted Garlic	½ cup (4.3 oz)	45	0	0	0	1	10	7	tr	60	560	—	—	15
Stewed	½ cup	35	0	0	0	1	9	6	1	40	220	—	—	9
Stewed w/ Celery & Green Peppers	½ cup	35	0	0	0	1	9	6	1	40	220	—	—	9
DEL MONTE														
Chunky Chili Style	½ cup (4.5 oz)	30	0	0	0	1	8	6	2	20	670	—	—	9
Chunky Pasta Style	½ cup (4.5 oz)	45	0	0	0	1	11	8	2	20	560	—	—	9
Crushed Italian Recipe	½ cup (4.4 oz)	45	0	0	0	2	9	5	1	0	390	—	—	9
Crushed Original Recipe	½ cup (4.4 oz)	45	0	0	0	2	9	5	1	0	390	—	—	6
Crushed w/ Garlic	½ cup (4.4 oz)	50	0	0	0	2	11	1	1	0	510	—	—	6
Diced	½ cup (4.4 oz)	25	0	0	0	1	6	4	2	20	160	—	—	9
Diced No Salt Added	½ cup (4.4 oz)	25	0	0	0	1	6	4	2	20	50	—	—	9
Diced w/ Basil Garlic & Oregano	½ cup	50	0	0	0	2	11	8	tr	80	650	—	—	9
Diced w/ Garlic & Onion	½ cup (4.4 oz)	40	1	—	0	2	8	6	1	20	610	—	—	9
Diced w/ Green Pepper & Onion	½ cup (4.4 oz)	40	0	0	0	1	9	7	2	20	480	—	—	15
Paste	2 tbsp (1.2 oz)	30	0	0	0	1	7	5	2	0	25	—	—	6
Petite Cut Garlic & Olive Oil	½ cup	45	1	0	0	1	10	7	1	20	620	—	—	9
Sauce	¼ cup (2.1 oz)	20	0	0	0	1	4	4	1	0	340	—	—	5

FOOD	PORTION	CALS	FAT	SAT FAT	CHOL	PROT	CARB	SUGAR	FIBER	CALCI	SOD	POTAS	FOLIC	VIT C
DEL MONTE (CONT.)														
Sauce No Salt Added	¼ cup (2.1 oz)	20	0	0	0	0	4	4	1	0	20	—	—	5
Stewed Cajun Recipe	½ cup (4.4 oz)	35	0	0	0	1	9	7	2	20	460	—	—	9
Stewed Italian Recipe	½ cup (4.4 oz)	30	0	0	0	1	8	6	2	20	420	—	—	9
Stewed Mexican Recipe	½ cup (4.4 oz)	35	0	0	0	1	9	7	2	20	400	—	—	9
Stewed Original	½ cup (4.4 oz)	35	0	0	0	1	9	7	2	20	360	—	—	9
Stewed Original No Salt Added	½ cup (4.4 oz)	35	0	0	0	1	9	7	2	20	50	—	—	9
Wedges	½ cup (4.4 oz)	35	0	0	0	1	9	7	2	20	380	—	—	9
Zesty Diced w/ Mild Green Chilies	½ cup (4.4 oz)	30	0	0	0	1	6	3	1	20	550	—	—	15
EDEN														
Organic Diced	½ cup	30	0	0	0	1	6	4	2	20	5	330	0	18
Organic Diced w/ Green Chilies	½ cup	30	0	0	0	2	5	3	2	20	35	250	0	9
HUNT'S														
Crushed	½ cup	30	0	0	0	2	7	5	2	0	350	400	—	12
Diced Original	½ cup	20	0	0	0	1	5	4	tr	40	380	260	—	21
Diced w/ Balsamic Vinegar Basil & Oil	½ cup	60	3	0	0	1	8	6	1	60	460	290	—	12
Diced w/ Basil Garlic & Oregano	½ cup	24	0	0	0	1	6	5	1	40	360	320	—	9
Diced w/ Green Pepper Celery & Onions	½ cup	45	0	0	0	1	10	8	1	40	340	240	—	5
Diced w/ Mild Green Chilies	½ cup	30	0	0	0	2	6	5	2	40	360	320	—	9
Diced w/ Roasted Garlic	½ cup	30	0	0	0	1	6	5	1	40	480	250	—	9
Diced w/ Sweet Onion	½ cup	45	0	0	0	1	10	7	tr	60	460	280	—	12
Family Favorites Meatloaf	¼ cup	30	0	0	0	1	7	4	2	0	390	200	—	4
Paste	2 tbsp	25	0	0	0	1	6	4	2	0	90	—	—	6
Paste No Salt Added	2 tbsp	30	0	0	0	1	6	4	2	0	15	—	—	4
Paste w/ Basil Garlic & Oregano	2 tbsp	25	0	0	0	1	6	4	2	0	260	—	—	5
Petite Diced	½ cup	20	0	0	0	1	5	3	1	40	330	—	—	15
Petite Diced w/ Mushrooms	½ cup	40	1	0	0	1	6	5	tr	40	380	—	—	9

FOOD	PORTION	CALS	FAT	SAT FAT	CHOL	PROT	CARB	SUGAR	FIBER	CALCI	SOD	POTAS	FOLIC	VIT C
HUNT'S (CONT.)														
Puree	½ cup	30	0	0	0	1	7	4	2	60	450	320	—	18
Sauce	¼ cup	15	0	0	0	tr	3	2	tr	0	360	—	—	5
Sauce Garlic & Herb	½ cup	40	1	0	0	2	8	5	3	20	610	390	—	9
Sauce No Salt Added	¼ cup	60	0	0	0	2	14	8	4	0	30	—	—	7
Sauce Roasted Garlic	¼ cup	15	0	0	0	tr	3	2	tr	0	380	160	—	5
Stewed	½ cup	35	0	0	0	1	8	6	1	60	390	—	—	12
Stewed No Salt Added	½ cup	40	0	0	0	2	9	6	1	40	30	—	—	9
Whole	½ cup	20	0	0	0	1	4	3	1	40	190	—	—	12
Whole No Salt Added	2 oz	20	0	0	0	tr	4	3	1	0	15	150	—	6
MUIR GLEN														
Diced Fire Roasted	¼ cup	30	0	0	0	1	6	4	1	20	290	—	—	15
Diced w/ Green Chilies	½ cup (4.5 oz)	25	0	0	0	1	4	4	1	0	290	—	—	15
Organic Chunky Sauce	¼ cup (2.3 oz)	20	0	0	0	tr	4	2	1	0	160	—	—	2
Organic Crushed Fire Roasted	¼ cup	20	0	0	0	1	5	4	1	0	160	—	—	9
Organic Diced	½ cup (4.5 oz)	25	0	0	0	1	4	4	1	0	290	—	—	15
Organic Diced No Salt Added	½ cup (4.5 oz)	25	0	0	0	1	4	4	1	0	45	—	—	15
Organic Diced w/ Basil & Garlic	½ cup (4.5 oz)	25	0	0	0	1	4	4	1	0	290	—	—	15
Organic Diced w/ Italian Herbs	½ cup (4.4 oz)	25	0	0	0	1	4	4	1	0	290	—	—	15
Organic Ground Peeled	¼ cup (2.3 oz)	10	0	0	0	tr	2	2	1	0	100	—	—	1
Organic Paste	2 tbsp (1.2 oz)	30	0	0	0	2	6	3	1	0	20	—	—	6
Organic Puree	¼ cup (2.2 oz)	20	0	0	0	1	5	3	1	0	20	—	—	4
Organic Sauce	¼ cup (2.2 oz)	20	0	0	0	tr	5	3	1	0	310	—	—	2
Organic Sauce No Salt Added	¼ cup (2.2 oz)	20	0	0	0	tr	5	3	1	0	30	—	—	2
Organic Stewed	½ cup (4.5 oz)	30	0	0	0	1	7	3	tr	40	290	—	—	15
Organic Whole Peeled	½ cup (4.6 oz)	30	0	0	0	1	5	4	1	0	260	—	—	15
Whole Peeled w/ Basil	½ cup (4.6 oz)	30	0	0	0	1	5	4	1	0	260	—	—	15
PROGRESSO														
Crushed w/ Added Puree	¼ cup (2.1 oz)	20	0	0	0	tr	3	2	0	20	95	—	—	6
Italian Style Peeled	½ cup (4.2 oz)	20	0	0	0	1	4	3	1	20	220	—	—	12

FOOD	PORTION	CALS	FAT	SAT FAT	CHOL	PROT	CARB	SUGAR	FIBER	CALCI	SOD	POTAS	FOLIC	VIT C
Paste	2 tbsp (1.2 oz)	30	0	0	0	2	6	3	1	0	20	—	—	6
Puree	¼ cup (2.2 oz)	25	0	0	0	1	5	3	1	0	15	—	—	9
Puree Thick Style	¼ cup (2.2 oz)	20	0	0	0	tr	5	3	1	0	15	—	—	15
Sauce	¼ cup (2.1 oz)	20	0	0	0	1	4	2	1	0	260	—	—	2
Whole Peeled	½ cup (4.2 oz)	25	0	0	0	1	5	3	1	20	220	—	—	9
REDPACK														
Chunky Style In Puree	½ cup	30	0	0	0	1	6	2	1	0	270	—	—	9
Crushed In Puree	¼ cup	20	0	0	0	0	4	2	1	20	120	—	—	6
Paste	2 tbsp	0	0	0	0	2	6	3	1	0	20	—	—	6
Puree	¼ cup (2.2 oz)	25	0	0	0	1	5	3	1	0	10	—	—	5
TUTTOROSSO														
Puree	¼ cup	20	0	0	0	1	4	3	1	0	15	—	—	5
DRIED														
sun dried	1 cup	140	2	tr	0	8	30	—	—	60	1131	1851	37	21
sun dried	1 piece	5	tr	tr	0	tr	1	—	—	2	42	69	1	1
sun dried in oil	1 cup (4 oz)	235	15	2	0	6	26	—	—	51	293	1721	25	112
sun dried in oil	1 piece (3 g)	6	tr	tr	0	tr	1	—	—	1	8	47	1	3
FRESH														
bruschetta	¼ cup	50	3	0	0	2	6	4	tr	0	360	—	—	8
cooked	½ cup	32	1	tr	0	1	7	—	—	7	13	335	16	27
grape tomatoes	20	30	0	0	0	1	6	4	1	0	0	250	—	27
green	1	30	tr	tr	0	1	6	—	—	16	16	251	—	29
red	1 (4.5 oz)	26	tr	tr	0	1	6	—	2	6	11	273	18	24
red chopped	1 cup	35	tr	tr	0	2	8	—	2	12	16	372	17	32
CHIQUITA														
Tomato	1 med (5.2 oz)	35	1	0	0	1	7	4	1	0	5	—	—	24
EUROFRESH														
Tomatoes On The Vine	1 med (5.2 oz)	35	1	0	0	1	—	4	1	0	5	—	—	21
TAKE-OUT														
bruschetta on toasted italian bread	1 slice	106	3	0	0	4	18	2	tr	23	355	—	—	4
stewed	1 cup	80	3	1	0	2	13	—	—	27	460	249	11	18

TOMATO JUICE

FOOD	PORTION	CALS	FAT	SAT FAT	CHOL	PROT	CARB	SUGAR	FIBER	CALCI	SOD	POTAS	FOLIC	VIT C
beef broth & tomato	5½ oz	61	tr	tr	—	1	14	—	—	19	220	162	—	2
clam & tomato	1 can (5½ oz)	77	tr	tr	—	1	18	—	—	21	664	149	—	7
tomato juice	6 oz	32	tr	tr	0	1	8	—	—	16	658	400	36	33
tomato juice	½ cup	21	tr	tr	0	1	5	—	—	10	441	268	24	22
CAMPBELL'S														
Juice	8 oz	51	1	tr	—	2	10	8	2	29	683	549	—	29
DEL MONTE														
Juice	8 fl oz	50	0	0	0	2	10	7	1	40	760	—	—	60

FOOD	PORTION	CALS	FAT	SAT FAT	CHOL	PROT	CARB	SUGAR	FIBER	CALCI	SOD	POTAS	FOLIC	VIT C
DEL MONTE (CONT.)														
Snap-E-Tom Chile Cocktail	6 fl oz	40	0	0	0	2	8	4	1	0	500	—	—	12
DOLE														
Juice	1 bottle (12 oz)	85	0	0	0	4	17	—	2	20	1000	900	—	30
HUNT'S														
Juice	1 can (6 oz)	22	tr	0	0	1	5	4	1	13	452	—	—	15
No Salt Added	8 fl oz	34	tr	0	0	2	8	7	2	10	12	—	—	22
MOTT'S														
Tomato Juice	8 fl oz	40	0	0	0	2	9	—	—	—	850	—	—	—
MUIR GLEN														
Organic	5.5 oz	40	0	0	0	1	8	3	4	20	420	—	—	14
TONGUE														
beef simmered	3 oz	241	18	8	91	19	tr	—	—	6	51	153	4	tr
lamb braised	3 oz	234	17	7	161	18	0	—	—	8	57	134	2	6
pork braised	3 oz	230	16	5	124	20	0	—	0	16	93	—	3	1
TORTILLA														
corn	1 (6 in diam)	56	1	tr	0	1	12	—	1	44	40	39	4	0
corn w/o salt	1 (6 in diam) (.9 oz)	56	1	tr	0	1	12	—	1	44	3	39	4	0
flour w/o salt	1 (8 in diam) (1.2 oz)	114	3	tr	0	3	20	—	1	44	167	46	4	0
CARBOLE														
Low-Carb	1 (2 oz)	100	4	0	0	11	14	0	9	20	310	—	—	0
LA MEXICANA														
Corn	1 (0.8 oz)	50	1	0	0	1	10	0	1	60	0	—	—	0
Flour	1 (0.8 oz)	80	3	1	0	2	13	1	1	40	260	—	—	0
Tortillas de Trigo	1 (1 oz)	140	7	1	0	2	18	0	1	40	75	—	—	—
LA TORTILLA FACTORY														
Low Carb Whole Wheat	1 reg	60	2	—	—	5	12	0	9	—	—	—	—	—
Low Carb Whole Wheat	1 lg	100	3	—	—	8	21	1	15	—	—	—	—	—
MARIACHI														
Tortilla	1	112	3	—	—	3	20	—	—	—	174	—	—	—
OLD EL PASO														
Flour	1 (1.4 oz)	130	4	1	0	3	21	0	0	60	290	—	—	0
TUMARO'S														
Low In Carb Green Onion	1 (8 inch)	100	3	0	0	6	13	0	8	100	120	—	—	0
Low In Carb Multi-grain	1 (8 inch)	100	3	0	—	6	13	tr	8	100	120	—	—	0
Low In Carb Sour Cream & Salsa	1 (8 inch)	100	3	0	0	6	13	—	8	80	125	—	—	0
Low In Carb Garden Vegetable	1 (8 inch)	100	3	0	0	6	13	tr	8	80	125	—	—	0

FOOD	PORTION	CALS	FAT	SAT FAT	CHOL	PROT	CARB	SUGAR	FIBER	CALCI	SOD	POTAS	FOLIC	VIT C
TYSON														
Flour	1 (1.7 oz)	150	4	1	0	3	24	1	1	0	310	—	—	0
Flour Heat Pressed	2 (2 oz)	170	4	1	0	4	30	1	2	40	410	—	—	0
White Corn	2 (1.8 oz)	100	1	0	0	2	21	0	3	0	70	—	—	0
Whole Wheat Heat Pressed	1 (1.4 oz)	120	3	1	0	4	20	2	3	20	240	—	—	0
Yellow Corn	3 (1.9 oz)	140	2	0	0	3	27	0	3	40	20	—	—	0
TREE FERN														
chopped cooked	½ cup	28	tr	—	0	tr	8	—	—	6	3	3	—	21
TRITICALE														
dry	1 cup (6.7 oz)	645	4	1	0	25	138	—	—	71	10	637	140	0
triticale not prep	1 oz	94	tr	—	—	4	18	—	2	11	7.4	127	5	—
TROUT														
baked	3 oz	162	7	1	63	23	0	—	—	47	57	393	13	tr
rainbow cooked	3 oz	129	4	1	62	22	0	—	—	73	29	539	—	3
sea trout baked	3 oz	113	4	1	90	18	0	—	—	19	63	372	—	—
TRUFFLES														
fresh	0.5 oz	4	tr	—	0	2	9	—	2	12	39	263	—	—
TUNA														
CANNED														
light in oil	3 oz	169	7	1	15	25	0	—	—	11	301	176	5	—
light in oil	1 can (6 oz)	399	14	3	30	50	0	—	—	23	606	354	9	—
light in water	3 oz	99	1	tr	25	22	0	—	—	10	287	202	3	0
light in water	1 can (5.8 oz)	192	1	tr	49	42	0	—	—	19	558	391	6	0
white in oil	1 can (6.2 oz)	331	14	—	55	47	0	—	—	8	704	593	8	—
white in oil	3 oz	158	7	—	26	23	0	—	—	4	336	283	4	—
white in water	3 oz	116	2	1	35	23	0	—	—	—	333	241	4	—
white in water	1 can (6 oz)	234	4	1	72	46	0	—	—	—	673	487	7	—
BUMBLE BEE														
Chunk Light In Water	¼ cup (2 oz)	60	1	0	30	13	0	0	0	0	250	—	—	0
Chunk Light In Water Pouch	2 oz	60	1	0	30	13	0	0	0	0	250	—	—	0
Chunk Light In Water Touch Of Lemon	2 oz	60	1	0	30	13	0	0	0	0	250	—	—	0
Solid White Albacore In Water	2 oz	70	1	0	25	15	0	0	0	0	250	—	—	0
Solid White Albacore In Oil	¼ cup	90	3	1	25	14	0	0	0	0	250	—	—	0
Solid White In Water	2 oz	70	1	0	25	15	0	0	0	0	250	—	—	0
CHICKEN OF THE SEA														
Albacore In Spring Water	2 oz	60	1	0	25	13	0	0	0	0	250	—	—	0

FOOD	PORTION	CALS	FAT	SAT FAT	CHOL	PROT	CARB	SUGAR	FIBER	CALCI	SOD	POTAS	FOLIC	VIT C
CHICKEN OF THE SEA (CONT.)														
Chunk Light In Water	¼ cup (2 oz)	60	1	0	30	13	0	0	0	0	125	—	—	0
PROGRESSO														
In Olive Oil drained	¼ cup (2 oz)	160	12	2	30	13	0	0	0	0	250	—	—	0
STARKIST														
Chunk Light In Water	¼ cup (2 oz)	60	1	0	30	13	0	0	0	0	250	—	—	0
Chunk Light No Drain Package	¼ cup (2 oz)	60	1	0	30	13	0	0	0	0	250	—	—	0
Low Sodium Chunk White In Water	2 oz	60	1	0	25	14	0	0	0	—	35	—	—	—
Solid White Albacore In Water	¼ cup	70	1	0	25	15	0	0	0	0	250	—	—	0
Tuna Fillet In Spring Water	¼ cup (2 oz)	60	1	0	30	13	0	0	0	0	250	—	—	0
FRESH														
bluefin cooked	3 oz	157	5	1	42	25	0	—	—	—	43	275	—	—
bluefin raw	3 oz	122	4	1	32	20	0	—	—	—	33	214	—	—
skipjack baked	3 oz	112	1	tr	51	24	0	—	—	32	40	444	—	—
yellowfin baked	3 oz	118	1	tr	49	25	0	—	—	17	40	—	—	—

TUNA DISHES

MIX

TUNA HELPER

FOOD	PORTION	CALS	FAT	SAT FAT	CHOL	PROT	CARB	SUGAR	FIBER	CALCI	SOD	POTAS	FOLIC	VIT C
AuGratin 50% Less Fat Recipe as prep	1 cup	240	6	2	15	13	37	5	1	100	840	250	60	0
AuGratin as prep	1 cup	300	11	3	20	13	37	5	1	100	890	250	60	0
Cheesy Broccoli 50% Less Fat Recipe as prep	1 cup	240	5	2	15	15	38	6	1	100	820	350	60	0
Cheesy Broccoli as prep	1 cup	290	9	3	20	15	38	6	1	100	860	350	60	0
Cheesy Pasta 50% Less Fat Recipe as prep	1 cup	230	5	2	15	14	32	5	tr	100	850	270	60	0
Cheesy Pasta as prep	1 cup	280	11	3	20	14	32	5	tr	100	890	270	60	0
Creamy Broccoli 50% Less Fat Recipe as prep	1 cup	240	5	2	15	14	35	6	1	80	820	290	60	0
Creamy Broccoli as prep	1 cup	310	12	3	20	14	35	6	1	80	880	290	60	0
Creamy Pasta 50% Less Fat Recipe as prep	1 cup	230	6	2	15	14	31	4	1	80	840	290	40	0

FOOD	PORTION	CALS	FAT	SAT FAT	CHOL	PROT	CARB	SUGAR	FIBER	CALCI	SOD	POTAS	FOLIC	VIT C
TUNA HELPER (CONT.)														
Creamy Pasta as prep	1 cup	300	13	4	20	14	31	4	1	80	910	290	40	0
Fettuccine Alfredo 50% Less Fat Recipe as prep	1 cup	240	6	2	15	14	32	6	1	80	870	260	60	0
Fettuccine Alfredo as prep	1 cup	310	14	4	15	14	32	6	1	80	950	260	60	0
Garden Cheddar 50% Less Fat Recipe as prep	1 cup	240	5	2	15	13	36	7	1	100	980	290	80	0
Garden Cheddar as prep	1 cup	290	11	3	20	13	36	7	1	100	1030	280	80	0
Pasta Salad as prep	⅔ cup	380	27	3	10	10	26	4	1	20	730	160	40	0
Pasta Salad Low Fat Recipe as prep	⅔ cup	230	2	0	10	10	26	4	1	20	790	160	40	0
Tetrazzini 50% Less Fat Recipe as prep	1 cup	230	5	2	20	14	34	3	1	60	980	250	100	0
Tetrazzini as prep	1 cup	300	12	4	20	14	34	3	1	60	1040	250	100	0
Tuna Melt as prep	1 cup	300	12	4	20	12	34	9	1	100	900	290	80	0
Tuna Melt Reduced Fat Recipe as prep	1 cup	240	6	2	15	12	34	9	1	100	850	290	80	0
Tuna Pot Pie as prep	1 cup	440	24	7	110	18	40	9	1	150	1080	390	60	0
Tuna Romanoff 50% Less Fat Recipe as prep	1 cup	240	3	1	20	15	38	3	1	40	740	270	60	0
Tuna Romanoff as prep	1 cup	280	8	2	20	15	38	3	1	40	800	270	60	0
READY-TO-EAT														
BUMBLE BEE														
Tuna Salad Fat Free	1 pkg (3.5 oz)	190	2	0	15	9	25	7	0	80	510	—	—	0
Tuna Salad Kit	1 pkg (3.8 oz)	250	13	2	45	17	15	2	0	40	550	—	—	0
STARKIST														
Lunch To-Go	1 pkg	310	13	3	40	22	26	11	tr	40	690	—	—	1
Ready-Mixed Tuna Salad Kit	1 pkg (3.5 oz)	190	6	3	5	9	25	11	2	—	420	—	—	—
Tuna Salad Lunch Kit	1 pkg (4.3 oz)	230	9	2	35	20	17	4	1	—	730	—	—	—
WAMPLER														
Salad	⅓ cup	180	12	—	20	6	9	—	—	—	450	—	—	—
Salad Chunky	⅓ cup	180	13	—	20	8	8	—	—	—	380	—	—	—

FOOD	PORTION	CALS	FAT	SAT FAT	CHOL	PROT	CARB	SUGAR	FIBER	CALCI	SOD	POTAS	FOLIC	VIT C
TAKE-OUT														
tuna salad	3 oz	159	8	1	11	14	8	—	—	15	342	151	6	1
tuna salad	1 cup	383	19	3	27	33	19	—	—	35	824	365	15	5
TURBOT														
european baked	3 oz	104	3	—	—	17	0	—	—	20	163	259	—	—
TURKEY														
(*see also* TURKEY DISHES, TURKEY SUBSTITUTES)														
CANNED														
w/ broth	½ can (2.5 oz)	116	5	1	—	17	0	—	—	9	332	—	—	1
w/ broth	1 can (5 oz)	231	10	3	—	34	0	—	—	17	663	—	—	3
MARY KITCHEN														
Roast Turkey Hash	1 can (14.9 oz)	420	11	3	110	39	42	4	3	40	1800	—	—	2
FRESH														
back w/ skin roasted	½ back (9 oz)	637	38	11	238	70	0	—	—	87	191	682	21	0
breast w/ skin roasted	4 oz	212	8	2	83	32	0	—	—	24	70	323	7	0
dark meat w/ skin roasted	3.6 oz	230	12	4	93	29	0	—	—	34	79	285	9	0
dark meat w/o skin roasted	1 cup (5 oz)	262	10	3	119	40	0	—	—	45	110	406	13	0
dark meat w/o skin roasted	3 oz	170	7	2	78	26	0	—	—	19	72	264	9	0
ground cooked	3 oz	188	11	3	57	20	0	—	—	21	68	222	5	0
leg w/ skin roasted	1 (1.2 lbs)	1133	54	17	466	152	0	—	—	176	420	1530	49	0
leg w/ skin roasted	2.5 oz	147	7	2	61	20	0	—	—	23	55	199	6	0
light meat w/ skin roasted	from ½ turkey (2.3 lbs)	2069	87	25	794	87	0	—	—	225	658	2996	61	0
light meat w/ skin roasted	4.7 oz	268	11	3	103	39	0	—	—	29	85	388	8	0
light meat w/o skin roasted	4 oz	183	4	1	81	35	0	—	—	23	75	356	7	0
neck simmered	1 (5.3 oz)	274	11	4	186	41	0	—	—	56	84	226	12	0
skin roasted	1 oz	141	13	3	36	13	0	—	—	11	17	51	1	0
skin roasted	from ½ turkey (9 oz)	1096	98	26	281	49	0	—	—	87	132	396	10	0
w/ skin roasted	½ turkey (4 lbs)	3857	181	53	1514	522	0	—	—	488	1269	5207	130	0
w/ skin roasted	8.4 oz	498	23	7	196	67	0	—	—	63	164	673	17	0
w/ skin neck & giblets roasted	½ turkey (8.8 lbs)	4123	190	56	1920	190	1	—	—	525	1358	5473	409	1
w/o skin roasted	1 cup (5 oz)	238	7	2	107	41	0	—	—	35	99	418	10	0

FOOD	PORTION	CALS	FAT	SAT FAT	CHOL	PROT	CARB	SUGAR	FIBER	CALCI	SOD	POTAS	FOLIC	VIT C
w/o skin roasted	7.3 oz	354	10	3	159	61	0	—	—	52	147	621	16	0
wing w/ skin roasted	1 (6.5 oz)	426	23	6	150	51	0	—	—	44	114	494	10	0
JENNIE-O														
Ground	4 oz	160	8	3	80	23	0	0	0	40	80	—	—	—
LOUIS RICH														
Ground	4 oz	190	12	4	90	20	0	0	0	20	140	—	—	0
Patties White	1 (4 oz)	170	10	3	65	19	0	0	0	0	440	—	—	0
PERDUE														
Breast Tenderloins Butter Garlic	3 oz	100	1	—	45	20	2	—	—	—	830	—	—	—
Burger Cooked	1 (4 oz)	160	9	3	85	20	0	—	—	60	85	—	—	—
Dark Cooked	3 oz	180	11	4	85	20	0	—	—	40	65	—	—	—
Drumsticks Cooked	1 (2.2 oz)	110	6	2	80	14	0	—	—	—	65	—	—	—
Ground Cooked	3 oz	160	9	3	85	20	0	—	—	—	85	—	—	—
Tenderloins Black Pepper Cooked	3 oz	90	1	—	45	20	1	—	—	—	690	—	—	—
Thighs Cooked	1 (3.2 oz)	240	19	6	115	17	0	—	—	—	65	—	—	—
White Cooked	3 oz	150	7	2	65	22	0	—	—	0	45	—	—	—
SHADY BROOK														
Cutlets	4 oz	110	1	0	60	25	0	0	0	20	240	—	—	—
Drumstick	4 oz	170	9	3	70	22	—	—	—	—	80	—	—	—
Ground	4 oz	160	8	3	80	22	0	0	0	—	85	—	—	—
Ground Breast	4 oz	120	1	0	70	28	0	—	—	—	55	—	—	—
Ground Turkey 85%	4 oz	220	15	5	75	21	—	—	—	—	75	—	—	—
Mesquite Seasoned Tenderloin	4 oz	110	1	0	50	23	—	—	—	—	360	—	—	—
OnlyOne Boneless Breast Roast	4 oz	130	1	0	70	28	—	—	—	—	55	—	—	—
Split Breast	4 oz	190	9	3	70	24	—	—	—	—	60	—	—	—
Tenderloin	4 oz	130	1	0	70	28	—	—	—	—	55	—	—	—
Teriyaki Seasoned Tenderloin	4 oz	120	1	0	50	24	—	—	—	—	460	—	—	—
Thigh	4 oz	220	15	5	75	21	—	—	—	—	75	—	—	—
Turkey Burgers	4 oz	170	9	3	90	20	—	—	—	—	105	—	—	—
Turkey Meatloaf Lean	4 oz	150	7	2	95	18	—	—	—	—	400	—	—	—
Whole Breast	4 oz	190	9	3	70	24	—	—	—	—	60	—	—	—
Whole Turkey	4 oz	180	9	3	75	23	—	—	—	—	75	—	—	—
Wing	4 oz	220	14	4	80	23	—	—	—	—	60	—	—	—

FOOD	PORTION	CALS	FAT	SAT FAT	CHOL	PROT	CARB	SUGAR	FIBER	CALCI	SOD	POTAS	FOLIC	VIT C
SHADY BROOK (CONT.)														
Zesty Lemon Seasoned Tenderloin	4 oz	120	1	0	50	24	—	—	—	—	200	—	—	—
TURKEY STORE														
Lean Ground Italian Style	4 oz	190	10	4	80	20	4	—	—	20	530	—	—	—
WAMPLER														
Boneless Breast Roast	4 oz	160	6	1	35	25	0	—	—	20	25	—	—	—
Breast Half	4 oz	160	6	1	35	25	0	—	—	20	25	—	—	—
Breast Steaks	4 oz	120	1	—	70	28	0	—	—	20	55	—	—	—
Drumsticks	4 oz	180	10	3	75	22	0	—	—	40	45	—	—	—
Ground	4 oz	210	15	3	100	18	0	—	—	100	70	—	—	—
Ground Breast	4 oz	130	1	0	70	28	0	—	—	20	55	—	—	—
Ground Lean	4 oz	160	8	2	90	20	0	—	—	20	70	—	—	—
Thighs	4 oz	170	10	2	80	22	0	—	—	—	40	—	—	—
Wings	4 oz	220	14	4	80	23	0	—	—	20	60	—	—	—
Woodfire Grill Burger	1 (3 oz)	180	9	3	65	21	2	—	—	20	360	—	—	—
FROZEN														
roast boneless seasoned light & dark meat roasted	1 pkg (1.7 lbs)	1213	45	—	413	167	24	—	—	40	5320	2332	—	—
WAMPLER														
Burger BBQ	1 (4 oz)	240	17	—	140	19	3	—	—	—	240	—	—	—
Burgers Cracked Peppercorn & Garlic	1 (3 oz)	170	9	3	65	21	0	—	—	20	380	—	—	—
Seasoned Burgers Cracked Peppercorn & Garlic	1 (3 oz)	170	9	3	65	21	0	—	—	20	380	—	—	—
READY-TO-EAT														
bologna	1 oz	57	4	—	28	4	tr	—	—	24	249	56	—	—
breast	1 slice (0.75 oz)	23	tr	tr	9	5	0	—	—	1	301	58	—	0
diced light & dark seasoned	1 oz	39	2	1	—	5	tr	—	—	0	241	88	—	—
diced light & dark seasoned	½ lb	313	14	4	—	42	2	—	—	2	1928	703	—	—
ham thigh meat	1 pkg (8 oz)	291	12	4	—	43	1	—	—	22	2260	738	—	—
ham thigh meat	2 oz	73	3	1	—	11	tr	—	—	5	565	184	—	—
pastrami	1 pkg (8 oz)	320	14	4	—	42	4	—	—	20	2372	589	—	—
pastrami	2 oz	80	4	1	—	10	1	—	—	5	698	147	—	—

FOOD	PORTION	CALS	FAT	SAT FAT	CHOL	PROT	CARB	SUGAR	FIBER	CALCI	SOD	POTAS	FOLIC	VIT C
patties battered & fried	1 (2.3 oz)	181	12	—	—	9	10	—	—	9	512	176	—	—
patties battered & fried	1 (3.3 oz)	266	17	—	—	13	15	—	—	13	752	259	—	—
patties breaded & fried	1 (3.3 oz)	266	17	—	—	13	15	—	—	13	752	259	—	—
patties breaded & fried	1 (2.3 oz)	181	12	—	—	9	10	—	—	9	512	176	—	—
poultry salad sandwich spread	1 oz	238	4	1	9	4	2	—	—	3	107	52	1	0
poultry salad sandwich spread	1 tbsp	109	2	tr	4	2	1	—	—	1	49	24	1	0
prebasted breast w/ skin roasted	½ breast (1.9 lbs)	1087	30	8	359	191	0	—	—	75	3434	2141	—	0
prebasted breast w/ skin roasted	1 breast (3.8 lbs)	2175	60	17	718	383	0	—	—	149	6868	4281	—	0
prebasted thigh w/ skin roasted	1 thigh (11 oz)	494	27	8	194	59	0	—	—	25	1371	758	—	—
roll light & dark meat	1 oz	42	2	1	16	5	1	—	—	9	166	77	—	—
roll light meat	1 oz	42	2	1	12	5	2	—	—	11	139	71	—	—
salami cooked	2 oz	111	8	—	46	9	tr	—	—	11	569	138	—	—
salami cooked	1 pkg (8 oz)	446	31	—	186	37	1	—	—	44	2278	553	—	—
turkey loaf breast meat	1 pkg (6 oz)	187	3	1	69	38	0	—	—	12	2433	473	—	0
turkey loaf breast meat	2 slices (1.5 oz)	47	1	tr	17	10	0	—	—	3	608	118	—	0
turkey sticks battered & fried	1 stick (2.3 oz)	178	11	—	—	9	11	—	—	9	536	166	—	—
turkey sticks breaded & fried	1 stick (2.3 oz)	178	11	—	—	9	11	—	—	9	536	166	—	—
ALPINE LACE														
Breast Fat Free	2 oz	45	0	0	25	10	0	0	0	—	350	—	—	
BOAR'S HEAD														
Breast Cracked Pepper Smoked	2 oz	60	1	0	30	13	1	0	0	0	460	—	—	0
Breast Golden Skin On	2 oz	60	2	1	25	11	0	0	0	0	340	—	—	0
Breast Golden Skinless	2 oz	60	1	0	25	12	tr	0	0	0	350	—	—	0
Breast Hickory Smoked	2 oz	70	2	1	25	12	tr	0	0	0	340	—	—	0
Breast Low Sodium Skinless	2 oz	60	1	0	25	12	tr	0	0	0	340	—	—	0

FOOD	PORTION	CALS	FAT	SAT FAT	CHOL	PROT	CARB	SUGAR	FIBER	CALCI	SOD	POTAS	FOLIC	VIT C
BOAR'S HEAD (CONT.)														
Breast Lower Sodium Skin On	2 oz	60	2	1	25	11	tr	0	0	0	310	—	—	0
Breast Maple Glazed Honey Coat	2 oz	70	1	0	30	14	2	2	0	0	440	—	—	0
Breast Ovengold Skin On	2 oz	60	2	0	35	12	1	0	0	0	360	—	—	0
Breast Ovengold Skinless	2 oz	60	1	0	20	13	0	0	0	0	350	—	—	0
Breast Roasted Mesquite Smoked Skinless	2 oz	60	1	0	25	13	0	0	0	0	440	—	—	0
Breast Roasted Salsalito	2 oz	60	1	0	25	13	1	0	0	0	460	—	—	0
Pastrami Seasoned	2 oz	60	1	0	25	13	1	0	0	0	440	—	—	0
CARL BUDDIG														
Honey Roasted Turkey Breast	1 pkg (2.5 oz)	120	7	3	40	12	3	3	—	—	780	—	—	—
Lean Slices Honey Roasted Breast	1 pkg (2.5 oz)	70	1	1	30	13	4	4	—	—	980	—	—	—
Lean Slices Oven Roasted Breast	1 pkg (2.5 oz)	70	1	1	30	15	1	1	—	—	980	—	—	—
Lean Slices Smoked Breast	1 pkg (2.5 oz)	70	1	1	30	15	1	1	—	—	880	—	—	—
Oven Roasted Breast	1 pkg (2.5 oz)	110	7	3	40	12	1	1	—	—	780	—	—	—
Smoked Breast	1 pkg (2.5 oz)	110	7	3	40	12	1	1	—	—	780	—	—	—
Turkey Ham	1 pkg (2.5 oz)	100	5	2	40	13	1	1	—	—	1020	—	—	—
HEALTHY CHOICE														
Smoked Breast	4 slices (1.8 oz)	60	2	1	25	9	2	0	0	0	450	—	—	0
HORMEL														
Light & Lean 97 Breast Sliced	1 slice (1 oz)	30	1	0	15	5	0	0	0	0	380	—	—	0
Light & Lean 97 Mesquite Smoked Breast	1 slice (1 oz)	30	1	0	15	5	0	0	0	0	370	—	—	0
Turkey Pepperoni	17 slices (1 oz)	80	4	2	40	9	0	0	0	0	550	—	—	0
JENNIE-O														
Turkey Breast Golden Roast	3 oz	100	3	1	35	19	2	—	—	—	740	—	—	—
JORDAN'S														
Fat Free Turkey Breast	1 slice (1 oz)	25	0	0	10	5	1	—	—	—	250	—	—	—
LOUIS RICH														
Bologna	1 slice (28 g)	50	4	1	20	3	1	0	0	40	270	—	—	0
Breaded Nuggets	4 (3.2 oz)	260	16	3	35	13	15	0	0	0	640	—	—	0

FOOD	PORTION	CALS	FAT	SAT FAT	CHOL	PROT	CARB	SUGAR	FIBER	CALCI	SOD	POTAS	FOLIC	VIT C
LOUIS RICH (CONT.)														
Breaded Patties	1 (3 oz)	220	13	3	35	12	13	0	0	0	530	—	—	0
Breaded Sticks	3 (3 oz)	230	15	3	35	12	12	0	0	0	580	—	—	0
Breast Skinless Hickory Smoked	2 oz	50	0	0	25	11	1	0	0	0	720	—	—	0
Breast Skinless Honey Roasted	2 oz	60	0	0	20	11	3	2	0	0	660	—	—	0
Breast Skinless Oven Roasted	2 oz	50	0	0	20	11	1	0	0	0	660	—	—	0
Breast Skinless Rotisserie	2 oz	50	0	0	20	11	1	1	0	0	670	—	—	0
Breast Slices Hickory Smoked	1 slice (2 oz)	50	0	0	25	11	1	0	0	0	720	—	—	0
Breast Slices Honey Roasted	1 slice (2 oz)	60	0	0	20	11	3	2	0	0	660	—	—	0
Breast Slices Oven Roasted	1 slice (2 oz)	50	0	0	20	11	1	0	0	0	660	—	—	0
Breast Slices Rotisserie	1 slice (2 oz)	50	0	0	20	11	1	1	0	0	670	—	—	0
Carving Board Hickory Smoked	2 slices (1.6 oz)	40	1	0	20	9	0	0	0	0	540	—	—	0
Carving Board Oven Roasted Thin	6 slices (2.1 oz)	60	1	0	25	12	1	0	0	0	710	—	—	0
Carving Board Oven Roasted Traditional	2 slices (1.6 oz)	40	1	0	20	9	0	0	0	0	540	—	—	0
Carving Board Rotisserie	2 slices (1.6 oz)	40	1	0	20	9	0	0	0	0	460	—	—	0
Cotto Salami	1 slice (28 g)	40	3	1	25	4	0	0	0	0	280	—	—	0
Deli-Thin Oven Roasted	4 slices (1.8 oz)	50	1	0	20	9	2	0	0	0	580	—	—	0
Deli-Thin Smoked	4 slices (1.8 oz)	50	2	1	20	9	1	tr	0	0	480	—	—	0
Fat Free Hickory Smoked Breast	1 slice (1 oz)	25	0	0	10	4	1	0	0	0	300	—	—	0
Fat Free Oven Roasted Breast	1 slice (1 oz)	25	0	0	10	4	1	tr	0	0	330	—	—	0
Fat Free Oven Roasted Deli-Thin Breast	4 slices (1.8 oz)	45	0	0	15	8	2	tr	0	0	620	—	—	0
Fat Free Turkey Ham Honey	2 slices (1.7 oz)	35	0	0	15	7	2	1	0	0	600	—	—	0
Fat Free Turkey Ham Smoked	2 slices (1.7 oz)	35	0	0	15	7	1	tr	0	0	580	—	—	0
Hickory Smoked	1 slice (1 oz)	30	1	0	10	5	1	0	0	0	260	—	—	0
Oven Roasted	1 slice (1 oz)	30	1	0	10	5	1	0	0	0	310	—	—	0
Pastrami	1 slice (1 oz)	30	1	0	20	5	1	0	0	0	380	—	—	0
Smoked	1 slice (1 oz)	30	1	0	15	5	0	0	0	0	280	—	—	0

FOOD	PORTION	CALS	FAT	SAT FAT	CHOL	PROT	CARB	SUGAR	FIBER	CALCI	SOD	POTAS	FOLIC	VIT C
LOUIS RICH (CONT.)														
Turkey Ham	1 slice (1 oz)	30	1	0	20	5	1	0	0	0	380	—	—	0
Turkey Ham Chopped	1 slice (1 oz)	45	3	1	20	5	1	0	0	0	350	—	—	0
Turkey Ham Honey Cured	1 slice (1 oz)	30	1	0	20	5	1	tr	0	0	350	—	—	0
OSCAR MAYER														
Lunchables Turkey Bagels	1 pkg	420	10	4	35	16	54	27	2	250	830	—	—	60
Smoked White	3 slices (3 oz)	90	3	1	30	12	2	tr	—	—	950	—	—	—
Smoked White Turkey	3 slices (3 oz)	90	3	1	30	12	2	tr	—	—	950	—	—	—
Turkey Bologna	3 slices (3 oz)	160	12	3	55	10	4	1	—	100	810	—	—	—
Turkey Cotto Salami	3 slices (3 oz)	130	8	3	65	13	tr	tr	—	20	850	—	—	—
PERDUE														
Breast Sliced Cajun Style	2 oz	50	1	—	20	9	1	—	—	—	800	—	—	—
Breast Sliced Honey Smoked	2 oz	50	0	—	20	10	2	2	—	—	510	—	—	—
Breast Sliced Pan Roasted	2 oz	70	2	1	30	14	0	—	—	—	390	—	—	—
Ham Hickory Smoked	2 oz	60	3	1	40	9	1	—	—	—	770	—	—	—
Healthsense Breast Sliced Oven Roasted	2 oz	60	0	—	20	10	3	1	—	—	290	—	—	—
Pastrami Hickory Smoked	2 oz	70	3	1	40	9	2	—	—	—	670	—	—	—
SHADY BROOK														
Black Forest Turkey Ham	2 oz	70	3	1	30	10	—	—	—	—	470	—	—	—
Browned Homestyle Oven Roasted Breast	2 oz	60	1	0	20	11	—	—	—	—	400	—	—	—
Browned Slow Roasted Breast	2 oz	60	0	0	20	11	—	—	—	—	400	—	—	—
Carved Breast Italian Seasoned	2 oz	60	0	0	20	12	—	—	—	—	490	—	—	—
Carved Breast Natural Roast	2 oz	60	0	0	20	12	—	—	—	—	470	—	—	—
Carved Breast Peppered	2 oz	60	0	0	20	12	—	—	—	—	450	—	—	—
Hickory Smoked Breast	2 oz	50	0	0	25	11	—	—	—	—	470	—	—	—
Honey Roasted Breast	2 oz	60	1	0	30	11	—	—	—	—	400	—	—	—

FOOD	PORTION	CALS	FAT	SAT FAT	CHOL	PROT	CARB	SUGAR	FIBER	CALCI	SOD	POTAS	FOLIC	VIT C
SHADY BROOK (CONT.)														
Honey Roasted Breast Covered w/ Cracked Pepper	2 oz	60	0	0	25	11	—	—	—	—	470	—	—	—
Meatballs Italian Style	3 (3 oz)	130	7	3	45	12	5	1	1	80	350	—	—	—
Smoked Drumstick	3 oz	180	8	3	70	22	—	—	—	—	620	—	—	—
Smoked Neck	3 oz	150	6	2	65	22	—	—	—	—	700	—	—	—
Smoked Whole Turkey	3 oz	150	4	2	60	24	—	—	—	—	660	—	—	—
Smoked Wing	3 oz	200	10	3	65	22	—	—	—	—	680	—	—	—
WAMPLER														
Bologna	2 oz	130	11	—	50	8	1	—	—	—	550	—	—	—
Dark Cured	2 oz	80	5	—	30	8	2	—	—	—	600	—	—	—
Deli Roast Breast	2 oz	50	1	—	25	12	0	—	—	—	250	—	—	—
Deli Roast Classic Spiced Breast	2 oz	70	1	—	25	16	1	—	—	—	380	—	—	—
Deli Roast Pan Roasted Breast	2 oz	70	2	—	20	13	1	—	—	—	400	—	—	—
Deli Roast Pan Roasted Skinless Breast	2 oz	50	0	—	20	12	1	—	—	—	400	—	—	—
Deli Roast Peppered Breast	2 oz	40	0	—	20	8	1	—	—	—	520	—	—	—
Deli Roast Rotisserie Breast	2 oz	50	2	—	20	9	1	—	—	—	500	—	—	—
Pastrami	2 oz	90	5	—	40	9	1	—	—	—	220	—	—	—
Salami	2 oz	90	6	—	55	9	1	—	—	—	560	—	—	—
Turkey Ham	2 oz	60	3	—	40	10	0	—	—	—	590	—	—	—
TURKEY DISHES														
CANNED														
DINTY MOORE														
Microwave Cup Stew	1 pkg (7.5 oz)	130	3	1	10	9	16	3	2	20	760	—	—	4
Stew	1 cup (8.5 oz)	140	3	1	20	10	19	3	2	20	910	—	—	2
FROZEN														
gravy & turkey	1 cup (8.4 oz)	160	6	2	—	14	11	—	—	33	1328	—	—	—
gravy & turkey	1 pkg (5 oz)	95	4	1	—	8	7	—	—	20	786	—	—	—
BANQUET														
Homestyle Gravy & Sliced Turkey	2 slices + gravy	130	9	3	45	8	3	1	1	20	550	—	—	0
Sandwich Toppers Gravy & Sliced Turkey	1 pkg (5 oz)	160	11	4	30	8	6	1	0	20	670	—	—	0

FOOD	PORTION	CALS	FAT	SAT FAT	CHOL	PROT	CARB	SUGAR	FIBER	CALCI	SOD	POTAS	FOLIC	VIT C
READY-TO-EAT														
JENNIE-O														
Stuffed Breast Cheddar Cheese & Broccoli	1 serv (6 oz)	240	9	5	85	36	3	1	0	150	1350	—	—	9
Stuffed Turkey Breast Pepper Cheese & Rice	1 piece (6 oz)	250	7	4	70	32	13	1	0	150	1290	—	—	1
Turkey Breast Roast In Homestyle Gravy	1 serv (5 oz)	110	1	0	40	20	3	1	0	20	680	—	—	1
MOSEY'S														
Turkey Breast w/ Gravy	1 serv (5 oz)	140	1	0	90	30	4	0	0	20	540	—	—	1
SHADY BROOK														
Meatloaf	1 serv (16 oz)	470	17	10	175	38	—	—	—	—	900	—	—	—
WAMPLER														
Turkey Ham Salad	⅓ cup	150	10	—	30	7	9	—	—	—	500	—	—	—
TAKE-OUT														
boneless breast w/ cranberry apple stuffing	1 serv (5 oz)	260	9	2	80	32	10	2	1	30	250	—	—	1

TURKEY SUBSTITUTES

FOOD	PORTION	CALS	FAT	SAT FAT	CHOL	PROT	CARB	SUGAR	FIBER	CALCI	SOD	POTAS	FOLIC	VIT C
LIGHTLIFE														
Smart Deli Turkey	3 slices (1.5 oz)	40	0	0	0	9	1	0	0	—	290	—	—	—
TOFURKEY														
Deli Slices Hickory	1.5 oz	120	2	0	0	13	14	0	2	20	286	—	—	0
Deli Slices Original	1.5 oz	120	2	0	0	13	14	0	2	20	286	—	—	0
Deli Slices Peppered	1.5 oz	120	2	0	0	13	14	0	2	20	286	—	—	0
Drummettes	1 (3 oz)	105	2	1	0	11	11	2	4	20	380	—	—	0
Giblet Gravy	1 serv (3.5 oz)	42	2	0	0	4	5	2	1	20	340	—	—	0
Stuffed Tofu Roast	1 serv (4 oz)	193	5	0	0	26	10	1	2	150	310	—	—	0
WORTHINGTON														
Smoked Turkey Meatless	3 slices (2 oz)	140	10	2	0	10	3	tr	2	0	620	70	—	0
Turkee Slices	3 slices (3.3 oz)	130	14	3	0	13	3	tr	2	0	580	45	—	0
YVES														
Veggie Turkey Deli Slices	1 serv (2.2 oz)	85	0	0	0	18	4	2	1	40	480	169	—	1

TURMERIC

FOOD	PORTION	CALS	FAT	SAT FAT	CHOL	PROT	CARB	SUGAR	FIBER	CALCI	SOD	POTAS	FOLIC	VIT C
ground	1 tsp	8	tr	—	0	tr	1	—	—	4	1	56	—	1

FOOD	PORTION	CALS	FAT	SAT FAT	CHOL	PROT	CARB	SUGAR	FIBER	CALCI	SOD	POTAS	FOLIC	VIT C
TURNIPS														
canned greens	½ cup	17	tr	tr	0	2	3	—	—	138	325	165	48	18
cooked mashed	½ cup (4.2 oz)	47	tr	tr	0	2	10	—	—	58	25	391	19	23
cubed cooked	½ cup (3 oz)	33	tr	tr	0	1	7	—	—	41	17	277	13	17
frzn greens cooked	½ cup	24	tr	tr	0	3	4	—	2	125	12	184	32	18
greens chopped cooked	½ cup	15	tr	tr	0	1	3	—	2	99	21	146	85	20
greens raw chopped	½ cup	7	tr	tr	0	tr	2	—	1	53	11	83	54	17
raw cubed	½ cup (2.4 oz)	25	tr	tr	0	1	6	—	—	39	14	236	14	18
BIRDS EYE														
Greens w/ Diced Turnip	1 cup	25	0	0	0	2	2	1	2	60	20	—	—	12
TURTLE														
raw	3.5 oz	85	1			18	0	—	—	107	—	235	—	—
TUSK FISH														
raw	3.5 oz	79	tr	—	—	17	0	—	—	17	113	328	tr	—
VANILLA														
STEEL'S														
Sugar Free	1 tbsp	24	0	0	0	0	6	0	0	—	0	—	—	—
VIRGINIA DARE														
Extract	1 tsp	10	0	—	0	—	—	—	—	0	—	—	—	—
VEAL														
(*see also* VEAL DISHES)														
cutlet lean only braised	3 oz	172	4	2	115	31	0	—	—	7	57	329	15	—
cutlet lean only fried	3 oz	156	4	1	91	28	0	—	—	6	65	375	14	—
ground broiled	3 oz	146	6	3	87	21	0	—	—	14	70	287	10	—
loin chop w/ bone lean & fat braised	1 chop (2.8 oz)	227	14	5	94	24	0	—	—	22	64	224	11	—
loin chop w/ bone lean only braised	1 chop (2.4 oz)	155	6	2	86	23	0	—	—	22	58	205	10	—
shoulder w/ bone lean only braised	3 oz	169	5	1	110	29	0	—	—	31	83	271	14	—
sirloin w/ bone lean & fat roasted	3 oz	171	9	4	87	21	0	—	—	11	71	299	13	—
sirloin w/ bone lean only roasted	3 oz	143	5	2	89	22	0	—	—	12	72	310	13	—
VEAL DISHES														
TAKE-OUT														
parmigiana	4.2 oz	279	18	10	136	22	6	—	2	137	545	531	11	15
scallopini	1 serv (8 oz)	608	146	13	46	—	—	—	—	—	900	—	—	—

FOOD	PORTION	CALS	FAT	SAT FAT	CHOL	PROT	CARB	SUGAR	FIBER	CALCI	SOD	POTAS	FOLIC	VIT C
VEGETABLE JUICE														
vegetable juice cocktail	6 fl oz	34	tr	tr	0	1	8	—	—	20	664	351	—	50
vegetable juice cocktail	½ cup	22	tr	tr	0	1	6	—	—	13	442	234	—	34
DOLE														
Vegetable Blend	1 bottle (12 oz)	90	0	0	0	4	19	—	2	40	820	1070	—	120
HUNT'S														
Cocktail	1 can (6 oz)	20	0	0	0	2	7	3	2	2	630	—	—	48
MUIR GLEN														
Organic	5.5 oz	50	0	0	0	1	10	7	2	80	420	—	—	48
V8														
Lightly Tangy	8 oz	58	1	0	—	2	11	9	2	39	345	615	—	112
Low Sodium	8 oz	53	tr	tr	—	2	11	8	2	41	95	659	—	68
Original	8 oz	51	1	0	—	2	10	8	2	36	615	542	—	98
Picante Vegetable	8 oz	51	tr	0	—	2	10	7	2	39	673	535	—	84
Spicy Hot	8 oz	49	tr	0	—	2	10	7	2	36	780	518	—	48
Splash Tropical Blend	8 fl oz	120	0	0	0	0	30	27	—	—	20	—	—	60
VEGETABLES MIXED														
CANNED														
mixed vegetables	½ cup	39	tr	tr	0	2	8	—	—	22	122	239	19	4
peas & carrots	½ cup	48	tr	tr	0	3	11	—	—	29	332	128	24	8
peas & carrots low sodium	½ cup	48	tr	tr	0	3	11	—	—	29	332	128	24	8
peas & onions	½ cup	30	tr	tr	0	2	5	—	—	10	265	57	—	2
succotash	½ cup	102	1	tr	0	4	23	—	—	15	325	243	59	9
CHI-CHI'S														
Diced Tomatoes & Green Chilies	¼ cup (2.5 oz)	20	0	0	0	0	4	3	0	20	340	—	—	1
CHUN KING														
Chow Mein Vegetables	⅔ cup (3 oz)	14	tr	0	0	1	3	0	1	50	323	—	—	6
DEL MONTE														
Mixed	½ cup (4.4 oz)	40	0	0	0	2	8	3	2	20	360	—	—	2
Mixed No Salt Added	½ cup (4.4 oz)	40	0	0	0	2	8	3	2	20	25	—	—	2
Peas And Carrots	½ cup (4.5 oz)	60	0	0	0	2	11	4	2	20	360	—	—	4
GREEN GIANT														
Garden Medley	½ cup (4.2 oz)	40	0	0	0	1	9	3	2	0	360	—	—	0
Mixed	½ cup (4.3 oz)	60	0	0	0	2	12	4	2	0	460	—	—	5
Sweet Peas & Carrots	½ cup (4.3 oz)	50	0	0	0	2	11	4	3	0	410	—	—	5
Sweet Peas & Tiny Pearl Onion	½ cup (4.4 oz)	60	0	0	0	4	11	3	4	20	520	—	—	6

FOOD	PORTION	CALS	FAT	SAT FAT	CHOL	PROT	CARB	SUGAR	FIBER	CALCI	SOD	POTAS	FOLIC	VIT C
HOUSE OF TSANG														
Vegetables & Sauce Cantonese Classic	½ cup (4.2 oz)	70	1	0	0	1	14	8	1	0	960	—	—	0
Vegetables & Sauce Hong Kong Sweet & Sour	½ cup (4.5 oz)	160	0	0	0	0	40	35	0	0	580	—	—	1
Vegetables & Sauce Szechuan Hot & Spicy	½ cup (4.2 oz)	70	1	0	0	1	14	8	1	20	1130	—	—	1
Vegetables & Sauce Tokyo Teriyaki	½ cup (4.4 oz)	100	0	0	0	1	23	19	1	20	1240	—	—	1
LA CHOY														
Chop Suey Vegetables	½ cup (2.2 oz)	10	tr	0	0	1	2	0	1	37	241	—	—	4
LESUEUR														
Early Peas w/ Mushrooms & Pearl Onions	½ cup (4.3 oz)	60	0	0	0	3	11	4	2	20	380	—	—	9
S&W														
Mixed	½ cup (4.4 oz)	35	0	0	0	1	7	3	2	20	370	—	—	4
Peas & Carrots	½ cup (4.5 oz)	60	0	0	0	2	11	4	2	20	360	—	—	4
Peas & Onions	½ cup (4.3 oz)	40	0	0	0	3	11	1	3	0	530	—	—	9
VEG-ALL														
Cajun Mixed	½ cup	50	0	0	0	2	10	2	3	20	410	—	—	1
FROZEN														
mixed vegetables cooked	½ cup	54	tr	tr	0	3	12	—	2	22	32	154	17	3
peas & carrots cooked	½ cup	38	tr	tr	0	3	8	—	—	18	55	127	21	7
peas & onions cooked	½ cup	40	tr	tr	0	2	8	—	—	13	—	—	—	6
succotash cooked	½ cup	79	1	tr	0	4	17	—	—	13	38	225	28	5
BIRDS EYE														
Baby Sweet Peas & Pearl Onions	⅔ cup	60	1	0	0	4	12	6	4	0	85	—	—	9
Bavarian Vegetables	1 cup (5.5 oz)	150	8	4	30	5	15	3	3	60	460	0	—	1
Broccoli Cauliflower & Carrots	½ cup	25	0	0	0	2	5	3	2	20	30	—	—	42
Broccoli Cauliflower & Carrots In Cheese Sauce	½ cup	70	4	1	5	3	7	3	2	60	460	—	—	18
Broccoli Cauliflower & Red Peppers	½ cup	20	0	0	0	2	5	3	2	20	20	—	—	54

FOOD	PORTION	CALS	FAT	SAT FAT	CHOL	PROT	CARB	SUGAR	FIBER	CALCI	SOD	POTAS	FOLIC	VIT C
BIRDS EYE (CONT.)														
Broccoli & Cauliflower	½ cup	20	0	0	0	2	4	2	2	20	20	—	—	54
Broccoli Carrots & Water Chestnuts	½ cup	30	0	0	0	2	7	3	3	20	30	—	—	30
Broccoli Corn & Red Peppers	½ cup	50	0	0	0	3	12	3	3	20	15	—	—	36
Broccoli Red Peppers Onions & Mushrooms	½ cup	25	0	0	0	2	5	3	2	20	20	—	—	48
Brussels Sprouts Cauliflower & Carrots	½ cup	30	0	0	0	2	7	3	3	20	20	—	—	42
California Style Vegetables	½ cup	100	5	2	10	3	9	4	3	20	240	—	—	6
Cauliflower Nuggets Corn Carrots & Snow Peaspods	½ cup	30	0	0	0	2	6	3	2	20	25	—	—	24
Gumbo Blend	¾ cup	40	0	0	0	2	10	3	2	40	30	—	—	2
Italian Style Vegetables & Bow Tie Pasta	1 cup	150	9	3	10	3	13	3	2	40	380	—	—	18
Mixed Vegetables	⅓ cup	50	0	0	0	—	—	—	3	0	35	—	—	6
New England Style Vegetables & Pasta Shells	1 pkg (9 oz)	260	14	5	15	6	29	6	3	—	480	—	—	—
Oriental Style Vegetables	½ cup	60	4	2	10	2	4	3	2	20	260	—	—	18
Peas & Pearl Onions	⅔ cup	90	1	0	0	5	18	9	5	0	520	—	—	12
Peas & Potatoes In Real Cream Sauce	½ cup	90	3	1	10	4	13	5	2	60	350	—	—	6
Radiatore Pasta & Vegetables	1 cup	200	8	2	5	6	27	5	1	60	430	—	—	9
Roasted Potatoes & Broccoli	⅔ cup (3.9 oz)	100	4	1	5	3	15	2	1	40	470	—	—	18
Roletti Pasta & Vegetables	1 cup (4.4 oz)	190	8	2	5	5	11	5	1	40	350	—	—	9
Simply Grillin' Garden Herb	1 cup	140	6	1	0	3	19	6	4	40	490	—	—	24
Stir Fry Asparagus	2 cups	90	1	0	0	5	16	4	3	40	35	—	—	21
Stir Fry Broccoli	1 cup	30	0	0	0	2	5	3	2	0	30	—	—	21
Stir Fry Pepper	1 cup	25	0	0	0	1	5	4	2	0	15	—	—	15
Stir Fry Sugar Snap	¾ cup	35	0	0	0	1	5	3	1	0	20	—	—	1

FOOD	PORTION	CALS	FAT	SAT FAT	CHOL	PROT	CARB	SUGAR	FIBER	CALCI	SOD	POTAS	FOLIC	VIT C
BIRDS EYE (CONT.)														
Stir Fry Whole Green Bean	1¾ cups	100	1	0	0	4	19	4	2	20	25	—	—	18
Stir Fry Style Vegetables	½ cup	60	4	2	10	2	5	4	1	0	270	—	—	9
Vegetables For Soup	⅔ cup	45	0	0	0	—	—	—	2	0	45	—	—	2
Vegetables For Stew	⅔ cup	40	0	0	0	1	9	2	1	0	40	—	—	1
Voilà! Italian Pesto Chicken	2 cups	240	9	3	25	15	24	5	1	100	690	—	—	12
Voilà! Three Cheese Chicken	1¾ cups	220	8	3	20	14	24	6	1	100	570	—	—	15
FRESH LIKE														
California Blend	3.5 oz	31	tr	—	—	2	7	—	1	38	21	206	—	40
Midwestern Blend	3.5 oz	42	tr	—	—	2	9	—	1	33	32	224	—	32
Mixed	3.5 oz	69	tr	—	—	30	14	—	1	24	48	212	—	10
Oriental Blend	3.5 oz	26	tr	—	—	3	5	—	1	43	11	214	—	55
Winter Blend	3.5 oz	26	tr	—	—	3	5	—	1	43	26	214	—	55
GREEN GIANT														
Alfredo Vegetables	¾ cup	70	2	1	5	4	8	3	2	80	360	—	—	12
American Mixtures Broccoli Carrots Cauliflower	¾ cup (2.6 oz)	25	0	0	0	1	5	2	2	20	30	—	—	15
American Mixtures Broccoli Carrots Waterchestnuts	¾ cup (3 oz)	30	0	0	0	1	6	2	3	20	30	—	—	15
American Mixtures Cauliflower Broccoli Sugar Snap & Sweet Pea	¾ cup (2.8 oz)	35	0	0	0	2	7	2	3	20	45	—	—	12
American Mixtures Corn Broccoli Red Pepper	¾ cup (3.1 oz)	60	0	0	0	2	13	3	2	0	10	—	—	12
American Mixtures Green Beans Potatoes Onions Red Peppers	¾ cup (2.8 oz)	45	1	0	0	1	8	2	2	20	15	—	—	6
American Mixtures Sweet Peas Potatoes Carrots	⅔ cup (3 oz)	70	2	0	0	2	12	2	3	0	70	—	—	6
Butter Sauce Broccoli Cauliflower Carrots Corn Sweet Peas	¾ cup (3.6 oz)	60	2	2	<5	2	8	3	2	20	300	—	—	18

FOOD	PORTION	CALS	FAT	SAT FAT	CHOL	PROT	CARB	SUGAR	FIBER	CALCI	SOD	POTAS	FOLIC	VIT C
GREEN GIANT (CONT.)														
Butter Sauce Broccoli Pasta Sweet Peas Corn Red Peppers	¾ cup (3.5 oz)	70	2	2	<5	3	11	3	2	20	280	—	—	21
Butter Sauce Mixed	¾ cup (3.6 oz)	70	2	1	<5	2	11	3	3	20	240	—	—	2
Cheese Sauce Broccoli Cauliflower Carrots	1 cup (4.1 oz)	60	3	1	5	3	7	3	2	40	460	—	—	18
Harvest Fresh Broccoli Cauliflower Carrots	1 cup (3.4 oz)	30	0	0	0	2	5	2	3	20	125	—	—	24
Harvest Fresh Mixed Vegetables	⅔ cup (3.1 oz)	50	0	0	0	2	10	3	3	0	125	—	—	5
Harvest Fresh Sweet Peas & Pearl Onions	½ cup (2.7 oz)	55	0	0	0	3	10	2	3	0	170	—	—	9
Mixed	¾ cup (2.9 oz)	50	0	0	0	2	11	1	3	20	35	—	—	6
Seasoned Broccoli & Carrots w/ Garlic & Herbs	½ cup	45	1	0	0	2	8	2	3	40	200	—	—	30
Select Sweet Peas & Pearl Onions	⅔ cup (3.1 oz)	60	0	0	0	4	12	2	4	20	125	—	—	12
HEALTH IS WEALTH														
Veggie Munchees	2 (1 oz)	50	1	0	0	2	9	0	1	0	170	—	—	2
LA CHOY														
Fancy Chinese Mixed Vegetables	½ cup (2.9 oz)	9	tr	0	0	1	1	0	1	18	31	—	—	7
MCKENZIE'S														
Gumbo Mixture	1 serv (2.9 oz)	35	0	0	0	1	8	3	2	—	30	—	—	—
TREE OF LIFE														
Mixed	½ cup (3 oz)	65	0	0	0	3	13	3	3	20	60	—	—	6
SHELF-STABLE														
TASTYBITE														
Curry Bangkok Red	½ pkg (5.3 oz)	88	6	5	0	2	7	0	1	60	825	—	—	0
Curry Patong Yellow	½ pkg (5.3 oz)	118	7	6	0	2	12	0	1	40	489	—	—	0
Curry Siam Green	½ pkg (5.3 oz)	63	3	3	0	2	6	0	1	40	522	—	—	0
Jaipur Vegetables	½ pkg (5 oz)	220	15	4	25	9	13	3	7	90	680	—	—	0
Malabar Mixed	½ pkg (5 oz)	67	1	1	0	1	15	1	1	120	475	—	—	8
TAKE-OUT														
buddha's delight	1 serv (16 oz)	174	5	1	35	17	17	8	3	109	1368	668	161	64
caponata	¼ cup	28	1	—	0	—	—	—	—	16	—	—	—	—

FOOD	PORTION	CALS	FAT	SAT FAT	CHOL	PROT	CARB	SUGAR	FIBER	CALCI	SOD	POTAS	FOLIC	VIT C
curry	1 serv (7.7 oz)	398	33	—	—	4	22	—	—	86	—	—	—	26
gyoza potstickers vegetable	8 (4.9 oz)	210	4	1	0	8	34	7	5	40	500	—	—	0
pakoras	1 (2 oz)	108	5	—	—	5	12	—	3	56	—	—	—	3
ratatouille	1 serv (3.5 oz)	96	7	1	0	2	7	7	4	32	812	468	36	50
samosas	2 (4 oz)	519	46	—	—	3	25	—	3	35	—	—	—	4
succotash	½ cup	111	1	tr	0	5	23	—	—	16	16	393	—	8
tapenade grilled vegetables	¼ cup	40	3	0	0	0	4	2	tr	0	150	—	—	19

VENISON

roasted	3 oz	134	3	1	95	26	0	—	—	6	46	285	—	—

VINEGAR

FOOD	PORTION	CALS	FAT	SAT FAT	CHOL	PROT	CARB	SUGAR	FIBER	CALCI	SOD	POTAS	FOLIC	VIT C
balsamic	1 tbsp (0.5 oz)	5	0	0	0	0	2	2	—	0	0	—	—	0
cider	1 tbsp	tr	0	0	0	tr	1	—	—	1	tr	15	—	0
EDEN														
Organic Brown Rice	1 tbsp	2	0	0	0	0	0	0	0	0	0	0	0	0
Ume Plum	1 tsp	2	0	0	0	0	0	0	0	0	1050	18	—	0
HEINZ														
White	1 tbsp	2	0	0	0	0	0	0	0	—	0	—	—	—
PROGRESSO														
Balsamic	2 tbsp (0.5 oz)	10	0	0	0	0	2	2	0	0	0	—	—	0
VICTORIA														
Balsamic	1 tbsp (0.5 oz)	5	0	0	0	0	2	2	—	0	0	—	—	0
WHITE HOUSE														
Apple Cider	1 tbsp (0.5 oz)	0	0	0	0	0	0	0	0	—	0	—	—	—
White	1 tbsp (0.5 oz)	0	0	0	0	0	0	0	—	—	0	—	—	—
WILD THYME FARMS														
Balsamic Red Raspberry	1 tbsp	13	0	0	0	0	3	3	—	—	0	—	—	—

WAFFLES

FOOD	PORTION	CALS	FAT	SAT FAT	CHOL	PROT	CARB	SUGAR	FIBER	CALCI	SOD	POTAS	FOLIC	VIT C
FROZEN														
buttermilk	1 (4 in sq)	88	3	tr	—	2	14	—	1	77	262	43	17	0
plain (1.2 oz)	1 4 in sq (1.2 oz)	88	3	tr	—	2	14	—	1	77	262	43	17	0
EGGO														
Apple Cinnamon	2 (2.7 oz)	220	8	2	20	5	33	5	1	40	450	40	40	0
Banana Bread	2 (2.7 oz)	200	7	1	0	5	32	5	2	40	280	140	40	0
Blueberry	2 (2.7 oz)	220	9	2	20	5	32	6	1	40	460	40	40	0
Buttermilk	2 (2.7 oz)	220	8	2	25	5	31	3	1	40	460	90	40	0
Golden Oat	2 (2.7 oz)	150	3	1	0	6	29	3	3	20	340	20	32	0
Homestyle	2 (2.7 oz)	220	8	2	25	5	32	3	1	40	480	100	40	0

FOOD	PORTION	CALS	FAT	SAT FAT	CHOL	PROT	CARB	SUGAR	FIBER	CALCI	SOD	POTAS	FOLIC	VIT C
EGGO (CONT.)														
Minis Cinnamon Toast	12 (3.2 oz)	290	10	2	25	5	45	17	2	40	470	100	40	0
Minis Homestyle	12 (3.3 oz)	260	9	2	25	7	38	3	2	60	600	130	60	0
Nut & Honey	2 (2.7 oz)	240	10	2	25	6	31	5	2	40	450	125	40	0
Nutri-Grain	2 (2.7 oz)	190	6	1	0	5	30	4	4	40	450	150	40	0
Nutri-Grain Multi-Bran	2 (2.7 oz)	180	6	1	0	5	32	4	6	40	410	160	20	0
Nutri-Grain Raisin & Bran	2 (2.9 oz)	210	6	1	0	5	36	10	5	40	430	210	20	0
Special K	2 (2 oz)	120	0	0	0	6	26	4	1	40	280	130	40	0
Strawberry	2 (2.7 oz)	220	8	2	20	6	32	5	1	40	460	110	40	0
KELLOGG'S														
Homestyle Low Fat	2 (2.7 oz)	180	3	1	20	6	34	5	1	40	340	110	60	0
Nutri-Grain Low Fat	2 (2.7 oz)	160	3	0	0	5	31	4	3	40	480	60	40	0
Nutri-Grain Low Fat Blueberry	2 (2.7 oz)	160	2	0	0	5	33	7	3	40	460	50	40	0
KID CUISINE														
Wave Rider Waffle Sticks	1 meal (6.6 oz)	380	8	2	30	3	75	38	3	20	580	—	—	0
MIX														
plain as prep	1 7 in diam (2.6 oz)	218	10	2	39	5	26	—	1	93	458	134	9	tr
READY-TO-EAT														
GOL D LITE														
Low Carb Belgian	1 (0.9 oz)	100	5	0	0	2	15	0	5	—	0	—	—	—
Low Carb Belgian Chocolate Covered	1 (1.1 oz)	130	8	0	0	2	18	0	1	—	0	—	—	—
KASHI														
GoLean Blueberry	2	170	3	0	0	8	33	4	6	60	300	130	—	0
GoLean Original	2	170	3	0	0	8	33	4	6	60	330	130	—	0
THOMAS'														
Buttermilk	1 (1.6 oz)	130	5	1	0	3	18	7	tr	400	490	—	40	0
Homestyle	1 (1.6 oz)	140	5	1	0	3	19	7	tr	300	390	—	40	0
TAKE-OUT														
plain	1 (7 in diam)	218	11	2	52	6	25	—	—	191	383	119	—	tr
WALNUTS														
black dried chopped	1 cup	759	71	5	0	30	15	—	—	72	2	655	—	—
english dried	1 oz	182	18	2	0	4	5	—	1	27	3	142	19	1

FOOD	PORTION	CALS	FAT	SAT FAT	CHOL	PROT	CARB	SUGAR	FIBER	CALCI	SOD	POTAS	FOLIC	VIT C
english dried chopped	1 cup	770	74	7	0	17	22	—	6	113	12	602	79	4
halves	14 (1 oz)	190	19	2	0	4	4	1	2	40	tr	130	24	—
SWEET DELIGHTS														
Walnut Roasters	⅓ pkg (1 oz)	210	20	2	0	5	3	0	2	—	200	—	—	—

WASABI (*see* HORSERADISH)

WATER

FOOD	PORTION	CALS	FAT	SAT FAT	CHOL	PROT	CARB	SUGAR	FIBER	CALCI	SOD	POTAS	FOLIC	VIT C
ice cubes	3	0	0	0	0	0	0	—	—	1	2	0	0	0
tap water	8 oz	0	0	0	0	0	0	—	—	5	7	0	0	0
ABSOPURE														
Natural Spring	8 fl oz	0	0	0	0	0	0	—	—	20	0	—	—	—
AQUAFINA														
Essentials B-Power Wild Berry	8 fl oz	40	0	0	0	0	11	11	—	—	10	—	—	—
Essentials Calcium + Tangerine Pineapple	8 fl oz	40	0	0	0	0	11	10	—	100	15	—	40	—
Essentials Daily C Citrus	8 fl oz	40	0	0	0	0	11	11	—	—	15	—	—	24
Essentials Multi-V Watermelon	8 fl oz	40	0	0	0	0	11	11	—	—	10	—	—	6
Water	8 fl oz	0	0	0	0	0	0	0	—	—	0	—	—	—
AQUESS														
Purified Water w/ Soluble Fiber	1 bottle (18 oz)	30	0	0	0	0	8	2	5	—	0	—	—	—
BASE ENERGY + WATER														
All Flavors	8 oz	28	0	0	0	0	7	—	—	—	45	25	—	—
BLU ITALY														
Sparkling Lemon	8 oz	0	0	0	0	0	0	0	0	20	25	—	—	—
CALABRIA														
Mineral	8 oz	0	0	0	0	0	0	0	0	0	0	—	—	—
CASTELLINA														
Sparking Spring	8 fl oz	0	0	0	0	0	0	0	0	14	<5	tr	—	—
CLEARLY CANADIAN														
Sparkling All Flavors	8 oz	45	0	0	0	0	10	10	—	—	10	—	—	—
CRYSTAL GEYSER														
Spring Water	8 fl oz	0	0	0	0	0	0	0	0	10	0	—	—	—
DASANI														
Purfied Water	8 oz	0	0	0	0	0	0	0	—	—	0	—	—	—
EVAMOR														
Artesian Water	8 fl oz	0	0	0	0	0	0	0	0	—	12	3	—	—
EVIAN														
Spring Water	1 bottle (11.5 oz)	0	0	0	0	0	0	0	0	20	<5	—	—	—

FOOD	PORTION	CALS	FAT	SAT FAT	CHOL	PROT	CARB	SUGAR	FIBER	CALCI	SOD	POTAS	FOLIC	VIT C
FERRARELLE														
Sparkling	8 fl oz	0	0	0	0	0	0	0	1	90	10	—	—	—
FLAVH20														
All Flavors	1 can (12.3 oz)	80	0	0	0	0	21	20	—	—	0	—	—	—
GEROLSTEINER														
Sparling Mineral	8 fl oz	0	0	0	0	0	0	0	0	80	30	—	—	—
GLACEAU VITAMIN WATER														
Balance	8 oz	50	0	0	0	0	13	12	—	>20	0	—	—	24
Defense	8 oz	40	0	0	0	0	9	8	—	—	0	—	—	60
Endurance	8 oz	50	0	0	0	0	13	13	—	—	0	—	—	36
Energy	8 oz	40	0	0	0	0	9	8	—	—	0	—	—	60
Essential	8 oz	40	0	0	0	0	9	8	—	20	0	50	—	15
Focus	8 oz	40	0	0	0	0	9	8	—	—	0	—	—	60
Multi-V	8 oz	40	0	0	0	0	9	8	—	20	0	—	—	60
Power-C	8 oz	40	0	0	0	0	9	8	—	—	5	—	—	150
Rescue	8 oz	40	0	0	0	0	9	8	—	—	0	—	—	60
Revive	8 oz	50	0	0	0	0	13	12	—	—	0	—	—	36
Stress-B	8 oz	40	0	0	0	0	9	8	—	—	0	—	—	36
GLACIER SPRINGS														
Drinking Water	8 fl oz	0	0	0	0	0	0	0	0	—	0	—	—	—
HANSEN'S														
Energy Water Lemon	8 oz	10	0	0	0	0	3	3	—	—	0	40	—	—
ICELAND SPRING														
Spring Water	1 liter	0	0	0	0	0	0	0	0	5	10	1	—	—
LACROIX														
Spring	1 bottle (12 oz)	0	0	0	0	0	0	0	0	—	<8	—	—	—
MERIDIAN														
Clear All Flavors	8 oz	100	0	0	0	0	25	25	—	—	0	—	—	—
METROMINT														
Peppermint Water	8 oz	0	0	0	0	0	0	0	0	—	0	—	—	—
MT SHASTA														
Natural Spring	1 bottle (20 oz)	0	0	0	0	0	0	0	0	—	<13	—	—	—
PARADISO														
Sligtly Sparkling	8 oz	0	0	0	0	0	0	0	0	10	1	—	—	—
PROPEL														
Fitness Water Berry	8 fl oz	10	0	0	0	0	3	2	—	—	35	40	—	6
Fitness Water Black Cherry	8 fl oz	10	0	0	0	0	3	2	—	—	35	40	—	6
REEBOK														
Fitness Water Berry	1 bottle (24 oz)	30	0	0	0	0	0	0	0	50	0	70	100	0
Fitness Water Natural	1 bottle (24 oz)	0	0	0	0	0	0	0	0	50	0	70	100	0

FOOD	PORTION	CALS	FAT	SAT FAT	CHOL	PROT	CARB	SUGAR	FIBER	CALCI	SOD	POTAS	FOLIC	VIT C
REPLENISH														
Elements Enhanced Water Orange	8 oz	40	0	0	0	0	10	10	—	—	80	—	—	—
SAN BENEDETTO														
Natural Mineral Water	1 liter	0	0	0	0	0	0	0	0	46	7	1	—	—
SAN PELLEGRINO														
Acqua Panna	8 fl oz	0	0	0	0	0	0	0	0	3	0	—	—	—
Mineral Water	1 liter (33.8 oz)	0	0	0	0	0	0	—	—	204	41	3	—	—
SANFAUSTINO														
Mineral	8 oz	0	0	0	0	0	0	0	0	100	4	—	—	—
SARATOGA														
Spring	8 oz	0	0	0	0	0	0	—	—	20	0	—	—	—
SPA														
Mineral Water Reine	1 bottle (17.5 oz)	0	0	0	0	0	0	—	—	3	2	tr	—	—
SPEEDO SPORTSWATER														
All Flavors	8 oz	10	0	0	0	0	3	2	—	—	40	35	100	15
TY NANT														
Mineral Water	1 liter	0	0	0	0	0	0	0	0	23	22	1	—	—
VASA														
Natural Spring	8 oz	0	0	0	0	0	0	0	0	—	0	—	—	—
VERYFINE														
Fruit 2 O Lemon	8 oz	0	0	0	0	0	0	0	—	—	5	—	—	—
Fruit 2 O Lemon Lime	8 fl oz	0	0	0	0	0	0	0	—	—	5	—	—	—
Fruit 2 O Orange	8 fl oz	0	0	0	0	0	0	0	—	—	5	—	—	—
Fruit 2 O Raspberry	8 fl oz	0	0	0	0	0	0	0	—	—	5	—	—	—
VITAZEST														
All Flavors	8 oz	0	0	0	0	0	0	0	0	20	10	—	—	30
VITTEL														
Mineral Water	1 bottle (18 oz)	0	0	0	0	0	0	—	—	202	5	1	—	—
VOLVIC														
Spring Water	8 oz	0	0	0	0	0	0	0	0	—	<5	—	—	—
VOSS														
Artesian	8 oz	0	0	0	0	0	0	0	0	1	—	0	—	—
WATER CHESTNUTS														
chinese sliced canned	½ cup	35	tr	—	0	1	9	—	—	3	6	82	—	1
fresh sliced	½ cup	66	tr	—	0	1	15	—	—	7	9	362	—	3
CHUN KING														
Sliced	2 tbsp (0.8 oz)	11	tr	0	0	tr	3	tr	1	1	3	—	—	0
Whole	2 (0.7 oz)	10	tr	0	0	tr	2	tr	1	1	2	—	—	0

FOOD	PORTION	CALS	FAT	SAT FAT	CHOL	PROT	CARB	SUGAR	FIBER	CALCI	SOD	POTAS	FOLIC	VIT C
LA CHOY														
Chopped	2 tbsp (0.6 oz)	9	tr	0	0	tr	2	tr	1	1	2	—	—	0
Sliced	2 tbsp (0.8 oz)	11	tr	0	0	tr	3	tr	1	1	3	—	—	0
Whole	2 (0.7 oz)	10	tr	0	0	tr	2	tr	1	1	2	—	—	0
WATERCRESS														
fresh chopped	½ cup	2	tr	tr	0	tr	tr	—	tr	20	7	56	—	7
garden fresh	½ cup	8	tr	tr	0	tr	1	—	—	20	4	152	—	17
garden fresh cooked	½ cup	16	tr	tr	0	1	3	—	—	41	5	240	—	16
WATERMELON														
cut up	1 cup	50	1	—	0	1	11	—	1	13	3	186	3	15
seeds dried	1 cup	602	51	3	0	8	17	—	—	15	28	184	16	0
seeds dried	1 oz	158	13	3	0	8	4	—	—	15	28	184	16	—
wedge	¹⁄₁₆	152	2	—	0	3	35	—	2	38	10	560	10	47
WATERMELON JUICE														
KOOL-AID														
Splash Drink	1 serv (8 oz)	110	0	0	0	0	30	30	0	0	35	15	—	0
SNAPPLE														
What-A-Melon	8 oz	90	0	0	0	0	25	23	—	—	40	—	—	—
SQUEEZIT														
Watermelon	1 bottle (7 oz)	110	0	0	0	0	28	27	0	0	0	—	—	0
WAX BEANS														
CANNED														
DEL MONTE														
Cut Golden	½ cup (4.2 oz)	20	0	0	0	1	4	2	2	20	360	—	—	4
S&W														
Cut	½ cup (4.2 oz)	20	0	0	0	1	4	2	2	20	360	—	—	4
WHALE														
raw	3.5 oz	134	3	—	—	23	0	—	—	12	100	300	—	—
WHEAT														
sprouted	1 cup (3.8 oz)	214	1	tr	0	8	46	—	1	30	17	183	41	3
starch	3.5 oz	348	tr	—	—	tr	86	—	—	0	2	16	—	0
BOB'S RED MILL														
Vital Wheat Gluten	¼ cup	120	1	—	0	23	6	0	0	—	9	—	—	—
LIGHTLIFE														
Savory Seitan Barbecue	4 oz	160	2	1	0	24	12	3	0	—	360	—	—	—
Savory Seitan Teriyaki	4 oz	160	2	1	0	26	10	2	0	—	320	—	—	—
NEAR EAST														
Pilaf Mix Wheat as prep	1 cup	220	5	2	9	7	40	2	9	20	640	—	—	0

FOOD	PORTION	CALS	FAT	SAT FAT	CHOL	PROT	CARB	SUGAR	FIBER	CALCI	SOD	POTAS	FOLIC	VIT C
NEAR EAST (CONT.)														
Taboule Salad Mix as prep	⅔ cup	110	3	tr	0	3	21	1	5	0	270	—	—	9
NOW														
Wheat Gluten Flour	¼ cup	125	0	0	0	23	5	0	—	—	40	—	—	—
WHEAT GERM														
plain toasted	1 cup	431	12	2	0	33	56	—	—	50	4	1070	398	7
plain toasted	¼ cup (1 oz)	108	3	1	0	8	14	—	4	13	1	268	100	2
w/ brown sugar & honey toasted	1 cup	426	9	2	—	25	69	—	—	38	3	803	298	—
w/ brown sugar & honey toasted	1 oz	107	2	tr	—	6	17	—	—	9	1	201	75	—
HODGSON MILL														
Untoasted	2 tbsp	55	1	0	0	4	7	0	4	0	0	40	40	—
KRETSCHMER														
Original Toasted	2 tbsp (0.5 oz)	50	1	0	0	4	6	1	2	—	0	140	40	—
MOTHER'S														
Toasted	2 tbsp	50	1	0	0	4	6	1	2	—	0	—	80	—
WHEY														
acid dry	1 tbsp (3 g)	10	tr	tr	—	tr	2	—	—	59	28	66	1	tr
acid fluid	1 cup (8 fl oz)	59	tr	tr	—	25	13	—	—	253	118	352	5	tr
sweet dry	1 tbsp (8 g)	26	tr	tr	—	1	6	—	—	59	80	155	1	tr
sweet fluid	1 cup (8 fl oz)	66	1	1	—	2	13	—	—	115	132	396	2	tr
whey cheese	1 oz	126	8	5	—	4	9	0	0	97	146	—	—	tr
WHIPPED TOPPINGS														
cream pressurized	1 cup (2.1 oz)	154	13	8	46	2	7	—	—	61	78	88	—	0
cream pressurized	1 tbsp (3 g)	8	tr	tr	2	tr	tr	—	—	3	4	4	—	0
nondairy frzn	1 tbsp	13	1	1	0	tr	1	—	—	tr	1	1	0	0
nondairy powdered as prep w/ whole milk	1 cup	151	10	9	8	3	13	—	—	72	53	121	3	1
nondairy powdered as prep w/ whole milk	1 tbsp (4 g)	8	tr	tr	tr	tr	1	—	—	4	3	6	tr	tr
nondairy pressurized	1 tbsp (4 g)	11	1	1	0	tr	1	—	—	tr	2	1	0	0
nondairy pressurized	1 cup	184	16	13	0	1	11	—	—	4	43	13	0	0
COOL WHIP														
Extra Creamy	2 tbsp (0.3 oz)	25	2	2	0	0	2	2	0	0	5	0	—	0
Free	2 tbsp (0.3 oz)	15	0	0	0	0	3	1	0	0	5	0	—	0
Lite	2 tbsp (0.3 oz)	20	1	1	0	0	2	1	0	0	0	0	—	0
Original	2 tbsp (0.3 oz)	25	2	2	0	0	2	1	0	0	0	0	0	—
DREAM WHIP														
Mix as prep	2 tbsp (0.3 oz)	20	1	1	0	0	2	2	0	0	5	15	—	0

FOOD	PORTION	CALS	FAT	SAT FAT	CHOL	PROT	CARB	SUGAR	FIBER	CALCI	SOD	POTAS	FOLIC	VIT C
ESTEE														
Whipped Topping	1 serv	10	1	0	0	0	1	0	0	—	5	10	—	—
KRAFT														
Dairy Whip Light Cream	2 tbsp (0.2 oz)	10	1	1	<5	0	tr	tr	0	0	0	5	—	0
Fat Free	1 tbsp (0.3 oz)	15	0	0	0	0	2	2	0	0	5	10	—	0

WHITE BEANS

FOOD	PORTION	CALS	FAT	SAT FAT	CHOL	PROT	CARB	SUGAR	FIBER	CALCI	SOD	POTAS	FOLIC	VIT C
canned	1 cup	306	1	tr	0	19	58	—	—	191	13	1189	171	0
dried regular cooked	1 cup	249	1	tr	0	17	45	—	—	161	11	1003	145	0
dried small cooked	1 cup	253	1	tr	0	16	46	—	—	131	4	828	245	0
PROGRESSO														
Cannellini	½ cup (4.6 oz)	100	1	0	0	5	18	0	5	40	270	—	—	0

WHITEFISH

FOOD	PORTION	CALS	FAT	SAT FAT	CHOL	PROT	CARB	SUGAR	FIBER	CALCI	SOD	POTAS	FOLIC	VIT C
baked	3 oz	146	6	1	65	21	0	—	—	—	56	345	—	—
smoked	1 oz	39	tr	tr	9	7	0	—	—	5	285	118	2	—
smoked	3 oz	92	1	tr	28	20	0	—	—	15	866	360	6	—

WHITING

FOOD	PORTION	CALS	FAT	SAT FAT	CHOL	PROT	CARB	SUGAR	FIBER	CALCI	SOD	POTAS	FOLIC	VIT C
cooked	3 oz	98	1	tr	71	20	0	—	—	53	113	369	13	—
raw	3 oz	77	1	tr	57	16	0	—	—	41	61	212	11	—

WILD RICE

FOOD	PORTION	CALS	FAT	SAT FAT	CHOL	PROT	CARB	SUGAR	FIBER	CALCI	SOD	POTAS	FOLIC	VIT C
cooked	1 cup (5.7 oz)	166	1	tr	0	7	35	—	3	5	5	166	43	0
GOURMET HOUSE														
Cracked not prep	¼ cup	170	0	0	0	6	35	0	2	20	0	120	—	0
Hand Harvested not prep	¼ cup	170	0	0	0	6	35	0	2	20	0	120	—	0
Quick Cooking not prep	½ cup	170	0	0	0	6	25	0	2	20	0	120	—	0
White & Wild not prep	¼ cup	170	0	0	0	4	35	1	1	20	0	90	—	0
Wild & Rice Garden Blend not prep	¼ cup	190	1	0	0	5	40	1	1	60	15	120	—	5

WINE

FOOD	PORTION	CALS	FAT	SAT FAT	CHOL	PROT	CARB	SUGAR	FIBER	CALCI	SOD	POTAS	FOLIC	VIT C
beaujolais	4 oz	95	—	—	—	—	—	—	—	—	—	—	—	—
bordeaux red	4 oz	95	—	—	—	—	—	—	—	—	—	—	—	—
chianti	4 oz	101	—	—	—	—	—	—	—	—	—	—	—	—
haiku	1 serv	93	0	0	0	tr	3	—	0	3	2	17	—	—
japanese plum	3 oz	139	tr	—	0	tr	16	—	0	1	—	—	—	0
japanese sake	1 oz	33	0	0	0	tr	2	—	0	1	1	1	—	0
kir	1 serv	78	0	0	0	tr	3	—	0	8	4	71	tr	—
liebfraumilch	4 oz	86	—	—	—	—	—	—	—	—	—	—	—	—
madeira	3.5 oz	169	0	—	0	0	10	10	0	8	—	—	—	—
marsala	4 oz	80	—	—	—	—	—	—	—	—	—	—	—	—
merlot	4 oz	95	—	—	—	—	—	—	—	—	—	—	—	—
muscatel	4 oz	160	—	—	—	—	—	—	—	—	—	—	—	—

FOOD	PORTION	CALS	FAT	SAT FAT	CHOL	PROT	CARB	SUGAR	FIBER	CALCI	SOD	POTAS	FOLIC	VIT C
port	3.5 oz	156	0	—	—	tr	11	11	0	4	4	—	—	0
red	3.5 oz	74	0	0	0	tr	2	—	0	8	6	115	2	0
rosé	3.5 oz	73	0	0	0	tr	2	—	0	9	5	102	1	0
sake screwdriver	1 serv	175	tr	tr	0	2	23	—	tr	24	3	389	56	93
sangria	1 serv	88	tr	0	0	tr	6	—	tr	7	4	95	5	7
sangria blanco	1 serv	155	tr	tr	0	1	24	—	3	70	13	267	23	27
sherry	2 oz	84	0	0	0	tr	5	—	—	—	—	—	—	—
sweet dessert	3.5 oz	158	0	0	0	tr	12	—	0	8	9	95	0	0
vermouth dry	3.5 oz	105	0	0	0	—	1	—	—	—	—	—	—	—
vermouth sweet	3.5 oz	167	0	0	0	—	12	—	—	—	—	—	—	—
wassail wine	1 serv	142	tr	tr	0	1	22	—	2	50	6	190	17	23
white	3.5 oz	70	0	0	0	tr	1	—	0	9	5	82	tr	0
wine cooler	1 serv	218	tr	tr	0	1	8	—	0	20	10	276	8	23
wine spritzer	1 serv	60	0	0	0	tr	1	—	0	9	11	71	tr	—
BOONE'S														
Country Kwencher	4 fl oz	96	0	0	0	0	12	—	—	—	—	4	—	—
Delicious Apple	4 fl oz	84	0	0	0	0	12	—	—	—	—	4	—	—
Sangria	4 fl oz	88	0	0	0	0	12	—	—	—	—	4	—	—
Snow Creek Berry	4 fl oz	72	0	0	0	0	12	—	—	—	—	tr	—	—
Strawberry Hill	4 fl oz	88	0	0	0	0	12	—	—	—	—	4	—	—
Sun Peak Peach	4 fl oz	72	0	0	0	0	12	—	—	—	—	4	—	—
Wild Island	4 fl oz	72	0	0	0	0	12	—	—	—	—	tr	—	—
CARLO ROSSI														
Blush	4 fl oz	84	0	0	0	0	4	—	—	—	—	4	—	—
Burgundy	4 fl oz	88	0	0	0	0	tr	—	—	—	—	4	—	—
Chablis	4 fl oz	84	0	0	0	0	tr	—	—	—	—	4	—	—
Paisano	4 fl oz	92	0	0	0	0	tr	—	—	—	—	12	—	—
Red Sangria	4 fl oz	92	0	0	0	0	8	—	—	—	—	4	—	—
Rhine	4 fl oz	84	0	0	0	0	4	—	—	—	—	4	—	—
Vin Rosé	4 fl oz	84	0	0	0	0	4	—	—	—	—	4	—	—
White Grenache	4 fl oz	80	0	0	0	0	4	—	—	—	—	tr	—	—
EDEN														
Mirin Rice Cooking Wine	1 tbsp	25	0	0	0	0	7	4	0	0	130	—	—	0
FAIRBANKS														
Cream Sherry	4 fl oz	168	0	0	0	0	16	—	—	—	4	—	—	—
Port	4 fl oz	176	0	0	0	0	16	—	—	—	4	—	—	—
Sherry	4 fl oz	136	0	0	0	0	8	—	—	—	8	—	—	—
White Port	4 fl oz	136	0	0	0	0	16	—	—	—	4	—	—	—
GALLO														
Blush Chablis	4 fl oz	88	0	0	0	0	4	—	—	—	—	8	—	—
Burgundy	4 fl oz	88	0	0	0	0	tr	—	—	—	—	4	—	—
Cabernet Sauvignon	4 fl oz	88	0	0	0	0	0	—	—	—	—	tr	—	—
Chablis Blanc	4 fl oz	80	0	0	0	0	tr	—	—	—	—	4	—	—

FOOD	PORTION	CALS	FAT	SAT FAT	CHOL	PROT	CARB	SUGAR	FIBER	CALCI	SOD	POTAS	FOLIC	VIT C
GALLO (CONT.)														
Chardonnay	4 fl oz	92	0	0	0	0	tr	—	—	—	4	—	—	—
Classic Burgundy	4 fl oz	84	0	0	0	0	0	—	—	—	tr	—	—	—
French Colombard	4 fl oz	84	0	0	0	0	4	—	—	—	4	—	—	—
Hearty Burgundy	4 fl oz	88	0	0	0	0	tr	—	—	—	4	—	—	—
Pink Chablis	4 fl oz	80	0	0	0	0	4	—	—	—	4	—	—	—
Red Rosé	4 fl oz	92	0	0	0	0	4	—	—	—	8	—	—	—
Rhine	4 fl oz	88	0	0	0	0	4	—	—	—	4	—	—	—
SHEFFIELD CELLARS														
Sherry	4 fl oz	136	0	0	0	0	16	—	—	—	4	—	—	—
Tawny Port	4 fl oz	180	0	0	0	0	16	—	—	—	8	—	—	—
Vermouth Extra Dry	1 fl oz	28	0	0	0	0	1	—	—	—	1	—	—	—
Vermouth Sweet	1 fl oz	43	0	0	0	0	4	—	—	—	2	—	—	—
Very Dry Sherry	4 fl oz	128	0	0	0	0	4	—	—	—	8	—	—	—
WINGED BEANS														
dried cooked	1 cup	252	10	1	0	18	26	—	—	244	22	481	18	0
WOLFFISH														
atlantic baked	3 oz	105	3	tr	50	19	0	—	—	—	93	—	—	—
WRAPS														
(*see* BREAD)														
XANTHAN GUM														
BOB'S RED MILL														
Xanthan Gum	1 tbsp	8	0	0	0	0	9	0	8	—	10	—	—	—
YAM														
(*see also* SWEET POTATO)														
CANNED														
S&W														
Candied	½ cup (4.9 oz)	170	0	0	0	2	46	21	4	20	360	210	—	5
FRESH														
mountain yam hawaii cooked	½ cup	59	tr	tr	0	1	14	—	—	6	9	356	—	0
yam cubed cooked	½ cup	79	tr	tr	0	1	19	—	—	9	6	455	11	8
YAMBEAN														
cooked	¾ cup	38	tr	—	0	1	9	—	—	11	4	135	8	14
YARDLONG BEANS														
dried cooked	1 cup	202	1	tr	0	14	36	—	—	72	9	539	249	1
YAUTIA (TANNIER)														
fresh sliced	1 cup (4.7 oz)	132	1	—	0	2	32	—	2	12	28	807	23	16
root raw	1 (10.7 oz)	299	1	—	0	4	72	—	5	27	64	1824	52	16
YEAST														
baker's compressed	1 cake (0.6 oz)	18	tr	tr	0	1	3	—	2	3	5	102	133	—
baker's dry	1 tbsp	35	1	tr	0	5	5	—	3	8	—	240	—	—

FOOD	PORTION	CALS	FAT	SAT FAT	CHOL	PROT	CARB	SUGAR	FIBER	CALCI	SOD	POTAS	FOLIC	VIT C
baker's dry	1 pkg (¼ oz)	21	tr	tr	0	3	3	—	—	5	—	140	—	—
brewer's dry	1 tbsp	25	tr	tr	0	3	3	—	—	17	10	152	—	tr
FLEISCHMANN'S														
Active Dry	1 pkg (7 g)	23	3	—	—	—	—	—	—	2	10	—	—	0
Bread Machine	1 pkg (7 g)	26	2	—	—	—	—	—	—	2	10	—	—	13
RapidRise	1 pkg (7 g)	26	2	—	—	—	—	—	—	2	10	—	—	13
HODGSON MILL														
Fast Rise	1 tsp (9 g)	25	0	0	0	3	4	0	1	0	0	—	—	0

YELLOW BEANS

FOOD	PORTION	CALS	FAT	SAT FAT	CHOL	PROT	CARB	SUGAR	FIBER	CALCI	SOD	POTAS	FOLIC	VIT C
canned	½ cup	13	tr	tr	0	1	3	—	1	18	170	74	22	3
canned low sodium	½ cup	13	tr	tr	0	1	3	—	1	18	1	74	22	3
dried cooked	1 cup	254	2	tr	0	16	45	—	—	110	8	576	143	3
fresh cooked	½ cup	22	tr	tr	0	1	5	—	—	29	2	185	21	6
fresh raw	½ cup	17	tr	tr	0	1	4	—	—	21	3	115	20	9
frozen cooked	½ cup	18	tr	tr	0	1	4	—	—	31	9	76	—	6

YELLOWTAIL

FOOD	PORTION	CALS	FAT	SAT FAT	CHOL	PROT	CARB	SUGAR	FIBER	CALCI	SOD	POTAS	FOLIC	VIT C
baked	3 oz	159	6	—	—	25	0	—	—	—	42	—	3	2

YOGURT

(*see also* YOGURT DRINKS, YOGURT FROZEN)

FOOD	PORTION	CALS	FAT	SAT FAT	CHOL	PROT	CARB	SUGAR	FIBER	CALCI	SOD	POTAS	FOLIC	VIT C
coffee lowfat	8 oz	194	3	2	11	11	31	—	—	389	149	498	24	2
fruit lowfat	8 oz	225	3	2	10	9	42	—	—	314	121	402	19	1
fruit lowfat	4 oz	113	1	1	5	5	21	—	—	157	60	201	10	1
plain	8 oz	139	7	5	29	8	11	—	—	274	105	351	17	1
plain lowfat	8 oz	144	4	2	14	12	16	—	—	415	159	531	25	2
plain no fat	8 oz	127	tr	tr	4	13	17	—	—	452	174	579	28	2
vanilla lowfat	8 oz	194	3	2	11	11	31	—	—	389	149	498	24	2
AXELROD														
Fat Free Lemon	1 pkg (6 oz)	90	0	0	<5	5	17	12	0	200	95	—	—	0
Fat Free Raspberry	6 oz	90	0	0	<5	5	17	11	0	200	95	—	—	0
Fat Free Vanilla	1 pkg (6 oz)	90	0	0	<5	5	17	11	0	200	95	—	—	0
BREYERS														
Blended Blueberry	4.4 oz	130	1	1	10	4	25	23	0	100	60	180	—	0
Blended Peach	4.4 oz	130	1	1	10	4	26	22	0	100	65	180	—	0
Blended Strawberry	4.4 oz	130	1	1	10	4	26	23	0	100	60	180	—	0
Light Nonfat Apple Pie A La Mode	8 oz	120	0	0	10	7	22	16	0	200	105	300	—	0
Light Nonfat Berry Banana Split	8 oz	120	0	0	10	8	21	16	0	200	105	320	—	0
Light Nonfat Black Cherry Jubilee	8 oz	120	0	0	10	8	23	17	0	200	100	330	—	0

FOOD	PORTION	CALS	FAT	SAT FAT	CHOL	PROT	CARB	SUGAR	FIBER	CALCI	SOD	POTAS	FOLIC	VIT C
BREYERS (CONT.)														
Light Nonfat Blueberries N' Cream	8 oz	120	0	0	10	8	23	17	0	200	100	310	—	0
Light Nonfat Cherry Bon-Bon	8 oz	120	0	0	10	8	22	17	0	200	105	300	—	0
Light Nonfat Cherry Vanilla Cream	8 oz	120	0	0	10	8	22	17	0	200	105	320	—	0
Light Nonfat Classic Strawberry	8 oz	120	0	0	10	8	22	17	0	200	100	320	—	0
Light Nonfat Key Lime Pie	8 oz	120	0	0	10	8	22	15	0	200	100	300	—	0
Light Nonfat Lemon Chiffon	8 oz	120	0	0	10	7	22	17	0	200	100	310	—	0
Light Nonfat Peaches N' Cream	8 oz	120	0	0	10	8	22	17	0	200	115	340	—	0
Light Nonfat Raspberries N' Cream	8 oz	120	0	0	10	8	22	17	0	200	105	330	—	0
Light Nonfat Strawberry Cheesecake	8 oz	120	0	0	10	8	22	17	tr	200	100	320	—	0
Lowfat Black Cherry	8 oz	240	3	2	15	9	44	43	0	300	125	450	—	0
Lowfat Blueberry	8 oz	230	3	2	15	9	43	42	0	300	125	430	—	0
Lowfat Mixed Berry	8 oz	320	3	2	15	9	43	42	0	300	125	440	—	0
Lowfat Peach	8 oz	240	3	2	15	9	43	43	0	300	125	440	—	0
Lowfat Pineapple	8 oz	240	3	2	15	9	45	44	0	300	125	430	—	0
Lowfat Red Raspberry	8 oz	230	3	2	15	9	43	42	2	300	125	450	—	0
Lowfat Strawberry	8 oz	230	3	2	15	9	43	43	0	300	125	440	—	0
Lowfat Strawberry Banana	8 oz	240	3	2	15	9	44	43	tr	300	125	470	—	0
Smooth & Creamy Apple Cobbler	8 oz	230	2	1	20	8	46	40	0	250	140	390	—	0
Smooth & Creamy Black Cherry Parfait	8 oz	240	2	1	20	9	46	41	0	250	130	390	—	0
Smooth & Creamy Black Cherry Parfait	4.4 oz	130	1	1	10	5	26	23	0	150	70	210	—	0
Smooth & Creamy Blueberries 'N Cream	8 oz	240	2	1	20	9	46	40	0	250	125	380	—	0
Smooth & Creamy Blueberries 'N Cream	4.4 oz	130	1	1	10	5	26	22	0	150	70	210	—	0

FOOD	PORTION	CALS	FAT	SAT FAT	CHOL	PROT	CARB	SUGAR	FIBER	CALCI	SOD	POTAS	FOLIC	VIT C
BREYERS (CONT.)														
Smooth & Creamy Classic Strawberry	4.4 oz	130	1	1	10	5	25	22	0	150	70	220	—	0
Smooth & Creamy Classic Strawberry	8 oz	230	2	1	20	9	45	39	0	250	125	400	—	0
Smooth & Creamy Orange Vanilla Cream	8 oz	230	2	1	20	9	45	39	0	250	125	380	—	0
Smooth & Creamy Peaches 'N Cream	4.4 oz	130	1	1	10	5	25	22	0	150	70	220	—	0
Smooth & Creamy Peaches 'N Cream	8 oz	230	2	1	20	9	46	40	0	250	125	390	—	0
Smooth & Creamy Raspberries 'N Cream	8 oz	230	2	1	20	9	45	40	0	250	135	400	—	0
Smooth & Creamy Strawberry Banana Split	8 oz	240	2	1	10	8	48	41	tr	250	125	390	—	0
Smooth & Creamy Strawberry Cheesecake	8 oz	240	2	1	20	9	46	39	0	250	125	400	—	0
Vanilla 98% Fat Free	½ cup	90	2	1	5	2	21	14	4	80	50	—	—	0
CABOT														
Non Fat	8 oz	100	0	0	0	10	19	13	0	300	135	—	—	12
Non Fat Berry Banana	8 oz	130	0	0	5	8	24	19	0	250	120	—	—	12
Non Fat Blueberry	8 oz	130	0	0	5	8	24	19	0	250	115	—	—	12
Non Fat Lemon	8 oz	130	0	0	5	8	24	19	0	250	115	—	—	12
Non Fat Raspberry	8 oz	130	0	0	5	8	24	19	0	250	115	—	—	12
Non Fat Very Berry	8 oz	130	0	0	5	8	24	19	0	250	115	—	—	12
COLOMBO														
Fat Free Plain	8 oz	100	0	0	10	10	16	10	0	300	160	440	—	—
Fat Free Vanilla	8 oz	160	0	0	5	8	32	26	0	250	140	410	—	—
French Vanilla	8 oz	180	2	2	15	8	42	32	0	250	120	370	—	—
Fruit On The Bottom Strawberry Banana	8 oz	230	2	2	15	7	47	42	0	200	90	330	—	—
Lowfat Plain	8 oz	130	3	2	15	10	16	10	0	300	125	440	—	—
Multipack Blended All Flavors	4 oz	110	1	1	5	3	22	19	0	100	60	190	—	0
Strawberry	8 oz	190	3	2	15	8	42	33	—	250	130	—	—	—
DANNON														
Chunky Fruit Nonfat Apple Cinnamon	6 oz	160	0	0	5	7	33	29	0	200	100	320	—	2

FOOD	PORTION	CALS	FAT	SAT FAT	CHOL	PROT	CARB	SUGAR	FIBER	CALCI	SOD	POTAS	FOLIC	VIT C
DANNON (CONT.)														
Chunky Fruit Nonfat Blueberry	6 oz	160	0	0	5	7	32	29	0	200	110	310	—	2
Chunky Fruit Nonfat Cherry Vanilla	6 oz	160	0	0	5	7	31	28	0	200	100	360	—	5
Chunky Fruit Nonfat Peach	6 oz	160	0	0	5	7	33	29	0	200	100	330	—	2
Chunky Fruit Nonfat Strawberry	6 oz	160	0	0	5	7	32	28	0	200	105	350	—	12
Chunky Fruit Nonfat Strawberry Banana	6 oz	160	0	0	5	7	32	28	0	200	105	350	—	12
Creamy Fruit Blends Raspberry	6 oz	170	2	2	10	6	31	28	tr	150	115	—	—	—
Danimals Lowfat Tropical Punch	4.4 oz	130	1	1	5	6	25	22	0	200	95	250	—	1
Danimals Lowfat Blueberry	4.4 oz	130	1	1	5	6	24	21	0	200	100	250	—	1
Danimals Lowfat Grape Lemonade	4.4 oz	120	1	1	5	6	22	20	0	200	90	270	—	1
Danimals Lowfat Lemon Ice	4.4 oz	120	1	1	5	6	22	19	0	200	100	270	—	4
Danimals Lowfat Orange Banana	4.4 oz	130	1	1	5	6	24	21	0	200	90	260	—	2
Danimals Lowfat Strawberry	4.4 oz	130	1	1	5	6	24	21	0	200	90	250	—	4
Danimals Lowfat Vanilla	4.4 oz	120	1	1	5	6	23	21	0	200	90	270	—	1
Danimals Lowfat Wild Raspberry	4.4 oz	120	1	1	5	6	22	19	0	200	90	270	—	2
Double Delights Banana Creme Strawberry	6 oz	160	1	1	10	7	32	28	0	200	100	330	—	15
Double Delights Bavarian Creme Raspberry	6 oz	170	1	1	10	7	34	31	0	200	125	330	—	6
Double Delights Cheesecake Cherry	6 oz	170	1	1	10	7	34	30	0	200	100	340	—	4
Double Delights Cheesecake Strawberry	6 oz	170	1	1	10	7	33	39	0	200	100	340	—	15
Double Delights Chocolate Cheesecake	6 oz	220	1	1	10	8	45	42	0	250	150	350	—	6
Double Delights Chocolate Dipped Strawberry	6 oz	210	1	1	10	8	45	41	0	250	150	350	—	15

FOOD	PORTION	CALS	FAT	SAT FAT	CHOL	PROT	CARB	SUGAR	FIBER	CALCI	SOD	POTAS	FOLIC	VIT C
DANNON (CONT.)														
Double Delights Chocolate Eclair	6 oz	220	1	1	10	8	45	42	0	250	150	350	—	6
Double Delights Vanilla Strawberry	6 oz	170	1	1	10	7	33	29	0	200	100	340	—	15
Double Delights Vanilla Peach & Apricot	6 oz	170	1	1	10	7	33	29	0	200	100	330	—	2
Fruit On The Bottom Lowfat Apple Cinnamon	8 oz	240	3	2	15	9	46	45	1	350	140	460	—	2
Fruit On The Bottom Lowfat Blueberry	8 oz	240	3	2	15	9	46	44	1	350	140	460	—	5
Fruit On The Bottom Lowfat Boysenberry	8 oz	240	3	2	15	9	45	42	1	350	150	450	—	4
Fruit On The Bottom Lowfat Cherry	8 oz	240	3	2	15	9	46	44	1	350	135	500	—	6
Fruit On The Bottom Lowfat Minipack Mixed Berry	4.4 oz	130	2	1	10	5	25	24	tr	200	80	250	—	4
Fruit On The Bottom Lowfat Minipack Strawberry	4.4 oz	130	2	1	10	5	25	24	tr	200	75	260	—	6
Fruit On The Bottom Lowfat Mixed Berries	8 oz	240	3	2	15	9	45	43	1	350	150	450	—	6
Fruit On The Bottom Lowfat Orange	8 oz	240	3	2	15	9	45	44	0	350	135	470	—	15
Fruit On The Bottom Lowfat Peach	8 oz	240	3	2	15	9	45	44	1	350	140	450	—	2
Fruit On The Bottom Lowfat Strawberry	8 oz	240	3	2	15	9	46	44	1	350	135	470	—	12
Fruit On The Bottom Lowfat Strawberry Banana	8 oz	240	3	2	15	9	43	40	1	350	140	480	—	15
La Creme Strawberry	1 pkg (4 oz)	140	5	3	20	5	21	18	—	150	75	240	—	—
La Creme Vanilla	1 pkg (4 oz)	140	5	3	20	5	20	18	—	150	75	240	—	—
Light Duets Cherry Cheesecake	6 oz	90	0	0	0	5	18	12	0	260	70	260	—	4
Light Duets Peaches N' Cream	6 oz	90	0	0	0	5	18	13	0	150	70	260	—	4

FOOD	PORTION	CALS	FAT	SAT FAT	CHOL	PROT	CARB	SUGAR	FIBER	CALCI	SOD	POTAS	FOLIC	VIT C
DANNON (CONT.)														
Light Duets Raspberry Royale	6 oz	90	0	0	0	5	17	12	0	150	75	240	—	5
Light Duets Strawberry Cheesecake	6 oz	90	0	0	0	5	18	12	0	150	70	240	—	15
Light 'N Crunchy Mint Chocolate Chip	8 oz	140	0	0	5	8	27	14	0	250	150	330	—	0
Light 'N Crunchy Nonfat Caramel Apple Crunch	8 oz	140	0	0	<5	8	26	14	0	250	340	160	—	0
Light 'N Crunchy Nonfat Lemon Blueberry Cobbler	8 oz	140	0	0	<5	8	25	17	0	250	135	350	—	0
Light 'N Crunchy Nonfat Mocha Cappuccino	8 oz	140	0	0	<5	8	26	14	0	250	150	330	—	0
Light 'N Crunchy Nonfat Raspberry w/ Granola	8 oz	140	0	0	<5	9	26	13	2	250	120	340	—	2
Light 'N Crunchy Nonfat Vanilla Chocolate Crunch	8 oz	130	0	0	<5	8	23	13	0	250	140	340	—	0
Light 'N Fit Vanilla	6 oz	90	0	0	<5	6	16	12	—	150	95	—	—	—
Light Nonfat Banana Cream Pie	8 oz	100	0	0	<5	8	15	9	0	250	120	350	—	0
Light Nonfat Blueberry	8 oz	100	0	0	<5	8	18	12	0	250	115	360	—	0
Light Nonfat Cappuccino	8 oz	100	0	0	5	8	16	9	0	250	120	340	—	0
Light Nonfat Cherry Vanilla	8 oz	100	0	0	<5	8	18	13	0	250	120	390	—	0
Light Nonfat Coconut Cream Pie	8 oz	100	0	0	5	8	16	9	0	250	120	350	—	0
Light Nonfat Creme Caramel	8 oz	100	0	0	<5	8	15	9	0	250	120	350	—	0
Light Nonfat Lemon Chiffon	8 oz	100	0	0	5	8	15	9	0	250	120	340	—	0
Light Nonfat Mint Chocolate Cream Pie	8 oz	100	0	0	<5	8	17	9	0	250	120	350	—	0
Light Nonfat Peach	8 oz	100	0	0	<5	8	16	11	0	250	115	370	—	0
Light Nonfat Raspberry	8 oz	100	0	0	<5	8	17	11	0	250	120	350	—	2

FOOD	PORTION	CALS	FAT	SAT FAT	CHOL	PROT	CARB	SUGAR	FIBER	CALCI	SOD	POTAS	FOLIC	VIT C
DANNON (CONT.)														
Light Nonfat Strawberry	8 oz	100	0	0	<5	8	16	10	0	250	115	370	—	12
Light Nonfat Strawberry Banana	8 oz	100	0	0	<5	8	17	11	0	250	120	380	—	4
Light Nonfat Strawberry Kiwi	8 oz	100	0	0	5	8	16	10	0	250	120	360	—	9
Light Nonfat Tangerine Chiffon	8 oz	100	0	0	5	8	15	9	0	250	120	350	—	0
Lowfat Coffee	8 oz	210	3	2	15	10	36	34	0	400	160	510	—	2
Lowfat Cranberry Raspberry	8 oz	210	3	2	15	10	36	35	0	400	160	510	—	2
Lowfat Lemon	8 oz	210	3	2	15	10	36	35	0	400	160	510	—	2
Lowfat Vanilla	8 oz	210	3	2	15	10	36	34	0	400	160	510	—	2
Minipack Blended Nonfat Blueberry	4.4 oz	120	0	0	5	5	25	22	0	150	80	260	—	2
Minipack Blended Nonfat Cherry	4.4 oz	110	0	0	5	5	24	20	0	150	80	270	—	2
Minipack Blended Nonfat Peach	4.4 oz	120	0	0	5	5	23	21	0	150	80	260	—	4
Minipack Blended Nonfat Raspberry	4.4 oz	120	0	0	5	5	24	21	0	150	80	260	—	4
Minipack Blended Nonfat Strawberry	4.4 oz	120	0	0	5	5	23	20	0	150	85	240	—	1
Minipack Blended Nonfat Strawberry Banana	4.4 oz	120	0	0	5	5	23	20	0	150	85	250	—	4
Sprinkl'ins Cherry Vanilla	1 (4.1 oz)	130	2	1	5	5	24	20	0	150	85	250	—	2
Sprinkl'ins Strawberry	1 (4.1 oz)	130	2	1	5	5	24	20	0	150	85	250	—	2
Sprinkl'ins Strawberry Banana	1 (4.1 oz)	130	2	1	5	5	24	20	0	150	80	250	—	2
Sprinkl'ins Vanilla w/ Cherry Crystals	1 (4.1 oz)	110	1	1	5	5	21	19	0	150	85	240	—	9
Sprinkl'ins Vanilla w/ Orange Crystals	1 (4.1 oz)	110	1	1	5	5	21	19	0	150	85	240	—	9
HORIZON ORGANIC														
Fat Free Apricot Mango	¾ cup (6 oz)	120	0	0	<5	7	23	21	0	250	100	—	—	2
Fat Free Honey	1 cup (8 oz)	160	0	0	<5	9	32	31	0	300	135	—	—	2
JELL-O														
Lowfat Cherry	4.4 oz	130	1	1	10	4	25	22	0	100	65	200	—	0
Lowfat Grape	4.4 oz	130	1	1	10	4	25	22	0	100	65	200	—	0
Lowfat Raspberry	4.4 oz	130	1	1	10	4	25	22	0	100	65	200	—	0
Lowfat Tropical Berry Twist	4.4 oz	130	1	1	10	4	25	22	0	100	65	200	—	0

FOOD	PORTION	CALS	FAT	SAT FAT	CHOL	PROT	CARB	SUGAR	FIBER	CALCI	SOD	POTAS	FOLIC	VIT C
JELL-O (CONT.)														
Lowfat Tropical Punch	4.4 oz	130	1	1	10	4	25	22	0	100	65	200	—	0
Lowfat Watermelon	4.4 oz	130	1	1	10	4	25	22	0	100	65	200	—	0
Lowfat Wild Berry	4.4 oz	130	1	1	10	4	25	22	0	100	65	200	—	0
Lowfat Wild Strawberry	4.4 oz	130	1	1	10	4	25	22	0	100	65	200	—	0
LECARB														
YoCarb Plain	1 pkg (4 oz)	50	3	2	10	5	3	2	—	100	110		—	—
LIGHT N'LIVELY														
Free Blueberry	4.4 oz	70	0	0	5	4	13	10	0	100	55	170	—	0
Free Peach	4.4 oz	70	0	0	5	4	12	9	0	100	65	190	—	0
Free Strawberry	4.4 oz	70	0	0	5	4	12	9	0	100	55	180	—	0
Free Strawberry Banana Cream	4.4 oz	70	0	0	5	4	13	10	0	100	55	190	—	0
Free Strawberry Fruit Cup	4.4 oz	70	0	0	5	4	13	10	0	100	55	180	—	0
Lowfat Blueberry	4.4 oz	130	1	1	10	4	25	23	0	100	60	180	—	0
Lowfat Peach	4.4 oz	130	1	1	10	4	26	22	0	100	65	180	—	0
Lowfat Pineapple	4.4 oz	130	1	1	10	4	26	22	0	100	60	230	—	0
Lowfat Red Raspberry	4.4 oz	120	1	1	10	5	23	20	0	100	65	200	—	0
Lowfat Strawberry	4.4 oz	130	1	1	10	4	26	23	0	100	60	180	—	0
Lowfat Strawberry Banana Cream	4.4 oz	130	1	1	10	4	25	22	0	100	60	190	—	0
Lowfat Strawberry Fruit Cup	4.4 oz	130	1	1	10	4	25	22	0	100	60	200	—	0
OBERWEIS														
Peach	1 pkg (8 oz)	210	3	2	15	10	39	35	0	350	140		—	2
PASCUAL														
Nonfat Cherries & Berries	1 pkg (4.4 oz)	100	0	0	0	4	19	12	5	100	70		—	0
Nonfat Peach	1 pkg (4.4 oz)	100	0	0	0	4	19	12	5	100	70		—	8
SILK														
Organic Soy Strawberry	1 pkg (6 oz)	160	2	0	0	4	31	22	1	500	20		—	3
Soy Apricot Mango	1 pkg	160	2	0	0	4	30	20	1	500	20		—	2
Soy Banana Strawberry	1 pkg	160	2	0	0	4	30	20	1	500	20		—	1
Soy Black Cherry	1 pkg	160	2	0	0	4	29	20	1	500	20		—	0
Soy Blueberry	1 pkg	160	2	0	0	4	29	21	1	500	20		—	0
Soy Key Lime	1 pkg	170	2	0	0	4	30	21	1	500	20		—	0
Soy Lemon	1 pkg	160	2	0	0	4	31	22	1	500	20		—	0
Soy Lemon Kiwi	1 pkg	150	2	0	0	4	29	21	1	500	20		—	6

FOOD	PORTION	CALS	FAT	SAT FAT	CHOL	PROT	CARB	SUGAR	FIBER	CALCI	SOD	POTAS	FOLIC	VIT C
SILK (CONT.)														
Soy Peach	1 pkg	170	2	0	0	4	32	25	1	500	20	—	—	0
Soy Plain	8 oz	120	3	0	0	5	22	12	1	700	30	—	—	0
Soy Raspberry	1 pkg	160	2	0	0	4	30	22	1	500	20	—	—	0
Soy Vanilla	1 pkg (8 oz)	120	2	0	0	4	23	16	1	500	20	—	—	0
SPEGA														
La Natura Low Fat	1 pkg (5.2 oz)	80	1	1	5	6	11	8	0	200	70	—	—	0
STONYFIELD FARM														
Creamy Maple	1 pkg	160	6	4	25	6	19	18	0	250	90	334	—	1
Mocho-Ccino	1 pkg	170	6	4	20	6	23	22	0	250	95	392	—	2
Nonfat Apricot Mango	1 pkg (8 oz)	160	0	0	0	8	31	30	tr	450	125	427	—	4
Nonfat Black Cherry	1 pkg (8 oz)	160	0	0	0	8	31	29	tr	400	130	434	—	2
Nonfat Cappuccino	1 pkg (8 oz)	160	0	0	0	9	31	29	0	450	135	503	—	2
Nonfat Cherry Vanilla	1 pkg (8 oz)	190	0	0	0	7	43	41	tr	400	120	—	—	2
Nonfat Chocolate Underground	1 pkg (8 oz)	200	0	0	0	8	46	45	tr	350	135	—	—	2
Nonfat French Vanilla	1 pkg (8 oz)	180	0	0	0	9	30	29	0	450	135	459	—	4
Nonfat Lotsa Lemon	1 pkg (8 oz)	160	0	0	0	9	30	29	0	400	140	—	—	5
Nonfat Peach	1 pkg (8 oz)	150	0	0	0	8	30	30	tr	450	130	450	—	15
Nonfat Plain	1 pkg (8 oz)	100	08	0	<5	10	15	15	0	450	150	—	—	4
Nonfat Raspberry	1 pkg (8 oz)	160	0	0	0	8	31	28	tr	450	130	418	—	4
Nonfat Strawberry	1 pkg (8 oz)	180	0	0	0	8	32	30	tr	450	130	431	—	4
Organic French Vanilla	1 pkg	170	6	4	20	6	23	22	0	350	85	—	—	2
Organic Wild Blueberry	1 pkg	160	6	4	20	5	22	21	tr	200	85	281	—	1
Organic Lowfat Blueberry	1 pkg (6 oz)	130	2	1	5	5	23	22	1	250	90	295	—	1
Organic Lowfat Luscious Lemon	1 pkg (6 oz)	130	2	1	5	5	23	22	1	350	115	300	—	2
Organic Lowfat Maple Vanilla	1 pkg (6 oz)	120	2	1	6	6	19	19	0	300	90	343	—	1
Organic Lowfat Mocha Latte	1 pkg (6 oz)	120	2	1	5	6	20	19	0	300	85	—	—	2
Organic Lowfat Plain	1 cup (8 oz)	110	2	2	10	9	14	13	0	400	135	487	—	2
Organic Lowfat Raspberry	1 pkg (6 oz)	130	2	1	5	6	23	21	1	250	100	302	—	2
Organic Lowfat Strawberry	1 pkg (6 oz)	130	2	1	5	5	23	22	1	250	115	304	—	4

FOOD	PORTION	CALS	FAT	SAT FAT	CHOL	PROT	CARB	SUGAR	FIBER	CALCI	SOD	POTAS	FOLIC	VIT C
STONYFIELD FARM (CONT.)														
Organic Lowfat Vanilla	1 pkg (6 oz)	120	2	1	5	6	20	20	0	300	100	—	—	2
Strawberries & Cream	1 pkg	160	5	4	20	5	23	22	tr	200	110	290	—	2
Vanilla Truffle	1 pkg	220	5	3	20	7	37	34	tr	250	100	360	—	1
YoSelf Organic Chocolate	1 (4 oz)	110	1	1	0	4	21	19	2	200	65	—	—	0
YoSelf Organic Creme Carmel	1 (4 oz)	110	1	1	5	4	21	19	2	200	65	—	—	0
Yosqueeze Strawberry	1 tube (2 oz)	60	1	1	5	2	11	10	1	100	30	—	—	0
TOTAL														
Greek Yogurt	1 pkg (5 oz)	180	12	6	25	10	10	10	0	300	180	—	—	1
Greek Yogurt 0% Fat	1 pkg (5 oz)	80	0	0	0	15	6	6	0	160	110	—	—	0
Greek Yogurt 1% Fat	1 pkg (5 oz)	120	8	6	25	8	8	8	0	160	120	—	—	0
YOPLAIT														
99% Fat Free Blueberry	6 oz	180	2	1	10	6	34	31	0	200	80	250	—	0
99% Fat Free Boysenberry	6 oz	180	2	1	10	6	34	31	0	200	80	250	—	0
99% Fat Free Cherry	6 oz	180	2	1	10	6	34	31	0	200	80	250	—	0
99% Fat Free Harvest Peach	4 oz	120	1	1	5	4	23	20	0	100	55	170	—	0
99% Fat Free Harvest Peach	6 oz	180	2	1	10	6	34	31	0	200	80	250	—	—
99% Fat Free Key Lime Pie	6 oz	180	2	1	10	6	34	31	0	200	80	250	—	0
99% Fat Free Lemon	6 oz	180	2	1	10	6	34	31	0	200	80	250	—	0
99% Fat Free Mixed Berry	4 oz	120	1	1	5	4	23	20	0	100	55	170	—	0
99% Fat Free Mixed Berry	6 oz	180	2	1	10	6	34	31	0	200	80	250	—	0
99% Fat Free Orange	6 oz	180	2	1	10	6	34	31	0	200	80	250	—	0
99% Fat Free Piña Colada	6 oz	180	2	1	10	6	34	31	0	200	80	250	—	0
99% Fat Free Pineapple	6 oz	180	2	1	10	6	34	31	0	200	80	250	—	0
99% Fat Free Raspberry	6 oz	180	2	1	10	6	34	31	0	200	80	250	—	0
99% Fat Free Strawberry	4 oz	120	1	1	5	4	23	20	0	100	55	170	—	0

FOOD	PORTION	CALS	FAT	SAT FAT	CHOL	PROT	CARB	SUGAR	FIBER	CALCI	SOD	POTAS	FOLIC	VIT C
99% Fat Free Strawberry	6 oz	180	2	1	10	6	43	31	0	200	80	250	—	0
99% Fat Free Strawberry Banana	4 oz	120	1	1	5	4	23	20	0	100	55	170	—	0
99% Fat Free Strawberry Banana	6 oz	180	2	1	10	6	34	31	0	200	80	250	—	0
99% Fat Free Strawberry Cheesecake	6 oz	180	2	1	10	6	34	31	0	200	80	250	—	0
Custard Style Banana	6 oz	190	4	2	15	7	32	28	0	200	100	310	—	0
Custard Style Blueberry	6 oz	190	4	2	15	7	32	28	0	200	100	310	—	0
Custard Style Cherry Vanilla	6 oz	190	4	2	15	7	32	28	0	200	100	310	—	0
Custard Style Key Lime Pie	6 oz	190	4	2	15	7	32	28	0	200	100	310	—	0
Custard Style Lemon	6 oz	190	4	2	15	7	32	28	0	200	100	310	—	0
Custard Style Peaches'n Cream	6 oz	190	4	2	15	7	32	28	0	200	100	310	—	0
Custard Style Raspberry	6 oz	190	4	2	15	7	32	28	0	200	100	310	—	0
Custard Style Raspberry Cheesecake	6 oz	190	4	2	15	7	32	28	0	200	100	310	—	0
Custard Style Strawberry	6 oz	190	4	2	15	7	32	28	0	200	100	310	—	0
Custard Style Strawberry Banana	6 oz	190	4	2	15	7	32	28	0	200	100	310	—	0
Custard Style Strawberry Vanilla	4 oz	120	2	2	10	5	21	19	0	150	70	200	—	0
Custard Style Vanilla	6 oz	190	4	2	15	8	32	27	0	200	95	300	—	0
Go-Gurt Strawberry Banana Burst	1 pkg (2.25 oz)	80	2	1	5	2	12	10	0	100	40	105	—	0
Go-Gurt Watermelon Meltdown	1 pkg (2.25 oz)	80	2	1	5	2	12	10	0	100	40	105	—	0
Light Amaretto Cheesecake	6 oz	90	0	0	5	6	16	10	0	200	95	250	—	0
Light Apricot Mango	6 oz	90	0	0	5	5	16	10	0	200	75	240	—	0

FOOD	PORTION	CALS	FAT	SAT FAT	CHOL	PROT	CARB	SUGAR	FIBER	CALCI	SOD	POTAS	FOLIC	VIT C
YOPLAIT (CONT.)														
Light Banana Cream	6 oz	90	0	0	5	6	16	0	0	200	95	250	—	0
Light Blueberry	6 oz	90	0	0	5	5	16	10	0	200	75	240	—	0
Light Boston Cream Pie	6 oz	90	0	0	5	6	16	10	0	200	95	250	—	0
Light Caramel Apple	6 oz	90	0	0	5	6	16	10	0	200	95	250	—	0
Light Cherry	6 oz	90	0	0	5	5	16	10	0	200	75	240	—	0
Light Key Lime Pie	6 oz	90	0	0	5	6	16	10	0	200	95	250	—	0
Light Lemon Cream Pie	6 oz	90	0	0	5	6	16	10	0	200	95	250	—	0
Light Peach	6 oz	90	0	0	5	5	16	10	0	200	75	240	—	0
Light Peach Melba	6 oz	90	0	0	5	5	16	10	0	200	75	240	—	9
Light Raspberry	6 oz	90	0	0	5	5	16	10	0	200	75	240	—	0
Light Strawberry	6 oz	90	0	0	5	5	16	10	0	200	75	240	—	0
Light Strawberry Banana	6 oz	90	0	0	5	5	16	10	0	200	75	240	—	0
Light White Chocolate Strawberry	6 oz	90	0	0	5	5	16	10	0	200	75	240	—	0
Original Cafe Au Lait	6 oz	170	2	1	10	6	31	27	0	150	80	270	—	0
Original Coconut Cream Pie	6 oz	200	4	3	10	6	35	30	0	200	80	260	—	0
Original French Vanilla	6 oz	180	2	1	10	6	34	30	0	200	90	240	—	0
Trix Rainbow Punch	6 oz	190	2	1	10	6	36	31	0	200	85	270	—	0
Trix Raspberry Rainbow	6 oz	190	2	1	10	6	36	31	0	200	85	270	—	0
Trix Strawberry Banana Bash	6 oz	190	2	1	10	6	36	31	0	200	85	270	—	0
Trix Strawberry Punch	4 oz	130	2	1	5	4	24	20	0	100	55	180	—	0
Trix Triple Cherry	6 oz	190	2	1	10	6	36	31	0	200	85	270	—	0
Trix Watermelon Burst	4 oz	130	2	1	5	4	24	20	0	100	55	180	—	0
Trix Wild Berry Blue	4 oz	130	2	1	5	4	24	20	0	100	55	180	—	0
Whips! Orange Creme	1 pkg (4 oz)	140	3	2	10	5	23	21	—	150	75	220	—	—
Whips! Raspberry Mousse	1 pkg (4 oz)	140	3	2	10	5	23	21	—	150	75	220	—	—

YOGURT DRINKS

FOOD	PORTION	CALS	FAT	SAT FAT	CHOL	PROT	CARB	SUGAR	FIBER	CALCI	SOD	POTAS	FOLIC	VIT C
DANNON														
Frusion Smoothie Peach Passion Fruit	1 bottle (10 oz)	270	4	2	15	8	51	49	0	250	180	430	—	1
Frusion Smoothie Tropical Fruit	1 bottle (10 oz)	270	4	2	15	8	52	49	0	250	130	430	—	4
STONYFIELD														
Smoothie Lowfat Strawberry	1 bottle (8.8 oz)	250	3	2	10	10	46	41	4	400	160	510	—	0
YO-GOAT														
Blueberry	8 oz	150	8	5	30	8	13	7	—	287	135	—	—	2
YOPLAIT														
Nouriche All Flavors	1 bottle (11 oz)	290	0	0	5	10	60	46	6	300	290	580	100	15

YOGURT FROZEN

FOOD	PORTION	CALS	FAT	SAT FAT	CHOL	PROT	CARB	SUGAR	FIBER	CALCI	SOD	POTAS	FOLIC	VIT C
chocolate soft serve	½ cup (4 fl oz)	115	4	3	3	3	18	—	—	106	71	188	8	tr
vanilla soft serve	½ cup (4 fl oz)	114	4	2	2	3	17	16	—	103	63	152	4	1
BREYERS														
Chocolate	½ cup	150	5	3	15	3	23	17	tr	100	50	—	—	0
Vanilla	½ cup	140	5	3	15	3	21	16	0	100	45	—	—	0
Vanilla No Sugar Added	½ cup	100	5	3	20	3	13	6	0	100	60	—	—	0
EDY'S														
Black Cherry Vanilla Swirl	½ cup	90	0	0	0	3	20	14	—	300	45	—	—	—
Caramel Fudge Cosmo	½ cup	140	4	3	10	2	23	18	—	300	50	—	—	—
Caramel Praline Crunch	½ cup	100	0	0	0	3	23	17	—	300	60	—	—	—
Chocolate Decadence	½ cup	120	4	2	10	2	20	14	—	300	45	—	—	—
Chocolate Fudge	½ cup	100	0	0	0	3	22	14	—	300	55	—	—	—
Coffee Fudge Sundae	½ cup	100	0	0	0	3	22	15	—	300	60	—	—	—
Cookies'N Cream	½ cup	120	4	2	10	2	19	14	—	300	45	—	—	—
Heath Toffee Crunch	½ cup	120	4	2	10	2	18	15	—	300	45	—	—	—
Raspberry	½ cup	90	3	2	10	2	16	13	—	200	25	—	—	—
Ultimate Tin Roof Sundae	½ cup	130	4	2	5	3	20	15	—	300	50	—	—	—
Vanilla	½ cup	90	0	0	0	3	19	13	—	300	45	—	—	—
Vanilla Chocolate Swirl	½ cup	90	0	0	0	3	19	13	—	300	45	—	—	—

FOOD	PORTION	CALS	FAT	SAT FAT	CHOL	PROT	CARB	SUGAR	FIBER	CALCI	SOD	POTAS	FOLIC	VIT C
HAAGEN-DAZS														
Lowfat Dulce De Leche	½ cup	190	3	2	5	6	35	25	0	200	75	—	—	0
Nonfat Chocolate	½ cup	140	0	0	<5	7	28	16	tr	200	45	—	—	0
Nonfat Coffee	½ cup	140	0	0	<5	7	29	16	0	200	45	—	—	0
Nonfat Strawberry	½ cup	140	0	0	<5	5	31	20	0	150	40	—	—	6
Nonfat Vanilla	½ cup	140	0	0	<5	6	29	16	0	200	45	—	—	0
Nonfat Vanilla Raspberry Swirl	½ cup	130	0	0	<5	4	29	20	tr	100	30	—	—	1
Nonfat Vanilla Fudge	½ cup	160	0	0	<5	6	34	21	0	150	105	—	—	0
TURKEY HILL														
Black Raspberry	½ cup	110	3	—	10	—	20	—	—	—	60	—	—	—
Caramel Cashew Crunch	½ cup	160	9	—	25	—	18	—	—	—	60	—	—	—
Chocolate Chip Cookie Dough	½ cup	140	5	3	10	3	23	21	0	100	120	—	—	0
Clark Bar	½ cup	140	5	—	10	—	22	—	—	—	95	—	—	—
Fat Free Chocolate Cherry Cordial	½ cup	100	0	0	0	4	24	21	0	100	70	—	—	0
Fat Free Chocolate Marshmallow	½ cup	130	0	0	0	3	30	21	0	80	40	—	—	0
Fat Free Mint Cookie 'N Cream	½ cup	110	0	0	0	4	24	18	0	100	80	—	—	0
Fat Free Neapolitan	½ cup	100	0	0	0	3	22	19	0	100	50	—	—	0
Fat Free Orange Swirl	½ cup	100	0	0	0	—	22	—	—	—	40	—	—	—
Fat Free Vanilla Fudge	½ cup	110	0	0	0	3	24	21	0	100	80	—	—	0
Peach Raspberry	½ cup	110	2	2	10	3	20	20	0	100	60	—	—	0
Tin Roof Sundae	½ cup	140	5	3	10	4	21	20	0	100	100	—	—	0
Vanilla & Chocolate	½ cup	110	3	2	10	3	19	18	0	100	70	—	—	0
Vanilla Bean	½ cup	110	3	2	10	4	17	17	0	100	70	—	—	0
ZUCCHINI														
baby raw	1 (0.5 oz)	3	tr	tr	0	tr	1	—	tr	3	0	73	3	6
canned italian style	½ cup	33	tr	tr	0	1	8	—	—	19	427	312	—	3
frzn cooked	½ cup	19	tr	tr	0	1	4	—	—	19	2	218	9	4
raw sliced	½ cup	9	tr	tr	0	1	2	—	1	10	2	161	14	6
sliced cooked	½ cup	14	tr	tr	0	1	4	—	1	12	2	228	15	4
PROGRESSO														
Italian Style	½ cup (4.2 oz)	50	2	0	0	2	7	4	2	20	400	—	—	6
TAKE-OUT														
indian paalkora	1 serv	46	2	tr	1	2	7	—	2	—	141	—	—	—

PART TWO

RESTAURANT CHAINS

Smart Stuff

Bigger isn't always better.

Supersizing, add-ons, toppings, extras, stuffed, doubles, and "buy one get one free" may cost little, but the extra calories, fat, and sodium you'll be tempted to eat are no bargain.

FOOD	PORTION	CALS	FAT	SAT FAT	CHOL	PROT	CARB	SUGAR	FIBER	CALCI	SOD	POTAS	FOLIC	VIT C
APPLEBEE'S														
DESSERTS														
Apple Betty Cobbler Ala Mode	1 serv	598	22	—	31	7	94	57	2	—	197	—	—	—
Berry Lemon Cheesecake	1 slice	230	7	—	—	—	—	—	2	—	—	—	—	—
Chocolate Raspberry Cake	1 slice	230	3	—	—	—	—	—	3	—	—	—	—	—
Fudge Brownie Sundae	1 serv	739	40	—	66	9	87	39	6	—	332	—	—	—
Low Fat Bikini Banana Strawberry Shortcake	1 serv	248	2	tr	8	6	48	27	2	—	223	—	—	—
Low Fat Brownie Sundae	1 serv	415	2	tr	3	11	82	57	3		417	—	—	—
Low Fat Marble Cheesecake	1 serv	261	2	1	10	10	50	37	4	—	378	—	—	—
MAIN MENU SELECTIONS														
Applebee's Burger w/ Fries	1 serv	1274	79	—	263	55	90	10	7	—	2713	—	—	—
Baja Chicken Rollup	1 serv	490	10	—	—	—	—	—	10	—	—	—	—	—
Basic Hamburger w/ Fries	1 serv	980	58	—	118	31	86	8	6	—	1814	—	—	—
Beef Fajita Quesadilla	1 serv	1205	86	—	159	51	58	5	6	—	2969	—	—	—
Bourbon Street Steak w/ Fried New Potatoes	1 serv	1115	94	—	168	60	50	3	—	—	3542	—	—	—
Grilled Citrus Chicken Salad	1 serv	240	6	—	—	—	—	—	4	—	—	—	—	—
Grilled Tilapia w/ Mango Salsa	1 serv	340	8	—	—	—	—	—	4	—	—	—	—	—
Low Fat Asian Chicken Salad	1 serv (5 oz)	623	9	2	76	35	107	—	14	—	2487	—	—	—
Low Fat Asian Chicken Salad	1 med serv (2.5 oz)	370	6	1	40	19	64	—	7	—	1431	—	—	—
Low Fat Blackened Chicken Salad	1 med serv (2.5 oz)	287	3	1	43	40	27	—	6	—	1763	—	—	—
Low Fat Blackened Chicken Salad	1 serv (5 oz)	411	5	1	82	56	39	—	11	—	2188	—	—	—
Low Fat Garlic Chicken Pasta	1 serv	587	8	2	39	41	89	7	9	—	1551	—	—	—
Low Fat Lemon Chicken Pasta	1 serv	528	11	4	50	33	78	12	8	—	2438	—	—	—

FOOD	PORTION	CALS	FAT	SAT FAT	CHOL	PROT	CARB	SUGAR	FIBER	CALCI	SOD	POTAS	FOLIC	VIT C
Low Fat Quesadilla Chicken Fajita	1 serv	518	11	tr	35	42	63	6	2	—	2244	—	—	—
Low Fat Quesadilla Veggie	1 serv	344	8	tr	8	27	46	4	3	—	1138	—	—	—
Mesquite Chicken Salad	1 serv	200	4	—	—	—	—	—	5	—	—	—	—	—
Mozzarella Stix	8 pieces	963	57	—	64	41	74	—	1	—	1990	—	—	—
Onion Soup Au Gratin	1 serv	150	8	—	—	—	—	—	1	—	—	—	—	—
Quesadillas	1 serv	684	46	—	99	31	40	5	4	—	2175	—	—	—
Riblet Basket w/ Fries	1 serv	1317	92	—	219	78	45	tr	7	—	2697	—	—	—
Salad Dinner w/o Dressing	1 serv	303	18	—	277	22	13	4	3	—	661	—	—	—
Salad Santa Fe Chicken	1 med	724	42	—	96	33	56	12	7	—	2409	—	—	—
Sandwich Bacon Cheese Chicken Grill w/o Fries	1	746	46	—	133	46	36	1	1	—	1722	—	—	—
Sandwich Gyro	1	880	69	—	15	24	44	5	3	—	2015	—	—	—
Sizzling Chicken Skillet	1 serv	360	4	—	—	—	—	—	10	—	—	—	—	—
Stir Fry Chicken	1 serv	566	7	—	76	38	89	24	5	—	2470	—	—	—
Teriyaki Shrimp Skewers	1 serv	260	2	—	—	—	—	—	6	—	—	—	—	—
Tortilla Chicken Melt	1 serv	480	13	—	—	—	—	—	6	—	—	—	—	—

ARBY'S

BEVERAGES

FOOD	PORTION	CALS	FAT	SAT FAT	CHOL	PROT	CARB	SUGAR	FIBER	CALCI	SOD	POTAS	FOLIC	VIT C
Chocolate Shake	1 (14 oz)	480	16	8	45	10	84	—	0	500	370	—	—	2
Hot Chocolate	1 serv (8.6 oz)	110	1	1	0	2	23	—	0	50	120	—	—	0
Jamocha Shake	1 (14 oz)	470	15	7	45	10	82	—	0	500	390	—	—	2
Milk	1 serv (8 oz)	120	5	3	20	8	12	—	0	300	120	—	—	2
Orange Juice	1 serv (10 oz)	140	0	0	0	1	34	—	0	0	0	—	—	78
Strawberry Shake	1 (14 oz)	500	13	8	15	11	87	—	0	350	340	—	—	1
Vanilla Shake	1 (14 oz)	470	15	7	45	10	83	—	0	500	360	—	—	2

BREAKFAST SELECTIONS

FOOD	PORTION	CALS	FAT	SAT FAT	CHOL	PROT	CARB	SUGAR	FIBER	CALCI	SOD	POTAS	FOLIC	VIT C
Add Egg	1 serv (2 oz)	110	9	2	175	5	2	—	0	20	170	—	—	0
Add Swiss Cheese Slice	1 slice (0.5 oz)	45	3	2	10	3	0	—	0	100	220	—	—	0
Biscuit w/ Bacon	1 (3.2 oz)	320	21	5	10	7	27	—	1	40	930	—	—	0
Biscuit w/ Butter	1 (2.9 oz)	280	17	4	0	5	27	—	1	40	780	—	—	0
Biscuit w/ Ham	1 (4.3 oz)	330	20	5	30	12	28	—	1	40	1610	—	—	0
Biscuit w/ Sausage	1 (4.2 oz)	460	33	9	30	10	27	—	1	0	1150	—	—	0

FOOD	PORTION	CALS	FAT	SAT FAT	CHOL	PROT	CARB	SUGAR	FIBER	CALCI	SOD	POTAS	FOLIC	VIT C
Croissant w/ Bacon	1 (2.5 oz)	300	20	11	30	8	28	—	0	0	450	—	—	0
Croissant w/ Ham	1 (3.7 oz)	310	19	11	50	13	29	—	0	—	1130	—	—	—
Croissant w/ Sausage	1 (3.6 oz)	420	32	15	50	11	28	—	0	0	670	—	—	0
French Toast Syrup	1 serv (0.5 oz)	130	0	0	0	0	32	—	0	0	45	—	—	0
Sourdough w/ Bacon	1 (5 oz)	380	7	2	10	14	29	—	2	80	890	—	—	0
Sourdough w/ Ham	1 (4 oz)	220	7	2	30	12	30	—	1	80	1270	—	—	0
Sourdough w/ Sausage	1 (4 oz)	330	19	6	30	10	29	—	1	80	810	—	—	0
Toastix w/o Syrup	1 serv (4.4 oz)	370	17	4	0	7	48	—	4	70	440	—	—	0
DESSERTS														
Apple Turnover Iced	1 (4.5 oz)	420	16	5	0	4	65	—	2	10	230	—	—	3
Cherry Turnover Iced	1 (4.5 oz)	410	16	5	0	4	63	—	1	10	250	—	—	7
MAIN MENU SELECTIONS														
Arby's Sauce	1 serv (0.5 oz)	15	0	0	0	0	4	—	0	0	180	—	—	1
Au Jus Sauce	1 serv (3 oz)	5	1	tr	0	tr	1	—	tr	0	386	—	—	0
Baked Potato Broccoli'N Cheddar	1 (14 oz)	540	24	12	50	12	71	—	7	250	680	—	—	72
Baked Potato Deluxe	1 (13 oz)	650	34	20	90	20	67	—	6	100	750	—	—	36
Baked Potato w/ Butter & Sour Cream	1 (11.2 oz)	500	24	15	55	8	65	—	6	100	170	—	—	30
BBQ Dipping Sauce	1 serv (1 oz)	40	0	0	0	0	10	—	0	0	350	—	—	2
Bronco Berry Sauce	1 serv (1.5 oz)	90	0	0	0	0	23	—	0	0	35	—	—	2
Chicken Finger 4-Pak	1 serv (6.77 oz)	640	38	8	70	31	42	—	0	20	1590	—	—	0
Chicken Finger Snack w/ Curly Fries	1 serv (6.4 oz)	580	32	7	35	19	55	—	3	0	1450	—	—	9
Curly Fries	1 lg (7 oz)	620	30	7	0	8	78	—	7	0	1540	—	—	21
Curly Fries	1 med (4.5 oz)	400	20	5	0	5	50	—	4	0	990	—	—	15
Curly Fries	1 sm (3.8 oz)	310	15	4	0	4	39	—	3	0	770	—	—	12
Curly Fries Cheddar	1 serv (6 oz)	460	24	6	5	6	54	—	4	60	1290	—	—	15
German Mustard	1 pkg (0.25 oz)	5	0	0	0	0	0	—	0	0	60	—	—	0
Homestyle Fries	1 lg (7.5 oz)	560	24	6	0	6	79		6	0	1070	—	—	30
Homestyle Fries	1 med (5 oz)	370	16	4	0	4	53	—	4	0	710	—	—	21
Homestyle Fries	1 sm (4 oz)	300	13	4	0	3	42	—	3	0	570	—	—	15

FOOD	PORTION	CALS	FAT	SAT FAT	CHOL	PROT	CARB	SUGAR	FIBER	CALCI	SOD	POTAS	FOLIC	VIT C
Homestyle Fries Child-Size	1 serv (3 oz)	220	10	3	0	3	32	—	3	0	430	—	—	12
Honey Mustard	1 serv (1 oz)	130	12	2	10	0	5	—	0	0	160	—	—	0
Horsey Sauce	1 pkg (0.5 oz)	60	5	1	5	0	3	—	0	0	150	—	—	0
Jalapeño Bites	1 serv (4 oz)	330	21	9	40	7	30	—	2	40	670	—	—	1
Ketchup	1 pkg (0.3 oz)	10	0	0	0	0	2	—	0	0	100	—	—	0
Marinara Sauce	1 serv (1.5 oz)	35	1	0	0	1	4	—	0	0	260	—	—	6
Mayonnaise	1 pkg (0.4 oz)	90	10	2	10	0	0	—	0	0	65	—	—	0
Mayonnaise Light Cholesterol Free	1 pkg (0.4 oz)	20	2	0	0	0	1	—	0	0	110	—	—	0
Mozzarella Sticks	4 (4.8 oz)	470	29	14	60	18	34	—	2	400	1330	—	—	1
Onion Petals	1 serv (4 oz)	410	24	4	0	4	43	—	2	40	300	—	—	0
Potato Cakes	2 (3.5 oz)	250	16	4	0	2	26	—	3	0	490	—	—	6
Sandwich Chicken Bacon'N Swiss	1 (7.4 oz)	610	33	8	110	31	49	—	2	150	1550	—	—	2
Sandwich Chicken Breast Fillet	1 (7.2 oz)	540	30	5	90	24	47	—	2	80	1160	—	—	4
Sandwich Chicken Cordon Bleu	1 (8.4 oz)	630	35	8	120	34	47	—	2	150	1820	—	—	1
Sandwich Grilled Chicken Deluxe	1 (8.7 oz)	450	22	4	110	29	37	—	2	60	1050	—	—	1
Sandwich Hot Ham 'N Swiss	1 (5.9 oz)	340	13	5	90	23	35	—	1	150	1450	—	—	1
Sandwich Market Fresh Roast Beef & Swiss	1 (12.5 oz)	810	42	13	130	37	73	—	5	350	1780	—	—	2
Sandwich Market Fresh Roast Beef Ranch & Bacon	1 (13.5 oz)	880	44	10	155	48	74	—	5	900	2320	—	—	2
Sandwich Market Fresh Roast Chicken Caesar	1 (12.7 oz)	820	38	9	140	43	75	—	5	350	2160	—	—	9
Sandwich Market Fresh Roast Ham & Swiss	1 (12.5 oz)	730	34	8	125	36	74	—	5	350	2180	—	—	4
Sandwich Market Fresh Roast Turkey & Swiss	1 (12.5 oz)	760	33	6	130	43	75	—	5	350	1920	—	—	2
Sandwich Market Fresh Ultimate BLT	1 (10.5 oz)	820	49	11	110	24	72	—	5	40	1480	—	—	15
Sandwich Roast Beef Arby-Q	1 (6.4 oz)	360	14	4	70	16	40	—	2	80	1530	—	—	5

FOOD	PORTION	CALS	FAT	SAT FAT	CHOL	PROT	CARB	SUGAR	FIBER	CALCI	SOD	POTAS	FOLIC	VIT C
Sandwich Roast Beef Beef'N Cheddar	1 (6.9 oz)	480	24	8	90	23	43	—	2	100	1240	—	—	1
Sandwich Roast Beef Big Montana	1 (11 oz)	630	32	15	155	47	41	—	3	80	2080	—	—	0
Sandwich Roast Beef Giant	1 (7.9 oz)	480	23	10	110	32	41	—	3	60	1440	—	—	0
Sandwich Roast Beef Junior	1 (4.4 oz)	310	13	5	70	16	34	—	2	60	740	—	—	0
Sandwich Roast Beef Melt w/ Cheddar	1 (5.2 oz)	340	15	5	70	16	36	—	2	80	890	—	—	0
Sandwich Roast Beef Regular	1 (5.4 oz)	350	16	6	85	21	34	—	2	60	950	—	—	0
Sandwich Roast Beef Super	1 (8.5 oz)	470	23	7	85	22	47	—	3	80	1130	—	—	1
Sandwich Roast Chicken Club	1 (8.4 oz)	520	28	7	115	29	38	—	2	150	1440	—	—	2
Sub Sandwich French Dip	1 (10 oz)	440	18	8	100	28	42	—	2	80	1680	—	—	1
Sub Sandwich Hot Ham'N Swiss	1 (9.7 oz)	530	27	8	110	29	45	—	3	300	1860	—	—	2
Sub Sandwich Italian	1 (11 oz)	780	53	15	120	29	49	—	3	250	2440	—	—	2
Sub Sandwich Philly Beef'N Swiss	1 (10.8 oz)	700	42	15	130	36	46	—	4	300	1940	—	—	9
Sub Sandwich Roast Beef	1 (11.6 oz)	760	48	16	130	35	47	—	3	300	2230	—	—	4
Sub Sandwich Turkey	1 (10.6 oz)	630	37	9	100	26	51	—	2	200	2170	—	—	2
Tangy Southwest Sauce	1 serv (1.5 oz)	250	26	5	30	0	3	—	0	0	790	—		0
SALAD DRESSINGS														
Bleu Cheese	1 serv (2 oz)	300	31	6	45	2	3	—	0	20	580	—	—	0
Buttermilk Ranch	1 serv (2 oz)	290	30	5	25	1	3	—	0	40	580	—	—	0
Buttermilk Ranch Light	1 serv (2 oz)	100	6	1	0	1	12	—	1	0	480	—	—	0
Caesar	1 serv (2 oz)	310	34	5	60	1	1	—	0	0	470	—	—	1
Honey French	1 serv (2 oz)	290	24	4	0	0	18	—	tr	0	410	—	—	0
Italian Reduced Calorie	1 serv (2 oz)	25	1	1	0	0	3	—	tr	0	1030	—	—	0
Italian Parmesan	1 serv (2 oz)	240	24	4	0	1	4	—	0	20	950	—	—	1
Thousand Island	1 serv (2 oz)	290	28	5	35	1	9	—	0	0	480	—	—	0

FOOD	PORTION	CALS	FAT	SAT FAT	CHOL	PROT	CARB	SUGAR	FIBER	CALCI	SOD	POTAS	FOLIC	VIT C
SALADS AND SALAD BARS														
Caesar Side Salad	1 (5 oz)	45	2	1	5	4	4	—	2	40	95	—	—	27
Caesar Salad w/o Dressing	1 serv (8 oz)	90	4	3	10	7	8	—	3	200	170	—	—	42
Chicken Finger w/o Dressing	1 serv (13 oz)	570	34	9	65	30	39	—	3	60	1300	—	—	42
Croutons Seasoned	1 serv (0.25 oz)	30	1	0	0	1	5	—	1	0	70	—	—	0
Croutons Cheese & Garlic	1 serv (0.63 oz)	100	6	—	—	3	10	—	0	—	138	—	—	—
Garden Salad	1 (12.3 oz)	70	1	0	0	4	14	—	6	80	45	—	—	42
Grilled Chicken	1 serv (16.3 oz)	210	5	2	65	30	14	—	6	80	800	—	—	42
Grilled Chicken Caesar w/o Dressing	1 serv (12 oz)	230	8	4	80	33	8	—	3	200	920	—	—	42
Roast Chicken	1 serv (14.8 oz)	160	3	0	40	20	15	—	6	80	700	—	—	42
Side Salad	1 (5.7 oz)	25	0	0	0	2	5	—	2	20	20	—	—	9
Turkey Club Salad w/o Dressing	1 serv (12 oz)	350	21	10	90	33	9	—	3	350	920	—	—	42

AU BON PAIN

FOOD	PORTION	CALS	FAT	SAT FAT	CHOL	PROT	CARB	SUGAR	FIBER	CALCI	SOD	POTAS	FOLIC	VIT C
BAKED SELECTIONS														
Bagel Cinnamon Crisp	1 (6 oz)	540	7	1	0	12	123	44	4	100	470	—	—	1
Baguette	1 loaf (10.6 oz)	680	3	0	0	28	136	2	6	100	1820	—	—	24
Bread Stick	1 (2.3 oz)	200	3	0	0	7	37	3	2	20	610	—	—	0
Cinnamon Roll	1 (4 oz)	300	5	2	20	7	60	25	2	60	280	—	—	6
Cookie Chocolate Chip	1 (2 oz)	230	7	4	20	3	39	23	1	40	125	—	—	0
Cookie Chocolate Chunk Macadamia	1 (2 oz)	250	13	4	25	3	31	17	1	40	230	—	—	0
Cookie Gingerbread Man w/ Raisins & Icing	1 (2.7 oz)	280	7	2	30	4	52	28	tr	20	250	—	—	0
Cookie Oatmeal Raisin	1 (2 oz)	210	6	2	20	3	38	13	2	20	190	—	—	0
Cookie Peanut Butter	1 (2 oz)	240	12	3	20	6	21	16	2	20	250	—	—	0
Cookie Shortbread	1 (2.3 oz)	240	7	4	15	5	44	12	1	40	260	—	—	0
Cookie Walnut Raisin	1 (2 oz)	250	13	4	20	4	31	17	2	20	210	—	—	0
Cookie English Toffee	1 (2 oz)	230	7	4	35	3	38	22	tr	20	200	—	—	0
Creme De Fleur	1 serv (5.55 oz)	470	19	11	70	12	69	23	2	60	530	—	—	9
Croissant Almond	1 (4.7 oz)	480	25	9	95	12	58	18	3	100	400	—	—	9
Croissant Apple	1 (3.5 oz)	200	3	2	20	5	40	16	2	40	200	—	—	30

FOOD	PORTION	CALS	FAT	SAT FAT	CHOL	PROT	CARB	SUGAR	FIBER	CALCI	SOD	POTAS	FOLIC	VIT C
Croissant Chocolate	1 (3.1 oz)	330	10	6	20	8	53	23	3	60	250	—	—	6
Croissant Cinnamon Raisin	1 (3.8 oz)	300	5	3	20	8	60	13	2	60	300	—	—	6
Croissant Raspberry Cheese	1 (3.6 oz)	290	9	5	45	8	47	17	1	40	310	—	—	6
Croissant Sweet Cheese	1 (3.6 oz)	320	12	7	60	8	46	15	1	40	350	—	—	6
Danish Cranberry	1 (4.5 oz)	350	9	4	45	7	59	25	2	60	360	—	—	9
Danish Lemon	1 (4.3 oz)	340	9	4	45	8	59	23	5	80	320	—	—	18
Danish Sweet Cheese	1 (4.2 oz)	390	16	7	70	9	55	21	1	60	380	—	—	9
Focaccia	1 piece (5.4 oz)	430	16	2	0	12	61	2	3	20	760	—	—	2
Four Grain Bread	1 serv (4.7 oz)	400	4	1	0	18	74	2	3	80	1110	—	—	24
French Roll	1 (4.2 oz)	260	1	0	0	11	53	0	2	60	710	—	—	15
French Roll Roast Beef	1 (11 oz)	540	19	4	80	39	58	1	3	100	1600	—	—	30
Hearth Roll	1 (3 oz)	210	2	1	0	10	38	1	2	20	430	—	—	6
Holiday Cookie w/ Icing & Sprinkles	1 (1.6 oz)	150	3	1	10	2	31	14	0	20	70	—	—	0
Loaf Multigrain	1 slice (1.8 oz)	130	1	0	0	6	24	0	1	40	360	—	—	12
Muffin Banana Walnut	1 (5.4 oz)	430	21	4	45	8	57	27	2	20	380	—	—	4
Muffin Blueberry	1 (5.6 oz)	470	15	3	90	8	79	44	2	40	450	—	—	1
Muffin Bran Raisin	1 (5.5 oz)	400	12	5	50	9	77	31	8	80	1060	—	—	1
Muffin Carrot	1 (5.8 oz)	520	25	5	55	9	67	38	4	60	780	—	—	5
Muffin Corn	1 (5.7 oz)	390	16	3	60	7	56	26	2	20	500	—	—	2
Muffin Cranberry Walnut	1 (5.4 oz)	500	27	5	50	9	57	26	3	60	430	—	—	4
Muffin Milk Chocolate Chunk	1 (5.3 oz)	530	23	8	65	9	77	42	3	80	390	—	—	0
Muffin Pumpkin	1 (6 oz)	510	18	3	65	9	74	38	3	80	350	—	—	2
Muffin Low Fat 3 Berry	1 (4.4 oz)	270	3	0	25	4	58	29	2	60	300	—	—	5
Muffin Low Fat Chocolate Cake	1 (4.2 oz)	470	0	0	0	0	117	113	0	0	—	—	—	0
Parisienne Loaf	1 loaf (19 oz)	1210	5	1	0	50	244	2	11	400	3220	—	—	66
Petit Pain	1 (2.9 oz)	180	1	0	0	7	37	0	2	40	490	—	—	12
Roll Braided w/ Topping	1 (10 oz)	430	14	3	40	13	63	8	3	80	730	—	—	9
Roll Pecan	1 (6 oz)	620	24	6	15	11	94	40	3	100	470	—	—	9
Sandwich Loaf Country White	1 serv (1.75 oz)	110	1	0	0	5	23	0	1	0	290	—	—	0
Sandwich Loaf Tomato Herb	1 serv (1.75 oz)	120	1	0	0	5	27	0	1	20	300	—	—	6

FOOD	PORTION	CALS	FAT	SAT FAT	CHOL	PROT	CARB	SUGAR	FIBER	CALCI	SOD	POTAS	FOLIC	VIT C
Scone Chocolate Walnut	1 (4 oz)	420	19	8	55	8	56	27	3	60	125	—	—	0
Scone Cranberry Orange Almond	1 (4 oz)	400	15	7	77	8	60	26	3	60	190	—	—	4
Scone Maple Oat Pecan Date	1 (4 oz)	410	17	8	60	7	58	27	3	40	170	—	—	0
Scone Orange	1 (4.2 oz)	370	13	7	115	10	56	11	2	80	310	—	—	2
Shortbread Heart ½ Chocolate	1 (2.7 oz)	290	10	6	20	6	51	13	1	40	280	—	—	0
Shortbread Heart w/ Red Sugar	1 (2.5 oz)	270	7	4	15	5	51	19	1	40	260	—	—	0
Sourdough Bagel Asiago Cheese	1 (4.8 oz)	340	5	3	15	16	57	5	2	150	560	—	—	0
Sourdough Bagel Cheddar Scallion	1 (4.1 oz)	310	5	3	10	15	51	5	2	200	610	—	—	1
Sourdough Bagel Cinnamon Crisp	1 (4.6 oz)	360	5	1	0	11	52	13	3	40	430	—	—	0
Sourdough Bagel Cinnamon Raisin	1 (4.5 oz)	300	1	0	0	11	65	4	3	40	440	—	—	1
Sourdough Bagel Cranberry Nut	1 (4.7 oz)	400	7	1	0	12	73	15	6	40	440	—	—	5
Sourdough Bagel Double Cheddar Jalapeño	1 serv (4.1 oz)	320	6	4	20	14	50	5	2	140	580	—	—	0
Sourdough Bagel Dutch Apple	1 (4.7 oz)	380	3	1	0	11	80	22	4	40	440	—	—	0
Sourdough Bagel Everything	1 (4.4 oz)	330	3	0	0	13	54	5	3	40	710	—	—	0
Sourdough Bagel Focaccia	1 (4.1 oz)	320	5	1	0	12	61	5	3	40	990	—	—	1
Sourdough Bagel Honey 9 Grain	1 (4.8 oz)	310	2	0	0	12	66	5	6	20	490	—	—	0
Sourdough Bagel Onion	1 (4.4 oz)	320	1	0	0	12	67	8	3	40	480	—	—	5
Sourdough Bagel Plain	1 (4 oz)	300	1	0	0	12	61	5	3	20	480	—	—	0
Sourdough Bagel Poppy Seed	1 (4.4 oz)	330	3	0	0	13	64	5	3	100	480	—	—	0
Sourdough Bagel Sesame	1 (4.4 oz)	340	4	1	0	13	64	5	3	80	480	—	—	0
Sourdough Bagel Wild Blueberry	1 (4.1 oz)	280	1	0	0	10	58	7	3	20	410	—	—	2
Streudel Cherry	1 serv (4 oz)	380	23	2	0	4	37	—	tr	20	90	—	—	0
Streudel Apple	1 serv (4.35 oz)	400	23	0	0	4	48	18	tr	0	110	—	—	0

FOOD	PORTION	CALS	FAT	SAT FAT	CHOL	PROT	CARB	SUGAR	FIBER	CALCI	SOD	POTAS	FOLIC	VIT C
SALADS AND SALAD BARS														
Caesar w/o Dressing	1 serv (7.8 oz)	240	12	6	30	13	19	2	4	350	370	—	—	42
Chef's	1 serv (10.3 oz)	290	15	7	65	27	11	7	3	300	1290	—	—	12
Chicken Caesar	1 serv (10.2 oz)	380	18	8	85	34	19	2	4	350	420	—	—	42
Chicken Oriental	1 serv (8.6 oz)	220	6	2	60	24	16	8	5	40	75	—	—	21
Chicken Pesto Salad	1 serv (8 oz)	400	23	6	105	40	7	2	2	250	310	—	—	5
Garden	1 serv (9.3 oz)	160	5	1	0	6	26	5	5	60	320	—	—	15
Garden Side	1 serv (5.1 oz)	90	2	1	0	3	14	3	3	40	160	—	—	9
Gorgonzola & Walnut	1 serv (5 oz)	330	28	7	25	11	8	3	5	200	410	—	—	5
Mozzarella & Red Pepper Salad	1 serv (10.5 oz)	360	25	16	90	23	10	6	2	700	380	—	—	66
Tuna	1 serv (13.2 oz)	440	24	4	35	27	28	7	5	80	710		—	18
SANDWICHES AND FILLINGS														
Chicken Tarragon	1 serv (4 oz)	240	17	3	65	20	1	1	0	20	170	—	—	0
Club Hot Roasted Turkey	1 (11.7 oz)	630	28	9	80	43	53	3	3	350	2290	—	—	21
Country Ham	1 serv (3.7 oz)	150	7	3	55	21	1	1	0	0	1370	—	—	1
Cracked Pepper Chicken	1 serv (3.9 oz)	140	2	0	72	27	2	0	0	0	184	—	—	19
Cream Cheese Plain	1 serv (2 oz)	190	10	11	55	4	0	0	0	0	210	—	—	0
Cream Cheese Reduced Fat Honey Walnut	1 serv (2 oz)	150	10	7	35	4	10	10	0	40	180	—	—	0
Cream Cheese Reduced Fat Sundried Tomato	1 serv (2 oz)	140	12	7	40	5	3	2	0	40	410	—	—	1
Cream Cheese Reduced Fat Veggie	1 serv (2 oz)	140	12	7	40	6	3	1	0	40	360	—	—	0
Croissant Spinach & Cheese	1 (3.6 oz)	220	9	5	35	9	29	4	2	150	360	—	—	6
Croque Madame	1 (11 oz)	570	22	15	75	40	53	5	3	700	1580	—	—	9
Croque Monsieur	1 (11 oz)	590	25	16	85	39	53	5	3	700	1740	—	—	12
Egg On A Bagel	1 serv (7.1 oz)	500	5	1	120	29	64	6	4	40	880	—	—	0
Egg On A Bagel w/ Bacon	1 serv (7.6 oz)	580	12	4	130	34	84	6	4	60	1110	—	—	0
Egg On A Bagel w/ Cheese	1 serv (7.85 oz)	590	12	5	145	25	84	6	4	200	1020	—	—	0
Egg On A Bagel w/ Cheese & Bacon	1 serv (8.35 oz)	670	19	7	155	39	84	6	4	200	1250	—	—	0
Focaccia Chicken & Mozzarella	1 serv (13.75 oz)	800	14	2	125	93	73	4	6	600	2430	—	—	18

FOOD	PORTION	CALS	FAT	SAT FAT	CHOL	PROT	CARB	SUGAR	FIBER	CALCI	SOD	POTAS	FOLIC	VIT C
Focaccia Chicken Tarragon w/ Field Greens	1 (12.5 oz)	870	47	8	115	47	54	3	4	60	1080	—	—	15
Focaccia Garden Vegetable Goat Cheese w/ Artichoke Spread	1 (14.25 oz)	570	21	6	25	20	75	5	5	150	1210	—	—	66
Focaccia Hickory Smoked Ham & Brie	1 (13.3 oz)	620	27	9	100	51	72	5	5	200	2320	—	—	21
Focaccia Smoked Turkey & Swiss w/ Cilantro	1 (13.25 oz)	810	40	14	90	42	68	4	4	450	2280	—	—	15
Fo-Ca-Cha-Cha Chicken	1 serv (11.15 oz)	730	17	3	110	68	75	5	9	100	2030	—	—	444
French Roll Ham	1 (11 oz)	390	16	3	65	32	58	3	3	80	2430	—	—	30
French Roll Hot Grilled Chicken	1 (11 oz)	620	23	5	100	46	57	1	3	100	1220	—	—	30
French Roll Hot Roast Turkey	1 (11 oz)	500	15	2	55	33	59	1	3	80	2020	—	—	30
French Roll Tuna	1 (10.6 oz)	550	21	3	35	33	58	3	4	100	1100	—	—	36
Grilled Chicken	1 serv (3.9 oz)	140	2	0	72	27	2	0	0	0	184	—	—	19
Hot Croissant Spinach & Cheese	1 (4 oz)	290	9	5	45	15	39	5	1	150	630	—	—	6
Pane Bagniate	1 (12 oz)	670	28	5	30	34	71	6	6	150	1220	—	—	15
Roast Beef	1 serv (3.7 oz)	140	5	0	50	22	1	0	0	20	550	—	—	0
Sandwich Arizona Chicken	1 (12 oz)	600	15	6	120	61	56	2	4	400	1390	—	—	30
Sandwich Cheese	1 (7.2 oz)	590	26	18	60	35	54	0	2	800	920	—	—	15
Sandwich Fresh Mozzarella Tomato & Pesto	1 (11 oz)	790	43	21	100	38	60	4	3	1000	1140	—	—	30
Sandwich Honey Dijon Chicken	1 (13.6 oz)	750	24	9	145	66	65	11	3	300	2410	—	—	30
Sandwich Thai Chicken	1 (11.4 oz)	550	12	3	95	47	62	4	3	100	1080	—	—	24
Tuna Salad	1 serv (4.5 oz)	360	29	5	50	21	3	2	1	20	520	—	—	1
Turkey Breast	1 serv (3.7 oz)	120	1	0	20	24	1	0	0	0	1110	—	—	0
Wrap Chicken Caesar	1 (10.5 oz)	640	26	9	115	43	61	2	5	350	920	—	—	15
Wrap Fields & Feta	1 (13.5 oz)	620	19	5	15	22	100	6	14	150	950	—	—	552
Wrap Honey Smoked Turkey	1 (15 oz)	520	7	1	35	36	85	14	11	60	1460	—	—	492

FOOD	PORTION	CALS	FAT	SAT FAT	CHOL	PROT	CARB	SUGAR	FIBER	CALCI	SOD	POTAS	FOLIC	VIT C
Wrap Roast Beef & Brie	1 (14 oz)	570	28	11	125	47	64	3	6	150	1160	—	—	24
SOUPS														
Autumn Pumpkin	1 serv (8 oz)	170	9	5	20	3	18	2	5	40	770	—	—	1
Black Bean	1 serv (8 oz)	180	1	0	0	11	33	2	18	—	910	—	—	—
Chicken Florentine	1 serv (8 oz)	140	8	4	30	4	14	2	1	—	660	—	—	—
Chicken Noodle	1 serv (8 oz)	100	2	1	15	8	12	2	1	—	760	—	—	—
Clam Chowder	1 serv (8 oz)	220	15	6	35	8	16	1	1	—	780	—	—	—
Corn & Green Chili Bisque	1 serv (8 oz)	200	10	6	30	5	21	4	2	—	1130	—	—	—
Corn Chowder	1 serv (8 oz)	270	15	9	40	6	28	4	2	—	580	—	—	—
Curried Rice & Lentil	1 serv (8 oz)	140	2	0	0	7	24	2	5	—	1220	—	—	—
French Moroccan Tomato Lentil	1 serv (8 oz)	130	2	1	0	7	22	4	7	—	550	—	—	—
Garden Vegetable	1 serv (8 oz)	50	1	0	0	2	8	3	2	—	720	—	—	—
Low Sodium Mediterranean Pepper	1 serv (12 oz)	280	6	0	0	12	44	4	10	80	640	—	—	468
Low Sodium Southwest Vegetable	1 serv (12 oz)	220	5	0	0	8	34	4	6	160	380	—	—	246
Old Fashioned Tomato	1 serv (8 oz)	140	6	2	10	4	19	11	2	—	1080	—	—	—
Pasta E Fagioli	1 serv (8 oz)	240	7	2	5	10	36	3	7	—	780	—	—	—
Potato Cheese	1 serv (8 oz)	190	10	1	5	5	21	2	1	60	910	—	—	12
Potato Leek	1 serv (8 oz)	200	13	8	45	4	18	2	2	—	1060	—	—	12
Red Beans & Rice	1 serv (8 oz)	200	5	1	10	11	31	2	12	—	690	—	—	—
Soup Bread Bowl	1 (9.25 oz)	600	3	0	0	26	118	3	5	150	1700	—	—	36
Southern Black Eyed Pea	1 serv (8 oz)	320	2	0	5	19	56	4	20	—	670	—	—	—
Split Pea	1 serv (8 oz)	160	1	0	5	12	27	2	9	—	800	—	—	—
Tomato Florentine	1 serv (8 oz)	120	3	1	5	5	17	5	2	—	1050	—	—	—
Tuscan Vegetable	1 serv (8 oz)	140	4	2	5	6	22	2	3	—	750	—	—	—
Vegetable Beef Barley	1 serv (8 oz)	110	3	1	10	7	14	2	3	—	1070	—	—	—
Vegetarian Lentil	1 serv (8 oz)	120	1	0	0	7	21	2	8	—	860	—	—	—
Vegetarian Chili	1 serv (8 oz)	170	2	0	0	9	31	3	15	—	940	—	—	—
Wild Mushroom Bisque	1 serv (8 oz)	140	7	2	5	4	16	3	2	—	1190	—	—	—

AUNTIE ANNE'S

FOOD	PORTION	CALS	FAT	SAT FAT	CHOL	PROT	CARB	SUGAR	FIBER	CALCI	SOD	POTAS	FOLIC	VIT C
BEVERAGES														
Dutch Smoothie Piña Colada	1 (14 oz)	260	8	5	30	3	44	41	0	80	90	—	—	5

FOOD	PORTION	CALS	FAT	SAT FAT	CHOL	PROT	CARB	SUGAR	FIBER	CALCI	SOD	POTAS	FOLIC	VIT C
Dutch Ice Blue Raspberry	1 (14 oz)	165	0	0	0	0	38	35	0	20	20	—	—	0
Dutch Ice Grape	1 (14 oz)	180	0	0	0	0	43	41	0	0	20	—	—	0
Dutch Ice Kiwi Banana	1 (14 oz)	190	0	0	0	0	44	41	0	10	30	—	—	2
Dutch Ice Lemonade	1 (14 oz)	315	0	0	0	0	77	77	0	0	0	—	—	7
Dutch Ice Mocha	1 (14 oz)	400	10	9	0	0	74	52	0	0	100	—	—	0
Dutch Ice Orange Creme	1 (14 oz)	280	0	0	0	0	64	59	0	10	35	—	—	11
Dutch Ice Piña Colada	1 (14 oz)	220	0	0	0	0	53	50	0	0	15	—	—	10
Dutch Ice Strawberry	1 (14 oz)	220	0	0	0	0	50	48	0	10	40	—	—	4
Dutch Ice Wild Cherry	1 (14 oz)	210	0	0	0	0	48	45	0	0	25	—	—	0
Dutch Shake Chocolate	1 (14 oz)	580	27	18	105	10	75	67	0	300	380	—	—	0
Dutch Shake Coffee	1 (14 oz)	590	27	18	105	10	77	70	0	300	304	—	—	0
Dutch Shake Strawberry	1 (14 oz)	610	27	18	105	10	78	74	0	300	304	—	—	0
Dutch Shake Vanilla	1 (14 oz)	510	27	17	105	10	58	54	0	300	300	—	—	0
Dutch Smoothie Blue Raspberry	1 (14 oz)	230	8	5	30	3	34	33	0	100	100	—	—	0
Dutch Smoothie Grape	1 (14 oz)	230	8	5	30	3	36	35	0	80	100	—	—	0
Dutch Smoothie Kiwi Banana	1 (14 oz)	240	8	5	30	3	38	35	0	100	100	—	—	1
Dutch Smoothie Lemonade	1 (14 oz)	300	8	5	30	3	53	51	0	80	80	—	—	4
Dutch Smoothie Mocha	1 (14 oz)	330	13	9	30	3	50	39	0	80	130	—	—	0
Dutch Smoothie Orange Creme	1 (14 oz)	280	8	5	30	3	46	44	0	100	100	—	—	5
Dutch Smoothie Strawberry	1 (14 oz)	250	8	5	30	3	40	39	0	100	100	—	—	1
Dutch Smoothie Wild Cherry	1 (14 oz)	250	8	5	30	3	41	39	0	80	90	—	—	0
Lemonade	1 (22 oz)	180	0	0	0	0	43	43	0	0	0	—	—	7
Lemonade Strawberry	1 (22 oz)	190	0	0	0	0	48	48	0	0	0	—	—	6
DIPPING SAUCES														
Caramel Dip	1 serv (1.5 oz)	135	3	2	5	1	27	21	0	20	110	—	—	0
Cheese Sauce	1 serv (1.25 oz)	100	8	4	10	3	4	3	0	100	510	—	—	0
Chocolate Dip	1 serv (1.25 oz)	130	4	2	2	1	24	12	1	20	65	—	—	0

FOOD	PORTION	CALS	FAT	SAT FAT	CHOL	PROT	CARB	SUGAR	FIBER	CALCI	SOD	POTAS	FOLIC	VIT C
Cream Cheese Light	1 serv (1.25 oz)	70	6	4	25	3	1	1	0	20	140	—	—	0
Cream Cheese Strawberry	1 serv (1.25 oz)	110	10	6	35	2	4	3	0	20	105	—	—	1
Hot Salsa Cheese	1 serv (1.25 oz)	100	8	4	10	2	4	4	0	100	550	—	—	1
Marinara Sauce	1 serv (1.25 oz)	10	0	0	0	0	4	2	0	0	180	—	—	0
Sweet Mustard	1 serv (1.25 oz)	60	2	1	40	tr	8	8	0	0	120	—	—	0
PRETZELS														
Almond	1	400	8	5	20	9	72	15	2	20	400	—	—	0
Almond w/o Butter	1	350	2	1	0	9	72	15	2	20	390	—	—	0
Cinnamon Raisin w/o Butter	1	350	2	0	0	9	74	16	2	20	410	—	—	0
Cinnamon Sugar	1	450	9	5	25	8	83	26	3	30	430	—	—	0
Garlic	1	350	5	3	10	9	68	9	2	20	850	—	—	0
Garlic w/o Butter	1	320	1	0	0	9	66	9	2	20	830	—	—	0
Glazin' Raisin	1	510	4	2	10	11	107	38	4	30	480	—	—	0
Glazin' Raisin w/o Butter	1	470	1	0	0	11	104	37	3	30	460	—	—	0
Jalapeño	1	310	5	3	10	8	59	9	2	20	940	—	—	0
Jalapeño w/o Butter	1	270	1	0	0	8	58	8	2	20	780	—	—	0
Maple Crumb	1	550	6	2	10	10	112	42	3	30	550	—	—	0
Maple Crumb w/o Butter	1	520	3	0	0	10	112	42	3	30	550	—	—	0
Original	1	370	4	2	10	10	72	10	2	30	930	—	—	0
Original w/o Butter	1	340	1	0	0	10	72	10	3	30	900	—	—	0
Parmesan Herb	1	440	13	7	30	10	72	10	9	60	660	—	—	1
Parmesan Herb w/o Butter	1	390	5	3	10	11	74	10	4	80	780	—	—	1
Sesame	1	410	12	4	15	12	64	9	7	20	860	—	—	0
Sesame w/o Butter	1	350	6	1	0	11	63	9	3	20	840	—	—	0
Sour Cream & Onion w/o Butter	1	310	1	0	0	9	66	9	2	20	920	—	—	0
Sour Cream & Onion	1	340	5	3	10	9	66	10	2	40	930	—	—	0
Stixs	4	247	3	1	7	7	48	7	2	20	620	—	—	0
Stixs w/o Butter	4	227	1	0	0	7	48	7	2	20	600	—	—	0
Whole Wheat	1	370	5	2	10	11	72	10	7	30	1120	—	—	0
Whole Wheat w/o Butter	1	350	2	0	0	11	72	10	7	30	1100	—	—	0

BAJA FRESH

FOOD	PORTION	CALS	FAT	SAT FAT	CHOL	PROT	CARB	SUGAR	FIBER	CALCI	SOD	POTAS	FOLIC	VIT C
Baja Burrito Chicken	1 serv	820	35	14	130	54	75	—	11	—	—	—	—	—

FOOD	PORTION	CALS	FAT	SAT FAT	CHOL	PROT	CARB	SUGAR	FIBER	CALCI	SOD	POTAS	FOLIC	VIT C
Baja Burrito Steak	1 serv	920	42	17	155	59	75	—	9	—	—	—	—	—
Black Beans	1 serv	360	3	1	5	23	61	—	26	—	1120	—	—	—
Burrito Bean & Cheese Chicken	1 serv	1000	33	15	145	69	104	—	21	—	2080	—	—	—
Burrito Bean & Cheese Steak	1 serv	1100	41	19	170	74	104	—	20	—	2090	—	—	—
Burrito Bean & Cheese Vegetarian	1 serv	870	31	15	70	41	104	—	20	—	1640	—	—	—
Burrito Dos Manos Chicken	1 full serv	1480	40	16	130	76	202	—	28	—	3680	—	—	—
Burrito Dos Manos Steak	1 full serv	1580	48	18	160	42	202	—	26	—	3680	—	—	—
Burrito Mexicano Chicken	1 serv	830	13	3	75	51	124	—	20	—	2110	—	—	—
Burrito Mexicano Steak	1 serv	920	20	6	100	56	124	—	19	—	2120	—	—	—
Burrito Ultimo Chicken	1 serv	860	30	13	130	55	90	—	10	—	2000	—	—	—
Burrito Ultimo Steak	1 serv	950	37	16	155	59	90	—	8	—	2010	—	—	—
Cebollitas	1 serv	40	2	0	0	1	5	—	3	—	160	—	—	—
Chips & Salsa Baja	1 serv	1100	50	5	0	17	134	—	17	—	1210	—	—	—
Enchiladas Cheese	1 serv	850	37	17	90	39	92	—	19	—	2310	—	—	—
Enchiladas Chicken	1 serv	780	25	10	100	48	91	—	20	—	2340	—	—	—
Enchiladas Steak	1 serv	890	33	15	125	51	94	—	20	—	2530	—	—	—
Enchiladas Verde Cheese	1 serv	840	35	17	90	39	91	—	19	—	2440	—	—	—
Enchiladas Verde Chicken	1 serv	770	23	10	100	48	91	—	20	—	2630	—	—	—
Enchiladas Verde Vegetarian	1 serv	720	22	10	50	30	100	—	21	—	2450	—	—	—
Fajitas Chicken Corn Tortillas	1 serv	1200	29	9	155	77	164	—	36	—	2780	—	—	—
Fajitas Chicken Flour Tortillas	1 serv	1360	37	12	155	82	176	—	32	—	3310	—	—	—
Fajitas Steak Corn Tortillas	1 serv	1360	42	15	205	87	164	—	33	—	2830	—	—	—
Fajitas Steak Flour Tortillas	1 serv	1530	50	18	205	92	176	—	30	—	3350	—	—	—
Grilled Vegetarian	1 serv	770	27	12	60	32	100	—	16	—	1680	—	—	—
Mini Quesa-Dita Cheese	1 serv	620	20	9	45	27	81	—	15	—	1480	—	—	—
Mini Quesa-Dita Chicken	1 serv	670	21	9	70	37	81	—	16	—	1640	—	—	—

FOOD	PORTION	CALS	FAT	SAT FAT	CHOL	PROT	CARB	SUGAR	FIBER	CALCI	SOD	POTAS	FOLIC	VIT C
Mini Quesa-Dita Steak	1 serv	700	23	11	80	38	81	—	15	—	1630	—	—	—
Mini Tosta-Dita Chicken	1 serv	570	17	4	55	32	67	—	13	—	1550	—	—	—
Mini Tosta-Dita Steak	1 serv	630	22	6	75	35	67	—	12	—	1560	—	—	—
Nachos Cheese	1 serv	1880	103	37	175	65	166	—	33	—	2590	—	—	—
Nachos Chicken	1 serv	2010	105	38	245	93	166	—	34	—	3030	—	—	—
Nachos Steak	1 serv	2100	113	41	275	98	166	—	33	—	3050	—	—	—
Pinto Beans	1 serv	320	1	0	5	19	56	—	21	—	840	—	—	—
Quesadilla	1 serv	1180	70	35	175	49	92	—	12	—	2330	—	—	—
Quesadilla Cheese	1 serv	1130	69	35	170	48	80	—	9	—	2170	—	—	—
Quesadilla Chicken	1 serv	1260	71	35	245	76	80	—	10	—	2170	—	—	—
Quesadilla Steak	1 serv	1350	79	39	270	81	80	—	9		2620	—	—	—
Rice	1 serv	280	4	1	0	5	55	—	4	—	980	—	—	—
Taco Baja Style Chicken	1 serv	190	5	1	25	13	26	—	4	—	310	—	—	—
Taco Baja Style Steak	1 serv	220	7	2	30	14	26	—	3	—	300	—	—	—
Taco Baja Style Wild Gulf Shrimp	1 serv	190	5	1	90	12	26	—	3	—	350	—	—	—
Taco Chilio Chicken	1 serv	320	10	4	40	20	38	—	9	—	600	—	—	—
Taco Chilito Steak	1 serv	340	12	5	45	21	38	—	8	—	600	—	—	—
Taco Fish	1 serv	270	13	2	15	9	31	—	3	—	480	—	—	—
Taco Mahi Mahi	1 serv	260	10	2	20	13	32	—	6	—	460	—	—	—
Taquitos Chicken w/ Beans	1 serv	750	36	12	85	30	64	—	9	—	—	—	—	—
Taquitos Chicken w/ Rice	1 serv	710	36	11	80	30	64	—	9	—	—	—	—	—
Taquitos Steak w/ Beans	1 serv	820	42	16	105	40	69	—	20	—	—	—	—	—
Taquitos Steak w/ Rice	1 serv	790	42	15	105	32	67	—	10	—	—	—	—	—
Tostada Chicken	1 serv	1140	52	14	120	61	102	—	30	—	2430	—	—	—
Tostada Steak	1 serv	1230	60	17	145	66	102	—	28	—	2440	—	—	—
Tostada Vegetarian	1 serv	1010	50	14	45	33	102	—	28	—	1990	—	—	—
SALAD DRESSINGS														
Fat Free Salsa Verde	1 serv (2.6 oz)	15	0	0	0	0	3	—	0	—	290	—	—	—
Guacamole	2 oz	70	6	1	0	1	5	—	4	—	190	—	—	—
Olive Oil Vinaigrette	1 serv (2.6 oz)	230	25	4	0	0	1	—	0	—	230	—	—	—
Pico De Gallo	1 serv	50	1	0	0	2	12	—	3	—	890	—	—	—

FOOD	PORTION	CALS	FAT	SAT FAT	CHOL	PROT	CARB	SUGAR	FIBER	CALCI	SOD	POTAS	FOLIC	VIT C
Pronto Guacamole	1 serv	550	30	4	0	8	61	—	11	—	380	—	—	—
Ranch	1 serv (2.6 oz)	220	19	4	15	1	6	—	0	—	440	—	—	—
Salsa Baja	1 serv	70	3	0	0	2	7	—	4	—	970	—	—	—
Salsa Roja	1 serv	70	1	0	0	3	13	—	4	—	1080	—	—	—
Salsa Verde	1 serv	50	0	0	0	2	11	—	3	—	1170	—	—	—
Sour Cream	1 oz	60	5	4	15	1	2	—	0	—	50	—	—	—
SALADS AND SALAD BARS														
Baja Ensalada Chicken	1 serv	310	18	2	110	47	17	—	7	—	1210	—	—	—
Baja Ensalada Fish	1 serv	360	15	4	70	35	27	—	10	—	1030	—	—	—
Baja Ensalada Steak	1 serv	460	18	7	150	55	17	—	5	—	1250	—	—	—
Side Salad	1 serv	70	3	1	5	4	10	—	3	—	240	—	—	—

BASKIN-ROBBINS

FOOD	PORTION	CALS	FAT	SAT FAT	CHOL	PROT	CARB	SUGAR	FIBER	CALCI	SOD	POTAS	FOLIC	VIT C
FROZEN YOGURT														
Cafe Mocha Truly Free Soft Serve	1 reg	140	1	1	5	—	27	11	—	—	130	—	—	—
Chocolate Nonfat Soft Serve	1 reg	190	1	0	5	—	39	36	—	—	125	—	—	—
Lowfat Maui Brownie Madness	1 reg	250	9	4	20	38	34	—	—	—	130	—	—	—
ICE CREAM														
Cappuccino Blast w/ Whipped Cream	1 reg	340	16	10	70	—	44	43	—	—	120	—	—	—
Chocolate	1 reg	270	16	10	55	—	31	29	—	—	105	—	—	—
Chocolate Chip	1 reg	270	17	11	60	—	26	25	—	—	80	—	—	—
Espresso'n Cream Lowfat	1 reg	180	3	2	10	—	31	29	—	—	100	—	—	—
Jamoca Almond Fudge	1 reg	280	16	8	45	—	30	29	—	—	70	—	—	—
Peach Crumb Pie No Sugar Added	1 reg	180	5	3	10	—	27	7	—	—	170	—	—	—
Pralines'n Cream	1 reg	280	15	8	50	—	33	32	—	—	160	—	—	—
Shake Chocolate	16 oz	750	43	21	115	—	80	69	—	—	290	—	—	—
Shake Vanilla	16 oz	630	35	22	170	—	69	61	—	—	220	—	—	—
Smoothie Very Strawberry w/ Soft Serve Ice Cream	1 reg	320	1	1	5	—	70	47	—	—	160	—	—	—
Thin Mint No Sugar Added	1 reg	160	4	3	10	—	27	7	—	—	110	—	—	—
Vanilla	1 reg	270	16	10	80	—	24	23	—	—	60	—	—	—
ICES														
Daiquiri Ice	1 reg	130	0	0	0	0	33	32	—	—	10	—	—	—

FOOD	PORTION	CALS	FAT	SAT FAT	CHOL	PROT	CARB	SUGAR	FIBER	CALCI	SOD	POTAS	FOLIC	VIT C
Sherbet Rainbow	1 reg	160	2	2	10	—	34	32	—	—	35	—	—	—
Sorbet Peachy Keen	1 reg	110	0	0	0	—	29	26	—	—	10	—	—	—

BEAR ROCK CAFE

BAKED SELECTIONS

FOOD	PORTION	CALS	FAT	SAT FAT	CHOL	PROT	CARB	SUGAR	FIBER	CALCI	SOD	POTAS	FOLIC	VIT C
Almond French Horn	1	491	23	5	5	8	68	38	4	37	471	—	—	6
Bear Claw	1	260	6	1	20	8	43	11	1	20	350	—	—	0
Cinnamon Roll w/ Cream Cheese Icing	1	540	26	10	25	9	68	34	2	40	540	—	—	0
English Muffin	1	120	1	0	0	4	25	1	1	80	200	—	—	0
Pecan Sticky Bun	1	555	33	9	25	6	52	26	2	40	500	—	—	1

SALAD DRESSINGS

FOOD	PORTION	CALS	FAT	SAT FAT	CHOL	PROT	CARB	SUGAR	FIBER	CALCI	SOD	POTAS	FOLIC	VIT C
Balsamic Vinaigrette	1 serv (1.5 oz)	156	17	2	0	0	1	1	0	0	397	—	—	0
Blue Cheese	1 serv (1.5 oz)	230	25	5	25	1	2	2	0	20	380	—	—	0
Caesar	1 serv (1.5 oz)	198	21	4	21	3	3	3	0	85	595	—	—	0
Creamy Italian	1 serv (1.5 oz)	180	18	3	0	0	4	3	0	0	420	—	—	0
Fat Free Ranch	1 serv (1.5 oz)	40	0	0	0	0	11	4	1	0	560	—	—	0
Fat Free Vidalia Onion	1 serv (1.5 oz)	56	tr	tr	0	tr	12	11	tr	3	166	—	—	tr
Honey Mustard	1 serv (1.5 oz)	184	16	2	21	0	10	10	0	0	298	—	—	0
Oil & Vinegar	1 serv (1.5 oz)	250	28	2	0	0	1	1	0	1	0	—	—	0
Ranch	1 serv (1.5 oz)	213	23	4	7	0	3	1	0	28	425	—	—	0
Red Wine Vinaigrette	1 serv (1.5 oz)	198	21	3	0	0	4	3	0	0	468	—	—	0
Sesame Oriental	1 serv (1.5 oz)	128	6	1	0	0	17	13	0	0	482	—	—	0
Sweet Vidalia Onion	1 serv (1.5 oz)	170	13	2	0	0	14	14	0	0	106	—	—	0
Thousand Island	1 serv (1.5 oz)	184	18	3	21	0	6	4	0	0	425	—	—	0

SALADS

FOOD	PORTION	CALS	FAT	SAT FAT	CHOL	PROT	CARB	SUGAR	FIBER	CALCI	SOD	POTAS	FOLIC	VIT C
Almond Citrus Chicken w/o Dressing	1 serv	443	25	8	85	33	26	18	4	298	967	—	—	49
BLT Chicken w/o Dressing	1 serv	394	22	7	124	44	9	6	4	81	1755	—	—	52
BLT w/o Dressing	1 sm	146	10	3	34	13	4	4	2	46	530	—	—	33
BLT w/o Dressing	1 lg	285	19	7	68	24	7	6	4	71	1057	—	—	52
Caesar Chicken w/ Dressing	1 serv	580	43	11	107	39	12	9	3	576	2056	—	—	41
Caesar w/ Dressing	1 sm	236	20	5	26	10	7	5	2	293	688	—	—	27
Caesar w/ Dressing	1 lg	451	40	11	51	19	11	9	3	566	1380	—	—	41
Dusk Mountain Blackened Chicken w/o Dressing	1 serv	304	19	7	85	30	13	7	3	266	915	—	—	38

FOOD	PORTION	CALS	FAT	SAT FAT	CHOL	PROT	CARB	SUGAR	FIBER	CALCI	SOD	POTAS	FOLIC	VIT C
Fruit Salad	1 serv (4 oz)	61	tr	tr	0	tr	15	14	1	2	5	—	—	19
Lodge	1 sm	55	5	tr	0	2	7	4	2	36	33	—	—	22
Lodge w/o Dressing	1 lg	82	7	tr	0	3	12	6	3	54	49	—	—	38
Low Carb BLT	1 serv	721	63	13	92	29	13	9	4	130	2080	—	—	52
Low Carb Side Salad w/ Dressing	1 serv	316	31	5	9	2	10	6	2	73	581	—	—	22
Low Carb w/ Chicken w/ Dressing	1 serv	567	49	8	70	23	14	8	3	117	1662	—	—	33
Low Fat Grilled Chicken w/o Dressing	1 serv	151	4	1	56	23	9	5	3	60	811	—	—	33
Mount Fuji w/ Dressing	1 serv	554	31	4	56	26	62	33	4	60	1893	—	—	23
SANDWICHES														
Bagel & Cream Cheese	1	378	11	6	30	13	59	4	2	42	593	—	—	0
Bear Cristo	1	310	32	11	91	36	48	15	6	419	2026	—	—	7
BLT	1	585	42	11	61	19	34	5	2	15	1147	—	—	11
Coop's Chicken Salad Croissant	1	439	31	6	44	24	46	12	5	86	375	—	—	10
Fajita Chicken	1	659	40	10	95	36	47	2	2	256	1767	—	—	24
Fireside Jack	1	699	42	10	98	36	53	12	6	444	1428	—	—	9
Garden	1	390	24	9	44	12	35	7	2	168	833	—	—	26
Giant Panda Wrap	1	556	23	4	58	31	68	21	23	151	2045	—	—	25
Grilled Cheese	1	480	32	14	52	17	29	2	1	345	1100	—	—	0
Ham & Swiss On Rye	1	394	13	7	76	31	38	10	2	278	2140	—	—	8
Hoot Owl	1	641	42	12	92	34	32	3	2	159	1618	—	—	9
Italian Asiago Focaccia	1	901	60	17	107	40	60	6	3	426	2360	—	—	13
Low Carb Wrap	1	308	11	2	56	33	28	5	19	68	1232	—	—	31
Low Fat Ham	1	309	7	2	50	24	39	11	2	9	1997	—	—	8
Low Fat Turkey	1	280	3	tr	40	29	35	6	3	14	1537	—	—	9
Mountain Bird	1	691	38	10	98	36	51	11	6	441	1284	—	—	8
Peanut Butter & Jelly	1	387	15	3	0	12	53	23	3	14	440	—	—	2
Reuben's Peak	1	540	23	9	76	36	49	3	3	285	3575	—	—	4
Rising Sunflower	1	591	41	9	93	35	34	7	2	236	1619	—	—	22
Roast Turkey & Bacon	1	522	30	6	71	32	31	2	2	15	1665	—	—	8
Rockside Focaccia	1	958	52	17	129	43	57	2	3	417	2546	—	—	11
Sasquash	1	408	26	7	19	14	41	12	3	239	632	—	—	12
The Early Bear Bagel + Bacon	1	530	21	10	254	27	59	3	2	218	1350	—	—	tr

FOOD	PORTION	CALS	FAT	SAT FAT	CHOL	PROT	CARB	SUGAR	FIBER	CALCI	SOD	POTAS	FOLIC	VIT C
The Early Bear English Muffin + Bacon	1	344	19	8	248	19	26	1	1	236	1087	—	—	tr
The Early Bear English Muffin + Sausage	1	514	34	14	288	24	25	1	1	236	1407	—	—	tr
The Moose	1	976	54	18	142	54	54	17	7	633	2565	—	—	8
Turkey On Whole Wheat	1	602	41	10	102	34	36	6	2	160	1667	—	—	9
SOUPS														
Aztec Black Bean	1 serv	162	1	0	0	9	28	5	9	40	1180	—	—	0
Baked Potato Mountain Chowder	1 serv	352	16	6	27	13	42	5	4	79	1179	—	—	12
Chicken & Dumpling	1 serv	249	7	3	73	16	28	6	4	4	1427	—	—	0
Chicken Gumbo	1 serv	123	3	1	14	8	10	5	3	4	1750	—	—	0
Chicken Noodle	1 serv	165	3	1	28	10	25	6	1	5	1176	—	—	0
Chicken w/ Wild Rice	1 serv	313	16	3	41	14	29	3	3	4	1655	—	—	0
Cream Of Broccoli w/ Cheddar	1 serv	264	17	7	21	8	21	0	4	4	1313	—	—	0
French Onion	1 serv	121	5	1	0	3	17	9	2	5	1556	—	—	0
Grande Chili	1 serv	351	12	6	35	25	36	10	19	2	1714	—	—	0
In Bread Bowl Aztec Black Bean	1 serv	545	3	0	0	23	105	8	12	4	2001	—	—	0
In Bread Bowl Baked Potato Mountain Chowder	1 serv	735	17	6	27	27	119	7	7	79	2000	—	—	12
In Bread Bowl Chicken & Dumplings	1 serv	632	9	3	73	29	104	8	7	4	2248	—	—	0
In Bread Bowl Chicken Gumbo	1 serv	506	4	1	14	22	86	8	5	4	2571	—	—	0
In Bread Bowl Chicken Noodle	1 serv	548	5	1	28	23	101	8	4	5	1997	—	—	0
In Bread Bowl Chicken w/ Wild Rice	1 serv	696	18	3	41	27	105	5	5	4	2475	—	—	0
In Bread Bowl Cream Of Broccoli w/ Cheddar	1 serv	647	18	7	21	22	97	2	7	4	2133	—	—	0
In Bread Bowl French Onion	1 serv	504	7	1	0	17	93	11	4	5	2377	—	—	0
In Bread Bowl Grande Chili	1 serv	734	14	6	35	39	113	12	22	2	2535	—	—	0

FOOD	PORTION	CALS	FAT	SAT FAT	CHOL	PROT	CARB	SUGAR	FIBER	CALCI	SOD	POTAS	FOLIC	VIT C
In Bread Bowl New England Clam Chowder	1 serv	653	9	4	15	15	113	16	4	210	2411	—	—	8
In Bread Bowl Normandy Vegetable Cheddar	1 serv	728	22	11	38	30	102	14	4	395	2771	—	—	18
In Bread Bowl Tomato Florentine	1 serv	533	4	0	5	20	104	14	4	5	2066	—	—	5
New England Clam Chowder	1 serv	270	8	4	15	1	36	14	1	210	1590	—	—	8
Normandy Vegetable Cheddar	1 serv	345	21	11	38	17	26	12	2	395	1950	—	—	18
Tomato Florentine	1 serv	150	2	0	5	6	27	12	2	5	1245	—	—	5

BEN & JERRY'S

FOOD	PORTION	CALS	FAT	SAT FAT	CHOL	PROT	CARB	SUGAR	FIBER	CALCI	SOD	POTAS	FOLIC	VIT C
Sugar Cone	1	48	tr	tr	0	1	10	3	tr	1	42	—	—	0
FROZEN YOGURT														
Black Raspberry Low Fat	½ cup	140	2	1	15	3	28	21	tr	150	60	—	—	2
Cherry Garcia	½ cup	170	3	2	20	4	32	27	0	150	80	—	—	0
Chocolate Fudge Brownie	½ cup	190	3	2	15	6	36	31	1	200	105	—	—	0
Half Baked	½ cup	210	4	2	20	5	30	29	tr	200	125	—	—	0
Phish Food	½ cup	230	5	4	15	4	42	30	1	150	110	—	—	0
ICE CREAM														
Brownie Batter	½ cup	310	18	10	70	5	32	26	1	150	115	—	—	0
Butter Pecan	½ cup	290	21	10	70	4	20	18	1	150	80	—	—	0
Cherry Garcia	½ cup	250	15	11	70	4	26	23	0	150	60	—	—	0
Chocolate Chip Cookie Dough	½ cup	280	16	9	70	4	31	24	0	100	90	—	—	0
Chocolate Chocolate Cookie	½ cup	280	14	9	35	4	34	26	2	100	115	—	—	0
Chocolate For A Change	½ cup	270	17	11	55	4	36	23	2	150	50	—	—	0
Chocolate Fudge Brownie	½ cup	280	14	9	40	5	33	29	2	100	85	—	—	0
Chubby Hubby	½ cup	330	21	12	60	7	32	24	1	100	160	—	—	0
Chunky Monkey	½ cup	300	19	11	60	4	30	26	1	100	45	—	—	1
Coffee For A Change	½ cup	240	15	10	75	4	21	19	0	150	55	—	—	0
Coffee Heath Bar Crunch	½ cup	310	18	12	65	4	32	25	0	100	125	—	—	0
Everything But The	½ cup	320	19	12	60	5	30	27	1	150	80	—	—	0

FOOD	PORTION	CALS	FAT	SAT FAT	CHOL	PROT	CARB	SUGAR	FIBER	CALCI	SOD	POTAS	FOLIC	VIT C
Fudge Central	½ cup	300	18	12	55	4	31	27	1	150	60	—	—	0
Half Baked	½ cup	280	14	9	60	4	34	31	1	100	105	—	—	0
Karamel Sutra	½ cup	290	15	10	55	4	33	27	1	150	75	—	—	0
Makin' Whoopie Pie	½ cup	270	14	9	40	4	33	24	2	100	75	—	—	0
Mint Chocolate Cookie	½ cup	270	16	10	70	4	26	22	tr	150	120	—	—	0
New York Super Fudge Chunk	½ cup	270	20	11	40	5	30	25	2	100	55	—	—	0
Oatmeal Cookie Chunk	½ cup	280	16	10	55	4	32	23	1	100	120	—	—	0
One Sweet Whirled	½ cup	280	15	11	60	4	33	27	1	100	85	—	—	0
Organic Chocolate Fudge Brownie	½ cup	260	13	9	35	4	30	25	2	100	55	—	—	0
Organic Strawberry	½ cup	200	12	8	55	3	20	17	0	100	40	—	—	9
Organic Sweet Cream & Cookies	½ cup	240	15	9	60	3	23	18	0	100	90	—	—	0
Organic Vanilla	½ cup	220	14	10	65	3	18	16	0	100	50	—	—	0
Peanut Butter Cup	½ cup	380	26	13	70	8	29	25	2	150	140	—	—	0
Peanut Butter Me Up	½ cup	330	21	11	50	6	28	24	2	150	130	—	—	0
Phish Food	½ cup	280	13	10	35	4	38	23	2	100	90	—	—	0
Pistachio Pistachio	½ cup	280	19	12	70	6	21	18	0	150	125	—	—	0
Uncanny Cashew	½ cup	290	19	13	70	4	27	22	0	150	130	—	—	0
Vanilla Heath Bar Crunch	½ cup	300	19	11	70	4	29	27	0	150	120	—	—	0
Vanilla For A Change	½ cup	240	16	11	75	4	21	19	0	150	55	—	—	0
SORBETS														
Berry Berry Extraordinary	½ cup	100	0	0	0	0	25	22	tr	0	5	—	—	4
Mango Lime	½ cup	100	0	0	0	0	27	22	0	20	10	—	—	9
Strawberry Kiwi	½ cup	100	0	0	0	0	27	22	tr	20	10	—	—	15
BIG BOY														
DESSERTS														
Frozen Yogurt Fat Free	1 serv	118	0	—	0	3	27	—	—	—	60	—	—	—
Frozen Yogurt Shake	1	156	1	—	2	7	33	—	—	—	120	—	—	—
MAIN MENU SELECTIONS														
Baked Cod w/ Salad Baked Potato Roll & Margarine	1 meal	744	21	—	76	57	82	—	—	—	655	—	—	—

FOOD	PORTION	CALS	FAT	SAT FAT	CHOL	PROT	CARB	SUGAR	FIBER	CALCI	SOD	POTAS	FOLIC	VIT C
Baked Potato	1	163	2	—	0	6	37	—	—	—	7	—	—	—
Breast of Chicken Pita w/ Mozzarella & Ranch Dressing	1	361	11	—	84	41	23	—	—	—	369	—	—	—
Breast of Chicken w/ Mozzarella Salad Baked Potato Roll & Margarine	1 meal	697	20	—	76	50	80	—	—	—	613	—	—	—
Cabbage Soup	1 bowl	40	5	—	0	1	7	—	—	—	347	—	—	—
Cabbage Soup	1 cup	34	4	—	0	1	6	—	—	—	295	—	—	—
Cajun Cod w/ Salad Baked Potato Roll & Margarine	1 meal	736	21	—	76	56	80	—	—	—	745	—	—	—
Chicken & Pasta Primavera w/ Salad Roll & Margarine	1 meal	676	14	—	65	53	83	—	—	—	875	—	—	—
Chicken 'n Vegetable Stir Fry w/ Salad Baked Potato Roll & Margarine	1 meal	795	18	—	65	51	109	—	—	—	845	—	—	—
Dinner Roll	1	210	5	—	0	0	36	—	—	—	340	—	—	—
Plain Egg Beaters Omelette w/ Whole Wheat Bread & Margarine	1 meal	305	10	—	0	19	36	—	—	—	603	—	—	—
Promise Margarine	1 pat	25	3	—	0	0	0	—	—	—	35	—	—	—
Rice Pilaf	1 serv	153	4	—	10	3	25	—	—	—	688	—	—	—
Scrambled Egg Beaters w/ Whole Wheat Bread & Margarine	1 meal	305	10	—	0	19	36	—	—	—	603	—	—	—
Southwest Chicken w/ Salad Baked Potato Roll & Margarine	1 meal	702	18	—	76	50	85	—	—	—	948	—	—	—
Spaghetti Marinara w/ Salad Roll & Margarine	1 meal	754	11	—	8	17	105	—	—	—	754	—	—	—
Turkey Pita w/ Ranch Dressing	1	245	6	—	83	25	23	—	—	—	938	—	—	—

FOOD	PORTION	CALS	FAT	SAT FAT	CHOL	PROT	CARB	SUGAR	FIBER	CALCI	SOD	POTAS	FOLIC	VIT C
Vegetable Stir Fry w/ Salad Baked Potato Roll & Margarine	1 meal	616	14	—	0	17	109	—	—	—	774	—	—	—
Vegetarian Egg Beaters Omelette w/ Whole Wheat Bread & Margarine	1 meal	330	10	—	0	21	40	—	—	—	618	—	—	—
SALAD DRESSINGS														
Italian Fat Free	1 oz	11	0	—	0	0	3	—	—	—	191	—	—	—
Lo Cal Oriental	1 oz	20	2	—	0	1	4	—	—	—	189	—	—	—
Lo Cal Ranch	1 oz	41	3	—	8	1	3	—	—	—	151	—	—	—
SALADS AND SALAD BARS														
Chicken Breast Salad w/ Roll & Margarine	1 serv	523	16	—	73	44	50	—	—	—	654	—	—	—
Oriental Chicken Breast Salad w/ Dinner Roll & Margarine	1 serv	660	20	—	65	48	73	—	—	—	855	—	—	—
Tossed Salad	1	35	2	—	0	2	7	—	—	—	71	—	—	—

BLIMPIE

FOOD	PORTION	CALS	FAT	SAT FAT	CHOL	PROT	CARB	SUGAR	FIBER	CALCI	SOD	POTAS	FOLIC	VIT C
COOKIES														
Chocolate Chunk	1	200	10	6	15	2	26	16	1	0	210	—	—	0
Macadamia White Chunk	1	210	10	5	20	2	26	15	1	0	140	—	—	0
Oatmeal Raisin	1	190	8	2	10	3	27	16	1	0	200	—	—	0
Peanut Butter	1	220	12	5	15	4	23	14	1	4	210	—	—	0
Sugar	1	330	17	5	30	3	24	24	0	0	290	—	—	0
SALAD DRESSINGS AND TOPPINGS														
Caesar Dressing	1 serv (1.5 oz)	208	22	4	10	1	2	1	0	0	504	—	—	0
Cracked Peppercorn Dressing	1 serv (1.5 oz)	237	25	1	15	1	2	2	0	20	386	—	—	0
Frank's Red Hot Buffalo Sauce	1 serv (1 oz)	13	tr	tr	0	2	2	1	tr	3	836	—	—	21
French's Honey Mustard	1 tbsp	5	0	0	0	0	1	1	0	0	35	—	—	0
GourMayo Chipotle Chili	1 tbsp	50	5	1	10	0	1	0	0	0	100	—	—	0
GourMayo Sun Dried Tomato	1 tbsp	50	5	1	10	0	1	0	0	0	100	—	—	0
GourMayo Wasabi Horseradish	1 tbsp	50	5	1	10	0	1	0	0	0	100	—	—	0
Guacamole	1 serv (1.5 oz)	194	18	3	tr	2	7	6	1	8	468	—	—	0

FOOD	PORTION	CALS	FAT	SAT FAT	CHOL	PROT	CARB	SUGAR	FIBER	CALCI	SOD	POTAS	FOLIC	VIT C
Oil & Vinegar	1 serv	36	4	1	0	0	1	0	0	0	0	—	—	0
Pesto Dressing	1 serv (1 oz)	132	13	2	0	0	1	0	0	0	236	—	—	0
SALADS AND SALAD BARS														
Antipasto	1 reg serv	244	13	6	69	23	10	6	3	201	1217	—	—	20
Chef	1 reg serv	212	9	5	66	20	9	5	3	254	961	—	—	26
Chili Olé	1 reg serv	480	27	11	45	21	42	2	3	262	1240	—	—	28
Grilled Chicken w/ Caesar Dressing	1 reg serv	347	27	5	45	18	9	5	3	30	862	—	—	25
Grilled Chicken w/o Dressing	1 serv	139	5	2	35	17	7	4	3	30	358	—	—	26
Roast Beef 'N Blue	1 reg serv	390	16	10	70	31	29	0	0	157	1550	—	—	17
Seafood	1 reg serv	122	4	1	19	6	16	5	3	44	418	—	—	21
Tuna	1 reg serv	261	20	3	50	16	8	3	3	31	398	—	—	20
Zesto Pesto Turkey	1 reg serv	370	19	8	40	20	31	1	0	40	1410	—	—	18
SANDWICHES														
6 Inch Hot Sub BLT	1	588	32	10	41	28	49	8	3	40	1596	—	—	29
6 Inch Hot Sub Buffalo Chicken	1	400	13	7	61	32	50	7	3	221	2108	—	—	21
6 Inch Hot Sub Buffalo Chicken w/o Cheese	1	320	7	3	61	32	50	7	3	21	2108	—	—	21
6 Inch Hot Sub ChiliMax	1	511	13	2	0	29	71	10	8	71	1287	—	—	23
6 Inch Hot Sub Grilled Chicken	1	373	9	3	35	29	50	8	3	29	836	—	—	28
6 Inch Hot Sub Meatball	1	572	27	10	58	28	55	12	2	223	1145	—	—	11
6 Inch Hot Sub MexiMelt	1	425	9	2	0	23	65	9	7	90	1012	—	—	23
6 Inch Hot Sub Pastrami	1	507	17	7	74	36	53	11	3	251	1658	—	—	23
6 Inch Hot Sub Steak & Onion Melt	1	440	16	6	68	29	49	9	3	197	1056	—	—	25
6 Inch Hot Sub VegiMax	1	395	7	2	0	24	60	8	8	69	982	—	—	26
6 Inch Sub Blimpie Best	1	476	16	7	69	30	52	10	2	200	1690	—	—	23
6 Inch Sub Club	1	440	12	6	66	28	51	9	3	251	1437	—	—	23
6 Inch Sub Ham & Cheese	1	436	13	6	59	28	52	10	3	251	1302	—	—	23
6 Inch Sub Roast Beef	1	468	14	6	71	37	49	7	3	200	1384	—	—	23
6 Inch Sub Roast Beef w/o Cheese	1	388	8	2	51	30	49	7	3	25	1338	—	—	23

FOOD	PORTION	CALS	FAT	SAT FAT	CHOL	PROT	CARB	SUGAR	FIBER	CALCI	SOD	POTAS	FOLIC	VIT C
6 Inch Sub Seafood	1	355	8	2	19	14	58	9	4	42	895	—	—	24
6 Inch Sub Tuna	1	493	23	4	50	24	51	7	3	29	876	—	—	23
6 inch Sub Turkey	1	424	11	5	62	25	49	7	3	200	1597	—	—	23
6 Inch Sub Turkey w/o Cheese	1	344	5	1	42	18	49	7	3	25	1551	—	—	23
Cheddar	1 slice	52	5	3	10	3	0	0	0	101	250	—	—	0
Grilled Subs Beef Turkey & Cheddar	1	600	31	10	69	28	49	9	3	235	1836	—	—	21
Grilled Subs Cuban	1	462	12	6	67	30	50	9	3	243	1526	—	—	21
Grilled Subs Pastrami	1	462	14	6	44	32	52	11	3	251	1438	—	—	23
Grilled Subs Reuben	1	630	33	5	46	31	55	15	2	246	1914	—	—	4
Provolone	1 slice	80	6	4	20	6	0	0	0	170	200	—	—	0
Swiss	1 slice	80	6	4	20	7	0	0	0	222	46	—	—	0
Wraps Southwestern	1	674	35	8	56	26	54	4	3	204	2504	—	—	28
Wraps Beef & Cheddar	1	714	37	11	78	34	57	5	3	412	2183	—	—	22
Wraps Chicken Caesar	1	646	35	7	45	25	56	6	3	198	1635	—	—	31
Wraps Steak & Onions	1	716	37	10	78	30	64	7	3	381	1716	—	—	25
Wraps Ultimate BLT	1	831	50	15	78	34	60	7	3	417	2677	—	—	25
Wraps Zesty Italian	1	638	33	10	62	26	74	13	3	367	2374	—	—	34
SIDE ORDERS														
Cole Slaw	1 serv (5 oz)	180	13	2	<5	1	13	13	1	4	230		—	180
Macaroni Salad	1 serv (5 oz)	360	25	4	10	4	25	6	1	2	660	—	—	2
Mustard Potato Salad	1 serv (5 oz)	160	5	1	5	2	21	13	1	0	660	—	—	8
Potato Chips Cheddar & Sour Cream	1 bag	210	11	2	<5	3	25	0	1	20	220	—	—	5
Potato Chips Jalapeño	1 bag	210	11	2	0	2	25	0	2	20	250	—	—	6
Potato Chips Lea & Perrins Barbecue	1 bag	210	10	2	0	3	25	2	2	20	270	—	—	6
Potato Chips Regular	1 bag	210	11	2	0	3	25	0	2	0	190	—	—	6

FOOD	PORTION	CALS	FAT	SAT FAT	CHOL	PROT	CARB	SUGAR	FIBER	CALCI	SOD	POTAS	FOLIC	VIT C
Potato Chips Romano & Garlic	1 bag	210	11	2	<5	3	25	0	2	30	220	—	—	7
Potato Chips Sour Cream & Onion	1 bag	210	11	2	<5	2	25	1	1	30	250	—	—	9
Potato Salad	1 serv (5 oz)	270	19	3	10	2	19	10	1	2	560	—	—	8
SOUPS														
Chicken w/ White & Wild Rice	1 serv (8 oz)	230	12	2	30	10	21	2	2	66	1210	—	—	2
Cream Of Broccoli & Cheese	1 serv (8 oz)	190	12	5	15	6	15	5	3	158	940	—	—	19
Cream Of Potato	1 serv (8 oz)	190	9	3	<5	5	24	3	3	140	860	—	—	4
Garden Vegetable	1 serv (8 oz)	80	1	0	0	5	14	5	3	36	620	—	—	15
Grande Chili w/ Beans & Beef	1 serv (8 oz)	250	7	4	40	18	30	7	18	55	1230	—	—	17
Homestyle Chicken Noodle	1 serv (8 oz)	120	3	1	20	7	18	4	1	46	850	—	—	0
Tomato Basil w/ Raviolini	1 serv (8 oz)	110	1	0	10	4	22	5	tr	27	720	—	—	1
Vegetable Beef	1 serv (8 oz)	80	2	1	5	4	13	3	2	26	1010	—	—	7

BOB EVANS

BREAKFAST SELECTIONS

FOOD	PORTION	CALS	FAT	SAT FAT	CHOL	PROT	CARB	SUGAR	FIBER	CALCI	SOD	POTAS	FOLIC	VIT C
Bacon	1 piece	36	4	2	5	1	0	0	—	—	55	—	—	—
Belgian Waffle	1	351	10	2	0	7	58	17	—	—	834	—	—	—
Canadian Bacon	1 piece	21	1	0	9	4	0	0	—	—	261	—	—	—
Country Biscuit Breakfast	1 serv	841	41	14	267	31	71	22	—	—	2387	—	—	—
Egg Hardboiled	1	60	4	2	190	6	1	0	—	—	55	—	—	—
Egg Over Easy	1	93	7	2	213	6	1	1	—	—	63	—	—	—
Eggs Scrambled	1 serv	170	11	3	482	14	2	0	—	—	142	—	—	—
Eggs Benedict	1 serv	514	23	6	484	41	37	7	—	—	2311	—	—	—
French Toast	1 slice	135	2	0	25	3	14	4	—	—	175	—	—	—
Fruit Cup	1 serv	164	1	0	0	2	42	36	—	—	11	—	—	—
Grits	1 serv	187	7	3	0	3	29	0	—	—	186	—	—	—
Ham Smoked	1 slice	66	2	1	39	11	2	1	—	—	855	—	—	—
Home Fries	1 serv	193	7	1	0	4	28	14	—	—	577	—	—	—
Hotcake Blueberry	1	192	5	1	0	4	33	12	—	—	419	—	—	—
Hotcake Buttermilk	1	176	5	1	0	3	29	9	—	—	417	—	—	—
Hotcake Cinnamon	1	166	5	1	8	4	28	8	—	—	409	—	—	—
Hotcake Multigrain	1	208	6	2	10	5	34	10	—	—	505	—	—	—
Lite Sausage Breakfast	1 serv	479	21	5	42	32	50	24	—	—	1011	—	—	—

FOOD	PORTION	CALS	FAT	SAT FAT	CHOL	PROT	CARB	SUGAR	FIBER	CALCI	SOD	POTAS	FOLIC	VIT C
Mush	1 serv	73	1	0	0	1	14	0	—	—	194	—	—	—
Oatmeal Plain	1 serv	185	3	0	0	7	34	1	—	—	301	—	—	—
Omelette Border	1	847	60	21	571	33	60	4	—	—	1551	—	—	—
Omelette Cheese	1	457	40	15	530	25	3	0	—	—	428	—	—	—
Omelette Farmer's Market	1	634	49	19	558	32	11	3	—	—	1986	—	—	—
Pot Roast Hash Breakfast	1 serv	698	41	16	529	45	36	19	—	—	1207	—	—	—
Sausage	1 link	117	13	3	21	5	0	0	0	—	167	—	—	—
Sausage Lite	1 link	100	7	2	37	10	0	0	—	—	278	—	—	—
Strawberry Yogurt	1 serv	145	1	1	5	6	28	26	—	—	85	—	—	—
CHILDREN'S MENU SELECTIONS														
Colorful Cool Cakes	1 serv	542	17	5	1	9	87	30		—	1112	—	—	—
Garden Salad	1 kid serv	41	2	1	7	3	3	1		—	54	—	—	—
Hot Diggety Dog Plain	1	446	33	13	55	15	23	1	—	—	1214	—	—	—
L'il Homesteader	1 serv	414	25	6	262	16	34	13	—	—	781	—	—	—
Mac & Cheese	1 serv	330	12	4	20	11	45	9	—	—	610	—	—	—
Mini Cheeseburger	1 serv	252	14	4	25	9	20	3	—	—	288	—	—	—
Pizza Pizzazz	1 serv	520	20	7	31	27	58	5	—	—	883	—	—	—
Plenty O Pancakes	1 serv	515	17	6	0	9	81	26	—	—	1114	—	—	—
Quesadilla Chicken	1 serv	542	31	12	73	28	39	1	—	—	1238	—	—	—
Smiley Face Potatoes	1 serv	335	13	7	0	5	49	1	—	—	786	—	—	—
Spaghetti & Meatballs	1 serv	523	21	9	51	27	57	8	—	—	999	—	—	—
Sundae Fudge Blast	1 serv	254	10	7	30	3	37	28	—	—	92	—	—	—
Sundae Oreo Cookies 'n' Cream	1 serv	315	13	7	21	3	64	34	—	—	200	—	—	—
Sundae Rainbow	1 serv	320	14	9	30	4	46	24	—	—	92	—	—	—
Sundae Reese's I'm Smiling	1 serv	325	15	9	31	5	42	32	—	—	130	—	—	—
MAIN MENU SELECTIONS														
Catfish Grilled New Orleans	1 piece	255	19	3	58	22	4	1	—	—	896	—	—	—
Cheeseburger Bacon Plain	1	1005	76	34	153	45	31	3	—	—	1367	—	—	—
Cheeseburger Plain	1	691	46	19	104	38	31	3	—	—	792	—	—	—
Chicken Quesadilla	1 serv	502	36	16	61	25	50	6	—	—	1674	—	—	—
Chicken & Broccoli Alfredo	1 serv	826	29	7	112	58	90	7	—	—	1105	—	—	—

FOOD	PORTION	CALS	FAT	SAT FAT	CHOL	PROT	CARB	SUGAR	FIBER	CALCI	SOD	POTAS	FOLIC	VIT C
Chicken Fried	1 piece	291	30	6	154	31	9	1	—	—	1332	—	—	—
Chicken Grilled	1 piece	229	10	2	98	38	0	0	—	—	632	—	—	—
Chicken Pot Pie	1 serv	758	49	22	209	32	46	10	—	—	1754	—	—	—
Chicken Tenders Grilled	1 piece	103	7	1	33	12	0	0	—	—	220	—	—	—
Chicken-N-Noodle	1 serv	407	22	5	115	20	32	4	—	—	658	—	—	—
Country Fried Steak w/ Gravy	1 serv	535	37	13	60	20	31	2	—	—	1763	—	—	—
Country Fried Steak w/o Gravy	1 serv	481	33	12	60	20	26	0	—	—	1217	—	—	—
Fish Market Halibut	1 piece	209	12	2	32	12	13	0	—	—	327	—	—	—
Hamburger Patty	1	388	30	13	82	28	0	0	—	—	64	—	—	—
Hamburger Plain	1	585	36	14	82	34	30	3	—	—	407	—	—	—
Hamburger Shroomin' Onion Plain	1	695	44	19	104	38	32	4	—	—	938	—	—	—
Meat Loaf	1 serv	626	44	19	157	42	14	7	—	—	1006	—	—	—
Open Faced Roast Beef Dinner	1 serv	633	29	10	118	37	31	8	—	—	1331	—	—	—
Pork Chop Dinner	1 serv	466	28	9	129	48	2	2	—	—	829	—	—	—
Pork Chop Dinner w/ Garlic Herb Butter	1 serv	624	39	11	130	50	16	3	—	—	1227	—	—	—
Pork Chop Dinner w/ Wildfire Barbecue Sauce	1 serv	645	35	10	129	49	29	17	—	—	1099	—	—	—
Salmon	1 serv	334	18	4	109	43	0	0	—	—	109	—	—	—
Salmon w/ Garlic Herb Butter	1 serv	491	29	6	110	45	14	1	—	—	506	—	—	—
Salmon w/ Wildfire Barbecue Sauce	1 serv	512	25	5	109	44	27	15	—	—	379	—	—	—
Sandwich Bob's BLT	1	795	54	21	276	25	55	2	—	—	1435	—	—	—
Sandwich Chicken Salad	1	694	43	7	62	21	55	7	—	—	1329	—	—	—
Sandwich Fish Market Haddock	1	570	25	4	32	21	65	0	—	—	944	—	—	—
Sandwich Fried Chicken	1	508	23	4	77	36	39	17	—	—	1032	—	—	—
Sandwich Fried Chicken Club	1	994	70	26	155	49	40	18	—	—	2002	—	—	—
Sandwich Grilled Cheese	1	391	17	7	30	9	25	4	—	—	776	—	—	—
Sandwich Grilled Chicken	1	447	18	3	98	44	30	3	—	—	998	—	—	—

FOOD	PORTION	CALS	FAT	SAT FAT	CHOL	PROT	CARB	SUGAR	FIBER	CALCI	SOD	POTAS	FOLIC	VIT C
Sandwich Grilled Chicken Club	1	993	70	29	194	59	32	4	—	—	2259	—	—	—
Sandwich Pot Roast	1	728	35	15	113	38	68	11	—	—	1614	—	—	—
Sandwich Turkey Bacon Melt	1	872	52	23	166	47	55	1	—	—	1794	—	—	—
Seniors Chicken & Broccoli Alfredo	1 serv	513	21	5	77	37	49	4	—	—	935	—	—	—
Seniors Chicken Pot Pie	1 serv	758	49	22	209	32	46	10	—	—	1754	—	—	—
Seniors Spaghetti & Meatballs	1 serv	617	29	11	69	31	59	8	—	—	1166	—	—	—
Seniors Steak Tips & Noodles	1 serv	550	25	6	134	38	46	3	—	—	1654	—	—	—
Seniors Stir-Fry Grilled Chicken	1 serv	479	18	4	66	31	54	19		—	1292	—	—	—
Spaghetti & Marinara Sauce	1 serv	619	7	3	15	34	104	14	—	—	1128	—	—	—
Spaghetti w/ Meatballs	1 serv	1087	45	17	107	54	116	16	—	—	1964	—	—	—
Steak Monterey	1 serv	584	41	17	126	44	7	2	—	—	1671	—	—	—
Steak Tips & Noodles	1 serv	985	37	10	266	76	90	5	—	—	2972	—	—	—
Stir-Fry Grilled Chicken	1 serv	728	28	6	98	46	31	83	—	—	2048	—	—	—
Stir-Fry Grilled Shrimp	1 serv	713	17	3	334	52	98	39	—	—	1798	—	—	—
Stir-Fry Vegetable	1 serv	497	7	1	0	15	98	39	—	—	1413	—	—	—
T-Bone Steak Plain	1 serv	1335	92	35	261	111	7	2	—	—	4944	—	—	—
T-Bone Steak w/ Garlic Herb Butter	1 serv	1492	102	37	262	113	21	4	—	—	5342	—	—	—
Turkey & Dressing	1 serv	542	24	7	105	37	41	5	—	—	1400	—	—	—
SALAD DRESSINGS AND TOPPINGS														
Dressing Bleu Cheese	1 serv (1.5 oz)	220	23	4	22	1	3	1	—	—	337	—	—	—
Dressing Colonial	1 serv (1.5 oz)	232	21	3	0	0	12	12	—	—	193	—	—	—
Dressing French	1 serv (1.5 oz)	219	21	3	14	0	10	8	—	—	247	—	—	—
Dressing Honey Mustard	1 serv (1.5 oz)	192	18	3	21	0	8	7	—	—	247	—	—	—
Dressing Hot Bacon	1 serv (1.5 oz)	106	3	1	4	0	18	17	—	—	189	—	—	—
Dressing Lite Italian	1 serv (1.5 oz)	82	7	1	0	0	4	3	—	—	590	—	—	—
Dressing Oriental	1 serv (1.5 oz)	194	16	2	0	0	12	12	—	—	253	—	—	—
Dressing Ranch	1 serv (1.5 oz)	156	16	3	14	1	1	1	—	—	312	—	—	—

FOOD	PORTION	CALS	FAT	SAT FAT	CHOL	PROT	CARB	SUGAR	FIBER	CALCI	SOD	POTAS	FOLIC	VIT C
Dressing Ranch Lite	1 serv (1.5 oz)	103	10	2	11	1	2	1	—	—	377	—	—	—
Dressing Raspberry Vinaigrette	1 serv (1.5 oz)	155	13	2	0	0	12	12	—	—	90	—	—	—
Dressing Thousand Island	1 serv (1.5 oz)	212	20	3	21	0	7	7	—	—	354	—	—	—
Dressing Wildfire Ranch	1 serv (1.5 oz)	212	9	1	8	1	9	1	—	—	307	—	—	—
SALADS														
Chicken Salad Plate	1 serv	789	46	7	87	23	78	65	—	—	1137	—	—	—
Cobb Salad w/ Grilled Chicken	1 serv	778	54	22	373	68	14	7	—	—	1852	—	—	—
Country Spinach w/ Grilled Chicken	1 serv	532	38	10	282	43	11	4	—	—	1128	—	—	—
Frisco Salad w/ Fried Chicken	1 serv	672	40	14	98	40	39	7	—	—	1685	—	—	—
Frisco Salad w/ Grilled Chicken	1 serv	599	40	14	154	54	13	7	—	—	1380	—	—	—
Fruit & Yogurt	1 serv	414	2	1	5	9	96	83	—	—	106	—	—	—
Raspberry Grilled Chicken	1 serv	637	42	16	155	55	18	13	—	—	1657	—	—	—
Speciality Side	1 serv	174	9	4	22	9	16	3	—	—	449	—	—	—
Wildfire Fried Chicken Salad	1 serv	806	31	9	66	36	100	22	—	—	1237	—	—	—
Wildfire Grilled Chicken Salad	1 serv	733	30	9	123	50	74	22	—	—	932	—	—	—
BOJANGLES														
Biscuit	1	243	12	3	2	4	29	—	2	—	663	—	—	—
Biscuit + Bacon	1	290	17	5	10	8	26	—	1	—	810	—	—	—
Biscuit + Bacon Egg Cheese	1	550	42	14	160	17	27	—	1	—	1250	—	—	—
Biscuit + Cajun Filet	1	454	21	6	41	20	46	—	1	—	949	—	—	—
Biscuit + Country Ham	1	270	15	4	20	9	26	—	1	—	1010	—	—	—
Biscuit + Egg	1	400	30	6	120	8	26	—	1	—	630	—	—	—
Biscuit + Sausage	1	350	23	7	20	9	26	—	1	—	810	—	—	—
Biscuit + Smoked Sausage	1	380	26	9	20	10	27	—	1	—	940	—	—	—
Biscuit + Steak	1	649	49	13	34	14	37	—	1	—	1126	—	—	—
Botato Rounds	1 serv	235	11	4	13	3	31	—	3	—	328	—	—	—
Buffalo Bites	1 serv	180	5	2	105	27	5	—	0	—	720	—	—	—
Cajun Pintos	1 serv	110	0	0	0	6	18	—	6	—	480	—	—	—

FOOD	PORTION	CALS	FAT	SAT FAT	CHOL	PROT	CARB	SUGAR	FIBER	CALCI	SOD	POTAS	FOLIC	VIT C
Cajun Spiced Breast	1 serv	278	17	—	75	18	12	—	tr	—	565	—	—	—
Cajun Spiced Leg	1 serv	284	19	—	96	19	11	—	tr	—	530	—	—	—
Cajun Spiced Thigh	1 serv	310	23	—	67	15	11	—	tr	—	465	—	—	—
Cajun Spiced Wing	1 serv	355	25	—	94	21	11	—	tr	—	630	—	—	—
Chicken Supremes	1 serv	337	16	6	58	21	26	—	1	—	629	—	—	—
Corn On The Cob	1 serv	140	2	0	0	5	34	—	2	—	20	—	—	—
Dirty Rice	1 serv	166	6	2	10	5	24	—	1	—	762	—	—	—
Green Beans	1 serv	25	0	0	0	0	5	—	2	—	710	—	—	—
Macaroni & Cheese	1 serv	198	14	5	26	7	12	—	tr	—	418	—	—	—
Marinated Cole Slaw	1 serv	136	3	0	0	1	26	—	3	—	454	—	—	—
Potatoes w/o Gravy	1 serv	80	1	0	0	2	16	—	1	—	380	—	—	—
Sandwich Cajun Filet w/o Mayo	1	337	11	5	45	22	41	—	3	—	401	—	—	—
Sandwich Cajun Filet w/ Mayo	1	437	22	7	55	22	41	—	3	—	506	—	—	—
Sandwich Grilled Filet w/ Mayo	1	335	16	5	61	23	25	—	2	—	645	—	—	—
Sandwich Grilled Filet w/o Mayo	1 serv	235	5	3	51	23	25	—	2	—	540	—	—	—
Seasoned Fries	1 serv	344	19	5	13	5	39	—	4	—	480	—	—	—
Southern Style Breast	1 serv	261	16	—	76	16	12	—	tr	—	702	—	—	—
Southern Style Leg	1 serv	254	15	—	94	19	11	—	tr	—	446	—	—	—
Southern Style Thigh	1 serv	308	21	—	78	16	14	—	tr	—	630	—	—	—
Southern Style Wing	1 serv	337	21	—	86	17	19	—	tr	—	684	—	—	—
Sweet Biscuit Bo Berry	1	220	10	3	tr	3	29	—	1	—	410	—	—	—
Sweet Biscuit Cinnamon	1	320	18	4	tr	4	37	—	1	—	560	—	—	—

BOSTON MARKET

BAKED SELECTIONS

FOOD	PORTION	CALS	FAT	SAT FAT	CHOL	PROT	CARB	SUGAR	FIBER	CALCI	SOD	POTAS	FOLIC	VIT C
Brownie	1 (3.3 oz)	450	27	7	80	6	47	32	3	20	190	—	—	0
Cinnamon Apple Pie	⅕ pie (4.8 oz)	390	23	4	0	2	46	2	2	0	250	—	—	0
Cookie Chocolate Chip	1 (2.8 oz)	340	17	6	25	4	48	29	1	40	240	—	—	0
MAIN MENU SELECTIONS														
½ Chicken w/ Skin	1 serv (9.7 oz)	590	33	10	280	70	4	4	0	0	1010	—	—	0

FOOD	PORTION	CALS	FAT	SAT FAT	CHOL	PROT	CARB	SUGAR	FIBER	CALCI	SOD	POTAS	FOLIC	VIT C
¼ Dark Meat Chicken No Skin	1 serv (3.3 oz)	190	10	3	115	22	1	1	0	0	440	—	—	0
¼ Dark Meat Chicken w/ Skin	1 serv (4.4 oz)	320	21	6	155	30	2	2	0	0	500	—	—	0
¼ White Meat Chicken No Skin Or Wing	1 serv (4.9 oz)	170	4	1	85	23	2	1	0	0	480	—	—	0
¼ White Meat Chicken w/ Skin And Wing	1 serv (5.3 oz)	280	12	4	135	40	2	2	0	0	510	—	—	0
Baked Sweet Potato Low Fat	1 (12.5 oz)	460	7	1	0	6	94	49	10	100	510	—	—	60
BBQ Baked Beans	¾ cup (7.1 oz)	270	5	2	0	8	48	20	12	100	540	—	—	6
BBQ Chicken Sandwich	1 (9.9 oz)	540	9	3	75	30	84	33	3	80	1690	—	—	0
Black Beans And Rice	1 cup (8 oz)	300	10	2	0	8	45	3	5	40	1050	—	—	4
Boston Hearth Ham Lean	1 serv (5 oz)	210	9	4	75	25	9	7	0	0	1490	—	—	0
Broccoli Cauliflower Au Gratin	¾ cup (6.1 oz)	200	11	7	20	9	14	4	3	200	600	—	—	42
Broccoli Rice Casserole	¾ cup (6 oz)	240	12	8	40	5	26	2	2	100	800	—	—	24
Broccoli w/ Red Peppers	¾ cup (3.4 oz)	60	4	1	0	3	5	1	3	20	130	—	—	66
Butternut Squash Low Fat	¾ cup (6.8 oz)	160	6	4	15	2	25	13	3	80	580	—	—	24
Chicken Gravy	1 serv (1 oz)	15	1	0	0	0	2	0	0	0	170	—	—	0
Chicken Salad Sandwich	1 (11.5 oz)	680	30	5	120	39	63	12	4	100	1360	—	—	12
Chicken Sandwich w/ Cheese & Sauce	1 (12.4 oz)	750	33	12	135	41	72	13	5	400	1860	—	—	9
Chicken Sandwich w/o Cheese & Sauce Low Fat	1 (10 oz)	430	5	1	65	34	62	12	4	100	910	—	—	3
Chunky Chicken Salad	¾ cup (5.5 oz)	370	27	5	120	28	3	1	1	20	800	—	—	4
Chunky Cinnamon Apple Sauce No Fat	¾ cup (6.4 oz)	250	0	0	0	1	62	55	2	20	30	—	—	90
Cole Slaw	¾ cup (6.5 oz)	300	19	3	20	2	30	26	3	60	540	—	—	36
Corn Bread	1 (2.4 oz)	200	6	2	25	3	33	13	1	0	390	—	—	0
Coyote Bean Salad	¾ cup (5.3 oz)	190	9	1	0	4	24	2	9	60	210	—	—	48
Cranberry Relish Low Fat	¾ cup (7.9 oz)	370	5	1	0	2	84	72	5	20	5	—	—	0
Creamed Spinach	¾ cup (6.4 oz)	260	20	13	55	9	11	2	2	250	740	—	—	9

FOOD	PORTION	CALS	FAT	SAT FAT	CHOL	PROT	CARB	SUGAR	FIBER	CALCI	SOD	POTAS	FOLIC	VIT C
Fruit Salad Low Fat	¾ cup (5.5 oz)	70	1	0	0	1	15	14	1	20	10	—	—	30
Green Bean Casserole	¾ cup (6 oz)	130	9	5	20	2	10	3	2	40	440	—	—	5
Green Beans	¾ cup (3 oz)	80	6	1	0	1	5	2	3	40	200	—	—	5
Ham Sandwich w/ Cheese & Sauce	1 (11.8 oz)	760	34	12	100	38	72	20	5	150	1730	—	—	30
Ham Sandwich w/o Cheese & Sauce	1 (9.3 oz)	440	8	3	45	25	66	16	4	80	1450	—	—	9
Homestyle Mashed Potatoes & Gravy	¾ cup (6.6 oz)	210	10	6	25	4	26	4	1	60	740	—	—	6
Honey Glazed Carrots	¾ cup (5.4 oz)	280	15	3	0	1	35	9	4	40	80	—	—	1
Hot Cinnamon Apples	¾ cup (6.4 oz)	250	5	1	0	0	56	48	3	20	45	—	—	0
Macaroni & Cheese	¾ cup (6.7 oz)	280	11	6	30	13	32	8	1	300	830	—	—	0
Mashed Potatoes	⅔ cup (5.6 oz)	190	9	6	25	3	24	4	1	60	570	—	—	6
Meat Loaf & Brown Gravy	1 serv (7 oz)	390	22	8	120	30	19	4	1	20	1040	—	—	5
Meat Loaf & Chunky Tomato Sauce	1 serv (8 oz)	370	18	8	120	30	22	5	2	40	1170	—	—	18
Meat Loaf Sandwich w/ Cheese	1 (13.8 oz)	860	33	16	165	46	95	21	6	400	2270	—	—	15
Meat Loaf Sandwich w/o Cheese	1 (12.3 oz)	690	21	7	120	40	86	21	6	100	1610	—	—	15
New Potatoes Low Fat	¾ cup (4.6 oz)	130	3	0	0	3	25	2	2	0	150	—	—	12
Old Fashioned Potato Salad	¾ cup (6.2 oz)	340	24	4	30	2	30	8	2	0	870			12
Open Face Turkey Sandwich	1 (13.4 oz)	500	12	2	80	37	61	13	3	100	2170	—	—	1
Original Chicken Pot Pie	1 pie (14.9 oz)	780	46	13	135	32	61	5	4	40	1480	—	—	4
Oven Roasted Potato Planks Low Fat	5 pieces (5.8 oz)	180	5	1	0	3	32	3	3	0	370	—	—	15
Pastry Sandwich BBQ Chicken	1 (7.2 oz)	640	39	12	60	17	56	13	1	100	1260	—	—	0
Pastry Sandwich Broccoli Chicken Cheddar	1 (7.2 oz)	690	47	13	85	21	45	2	2	150	1050	—	—	9
Pastry Sandwich Ham & Cheddar	1 (6.6 oz)	640	41	13	60	19	47	5	1	100	1560	—	—	0

FOOD	PORTION	CALS	FAT	SAT FAT	CHOL	PROT	CARB	SUGAR	FIBER	CALCI	SOD	POTAS	FOLIC	VIT C
Pastry Sandwich Italian Chicken	1 (7.2 oz)	630	41	12	60	21	43	3	2	200	910	—	—	5
Red Beans And Rice Low Fat	1 cup (8 oz)	260	5	0	5	8	45	2	4	60	1050	—	—	12
Rice Pilaf	⅔ cup (5.1 oz)	180	5	1	0	5	32	0	2	40	600	—	—	5
Rotisserie Turkey Breast Skinless Low Fat	1 serv (5 oz)	170	1	1	100	36	1	0	0	20	850	—	—	0
Savory Stuffing	¾ cup (6.1 oz)	310	12	2	0	6	44	3	3	60	1140	—	—	1
Southwest Savory Chicken	1 serv (9.6 oz)	400	15	5	100	40	26	4	4	80	1670	—	—	1
Squash Casserole	¾ cup (6.6 oz)	330	24	13	70	7	20	8	3	200	1110	—	—	5
Steamed Vegetables Low Fat	⅔ cup (3.7 oz)	35	1	0	0	2	7	3	3	20	35	—	—	21
Sweet Potato Casserole	¾ cup (6.4 oz)	280	18	5	10	3	39	23	2	40	190	—	—	9
Tabasco BBQ Drumstick	1 (2.4 oz)	130	6	2	50	14	4	4	0	0	190	—	—	0
Tabasco BBQ Wing	1 (1.8 oz)	110	7	2	30	9	4	4	0	0	170	—	—	0
Teriyaki Chicken ¼ w/ Skin	1 serv (5.9 oz)	380	21	6	155	30	17	15	0	0	870	—	—	0
Teriyaki Chicken ¼ White w/ Skin	1 serv (6.8 oz)	340	12	4	135	40	17	14	0	0	890	—	—	0
Triple Topped Chicken	1 serv (9.2 oz)	470	22	12	155	50	20	5	1	300	1350	—	—	0
Turkey Club Sandwich	1 (11.1 oz)	650	26	8	105	39	64	16	4	250	1590	—	—	12
Turkey Sandwich w/ Cheese & Sauce	1 (11.8 oz)	710	28	10	110	45	68	17	4	500	1390	—	—	9
Turkey Sandwich w/o Cheese & Sauce	1 (9.3 oz)	400	4	1	60	45	61	12	4	100	1070	—	—	9
Whole Kernel Corn	¾ cup (5.8 oz)	180	4	1	0	5	30	13	2	0	170	—	—	5
Zucchini Marinara Low Fat	¾ cup (6.6 oz)	60	3	0	0	1	7	3	2	20	330	—	—	9
SALADS AND SALAD BARS														
Caesar Salad Entree	1 serv (10 oz)	510	42	11	35	17	17	5	3	500	1130	—	—	30
Caesar Salad w/o Dressing	1 serv (8 oz)	230	12	6	20	16	14	4	3	500	500	—	—	30
Caesar Side Salad	1 (4 oz)	200	17	5	15	7	7	2	1	200	450	—	—	12
Chicken Caesar Salad	1 serv (13 oz)	650	45	12	105	43	17	5	3	500	1580	—	—	30

FOOD	PORTION	CALS	FAT	SAT FAT	CHOL	PROT	CARB	SUGAR	FIBER	CALCI	SOD	POTAS	FOLIC	VIT C
Tossed Salad w/ Caesar Dressing	1 serv (8 oz)	380	31	5	15	5	18	6	3	60	810	—	—	36
Tossed Salad w/ Fat Free Ranch	1 serv (8 oz)	160	3	0	0	5	29	9	4	60	940	—	—	36
Tossed Salad w/ Old Venice Dressing	1 serv (8 oz)	340	27	4	0	4	20	6	3	40	1110	—	—	36
SOUPS														
Chicken Chili	1 cup (8.7 oz)	220	7	2	40	18	21	4	6	40	1000	—	—	21
Chicken Noodle	1 cup (8.4 oz)	130	5	1	40	11	12	2	2	20	1310	—	—	2
Chicken Tortilla	1 cup (8.4 oz)	220	11	4	35	10	19	2	2	30	1410	—	—	12
Potato	1 cup (8 oz)	270	16	8	40	8	24	5	2	150	1020	—	—	9
Tomato Bisque	1 cup (8 oz)	280	23	10	50	4	16	12	2	60	1280	—	—	21

BOSTON PIZZA

CHILDREN'S MENU SELECTIONS

FOOD	PORTION	CALS	FAT	SAT FAT	CHOL	PROT	CARB	SUGAR	FIBER	CALCI	SOD	POTAS	FOLIC	VIT C
Corkscrews n' Cheese	1 serv	870	33	—	—	30	112	—	—	—	760	—	—	—
Dino Fingers & Fries w/ Ketchup	1 serv	680	35	—	—	22	87	—	—	—	1270	—	—	—
Grill Cheese Sandwich w/ Fries & Ketchup	1 serv	770	32	—	—	25	103	—	—	—	1450	—	—	—
Mini Lasagna	1 serv	400	14	—	—	19	48	—	—	—	630	—	—	—
Pint Sized Ham Pizza	1 serv	430	8	—	—	22	66	—	—	—	850	—	—	—
Potato Smiles	1 serv	580	30	—	—	8	84	—	—	—	1470	—	—	—
Stuffed Pizza w/ Fries & Ketchup	1 serv	850	31	—	—	30	124	—	—	—	1520	—	—	—
Super Spaghetti	1 serv	340	6	—	—	10	61	—	—	—	660	—	—	—
MAIN MENU SELECTIONS														
Baked Onion Soup	1 serv	210	7	—	—	11	28	—	—	—	1130	—	—	—
Bayou Chicken Strips w/ Dipping Sauce	1 serv	370	16	—	—	43	6	—	—	—	3740	—	—	—
BBQ Ribs w/ Fries	1 serv	2220	148	—	—	71	140	—	—	—	2420	—	—	—
BBQ Ribs w/ Garlic Mashed Potatoes	1 serv	1760	122	—	—	65	94	—	—	—	3090	—	—	—
BBQ Ribs w/ Spaghetti	1 serv	1870	121	—	—	74	113	—	—	—	2570	—	—	—
Boston's Extreme Double Order	1 serv	1660	107	—	—	159	15	—	—	—	7990	—	—	—
Boston's Extreme Starter Order	1 serv	940	61	—	—	90	10	—	—	—	5400	—	—	—
Bruschetta	1 serv	640	39	—	—	17	55	—	—	—	1590	—	—	—

FOOD	PORTION	CALS	FAT	SAT FAT	CHOL	PROT	CARB	SUGAR	FIBER	CALCI	SOD	POTAS	FOLIC	VIT C
Buffalo Chicken Fingers w/ Caesar Salad	1 serv	650	38	—	—	37	42	—	—	—	2790	—	—	—
Buffalo Chicken Fingers w/ Fries	1 serv	1430	82	—	—	45	122	—	—	—	3440	—	—	—
Buffalo Chicken Fingers w/ Light Ranch	1 serv	600	34	—	—	35	40	—	—	—	3260	—	—	—
Cactus Cuts & Dip	1 serv	1380	83	—	—	21	136	—	—	—	1110	—	—	—
Carne Amore	1 full order	1250	50	—	—	50	144	—	—	—	2970	—	—	—
Cheese Toast	1 serv	400	21	—	—	18	32	—	—	—	670	—	—	—
Cheese Toast	1 basket	800	41	—	—	36	64	—	—	—	1310	—	—	—
Chicken & Rib Combo	1 serv	1470	90	—	—	68	94	—	—	—	2910	—	—	—
Chicken & Rib Combo w/ Fries	1 serv	1920	116	—	—	74	140	—	—	—	2250	—	—	—
Chicken & Rib Combo w/ Spaghetti	1 serv	1590	90	—	—	78	113	—	—	—	2440	—	—	—
Chicken Fingers w/ Caesar Salad	1 serv	640	38	—	—	37	38	—	—	—	980	—	—	—
Chicken Fingers w/ Fries	1 serv	1420	82	—	—	45	118	—	—	—	1630	—	—	—
Chicken Fingers w/ Light Ranch	1 serv	590	34	—	—	34	36	—	—	—	1440	—	—	—
Chips & Salsa	1 serv	830	41	—	—	11	109	—	—	—	1620	—	—	—
Deluxe Cheese Bread	1 basket	890	42	—	—	37	84	—	—	—	6450	—	—	—
Deluxe Cheese Toast	1 serv	420	21	—	—	19	35	—	—	—	1140	—	—	—
Fettuccini Cajun Shrimp	1 full order	1200	43	—	—	53	144	—	—	—	3260	—	—	—
Fettuccini Four Cheese	1 full order	1370	64	—	—	54	140	—	—	—	2280	—	—	—
Fettuccini Jambalaya	1 full order	1360	50	—	—	68	151	—	—	—	5640	—	—	—
Fettuccini Spicy Chicken & Spinach	1 full order	1330	53	—	—	53	146	—	—	—	4520	—	—	—
Fries	1 serv	700	33	—	—	10	87	—	—	—	450	—	—	—
Garlic Toast w/ Garlic Margarine	1 slice	170	6	—	—	4	22	—	—	—	240	—	—	—
Garlic Twist Bread	1 basket	1080	30	—	—	33	168	—	—	—	1180	—	—	—
Garlic Twist Bread	1 serv	540	15	—	—	17	84	—	—	—	590	—	—	—
Homestyle Macaroni	1 full order	1490	83	—	—	62	119	—	—	—	2490	—	—	—

FOOD	PORTION	CALS	FAT	SAT FAT	CHOL	PROT	CARB	SUGAR	FIBER	CALCI	SOD	POTAS	FOLIC	VIT C
Italian Pizza Bread w/ Dip	1 serv	1000	53	—	—	32	98	—	—	—	830	—	—	—
Ketchup	1 serv (2 oz)	20	1	—	—	1	16	—	—	—	490	—	—	—
Lasagna Boston's	1 full order	820	30	—	—	40	95	—	—	—	1610	—	—	—
Lasagna Mediterranean	1 full order	870	35	—	—	41	97	—	—	—	2050	—	—	—
Lasagna Seafood	1 full order	970	45	—	—	41	95	—	—	—	1750	—	—	—
Linguini Chicken & Mushroom	1 full order	1320	53	—	—	59	144	—	—	—	2430	—	—	—
Mashed Potatoes	1 serv	240	8	—	—	4	41	—	—	—	1110	—	—	—
Mexican Beef w/ Sour Cream	1 serv	970	57	—	—	49	66	—	—	—	1820	—	—	—
Mini Tortellini	1 serv	490	15	—	—	17	73	—	—	—	850	—	—	—
Nachos	1 full order	1540	95	—	—	52	127	—	—	—	2370	—	—	—
Nachos Beef	1 full order	1760	106	—	—	73	129	—	—	—	2720	—	—	—
Nachos Chicken	1 full order	1630	96	—	—	68	129	—	—	—	3720	—	—	—
NY Steak Sandwich w/ Fries	1 serv	1580	96	—	—	54	118	—	—	—	970	—	—	—
Penne Baked 3 Cheese	1 full order	990	37	—	—	43	118	—	—	—	1860	—	—	—
Penne Italiano	1 full order	1160	46	—	—	50	137	—	—	—	3820	—	—	—
Penne Pisa Pesto	1 full order	1270	63	—	—	49	110	—	—	—	2260	—	—	—
Penne Roast Veggie	1 full order	900	31	—	—	25	146	—	—	—	2330	—	—	—
Pizza Bread w/o Meat Sauce	1 serv	520	14	—	—	15	84	—	—	—	520	—	—	—
Plain Pasta w/ Alfredo Sauce	1 full order	1200	52	—	—	36	141	—	—	—	1940	—	—	—
Plain Pasta w/ Creamy Tomato Sauce	1 full order	1070	38	—	—	33	142	—	—	—	1850	—	—	—
Plain Pasta w/ Marinara Sauce	1 full order	870	20	—	—	26	144	—	—	—	1730	—	—	—
Plain Pasta w/ Meatsauce	1 full order	910	22	—	—	33	142	—	—	—	1600	—	—	—
Plain Pasta w/ Seafood Sauce	1 full order	1050	36	—	—	34	141	—	—	—	1650	—	—	—
Plain Pasta w/ Spicy Tomato Sauce	1 full order	880	20	—	—	27	145	—	—	—	1770	—	—	—
Plain Pasta w/ Tex Mex Sauce	1 full order	940	23	—	—	37	141	—	—	—	1790	—	—	—
Potato Skins	1 full order	860	53	—	—	28	70	—	—	—	610	—	—	—
Quesadilla Chicken w/ Sour Cream	1 serv	770	40	—	—	36	67	—	—	—	1890	—	—	—

FOOD	PORTION	CALS	FAT	SAT FAT	CHOL	PROT	CARB	SUGAR	FIBER	CALCI	SOD	POTAS	FOLIC	VIT C
Quesadilla Garden Veggie w/ Sour Cream	1 serv	750	40	—	—	29	70	—	—	—	1560	—	—	—
Quesadilla Sundried Tomato w/ Sour Cream	1 serv	890	50	—	—	67	39	—	—	—	1870	—	—	—
Shrimp Dinner w/ Fries	1 serv	1510	82	—	—	51	135	—	—	—	1330	—	—	—
Shrimp Dinner w/ Garlic Mashed Potatoes	1 serv	1050	57	—	—	45	89	—	—	—	1990	—	—	—
Shrimp Dinner w/ Spaghetti	1 serv	1180	56	—	—	55	108	—	—	—	1520	—	—	—
Side Tossed Salad w/ House Dressing	1 serv	170	14	—	—	2	10	—	—	—	340	—	—	—
Sirloin Steak Dinner w/ Fries	1 serv	1910	113	—	—	95	117	—	—	—	790	—	—	—
Sirloin Steak Dinner w/ Garlic Mashed Potatoes	1 serv	1450	88	—	—	89	71	—	—	—	1450	—	—	—
Sirloin Steak Dinner w/ Spaghetti	1 serv	1580	87	—	—	100	90	—	—	—	980	—	—	—
Smokey Mountain Spaghetti	1 full order	1860	71	—	—	83	211	—	—	—	2590	—	—	—
Spaghetti w/ Meatsauce	1 serv	370	8	—	—	14	60	—	—	—	650	—	—	—
Spinach & Artichoke Dip w/ Tortilla Chips	1 serv	890	57	—	—	21	81	—	—	—	1290	—	—	—
Steak & Shrimp Dinner w/ Fries	1 serv	1760	108	—	—	65	129	—	—	—	1550	—	—	—
Steak & Shrimp Dinner w/ Garlic Mashed Potatoes	1 serv	1310	83	—	—	59	83	—	—	—	2210	—	—	—
Steak & Shrimp Dinner w/ Spaghetti	1 serv	1430	82	—	—	69	102	—	—	—	1740	—	—	—
The Ribber w/ Fries	1 serv	1470	85	—	—	46	121	—	—	—	1650	—	—	—
The Ribber w/ Garlic Mashed Potatoes	1 serv	1010	60	—	—	40	74	—	—	—	2310	—	—	—
The Ribber w/ Spaghetti	1 serv	1140	60	—	—	50	94	—	—	—	1850	—	—	—
Tortellini w/ Alfredo Sauce	1 full order	1220	40	—	—	46	165	—	—	—	1820	—	—	—

FOOD	PORTION	CALS	FAT	SAT FAT	CHOL	PROT	CARB	SUGAR	FIBER	CALCI	SOD	POTAS	FOLIC	VIT C
Tortellini w/ Creamy Tomato Sauce	1 full order	1370	57	—	—	46	166	—	—	—	2070	—	—	—
Tortellini w/ Marinara Sauce	1 full order	1180	39	—	—	40	167	—	—	—	1950	—	—	—
Tortellini w/ Meatsauce	1 full order	1500	71	—	—	50	164	—	—	—	2150	—	—	—
Tortellini w/ Seafood Sauce	1 full order	1360	55	—	—	48	164	—	—	—	1860	—	—	—
Tortellini w/ Spicy Tomato Sauce	1 full order	1180	39	—	—	40	168	—	—	—	1990	—	—	—
Tortellini w/ Tex Mex Sauce	1 full order	1240	42	—	—	51	164	—	—	—	2010	—	—	—
Veal Parmigan w/ Fries	1 serv	1550	88	—	—	46	138	—	—	—	1430	—	—	—
Veal Parmigan w/ Garlic Mashed Potatoes	1 serv	1090	63	—	—	40	92	—	—	—	2100	—	—	—
Veal Parmigan w/ Spaghetti	1 serv	1220	62	—	—	50	112	—	—	—	1450	—	—	—
Wings BBQ Double Order	1 serv	1700	107	—	—	159	26	—	—	—	3200	—	—	—
Wings BBQ Starter Size	1 serv	960	61	—	—	90	13	—	—	—	1810	—	—	—
Wings Cajun Double Order	1 serv	1610	107	—	—	158	5	—	—	—	4940	—	—	—
Wings Cajun Starter Size	1 serv	910	60	—	—	89	3	—	—	—	2680	—	—	—
Wings Honey Garlic Double Order	1 serv	1720	107	—	—	158	32	—	—	—	3370	—	—	—
Wings Honey Garlic Starter Size	1 serv	970	60	—	—	89	17	—	—	—	1890	—	—	—
Wings Screamin' Hot Double Order	1 serv	1630	107	—	—	158	10	—	—	—	5620	—	—	—
Wings Screamin' Hot Starter Size	1 serv	920	60	—	—	89	5	—	—	—	3020	—	—	—
Wings Teriyaki Double Order	1 serv	1690	107	—	—	159	21	—	—	—	4660	—	—	—
Wings Teriyaki Starter Size	1 serv	950	60	—	—	90	11	—	—	—	2540	—	—	—
Wings Thai Double Order	1 serv	1870	123	—	—	164	27	—	—	—	3200	—	—	—
Wings Thai Starter Size	1 serv	1040	69	—	—	92	14	—	—	—	1810	—	—	—

FOOD	PORTION	CALS	FAT	SAT FAT	CHOL	PROT	CARB	SUGAR	FIBER	CALCI	SOD	POTAS	FOLIC	VIT C
PIZZA
Bacon Double Cheeseburger Individual	1 pie	1210	56	—	—	77	94	—	—	—	2170	—	—	—
Bacon Double Cheeseburger Large	1 slice	350	15	—	—	23	30	—	—	—	650	—	—	—
Bacon Double Cheeseburger Medium	1 slice	300	13	—	—	19	25	—	—	—	550	—	—	—
Boston Royal Individual	1 pie	770	23	—	—	45	96	—	—	—	1980	—	—	—
Boston Royal Large	1 slice	230	6	—	—	13	31	—	—	—	590	—	—	—
Boston Royal Medium	1 slice	200	6	—	—	11	26	—	—	—	540	—	—	—
Cajun Chicken Individual	1 pie	780	25	—	—	41	99	—	—	—	2140	—	—	—
Cajun Chicken Large	1 slice	250	8	—	—	13	31	—	—	—	610	—	—	—
Cajun Chicken Medium	1 slice	200	7	—	—	10	26	—	—	—	530	—	—	—
Californian Individual	1 pie	580	8	—	—	23	109	—	—	—	960	—	—	—
Californian Large	1 slice	190	3	—	—	8	35	—	—	—	320	—	—	—
Californian Medium	1 slice	160	2	—	—	6	30	—	—	—	290	—	—	—
Four Cheese Individual	1 pie	800	29	—	—	45	89	—	—	—	1580	—	—	—
Four Cheese Large	1 slice	260	10	—	—	14	29	—	—	—	540	—	—	—
Four Cheese Medium	1 slice	240	10	—	—	14	24	—	—	—	510	—	—	—
Great White Individual	1 pie	880	34	—	—	53	89	—	—	—	1820	—	—	—
Great White Large	1 slice	260	9	—	—	16	29	—	—	—	560	—	—	—
Great White Medium	1 slice	220	8	—	—	13	24	—	—	—	490	—	—	—
Hawaiian Individual	1 pie	690	16	—	—	39	97	—	—	—	1460	—	—	—
Hawaiian Large	1 slice	220	5	—	—	13	31	—	—	—	490	—	—	—
Hawaiian Medium	1 slice	180	4	—	—	10	26	—	—	—	420	—	—	—
Meat Lovers Individual	1 pie	1120	55	—	—	64	89	—	—	—	2450	—	—	—
Meat Lovers Large	1 slice	330	15	—	—	19	28	—	—	—	680	—	—	—
Meat Lovers Medium	1 slice	280	14	—	—	15	24	—	—	—	600	—	—	—
Pepperoni Individual	1 pie	760	27	—	—	39	89	—	—	—	1500	—	—	—
Pepperoni Large	1 slice	240	9	—	—	13	28	—	—	—	490	—	—	—

FOOD	PORTION	CALS	FAT	SAT FAT	CHOL	PROT	CARB	SUGAR	FIBER	CALCI	SOD	POTAS	FOLIC	VIT C
Pepperoni Medium	1 slice	200	7	—	—	10	24	—	—	—	430	—	—	—
Pepperoni & Mushroom Individual	1 pie	760	27	—	—	90	40	—	—	—	1500	—	—	—
Pepperoni & Mushroom Large	1 slice	250	9	—	—	13	29	—	—	—	490	—	—	—
Pepperoni & Mushroom Medium	1 slice	200	7	—	—	10	24	—	—	—	430	—	—	—
Perogy Individual	1 pie	1010	45	—	—	50	102	—	—	—	1020	—	—	—
Perogy Large	1 slice	330	15	—	—	16	33	—	—	—	340	—	—	—
Perogy Medium	1 slice	280	13	—	—	13	28	—	—	—	280	—	—	—
Popeye Individual	1 pie	730	21	—	—	41	94	—	—	—	1390	—	—	—
Popeye Large	1 slice	240	7	—	—	11	30	—	—	—	490	—	—	—
Popeye Medium	1 slice	200	6	—	—	11	26	—	—	—	420	—	—	—
Rustic Italian Individual	1 pie	940	37	—	—	50	102	—	—	—	4250	—	—	—
Rustic Italian Large	1 slice	310	12	—	—	16	33	—	—	—	1420	—	—	—
Rustic Italian Medium	1 slice	250	10	—	—	13	28	—	—	—	1250	—	—	—
Sante Fe Chicken Individual	1 pie	800	27	—	—	47	94	—	—	—	1650	—	—	—
Sante Fe Chicken Large	1 slice	260	9	—	—	15	30	—	—	—	550	—	—	—
Sante Fe Chicken Medium	1 slice	220	7	—	—	12	25	—	—	—	470	—	—	—
Super Veggie Individual	1 pie	850	29	—	—	42	108	—	—	—	2020	—	—	—
Super Veggie Large	1 slice	280	10	—	—	14	35	—	—	—	670	—	—	—
Super Veggie Medium	1 slice	230	7	—	—	11	30	—	—	—	580	—	—	—
Thai Chicken Individual	1 pie	870	29	—	—	45	106	—	—	—	850	—	—	—
Thai Chicken Large	1 slice	280	10	—	—	15	34	—	—	—	280	—	—	—
Thai Chicken Medium	1 slice	240	8	—	—	12	29	—	—	—	230	—	—	—
The Basic Individual	1 pie	620	15	—	—	34	89	—	—	—	1050	—	—	—
The Basic Large	1 slice	200	5	—	—	11	28	—	—	—	350	—	—	—
The Basic Medium	1 slice	160	4	—	—	9	24	—	—	—	290	—	—	—
The Deluxe Individual	1 pie	780	26	—	—	43	92	—	—	—	1830	—	—	—

FOOD	PORTION	CALS	FAT	SAT FAT	CHOL	PROT	CARB	SUGAR	FIBER	CALCI	SOD	POTAS	FOLIC	VIT C
The Deluxe Large	1 slice	240	7	—	—	14	30	—	—	—	540	—	—	—
The Deluxe Medium	1 slice	190	6	—	—	11	25	—	—	—	460	—	—	—
Tropical Chicken Individual	1 pie	1060	50	—	—	57	94	—	—	—	1930	—	—	—
Tropical Chicken Large	1 slice	340	16	—	—	18	30	—	—	—	610	—	—	—
Tropical Chicken Medium	1 slice	280	13	—	—	15	25	—	—	—	520	—	—	—
Tuscan Individual	1 pie	900	32	—	—	49	108	—	—	—	2060	—	—	—
Tuscan Large	1 slice	290	11	—	—	16	35	—	—	—	690	—	—	—
Tuscan Medium	1 slice	240	8	—	—	13	30	—	—	—	590	—	—	—
Vegetarian Individual	1 pie	670	15	—	—	36	100	—	—	—	1060	—	—	—
Vegetarian Large	1 slice	220	5	—	—	12	31	—	—	—	350	—	—	—
Vegetarian Medium	1 slice	170	4	—	—	9	26	—	—	—	300	—	—	—
Zorba The Greek Individual	1 pie	810	27	—	—	43	99	—	—	—	1780	—	—	—
Zorba The Greek Large	1 slice	270	9	—	—	14	32	—	—	—	610	—	—	—
Zorba The Greek Medium	1 slice	220	7	—	—	11	27	—	—	—	510	—	—	—
SALADS AND SALAD BARS														
Boston's Cobb Salad	1 serv	1100	80	—	—	25	66	—	—	—	2280	—	—	—
Caesar Salad	1 reg	260	21	—	—	5	15	—	—	—	410	—	—	—
Caesar Salad Meal Sized	1 serv	690	48	—	—	13	52	—	—	—	1060	—	—	—
Greek Salad	1 serv	500	44	—	—	10	19	—	—	—	2380	—	—	—
Greek Salad Meal Sized	1 serv	1110	90	—	—	22	53	—	—	—	3680	—	—	—
House Dressing	1 serv (2 oz)	136	13	—	—	tr	4	—	—	—	340	—	—	—
Spinach Salad	1 serv	190	14	—	—	10	6	—	—	—	470	—	—	—
Spinach Salad Meal Sized	1 serv	500	31	—	—	20	32	—	—	—	1050	—	—	—
Taco Salad Beef w/ Sour Cream & Salsa	1 serv	640	41	—	—	33	40	—	—	—	1130	—	—	—
Taco Salad Chicken w/ Sour Cream & Salsa	1 serv	520	28	—	—	28	39	—	—	—	2130	—	—	—
Thai Chicken Salad	1 serv	730	21	—	—	44	90	—	—	—	1150	—	—	—
Tossed Garden Greens w/ House Dressing	1 serv	170	14	—	—	2	10	—	—	—	350	—	—	—

FOOD	PORTION	CALS	FAT	SAT FAT	CHOL	PROT	CARB	SUGAR	FIBER	CALCI	SOD	POTAS	FOLIC	VIT C
Veggie Plate w/ Low Fat Ranch Dressing	1 serv	180	7	—	—	6	26	—	—	—	115	—	—	—
SANDWICHES														
BBQ Beef w/ Fries	1 serv	1580	62	—	—	66	179	—	—	—	2220	—	—	—
Beef Dip w/ Fries & Au Jus	1 serv	1560	72	—	—	64	151	—	—	—	1360	—	—	—
Boston Cheesesteak w/ Fries & Au Jus	1 serv	1790	87	—	—	80	172	—	—	—	2200	—	—	—
Boston Brute w/ Fries	1 serv	1420	60	—	—	48	163	—	—	—	3260	—	—	—
Buffalo Chicken w/ Fries	1 serv	1720	80	—	—	85	187	—	—	—	4470	—	—	—
Chicken Foccacia w/ Fries	1 serv	1350	65	—	—	45	140	—	—	—	1320	—	—	—
Spicy Italian Sausage w/ Caesar Salad	1 serv	1070	51	—	—	47	104	—	—	—	1580	—	—	—
Stromboli Chicken w/ Caesar Salad	1 serv	1020	44	—	—	53	101	—	—	—	1490	—	—	—
Stromboli Perogy w/ Caesar Salad	1 serv	1120	58	—	—	41	109	—	—	—	1550	—	—	—
Stromboli Santa Fe w/ Caesar Salad	1 serv	1000	45	—	—	44	104	—	—	—	2000	—	—	—
Super Ham & Cheese w/ Fries	1 serv	1370	71	—	—	39	137	—	—	—	2130	—	—	—
Tango Chicken Wrap w/ Caesar Salad	1 serv	740	42	—	—	37	55	—	—	—	1460	—	—	—

BROWN'S CHICKEN

FOOD	PORTION	CALS	FAT	SAT FAT	CHOL	PROT	CARB	SUGAR	FIBER	CALCI	SOD	POTAS	FOLIC	VIT C
Breadsticks w/ Garlic Butter	1	199	4		tr	6	36	—	—	—	2213	—	—	—
Breast	3.5 oz	284	15	—	67	26	12	—	—	—	529	—	—	tr
Coleslaw	3.5 oz	131	10	—	6	2	9	—	—	—	211	—	—	32
Corn Fritters	3.5 oz	415	25	—	4	5	42	—	—	—	552	—	—	tr
Corn On Cob	1 ear (3 inch)	126	3	—	1	3	22	—	—	—	23	—	—	8
Fettucini Alfredo	1 serv (12 oz)	1507	64	—	51	56	173	—	—	—	3018	—	—	—
French Fries	3.5 oz	503	22	—	1	5	44	—	—	—	235	—	—	8
Gizzard	3.5 oz	387	20	—	88	24	26	—	—	—	795	—	—	tr
Leg	3.5 oz	287	16	—	52	26	9	—	—	—	542	—	—	tr
Liver	3.5 oz	341	19	—	147	23	19	—	—	—	704	—	—	11
Mostaccioli w/ Meat	1 serv (12 oz)	835	14	—	17	27	44	—	—	—	898	—	—	—
Mostaccioli w/o Meat	1 serv (12 oz)	792	10	—	0	24	146	—	—	—	842	—	—	—

FOOD	PORTION	CALS	FAT	SAT FAT	CHOL	PROT	CARB	SUGAR	FIBER	CALCI	SOD	POTAS	FOLIC	VIT C
Mushrooms	3.5 oz	289	16	—	1	6	30	—	—	—	671	—	—	4
Potato Salad	3.5 oz	94	4	—	11	2	13	—	—	—	639	—	—	6
Ravioli w/ Meat	1 serv (12 oz)	865	20	—	17	30	138	—	—	—	934	—	—	—
Ravioli w/o Meat	1 serv (12 oz)	822	16	—	0	27	140	—	—	—	878	—	—	—
Shrimp	3.5 oz	277	10	—	31	13	34	—	—	—	778	—	—	tr
Thigh	3.5 oz	355	24	—	63	21	13	—	—	—	574	—	—	tr
Wing	3.5 oz	385	25	—	81	23	17	—	—	—	654	—	—	tr

BRUEGGER'S BAGELS

BAGELS

FOOD	PORTION	CALS	FAT	SAT FAT	CHOL	PROT	CARB	SUGAR	FIBER	CALCI	SOD	POTAS	FOLIC	VIT C
Blueberry	1	330	2	0	0	11	68	14	4	20	530	—	—	0
Chocolate Chip	1	310	5	2	0	11	69	19	4	20	500	—	—	0
Cinnamon Raisin	1	320	2	0	0	11	68	16	4	20	510	—	—	0
Cinnamon Sugar	1	340	2	0	0	12	71	15	6	60	540	—	—	0
Everything	1	310	2	0	0	12	62	8	4	40	710	—	—	0
Garlic	1	310	2	0	0	12	62	7	4	40	540	—	—	0
Honey Grain	1	330	3	0	0	13	64	10	5	40	500	—	—	0
Jalapeño Bagel	1	310	2	0	0	12	63	7	4	20	550	—	—	2
Onion	1	310	2	0	0	12	62	8	4	20	540	—	—	1
Orange Cranberry	1	330	2	0	0	11	68	17	4	20	510	—	—	1
Plain	1	300	2	0	0	12	61	7	4	20	540	—	—	0
Poppy Seed	1	310	3	0	0	12	61	7	4	20	540	—	—	0
Pumpernickel	1	320	3	0	0	12	64	11	5	20	600	—	—	0
Rosemary Olive Oil	1	350	6	1	0	11	62	10	4	20	530	—	—	0
Salt	1	300	2	0	0	12	61	7	4	20	1540	—	—	0
Sesame	1	320	2	0	0	12	61	7	4	20	540	—	—	0
Sun Dried Tomato	1	320	2	0	0	11	65	11	4	20	630	—	—	1

DESSERTS

FOOD	PORTION	CALS	FAT	SAT FAT	CHOL	PROT	CARB	SUGAR	FIBER	CALCI	SOD	POTAS	FOLIC	VIT C
Blondies	1	370	23	6	25	5	42	29	2	40	220	—	—	0
Brownie Chocolate Chunk	1	330	19	7	55	4	39	26	2	20	150	—	—	0
Brownie Mint	1	300	17	7	40	3	34	27	0	60	95	—	—	0
Bruegger Bar	1	420	24	11	15	6	47	31	3	60	240	—	—	0
Cappuccino Bar	1	420	25	9	60	5	45	32	1	20	125	—	—	0
Luscious Lemon Bar	1	350	20	7	85	4	39	24	0	40	260	—	—	0
Oatmeal Cranberry Mountains	1	430	24	13	60	7	49	22	3	40	320	—	—	0
Raspberry Sammies	1	270	13	8	35	3	36	18	1	0	130	—	—	0

SANDWICH FILLINGS

FOOD	PORTION	CALS	FAT	SAT FAT	CHOL	PROT	CARB	SUGAR	FIBER	CALCI	SOD	POTAS	FOLIC	VIT C
Atlantic Smoked Salmon	2 oz	90	3	1	30	15	tr	tr	0	0	840	—	—	0

FOOD	PORTION	CALS	FAT	SAT FAT	CHOL	PROT	CARB	SUGAR	FIBER	CALCI	SOD	POTAS	FOLIC	VIT C
Cream Cheese Bacon Scallion	2 tbsp	100	8	5	30	2	4	1	0	40	105	—	—	0
Cream Cheese Chive	2 tbsp	100	9	5	30	2	2	1	0	40	90	—	—	0
Cream Cheese Garden Veggie	2 tbsp	90	8	5	25	2	3	2	0	40	95	—	—	4
Cream Cheese Garden Veggie Light	2 tbsp	60	4	3	15	4	2	1	0	60	75	—	—	2
Cream Cheese Herb Garlic Light	2 tbsp	70	5	3	15	4	3	2	0	60	85	—	—	0
Cream Cheese Honey Walnut	2 tbsp	110	8	5	25	2	5	2	0	40	85	—	—	0
Cream Cheese Jalapeño	2 tbsp	100	9	5	30	2	3	2	0	40	100	—	—	0
Cream Cheese Light Strawberry	2 tbsp	70	4	3	15	4	4	3	0	60	85	—	—	0
Cream Cheese Olive Pimento	2 tbsp	100	9	4	30	2	2	1	0	40	90	—	—	0
Cream Cheese Plain	2 tbsp	90	8	5	25	2	4	1	0	40	85	—	—	0
Cream Cheese Plain Light	2 tbsp	70	5	2	15	2	3	2	0	60	90	—	—	0
Cream Cheese Smoked Salmon	2 tbsp	100	9	5	25	2	2	1	0	40	105	—	—	0
Cream Cheese Wildberry	2 tbsp	100	9	5	25	2	4	2	0	40	85	—	—	0
Hummus	2 tbsp	60	4	1	0	2	4	0	2	0	85	—	—	0
Tuna Salad	1 serv (2.5 oz)	180	14	2	20	8	6	4	0	20	440	—	—	1
SANDWICHES														
Atlantic Smoked Salmon	1	470	12	6	55	26	66	10	4	40	590	—	—	0
Chicken Breast	1	440	6	2	60	37	62	7	4	20	1230	—	—	0
Chicken Fajita	1	500	12	5	85	28	74	15	5	60	970	—	—	21
Chicken Salad w/ Mayo	1	460	12	2	55	24	67	11	4	40	820	—	—	4
Deli-Style Ham w/ Honey Mustard	1	440	5	1	30	24	77	21	4	20	1440	—	—	9
Egg Cheese	1	480	15	6	190	22	66	10	4	200	840	—	—	0
Egg Cheese Sausage	1	680	33	12	235	33	66	11	4	200	1570	—	—	1
Egg Cheese Bacon	1	560	22	9	200	26	66	10	4	200	1070	—	—	0
Egg Cheese Ham	1	520	17	7	205	28	66	10	4	200	1350	—	—	0
Garden Veggie	1	390	3	0	0	16	80	15	7	60	610	—	—	36
Herby Turkey	1	530	14	7	55	28	73	11	4	60	1180	—	—	9
Leonardo Da Veggie	1	460	11	6	40	19	69	11	4	200	740	—	—	18

FOOD	PORTION	CALS	FAT	SAT FAT	CHOL	PROT	CARB	SUGAR	FIBER	CALCI	SOD	POTAS	FOLIC	VIT C
Santa Fe Turkey	1	480	10	4	55	29	71	13	4	60	1630	—	—	42
Turkey w/ Mayo	1	480	14	2	35	25	65	10	4	40	1220	—	—	9

BURGER KING

BEVERAGES

FOOD	PORTION	CALS	FAT	SAT FAT	CHOL	PROT	CARB	SUGAR	FIBER	CALCI	SOD	POTAS	FOLIC	VIT C
Aquafina Water	1 bottle	0	0	0	0	0	0	0	0	0	0	—	—	0
Coffee Black	1 lg	10	0	0	0	0	2	0	0	0	10	—	—	0
Coffee Black	1 sm	0	0	0	0	0	1	0	0	0	0	—	—	0
Coke Classic	1 lg	330	0	0	0	0	82	82	0	—	—	—	—	—
Coke Classic	1 sm	160	0	0	0	0	41	41	0	—	—	—	—	—
Coke Classic frzn	1 sm	370	0	0	0	0	92	92	0	—	—	—	—	—
Diet Coke	1 sm	0	0	0	0	0	0	0	0	—	—	—	—	—
Dr Pepper	1 lg	410	0	0	0	0	104	104	0	—	—	—	—	—
Dr Pepper	1 sm	160	0	0	0	0	39	39	0	—	—	—	—	—
Milk 1%	1	100	3	2	10	8	12	12	0	300	125	—	—	2
Minute Maid Cherry frzn	1 sm	370	0	0	0	0	92	92	0	—	—	—	—	—
Minute Maid Orange Juice	1 serv	140	0	0	0	2	33	30	0	0	25	—	—	42
Shake Chocolate	1 sm	620	32	21	95	12	72	61	2	350	310	—	—	0
Shake Strawberry	1 sm	620	32	21	95	11	71	61	1	350	230	—	—	0
Shake Vanilla	1 sm	560	32	21	95	11	56	46	1	300	220	—	—	0
Sprite	1 sm	160	0	0	0	0	40	40	0	—	—	—	—	—
Sprite	1 lg	320	0	0	0	0	80	80	0	—	—	—	—	—

BREAKFAST SELECTIONS

FOOD	PORTION	CALS	FAT	SAT FAT	CHOL	PROT	CARB	SUGAR	FIBER	CALCI	SOD	POTAS	FOLIC	VIT C
Croissan'wich Bacon Egg & Cheese	1	360	22	8	195	15	25	4	tr	300	950	—	—	0
Croissan'wich Egg & Cheese	1	320	19	7	185	12	24	3	tr	300	730	—	—	0
Croissan'wich Ham Egg & Cheese	1	360	20	8	200	18	25	3	tr	300	1500	—	—	1
Croissan'wich Sausage Egg & Cheese	1	520	39	14	210	19	24	4	1	300	1090	—	—	0
Croissan'wich w/ Sausage & Cheese	1	420	31	11	45	14	23	4	tr	100	840	—	—	0
French Toast Sticks	5 pieces	390	20	5	0	7	46	11	2	60	440	—	—	0
Hash Browns	1 lg	390	25	7	0	3	38	0	4	20	760	—	—	1
Hash Browns	1 sm	230	15	4	0	2	23	0	2	0	450	—	—	1
Sourdough Breakfast Sandwich Bacon Egg & Cheese	1	380	22	8	190	16	30	3	2	250	990	—	—	1

FOOD	PORTION	CALS	FAT	SAT FAT	CHOL	PROT	CARB	SUGAR	FIBER	CALCI	SOD	POTAS	FOLIC	VIT C
Sourdough Breakfast Sandwich Ham Egg & Cheese	1	380	20	7	195	19	30	3	2	250	1560	—	—	1
Sourdough Breakfast Sandwich Sausage Egg & Cheese	1	540	39	13	210	20	30	3	2	250	1140	—	—	0
DESSERTS														
Chocolate Chip Cookies	2	440	16	5	20	5	68	32	0	80	360	—	—	1
Hershey Sundae Pie	1	300	18	10	10	3	31	23	1	40	190	—	—	0
MAIN MENU SELECTIONS														
Bacon Cheeseburger	1	400	20	9	60	22	32	6	2	150	1010	—	—	1
Bacon Double Cheeseburger	1	580	34	17	110	35	32	6	2	250	1270	—	—	1
Baguette Santa Fe Fire Grilled Chicken	1	350	5	2	45	29	47	4	4	40	1220	—	—	12
Baguette Savory Mustard Fire Grilled Chicken	1	350	5	1	45	28	47	5	3	40	1110	—	—	9
Baguette Smokey BBQ Fire Grilled Chicken	1	350	5	2	45	29	48	5	4	40	1450	—	—	9
Baja BBQ Sauce	1 serv	14	tr	tr	0	tr	3	2	tr	—	351	—	—	—
BK Veggie Burger	1	340	10	2	0	14	47	8	4	80	950	—	—	4
Cheeseburger	1	360	17	8	50	19	31	6	2	150	790	—	—	1
Chicken Tenders	8 pieces	340	19	5	50	22	20	0	tr	20	840	—	—	0
Chicken Tenders	5 pieces	210	12	4	30	14	13	0	tr	20	530	—	—	0
Chili	1 serv	190	8	3	25	13	17	5	5	80	1040	—	—	33
Dipping Sauce Sweet And Sour	1 serv	40	0	0	0	0	10	5	0	—	65	—	—	—
Double Cheeseburger	1	540	31	15	100	32	32	6	2	250	1050	—	—	1
Double Hamburger	1	450	24	10	75	28	31	6	2	100	620	—	—	1
Double Whopper	1	980	62	22	160	52	52	11	4	150	1070	—	—	9
Double Whopper w/ Cheese	1	1070	70	27	185	57	53	11	4	300	1500	—	—	9
Dutch Apple Pie	1 serv	340	14	3	0	2	52	23	1	0	470	—	—	0
French Fries No Salt Added	1 lg	500	25	7	0	6	63	tr	5	20	510	—	—	12
French Fries No Salt Added	1 sm	230	11	3	0	3	29	0	2	20	240	—	—	5

FOOD	PORTION	CALS	FAT	SAT FAT	CHOL	PROT	CARB	SUGAR	FIBER	CALCI	SOD	POTAS	FOLIC	VIT C
French Fries Salted	1 lg	500	25	7	0	6	63	tr	5	20	880	—	—	12
French Fries Salted	1 sm	230	11	3	0	3	29	0	2	20	410	—	—	5
Hamburger	1	310	14	5	40	17	31	6	2	80	580	—	—	1
Onion Rings	1 lg	480	23	6	<5	7	60	7	5	150	690	—	—	0
Onion Rings	1 sm	180	9	2	0	2	22	3	2	60	280	—	—	0
Sandwich BK Fish Filet	1	520	30	8	55	18	44	4	2	150	840	—	—	1
Sandwich Grilled Chicken Caesar Club	1	540	27	6	65	34	40	5	3	150	1510	—	—	6
Sandwich Original Chicken	1	560	28	6	60	25	52	5	3	60	1270	—	—	0
Sandwich Whopper	1	580	26	5	75	39	48	7	4	80	1370	—	—	6
Whopper	1	710	43	13	85	31	52	11	4	150	980	—	—	9
Whopper Jr.	1	390	22	7	45	17	32	6	2	80	570	—	—	4
Whopper Jr. w/ Cheese	1	440	26	9	55	19	32	6	2	150	790	—	—	4
Whopper w/ Cheese	1	800	50	18	110	36	53	11	4	250	1420	—	—	9
SALAD DRESSINGS AND TOPPINGS														
Breakfast Syrup	1 serv	80	0	0	0	0	21	14	0	—	20	—	—	—
Dipping Sauce Barbecue	1 serv	35	0	0	0	0	9	7	0	—	390	—	—	—
Dipping Sauce Honey	1 serv	90	0	0	0	0	23	22	0	—	0	—	—	—
Dipping Sauce Honey Mustard	1 serv	90	6	1	10	0	9	4	0	—	150	—	—	—
Dipping Sauce Ranch	1 serv	140	15	3	<5	tr	tr	tr	—	—	95	—	—	—
Dipping Sauce Zesty Onion Ring	1 serv	150	15	3	15	0	3	2	tr	—	210	—	—	—
Dressing Kraft Catalina	1 serv	180	16	3	0	0	10	9	0	—	530	—	—	—
Dressing Kraft Fat Free Ranch	1 serv	60	0	0	0	0	6	1	0	—	430	—	—	—
Dressing Kraft Ranch	1 serv	220	23	4	10	0	2	2	0	—	410	—	—	—
Dressing Light Done Right Light Italian	1 serv	50	5	1	0	0	4	3	0	—	360	—	—	—
Dressing Signature Creamy Caesar	1 serv	140	13	2	10	tr	4	2	0	—	340	—	—	—
Fire Roasted Sauce	1 serv	9	tr	0	0	tr	2	tr	tr	—	129	—	—	—
Grape Jam	1 serv	30	0	0	0	0	7	6	0	—	0	—	—	—

FOOD	PORTION	CALS	FAT	SAT FAT	CHOL	PROT	CARB	SUGAR	FIBER	CALCI	SOD	POTAS	FOLIC	VIT C
Peppers & Onions Flame Roasted	1 serv	18	tr	tr	0	tr	3	2	2	—	81	—	—	—
Savory Mustard Sauce	1 serv	21	tr	tr	2	tr	4	3	tr	—	92	—	—	—
Strawberry Jam	1 serv	30	0	0	0	0	7	6	0	—	0	—	—	—
SALADS														
Chicken Caesar w/o Dressing And Croutons	1 serv	230	7	3	60	36	5	3	3	200	1040	—	—	6
Side Salad w/o Dressing	1 srv	25	0	0	0	1	5	3	2	20	15	—	—	15

BURGERVILLE

FOOD	PORTION	CALS	FAT	SAT FAT	CHOL	PROT	CARB	SUGAR	FIBER	CALCI	SOD	POTAS	FOLIC	VIT C
BEVERAGES														
Milkshake Black Forest	1 (16 oz)	600	20	—	75	9	103	—	—	—	170	—	—	—
Milkshake Blackberry	1 (16 oz)	610	25	—	100	9	95	—	—	—	180	—	—	—
Milkshake Caramel Apple	1 (16 oz)	540	26	—	110	9	69	—	—	—	230	—	—	—
Milkshake Chocolate	1 (16 oz)	520	23	—	95	9	73	—	—	—	220	—	—	—
Milkshake Fresh Strawberry	1 (16 oz)	560	21	—	85	8	88	—	—	—	160	—	—	—
Milkshake Mocha Perk	1 (16 oz)	590	25	—	100	11	83	—	—	—	210	—	—	—
Milkshake Pumpkin	1 (16 oz)	460	22	—	90	10	60	—	—	—	170	—	—	—
Milkshake Vanilla	1 (16 oz)	500	20	—	85	8	74	—	—	—	180	—	—	—
Smoothies Chocolate Monkey	1 (16 oz)	470	1	—	0	9	105	—	—	—	180	—	—	—
Smoothies Fresh Blackberry	1 (16 oz)	420	0	0	0	9	94	—	—	—	200	—	—	—
Smoothies Fresh Raspberry	1 (16 oz)	470	0	0	0	9	103	—	—	—	220	—	—	—
Smoothies Fresh Strawberry	1 (16 oz)	390	0	0	0	9	86	—	—	—	170	—	—	—
Smoothies Strawberry Splash	1 (16 oz)	310	1	—	0	7	70	—	—	—	125	—	—	—
Smoothies Triple Berry Blast	1 (16 oz)	360	0	0	0	8	77	—	—	—	160	—	—	—
BREAKFAST SELECTIONS														
American Cheese	2 slices	90	7	—	20	5	0	0	—	—	450	—	—	—
Bagel Bacon Egg	1	450	11	—	250	23	64	—	—	—	1070	—	—	—
Bagel Cheese	1	290	6	—	10	12	53	—	—	—	580	—	—	6
Bagel Ham Egg	1	450	8	—	260	28	65	—	—	—	1380	—	—	—
Bagel Plain	1	310	1	—	0	12	63	—	—	—	700	—	—	—

FOOD	PORTION	CALS	FAT	SAT FAT	CHOL	PROT	CARB	SUGAR	FIBER	CALCI	SOD	POTAS	FOLIC	VIT C
Bagel Sausage Egg	1	640	29	—	280	29	65	—	—	—	1210	—	—	—
Biscuit Bacon Egg	1	400	23	—	250	16	32	—	—	—	580	—	—	—
Biscuit Ham Egg	1	400	20	—	260	21	33	—	—	—	890	—	—	—
Biscuit Sausage Egg	1	590	41	—	280	22	33	—	—	—	720	—	—	—
Tillamook Cheese	1 slice	120	10	—	40	7	1	—	—	—	170	—	—	—
MAIN MENU SELECTIONS														
Cheeseburger	1	370	20	—	45	17	29	—	—	—	720	—	—	—
Cheeseburger Double Beef	1	470	27	—	75	27	29	—	—	—	760	—	—	—
Cheeseburger Pepper Bacon	1	680	45	—	75	38	28	—	—	—	1120	—	—	—
Cheeseburger Tillamook	1	630	40	—	65	34	32	—	—	—	970	—	—	—
Cheeseburger Walla Walla Onion	1	679	44	—	80	31	39	—	—	—	1660	—	—	—
Chicken Strips	5 pieces	550	30	—	20	33	36	—	—	—	1330	—	—	—
Colossal	1	530	30	—	35	30	31	—	—	—	1050	—	—	—
French Fries	1 reg	390	22	—	—	5	44	—	—	—	440	—	—	—
French Fries	1 kid size	220	12	—	—	3	24	—	—	—	240	—	—	—
Gardenburger	1	460	19	—	30	18	53	—	—	—	1500	—	—	—
Gardenburger Spicy Black Bean	1	550	32	—	40	24	45	—	—	—	1140	—	—	—
Halibut	3 pieces	230	14	—	15	17	10	—	—	—	300	—	—	—
Hamburger	1	320	16	—	35	15	29	—	—	—	490	—	—	—
Onion Rings Walla Walla	3 pieces	485	29	—	0	7	50	—	—	—	758	—	—	—
Roasted Turkey Salad w/o Hazelnuts	1 serv	375	19	—	65	30	22	—	—	—	880	—	—	—
Rogue River Blue Cheese Bacon Burger	1	510	56	—	70	36	29	—	—	—	1160	—	—	—
Sandwich Crispy Chicken	1	450	18	—	40	20	55	—	—	—	1050	—	—	—
Sandwich Deluxe Crispy Chicken	1	610	30	—	85	30	56	—	—	—	1380	—	—	—
Sandwich Grilled Chicken	1	350	3	—	5	37	45	—	—	—	1100	—	—	—
Sandwich Halibut	1	490	30	—	35	20	35	—	—	—	680	—	—	—
Sandwich Turkey Club	1	490	32	—	55	25	27	—	—	—	910	—	—	—
Side Salad w/o Dressing	1 serv	70	4	—	10	5	5	—	—	—	100	—	—	—

FOOD	PORTION	CALS	FAT	SAT FAT	CHOL	PROT	CARB	SUGAR	FIBER	CALCI	SOD	POTAS	FOLIC	VIT C
Smoked Salmon Salad w/o Hazelnuts	1 serv	370	18	—	55	31	21	—	—	—	1250	—	—	—
Sweet Potato Fries	1 serv	530	29	—	0	4	60	—	—	—	510	—	—	—
Turkey Burger	1	470	21	—	75	35	32	—	—	—	850	—	—	—

CARIBOU COFFEE

FOOD	PORTION	CALS	FAT	SAT FAT	CHOL	PROT	CARB	SUGAR	FIBER	CALCI	SOD	POTAS	FOLIC	VIT C
Black Forest Mocha	1 med	553	19	—	—	12	83	73	—	—	—	—	—	—
Black Forest Wild Drink	1 med	553	19	—	—	12	86	73	—	—	—	—	—	—
Cappuccino	1 med (16 oz)	113	1	—	—	11	15	13	—	—	—	—	—	—
Cappuccino 2%	1 med (16 oz)	162	7	—	—	11	17	13	—	—	—	—	—	—
Caramel Hirise	1 med (16 oz)	414	13	—	—	11	59	56	—	—	—	—	—	—
Chai Latte 2%	1 med (16 oz)	286	5	—	—	8	50	47	—	—	—	—	—	—
Chai Skim	1 med (16 oz)	236	—	—	—	8	48	42	—	—	—	—	—	—
Cooler Caramel	1 med (12 oz)	450	10	—	—	3	83	77	—	—	—	—	—	—
Cooler Chocolate	1 med (12 oz)	257	3	—	—	4	54	44	—	—	—	—	—	—
Cooler Coffee	1 med (16 oz)	230	3	—	—	4	48	40	—	—	—	—	—	—
Cooler Espresso	1 med (16 oz)	193	2	—	—	3	40	33	—	—	—	—	—	—
Cooler Mint Oreo	1 med (12 oz)	614	19	—	—	10	108	89	—	—	—	—	—	—
Cooler Vanilla	1 med (16 oz)	257	4	—	—	3	52	45	—	—	—	—	—	—
Glacier Gum	2 pieces	5	0	0	0	0	2	0	—	—	—	—	—	—
Hot Apple Blast	1 med	379	8	—	—	—	76	41	—	—	—	—	—	—
Latte 2%	1 med (16 oz)	171	6	—	—	11	17	14	—	—	—	—	—	—
Latte Skim	1 med (16 oz)	121	1	—	—	12	17	13	—	—	—	—	—	—
Latte Skinny Bou Low Cal	1 med	120	1	—	—	12	17	17	—	—	—	—	—	—
Lite White Berry	1 med (16 oz)	311	5	—	—	9	57	51	—	—	—	—	—	—
Mint Condition	1 med (16 oz)	520	19	—	—	10	75	69	—	—	—	—	—	—
Mints All Flavors	3 pieces	5	0	0	0	0	1	0	—	—	—	—	—	—
Mocha 2%	1 med (16 oz)	347	16	—	—	10	41	28	—	—	—	—	—	—
Mocha Skim	1 med (16 oz)	302	12	—	—	13	34	33	—	—	—	—	—	—
Mocha Turtle	1 med (16 oz)	559	19	—	—	10	82	75	—	—	—	—	—	—
Smoothie Passion Green Tea	1 med (16 oz)	252	tr	—	—	2	61	58	—	—	—	—	—	—
Smoothie Raspberry	1 med (12 oz)	293	tr	—	—	2	70	54	—	—	—	—	—	—
Smoothie Strawberry Banana	1 med (16 oz)	253	tr	—	—	2	61	50	—	—	—	—	—	—
Smoothie Wild Berry	1 med (16 oz)	235	tr	—	—	2	56	45	—	—	—	—	—	—

CARL'S JR.

BAKED SELECTIONS

FOOD	PORTION	CALS	FAT	SAT FAT	CHOL	PROT	CARB	SUGAR	FIBER	CALCI	SOD	POTAS	FOLIC	VIT C
Cheese Danish	1	400	23	6	15	5	49	21	1	60	390	—	—	0

FOOD	PORTION	CALS	FAT	SAT FAT	CHOL	PROT	CARB	SUGAR	FIBER	CALCI	SOD	POTAS	FOLIC	VIT C
Cheesecake Strawberry Swirl	1 serv	290	17	9	55	6	30	20	2	100	230	—	—	1
Chocolate Cake	1 serv	300	12	3	30	3	48	37	1	20	350	—	—	0
Chocolate Chip Cookie	1	350	18	7	20	3	46	27	1	0	330	—	—	0
Muffin Blueberry	1	340	14	2	40	5	49	29	1	150	340	—	—	1
Muffin Bran Raisin	1	370	13	2	45	6	61	35	6	100	410	—	—	—
BEVERAGES														
Coca-Cola Classic	1 reg (21 oz)	220	0	0	0	0	54	54	0	0	30	—	—	0
Coffee	1 reg (12 oz)	2	tr	0	0	0	tr	0	0	0	<5	—	—	0
Diet Coke	1 reg (21 oz)	tr	0	0	0	0	tr	0	0	0	40	—	—	0
Dr. Pepper	1 reg (21 oz)	200	0	0	0	0	53	53	0	0	95	—	—	0
Hot Chocolate	1 serv (12 oz)	120	2	2	0	2	22	21	1	100	125	—	—	0
Iced Tea	1 reg (12 oz)	5	0	0	0	0	0	0	0	0	0	—	—	0
Lemonade Minute Maid Orange	1 reg (21 oz)	200	0	0	0	0	52	52	0	0	100	—	—	0
Milk 1%	1 (10 fl oz)	150	3	2	15	14	18	18	0	400	180	—	—	2
Minute Maid Orange Soda	1 reg (21 oz)	200	0	0	0	0	52	52	0	0	100	—	—	0
Nestea Raspberry	1 reg (21 oz)	160	0	0	0	0	42	42	0	0	40	—	—	0
Orange Juice	1 (10 oz)	150	0	0	0	1	37	35	0	20	0	—	—	96
Ramblin' Root Beer	1 reg (21 oz)	220	0	0	0	0	60	60	0	0	70	—	—	0
Shake Chocolate	1 reg (32 oz)	770	15	10	65	21	140	121	tr	800	520	—	—	0
Shake Strawberry	1 reg (32 oz)	750	15	10	65	20	133	117	0	800	490	—	—	0
Shake Vanilla	1 reg (32 oz)	700	16	11	70	22	115	98	0	900	530	—	—	0
Sprite	1 reg (21 oz)	200	0	0	0	0	52	52	0	0	65	—	—	0
BREAKFAST SELECTIONS														
Bacon	2 strips	45	4	2	10	3	0	0	0	0	150	—	—	0
Breakfast Burrito	1	560	32	11	495	29	36	2	1	350	980	—	—	0
Breakfast Quesadilla	1	370	17	5	240	16	36	3	1	250	910	—	—	1
English Muffin w/ Margarine	1	210	9	2	0	5	28	2	2	80	300	—	—	0
French Toast Dips w/o Syrup	1 serv	370	20	3	0	6	42	11	1	40	430	—	—	0
Grape Jelly	1 serv (0.5 oz)	40	0	0	0	0	9	7	0	0	15	—	—	0
Hash Brown Nuggets	1 serv	330	21	5	0	3	32	1	2	20	470	—	—	9
Sausage	1 patty	190	18	6	40	7	2	0	0	—	480	—	—	0
Scrambed Eggs	1 serv	180	14	3	455	13	1	1	0	40	110	—	—	0
Sourdough Breakfast	1 serv	410	20	10	275	26	33	4	1	250	930	—	—	0
Strawberry Jam	1 serv (0.5 oz)	40	0	0	0	0	9	7	0	0	15	—	—	0

FOOD	PORTION	CALS	FAT	SAT FAT	CHOL	PROT	CARB	SUGAR	FIBER	CALCI	SOD	POTAS	FOLIC	VIT C
Sunrise Sandwich w/o Meat	1	360	21	8	245	13	28	5	tr	100	470	—	—	0
Table Syrup	1 serv (1 oz)	90	0	0	0	0	21	16	0	0	0	—	—	0
MAIN MENU SELECTIONS														
American Cheese	1 sm	50	4	3	10	3	1	1	0	60	200	—	—	0
BBQ Sauce	1 serv (1.1 oz)	50	0	0	0	1	11	7	0	0	270	—	—	0
Breadstick	1 (0.3 oz)	35	1	0	0	1	7	0	tr	0	60	—	—	0
Carl's Famous Star	1	590	32	9	70	24	50	8	3	100	910	—	—	6
Chicken Stars	6 pieces	260	16	5	40	13	14	1	tr	20	480	—	—	0
CrissCut Fries	1 serv	410	24	5	0	5	43	0	4	20	950	—	—	12
Croutons	1 serv (0.5 oz)	30	1	0	0	1	5	0	0	0	105	—	—	0
Double Sourdough Bacon Cheeseburger	1	880	59	24	165	50	37	7	2	250	1010	—	—	6
Double Western Bacon Cheeseburger	1	920	50	21	155	51	65	15	3	300	1770	—	—	1
Famous Bacon Cheeseburger	1	700	41	13	95	31	51	9	3	200	1310	—	—	6
French Fries	1 med	460	22	5	0	7	59	1	5	—	280	—	—	36
French Fries	1 kid size	250	12	3	0	4	32	tr	2	0	150	—	—	18
Hamburger	1	280	9	4	35	14	36	5	1	80	480	—	—	1
Honey Sauce	1 serv (1 oz)	90	0	0	0	0	22	20	0	0	0	—	—	0
Mustard Sauce	1 serv (1 oz)	50	0	0	0	0	11	8	0	0	210	—	—	0
Onion Rings	1 serv	430	22	5	0	7	53	5	3	20	700	—	—	4
Potato Bacon & Cheese	1	640	29	9	40	21	75	7	6	150	1660	—	—	40
Potato Broccoli & Cheese	1 serv	530	21	5	15	11	76	6	6	100	940	—	—	48
Potato Plain w/o Margarine	1	290	0	0	0	6	68	4	6	20	20	—	—	33
Potato Sour Cream & Chives	1	430	14	4	10	7	70	6	6	60	180	—	—	36
Salsa	1 serv (0.9 oz)	10	0	0	0	0	2	1	0	0	160	—	—	1
Sandwich Bacon Swiss Crispy Chicken	1	760	38	11	90	31	72	8	3	200	1550	—	—	6
Sandwich Carl's Catch Fish	1	530	28	7	80	18	55	8	2	150	1030	—	—	2
Sandwich Charbroiled Sirloin Steak	1	550	24	5	80	30	52	6	2	80	1080	—	—	9
Sandwich Chargrilled Chicken Club	1	470	23	7	95	31	37	6	2	250	1110	—	—	6

FOOD	PORTION	CALS	FAT	SAT FAT	CHOL	PROT	CARB	SUGAR	FIBER	CALCI	SOD	POTAS	FOLIC	VIT C
Sandwich Chargrilled Santa Fe Chicken	1	540	31	8	95	28	37	7	2	200	1210	—	—	6
Sandwich Chargrilled BBQ Chicken	1	290	4	1	60	25	41	9	2	100	840	—	—	5
Sandwich Ranch Crispy Chicken	1	660	31	7	70	24	71	8	3	80	1180	—	—	6
Sandwich Southwest Spicy Chicken	1	620	41	10	65	16	48	7	2	200	1640	—	—	6
Sandwich Spicy Chicken	1	480	26	5	40	14	47	6	2	100	1220	—	—	6
Sandwich Western Bacon Crispy Chicken	1	750	28	11	80	31	91	15	3	200	1900	—	—	1
Sourdough Bacon Cheeseburger	1	640	41	15	95	30	37	6	2	150	690	—	—	5
Sourdough Ranch Bacon Cheeseburger	1	720	46	16	95	33	43	5	3	200	800	—	—	6
Super Star	1	790	47	15	130	41	51	9	3	100	980	—	—	9
Sweet N'Sour Sauce	1 serv (1 oz)	50	0	0	0	0	12	9	0	0	80	—	—	2
Swiss Cheese	1 serv	50	4	3	15	4	0	0	0	100	230	—	—	0
Western Bacon Cheeseburger	1	660	30	12	85	31	64	15	3	200	1410	—	—	1
Zucchini	1 serv	320	19	5	0	6	31	3	2	40	860	—	—	—
SALAD DRESSINGS														
1000 Island	1 serv (2 oz)	230	23	4	20	tr	5	3	0	0	420	—	—	—
Blue Cheese	1 serv (2 oz)	320	35	7	25	2	1	1	0	40	370	—	—	0
French Fat Free	1 serv (2 oz)	60	0	0	0	0	16	12	tr	0	660	—	—	0
House	1 serv (2 oz)	220	22	4	25	1	1	2	0	40	450	—	—	0
Italian Fat Free	1 serv (2 oz)	15	0	0	0	0	4	2	0	0	770	—	—	0
SALADS AND SALAD BARS														
Salad-To-Go Charbroiled Chicken	1 serv	200	7	3	75	25	12	3	4	150	440	—	—	5
Salad-To-Go Garden	1	50	3	2	5	3	4	2	2	60	60	—	—	1

CARVEL

BEVERAGES														
Carvelanche w/ Topping	1 (16 oz)	600	30	18	95	21	71	—	tr	400	280	—	—	5
Regular Fizzlers	1 (16 oz)	340	5	3	10	2	75	—	1	100	105	—	—	9
Thick Shake Chocolate	1 (16 oz)	720	31	18	115	18	96	70	0	600	420	689	9	5

FOOD	PORTION	CALS	FAT	SAT FAT	CHOL	PROT	CARB	SUGAR	FIBER	CALCI	SOD	POTAS	FOLIC	VIT C
Thick Shake Reduced Fat Chocolate	1 (16 oz)	520	8	5	35	17	100	—	tr	600	350	—	—	4
Thick Shake Reduced Fat Vanilla	1 (16 oz)	460	7	4	35	16	84	—	tr	500	280	—	—	4
Thick Shake Vanilla	1 (16 oz)	657	30	18	116	17	79	73	tr	603	350	581	9	5
ICE CREAM														
Cake Butterscotch Dream	1 slice (4 oz)	260	10	6	25	5	37	—	0	150	180	—	—	1
Cake Celebration	1 slice (4 oz)	200	10	7	25	4	24	—	tr	100	115	—	—	1
Cake Cookies & Cream	1 serv (4 oz)	240	12	7	25	4	29	—	1	100	140	—	—	1
Cake Fudge Drizzle	1 slice (4 oz)	240	11	7	20	4	32	—	1	100	160	—	—	1
Cake Fudgie The Whale	1/11 cake (3.6 oz)	290	16	7	30	5	33	23	1	100	180	—	—	0
Cake Game Ball	1 slice (4 oz)	330	17	10	40	5	41	—	1	150	170	—	—	1
Cake Holiday	1 slice (4 oz)	200	10	7	25	4	24	—	tr	100	115	—	—	1
Cake Lil'Love	1 piece (4 oz)	200	10	7	25	4	24	—	tr	100	115	—	—	1
Cake Lil'Love All Vanilla	1 piece (4.4 oz)	330	16	10	35	6	41	27	tr	150	200	—	—	1
Cake Sinfully Chocolate	1 slice (4 oz)	240	10	6	20	5	34	—	1	100	170	—	—	1
Cake Strawberries & Cream	1 slice (4 oz)	270	10	6	30	5	40	—	1	100	160	—	—	1
Chocolate	4 oz	190	10	6	25	4	22	19	0	150	100	—	—	1
Chocolate No Fat	4 oz	120	0	0	0	2	28	25	0	80	40	—	—	0
Flying Saucer 98% Fat Free Black Raspberry	1	170	2	0	5	4	40	24	tr	—	170	—	—	—
Flying Saucer 98% Fat Free Chocolate	1	170	2	0	0	4	34	17	1	—	170	—	—	—
Flying Saucer 98% Fat Free Coffee	1	190	2	0	5	5	40	26	tr	—	170	—	—	—
Flying Saucer 98% Fat Free Maple	1	190	2	0	5	5	40	26	tr	—	170	—	—	—
Flying Saucer 98% Fat Free Mint	1	190	2	0	5	5	40	26	tr	—	170	—	—	—

FOOD	PORTION	CALS	FAT	SAT FAT	CHOL	PROT	CARB	SUGAR	FIBER	CALCI	SOD	POTAS	FOLIC	VIT C
Flying Saucer 98% Fat Free Pistachio	1	190	2	0	5	5	40	26	tr	—	170	—	—	—
Flying Saucer 98% Fat Free Strawberry	1	190	2	0	5	5	40	27	1	—	170	—	—	—
Flying Saucer 98% Fat Free Vanilla	1	190	2	0	5	5	40	26	tr	100	170	—	—	1
Flying Saucer Chocolate	1	230	9	5	30	5	33	19	2	100	140	—	—	1
Flying Saucer Vanilla	1	240	10	5	30	5	33	19	tr	100	180	—	—	1
Vanilla	4 oz	200	10	6	40	5	21	19	0	150	110	—	—	1
Vanilla No Fat	4 oz	120	0	0	0	4	25	22	0	150	55	—	—	1
Vanilla No Sugar Added	4 oz	130	3	2	15	5	25	7	0	150	85	—	—	0
ICES														
Italian Ice Blue Raspberry	4 oz	70	0	0	0	0	19	18	0	0	0	—	—	0
Italian Ice Bubble Gum	4 oz	70	0	0	0	0	19	18	0	0	0	—	—	0
Italian Ice Cherry	4 oz	100	0	0	0	0	25	21	0	0	0	—	—	0
Italian Ice Chocolate Ice Cream	4 oz	90	1	0	7	1	20	19	0	20	20	—	—	0
Italian Ice Cotton Candy	4 oz	70	0	0	0	0	19	18	0	0	0	—	—	0
Italian Ice Lemon	4 oz	70	0	0	0	0	19	18	0	0	0	—	—	1
Italian Ice Mango	4 oz	70	0	0	0	0	27	22	0	0	0	—	—	2
Italian Ice Orange	4 oz	70	0	0	0	0	19	18	0	0	0	—	—	0
Italian Ice Vanilla Ice Cream	4 oz	90	2	0	7	tr	20	20	0	20	20	—	—	0
Italian Ice Watermelon	4 oz	70	0	0	0	0	19	18	0	0	0	—	—	0
Sherbet All Flavors	4 oz	140	1	1	5	2	31	24	0	40	45	—	—	0

CHICKEN OUT ROTISSERIE

MAIN MENU SELECTIONS

FOOD	PORTION	CALS	FAT	SAT FAT	CHOL	PROT	CARB	SUGAR	FIBER	CALCI	SOD	POTAS	FOLIC	VIT C
Apple Cornbread Stuffing	1 serv (6 oz)	215	2	—	—	6	42	—	—	—	—	—	—	—
Baked Potato Wedges	1 serv (6 oz)	110	tr	—	—	2	26	—	—	—	—	—	—	—
Biscuit	1	150	4	—	—	4	29	—	—	—	—	—	—	—
Chicken Breast Skinless	1 serv (6 oz)	210	4	—	—	35	0	0	0	—	—	—	—	—
Chicken Burger w/o Cheese	1	285	7	—	—	50	36	—	—	—	—	—	—	—

FOOD	PORTION	CALS	FAT	SAT FAT	CHOL	PROT	CARB	SUGAR	FIBER	CALCI	SOD	POTAS	FOLIC	VIT C
Chunky Cinnamon Applesauce	1 serv (6 oz)	60	0	—	—	0	25	—	—	—	—	—	—	—
Creamed Spinach w/ Artichokes	1 serv (6 oz)	160	6	—	—	8	20	—	—	—	—	—	—	—
Farm Fresh Cole Slaw	1 serv (6 oz)	55	0	—	—	2	10	—	—	—	—	—	—	—
French Baguette	1	80	1	—	—	6	28	—	—	—	—	—	—	—
Fresh Fruit Salad	1 serv (6 oz)	77	tr	—	—	1	56	—	—	—	—	—	—	—
Mandarin Walnut Cranberry Relish	1 serv (6 oz)	240	1	—	—	0	66	—	—	—	—	—	—	—
Mashed Sweet Potatoes	1 serv (6 oz)	120	tr	—	—	0	40	—	—	—	—	—	—	—
Oriental Green Beans	1 serv (6 oz)	34	0	—	—	2	8	—	—	—	—	—	—	—
Pulled White Meat	1 serv (6 oz)	180	4		—	25	0	0	0	—	—	—	—	—
Real Cheese & Macaroni	1 serv (6 oz)	311	12	—	—	4	39	—	—	—	—	—	—	—
Red Skin Mashed Potatoes	1 serv (6 oz)	181	6	—	—	3	26	—	—	—	—	—	—	—
Rice Pilaf	1 serv (6 oz)	140	1	—	—	4	28	—	—	—	—	—	—	—
Roasted Peas Corn & Carrots	1 scrv (6 oz)	120	tr	—	—	8	22	—	—	—	—	—	—	—
Rotisserie Chicken Quarter Dark No Skin	1 serv	232	6	—	—	31	0	0	0	—	—	—	—	—
Rotisserie Chicken Quarter White No Skin	1 serv	196	4	—	—	35	0	0		—	—	—	—	—
Sandwich BBQ Pulled Chicken	1	406	8	—	—	47	42	—	—	—	—	—	—	—
Sandwich Grilled Chicken Breast	1	350	6	—	—	42	28	—	—	—	—	—	—	—
Sandwich Open Faced Pulled Chicken	1	682	18	—	—	37	80	—	—	—	—	—	—	—
Sandwich Pulled Chicken	1	320	6	—	—	32	28	—	—	—	—	—	—	—
Sandwich Signature Chicken Salad	1	370	5	—	—	42	31	—	—	—	—	—	—	—
Steamed Broccoli & Carrots	1 serv (6 oz)	30	0	—	—	9	6	—	—	—	—	—	—	—
Vegetarian Baked Beans	1 serv (6 oz)	150	1	—	—	7	26	—	—	—	—	—	—	—
Wrap Chinese Chicken Salad w/o Dressing	1	330	9	—	—	41	36	—	—	—	—	—	—	—

FOOD	PORTION	CALS	FAT	SAT FAT	CHOL	PROT	CARB	SUGAR	FIBER	CALCI	SOD	POTAS	FOLIC	VIT C
Wrap Fajita	1	360	10	—	—	43	38	—	—	—	—	—	—	—
Wrap Fresh Vegetable Salad w/o Dressing	1	170	4	—	—	5	32	—	—	—	—	—	—	—
Wrap Grilled Chicken Caesar	1	355	11	—	—	8	31	—	—	—	—	—	—	—
Wrap Pesto Chicken	1	405	11	—	—	39	25	—	—	—	—	—	—	—
Wrap Pulled Chicken	1	300	7	—	—	28	24	—	—	—	—	—	—	—
Wrap Skinless Grilled Chicken	1	330	7	—	—	38	24	—	—	—	—	—	—	—
SALAD DRESSINGS														
Balsamic Vinaigrette	1 oz	18	0	—	—	0	4	—	—	—	—	—	—	—
Caesar	1 oz	55	5	—	—	0	1	—	—	—	—	—	—	—
Chinese	1 oz	72	7	—	—	0	2	—	—	—	—	—	—	—
Low Fat Honey Mustard	1 oz	23	1	—	—	1	5	—	—	—	—	—	—	—
Ranch	1 oz	90	6	—	—	1	1	—	—	—	—	—	—	—
Southwestern	1 oz	85	7	—	—	1	3	—	—	—	—	—	—	—
SALADS														
Caesar w/ Grilled Chicken w/o Dressing	½ serv	235	8	—	—	5	7	—	—	—	—	—	—	—
Caesar w/o Dressing	½ serv	140	4	—	—	3	9	—	—	—	—	—	—	—
Chicken Salad Apricot	1 serv (6 oz)	300	8	—	—	39	1	—	—	—	—	—	—	—
Chicken Salad BBQ Pulled	1 serv (6 oz)	263	5	—	—	44	8	—	—	—	—	—	—	—
Chicken Salad Chinese w/o Dressing	½ serv	210	6	—	—	38	12	—	—	—	—	—	—	—
Chicken Salad Pesto	1 serv (6 oz)	285	8	—	—	36	1	—	—	—	—	—	—	—
Chicken Salad Pulled w/o Dressing	½ serv	204	4	—	—	37	5	—	—	—	—	—	—	—
Chicken Salad Santa Fe w/o Dressing	½ serv	240	7	—	—	40	14	—	—	—	—	—	—	—
Chicken Salad Signature	1 serv (6 oz)	230	5	—	—	37	1	—	—	—	—	—	—	—
Garden w/ Grilled Chicken w/o Dressing	½ serv	200	4	—	—	40	5	—	—	—	—	—	—	—

FOOD	PORTION	CALS	FAT	SAT FAT	CHOL	PROT	CARB	SUGAR	FIBER	CALCI	SOD	POTAS	FOLIC	VIT C
Garden w/o Dressing	½ serv	25	1	—	—	1	4	—	—	—	—	—	—	—
Young Spinach w/ Grilled Chicken w/o Dressing	½ serv	270	4	—	—	35	19	—	—	—	—	—	—	—
Young Spinach w/o Dressing	½ serv	180	2	—	—	5	19	—	—	—	—	—	—	—
SOUPS														
Chicken Noodle	1 serv (6 oz)	130	3	—	—	11	8	—	—	—	—	—	—	—
Vegetable Minestrone	1 serv (6 oz)	96	2	—	—	3	12	—	—	—	—	—	—	—

CHICK-FIL-A

FOOD	PORTION	CALS	FAT	SAT FAT	CHOL	PROT	CARB	SUGAR	FIBER	CALCI	SOD	POTAS	FOLIC	VIT C
BEVERAGES														
Coca-Cola Classic	1 sm	110	0	0	0	0	28	28	0	0	10	—	—	0
Diet Coke	1 sm	0	0	0	0	0	0	0	0	0	10	—	—	0
Diet Lemonade	1 sm	25	0	0	0	0	5	3	0	0	5	—	—	15
Ice Tea Sweetened	1 sm	80	0	0	0	0	19	19	0	0	0	—	—	0
Iced Tea Unsweetened	1 serv	0	0	0	0	0	0	0	0	0	0	—	—	0
Lemonade	1 sm	170	1	0	0	0	41	40	0	0	10	—	—	15
DESSERTS														
Cheesecake w/ Blueberry Topping	1 slice	370	21	12	90	6	39	32	2	60	280	—	—	0
Cheesecake w/ Strawberry Topping	1 slice	360	21	12	90	6	38	31	2	60	290	—	—	0
Fudge Nut Brownie	1	330	15	4	20	4	45	29	2	20	210	—	—	0
IceDream Cone	1 sm	160	4	2	15	4	28	24	0	100	80	—	—	0
IceDream Cup	1 sm	230	6	4	25	5	39	38	0	150	100	—	—	0
Lemon Pie	1 slice	320	10	4	110	7	51	39	3	150	220	—	—	4
MAIN MENU SELECTIONS														
Barbecue Sauce	1 pkg	45	0	0	0	0	11	9	0	20	180	—	—	1
Carrot & Raisin Salad	1 sm	130	6	1	0	1	22	15	2	20	90	—	—	4
Chargrilled Chicken Caesar Salad	1 serv	240	10	6	85	31	6	3	2	350	1170	—	—	0
Chargrilled Chicken Club Sandwich w/o Sauce	1	360	13	5	80	30	31	5	2	150	1370	—	—	4
Chargrilled Chicken Deluxe Sandwich	1	280	7	2	60	26	30	5	2	80	1010	—	—	4

FOOD	PORTION	CALS	FAT	SAT FAT	CHOL	PROT	CARB	SUGAR	FIBER	CALCI	SOD	POTAS	FOLIC	VIT C
Chargrilled Chicken Filet	1	100	2	0	60	20	1	1	0	0	690	—	—	0
Chargrilled Chicken Sandwich	1	280	7	2	60	25	29	4	1	80	1000	—	—	0
Chargrilled Chicken Sandwich w/o Butter	1	240	4	1	60	25	28	4	1	60	1000	—	—	0
Chicken Deluxe Sandwich	1	420	16	4	60	28	39	5	2	100	1300	—	—	2
Chicken Sandwich	1	410	16	4	60	28	38	5	1	100	1300	—	—	0
Chicken Sandwich w/o Butter	1	380	13	3	60	28	37	5	1	100	1290	—	—	0
Chicken Filet	1	230	11	3	60	23	10	2	0	40	990	—	—	0
Chicken Salad Sandwich On Whole Wheat	1	350	15	3	65	20	32	6	5	150	880	—	—	0
Chick-N-Strips	4	250	11	3	70	25	12	2	0	40	570	—	—	0
Cole Slaw	1 sm	210	17	3	20	1	14	9	2	40	180	—	—	27
Cool Wrap Chargrilled Chicken	1	390	7	8	70	31	53	6	3	200	1120	—	—	5
Cool Wrap Chicken Caesar	1	460	11	6	85	38	51	5	3	400	1540	—	—	0
Cool Wrap Spicy Chicken	1	390	7	4	70	31	51	5	3	200	1150	—	—	5
Dijon Honey Mustard Sauce	1 pkg	50	5	1	5	0	2	2	0	0	65	—	—	0
Hearty Breast of Chicken Soup	1 cup	100	2	0	50	9	13	2	1	40	940	—	—	0
Honey Mustard Sauce	1 pkg	45	0	0	0	0	10	10	0	0	150	—	—	0
Nuggets	8	260	12	3	70	26	12	3	tr	40	1090	—	—	0
Polynesian Sauce	1 pkg	110	6	1	0	0	13	13	0	0	210	—	—	0
Waffle Fries w/o Salt	1 sm	280	14	5	15	3	36	0	4	20	40	—	—	21
Waffle Potato Fries	1 sm	280	14	5	15	3	37	0	5	20	105	—	—	21
SALAD DRESSINGS														
Basil Vinaigrette	1 pkg	210	21	4	0	0	4	4	0	0	160	—	—	0
Blue Cheese	1 pkg	190	20	4	20	1	2	1	0	20	370	—	—	0
Buttermilk Ranch	1 pkg	190	20	3	10	1	2	1	0	20	350	—	—	0
Caesar	1 pkg	200	21	4	45	1	1	0	0	20	300	—	—	1
Fat Free Dijon Honey Mustard	1 pkg	60	0	0	0	0	14	11	0	0	200	—	—	0
Light Italian	1 pkg	20	1	0	0	0	3	2	0	0	640	—	—	0

FOOD	PORTION	CALS	FAT	SAT FAT	CHOL	PROT	CARB	SUGAR	FIBER	CALCI	SOD	POTAS	FOLIC	VIT C
Spicy	1 pkg	210	22	4	10	0	2	1	0	0	170	—	—	2
Thousand Island	1 pkg	170	16	3	10	0	6	5	0	0	300	—	—	0
SALADS AND SALAD BARS														
Chargrilled Chicken Garden Salad	1 serv	180	6	3	70	23	8	4	3	150	730	—	—	6
Chick-N-Strips Salad	1 serv	340	16	5	85	30	19	5	3	150	680	—	—	6
Croutons Garlic & Butter	1 pkg	90	4	0	0	2	11	0	0	0	140	—	—	0
Roasted Sunflower Kernels Unsalted	1 pkg	80	7	1	0	3	3	1	tr	0	0	—	—	0
Side Salad	1 serv	80	5	3	15	5	6	3	2	150	110	—	—	5

CHIPOTLE

FOOD	PORTION	CALS	FAT	SAT FAT	CHOL	PROT	CARB	SUGAR	FIBER	CALCI	SOD	POTAS	FOLIC	VIT C
Barbacoa	1 serv (5 oz)	285	16	4	74	43	1	—	—	—	680	—	—	—
Black Beans	1 serv (4 oz)	130	1	tr	0	9	22	—	—	—	318	—	—	—
Carnitas	1 serv (4 oz)	227	12	3	66	29	0	—	—	—	873	—	—	—
Cheese	1 serv (1 oz)	110	9	6	30	7	tr	0	0	200	180	—	—	0
Chicken	1 serv (4 oz)	219	11	2	96	29	0	—	—	—	431	—	—	—
Chips	1 serv (4 oz)	490	19	4	0	7	71	1	5	60	130	—	—	0
Crispy Taco Shells	4	240	9	2	0	4	34	0	2	40	40	—	—	0
Fajita Vegetables	1 serv (3 oz)	100	8	1	0	1	6	3	1	20	640	—	—	42
Flour Tortilla	1 (6 inch)	300	8	2	0	9	45	0	2	180	720	—	—	0
Flour Tortilla	1 (13 inch)	340	9	2	0	9	54	1	2	200	860	—	—	0
Guacamole	1 serv (4 oz)	170	15	3	0	2	8	1	5	20	370	—	—	9
Lettuce	1 serv (1 oz)	5	0	0	0	tr	tr	0	tr	10	0	—	—	7
Pinto Beans	1 serv (4 oz)	138	1	tr	0	9	23	—	—	—	374	—	—	—
Rice	1 serv (5 oz)	240	7	1	0	4	40	0	tr	20	610	—	—	2
Salsa Corn	1 serv (4 oz)	100	1	0	0	3	22	3	3	0	540	—	—	12
Salsa Tomato	1 serv (4 oz)	25	0	0	0	1	6	3	1	20	560	—	—	21
Sour Cream	1 serv (2 oz)	120	10	7	40	2	2	2	0	80	30	—	—	0
Steak	1 serv (4 oz)	230	12	4	51	29	2	—	—	—	306	—	—	—
Tomatillo Green	1 serv (2 oz)	15	tr	0	0	1	3	—	—	—	227	—	—	—
Tomatillo Red	1 serv (2 oz)	28	1	0	0	1	4	—	—	—	493	—	—	—

CHURCH'S CHICKEN

FOOD	PORTION	CALS	FAT	SAT FAT	CHOL	PROT	CARB	SUGAR	FIBER	CALCI	SOD	POTAS	FOLIC	VIT C
DESSERTS														
Apple Pie	1 pie	280	12	—	<5	2	41	13	1	0	340	—	—	0
Edward's Double Lemon Pie	1 pie	300	14	—	25	5	39	29	0	100	160	—	—	0
Edward's Strawberry Cream Cheese Pie	1 pie	280	15	—	15	4	32	22	2	40	130	—	—	0
MAIN MENU SELECTIONS														
Breast	1 serv	200	12	—	65	19	4	0	0	0	510	—	—	0
Cajun Rice	1 reg	130	7	—	5	1	16	0	tr	0	260	—	—	0

FOOD	PORTION	CALS	FAT	SAT FAT	CHOL	PROT	CARB	SUGAR	FIBER	CALCI	SOD	POTAS	FOLIC	VIT C
Chicken Fried Steak w/ White Gravy	1 serv	470	28	—	65	21	36	4	1	90	1615	—	—	0
Cole Slaw	1 reg	92	6	—	0	4	8	6	2	0	230	—	—	5
Collard Greens	1 reg	25	0	0	0	2	5	0	2	150	170	—	—	18
Corn On The Cob	1 ear	139	3	—	0	4	24	2	9	0	15	—	—	1
French Fries	1 reg	210	11	—	0	3	29	0	2	0	60	—	—	0
Honey Butter Biscuit	1	250	16	—	<5	2	26	3	1	40	640	—	—	0
Jalapeño Cheese Bombers	4 pieces	240	10	—	28	8	29	5	3	200	968	—	—	0
Krispy Tender Strips	1 piece	137	5	—	25	11	11	0	tr	0	431	—	—	1
Leg	1 serv	140	9	—	45	13	2	0	0	0	160	—	—	0
Macaroni & Cheese	1 reg	210	11	—	15	8	23	6	1	120	690	—	—	0
Mashed Potatoes & Gravy	1 reg	90	3	—	0	1	14	2	1	0	520	—	—	0
Okra	1 reg	210	16	—	0	3	19	tr	4	80	520	—	—	1
Sweet Corn Nuggets	1 reg	250	12	—	0	3	30	6	2	40	530	—	—	0
Tender Crunchers	6–8 pieces	411	15	—	74	34	32	0	1	30	1294	—	—	2
Thigh	1 serv	230	16	—	80	16	5	0	0	0	520	—	—	0
Whole Jalapeño Peppers	2	10	0	0	0	0	2	tr	1	0	390	—	—	0
Wing	1 serv	250	16	—	60	19	8	0	0	40	540	—	—	0
SAUCES														
BBQ	1 pkg	29	0	0	0	0	7	2	0	0	181	—	—	2
Creamy Jalapeño	1 pkg	102	11	—	10	0	1	0	0	0	137	—	—	0
Honey Mustard	1 pkg	111	11	—	10	0	4	1	0	10	130	—	—	0
Purple Pepper	1 pkg	21	0	0	0	0	12	6	0	0	26	—	—	0
Sweet & Sour	1 pkg	31	0	0	0	0	8	2	0	0	116	—	—	1

CINNABON

FOOD	PORTION	CALS	FAT	SAT FAT	CHOL	PROT	CARB	SUGAR	FIBER	CALCI	SOD	POTAS	FOLIC	VIT C
Caramel Pecanbon	1	890	41	13	—	—	—	48	—	—	—	—	—	—
Cinnabon	1 reg	670	34	14	—	—	—	49	—	—	—	—	—	—

COLOMBO FROZEN YOGURT

FOOD	PORTION	CALS	FAT	SAT FAT	CHOL	PROT	CARB	SUGAR	FIBER	CALCI	SOD	POTAS	FOLIC	VIT C
Strawberry Lowfat	½ cup	110	2	1	10	3	21	16	0	100	55	—	—	0
Strawberry Nonfat	½ cup	100	0	0	<5	3	20	16	0	100	55	—	—	0

DAIRY QUEEN

FOOD SELECTIONS

FOOD	PORTION	CALS	FAT	SAT FAT	CHOL	PROT	CARB	SUGAR	FIBER	CALCI	SOD	POTAS	FOLIC	VIT C
Chicken Breast Fillet Sandwich	1 (6.7 oz)	430	20	4	55	24	37	5	2	40	760	—	—	0
Chicken Strip Basket	1 serv (14.5 oz)	1000	50	13	55	35	102	3	5	60	2510	—	—	9

FOOD	PORTION	CALS	FAT	SAT FAT	CHOL	PROT	CARB	SUGAR	FIBER	CALCI	SOD	POTAS	FOLIC	VIT C
Chili 'n' Cheese Dog	1 (5 oz)	330	21	9	45	14	22	4	2	150	1090	—	—	4
DQ Homestyle Bacon Double Cheeseburger	1 (8.9 oz)	610	36	18	130	41	31	6	2	250	1380	—	—	6
DQ Homestyle Cheeseburger	1 (5.3 oz)	340	17	8	55	20	29	5	2	150	850	—	—	4
DQ Homestyle Double Cheeseburger	1 (7.7 oz)	540	31	16	115	35	30	5	2	250	1130	—	—	4
DQ Homestyle Hamburger	1 (4.8 oz)	290	12	5	45	17	29	5	2	60	630	—	—	4
DQ Ultimate Burger	1 (9.4 oz)	670	43	19	135	40	29	6	2	250	1210	—	—	9
French Fries	1 med (3.9 oz)	440	23	5	0	5	53	tr	4	40	1110	—	—	5
French Fries	1 sm (4 oz)	350	18	4	0	4	47	tr	3	20	880	—	—	4
Grilled Chicken Sandwich	1 (6.5 oz)	310	10	3	50	24	30	5	3	200	1040	—	—	0
Hot Dog	1 (3.5 oz)	240	14	5	25	9	19	4	1	60	730	—	—	4
Onion Rings	1 serv (4 oz)	320	16	4	0	5	39	4	3	20	180	—	—	0
The Great Steakmelt Basket	1 serv (13.2 oz)	770	38	13	75	32	72	7	5	250	2290	—	—	9
ICE CREAM														
Banana Split	1 (12.9 oz)	510	12	8	30	8	96	82	3	250	180	—	—	15
Blizzard Chocolate Sandwich Cookie	1 sm (12 oz)	520	18	9	40	10	79	61	1	350	380	—	—	1
Blizzard Chocolate Sandwich Cookie	1 med (11.4 oz)	640	23	11	45	12	97	74	1	400	500	—	—	1
Blizzard Chocolate Chip Cookie Dough	1 sm (12 oz)	660	24	13	55	12	99	74	1	350	440	—	—	1
Blizzard Chocolate Chip Cookie Dough	1 med (15.4 oz)	950	36	19	75	17	143	106	2	450	660	—	—	1
Breeze Heath	1 sm (10.2 oz)	470	10	6	10	11	85	70	1	350	380	—	—	2
Breeze Heath	1 med (14.2 oz)	710	18	11	20	15	123	103	1	450	580	—	—	2
Breeze Strawberry	1 med (13.4 oz)	460	1	1	10	13	99	79	1	450	270	—	—	9
Breeze Strawberry	1 sm (12 oz)	320	1	1	5	10	68	54	1	350	190	—	—	6
Buster Bar	1 (5.2 oz)	450	28	12	15	10	41	33	2	150	280	—	—	0
Chocolate Malt	1 med (19.9 oz)	880	22	14	70	19	153	131	0	600	500	—	—	2
Chocolate Malt	1 sm (14.7 oz)	650	16	10	55	15	111	95	0	450	370	—	—	2

FOOD	PORTION	CALS	FAT	SAT FAT	CHOL	PROT	CARB	SUGAR	FIBER	CALCI	SOD	POTAS	FOLIC	VIT C
Cone Chocolate	1 med (6.9 oz)	340	11	7	30	8	53	34	0	250	160	—	—	1
Cone Chocolate	1 sm (5 oz)	240	8	5	20	6	37	25	0	150	115	—	—	0
Cone Vanilla	1 lg (8.9 oz)	410	12	8	40	10	65	49	0	350	200	—	—	2
Cone Vanilla	1 med (6.9 oz)	330	9	6	30	8	53	38	0	250	160	—	—	2
Cone Vanilla	1 sm (5 oz)	230	7	5	20	6	38	27	0	200	115	—	—	1
Cone Yogurt	1 med (6.9 oz)	260	1	1	5	9	56	36	0	250	160	—	—	2
Cone Dipped	1 sm (5.5 oz)	340	17	9	20	6	42	31	1	200	130	—	—	1
Cone Dipped	1 med (7.7 oz)	490	24	13	30	9	59	43	1	250	190	—	—	2
Cup Of Yogurt	1 med (6.7 oz)	230	1	0	5	8	48	36	0	250	150	—	—	1
Dilly Bar Chocolate	1 (3 oz)	210	13	7	10	3	21	17	0	100	75	—	—	0
DQ 8 Inch Round Cake Undecorated	⅛ of cake (6.2 oz)	340	13	8	25	7	56	42	1	200	280	—	—	0
DQ Fudge Bar No Sugar Added	1 (2.3 oz)	50	0	0	0	4	13	3	0	100	70	—	—	0
DQ Lemon Freez'r	½ cup (3.2 oz)	80	0	0	0	0	20	20	0	0	10	—	—	0
DQ Nonfat Frozen Yogurt	½ cup (3 oz)	100	0	0	<5	3	21	16	0	100	70	—	—	0
DQ Sandwich	1 (2.1 oz)	200	6	3	10	4	31	18	1	80	140	—	—	0
DQ Soft Serve Chocolate	½ cup (3.3 oz)	150	5	4	15	4	22	17	0	100	75	—	—	0
DQ Soft Serve Vanilla	½ cup (3.3 oz)	140	5	3	15	3	22	19	0	150	70	—	—	0
DQ Treatzza Pizza Heath	⅛ of pie (2.3 oz)	180	7	4	5	3	28	18	1	60	160	—	—	0
DQ Treatzza Pizza M&M	⅛ of pie (2.4 oz)	190	7	4	5	3	29	20	1	60	160	—	—	0
DQ Vanilla Orange Bar No Sugar Added	1 (2.3 oz)	60	0	0	0	2	17	2	0	60	40	—	—	0
Frozen Hot Chocolate	1 (20.9 oz)	860	35	16	50	14	127	109	3	450	350	—	—	1
Misty Slush	1 sm (15.9 oz)	220	0	0	0	0	56	56	0	0	20	—	—	0
Misty Slush	1 med (20.9 oz)	290	0	0	0	0	74	74	0	0	30	—	—	0
Peanut Buster Parfait	1 (10.7 oz)	730	31	17	35	16	99	85	2	300	400	—	—	1
Pecan Mudslide Treat	1 (4.6 oz)	650	30	12	35	11	85	70	2	300	420	—	—	1
Shake Chocolate	1 med (18.9 oz)	770	20	13	70	17	130	113	0	600	420	—	—	2
Shake Chocolate	1 sm (13.9 oz)	560	15	10	50	13	94	81	0	450	310	—	—	2
S'more Galore Parfait	1 (10.7 oz)	730	30	10	30	11	111	86	3	300	340	—	—	0
Starkiss	1 (3 oz)	80	0	0	0	0	21	21	0	0	10	—	—	0

FOOD	PORTION	CALS	FAT	SAT FAT	CHOL	PROT	CARB	SUGAR	FIBER	CALCI	SOD	POTAS	FOLIC	VIT C
Strawberry Shortcake	1 (8.5 oz)	430	14	9	60	7	70	57	1	250	360	—	—	6
Sundae Chocolate	1 sm (5.7 oz)	280	7	5	20	5	49	42	0	200	140	—	—	0
Sundae Chocolate	1 med (8.2 oz)	400	10	6	30	8	71	61	0	250	210	—	—	0
Yogurt Sundae Strawberry	1 med (8.2 oz)	280	1	0	5	8	61	49	1	300	160	—	—	6

D'ANGELO'S SANDWICH SHOP

CHILDREN'S MENU SELECTIONS

FOOD	PORTION	CALS	FAT	SAT FAT	CHOL	PROT	CARB	SUGAR	FIBER	CALCI	SOD	POTAS	FOLIC	VIT C
D'Lite Turkey	1 kidz	217	3	0	14	19	30	2	3	—	369	—	—	—
Sub Cheeseburger	1 kidz	294	13	6	43	15	28	2	3	40	459	—	—	1
Sub Ham & Cheese	1 kidz	214	4	2	27	13	31	2	1	40	963	—	—	0
Sub Meatball	1 kidz	330	15	5	37	15	37	5	4	—	812	—	—	—
Sub Tuna	1 kidz	450	30	4	35	15	30	2	1	—	611	—	—	—

SALAD DRESSINGS AND TOPPINGS

FOOD	PORTION	CALS	FAT	SAT FAT	CHOL	PROT	CARB	SUGAR	FIBER	CALCI	SOD	POTAS	FOLIC	VIT C
Bacon	1 serv	64	5	2	15	5	0	0	0	—	247	—	—	—
Bleu Cheese	1 serv (1 oz)	152	15	3	15	1	3	2	0	—	283	—	—	—
Buffalo Sauce	1 serv (1 oz)	10	0	0	0	0	2	0	0	0	960	—	—	0
Caesar	1 serv (1 oz)	140	15	3	15	2	2	2	0	—	420	—	—	—
Caesar Fat Free	1 serv (1 oz)	20	0	0	0	0	3	3	0	—	590	—	—	—
Creamy Italian	1 serv (1 oz)	122	13	2	0	0	3	2	0	—	304	—	—	—
Cucumbers	3 slices	2	0	0	0	0	0	0	tr	—	0	—	—	—
Greek Dressing w/ Feta	1 serv (3 oz)	227	26	4	14	0	6	3	0	—	765	—	—	—
Honey Mustard Dressing	1 serv (1 oz)	150	142	2	0	0	7	6	0	—	210	—	—	—
Hot Peppers	1 serv	0	0	0	0	0	1	1	0	—	397	—	—	—
Mayonnaise	2 tbsp	236	26	3	21	0	0	0	0	0	141	—	—	0
Mayonnaise Fat Free	1 pkg	10	0	0	0	0	2	0	0	0	95	—	—	0
Mustard Honey Dijon	2 tbsp	60	0	0	0	0	18	18	0	—	180	—	—	—
Mustard Yellow	2 tbsp	20	1	0	0	1	2	0	1	20	336	—	—	tr
Olive Oil Vinaigrette	1 serv (3 oz)	170	17	3	0	0	9	6	0	—	652	—	—	—
Olive Oil Blend	2 tbsp	239	27	4	0	0	0	0	0	—	0	—	—	—
Ranch Lite	1 serv (3 oz)	240	19	3	20	2	6	4	1	—	961	—	—	—
Sesame Ginger	1 serv (1 oz)	170	7	1	0	0	10	10	0	—	420	—	—	—

SALADS

FOOD	PORTION	CALS	FAT	SAT FAT	CHOL	PROT	CARB	SUGAR	FIBER	CALCI	SOD	POTAS	FOLIC	VIT C
Antipasto Salad w/o Dressing	1 serv	275	16	6	38	16	15	5	6	260	1102	—	—	61
Asian Chicken w/o Dressing	1 serv	224	4	1	59	27	23	7	6	70	584	—	—	59
Caesar w/ Dressing	1 serv	474	39	7	29	14	20	2	3	240	1051	—	—	26
Chef w/o Dressing	1 serv	273	12	5	48	25	17	5	4	320	621	—	—	56

FOOD	PORTION	CALS	FAT	SAT FAT	CHOL	PROT	CARB	SUGAR	FIBER	CALCI	SOD	POTAS	FOLIC	VIT C
Chicken Caesar w/ Dressing	1 serv	532	38	8	86	34	13	2	3	240	1497	—	—	26
Chicken Stir Fry w/o Dressing	1 serv	166	3	1	59	25	10	5	4	50	588	—	—	61
Cobb w/o Dressing	1 serv	289	17	8	76	27	9	5	4	330	651	—	—	35
Greek w/o Dressing	1 serv	298	23	9	50	11	16	6	4	330	1099	—	—	56
Lobster w/o Dressing	1 serv	385	27	3	101	26	11	4	4	110	587	—	—	56
Roast Beef w/o Dressing	1 serv	146	3	1	49	23	9	4	4	50	243	—	—	56
Tossed Garden w/o Dressing	1 serv	47	1	tr	0	3	9	4	4	50	21	—	—	61
Turkey w/o Dressing	1 serv	157	2	tr	22	26	9	4	4	50	87	—	—	57
SANDWICHES														
D'Lite Chicken Stir Fry	1 sm	426	6	1	73	37	57	8	7	20	1240	—	—	41
D'Lite Fresh Veggie	1	348	7	3	13	13	62	14	7	160	650	—	—	43
D'Lite Grilled Chicken Breast	1 sm	387	7	1	67	31	52	5	6	10	952	—	—	13
D'Lite Ham & Cheese	1 sm	351	6	2	46	24	52	5	2	50	1666	—	—	13
D'Lite Roast Beef	1 sm	353	5	1	49	28	51	5	6	10	761	—	—	13
D'Lite Turkey	1 sm	364	4	0	22	32	51	5	6	10	605	—	—	13
D'Lite Turkey Cranberry	1 sm	460	4	0	22	32	75	22	6	10	605	—	—	13
Pokket Caesar Salad	1 sm	643	40	7	29	20	55	1	2	220	1473	—	—	20
Pokket Capacola & Cheese	1 sm	426	14	6	50	25	52	5	6	240	1522	—	—	8
Pokket Cheeseburger	1 sm	481	25	11	85	28	37	2	1	90	711	—	—	7
Pokket Chicken Caesar Salad	1 sm	701	39	1	88	40	48	2	2	220	1919	—	—	20
Pokket Chicken Club	1 sm	559	28	5	97	35	47	2	1	10	1197	—	—	17
Pokket Chicken Honey Dijon	1 sm	527	20	7	108	41	45	5	1	290	1285	—	—	17
Pokket Chicken Salad	1 sm	705	42	6	129	41	39	1	1	10	758	—	—	8
Pokket Chicken Stir Fry	1 sm	425	10	5	88	40	45	4	1	110	1474	—	—	28
Pokket Classic Veggie No Cheese	1 sm	238	2	tr	0	10	50	6	4	20	439	—	—	88

FOOD	PORTION	CALS	FAT	SAT FAT	CHOL	PROT	CARB	SUGAR	FIBER	CALCI	SOD	POTAS	FOLIC	VIT C
Pokket Greek	1 sm	812	61	14	50	18	54	6	3	320	2003	—	—	34
Pokket Grilled Chicken	1 sm	328	5	1	67	30	41	1	1	10	851	—	—	17
Pokket Ham & Cheese	1 sm	349	9	5	60	26	41	2	1	140	1891	—	—	8
Pokket Ham & Salami	1 sm	412	17	8	60	26	39	2	1	240	1557	—	—	8
Pokket Hamburger	1 sm	422	21	8	72	25	35	1	1	10	442	—	—	7
Pokket Italian	1 sm	574	33	13	88	30	42	2	1	240	1925	—	—	8
Pokket Lobster	1 sm	568	32	4	102	29	39	0	1	70	1004	—	—	2
Pokket Meatball	1 sm	600	31	10	73	27	56	9	3	—	1877	—	—	—
Pokket Mortadella & Cheese	1 sm	505	28	11	73	26	42	2	1	240	1488	—	—	8
Pokket Seafood Salad	1 sm	532	28	3	29	15	56	5	2	10	1320	—	—	1
Pokket Steak	1 sm	335	13	5	59	27	29	0	0	—	411	—	—	—
Pokket Steak & Cheese	1 sm	407	18	9	74	31	31	1	0	100	751	—	—	0
Pokket Tuna	1 sm	791	58	7	71	—	28	38	1	20	1013	—	—	1
Sub Cheeseburger	1 sm	542	27	11	86	29	47	5	5	90	811	—	—	7
Sub Chicken Club	1 sm	619	30	5	97	36	52	5	6	10	1299	—	—	14
Sub Chicken Honey Dijon	1 sm	587	22	7	108	42	56	8	6	280	1287	—	—	14
Sub Chicken Salad	1 sm	769	44	6	130	42	50	4	6	10	862	—	—	8
Sub Chicken Stir Fry	1 sm	487	11	5	88	41	57	8	6	110	1578	—	—	28
Sub Classic Veggie	1 sm	465	15	8	34	22	64	11	8	310	1161	—	—	88
Sub Grilled Chicken	1 sm	387	7	1	67	31	52	5	6	10	952	—	—	14
Sub Ham & Cheese	1 sm	412	11	5	60	27	53	5	2	140	1995	—	—	8
Sub Ham & Salami	1 sm	474	19	8	60	27	51	5	2	240	1661	—	—	8
Sub Hamburger	1 sm	482	22	8	73	26	45	4	5	10	540	—	—	7
Sub Italian	1 sm	637	34	13	88	31	54	5	3	240	2028	—	—	8
Sub Lobster	1 sm	628	33	4	102	30	50	3	5	70	1107	—	—	1
Sub Meatball	1 sm	663	33	10	73	28	70	13	8	—	1980	—	—	—
Sub Mortadella & Cheese	1 sm	568	29	11	73	27	54	5	6	240	1591	—	—	8
Sub Number 9	1 sm	475	19	9	74	33	44	6	5	110	834	—	—	22
Sub Pastrami	1 sm	526	27	9	91	26	51	3	5	—	1858	—	—	—
Sub Pepperoni	1 sm	614	34	13	76	27	53	5	6	240	1901	—	—	8
Sub Roast Beef	1 sm	350	5	1	49	28	50	4	5	10	780	—	—	8
Sub Salad	1 sm	298	3	tr	0	11	60	10	9	30	561	—	—	56

FOOD	PORTION	CALS	FAT	SAT FAT	CHOL	PROT	CARB	SUGAR	FIBER	CALCI	SOD	POTAS	FOLIC	VIT C
Sub Salami & Cheese	1 sm	597	32	13	75	27	51	5	6	240	1805	—	—	8
Sub Seafood Salad	1	595	29	3	29	16	67	9	7	10	1424	—	—	1
Sub Steak	1 sm	383	14	5	59	28	37	2	4	—	491	—	—	—
Sub Steak & Cheese	1 sm	455	19	9	74	32	40	4	4	100	832	—	—	0
Sub Steak Tip	1 sm	486	14	3	57	28	63	13	3	20	1229	—	—	15
Sub Stuffed Turkey	1 sm	1036	37	9	36	41	136	18	10	—	2717	—	—	—
Sub Tuna	1 sm	853	59	7	71	29	49	4	2	20	1115	—	—	2
Sub Turkey	1 sm	361	4	0	22	32	50	4	5	10	604	—	—	8
Sub Turkey Club	1 sm	360	8	2	54	34	37	4	3	10	692	—	—	17
Wrap Asian Chicken Salad	1	914	24	5	59	36	105	26	9	50	1930	—	—	49
Wrap BLT & Cheese	1	500	18	8	50	26	58	5	3	140	1249	—	—	9
Wrap Buffalo Chicken Salad	1	778	36	5	101	42	71	7	3	20	2624	—	—	10
Wrap Caesar Salad	1	669	37	7	29	21	64	3	4	210	1230	—	—	16
Wrap Capacola & Cheese	1	451	12	6	50	27	57	4	3	240	1297	—	—	8
Wrap Cheese	1	631	27	18	74	33	63	7	3	590	1754	—	—	8
Wrap Cheeseburger	1	569	26	11	86	32	52	4	3	90	611	—	—	7
Wrap Chef	1	832	40	9	72	34	82	18	5	300	1319	—	—	51
Wrap Chicken Caesar Salad	1	788	39	8	88	43	65	4	4	210	1798	—	—	16
Wrap Chicken Cobb	1	855	46	12	102	38	69	17	4	310	1469	—	—	25
Wrap Chicken Filet & Bacon	1	643	28	5	97	38	57	3	3	10	1074	—	—	14
Wrap Chicken Honey Dijon	1	619	20	7	106	45	63	8	4	300	1167	—	—	23
Wrap Chicken Salad	1	780	41	6	128	44	55	3	3	10	629	—	—	8
Wrap Chicken Stir Fry	1	511	10	5	88	43	61	7	3	110	1352	—	—	28
Wrap Classic Veggie	1	490	14	8	34	24	69	10	6	310	935	—	—	88
Wrap Greek	1	761	61	14	50	16	43	6	4	320	1722	—	—	34
Wrap Grilled Chicken	1	420	5	1	67	34	56	4	4	30	732	—	—	23
Wrap Ham & Cheese	1	436	9	5	60	29	58	4	3	140	1770	—	—	8
Wrap Ham & Salami	1	499	17	8	60	29	56	4	3	240	1435	—	—	8
Wrap Hamburger	1	509	21	8	74	28	50	3	3	10	340	—	—	7

FOOD	PORTION	CALS	FAT	SAT FAT	CHOL	PROT	CARB	SUGAR	FIBER	CALCI	SOD	POTAS	FOLIC	VIT C
Wrap Italian	1	654	32	13	88	33	59	4	3	240	1803	—	—	8
Wrap Lobster	1	766	44	5	112	32	56	2	3	70	949	—	—	2
Wrap Meatball	1	687	31	10	73	31	75	11	5	—	1755	—	—	—
Wrap Mortadella & Cheese	1	592	28	11	73	29	58	4	3	240	1366	—	—	8
Wrap Number 9	1	494	18	9	74	35	48	5	3	110	659	—	—	22
Wrap Pastrami	1	550	25	9	91	28	55	2	2	—	1632	—	—	—
Wrap Pepperoni	1	638	33	13	76	29	58	4	3	240	1675	—	—	8
Wrap Roast Beef	1	374	4	1	49	31	55	3	3	10	535	—	—	8
Wrap Salad	1	322	2	tr	0	13	65	8	6	30	336	—	—	56
Wrap Salami & Cheese	1	605	29	12	72	29	56	4	3	240	1509	—	—	8
Wrap Steak	1	402	13	5	59	29	41	2	2	—	316	—	—	—
Wrap Steak & Cheese	1	474	18	9	74	34	43	3	2	100	657	—	—	0
Wrap Steak Tip	1	374	12	3	57	25	40	11	2	20	845	—	—	15
Wrap Tuna	1	881	58	7	71	31	55	3	3	20	891	—	—	8
Wrap Turkey	1	385	3	0	22	34	55	3	3	10	379	—	—	8
Wrap Turkey Club	1	435	8	2	54	38	52	4	3	10	603	—	—	17
SOUPS														
#9 Steak & Cheese	1 sm	280	21	12	65	12	11	2	1	—	739	—	—	—
Chicken Noodle	1 sm	130	2	1	50	19	8	5	1	—	839	—	—	—
Hearty Vegetable	1 sm	40	0	0	0	2	7	4	2	—	270	—	—	—
Lobster Bisque	1 sm	360	29	18	105	8	16	3	0	—	849	—	—	—
New England Clam Chowder	1 sm	270	20	12	70	8	15	2	1	—	699	—	—	—
Santa Fe Chipotle Vegetable	1 sm	130	1	0	0	7	22	3	8	—	579	—	—	—
Shrimp & Roasted Corn	1 sm	250	16	8	65	7	23	6	2	—	669	—	—	—
Thanksgiving Everyday	1 sm	250	17	9	55	7	18	4	2	—	999	—	—	—

DELTACO

FOOD	PORTION	CALS	FAT	SAT FAT	CHOL	PROT	CARB	SUGAR	FIBER	CALCI	SOD	POTAS	FOLIC	VIT C
BEVERAGES														
Coffee	1 serv (8 oz)	0	0	0	0	0	1	0	0	5	5	—	—	0
Coke Classic	1 sm (10 oz)	120	0	0	0	0	29	29	0	10	10	—	—	0
Coke Classic	1 med (12 oz)	150	0	0	0	0	37	37	0	10	15	—	—	0
Coke Classic	1 lg (20 oz)	230	0	0	0	0	59	59	0	15	25	—	—	0
Coke Classic Best Value	1 serv (27 oz)	320	0	0	0	0	81	81	0	25	30	—	—	0
Diet Coke	1 lg (20 oz)	5	0	0	0	1	1	0	0	25	35	—	—	0
Diet Coke	1 sm (10 oz)	0	0	0	0	0	0	0	0	10	15	—	—	0
Diet Coke	1 med (12 oz)	0	0	0	0	0	0	0	0	0	15	—	—	0
Diet Coke Best Value	1 serv (27 oz)	10	0	0	0	1	1	0	0	30	45	—	—	0
Iced Tea	1 med (12 oz)	0	0	0	0	0	1	0	0	0	10	—	—	0

FOOD	PORTION	CALS	FAT	SAT FAT	CHOL	PROT	CARB	SUGAR	FIBER	CALCI	SOD	POTAS	FOLIC	VIT C
Iced Tea	1 lg (20 oz)	5	0	0	0	0	2	0	0	0	15	—	—	0
Iced Tea	1 sm (10 oz)	0	0	0	0	0	0	0	0	0	10	—	—	0
Iced Tea Best Value	1 serv (27 oz)	10	0	0	0	0	2	0	0	0	25	—	—	0
Milk 1% Lowfat	1 serv (11 oz)	130	3	2	10	10	15	15	0	380	150	—	—	3
Mr Pibb	1 sm (10 oz)	120	0	0	0	0	29	29	0	10	30	—	—	0
Mr Pibb	1 med (12 oz)	150	0	0	0	0	37	37	0	0	10	—	—	0
Mr Pibb	1 lg (20 oz)	230	0	0	0	0	59	59	0	15	55	—	—	0
Mr Pibb Best Value	1 serv (27 oz)	320	0	0	0	0	81	81	0	25	80	—	—	0
Orange Juice	1 serv (11 oz)	140	0	0	0	2	34	33	1	30	0	—	—	120
Shake Chocolate	1 lg (15 oz)	680	16	12	45	16	117	101	1	600	350	—	—	3
Shake Chocolate	1 sm (11.4 oz)	520	12	9	35	12	89	77	1	400	270	—	—	3
Shake Strawberry	1 lg (15 oz)	540	8	6	40	14	100	85	1	570	280	—	—	25
Shake Strawberry	1 sm (11.4 oz)	410	6	4	30	11	76	65	1	440	220	—	—	15
Shake Vanilla	1 lg (15 oz)	550	10	6	50	16	97	81	0	650	320	—	—	4
Shake Vanilla	1 sm (11.4 oz)	420	7	5	35	12	75	62	0	500	250	—	—	3
Sprite	1 sm (10 oz)	110	0	0	0	0	29	29	0	5	30	—	—	0
Sprite	1 lg (20 oz)	230	0	0	0	0	59	59	0	10	60	—	—	0
Sprite	1 med (12 oz)	140	0	0	0	0	37	37	0	0	40	—	—	0
Sprite Best Value	1 serv (27 oz)	310	0	0	0	0	81	81	0	15	85	—	—	0
BREAKFAST SELECTIONS														
Burrito Breakfast	1 (3.8 oz)	250	11	6	160	10	24	2	1	180	520	—	—	1
Burrito Egg & Cheese	1 (7.5 oz)	450	24	13	530	23	39	2	3	400	740	—	—	1
Burrito Macho Bacon & Egg	1 (15.9 oz)	1030	60	20	790	40	82	6	6	490	1760	—	—	16
Burrito Steak & Egg	1 (9 oz)	580	34	16	560	33	41	2	3	410	1270	—	—	2
Quesadilla Bacon & Egg	1 (6.1 oz)	450	23	12	260	21	40	2	2	320	920	—	—	4
Side of Bacon	2 strips (0.3 oz)	50	4	2	10	3	0	0	0	0	170	—	—	0
MAIN MENU SELECTIONS														
Beans 'n Cheese Cup	1 serv (7.7 oz)	260	3	2	5	16	44	4	16	140	1810	—	—	5
Burrito Combo	1 (8.2 oz)	490	21	13	55	26	53	3	8	370	1380	—	—	3
Burrito Del Beef	1 (8 oz)	550	30	17	90	31	42	2	3	350	1090	—	—	2
Burrito Del Classic Chicken	1 (8.5 oz)	580	38	13	70	24	42	4	3	370	1100	—	—	10
Burrito Deluxe Combo	1 (10.7 oz)	530	25	15	60	27	56	5	9	410	1390	—	—	15
Burrito Deluxe Del Beef	1 (10.5 oz)	590	33	19	95	32	45	4	4	390	1110	—	—	15
Burrito Green	1 (5 oz)	280	8	5	15	11	38	2	6	190	1030	—	—	4
Burrito Macho Beef	1 (18.9 oz)	1170	62	29	190	60	89	8	7	470	2190	—	—	20

FOOD	PORTION	CALS	FAT	SAT FAT	CHOL	PROT	CARB	SUGAR	FIBER	CALCI	SOD	POTAS	FOLIC	VIT C
Burrito Macho Combo	1 (19.4 oz)	1050	44	21	115	49	113	9	17	510	2760	—	—	20
Burrito Red	1 (5 oz)	270	8	5	15	11	38	2	6	190	1020	—	—	2
Burrito Red Regular	1 (7.5 oz)	390	12	9	20	18	59	3	11	380	1439	—	—	3
Burrito Regular Green	1 (7.5 oz)	400	12	9	10	18	59	3	10	380	1450	—	—	6
Burrito Spicy Chicken	1 (8.7 oz)	480	16	10	40	23	65	3	8	380	1620	—	—	4
Burrito The Works	1 (10.2 oz)	480	18	11	25	18	69	5	9	400	1500	—	—	9
Cheeseburger	1 (4.6 oz)	330	13	6	35	16	37	4	3	170	870	—	—	2
Del Cheeseburger	1 (5.6 oz)	430	25	7	45	16	35	3	4	180	710	—	—	6
Double Del Cheeseburger	1 (7.1 oz)	560	35	12	85	26	35	4	4	260	960	—	—	6
Fries	1 reg (5 oz)	350	23	4	0	3	34	1	3	10	270	—	—	15
Fries	1 sm (3 oz)	210	14	2	0	2	20	0	2	5	160	—	—	8
Fries Best Value	1 serv (7 oz)	490	32	5	0	5	47	1	5	10	380	—	—	20
Fries Chili Cheese	1 serv (10.5 oz)	670	46	15	45	17	51	2	5	230	880	—	—	20
Fries Deluxe Chili Cheese	1 serv (11.9 oz)	710	49	16	50	17	53	4	6	250	880	—	—	25
Get A Lot Meals #1 Combo Burrito Fries Drink	1 meal	980	44	16	55	29	124	41	11	300	1670	—	—	15
Get A Lot Meals #2 Del Classic Chicken Burrito Fries Drink	1 meal	1080	61	17	70	28	113	42	7	390	1390	—	—	25
Get A Lot Meals #3 Regular Red Burrito Fries Drink	1 meal	890	35	12	20	21	130	41	14	400	1710	—	—	15
Get A Lot Meals #4 Two Chicken Soft Tacos Fries Drink	1 meal	910	46	11	60	25	102	39	5	240	1330	—	—	20
Get A Lot Meals #5 Taco Combo Burrito Drink	1 meal	790	31	17	75	32	101	40	9	450	1540	—	—	5
Get A Lot Meals #6 Two Tacos Quesadilla Drink	1 meal	960	47	29	115	37	98	40	3	750	1170	—	—	10
Get A Lot Meals #7 Macho Combo Burrito Fries Drink	1 meal	1530	67	25	115	52	183	47	20	530	3050	—	—	35
Get A Lot Meals #8 Two Big Fat Tacos Fries Drink	1 meal	802	45	14	70	35	148	44	10	300	1640	—	—	25

FOOD	PORTION	CALS	FAT	SAT FAT	CHOL	PROT	CARB	SUGAR	FIBER	CALCI	SOD	POTAS	FOLIC	VIT C
Get A Lot Meals #9 Double Del Cheeseburger Fries Drink	1 meal	1050	58	16	85	29	106	41	7	280	1250	—	—	20
Nachos	1 serv (4 oz)	380	24	8	5	5	40	1	2	80	630	—	—	0
Nachos Macho	1 serv (17 oz)	1200	66	26	55	33	130	7	16	260	2720	—	—	10
Quesadilla Chicken	1 (6.8 oz)	580	31	21	104	33	41	2	2	610	1240	—	—	2
Quesadilla Regular	1 (5.3 oz)	500	27	20	75	23	39	2	2	600	860	—	—	2
Quesadilla Spicy Jack Chicken	1 (6.8 oz)	570	30	16	105	32	40	1	2	600	1300	—	—	5
Quesadilla Spicy Jack Regular	1 (5.3 oz)	490	26	17	75	23	38	1	2	590	920	—	—	5
Rice Cup	1 serv (4 oz)	150	2	1	2	3	28	2	1	20	600	—	—	1
Soft Taco	1 (2.8 oz)	160	8	4	20	8	16	1	1	110	330	—	—	4
Soft Taco Chicken	1 (3.3 oz)	210	12	4	30	11	16	1	1	110	520	—	—	4
Taco	1 (2.2 oz)	160	10	4	20	7	11	1	1	70	150	—	—	4
Taco Big Fat	1 (5.4 oz)	320	11	5	35	16	39	3	3	140	680	—	—	6
Taco Big Fat Chicken	1 (5.4 oz)	340	13	4	45	18	38	3	3	140	840	—	—	6
Taco Big Fat Steak	1 (5.4 oz)	390	19	6	45	18	38	3	3	140	960	—	—	5
Taco Salad Deluxe	1 (18.8 oz)	760	37	17	70	31	76	10	14	430	2010	—	—	45
Tostada Salad	1 (4.5 oz)	210	9	5	15	9	24	2	6	150	640	—	—	8

DENNY'S

BEVERAGES

FOOD	PORTION	CALS	FAT	SAT FAT	CHOL	PROT	CARB	SUGAR	FIBER	CALCI	SOD	POTAS	FOLIC	VIT C
2% Milk	10 oz	151	6	4	22	10	15	14	0	370	152	—	—	1
Apple Juice	1 reg	126	0	0	0	0	33	33	0	0	24	—	—	2
Cappuccino French Vanilla	8 oz	100	2	2	0	3	28	24	1	10	220	—	—	0
Cappuccino Original	8 oz	100	3	3	0	2	17	13	0	0	100	—	—	0
Chocolate Milk	10 oz	235	9	6	37	9	30	24	0	330	189	—	—	2
Grapefruit	1 serv (10 oz)	162	0	0	0	0	41	41	0	0	43	—	—	75
Hot Chocolate	8 oz	100	2	2	0	3	28	24	1	10	219	—	—	0
Lemonade	16 oz	150	0	0	0	0	35	35	0	0	38	—	—	0
Malted Milk Shake Chocolate Or Vanilla	12 oz	583	26	16	100	12	82	71	tr	310	278	—	—	2
Orange Juice	10 oz	126	0	0	0	2	31	24	0	20	31	—	—	105
Raspberry Ice Tea	16 oz	78	0	0	0	0	21	21	0	0	0	—	—	0
Tomato Juice	1 serv (10 oz)	56	0	0	0	2	11	0	2	10	921	—	—	29

BREAKFAST SELECTIONS

FOOD	PORTION	CALS	FAT	SAT FAT	CHOL	PROT	CARB	SUGAR	FIBER	CALCI	SOD	POTAS	FOLIC	VIT C
All American Slam	1 serv	816	67	24	828	45	3	0	1	240	1826	—	—	26
Applesauce	1 serv	60	0	0	0	0	15	15	1	0	13	—	—	0

FOOD	PORTION	CALS	FAT	SAT FAT	CHOL	PROT	CARB	SUGAR	FIBER	CALCI	SOD	POTAS	FOLIC	VIT C
Bacon	4 strips	162	18	5	36	12	1	1	0	0	640	—	—	1
Bagel Dry	1	235	1	0	0	9	46	0	0	0	495	—	—	0
Banana	1	110	0	0	0	1	29	21	4	0	0	—	—	9
Belgian Waffle	1	619	45	22	274	22	28	1	0	130	1638	—	—	0
Breakfast Dagwood	1 serv	1446	90	35	765	82	81	5	1	820	4003	—	—	0
Buttermilk Hotcakes	3	466	23	7	47	20	47	0	2	80	2077	—	—	0
Cantaloupe	¼	32	0	0	0	1	8	7	1	10	16	—	—	30
Chicken Fajita Skillet	1 serv	855	49	15	515	26	30	5	11	270	1863	—	—	27
Corned Beef Hash Slam	1 serv	668	55	19	535	32	11	2	1	70	816	—	—	3
Country Fish Potatoes	1 serv	394	20	6	9	3	23	2	10	0	938	—	—	0
Egg	1	120	10	3	210	6	tr	tr	0	0	120	—	—	4
English Muffin Dry	1	125	1	0	0	5	24	0	1	80	198	—	—	0
Fabulous French Toast	1 serv	1146	71	24	297	26	104	20	3	240	2441	—	—	0
Farmer's Slam	1 serv	1200	80	24	704	51	82	5	3	320	3204	—	—	17
French Slam	1 serv	1119	77	25	705	45	71	17	3	120	2265	—	—	0
Fruit Mix	1 serv	36	0	0	0	1	9	9	1	0	16	—	—	18
Grand Slam Slugger	1 serv	927	55	15	476	34	74	24	3	140	2399	—	—	82
Grapefruit	½	60	0	0	0	1	16	10	6	20	0	—	—	66
Grapes	1 serv	55	1	0	0	1	15	14	1	10	0	—	—	9
Grits	1 serv	80	0	0	0	2	18	0	0	0	520	—	—	0
Ham & Cheddar Omelette	1 serv	595	47	16	783	41	5	2	0	380	1200	—	—	0
Ham & Cheese Omelette w/ Eggbeaters	1 serv	468	32	11	58	37	5	2	0	70	1351	—	—	0
Ham Slice	1	94	3	1	23	15	2	0	0	0	761	—	—	0
Hashed Browns	1 serv	197	12	2	0	2	20	1	2	10	446	—	—	7
Hashed Browns Covered	1 serv	280	19	6	23	7	21	1	2	170	583	—	—	7
Hashed Browns Covered & Smothered	1 serv	493	25	9	29	14	54	12	3	230	3534	—	—	10
Honeydew	¼	31	0	0	0	1	8	7	1	0	22	—	—	16
Lumberjack Slam w/ Hash Browns	1 serv	1035	58	17	589	51	73	7	3	150	4462	—	—	9
Meat Lover's Skillet	1 serv	1031	74	24	528	39	27	3	10	240	2374	—	—	1
Moon Over My Hammy	1 serv	841	51	22	580	54	42	4	2	580	2699	—	—	0

FOOD	PORTION	CALS	FAT	SAT FAT	CHOL	PROT	CARB	SUGAR	FIBER	CALCI	SOD	POTAS	FOLIC	VIT C
Oatmeal	1 serv	100	2	0	0	5	18	0	3	10	175	—	—	0
Oatmeal Deluxe	1 serv	460	6	3	11	13	95	63	7	250	87	—	—	4
Original Grand Slam	1 serv	665	49	15	515	26	33	1	2	120	1106	—	—	1
Ready To Eat Cereal	1 serv	100	0	0	0	2	23	5	1	0	276	—	—	10
Sausage	4 links	354	32	2	64	16	0	4	0	10	944	—	—	0
Scram Slam	1 serv	827	68	21	801	45	8	4	1	260	1937	—	—	23
Senior Belgian Waffle Slam	1 serv	399	33	8	302	16	12	2	0	90	612	—	—	1
Senior Omelette	1 serv	429	20	12	515	25	8	6	2	200	755	—	—	9
Sirloin Steak & Eggs	1 serv	675	45	16	643	52	1	0	1	90	368	—	—	1
Slim Slam	1 serv	438	6	3	50	32	56	15	2	50	2417	—	—	0
T-Bone Steak & Eggs	1 serv	991	77	31	657	73	1	0	1	200	1003	—	—	2
Toast Dry	1 slice	92	1	0	0	3	17	1	1	30	166	—	—	0
Two Egg Breakfast w/ Hash Browns	1 serv	825	67	17	538	31	24	1	2	80	1765	—	—	8
Ultimate Omelette	1 serv	611	50	17	756	34	11	6	3	80	1007	—	—	55
Veggie Cheese Omelette	1 serv	494	39	12	747	30	11	6	2	280	719	—	—	16
CHILDREN'S MENU SELECTIONS														
Burgerlicious	1 serv	296	17	6	28	13	24	2	1	30	368	—	—	0
Burgerlicious w/ Cheese	1 serv	341	20	6	40	15	24	2	1	100	560	—	—	0
Dennysaur Chicken Nuggets	1 serv	190	13	4	30	9	9	0	0	20	340	—	—	0
Frenchtastic Slam	1 serv	452	33	9	311	19	22	3	1	50	664	—	—	0
Junior Grand Slam	1 serv	397	25	7	230	17	33	2	1	80	1118	—	—	0
Junior Shrimps Ahoy!	1 serv	411	18	4	66	13	50	4	4	30	792	—	—	9
Oreo Blender Blaster	1 serv	580	29	15	87	11	72	60	1	340	194	—	—	2
Pizza Party	1 serv	400	15	3	10	18	47	8	7	500	1090	—	—	2
Smiley-Face Hotcakes w/ Meat	1 serv	463	22	7	38	14	63	7	2	90	1410	—	—	0
Smiley-Face Hotcakes w/o Meat	1 serv	344	9	3	13	7	62	6	2	90	1014	—	—	0
The Big Cheese	1 serv	334	20	2	24	9	28	3	2	200	828	—	—	0
DESSERTS														
Apple Pie	1 serv	470	24	6	0	3	64	36	1	0	470	—	—	0
Banana Split	1	894	43	19	78	15	121	29	6	240	177	—	—	33
Carrot Cake	1 serv	799	45	13	125	9	99	75	2	80	630	—	—	4
Cheesecake	1 serv	580	38	24	174	8	51	36	0	110	380	—	—	2

FOOD	PORTION	CALS	FAT	SAT FAT	CHOL	PROT	CARB	SUGAR	FIBER	CALCI	SOD	POTAS	FOLIC	VIT C
Chocolate Topping	1 serv	317	25	0	0	2	27	27	0	0	83	—	—	0
Chocolate Peanut Butter Pie	1 serv	653	39	19	27	15	64	45	3	110	319	—	—	0
Double Scoop Sundae	1 serv	375	27	12	74	6	29	8	0	130	86	—	—	0
Float Rootbeer or Coke	12 oz	280	10	6	39	3	47	33	0	120	109	—	—	0
Hot Fudge Brownie A La Mode	1 serv	997	42	6	14	12	147	105	6	170	82	—	—	1
Milkshake Vanilla Or Chocolate	12 oz	560	26	16	100	11	76	71	tr	300	272	—	—	2
Oreo Blender Blaster	1 serv	895	46	23	135	16	112	93	2	480	280	—	—	2
Single Scoop Sundae	1 serv	188	14	6	37	3	14	4	0	60	43	—	—	0
MAIN MENU SELECTIONS														
Albacore Tuna Melt	1 serv	640	39	13	109	30	42	3	3	340	1436	—	—	10
Applesauce	1 serv	60	0	0	0	0	15	15	1	0	13	—	—	0
Bacon Lettuce & Tomato	1	610	38	9	35	15	50	5	2	70	862	—	—	17
Baked Potato Plain	1	220	0	0	0	5	51	3	5	20	16	—	—	27
BBQ Chicken Sandwich	1 serv	1089	62	14	103	48	86	20	5	450	1872	—	—	42
Bread Stuffing Plain	1 serv	100	1	0	0	3	19	3	1	20	405	—	—	2
Buffalo Chicken Sandwich	1 serv	708	28	6	74	37	80	20	5	190	1733	—	—	28
Buffalo Chicken Strips	5 pieces	734	42	4	96	48	43	0	0	20	1673	—	—	22
Buffalo Wings	12 pieces	856	54	17	500	92	1	0	1	190	5552	—	—	29
Burger Bacon Cheddar	1	875	52	19	163	53	58	9	5	380	1672	—	—	8
Burger BBQ	1 serv	953	52	21	136	52	72	12	4	440	2130	—	—	12
Burger Boca	1 serv	601	27	6	14	32	64	10	9	350	1446	—	—	8
Burger Classic	1	694	35	12	100	40	56	11	4	130	785	—	—	11
Burger Classic w/ Cheese	1	852	48	20	140	49	57	11	4	340	1385	—	—	11
Burger Mushroom Swiss	1 serv	880	49	19	137	51	63	14	5	170	1619	—	—	7
Carrots In Honey Glaze	1 serv	80	3	1	0	1	12	7	3	40	220	—	—	3
Chicken Strips	5 pieces	720	33	4	95	47	56	14	0	20	1666	—	—	0
Chicken Ranch Melt	1 serv	758	45	14	105	44	44	4	3	400	2195	—	—	9
Chicken Strips	1 serv	635	25	1	95	47	55	13	0	20	1510	—	—	0

FOOD	PORTION	CALS	FAT	SAT FAT	CHOL	PROT	CARB	SUGAR	FIBER	CALCI	SOD	POTAS	FOLIC	VIT C
Club Sandwich	1	718	38	7	75	32	62	6	3	120	1666	—	—	13
Coleslaw	1 serv	274	30	24	37	2	14	11	2	50	568	—	—.	33
Corn In Butter Sauce	1 serv	120	4	2	5	3	19	4	5	0	260	—	—	1
Cottage Cheese	1 serv	72	3	2	10	9	2	0	0	40	281	—	—	0
Country Fried Steak	1 serv	644	48	10	89	28	30	7	11	10	2149	—	—	0
Fish & Chips Dinner	1 serv	955	57	37	97	34	77	11	6	90	1497	—	—	60
French Fries Unsalted	1 serv	423	20	5	0	6	57	0	5	0	221	—	—	0
Fried Shrimp Dinner	1 serv	219	10	2	133	17	18	5	1	60	774	—	—	8
Fried Shrimp & Shrimp Scampi	1 serv	346	20	4	241	27	15	5	1	80	1104	—	—	26
Green Beans w/ Bacon	1 serv	60	4	2	5	1	6	2	3	40	390	—	—	6
Grilled Cheese Sandwich	1	510	30	14	54	19	40	2	3	400	1360	—	—	9
Grilled Chicken Dinner	1 serv	130	4	1	67	24	0	0	0	10	560	—	—	1
Grilled Chicken Sandwich	1	469	14	3	77	35	53	8	4	—	1392	—	—	5
Ham & Swiss On Rye	1	417	16	8	57	32	39	8	5	70	1763	—	—	8
Herb Toast	1 serv	170	11	2	tr	2	15	1	1	40	325	—	—	0
Hoagie Chicken Melt	1	751	44	12	93	46	43	2	2	400	1834	—	—	14
Hoagie Philly Melt	1 serv	874	50	16	114	47	58	14	5	530	2444	—	—	16
Mashed Potatoes Plain	1 serv	168	7	3	8	3	23	1	2	20	498	—	—	5
Mozzarella Sticks	8 pieces	710	41	24	48	36	49	0	6	780	5220	—	—	3
Onion Rings	1 serv	381	23	6	6	5	38	2	1	20	1003	—	—	2
Patty Melt	1	798	51	21	127	45	37	10	4	380	1285	—	—	1
Pot Roast Dinner w/ Gravy	1 serv	292	11	5	87	42	5	0	0	0	927	—	—	0
Roast Turkey & Stuffing w/ Gravy	1 serv	388	3	1	116	46	38	17	2	40	2467	—	—	6
Sampler	1 serv	1405	80	24	75	47	124	4	4	440	5305	—	—	6
Seasoned Fries	1 serv	261	12	3	0	5	35	0	0	10	556	—	—	0
Senior Chicken Strip Dinner	1 serv	285	10	0	37	19	31	13	0	10	969	—	—	0
Senior Club	1 serv	540	31	5	89	29	34	4	3	90	1499	—	—	8
Senior Country Fried Steak	1 serv	341	23	5	44	14	18	6	6	30	1464	—	—	3
Senior Fish & Chips	1 serv	756	47	35	67	20	64	11	6	70	1116	—	—	47

FOOD	PORTION	CALS	FAT	SAT FAT	CHOL	PROT	CARB	SUGAR	FIBER	CALCI	SOD	POTAS	FOLIC	VIT C
Senior French Slam	1 serv	820	65	22	432	28	40	8	1	130	777	—	—	0
Senior Fried Shrimp Dinner	1 serv	129	5	1	66	12	13	4	1	0	645	—	—	0
Senior Grilled Chicken Breast	1 serv	200	5	1	67	25	15	0	1	220	824	—	—	2
Senior Pot Roast	1 serv	160	6	3	48	25	3	0	0	20	512	—	—	6
Senior Starter	1 serv	544	42	11	245	16	23	1	2	40	631	—	—	7
Senior Turkey & Stuffing	1 serv	220	2	0	60	25	25	9	1	40	1378	—	—	4
Shrimp Scampi Skillet Dinner	1 serv	289	19	4	192	25	3	tr	tr	80	766	—	—	17
Sirloin Steak Dinner	1 serv	337	28	8	687	18	1	0	1	90	344	—	—	0
Sliced Tomatoes	3 slices	13	0	0	0	1	3	2	1	0	6	—	—	11
Smothered Cheese Fries	1 serv	767	48	17	78	27	69	1	0	410	875	—	—	4
Steak & Shrimp Dinner	1 serv	645	42	14	150	36	31	4	2	80	1143	—	—	0
T-Bone Steak Dinner	1 serv	860	65	29	196	65	0	0	0	120	867	—	—	tr
The Super Bird Sandwich	1	620	32	5	60	35	48	4	2	80	1880	—	—	12
Turkey Breast On Multigrain w/o Mayo	1	277	4	tr	15	23	41	6	5	90	1607	—	—	8
SALAD DRESSINGS AND TOPPINGS														
BBQ Sauce	1.5 oz	47	1	0	0	0	11	5	0	10	595	—	—	2
Bleu Cheese	1 oz	163	18	3	20	1	1	0	0	0	205	—	—	1
Blueberry Topping	1 serv	71	0	0	0	0	17	17	0	0	10	—	—	0
Caesar	1 oz	133	14	2	2	1	1	1	0	20	380	—	—	0
Cherry Topping	1 serv	57	0	0	0	0	14	6	0	0	3	—	—	0
Cream Cheese	1 oz	100	10	6	31	2	1	1	0	20	6	—	—	0
French	1 oz	106	10	2	7	0	3	3	0	0	274	—	—	0
Fudge Topping	1 serv	201	10	7	3	1	30	27	1	30	96	—	—	0
Gravy Brown	1 serv	13	0	0	0	0	2	1	0	0	184	—	—	0
Gravy Chicken	1 serv	14	1	0	2	0	2	1	0	0	139	—	—	0
Gravy Country	1 serv	17	1	0	0	0	2	0	0	0	93	—	—	0
Honey Mustard	1 serv	160	15	8	20	0	20	4	0	0	123	—	—	0
Low Calorie Italian	1 oz	15	1	0	0	0	3	2	0	0	390	—	—	1
Marinara Sauce	1 serv	48	2	1	0	1	7	5	1	10	206	—	—	5
Ranch	1 oz	129	14	2	8	0	1	0	0	0	189	—	—	0
Ranch Fat Free	1 serv	25	tr	0	0	0	6	2	0	0	300	—	—	0
Sour Cream	1.5 oz	91	9	6	19	1	2	0	0	40	23	—	—	0
Strawberry Topping	1 serv	77	1	0	0	1	17	13	1	0	8	—	—	1

FOOD	PORTION	CALS	FAT	SAT FAT	CHOL	PROT	CARB	SUGAR	FIBER	CALCI	SOD	POTAS	FOLIC	VIT C
Syrup	3 tbsp	143	0	0	0	0	36	36	0	0	26	—	—	0
Syrup Sugar Free	1 serv	23	0	0	0	0	9	0	0	0	71	—	—	0
Tartar Sauce	1 serv	225	23	4	15	0	3	3	0	0	157	—	—	0
Thousand Island	2 tbsp	170	18	3	15	0	2	—	0	—	110	—	—	—
Thousand Island	1 oz	118	11	2	15	0	5	5	0	0	170	—	—	1
Whipped Margarine	1 serv	87	10	2	0	0	0	0	0	0	117	—	—	0
Whipped Cream	2 tbsp	23	2	0	7	0	2	0	0	0	3	—	—	0
SALADS														
Garden Salad w/ Albacore Tuna	1 serv	444	29	8	81	35	12	6	4	230	824	—	—	22
Garden Salad w/ Fried Chicken Strips	1 serv	438	26	6	78	33	26	5	4	240	1030	—	—	35
Garden Salad w/ Grilled Chicken Breast	1 serv	264	11	5	89	32	10	5	4	220	714	—	—	20
Grilled Chicken Caesar Salad w/ Dressing	1 serv	600	41	10	101	37	19	3	4	300	1792	—	—	42
Side Caesar w/ Dressing	1 serv	362	26	7	23	11	20	2	3	250	913	—	—	27
Side Garden Salad w/o Dressing	1 serv	113	4	1	0	3	16	4	3	40	147	—	—	23
SOUPS														
Chicken Noodle	1 serv	60	2	0	10	2	8	0	0	10	640	—	—	0
Clam Chowder	1 serv	624	42	34	5	7	55	7	4	30	1474	—	—	2
Cream Of Broccoli	1 serv	574	43	34	0	6	41	6	2	100	1174	—	—	12
Vegetable Beef	1 serv	79	1	1	5	6	11	2	2	20	820	—	—	1

DOMINO'S PIZZA

12 INCH MEDIUM PIZZAS

FOOD	PORTION	CALS	FAT	SAT FAT	CHOL	PROT	CARB	SUGAR	FIBER	CALCI	SOD	POTAS	FOLIC	VIT C
Deep Dish Cheese Only	2 slices	482	22	8	30	19	56	6	3	241	1123	—	—	tr
Hand Tossed America's Favorite Feast	1 serv	508	22	9	49	22	57	5	4	202	1221	—	—	1
Hand Tossed Bacon Cheeseburger Feast	2 slices	549	26	12	60	25	55	5	3	293	1274	—	—	0
Hand Tossed Barbeque Feast	2 slices	506	20	9	46	22	62	9	3	292	1206	—	—	1
Hand Tossed Cheese Only	2 slices	375	11	5	23	15	55	5	3	187	776	—	—	0

FOOD	PORTION	CALS	FAT	SAT FAT	CHOL	PROT	CARB	SUGAR	FIBER	CALCI	SOD	POTAS	FOLIC	VIT C
Hand Tossed Deluxe Feast	2 slices	465	18	8	40	20	57	5	3	199	1063	—	—	1
Hand Tossed ExtravaganZZa Feast	2 slices	576	27	12	64	27	59	5	4	290	1511	—	—	1
Hand Tossed Hawaiian Feast	2 slices	450	16	7	41	21	58	7	3	274	1102	—	—	2
Hand Tossed MeatZZa Feast	2 slices	560	26	11	64	26	57	5	3	282	1463	—	—	tr
Hand Tossed Pepperoni Feast	2 slices	534	25	11	57	24	56	5	3	279	1349	—	—	tr
Hand Tossed Vegi Feast	2 slices	439	16	7	34	19	57	5	4	279	987	—	—	1
Thin Crust Cheese	¼ pie	273	12	4	23	12	31	4	2	225	835	—	—	0
Toppings Pineapple	1 serv	12	0	0	0	tr	3	3	tr	3	1	—	—	2
DESSERTS														
Cinna Stix	1 serv	111	5	1	0	2	15	3	1	6	105	—	—	tr
Sweet Icing	1 serv	283	5	3	0	0	60	51	0	1	4	—	—	0
MAIN MENU SELECTIONS														
Breadstick	1	116	4	1	0	3	18	1	1	6	152	—	—	tr
Buffalo Chicken Kickers	1 piece	47	2	tr	9	4	3	tr	tr	3	163	—	—	0
Buffalo Wings Barbeque	1 piece	50	2	1	25	6	2	1	tr	6	175	—	—	tr
Buffalo Wings Hot	1 piece	45	2	1	26	5	1	tr	tr	5	354	—	—	1
Cheesy Bread	1 piece	142	6	2	6	4	18	1	1	47	183	—	—	tr
TOPPINGS														
Blue Cheese	1 serv	223	23	4	20	1	2	2	tr	25	417	—	—	tr
Hot Sauce	1 serv	14	tr	0	0	tr	4	1	tr	6	1816	—	—	9
Medium Pizza Anchovies	1 serv	34	1	tr	14	6	0	0	0	37	593	—	—	0
Medium Pizza Bacon	1 serv	102	9	3	15	5	tr	tr	0	2	283	—	—	6
Medium Pizza Banana Peppers	1 serv	5	tr	0	0	tr	1	0	0	5	137	—	—	5
Medium Pizza Cheddar Cheese	1 serv	57	5	3	15	4	tr	tr	0	102	88	—	—	0
Medium Pizza Extra Cheese	1 serv	49	4	2	11	3	1	tr	tr	84	163	—	—	0
Medium Pizza Green Olives	1 serv	19	2	tr	0	tr	tr	tr	tr	10	283	—	—	0
Medium Pizza Green Peppers	1 serv	4	tr	0	0	tr	1	0	tr	1	tr	—	—	1
Medium Pizza Ham	1 serv	23	1	tr	9	3	tr	tr	0	2	215	—	—	tr

FOOD	PORTION	CALS	FAT	SAT FAT	CHOL	PROT	CARB	SUGAR	FIBER	CALCI	SOD	POTAS	FOLIC	VIT C
Medium Pizza Italian Sausage	1 serv	77	6	2	16	3	2	tr	tr	11	239	—	—	tr
Medium Pizza Mushrooms	1 serv	6	tr	tr	0	1	1	tr	tr	1	1	—	—	1
Medium Pizza Onion	1 serv	5	tr	0	0	tr	1	0	tr	4	tr	—	—	1
Medium Pizza Pepperoni	1 serv	74	7	3	15	3	tr	tr	tr	6	273	—	—	tr
Medium Pizza Ripe Olives	1 serv	21	2	tr	0	tr	1	tr	1	12	107	—	—	0
Ranch	1 serv	197	20	3	9	1	2	2	tr	10	380	—	—	tr

DONATOS PIZZA

PIZZA

FOOD	PORTION	CALS	FAT	SAT FAT	CHOL	PROT	CARB	SUGAR	FIBER	CALCI	SOD	POTAS	FOLIC	VIT C
Dessert Apple	¼ pie	722	20	4	21	12	137	66	15	70	926	—	—	0
Dessert Cherry	¼ pie	818	20	4	20	12	149	70	13	50	924	—	—	0
Original	¼ pie	660	33	14	54	30	58	6	6	250	1770	—	—	6
Original Chicken Vegy Medley	¼ pie	500	19	8	80	28	56	6	11	280	1768	—	—	22
Original Chicken Vegy Medley No Cheese	¼ pie	392	10	3	56	21	54	6	11	70	1536	—	—	22
Original Founders	¼ pie	737	42	17	134	38	71	6	10	430	2954	—	—	1
Original Hawaiian	¼ pie	620	30	10	60	30	58	16	4	520	1780	—	—	4
Original Hawaiian No Cheese	¼ pie	411	13	2	46	17	58	10	11	40	1379	—	—	3
Original Mariachi Beef	¼ pie	613	30	14	81	31	56	6	11	460	2324	—	—	23
Original Mariachi Chicken	¼ pie	580	25	12	94	35	56	6	11	450	2480	—	—	23
Original Serious Cheese	¼ pie	640	28	20	140	34	62	4	6	600	1640	—	—	5
Original Serious Meat	¼ pie	817	47	20	136	45	68	6	10	430	2535	—	—	1
Original Vegy	¼ pie	564	24	10	60	26	60	8	12	430	1674	—	—	38
Original Vegy No Cheese	¼ pie	370	9	2	21	12	59	7	12	40	1207	—	—	38
Original Works	¼ pie	729	41	17	106	35	75	6	12	440	2179	—	—	30
Traditional Chicken Vegy Medley	¼ pie	647	17	8	62	37	90	8	4	280	1997	—	—	22
Traditional Founders	¼ pie	900	40	17	112	48	107	11	3	260	3206	—	—	12
Traditional Hawaiian	¼ pie	794	30	12	74	42	98	17	4	520	2316	—	—	14
Traditional Mariachi Beef	¼ pie	797	31	15	68	41	95	11	4	560	2773	—	—	34

FOOD	PORTION	CALS	FAT	SAT FAT	CHOL	PROT	CARB	SUGAR	FIBER	CALCI	SOD	POTAS	FOLIC	VIT C
Traditional Mariachi Chicken	¼ pie	770	26	13	79	45	95	11	4	550	2911	—	—	34
Traditional Serious Meat	¼ pie	977	46	20	118	54	104	11	3	530	2881	—	—	12
Traditional Vegy	¼ pie	752	26	12	49	37	98	12	5	520	2104	—	—	44
Traditional Works	¼ pie	892	39	17	90	45	111	11	5	530	2536	—	—	37
Traditional Original	¼ pie	928	39	28	121	40	89	11	9	470	2076	—	—	5
Traditional Serious Cheese	¼ pie	830	36	30	123	40	123	8	12	660	1889	—	—	8
SALAD DRESSINGS														
Italian	1 serv (1.5 oz)	230	24	4	0	0	1	1	0	0	460	—	—	0
Italian Lite	1 serv (1.5 oz)	20	1	0	0	0	2	0	0	0	780	—	—	0
SALADS														
Grilled Chicken w/o Dressing	1 serv	314	18	7	71	28	12	8	5	280	903	—	—	21
Italian Chef w/o Dressing	1 serv	338	23	9	72	20	13	8	5	170	1856	—	—	21
Side w/o Dressing	1 serv	106	7	3	16	6	6	4	2	130	370	—	—	9
SIDE ORDERS														
Breadsticks	2	220	5	1	0	5	29	1	0	0	330	—	—	2
Chicken Wings Hot	5	449	29	—	286	41	6	—	tr	60	1766	—	—	1
Chicken Wings Mild	5	451	29	—	286	41	6	—	tr	60	1781	—	—	1
Three Cheese Garlic Bread	1 bun	605	28	8	38	24	66	3	3	340	689	—	—	4
SUBS														
Big Don Italian	1 serv	705	33	10	85	34	68	6	3	210	1982	—	—	12
Big Don Lite Italian	1 serv	631	25	9	84	34	69	6	3	200	2069	—	—	12
Grilled Chicken	1 serv	786	43	12	71	31	68	5	3	440	1184	—	—	14
Ham & Cheese Italian	1 serv	609	22	5	86	32	70	8	3	210	1659	—	—	12
Ham & Cheese Lite Italian	1 serv	534	14	4	85	32	70	8	3	200	1745	—	—	13
Southwest Turkey	1 serv	710	33	7	70	33	74	12	3	160	1519	—	—	6
Steak & Cheese	1 serv	929	52	18	111	43	107	4	3	230	907	—	—	16
Vegy Italian	1 serv	730	36	9	38	26	75	8	6	360	1267	—	—	42
Vegy Lite Italian	1 serv	661	28	8	38	26	78	6	6	360	1487	—	—	44

DUNKIN' DONUTS

FOOD	PORTION	CALS	FAT	SAT FAT	CHOL	PROT	CARB	SUGAR	FIBER	CALCI	SOD	POTAS	FOLIC	VIT C
BAGELS AND CREAM CHEESE														
Bagel Blueberry	1	340	1	0	0	10	75	7	tr	20	670	—	—	0
Bagel Cinnamon Raisin	1	340	1	0	0	10	74	11	1	40	480	—	—	0

FOOD	PORTION	CALS	FAT	SAT FAT	CHOL	PROT	CARB	SUGAR	FIBER	CALCI	SOD	POTAS	FOLIC	VIT C
Bagel Egg	1	350	2	0	25	11	72	3	0	20	610	—	—	0
Bagel Everything	1	360	2	0	0	11	74	3	0	40	710	—	—	0
Bagel Garlic	1	360	1	0	0	11	76	4	0	0	720	—	—	0
Bagel Onion	1	330	1	0	0	10	70	3	0	20	660	—	—	0
Bagel Plain	1	340	1	0	0	10	73	3	0	20	710	—	—	0
Bagel Poppyseed	1	360	3	0	0	11	74	3	tr	60	710	—	—	0
Bagel Pumpernickel	1	350	2	0	0	11	75	6	2	40	560	—	—	0
Bagel Salt	1	340	1	0	0	10	73	3	0	20	3030	—	—	0
Bagel Sesame	1	380	5	1	0	12	74	3	0	20	720	—	—	0
Bagel Wheat	1	330	2	0	0	12	73	6	4	20	670	—	—	0
Cream Cheese Chive	1 pkg	190	19	13	55	3	3	3	tr	60	220	—	—	0
Cream Cheese Garden Vegetable	1 pkg	180	17	11	45	3	3	2	tr	—	310	—	—	0
Cream Cheese Lite	1 pkg	130	11	7	30	5	3	2	0	—	250	—	—	0
Cream Cheese Plain	1 pkg	200	19	13	60	4	3	2	0	40	230	—	—	0
Cream Cheese Salmon	1 pkg	180	17	11	50	5	2	2	0	20	150	—	—	0
BAKED SELECTIONS														
Bow Tie Donut	1	300	17	4	0	4	34	10	tr	0	340	—	—	2
Cake Donut Blueberry	1	290	16	4	10	3	35	16	tr	0	400	—	—	0
Cake Donut Butternut	1	300	16	5	0	3	36	16	tr	20	360	—	—	1
Cake Donut Chocolate Coconut	1	300	19	6	0	4	31	12	1	20	370	—	—	4
Cake Donut Chocolate Frosted	1	300	16	3	0	3	38	18	tr	20	370	—	—	0
Cake Donut Chocolate Glazed	1	290	16	4	0	3	33	14	1	20	370	—	—	0
Cake Donut Cinnamon	1	270	15	3	0	3	31	12	tr	20	360	—	—	0
Cake Donut Coconut	1	290	17	5	0	3	33	13	tr	20	360	—	—	0
Cake Donut Double Chocolate	1	310	17	4	0	3	37	18	2	40	370	—	—	0
Cake Donut Glazed	1	270	15	3	0	3	33	14	tr	20	360	—	—	0
Cake Donut Old Fashioned	1	250	15	3	0	3	26	7	tr	20	360	—	—	0

FOOD	PORTION	CALS	FAT	SAT FAT	CHOL	PROT	CARB	SUGAR	FIBER	CALCI	SOD	POTAS	FOLIC	VIT C
Cake Donut Powdered	1	270	15	3	0	3	32	13	tr	20	350	—	—	0
Cake Donut Toasted Coconut	1	300	17	5	0	3	35	16	tr	20	370	—	—	0
Cake Donut Whole Wheat Glazed	1	310	19	4	0	4	32	14	2	20	380	—	—	0
Chocolate Frosted Donut	1	200	9	2	0	3	29	10	tr	0	260	—	—	0
Chocolate Kreme Filled Donut	1	270	13	3	0	3	35	16	tr	0	260	—	—	0
Cinnamon Bun	1	510	15	4	10	8	85	42	0	40	420	—	—	0
Coffee Roll	1	270	14	3	0	4	33	10	1	0	340	—	—	0
Coffee Roll Chocolate Frosted	1	290	15	3	0	4	36	12	1	0	340	—	—	0
Coffee Roll Maple Frosted	1	290	14	3	0	4	36	13	1	0	340	—	—	0
Coffee Roll Vanilla Frosted	1	290	14	3	0	4	36	13	1	0	340	—	—	0
Cookie Chocolate Chocolate Chunk	1	210	11	7	35	3	26	16	2	0	110	—	—	0
Cookie Chocolate Chunk	1	220	11	7	35	3	28	17	1	0	105	—	—	0
Cookie Chocolate Chunk w/ Nut	1	230	12	6	35	3	27	16	1	0	110	—	—	0
Cookie Chocolate White Chocolate Chunk	1	230	12	7	35	3	28	19	1	20	160	—	—	0
Cookie Oatmeal Raisin Pecan	1	220	10	5	30	3	29	18	1	0	110	—	—	0
Cookie Peanut Butter Chocolate Chunk w/ Nuts	1	240	14	6	25	4	24	16	2	0	125	—	—	0
Cookie Peanut Butter w/ Nuts	1	240	14	6	30	5	24	15	1	0	150	—	—	0
Croissant Almond	1	350	22	5	5	6	34	13	2	40	270	—	—	0
Croissant Chocolate	1	400	25	9	5	5	37	15	2	0	240	—	—	0
Croissant Plain	1	290	18	6	5	5	26	3	tr	0	270	—	—	0
Cruller Glazed	1	290	15	2	0	3	37	18	tr	20	350	—	—	0
Cruller Glazed Chocolate	1	280	15	3	0	3	35	16	1	20	360	—	—	0
Cruller Plain	1	240	15	3	0	3	25	6	tr	20	340	—	—	0
Cruller Powdered	1	270	15	3	0	3	30	11	tr	20	340	—	—	0
Cruller Sugar	1	250	15	3	0	3	27	8	tr	20	340	—	—	0

FOOD	PORTION	CALS	FAT	SAT FAT	CHOL	PROT	CARB	SUGAR	FIBER	CALCI	SOD	POTAS	FOLIC	VIT C
Donut Apple Crumb	1	230	10	3	0	3	34	12	tr	0	270	—	—	0
Donut Apple N' Spice	1	200	8	2	0	3	29	7	tr	0	270	—	—	0
Donut Bavarian Kreme	1	210	9	2	0	3	30	9	tr	0	270	—	—	0
Donut Black Raspberry	1	210	8	2	0	3	32	10	tr	0	280	—	—	0
Donut Blueberry Crumb	1	240	10	3	0	3	36	15	tr	0	260	—	—	0
Donut Boston Kreme	1	240	9	2	0	3	36	14	tr	0	280	—	—	0
Donut Chocolate Iced Bismarck	1	340	15	4	0	3	50	31	tr	0	290	—	—	0
Dunkin' Donut	1	240	15	3	0	3	25	6	tr	20	340	—	—	0
Eclair Donut	1	270	11	3	0	3	39	17	tr	0	290	—	—	0
Fritter Glazed	1	260	14	3	0	4	31	7	1	0	330	—	—	0
Glazed Donut	1	180	8	2	0	3	25	6	tr	0	250	—	—	0
Jelly Filled Donut	1	210	8	2	0	3	32	14	tr	0	280	—	—	0
Jelly Stick	1	290	12	3	0	3	44	24	tr	20	390	—	—	0
Lemon Donut	1	200	9	2	0	3	28	8	tr	0	270	—	—	0
Maple Frosted Donut	1	210	9	2	0	3	30	12	tr	0	260	—	—	0
Marble Frosted Donut	1	200	9	2	0	3	29	11	tr	0	260	—	—	0
Muffin Apple Cinnamon Pecan	1	510	21	6	70	8	74	41	1	80	590	—	—	0
Muffin Apple N'Spice	1	350	12	3	35	5	57	29	2	40	390	—	—	0
Muffin Banana Nut	1	360	15	3	35	7	52	29	3	40	490	—	—	0
Muffin Blueberry	1 (4 oz)	320	12	3	35	6	49	27	3	40	480	—	—	0
Muffin Blueberry	1 (6 oz)	490	17	6	75	8	78	41	2	60	610	—	—	0
Muffin Bran	1	390	12	2	20	11	60	34	3	40	620	—	—	0
Muffin Cherry	1	340	12	3	40	6	53	29	2	40	510	—	—	0
Muffin Chocolate Hazelnut	1	610	26	8	70	10	87	52	3	100	610	—	—	0
Muffin Chocolate Chip	1 (6 oz)	590	24	10	75	8	88	50	3	60	560	—	—	0
Muffin Chocolate Chip	1 (4 oz)	400	17	6	35	6	58	36	4	40	440	—	—	0
Muffin Corn	1 (6 oz)	500	16	5	80	10	78	34	1	60	920	—	—	—
Muffin Corn	1 (4 oz)	390	15	3	55	8	57	22	2	40	590	—	—	0
Muffin Cranberry Orange	1	470	15	5	75	8	76	41	2	20	600	—	—	0
Muffin Cranberry Orange Nut	1	350	15	3	35	6	52	27	3	40	500	—	—	0

FOOD	PORTION	CALS	FAT	SAT FAT	CHOL	PROT	CARB	SUGAR	FIBER	CALCI	SOD	POTAS	FOLIC	VIT C
Muffin Lemon Poppyseed	1	360	13	3	35	5	56	27	1	80	530	—	—	0
Muffin Oat Bran	1	370	13	2	20	11	55	29	3	40	620	—	—	0
Muffin Lowfat Apple & Spice	1	240	2	0	0	4	54	32	tr	0	460	—	—	0
Muffin Lowfat Banana	1	250	2	0	0	4	57	35	tr	0	430	—	—	0
Muffin Lowfat Blueberry	1	250	2	0	0	4	55	33	1	0	430	—	—	0
Muffin Lowfat Bran	1	240	1	0	0	4	57	32	4	40	430	—	—	0
Muffin Lowfat Cherry	1	250	2	0	0	4	56	34	tr	0	430	—	—	0
Muffin Lowfat Chocolate	1	250	3	1	0	4	53	29	2	40	470	—	—	0
Muffin Lowfat Corn	1	240	3	1	45	3	52	20	0	40	480	—	—	0
Muffin Lowfat Cranberry Orange	1	240	2	0	0	4	55	32	1	0	430	—	—	0
Muffin Reduced Fat Blueberry	1	450	12	9	65	8	77	42	2	60	590	—	—	0
Muffin Reduced Fat Corn	1	460	11	7	75	10	79	35	1	60	900	—	—	0
Munchkins Chocolate Cake Glazed	3	200	10	2	0	2	26	13	tr	0	250	—	—	0
Munchkins Cake Butternut	3	200	11	3	0	2	25	12	tr	0	240	—	—	0
Munchkins Cake Cinnamon	4	250	14	3	0	3	29	13	tr	20	350	—	—	0
Munchkins Cake Coconut	3	200	12	4	0	2	23	10	tr	0	240	—	—	0
Munchkins Cake Glazed	3	200	10	2	0	2	27	14	0	0	250	—	—	0
Munchkins Cake Plain	4	220	14	3	0	2	22	6	tr	20	310	—	—	0
Munchkins Cake Powdered	4	250	14	3	0	2	29	12	tr	20	310	—	—	0
Munchkins Cake Sugared	4	240	14	3	0	2	28	12	tr	20	310	—	—	0
Munchkins Cake Toasted Coconut	3	200	11	—	0	2	24	11	tr	0	—	—	—	0
Munchkins Yeast Glazed	5	200	9	2	0	3	27	12	tr	0	220	—	—	0
Munchkins Yeast Jelly Filled	5	210	9	2	0	3	30	15	tr	0	240	—	—	0

FOOD	PORTION	CALS	FAT	SAT FAT	CHOL	PROT	CARB	SUGAR	FIBER	CALCI	SOD	POTAS	FOLIC	VIT C
Munchkins Yeast Lemon Filled	4	170	8	2	0	2	23	9	0	0	190	—	—	0
Munchkins Yeast Sugar Raised	7	220	12	3	0	4	26	5	tr	0	290	—	—	0
Strawberry Frosted Donut	1	210	9	2	0	3	30	12	tr	0	260	—	—	0
Strawberry Donut	1	210	8	2	0	3	32	11	tr	0	260	—	—	0
Sugar Raised Donut	1	170	8	2	0	3	22	4	tr	0	250	—	—	0
Sugared Cake Donut	1	250	15	3	0	3	27	9	tr	20	350	—	—	0
Vanilla Frosted Donut	1	210	9	2	0	3	30	12	tr	0	260	—	—	0
Vanilla Kreme Filled Donut	1	270	13	3	0	3	36	17	tr	0	250	—	—	0
BEVERAGES														
Coffee Coolatta w/ 2% Milk	1 (16 oz)	240	2	2	10	4	52	51	0	150	80	—	—	0
Coffee Coolatta w/ Cream	1 (16 oz)	410	22	14	75	3	51	50	0	100	65	—	—	0
Coffee Coolatta w/ Milk	1 (16 oz)	260	4	3	15	4	52	51	0	150	75	—	—	0
Coffee Coolatta w/ Skim Milk	1 (16 oz)	230	0	0	<5	4	52	51	0	150	80	—	—	0
Coolatta Orange Mango Fruit	1 (16 oz)	290	0	0	0	tr	71	63	tr	0	30	—	—	42
Coolatta Pink Lemonade Fruit	1 (16 oz)	350	0	0	0	07	88	63	0	0	30	—	—	6
Coolatta Raspberry Lemonade	1 (16 oz)	280	0	0	0	0	68	64	0	0	35	—	—	15
Coolatta Strawberry Fruit	1 (16 oz)	280	0	0	0	0	70	63	1	0	30	—	—	27
Coolatta Vanilla	1 (16 oz)	450	7	4	0	1	94	80	0	30	170	—	—	0
Dunkaccino	1 (20 oz)	510	23	7	20	4	71	50	1	80	500	—	—	0
Dunkaccino	1 (10 oz)	250	11	4	10	2	34	25	tr	40	240	—	—	0
Dunkaccino	1 (14 oz)	360	17	5	15	3	51	36	1	60	360	—	—	0
Dunkaccino	1 (18.75 oz)	480	22	7	20	4	67	48	1	80	470	—	—	0
Hot Cocoa	1 (20 oz)	470	16	4	0	5	79	61	3	80	640	—	—	0
Hot Cocoa	1 (18.75 oz)	440	15	4	0	4	75	57	3	60	610	—	—	—
Hot Cocoa	1 (14 oz)	330	11	3	0	3	57	43	2	60	460	—	—	0
Hot Cocoa	1 (10 oz)	230	8	2	0	2	38	29	2	40	310	—	—	0
SANDWICHES														
Breakfast Sandwich Ham Egg Cheese	1	320	12	6	195	22	31	3	2	200	1340	—	—	0
Omwich Bagel Bacon Cheddar	1	600	21	8	295	26	79	5	tr	250	1630	—	—	5

FOOD	PORTION	CALS	FAT	SAT FAT	CHOL	PROT	CARB	SUGAR	FIBER	CALCI	SOD	POTAS	FOLIC	VIT C
Omwich Bagel Spanish Cheese	1	570	18	6	280	24	79	5	tr	200	1370	—	—	5
Omwich Bagel Three Cheese	1	610	22	9	305	25	78	5	tr	250	1630	—	—	5
Omwich Croissant Spanish Cheese	1	530	36	11	285	19	33	5	1	200	930	—	—	6
Omwich Croissant Bacon Cheddar	1	560	38	13	295	21	33	5	1	250	1190	—	—	6
Omwich Croissant Three Cheese	1	560	39	15	305	20	33	5	1	250	1200	—	—	6
Omwich English Muffin Bacon Cheddar	1	400	21	8	295	21	33	4	2	300	1440	—	—	0
Omwich English Muffin Spanish Cheese	1	370	18	6	280	18	34	4	2	250	1180	—	—	0
Omwich English Muffin Three Cheese	1	400	22	9	305	19	33	4	2	300	1450	—	—	0

EINSTEIN BROS BAGELS

BAGELS AND BREADS

FOOD	PORTION	CALS	FAT	SAT FAT	CHOL	PROT	CARB	SUGAR	FIBER	CALCI	SOD	POTAS	FOLIC	VIT C
Bagel Asiago Cheese	1	360	3	2	5	13	71	4	2	100	570	—	—	0
Bagel Cranberry Special	1	350	1	0	0	10	78	13	3	20	490	—	—	0
Bagel Egg	1	340	3	1	35	11	69	5	2	20	510	—	—	0
Bagel Honey Whole Wheat	1	320	1	0	0	10	71	11	3	20	470	—	—	0
Bagel Jalapeño	1	330	1	0	0	11	71	4	2	20	510	—	—	0
Bagel Lucky Gree	1	320	1	0	0	11	71	4	2	20	520	—	—	0
Bagel Mango	1	360	1	0	0	10	80	14	2	20	490	—	—	0
Bagel Marble Rye	1	340	2	0	0	11	73	3	3	40	690	—	—	0
Bagel Potato	1	350	5	1	0	10	69	5	2	0	590	—	—	0
Bagel Power	1	410	5	1	0	13	81	18	4	40	310	—	—	0
Bagel Power w/ Peanut Butter	1	750	34	6	0	27	92	22	7	60	780	—	—	0
Bagel Pumpkin	1	330	2	0	0	10	72	6	3	40	470	—	—	0
Bagel Roasted Red Pepper & Pesto	1	410	7	4	15	17	73	5	2	200	710	—	—	9
Bagel Six Cheese	1	390	6	3	15	16	72	4	2	200	650	—	—	0
Bagel Spicy Nacho	1	450	9	5	20	17	77	5	3	200	890	—	—	1
Bagel Spinach Florentine	1	410	7	4	20	17	72	5	3	250	620	—	—	4
Bagel Croutons	¼ cup	25	1	0	0	1	4	0	0	0	75	—	—	0
Bagel Twist	1	220	4	2	5	8	39	3	1	100	510	—	—	0
Bread Ciabatta	1 serv	320	3	1	0	12	64	0	3	60	460	—	—	0
Chocolate Chip	1	370	3	2	0	11	76	10	3	20	500	—	—	0

FOOD	PORTION	CALS	FAT	SAT FAT	CHOL	PROT	CARB	SUGAR	FIBER	CALCI	SOD	POTAS	FOLIC	VIT C
Chopped Garlic	1	380	3	1	0	13	79	3	4	40	600	—	—	0
Chopped Onion	1	330	1	0	0	11	71	4	2	40	500	—	—	0
Cinnamon Raisin Swirl	1	350	1	0	0	11	78	14	2	40	490	—	—	0
Cinnamon Sugar	1	330	1	0	0	10	74	10	2	40	490	—	—	0
Dark Pumpernickel	1	320	1	0	0	11	68	3	3	40	730	—	—	0
Everything	1	340	2	0	0	13	75	5	2	20	820	—	—	1
Focaccia Cheese Pizza	1 serv	500	11	7	35	25	75	6	3	350	1010	—	—	1
Focaccia Margherita	1 serv	400	17	2	5	14	76	6	3	100	580	—	—	12
Focaccia Pepperoni Pizza	1 serv	590	19	10	55	29	76	6	3	350	1380	—	—	1
Nutty Banana	1	360	3	1	0	11	74	5	2	20	510	—	—	0
Plain	1	320	1	0	0	11	71	4	2	20	520	—	—	0
Poppy Dip'd	1	350	2	0	0	12	74	3	2	60	680	—	—	0
Roll Challah	1	300	5	1	40	11	55	7	2	20	270	—	—	9
Salt	1	330	1	0	0	11	73	3	2	30	1790	—	—	0
Sesame Dip'd	1	380	5	1	0	11	75	3	3	20	680	—	—	0
Sun Dried Tomato	1	320	1	0	0	11	69	3	3	20	520	—	—	0
Wild Blueberry	1	350	1	0	0	11	77	9	3	20	510	—	—	0
BEVERAGES														
Americano	1 reg	1	0	0	0	0	0	0	0	0	0	—	—	0
Cafe Latte	1 reg	140	5	4	20	9	13	13	0	300	140	—	—	2
Cafe Latte Nonfat	1 reg	100	0	0	5	9	14	12	0	300	140	—	—	2
Cappuccino	1 reg	90	4	2	15	6	9	8	0	200	95	—	—	1
Cappuccino Nonfat	1 reg	60	0	0	5	6	9	8	0	200	95	—	—	1
Chai 2% Milk	1 reg	210	2	2	10	4	41	41	0	150	75	—	—	1
Chai Skim Milk	1 reg	190	0	0	0	4	41	41	0	150	75	—	—	1
Coffee	1 reg	0	0	0	0	0	0	0	0	0	0	—	—	0
Espresso	1 reg	1	0	0	0	0	0	0	0	0	0	—	—	0
Half & Half	2 tbsp	40	3	2	15	1	1	1	—	40	25	—	—	0
Hot Chocolate	1 reg	290	11	8	20	9	39	33	0	300	160	—	—	1
Hot Chocolate Lower Fat	1 reg	260	7	6	5	9	39	33	0	300	160	—	—	1
Hot Tea All Flavors	1 cup	0	0	0	0	0	0	0	0	0	0	—	—	0
Iced Americano	1 serv	1	0	0	0	0	0	0	0	0	0	—	—	0
Iced Coffee	1 serv	0	0	0	0	0	0	0	0	0	0	—	—	0
Iced Latte	1 serv	120	5	3	20	8	12	11	0	300	125	—	—	2
Iced Latte Nonfat	1 serv	90	0	0	5	8	12	11	0	300	130	—	—	2
Iced Mocha	1 serv	210	6	4	15	7	33	31	0	200	120	—	—	1
Iced Mocha Low Fat	1 serv	180	3	2	5	7	32	30	0	200	115	—	—	1

FOOD	PORTION	CALS	FAT	SAT FAT	CHOL	PROT	CARB	SUGAR	FIBER	CALCI	SOD	POTAS	FOLIC	VIT C
Mocha	1 reg	230	6	5	15	8	34	32	0	250	135	—	—	1
Mocha Low Fat	1 reg	190	3	2	5	8	34	31	0	250	130	—	—	1
DESSERTS														
Brownie Iced	1	550	24	6	35	5	81	56	3	20	310	—	—	0
Brownie Iced w/ Walnuts	1	600	29	6	35	6	82	57	4	20	310	—	—	0
Cherry Figure 8	1	400	18	6	40	7	51	26	1	20	380	—	—	1
Cinnamon Roll	1	810	32	9	45	13	118	50	4	80	580	—	—	0
Cookie Chocolate Chunk	1	640	31	10	50	7	87	48	3	50	350	—	—	0
Cookie Oatmeal Raisin	1	600	27	6	50	7	82	40	2	60	640	—	—	0
Cookie Peanut Butter	1	640	34	7	55	11	75	36	3	40	490	—	—	0
Muffin Banana Nut	1	640	32	4	80	10	81	32	2	80	430	—	—	0
Muffin Blueberry	1	540	22	4	95	8	80	35	1	80	510	—	—	0
Muffin Chocolate Chip	1	620	27	8	90	8	89	48	3	60	460	—	—	0
Pound Cake Lemon Iced	1 slice	540	25	13	155	7	74	50	0	20	420	—	—	2
Pound Cake Marble	1 slice	460	24	12	150	7	57	33	1	40	430	—	—	0
Rice Krispy Bar	1	420	8	2	0	5	83	29	1	0	610	—	—	12
Scone Blueberry w/ Icing	1	450	18	8	55	7	64	21	2	20	460	—	—	1
Scone Lemon Currant	1	430	15	5	40	7	69	25	4	20	450	—	—	4
Strudel Cinnamon Walnut	1 piece	550	31	11	30	7	63	25	3	40	380	—	—	0
Sweetie Pie	1	620	20	2	5	4	106	72	1	20	220	—	—	0
SALAD DRESSINGS														
Asian Sesame	2 tbsp	80	2	0	0	1	16	13	0	0	600	—	—	2
Caesar	2 tbsp	150	16	3	10	1	1	1	0	0	360	—	—	0
Chipotle Vinaigrette	2 tbsp	110	10	2	0	0	5	4	0	0	440	—	—	2
Horseradish Sauce	2 tbsp	170	18	3	20	0	1	0	0	0	190	—	—	0
Raspberry Vinaigrette	2 tbsp	160	14	2	0	0	8	8	0	0	80	—	—	0
Thousand Island	2 tbsp	110	9	20	10	0	5	4	0	40	210	—	—	0
SALADS														
Asian Chicken Salad	1 serv (14.5 oz)	550	9	2	55	29	88	23	5	100	1610	—	—	36
Bros Bistro	1 serv (9.5 oz)	520	43	10	25	10	25	18	2	200	480	—	—	6
Chicken Caesar	1 serv (12.5 oz)	750	53	11	90	33	26	8	2	200	1850	—	—	4
Chicken Chipotle Salad	1 serv	710	43	9	80	34	48	18	13	250	1890	—	—	42

FOOD	PORTION	CALS	FAT	SAT FAT	CHOL	PROT	CARB	SUGAR	FIBER	CALCI	SOD	POTAS	FOLIC	VIT C
Chicken Salad On Greens	1 serv (10.5 oz)	210	9	2	55	19	11	6	3	20	640	—	—	15
Egg Salad	1 serv (4 oz)	200	17	4	310	9	5	2	0	40	340	—	—	0
Fresh Fruit Cup	1 serv (8 oz)	110	1	0	0	1	25	24	2	20	10	—	—	48
Mixed Greens	1 serv (3.5 oz)	228	18	3	0	2	13	4	1	20	380	—	—	2
Potato	½ cup	290	21	3	15	3	21	1	2	0	600	—	—	4
Tuna Salad On Greens	1 serv (10.5 oz)	170	5	1	35	20	10	6	3	20	520	—	—	18
SANDWICHES														
12 Grain Bread Deli Chicken Salad	1	440	13	2	55	26	55	8	6	150	1090	—	—	12
12 Grain Bread Deli Egg Salad	1	490	21	4	315	18	57	8	5	150	800	—	—	9
12 Grain Bread Deli Ham	1	560	25	7	75	29	55	8	5	250	1680	—	—	9
12 Grain Bread Deli Roast Beef	1	560	24	7	80	34	56	8	5	250	1170	—	—	9
12 Grain Bread Deli Smoked Turkey	1	530	21	6	70	31	56	9	5	250	1700	—	—	9
12 Grain Bread Deli Tuna Salad	1	440	13	2	55	26	56	8	6	150	1090	—	—	12
12 Grain Bread Deli Turkey Pastrami	1	540	21	6	70	34	55	9	5	250	1900	—	—	9
12 Grain Bread Ultimate Toasted Cheese w/ Tomato	1	870	50	25	110	36	77	7	2	700	1530	—	—	9
Bagel Chicken Salad	1	500	10	2	55	28	78	8	4	60	1160	—	—	12
Bagel Egg Bacon	1	580	19	7	285	29	74	6	2	200	970	—	—	0
Bagel Egg Ham	1	530	13	5	295	31	74	6	2	150	1120	—	—	0
Bagel Egg Salad	1	560	18	5	315	20	79	7	3	80	860	—	—	12
Bagel Egg Sausage	1	550	14	5	295	33	74	6	2	150	1000	—	—	0
Bagel Ham	1	450	6	2	45	26	74	6	3	40	1390	—	—	12
Bagel Holey Cow	1	900	50	13	105	36	77	6	3	150	1450	—	—	9
Bagel Hummus & Feta	1	540	13	4	15	18	89	10	5	100	880	—	—	36
Bagel New York Lox	1	660	27	19	85	26	79	10	3	60	1150	—	—	6
Bagel Original	1	480	10	4	270	23	74	6	2	150	680	—	—	0
Bagel Roast Beef	1	460	4	2	45	31	76	6	3	40	880	—	—	12
Bagel Reuben Deli	1	660	19	6	65	39	83	8	4	300	2590	—	—	4

FOOD	PORTION	CALS	FAT	SAT FAT	CHOL	PROT	CARB	SUGAR	FIBER	CALCI	SOD	POTAS	FOLIC	VIT C
Bagel Salmon & Shmear	1	650	22	12	310	31	82	10	2	200	1040	—	—	9
Bagel Santa Fe	1	650	24	8	300	30	78	6	2	200	1210	—	—	1
Bagel Smoked Turkey	1	420	2	0	30	25	75	6	3	40	1270	—	—	12
Bagel Tasty Turkey	1	570	15	9	80	31	83	9	4	40	1420	—	—	12
Bagel The Veg Out	1	490	13	7	30	17	77	11	3	150	850	—	—	15
Bagel Tuna Salad	1	470	6	2	35	29	77	7	4	60	1040	—	—	15
Bagel Turkey Pastrami	1	440	2	0	40	31	76	7	3	40	1610	—	—	12
Challah Club Mex	1	750	45	14	135	39	47	3	2	150	2290	—	—	24
Challah Cobbie	1	630	33	12	110	37	45	5	4	100	1920	—	—	24
Challah Deli Chicken Salad	1	480	14	3	95	29	62	11	4	60	920	—	—	15
Challah Deli Egg Salad	1	430	20	5	345	18	45	7	2	60	540	—	—	9
Challah Deli Pastrami	1	480	21	7	100	34	43	8	2	150	1650	—	—	9
Challah Deli Roast Beef	1	500	23	8	110	34	44	7	2	150	920	—	—	9
Challah Deli Smoked Turkey	1	470	21	7	100	31	44	8	2	150	1450	—	—	9
Challah Deli Tuna Salad	1	370	10	3	60	30	42	6	2	60	740	—	—	9
Challah Deli Turkey Ham	1	500	25	8	105	29	43	7	2	150	1430	—	—	9
Challah BBQ Chicken	1	380	8	2	80	27	52	17	2	40	1000	—	—	9
Challah Roasted Chicken & Smoked Gouda	1	440	13	6	110	36	47	10	2	200	1010	—	—	9
Chicago Bagel Dog Asiago	1	740	34	15	80	29	78	6	2	200	1360	—	—	0
Chicago Bagel Dog Chili Cheese	1	810	38	17	105	33	83	9	4	200	1550	—	—	12
Chicago Bagel Dog Everything	1	730	34	12	70	26	80	6	3	40	1850	—	—	0
Chicago Bagel Dog Onion w/o Cheese	1	680	30	12	70	25	78	6	2	60	1220	—	—	0
Country White Deli Chicken Salad	1	540	15	4	55	30	75	8	4	100	1570	—	—	12
Country White Deli Egg Salad	1	590	23	6	315	22	77	8	3	100	1280	—	—	9
Country White Deli Ham	1	660	27	9	15	33	75	8	3	200	2160	—	—	9

FOOD	PORTION	CALS	FAT	SAT FAT	CHOL	PROT	CARB	SUGAR	FIBER	CALCI	SOD	POTAS	FOLIC	VIT C
Country White Deli Roast Beef	1	660	26	9	80	38	76	8	3	200	1650	—	—	9
Country White Deli Smoked Turkey	1	630	23	8	70	35	76	9	3	200	2180	—	—	9
Country White Deli Tuna Salad	1	510	11	3	35	30	74	7	4	100	1440	—	—	15
Country White Deli Turkey Pastrami	1	640	23	8	70	38	75	9	3	200	2380	—	—	9
Country White Ultimate Toasted Cheese w/ Tomato	1	870	51	26	110	36	73	7	2	700	1610	—	—	6
Panini Cali Club	1	730	24	9	75	47	90	15	9	450	2340	—	—	54
Panini Cuban Ham	1	700	31	11	90	40	68	2	4	500	2010	—	—	1
Panini Denver Omelet Breakfast	1	740	33	13	310	42	70	4	3	500	1380	—	—	12
Panini Italian Chicken	1	770	36	13	85	44	69	3	4	400	1840	—	—	24
Panini Taos Turkey	1	740	25	9	80	45	93	15	9	400	2140	—	—	84
Panini Ultimate Toasted Cheese	1	900	44	24	110	39	96	19	7	500	1910	—	—	84
Roll Ups Albuquerque Turkey	1	790	39	15	85	31	81	28	5	300	2040	—	—	15
Roll Ups Thai Vegetable w/ Chicken	1	670	18	1	40	27	99	26	4	250	1850	—	—	24
Roll Ups Thai Vegetables	1	630	21	2	0	24	97	17	5	250	1310	—	—	39
SOUPS														
Broccoli Sharp Cheddar	1 cup	230	15	8	40	11	13	8	1	300	490	—	—	27
Chicken & Wild Rice	1 cup	190	4	1	15	10	29	3	2	60	1440	—	—	4
Chicken Noodle	1 cup	220	9	3	60	16	17	2	2	40	980	—	—	5
Clam Chowda	1 cup	160	11	6	35	5	11	1	0	100	480	—	—	5
Minestroni Low Fat	1 cup	180	3	1	0	8	32	7	5	40	1410	—	—	9
Tomato Bisque	1 cup	190	10	3	15	5	23	9	3	40	1390	—	—	54
Tortilla	1 cup	90	3	0	0	2	14	5	2	40	1530	—	—	6
Turkey Chili	1 cup	140	5	1	20	10	14	4	2	40	930	—	—	21
SPREADS														
Butter	1 tbsp	100	11	8	30	0	0	0	0	0	115	—	—	0
Butter &	1 tbsp	60	7	2	0	0	0	0	0	0	75	—	—	0

FOOD	PORTION	CALS	FAT	SAT FAT	CHOL	PROT	CARB	SUGAR	FIBER	CALCI	SOD	POTAS	FOLIC	VIT C
Margarine Blend														
Cream Cheese Blueberry	1 tbsp	70	5	4	15	1	6	5	0	0	50	—	—	0
Cream Cheese Cappuccino	2 tbsp	70	5	4	15	1	4	4	0	0	50	—	—	0
Cream Cheese Garden Vegetable	2 tbsp	60	5	4	15	1	2	1	0	0	105	—	—	0
Cream Cheese Honey Almond Reduced Fat	2 tbsp	70	5	3	15	1	5	4	0	0	40	—	—	0
Cream Cheese Jalapeño Salsa	1 tbsp	60	5	3	15	1	3	1	0	0	95	—	—	0
Cream Cheese Maple Walnut Raisin	2 tbsp	60	5	4	15	1	4	3	0	0	45	—	—	0
Cream Cheese Onion & Chive	2 tbsp	70	6	4	20	4	3	1	0	0	55	—	—	0
Cream Cheese Plain	2 tbsp	60	7	5	20	1	1	1	0	0	65	—	—	0
Cream Cheese Plain Reduced Fat	2 tbsp	60	5	4	15	1	2	1	0	0	85	—	—	0
Cream Cheese Pumpkin	2 tbsp	100	8	6	25	1	6	5	0	20	80	—	—	0
Cream Cheese Smoked Salmon	2 tbsp	60	5	4	15	1	3	1	0	0	115	—	—	0
Cream Cheese Strawberry	2 tbsp	70	5	4	15	1	5	4	0	0	50	—	—	0
Cream Cheese Sun Dried Tomato & Basil	2 tbsp	60	5	4	15	1	2	1	0	0	50	—	—	0
Fruit Spread Apricot	1 serv	75	0	0	0	0	19	0	0	0	8	—	—	0
Fruit Spread Grape	1 serv (1 oz)	75	0	0	0	0	19	0	0	0	3	—	—	0
Fruit Spread Strawberry	1 serv (1 oz)	75	0	0	0	0	19	0	0	0	17	—	—	0
Honey Butter	1 tbsp	90	8	4	15	0	4	3	0	0	35	—	—	0
Hummus	1 serv	110	7	1	0	3	9	2	2	40	390	—	—	4
Mayo Ancho Lime	1 tbsp	50	5	1	5	0	1	0	0	0	160	—	—	0
Mustard French Dijon	1 tsp	10	0	0	0	0	0	0	0	0	130	—	—	0
Mustard Grain Dijon	1 tsp	5	0	0	0	0	0	0	0	0	105	—	—	0
Mustard Honey	1 tsp	15	0	0	0	0	2	0	0	0	45	—	—	0
Mustard Raspberry	2 tbsp	50	2	0	2	1	7	5	0	20	190	—	—	0
Mustard Yellow	1 tbsp	5	0	0	0	0	0	0	0	0	80	—	—	0
Peanut Butter	2 tbsp	190	15	2	0	7	8	3	2	20	140	—	—	0

FOOD	PORTION	CALS	FAT	SAT FAT	CHOL	PROT	CARB	SUGAR	FIBER	CALCI	SOD	POTAS	FOLIC	VIT C
Salsa Ancho Lime	¼ cup	20	1	0	0	0	3	0	0	0	670	—	—	9

EL POLLO LOCO

DESSERTS

FOOD	PORTION	CALS	FAT	SAT FAT	CHOL	PROT	CARB	SUGAR	FIBER	CALCI	SOD	POTAS	FOLIC	VIT C
Churro	1	179	11	3	5	3	18	0	1	10	221	—	—	0
Fosters Freeze Soft Serve	1 cup	180	5	3	20	4	30	26	0	150	100	—	—	0

MAIN MENU SELECTIONS

FOOD	PORTION	CALS	FAT	SAT FAT	CHOL	PROT	CARB	SUGAR	FIBER	CALCI	SOD	POTAS	FOLIC	VIT C
Bowl Chicken Caesar	1 serv	535	28	5	50	25	46	4	4	110	1450	—	—	29
Bowl Pollo	1 serv	545	10	1	40	31	84	1	12	100	2160	—	—	10
Bowl Veggie	1 serv	570	16	4	10	20	91	3	16	210	1705	—	—	127
Bowl Veggie w/o Cheese	1 serv	529	12	2	0	17	91	3	16	150	1608	—	—	127
Burrito BRC	1 (9.3 oz)	482	15	5	15	16	72	1	9	350	1250	—	—	16
Burrito Classic Chicken	1	580	22	7	108	17	66	1	6	320	1595	—	—	1
Burrito Twice Grilled	1 serv	835	39	16	150	59	60	3	2	640	2880	—	—	13
Burrito BRC	1 serv	530	15	5	15	17	79	1	6	320	1395	—	—	1
Burrito Caesar	1 serv	895	45	7	100	48	76	3	4	230	2680	—	—	10
Burrito Chicken Lover's	1 serv	525	18	6	100	34	55	2	2	310	1810	—	—	5
Burrito Spicy	1 serv	555	19	6	70	31	64	2	9	400	1980	—	—	26
Burrito Ultimate Chicken	1 serv	685	23	7	65	35	84	2	6	350	2250	—	—	8
Chicken Breast	1 piece	153	4	1	95	29	0	0	0	10	540	—	—	1
Chicken Leg	1 piece	86	3	0	80	14	0	0	0	0	206	—	—	0
Chicken Thigh	1 piece	120	7	2	82	14	0	0	0	30	225	—	—	0
Chicken Wing	1	83	3	1	58	13	0	0	0	20	334	—	—	1
Cole Slaw	1 serv	206	16	3	11	2	12	5	2	30	358	—	—	34
Corn Cobbette	1 serv	80	1	0	0	3	18	4	1	0	10	—	—	0
French Fries	1 serv	444	19	5	0	6	61	0	0	0	605	—	—	0
Fresh Vegetables	1 serv	70	4	1	0	3	6	2	4	60	80	—	—	106
Gravy	1 serv (1 oz)	107	4	1	8	3	15	4	0	60	1344	—	—	11
Mashed Potatoes	1 serv	97	1	0	0	3	21	1	2	20	369	—	—	4
Nachos Chicken	1 serv	1420	91	26	161	47	105	6	15	740	1506	—	—	11
Pinto Beans	1 serv	165	4	tr	0	8	26	0	10	70	715	—	—	3
Popcorn Chicken	1 serv	226	12	2	53	17	15	0	0	0	787	—	—	0
Potato Salad	1 serv	256	14	2	15	3	30	6	3	30	527	—	—	18
Quesadilla Cheese	1 serv	495	25	11	53	22	45	2	2	580	1008	—	—	0
Quesadilla Chicken	1 serv	593	29	12	107	36	48	2	0	590	1329	—	—	0
Smokey Black Beans	1 serv	306	16	6	13	7	35	19	5	0	731	—	—	0
Spanish Rice	1 serv	165	1	tr	0	3	34	0	1	20	425	—	—	5

FOOD	PORTION	CALS	FAT	SAT FAT	CHOL	PROT	CARB	SUGAR	FIBER	CALCI	SOD	POTAS	FOLIC	VIT C
Taco Al Carbon Chicken	1 serv	135	3	tr	30	9	18	0	1	70	225	—	—	1
Taco Soft Chicken	1	237	12	4	74	17	15	1	0	180	629	—	—	10
Taquitos Chicken	2	370	17	4	25	15	43	2	3	20	690	—	—	2
Tortilla Chips	1 serv	426	24	6	0	5	48	1	4	70	166	—	—	0
Tortilla Corn	1 (4.5 inch)	40	1	0	0	1	8	0	1	0	<5	—	—	0
Tortilla Corn	1 (6 inches)	70	1	0	0	1	14	0	1	10	35	—	—	0
Tortilla Flour	1 (6.5 inch)	110	4	0	0	3	13	0	0	80	16	—	—	0
Tortilla Flour	1 (12 inches)	325	8	2	0	8	51	1	2	180	815	—	—	0
Tortilla Spicy Tomato	1 (12 inches)	270	7	1	0	8	43	1	2	150	670	—	—	4
Tostada Salad	1 serv	700	32	9	65	32	76	8	10	290	1725	—	—	11
SALAD DRESSINGS AND TOPPINGS														
Bleu Cheese	1 serv (1.5 oz)	230	24	5	30	2	2	2	0	20	450	—	—	0
Buttermilk Ranch	1 serv (1.5 oz)	220	24	4	10	1	2	2	0	0	420	—	—	0
Creamy Chipotle	1 serv (0.5 oz)	75	8	1	5	0	1	0	0	10	100	—	—	1
Creamy Cilantro	1 serv (0.5 oz)	80	8	1	5	0	0	0	0	10	85	—	—	1
Guacamole	1 serv (1 oz)	30	2	0	0	0	3	0	0	20	160	—	—	3
Hot Sauce Jalapeño	1 pkg (0.5 oz)	5	0	0	0	0	1	0	0	0	110	—	—	0
Light Italian	1 serv (1.5 oz)	20	1	0	0	0	2	2	0	0	780	—	—	0
Salsa Avocado	1 serv (1 oz)	20	1	0	0	0	1	0	0	0	225	—	—	2
Salsa House	1 serv (1 oz)	6	tr	0	0	0	1	1	0	0	85	—	—	5
Salsa Pico De Gallo	1 serv (1 oz)	10	tr	0	0	0	1	1	0	0	135	—	—	5
Salsa Spicy Chipotle	1 serv (1 oz)	7	0	0	0	0	1	1	0	0	180	—	—	6
Sour Cream	1 serv (1 oz)	60	5	4	20	1	1	1	0	40	15	—	—	0
Thousand Island	1 serv (1.5 oz)	220	21	3	30	0	7	7	0	0	360	—	—	0
SALADS														
Caesar	1 serv	565	45	8	70	24	18	5	3	110	1305	—	—	12
Caesar w/o Dressing	1 serv	250	11	3	55	22	16	4	3	80	975	—	—	11
Fiesta Salad	1 serv	755	58	16	105	32	28	6	4	340	1680	—	—	17
Fiesta Salad w/o Dressing	1 serv	450	26	11	95	31	25	5	4	320	1275	—	—	16
Garden Salad	1 serv	110	7	3	15	5	8	2	2	130	270	—	—	5
Macaroni & Cheese	1 serv	381	26	16	65	11	25	3	2	200	891	—	—	0
Tostada Salad w/o Shell	1 serv	360	14	6	65	28	34	3	6	190	1365	—	—	11

FAZOLI'S

SALADS

DESSERTS

FOOD	PORTION	CALS	FAT	SAT FAT	CHOL	PROT	CARB	SUGAR	FIBER	CALCI	SOD	POTAS	FOLIC	VIT C
Cheesecake	1 slice	290	22	14	950	6	17	17	0	—	220	—	—	—
Cheesecake Turtle	1 slice	420	34	17	100	8	24	21	2	—	220	—	—	—

FOOD	PORTION	CALS	FAT	SAT FAT	CHOL	PROT	CARB	SUGAR	FIBER	CALCI	SOD	POTAS	FOLIC	VIT C
Cookie Milk Chocolate Chunk	1	360	15	12	30	6	54	33	0	—	350	—	—	—
Lemon Ice	1 serv	190	0	0	0	0	45	44	0	—	95	—	—	—
Specialty Cheesecake	1 serv	300	22	14	85	7	22	19	1	—	200	—	—	—
Strawberry Topping	1 serv	35	0	0	0	0	8	8	0	—	95	—	—	—
MAIN MENU SELECTIONS														
Baked Chicken Parmesan	1 serv	740	20	4	65	42	99	10	6	—	900	—	—	—
Baked Spaghetti Parmesan	1 serv	700	25	13	60	38	76	8	5	—	700	—	—	—
Baked Ziti	1 sm	490	17	7	35	23	56	7	4	—	570	—	—	—
Baked Ziti	1 reg	750	26	11	55	36	87	11	6	—	860	—	—	—
Breadstick	1	140	6	1	0	4	18	1	1	—	510	—	—	—
Breadstick Dry	1	90	1	0	0	4	17	1	1	—	170	—	—	—
Broccoli Fettuccine Alfredo	1 sm	560	15	4	15	19	85	5	6	—	190	—	—	—
Broccoli Fettuccine Alfredo	1 reg	830	23	6	20	27	125	5	6	—	250	—	—	—
Cheese Ravioli w/ Marinara Sauce	1 serv	480	15	7	65	21	65	9	4	—	530	—	—	—
Cheese Ravioli w/ Meat Sauce	1 serv	510	17	8	70	20	65	8	4	—	800	—	—	—
Classic Sampler	1 serv	710	21	6	85	26	97	9	6	—	710	—	—	—
Fettuccine Alfredo	1 reg	800	22	6	20	25	119	5	5	—	230	—	—	—
Fettuccine Alfredo	1 sm	530	15	4	15	17	80	3	3	—	170	—	—	—
Fettuccine w/ Shrimp & Scallop	1 serv	590	16	5	95	32	81	3	3	—	590	—	—	—
Homestyle Lasagna	1 serv	440	19	6	145	22	41	7	4	—	970	—	—	—
Homestyle Lasagna w/ Broccoli	1 serv	420	18	5	140	21	45	4	5	—	750	—	—	—
Minestrone Soup	1 serv	120	1	0	0	1	23	8	8	—	910	—	—	—
Peppery Chicken Alfredo	1 serv	610	16	4	50	31	80	3	3	—	410	—	—	—
Pizza Cheese	1 serv	460	15	8	40	24	58	6	2	—	970	—	—	—
Pizza Combination Double Slice	1 serv	570	25	12	60	29	63	7	3	—	1360	—	—	—
Pizza Pepperoni	1 serv	530	22	11	53	27	61	6	2	—	1230	—	—	—

FOOD	PORTION	CALS	FAT	SAT FAT	CHOL	PROT	CARB	SUGAR	FIBER	CALCI	SOD	POTAS	FOLIC	VIT C
Pizza Baked Spaghetti	1 serv	750	31	15	75	40	78	8	5	—	1000	—	—	—
Spaghetti w/ Marinara Sauce	1 sm	420	6	1	0	15	74	8	5	—	105	—	—	—
Spaghetti w/ Marinara Sauce	1 reg	620	8	1	0	21	111	12	7	—	140	—	—	—
Spaghetti w/ Meat Sauce	1 sm	450	8	2	10	14	74	8	5	—	370	—	—	—
Spaghetti w/ Meat Sauce	1 reg	670	11	3	10	21	111	11	8	—	530	—	—	—
Spaghetti w/ Meatballs	1 sm	730	31	11	60	28	80	9	6	—	730	—	—	—
Spaghetti w/ Meatballs	1 reg	1020	42	14	80	39	119	13	8	—	970	—	—	—
SALAD DRESSINGS														
Honey French	1 serv	150	12	2	0	0	9	9	0	—	210	—	—	—
House Italian	1 serv	110	9	2	0	0	5	5	0	—	510	—	—	—
Ranch	1 serv	150	17	3	3	0	1	1	0	—	210	—	—	—
Reduced Calorie Italian	1 serv	50	5	1	0	0	3	2	0	—	390	—	—	—
Thousand Island	1 serv	130	13	2	15	0	4	4	0	—	220	—	—	—
SALADS AND SALAD BARS														
Caesar Side Salad	1	220	17	4	5	7	13	3	3	—	690	—	—	—
Chicken & Pasta Caesar Salad	1	500	27	7	55	28	35	8	4	—	1430	—	—	—
Chicken Caesar Salad	1	420	29	6	45	22	17	5	4	—	1350	—	—	—
Chicken Finger Salad	1	190	9	3	45	20	8	4	2	—	540	—	—	—
Chicken Finger Salad w/ Bacon & Honey Mustard	1	400	28	7	50	20	17	13	2	—	950	—	—	—
Garden Salad	1	25	0	0	0	2	4	3	1	—	15	—	—	—
Garden Salad w/ Balsamic Vinaigrette	1	120	9	2	0	2	10	8	1	—	150	—	—	—
Italian Chef Salad	1	260	21	9	45	15	13	3	3	—	1450	—	—	—
Pasta Salad	1 serv	590	25	6	20	18	70	13	5	—	2010	—	—	—
SANDWICHES														
Panini Chicken Caesar Club	1	660	35	11	110	39	51	1	3	—	1670	—	—	—
Panini Chicken Pesto	1	510	20	6	60	33	51	1	3	—	1350	—	—	—
Panini Four Cheese & Tomato	1	720	43	16	75	28	55	3	3	—	1450	—	—	—
Panini Ham & Swiss	1	600	30	9	70	31	53	4	2	—	2000	—	—	—

FOOD	PORTION	CALS	FAT	SAT FAT	CHOL	PROT	CARB	SUGAR	FIBER	CALCI	SOD	POTAS	FOLIC	VIT C
Panini Italian Club	1	670	37	11	85	30	54	3	3	—	1970	—	—	—
Panini Italian Deli	1	660	35	13	90	34	61	1	4	—	2450	—	—	—
Panini Smoked Turkey	1	710	38	12	110	32	57	3	3	—	2110	—	—	—
Submarinos Club	half	1100	44	14	120	51	121	8	7	—	2890	—	—	—
Submarinos Ham & Swiss	1	1000	37	11	75	44	120	8	7	—	2350	—	—	—
Submarinos Meatball	half	1260	59	23	125	55	128	10	8	—	2340	—	—	—
Submarinos Original	half	1160	55	17	105	45	124	8	8	—	2530	—	—	—
Submarinos Pepperoni Pizza	half	1060	40	19	95	55	133	11	6	—	2700	—	—	—
Submarinos Turkey	half	990	34	10	90	43	121	8	7	—	2440	—	—	—

FOSTERS FREEZE

FOOD	PORTION	CALS	FAT	SAT FAT	CHOL	PROT	CARB	SUGAR	FIBER	CALCI	SOD	POTAS	FOLIC	VIT C
Soft Serve Vanilla	1 serv (4 oz)	152	4	—	9	—	—	—	—	172	100	—	—	—

FRULLATI CAFE

BEVERAGES

FOOD	PORTION	CALS	FAT	SAT FAT	CHOL	PROT	CARB	SUGAR	FIBER	CALCI	SOD	POTAS	FOLIC	VIT C
Smoothie	1 serv (14 oz)	195	3	2	0	1	41	27	tr	5	154	—	—	—

GODFATHER'S PIZZA

FOOD	PORTION	CALS	FAT	SAT FAT	CHOL	PROT	CARB	SUGAR	FIBER	CALCI	SOD	POTAS	FOLIC	VIT C
Golden Crust Cheese	⅛ med (3.1 oz)	212	8	—	12	10	26	—	—	170	311	51	—	2
Golden Crust Cheese	⅒ lg (3.5 oz)	242	9	—	14	12	28	—	—	200	363	57	—	3
Golden Crust Combo	⅛ med (4.4 oz)	271	12	—	22	13	28	—	—	180	562	154	—	3
Golden Crust Combo	⅒ lg (4.9 oz)	305	14	—	25	16	31	—	—	220	674	176	—	4
Original Crust Cheese	¼ mini (1.9 oz)	131	3	—	8	7	19	—	—	110	183	36	—	1
Original Crust Cheese	⅒ jumbo (5.8 oz)	382	9	—	27	22	53	—	—	360	580	106	—	4
Original Crust Cheese	⅛ med (3.5 oz)	231	5	—	14	13	24	—	—	190	338	64	—	2
Original Crust Cheese	⅒ lg (4 oz)	258	6	—	18	15	36	—	—	240	396	72	—	3
Original Crust Combo	¼ mini (2.9 oz)	176	7	—	16	10	21	—	—	130	382	127	—	1
Original Crust Combo	⅒ lg (5.6 oz)	338	12	—	31	19	38	—	—	270	740	217	—	4
Original Crust Combo	⅛ med (5.1 oz)	306	11	—	27	17	36	—	—	220	660	200	—	3
Original Crust Combo	⅒ jumbo (8.3 oz)	503	18	—	47	29	56	—	—	400	1096	325	—	5

FOOD	PORTION	CALS	FAT	SAT FAT	CHOL	PROT	CARB	SUGAR	FIBER	CALCI	SOD	POTAS	FOLIC	VIT C
GREAT STEAK & POTATO COMPANY														
Baked Potato w/ Broccoli & Cheese	1 serv (12 oz)	340	5	2	—	—	—	—	—	—	340	—	—	—
Chicken Philadelpia	1 serv (10 oz)	640	27	7	—	—	—	—	—	—	620	—	—	—
Chicken Teriyaki	1 serv (11 oz)	580	17	5	—	—	—	—	—	—	1470	—	—	—
Fresh Cut Fries	1 reg	540	29	7	—	—	—	—	—	—	440	—	—	—
Fresh Cut Fries	1 sm	460	24	6	—	—	—	—	—	—	380	—	—	—
Fresh Cut Fries	1 lg	920	48	12	—	—	—	—	—	—	760	—	—	—
Great Potato w/ Steak	1 serv (14 oz)	600	32	7	—	—	—	—	—	—	600	—	—	—
Great Potato w/ Turkey	1 serv (14 oz)	610	28	6	—	—	—	—	—	—	620	—	—	—
Great Salad Experience w/ Chicken w/o Dressing	1 serv (15 oz)	260	9	5	—	—	—	—	—	—	490	—	—	—
Great Steak	1 serv (11 oz)	660	34	10	—	—	—	—	—	—	400	—	—	—
Great Steak	1 lg (18 oz)	1070	55	16	—	—	—	—	—	—	610	—	—	—
Ham Delight	1 serv (11 oz)	710	33	9	—	—	—	—	—	—	1590	—	—	—
Turkey Philadelphia	1 serv (10 oz)	690	28	7	—	—	—	—	—	—	290	—	—	—
Veggi Delight	1 serv (7 oz)	570	29	7	—	—	—	—	—	—	440	—	—	—
HAAGEN-DAZS														
FROZEN YOGURT														
Pineapple Coconut	½ cup	230	13	8	90	4	25	24	0	100	55	—	—	0
Soft Serve Nonfat Chocolate	½ cup	110	0	0	0	4	23	20	0	150	65	—	—	0
Soft Serve Nonfat Chocolate Mousse	½ cup	80	0	0	0	5	24	7	1	150	65	—	—	0
Soft Serve Nonfat Coffee	½ cup	110	0	0	<5	5	22	21	0	150	70	—	—	0
Soft Serve Nonfat Strawberry	½ cup	110	0	0	0	4	24	23	0	150	60	—	—	5
Soft Serve Nonfat Vanilla	½ cup	110	0	0	<5	5	22	21	0	150	75	—	—	0
Soft Serve Nonfat Vanilla Mousse	½ cup	70	0	0	<5	4	23	7	0	150	65	—	—	0
Soft Serve Nonfat White Chocolate	½ cup	110	0	0	<5	5	22	21	0	150	75	—	—	0
Vanilla Fudge	½ cup	160	0	0	<5	6	34	22	0	150	100	—	—	0
Vanilla Raspberry Swirl	½ cup	130	0	0	<5	4	29	20	tr	100	30	—	—	1

FOOD	PORTION	CALS	FAT	SAT FAT	CHOL	PROT	CARB	SUGAR	FIBER	CALCI	SOD	POTAS	FOLIC	VIT C
ICE CREAM														
Bailey's Irish Cream	½ cup	270	17	10	115	5	23	22	0	150	70	—	—	0
Bar Chocolate	1 (2.7 oz)	200	12	8	85	4	16	15	tr	100	55	—	—	0
Bar Chocolate & Dark Chocolate	1 (3.6 oz)	350	24	15	85	5	28	24	2	100	45	—	—	0
Bar Coffee	1 (2.7 oz)	190	13	8	85	3	15	15	0	100	65	—	—	0
Bar Coffee & Almond Crunch	1 (3.7 oz)	370	27	15	90	5	27	26	tr	150	80	—	—	0
Bar Vanilla	1 (2.7 oz)	190	13	8	85	3	15	15	0	100	50	—	—	0
Bar Vanilla & Almonds	1 (3.7 oz)	380	28	14	90	6	26	24	1	150	70	—	—	0
Bar Vanilla & Milk Chocolate	1 (3.5 oz)	340	24	14	90	5	25	24	tr	150	65	—	—	0
Belgian Chocolate Chocolate	½ cup	330	21	12	85	5	29	26	2	100	85	—	—	0
Brownies A La Mode	½ cup	280	16	10	90	5	28	23	tr	100	135	—	—	0
Butter Pecan	½ cup	300	22	10	105	5	20	17	tr	100	110	—	—	0
Cappuccino Commotion	½ cup	310	21	12	100	5	25	23	1	100	90	—	—	0
Chocolate	½ cup	269	17	10	110	5	21	20	1	100	60	—	—	0
Chocolate Chocolate Chip	½ cup	300	19	11	100	5	26	23	2	100	55	—	—	0
Chocolate Chocolate Mint	½ cup	300	20	11	95	5	25	22	1	100	50	—	—	0
Chocolate Swiss Almond	½ cup	300	20	11	100	5	24	21	2	100	55	—	—	0
Coffee	½ cup	250	17	10	115	5	20	20	0	150	65	—	—	0
Coffee Mocha Chip	½ cup	270	19	12	105	4	24	21	tr	100	75	—	—	0
Cookie Dough Dynamo	½ cup	310	20	12	95	4	29	24	0	100	125	—	—	0
Cookies & Cream	½ cup	270	17	10	105	5	23	21	0	150	95	—	—	0
Cookies & Fudge	½ cup	180	3	2	15	7	33	20	tr	150	115	—	—	0
Deep Chocolate Peanut Butter	½ cup	350	24	11	80	8	26	21	4	100	85	—	—	0
Dulce De Leche Caramel	½ cup	270	16	10	95	5	27	27	0	150	90	—	—	0
Lowfat Coffee Fudge	½ cup	170	3	2	25	5	32	22	0	150	95	—	—	0
Macadamia Brittle	½ cup	280	19	11	105	4	24	23	0	100	105	—	—	0
Macadamia Nut	½ cup	320	24	12	110	5	20	19	0	150	100	—	—	0
Mint Chip	½ cup	280	18	12	105	4	25	22	tr	100	85	—	—	0
Pistachio	½ cup	280	19	10	110	5	21	18	tr	100	80	—	—	0
Pralines & Cream	½ cup	280	17	9	95	4	28	26	0	100	160	—	—	0
Rum Raisin	½ cup	260	17	10	105	4	21	20	0	100	55	—	—	0

FOOD	PORTION	CALS	FAT	SAT FAT	CHOL	PROT	CARB	SUGAR	FIBER	CALCI	SOD	POTAS	FOLIC	VIT C
Strawberry	½ cup	250	16	9	90	4	22	21	tr	150	90	—	—	6
Vanilla	½ cup	250	17	10	115	4	20	20	0	150	65	—	—	0
Vanilla Chocolate Chip	½ cup	290	19	12	100	5	25	22	tr	100	70	—	—	0
Vanilla Swiss Almond	½ cup	290	20	11	100	5	23	20	tr	100	70	—	—	0
SORBET														
Bar Raspberry & Vanilla	1 (2.5 oz)	90	0	0	0	2	21	15	tr	60	15	—	—	1
Mango	½ cup	120	0	0	0	0	31	29	tr	0	0	—	—	2
Orange	½ cup	120	0	0	0	0	30	24	tr	0	0	—	—	15
Raspberry	½ cup	120	0	0	0	0	30	26	2	0	0	—	—	2
Soft Serve Raspberry	½ cup	110	0	0	0	0	28	25	2	0	0	—	—	2
Strawberry	½ cup	120	0	0	0	0	30	27	1	0	0	—	—	9
Zesty Lemon	½ cup	120	0	0	0	0	31	27	tr	0	0	—	—	4

HARDEE'S

FOOD	PORTION	CALS	FAT	SAT FAT	CHOL	PROT	CARB	SUGAR	FIBER	CALCI	SOD	POTAS	FOLIC	VIT C
BEVERAGES														
Orange Juice	1 serv (11 oz)	140	tr	tr	0	2	34	—	—	—	5	—	—	—
Shake Chocolate	1 (12.2 oz)	370	5	3	30	13	67	—	—	—	270	—	—	—
Shake Peach	1 (12.1 oz)	390	4	3	25	10	77	—	—	—	290	—	—	—
Shake Strawberry	1 (12.7 oz)	420	4	3	20	11	83	—	—	—	270	—	—	—
Shake Vanilla	1 (12.2 oz)	350	5	3	20	12	65	—	—	—	300	—	—	—
BREAKFAST SELECTIONS														
Apple Cinnamon 'N' Raisin Biscuit	1 (2.18 oz)	200	8	2	0	2	30	—	—	—	350	—	—	—
Bacon & Egg Biscuit	1 (5.5 oz)	570	33	11	275	22	45	—	—	—	1400	—	—	—
Bacon Egg & Cheese Biscuit	1 (5.9 oz)	610	37	13	280	24	45	—	—	—	1630	—	—	—
Big Country Breakfast Bacon	1 serv (9.4 oz)	820	49	15	535	33	62	—	—	—	1870	—	—	—
Big Country Breakfast Sausage	1 serv (11.4 oz)	1000	66	38	570	41	62	—	—	—	3210	—	—	—
Biscuit 'N' Gravy	1 (7.8 oz)	510	28	9	15	10	55	—	—	—	1500	—	—	—
Country Ham Biscuit	1 (3.8 oz)	430	22	5	25	15	45	—	—	—	1930	—	—	—
Frisco Breakfast Sandwich Ham	1 (7.4 oz)	500	25	9	290	24	46	—	—	—	1370	—	—	—
Ham Biscuit	1 (4 oz)	400	20	6	15	9	47	—	—	—	1340	—	—	—
Ham Egg & Cheese Biscuit	1 (6.5 oz)	540	30	11	285	20	48	—	—	—	1660	—	—	—
Hash Rounds	1 serv (2.8 oz)	230	14	3	0	3	24	—	—	—	560	—	—	—
Jelly Biscuit	1 (3.5 oz)	440	21	6	0	6	57	—	—	—	1000	—	—	—

FOOD	PORTION	CALS	FAT	SAT FAT	CHOL	PROT	CARB	SUGAR	FIBER	CALCI	SOD	POTAS	FOLIC	VIT C
Rise 'N' Shine Biscuit	1 (2.9 oz)	390	21	6	0	6	44	—	—	—	1000	—	—	—
Sausage Biscuit	1 (4.1 oz)	510	31	10	25	14	44	—	—	—	1360	—	—	—
Sausage & Egg Biscuit	1 (6.3 oz)	630	40	22	285	23	45	—	—	—	1480	—	—	—
Three Pancakes	1 serv (4.8 oz)	280	2	1	15	8	56	—	—	—	890	—	—	—
Ultimate Omelet Biscuit	1 (5.8 oz)	570	33	12	120	22	45	—	—	—	1370	—	—	—
DESSERTS														
Big Cookie	1 (2.0 oz)	280	12	4	15	4	41	—	—	—	150	—	—	—
Cone Chocolate	1 (4.1 oz)	180	2	1	15	5	34	—	—	—	110	—	—	—
Cone Vanilla	1 (4.1 oz)	170	2	1	10	4	34	—	—	—	130	—	—	—
Cool Twist Cone Vanilla/Chocolate	1 (4.1 oz)	180	2	1	10	4	34	—	—	—	120	—	—	—
Peach Cobbler	1 serv (6 oz)	310	7	1	0	2	60	—	—	—	360	—	—	—
Sundae Hot Fudge	1 (5.5 oz)	290	6	3	20	7	51	—	—	—	310	—	—	—
Sundae Strawberry	1 (5.8 oz)	210	2	1	10	5	43	—	—	—	140	—	—	—
MAIN MENU SELECTIONS														
Baked Beans	1 serv (5 oz)	170	1	0	0	8	32	—	—	—	600	—	—	—
Big Roast Beef Sandwich	1 (6.5 oz)	460	24	9	70	26	35	—	—	—	1230	—	—	—
Cheeseburger	1 (4.3 oz)	310	14	6	40	16	30	—	—	—	890	—	—	—
Chicken Fillet Sandwich	1 (7.5 oz)	480	18	3	55	26	54	—	—	—	1280	—	—	—
Cole Slaw	1 serv (4 oz)	240	20	3	10	2	13	—	—	—	340	—	—	—
Fisherman's Fillet	1 (8.3 oz)	560	27	7	65	26	54	—	—	—	1330	—	—	—
French Fries	1 med (5 oz)	350	15	4	0	5	49	—	—	—	150	—	—	—
French Fries	1 sm (3.4 oz)	240	10	3	0	4	33	—	—	—	100	—	—	—
French Fries	1 lg (6 oz)	430	18	5	0	6	59	—	—	—	190	—	—	—
Fried Chicken Breast	1 piece (5.2 oz)	370	15	4	75	29	29	—	—	—	1190	—	—	—
Fried Chicken Leg	1 piece (2.4 oz)	170	7	2	45	13	15	—	—	—	570	—	—	—
Fried Chicken Thigh	1 piece (4.2 oz)	330	15	4	60	19	30	—	—	—	1000	—	—	—
Fried Chicken Wing	1 piece (2.3 oz)	200	8	2	30	10	23	—	—	—	740	—	—	—
Frisco Burger	1 (8.1 oz)	720	46	16	95	33	43	—	—	—	1340	—	—	—
Gravy	1 serv (1.5 oz)	20	tr	tr	0	tr	3	—	—	—	260	—	—	—
Grilled Chicken Sandwich	1 (7.1 oz)	350	11	2	65	25	38	—	—	—	950	—	—	—
Hamburger	1 (3.9 oz)	270	11	3	35	14	29	—	—	—	670	—	—	—
Hot Ham 'N' Cheese	1 (5.1 oz)	310	12	6	50	16	34	—	—	—	1410	—	—	—
Mashed Potatoes	1 serv (4 oz)	70	tr	tr	0	2	14	—	—	—	330	—	—	—

FOOD	PORTION	CALS	FAT	SAT FAT	CHOL	PROT	CARB	SUGAR	FIBER	CALCI	SOD	POTAS	FOLIC	VIT C
Mesquite Bacon Cheeseburger	1 (4.5 oz)	370	18	7	45	19	32	—	—	—	970	—	—	—
Monster Thickburger	1	1400	107	—	—	—	—	—	—	—	—	—	—	—
Mushroom 'N' Swiss Burger	1 (6.8 oz)	490	25	12	80	28	39	—	—	—	1100	—	—	—
Quarter Pound Double Cheeseburger	1 (6 oz)	470	27	11	80	27	31	—	—	—	1290	—	—	—
Regular Roast Beef	1 (4.3 oz)	320	16	6	43	17	26	—	—	—	820	—	—	—
The Boss	1 (7 oz)	570	33	12	85	37	42	—	—	—	910	—	—	—
The Works Burger	1 (8.1 oz)	530	30	12	80	25	41	—	—	—	1030	—	—	—
SALAD DRESSINGS														
French Fat Free	1 serv (2 oz)	70	0	0	0	0	18	13	0	0	300	—	—	0
Ranch	1 serv (2 oz)	290	29	4	25	1	6	—	—	—	510	—	—	—
Thousand Island	1 serv (2 oz)	250	23	3	35	1	9	—	—	—	540	—	—	—
SALADS AND SALAD BARS														
Garden Salad	1 (10.2 oz)	220	13	9	40	12	11	—	—	—	350	—	—	—
Grilled Chicken Salad	1 (11.5 oz)	150	3	1	60	20	11	—	—	—	610	—	—	—
Side Salad	1 (4.6 oz)	25	tr	tr	0	1	4	—	—	—	45	—	—	—

HOT SAM'S PRETZELS

FOOD	PORTION	CALS	FAT	SAT FAT	CHOL	PROT	CARB	SUGAR	FIBER	CALCI	SOD	POTAS	FOLIC	VIT C
Bavarian	1 lg (5.1 oz)	390	0	0	0	14	83	4	4	40	780	—	—	0
Bavarian	1 reg (2.5 oz)	200	0	0	0	7	42	2	2	20	390	—	—	0
Bavarian Stix	10 (5 oz)	390	0	0	0	14	83	4	4	40	780	—	—	0
Sweet Dough	1 (4.5 oz)	360	3	1	0	11	73	4	4	40	780	—	—	0
Sweet Dough Blueberry	1 (4.5 oz)	400	4	2	0	11	81	18	2	40	610	—	—	0

HUNGRY HOWIE'S

FOOD	PORTION	CALS	FAT	SAT FAT	CHOL	PROT	CARB	SUGAR	FIBER	CALCI	SOD	POTAS	FOLIC	VIT C
MAIN MENU SELECTIONS														
Howie Wings	6 (3 oz)	180	14	4	70	12	0	—	0	—	760	—	—	—
Three Cheeser Bread	1 serv	370	14	5	17	15	47	—	1	—	384	—	—	—
PIZZA														
Large Cheese	1 slice	175	4	3	11	10	24	—	1	—	387	—	—	—
Large Cheese + Bacon	1 slice	208	5	3	13	17	25	—	1	—	388	—	—	—
Large Cheese + Beef	1 slice	197	6	3	16	11	24	—	1	—	464	—	—	—
Large Cheese + Black Olives	1 slice	181	5	3	12	10	24	—	1	—	436	—	—	—
Large Cheese + Green Olives	1 slice	181	5	3	12	10	24	—	1	—	436	—	—	—
Large Cheese + Green Peppers	1 slice	175	4	3	11	10	24	—	1	—	387	—	—	—

FOOD	PORTION	CALS	FAT	SAT FAT	CHOL	PROT	CARB	SUGAR	FIBER	CALCI	SOD	POTAS	FOLIC	VIT C
Large Cheese + Ham	1 slice	179	6	3	14	11	24	—	1	—	452	—	—	—
Large Cheese + Mushrooms	1 slice	175	4	3	11	10	24	—	1	—	387	—	—	—
Large Cheese + Onions	1 slice	175	5	3	12	10	24	—	1	—	388	—	—	—
Large Cheese + Pepperoni	1 slice	191	4	3	16	11	24	—	1	—	450	—	—	—
Large Cheese + Pineapple	1 slice	388	5	3	12	11	25	—	1	—	388	—	—	—
Large Cheese + Sausage	1 slice	195	6	3	14	12	24	—	1	—	484	—	—	—
Medium Cheese	1 slice	153	5	2	9	9	21	—	1	—	350	—	—	—
Medium Cheese + Bacon	1 slice	179	5	3	10	14	21	—	1	—	351	—	—	—
Medium Cheese + Beef	1 slice	177	6	3	14	10	21	—	1	—	427	—	—	—
Medium Cheese + Black Olives	1 slice	159	5	3	11	9	21	—	1	—	388	—	—	—
Medium Cheese + Green Olives	1 slice	159	4	3	11	9	21	—	1	—	388	—	—	—
Medium Cheese + Green Peppers	1 slice	155	5	3	10	9	21	—	1	—	351	—	—	—
Medium Cheese + Ham	1 slice	159	6	2	12	10	21	—	1	—	415	—	—	—
Medium Cheese + Mushrooms	1 slice	155	5	2	9	9	21	—	1	—	350	—	—	—
Medium Cheese + Onions	1 slice	155	5	3	10	9	21	—	1	—	351	—	—	—
Medium Cheese + Pepperoni	1 slice	171	6	3	14	10	21	—	1	—	410	—	—	—
Medium Cheese + Pineapple	1 slice	158	5	3	10	9	22	—	1	—	351	—	—	—
Medium Cheese + Sausage	1 slice	175	6	2	12	10	21	—	1	—	447	—	—	—
Small Cheese	1 slice	121	3	2	8	7	37	—	1	—	278	—	—	—
Small Cheese + Bacon	1 slice	138	3	2	9	10	17	—	1	—	278	—	—	—
Small Cheese + Beef	1 slice	137	4	2	12	8	17	—	1	—	328	—	—	—
Small Cheese + Black Olives	1 slice	125	3	2	9	7	17	—	1	—	303	—	—	—
Small Cheese + Green Olives	1 slice	125	3	2	9	7	17	—	1	—	303	—	—	—
Small Cheese + Green Peppers	1 slice	122	3	2	8	7	17	—	1	—	278	—	—	—
Small Cheese + Ham	1 slice	126	3	2	11	8	17	—	1	—	331	—	—	—

FOOD	PORTION	CALS	FAT	SAT FAT	CHOL	PROT	CARB	SUGAR	FIBER	CALCI	SOD	POTAS	FOLIC	VIT C
Small Cheese + Mushrooms	1 slice	123	3	2	8	7	17	—	1	—	279	—	—	—
Small Cheese + Onions	1 slice	122	3	2	8	7	17	—	1	—	278	—	—	—
Small Cheese + Pepperoni	1 slice	136	4	3	12	8	17	—	1	—	329	—	—	—
Small Cheese + Pineapple	1 slice	124	3	2	8	7	18	—	1	—	278	—	—	—
Small Cheese + Sausage	1 slice	136	3	2	11	8	17	—	1	—	343	—	—	—
SALADS AND SALAD BARS														
Antipasto Salad w/o Dressing	1 lg	101	7	3	24	8	3	—	1	—	477	—	—	—
Chef Salad w/o Dressing	1 lg	99	6	3	24	8	4	—	2	—	341	—	—	—
Garden Salad w/o Dressing	1 lg	17	tr	0	0	1	3	—	2	—	9	—	—	—
Greek Salad w/o Dressing	1 lg	109	7	4	25	6	7	—	2	—	501	—	—	—
SANDWICHES														
Sub Deluxe Italian	½ sub	506	18	8	44	24	61	—	2	—	1005	—	—	—
Sub Ham & Cheese	½ sub	475	15	7	44	26	61	—	2	—	1020	—	—	—
Sub Pizza	½ sub	689	34	14	86	30	67	—	3	—	1722	—	—	—
Sub Pizza Special	½ sub	606	24	11	65	29	68	—	3	—	1584	—	—	—
Sub Steak Cheese Mushroom	½ sub	491	15	7	47	27	64	—	2	—	914	—	—	—
Sub Turkey	½ sub	466	13	6	38	25	63	—	2	—	1108	—	—	—
Sub Turkey Club	½ sub	556	18	8	44	42	62	—	2	—	1065	—	—	—
Sub Vegetarian	½ sub	530	21	11	39	22	64	—	3	—	895	—	—	—

IHOP

FOOD	PORTION	CALS	FAT	SAT FAT	CHOL	PROT	CARB	SUGAR	FIBER	CALCI	SOD	POTAS	FOLIC	VIT C
Pancake Buckwheat	1 (1.7 oz)	110	4	1	50	3	15	—	1	40	280	—	—	0
Pancake Buttermilk	1 (1.7 oz)	110	3	1	30	3	17	—	tr	100	450	—	—	0
Pancake Country Griddle	1 (2 oz)	120	4	1	35	3	19	—	tr	150	440	—	—	0
Pancake Harvest Grain 'N Nut	1 (2.25 oz)	180	9	2	40	5	20	—	2	150	410	—	—	0

JACK IN THE BOX

FOOD	PORTION	CALS	FAT	SAT FAT	CHOL	PROT	CARB	SUGAR	FIBER	CALCI	SOD	POTAS	FOLIC	VIT C
BEVERAGES														
Barq's Root Beer	1 serv (20 oz)	180	0	0	0	0	50	50	0	—	40	0	—	—
Coca-Cola Classic	1 serv (20 oz)	170	0	0	0	0	46	46	0	—	8	0	—	—
Coffee	1 serv (12 oz)	5	0	0	0	0	1	0	0	—	5	130	—	—
Diet Coke	1 serv (20 oz)	0	0	0	0	0	0	0	0	—	15	45	—	—
Dr Pepper	1 serv (20 oz)	190	0	0	0	0	50	50	0	—	25	0	—	—

FOOD	PORTION	CALS	FAT	SAT FAT	CHOL	PROT	CARB	SUGAR	FIBER	CALCI	SOD	POTAS	FOLIC	VIT C
Ice Cream Shake Caramel	1 serv (16 oz)	660	30	19	115	11	86	74	0	—	280	630	—	—
Ice Cream Shake Chocolate	1 (16 oz)	660	29	18	110	11	89	79	1	—	270	720	—	—
Ice Cream Shake Oreo	1 serv (16 oz)	670	33	19	110	11	81	62	1	—	350	660	—	—
Ice Cream Shake Strawberry	1 serv (16 oz)	640	28	18	110	10	84	71	0	—	220	610	—	—
Ice Cream Shake Strawberry Banana	1 serv (16 oz)	700	28	18	110	10	100	67	0	—	230	630	—	—
Ice Cream Shake Vanilla	1 (16 oz)	570	29	18	115	11	65	54	0	—	220	630	—	—
Iced Tea	1 serv (20 oz)	0	0	0	0	0	0	0	0	—	0	70	—	—
Lowfat Milk 2%	1 serv (8 oz)	140	5	3	20	10	14	13	0	—	140	460	—	—
Orange Juice	1 serv (10 oz)	140	0	0	0	2	32	27	2	—	25	220	—	—
Sprite	1 serv (20 oz)	160	0	0	0	0	41	41	0	—	40	0	—	—
BREAKFAST SELECTIONS														
Breakfast Sandwich Sourdough	1	440	26	8	215	17	36	3	2	—	880	210	—	—
Breakfast Sandwich Ultimate	1	730	40	11	440	30	66	9	2	—	1870	390	—	—
Breakfast Jack	1	310	14	5	205	13	33	4	1	—	720	200	—	—
Croissant Sausage	1	680	50	15	250	18	41	5	2	—	760	230	—	—
Croissant Supreme	1	570	37	9	240	19	41	5	1	—	1040	270	—	—
French Toast Sticks	4 pieces	430	18	4	10	8	57	11	2	—	460	140	—	—
Hash Brown	1 serv	150	10	3	0	1	13	0	2	—	230	190	—	—
Pancakes w/ Bacon	1 serv (5.6 oz)	400	12	3	30	13	59	12	3	80	980	280	—	0
Sandwich Extreme Sausage	1	720	53	18	280	25	35	5	2	—	1180	310	—	—
DESSERTS														
Cheesecake	1 serv	310	16	9	55	7	34	23	0	—	220	180	—	—
Double Fudge Cake	1 serv	310	11	3	25	3	49	37	4	—	270	0	—	—
MAIN MENU SELECTIONS														
American Cheese	1 slice	45	4	2	10	2	1	0	0	—	180	15	—	—
Bacon Cheddar Potato Wedges	1 serv	770	53	16	45	21	52	2	4	—	1330	950	—	—
Cheeseburger	1 (4 oz)	330	15	6	60	15	32	7	2	150	760	210	—	—
Cheeseburger Bacon Bacon	1	910	59	19	100	38	58	10	3	—	1780	460	—	—
Cheeseburger Bacon Ultimate	1	1120	75	28	160	52	59	12	2	—	2260	600	—	—

FOOD	PORTION	CALS	FAT	SAT FAT	CHOL	PROT	CARB	SUGAR	FIBER	CALCI	SOD	POTAS	FOLIC	VIT C
Cheeseburger Junior Bacon	1	540	36	10	75	22	31	6	1	—	940	160	—	—
Cheeseburger Ultimate	1	990	66	28	130	41	59	12	2	—	1620	480	—	—
Chicken Breast Pieces	4	360	17	3	80	27	24	0	1	—	970	430	—	—
Chicken Breast Strips	1 serv	500	25	6	80	35	36	1	3	—	1260	530	—	—
Chicken Fajita Pita	1	330	11	5	55	24	35	4	3	—	910	430	—	—
Chicken Sandwich	1	410	21	5	35	15	39	4	2	—	740	290	—	—
Dipping Sauce Barbeque	1 serv (1.6 oz)	45	0	0	0	0	11	4	0	—	330	65	—	—
Double Cheeseburger	1 (5.3 oz)	450	24	12	75	24	35	6	0	250	970	320	—	0
Egg Rolls	5 pieces (10 oz)	730	41	10	60	25	67	8	7	150	1700	830	—	18
Egg Rolls	1	130	6	2	5	5	15	1	2	—	310	140	—	—
Fish & Chips	1 serv	610	31	7	40	18	66	0	5	—	1240	660	—	—
French Fries	1 lg	580	28	6	0	6	77	0	6	—	960	770	—	—
French Fries	1 med	410	20	5	0	4	55	0	4	—	690	550	—	—
French Fries	1 sm	330	16	4	0	3	44	0	3	—	550	440	—	—
Hamburger	1	310	14	6	45	17	30	6	1	—	600	120	—	—
Hamburger w/ Cheese	1	360	18	8	60	19	31	6	1	—	740	130	—	—
Jumbo Jack	1	600	31	11	45	22	58	12	3	—	980	390	—	—
Jumbo Jack w/ Cheese	1	690	38	16	70	27	61	13	3	—	1360	470	—	—
Onion Rings	1 serv	500	30	5	0	6	51	3	3	—	420	140	—	—
Pilly Cheesesteak	1	580	22	11	90	35	55	6	3	—	1660	390	—	—
Salsa	1 serv (1 oz)	10	0	0	0	0	2	1	0	—	220	55	—	—
Sandwich Roasted Turkey	1	580	25	8	110	34	50	5	3	—	1600	500	—	—
Sandwich Ultimate Club	1	640	30	9	105	37	51	7	3	—	2000	440	—	—
Seasoned Curly Fries	1 serv	400	23	5	0	6	45	1	5	—	690	580	—	—
Sour Cream	1 serv (1 oz)	60	5	3	15	1	2	0	0	—	20	35	—	—
Sourdough Grilled Chicken Club	1	520	28	6	85	33	33	5	3	—	1330	540	—	—
Sourdough Jack	1	700	49	16	80	30	36	7	3	—	1220	450	—	—
Spicy Crispy Chicken	1	730	37	10	70	30	69	9	4	—	1480	490	—	—
Stuffed Jalapeño	3 pieces	230	13	6	20	7	22	2	2	—	690	105	—	—
Swiss Style Cheese	1 slice	40	3	2	10	2	1	0	0	—	150	10	—	—

FOOD	PORTION	CALS	FAT	SAT FAT	CHOL	PROT	CARB	SUGAR	FIBER	CALCI	SOD	POTAS	FOLIC	VIT C
Taco	1	170	9	3	20	6	15	2	2	—	210	190	—	—
Taco Monster	1	260	15	5	30	9	21	4	3	—	340	130	—	—
Turkey Jack	1	700	32	11	115	38	69	18	4	—	1930	710	—	—
SALAD DRESSINGS AND TOPPINGS														
Almonds Roasted Slivered	1 serv (0.7 oz)	130	11	1	0	5	4	1	2	—	5	150	—	—
Asian Sesame	1 serv (2.5 oz)	230	17	3	0	1	20	13	0	—	780	60	—	—
Bacon Ranch	1 serv (2.5 oz)	320	33	5	30	2	5	2	0	—	820	95	—	—
Balsamic Vinaigrette Low Fat	1 serv (2.5 oz)	40	2	0	0	0	6	3	0	—	600	30	—	—
Country Crock Spread	1 pkg	25	3	1	0	0	0	0	0	—	45	0	—	—
Creamy Southwest Dressing	1 serv (2.5 oz)	270	26	4	30	2	7	2	0	—	1080	115	—	—
Croutons	1 serv (0.5 oz)	60	2	0	0	2	10	1	0	—	130	20	—	—
Dipping Sauce Buttermilk House	1 serv (0.9 oz)	130	13	2	10	0	3	0	0	—	210	15	—	—
Dipping Sauce Frank's Red Hot Buffalo	1 serv (1 oz)	10	0	0	0	0	2	0	0	—	840	15	—	—
Dipping Sauce Sweet & Sour	1 serv (1 oz)	45	0	0	0	0	11	6	0	—	160	5	—	—
Grape Jelly	1 serv (0.5 oz)	35	0	0	0	0	9	9	0	—	10	0	—	—
Herb Mayo Sauce Low Fat	1 serv (1.5 oz)	45	4	1	0	1	3	1	1	—	370	15	—	—
Ketchup	1 pkg (0.3 oz)	10	0	0	0	0	2	2	0	—	105	30	—	—
Marinara Sauce	1 serv (0.9 oz)	15	0	0	0	0	3	3	0	—	210	85	—	—
Mustard	1 pkg	0	0	0	0	0	0	0	0	—	50	0	—	—
Ranch	1 serv (2.5 oz)	390	41	6	30	1	4	2	0	—	590	55	—	—
Ranch Lite	1 serv (2.5 oz)	190	18	3	25	1	3	2	0	—	700	50	—	—
Soy Sauce	1 serv (0.3 oz)	5	0	0	0	1	1	0	0	—	480	35	—	—
Syrup	1 serv (1.5 oz)	130	0	0	0	0	32	27	0	—	30	10	—	—
Taco Sauce	1 serv (0.3 oz)	0	0	0	0	0	0	0	0	—	80	20	—	—
Tartar Sauce	1 serv (1.5 oz)	210	22	4	20	0	2	1	0	—	370	30	—	—
Thousand Island	1 serv (2 oz)	160	12	2	15	0	12	10	0	—	490	45	—	—
Vingegar	1 serv	0	0	0	0	0	0	0	0	—	20	0	—	—
Wonton Strips	1 serv (0.7 oz)	110	6	2	0	2	13	1	2	—	45	—	—	—
SALADS														
Asian Salad	1 serv	140	2	0	25	15	18	11	6	—	470	890	—	—
Chicken Club Salad	1 serv	290	16	6	65	28	12	5	5	—	890	890	—	—
Side Salad	1 serv	50	3	2	10	3	4	2	2	—	65	280	—	—
Southwest Chicken	1 serv	320	13	6	60	28	28	6	8	—	920	890	—	—

FOOD	PORTION	CALS	FAT	SAT FAT	CHOL	PROT	CARB	SUGAR	FIBER	CALCI	SOD	POTAS	FOLIC	VIT C
JAMBA JUICE														
Jambolas Honey Nut Energy	1 serv	192	1	—	—	5	—	—	2	—	—	—	—	—
Jambolas Mighty Multi Grain	1 serv	208	3	—	—	8	—	—	5	—	—	—	—	—
Jambolas Mind Over Blueberry	1 serv	170	1	—	—	5	—	—	2	—	—	—	—	—
Jambolas Pizza Protein	1 serv	199	3	—	—	9	—	—	3	—	—	—	—	—
Mango-A-Go-Go	1 reg (24 oz)	460	2	—	—	2	—	—	3	—	—	—	—	—
Orchard Oasis	1 reg (24 oz)	440	2	—	—	2	—	—	4	—	—	—	—	—
Protein Berry Pizazz	1 reg (24 oz)	470	1	—	—	25	—	—	6	—	—	—	—	—
Razzmatazz	1 reg (24 oz)	440	2	—	—	3	—	—	4	—	—	—	—	—
JERSEY MIKE'S														
Ham On Wheat	1	240	4	2	35	20	31	—	2	—	1130	—	—	—
Ham On White	1	240	5	2	35	20	31	—	1	—	1230	—	—	—
Ham/Turkey Wheat	1	230	3	1	30	21	32	—	1	—	1130	—	—	—
Ham/Turkey White	1	240	4	1	30	20	32	—	2	—	960	—	—	—
Roast Beef Wheat	1	290	5	2	60	30	30	—	2	—	330	—	—	—
Roast Beef White	1	280	5	2	55	29	30	—	0	—	310	—	—	—
Turkey On Wheat	1	230	2	1	30	23	30	—	2	—	910	—	—	—
Turkey On White	1	230	3	1	30	32	18	—	1	—	860	—	—	—
Veggie On Wheat	1	170	2	0	0	7	32	—	2	—	340	—	—	—
Veggie On White	1	170	2	1	0	7	31	—	2	—	290	—	—	—
KENTUCKY FRIED CHICKEN														
BEVERAGES														
Diet Pepsi	1 sm	0	0	0	0	0	0	0	0	0	35	—	—	0
Mt. Dew	1 sm	150	0	0	0	0	43	43	0	0	50	—	—	0
Pepsi	1 sm (11 oz)	140	0	0	0	0	37	37	0	0	35	—	—	0
DESSERTS														
Cake Double Chocolate Chip	1 slice	400	29	5	45	4	31	27	2	40	230	—	—	0
Cherry Cheesecake Parfait	1 serv	300	11	5	4	3	46	37	2	20	130	—	—	0
Lil' Bucket Chocolate Creme	1 serv	270	13	8	0	2	37	28	2	20	190	—	—	0
Lil' Bucket Fudge Brownie	1	270	9	4	30	2	44	39	1	40	170	—	—	0
Lil' Bucket Lemon Creme	1 serv	400	14	7	5	4	65	51	2	200	210	—	—	0

FOOD	PORTION	CALS	FAT	SAT FAT	CHOL	PROT	CARB	SUGAR	FIBER	CALCI	SOD	POTAS	FOLIC	VIT C
Lil' Bucket Strawberry Shortcake	1 serv	200	6	4	20	2	34	34	0	20	110	—	—	0
Pie Apple	1 slice	270	9	2	0	3	45	22	4	0	200	—	—	24
Pie Lemon Meringue	1 slice	310	11	5	40	5	47	36	3	150	160	—	—	4
Pie Pecan	1 slice	370	15	3	40	4	55	20	2	0	190	—	—	0
Pie Strawberry Creme	1 slice	270	12	7	10	3	37	23	0	60	200	—	—	2
MAIN MENU SELECTIONS														
BBQ Beans	1 serv	230	1	1	0	8	46	22	7	150	720	—	—	5
Biscuit	1	190	10	2	2	2	23	1	0	0	580	—	—	0
Boneless Wings HBBQ Sauced	7 pieces	600	28	5	75	35	40	7	2	40	1950	—	—	0
Chicken Pot Pie	1 serv	770	40	15	115	33	70	2	5	0	1680	—	—	0
Cole Slaw	1 serv	190	11	2	5	1	22	13	3	40	300	—	—	24
Corn On The Cob	1 ear (3 inch)	70	2	1	0	2	13	5	3	40	5	—	—	4
Crispy Strips	3	400	24	5	75	29	17	0	0	0	1250	—	—	4
Extra Crispy Breast	1 serv	490	28	8	135	34	19	0	0	0	1230	—	—	0
Extra Crispy Drumstick	1	160	10	3	70	12	5	0	0	0	420	—	—	0
Extra Crispy Thigh	1	370	26	7	120	21	12	0	0	0	710	—	—	0
Extra Crispy Whole Wing	1	190	12	4	55	10	10	0	0	0	390	—	—	0
Green Beans	1 serv	50	2	1	5	5	5	2	2	0	480	—	—	1
Hot & Spicy Breast	1 serv	460	27	8	130	33	20	0	0	0	1450	—	—	0
Hot & Spicy Drumstick	1	150	9	3	65	13	4	0	0	0	380	—	—	0
Hot & Spicy Thigh	1	400	28	8	125	22	14	0	0	0	1240	—	—	0
Hot & Spicy Whole Wing	1	180	11	3	60	11	9	0	0	0	420	—	—	0
Hot Wings	6 pieces	450	29	6	145	24	23	1	1	80	1120	—	—	4
Mac & Cheese	1 serv	130	8	2	5	5	15	1	1	100	810	—	—	2
Mashed Potatoes w/o Gravy	1 serv	110	4	1	0	2	16	0	1	0	260	—	—	2
Mashed Potatoes w/ Gravy	1 serv	120	5	1	0	2	18	tr	1	0	380	—	—	2
Original Recipe Breast	1 serv	380	19	6	145	40	11	0	0	0	1150	—	—	0
Original Recipe Breast w/o Skin Or Breading	1 serv	140	3	1	95	29	0	0	0	0	410	—	—	0
Original Recipe Drumstick	1	140	8	2	75	14	4	0	0	0	440	—	—	0
Original Recipe Thigh	1	360	25	7	165	22	12	0	0	0	1060	—	—	0

FOOD	PORTION	CALS	FAT	SAT FAT	CHOL	PROT	CARB	SUGAR	FIBER	CALCI	SOD	POTAS	FOLIC	VIT C
Original Recipe Whole Wing	1	150	9	3	60	11	5	0	0	0	370	—	—	0
Popcorn Chicken	1 reg serv	450	30	7	50	19	25	0	0	20	1030	—	—	1
Potato Salad	1 serv	180	9	2	5	2	22	5	1	0	470	—	—	6
Potato Wedges	1 sm	240	12	3	0	4	30	0	3	20	830	—	—	4
Sandwich HBBQ	1	300	8	2	50	21	41	16	4	60	640	—	—	2
Sandwich Original Recipe w/ Sauce	1	450	27	6	65	29	22	0	0	40	1010	—	—	0
Sandwich Tender Roast w/ Sauce	1	390	19	4	70	31	24	0	1	40	810	—	—	0
Sandwich Tender Roast w/o Sauce	1	260	5	2	65	31	23	0	1	40	690	—	—	0
Sandwich Twister	1	670	38	7	60	27	55	7	3	150	1650	—	—	5
Sandwich Zinger w/ Sauce	1	680	41	8	90	35	42	3	1	60	1850	—	—	5
Sandwich Zinger w/o Sauce	1	540	26	6	75	35	41	2	1	60	1510	—	—	5
Sandwiches Original Recipe w/o Sauce	1	320	13	4	60	29	21	0	0	40	890	—	—	0
Wings HBBQ Sauced	6 pieces	540	33	7	150	25	36	15	1	60	1130	—	—	5
KOO-KOO-ROO														
Original Breast	1 piece	187	6	1	117	34	tr	—	0	—	422	—	—	—
Original Chicken Dark	3 pieces	320	16	5	101	39	5	—	0	—	659	—	—	—
Rotisserie Chicken Breast & Wing	1 serv	355	16	4	140	49	1	—	tr	—	675	—	—	—
Rotisserie Chicken Leg & Thigh	1 serv	300	18	5	114	31	1	—	tr	—	513	—	—	—
Rotisserie Half Chicken	1 serv	655	34	9	254	80	2	—	tr	—	1188	—	—	—
Sandwich BBQ Chicken	1	562	12	4	113	45	71	—	3	—	1398	—	—	—
Sandwich Chicken Caesar	1	781	36	11	138	56	63	—	2	—	1775	—	—	—
Sandwich Original Chicken	1	661	29	5	116	41	63	—	3	—	1144	—	—	—
Traditional Turkey Dinner	1 serv	692	29	10	127	42	67	—	8	—	3719	—	—	—
Turkey Pot Pie	1 serv	883	44	12	98	37	83	—	6	—	1287	—	—	—
Turkey Sandwich Hand Carved	1	599	32	8	122	46	31	—	5	—	786	—	—	—
Wrap Caesar Chicken	1	757	39	8	97	42	59	—	4	—	1890	—	—	—
Wrap Chipotle Chicken	1	924	43	15	123	42	89	—	6	—	2449	—	—	—

FOOD	PORTION	CALS	FAT	SAT FAT	CHOL	PROT	CARB	SUGAR	FIBER	CALCI	SOD	POTAS	FOLIC	VIT C
KRISPY KREME														
Apple Fritter	1	380	21	5	5	4	46	23	2	100	290	—	—	1
Caramel Kreme Crunch	1	350	19	5	5	4	43	25	tr	100	170	—	—	1
Chocolate Iced Glazed w/ Sprinkles	1	260	12	5	3	3	38	24	tr	60	100	—	—	1
Chocolate Malted Kreme	1	390	21	5	5	4	49	30	tr	100	180	—	—	1
Chocolate Iced	1	250	12	3	5	3	33	21	tr	60	100	—	—	1
Chocolate Iced Cake	1	270	14	3	20	3	36	20	tr	20	320	—	—	0
Chocolate Iced Creme Filled	1	350	21	5	5	3	39	23	tr	80	140	—	—	1
Chocolate Iced Cruller	1	290	15	4	15	2	37	25	tr	20	240	—	—	0
Chocolate Iced Custard Filled	1	300	17	4	5	3	35	17	tr	80	150	—	—	1
Chocolated Iced w/ Sprinkles	1	290	14	3	20	3	40	23	tr	20	320	—	—	0
Cinnamon Apple Filled	1	290	16	4	5	3	32	14	tr	100	150	—	—	1
Cinnamon Bun	1	260	16	4	5	3	28	13	tr	80	125	—	—	1
Cinnamon Sugar Cake	1	280	14	3	20	3	37	18	1	40	340	—	—	0
Cinnamon Twist	1	230	9	3	5	3	33	19	tr	80	85	—	—	1
Coffee & Kreme	1	360	20	5	5	3	43	27	tr	80	150	—	—	1
Dulce De Leche	1	290	18	5	5	3	30	12	tr	100	160	—	—	1
Glazed Blueberry	1	340	18	5	20	3	42	27	tr	20	310	—	—	0
Glazed Creme Filled	1	340	20	5	5	3	39	23	tr	80	140	—	—	1
Glazed Devil's Food	1	340	18	5	20	3	42	27	tr	20	310	—	—	0
Glazed Lemon Filled	1	290	16	4	5	3	34	18	tr	80	135	—	—	1
Glazed Raspberry Filled	1	300	16	4	5	3	39	21	tr	100	125	—	—	1
Glazed Sour Cream	1	340	18	5	20	3	42	27	tr	20	310	—	—	0
Glazed Strawberry Filled	1	290	16	4	5	3	35	17	tr	80	135	—	—	1
Glazed Cinnamon	1	210	12	3	5	2	24	12	tr	60	100	—	—	1
Glazed Cruller	1	240	14	4	15	2	26	14	tr	20	240	—	—	0
Glazed Custard Filled	1	290	16	4	5	3	34	17	tr	80	160	—	—	1
Glazed Blueberry Filled	1	290	16	4	5	3	35	18	tr	80	140	—	—	1

FOOD	PORTION	CALS	FAT	SAT FAT	CHOL	PROT	CARB	SUGAR	FIBER	CALCI	SOD	POTAS	FOLIC	VIT C
Glazed Twist	1	210	9	3	5	3	28	16	tr	60	80	—	—	0
Honey & Oat	1	340	18	5	20	3	42	27	tr	20	310	—	—	0
Key Lime Pie	1	330	18	5	5	3	40	23	tr	80	160	—	—	1
Maple Iced	1	240	12	3	5	2	32	20	tr	60	100	—	—	1
Maple Iced Cake	1	270	13	3	20	3	35	19	tr	20	320	—	—	0
New York Cheesecake	1	330	19	5	10	4	36	17	1	80	190	—	—	1
Original Glazed	1	200	12	3	5	2	22	10	tr	60	95	—	—	1
Powdered Blueberry Filled	1	290	16	4	5	3	32	14	tr	80	140	—	—	1
Powdered Strawberry Filled	1	260	16	4	5	3	26	9	tr	80	130	—	—	1
Powdered Cake	1	280	14	3	20	3	37	19	tr	40	320	—	—	0
Powdered Creme Filled	1	340	21	5	5	3	36	19	tr	80	140	—	—	1
Powdered Raspberry	1	300	16	4	5	3	36	17	tr	100	125	—	—	1
Pumpkin Spice Cake	1	340	18	5	20	3	42	27	tr	10	310	—	—	0
Sugar Coated	1	200	12	3	5	2	21	10	0	60	95	—	—	1
Traditional Cake	1	230	13	3	20	3	25	9	tr	20	320	—	—	0
Vanilla Iced Creme Filled	1	340	20	5	5	3	38	23	tr	80	135	—	—	1
Vanilla Iced Glazed	1	240	12	3	5	2	32	20	tr	60	95	—	—	1
Vanilla Iced Cake w/ Sprinkles	1	270	13	3	20	3	35	19	tr	20	320	—	—	0
Vanilla Iced Custard Filled	1	290	16	4	5	3	33	16	tr	80	150	—	—	1
Vanilla Iced Raspberry Glazed	1	350	16	4	5	3	50	31	tr	100	125	—	—	1
KRYSTAL														
BEVERAGES														
Coca-Cola Classic frzn	1 (16 oz)	130	0	0	0	0	36	36	0	0	12	—	—	0
Coca-Cola Classic	1 sm (16 oz)	129	0	0	0	0	40	40	0	0	9	—	—	0
Diet Coke	1 sm (16 oz)	tr	0	0	0	0	tr	0	0	0	15	—	—	0
Sprite	1 sm (16 oz)	126	0	0	0	0	39	39	0	0	33	—	—	0
BREAKFAST SELECTIONS														
Biscuit	1	270	13	3	0	5	33	2	0	40	660	—	—	—
Biscuit And Gravy	1	280	14	3	0	5	34	2	0	40	710	—	—	0
Biscuit Bacon Egg & Cheese	1	390	23	7	40	11	33	2	0	100	1090	—	—	0
Biscuit Chik	1	360	15	3	20	13	40	2	0	40	1030	—	—	—
Biscuit Sausage	1	480	33	10	40	12	33	2	0	60	980	—	—	—
Country Breakfast	1 serv	660	42	14	590	24	46	3	8	40	1450	—	—	5

FOOD	PORTION	CALS	FAT	SAT FAT	CHOL	PROT	CARB	SUGAR	FIBER	CALCI	SOD	POTAS	FOLIC	VIT C
Kryspers	1 serv	190	13	5	10	1	17	0	2	—	340	—	—	—
Krystal Sunriser	1	240	14	5	255	12	14	1	2	100	460	—	—	—
Scrambler	1 serv	440	26	11	255	20	33	tr	3	80	840	—	—	—
DESSERTS														
Fried Apple Turnover	1	220	10	4	<5	3	31	7	2	—	300	—	—	—
Lemon Icebox Pie	1 serv	260	9	2	25	5	41	37	2	150	180	—	—	1
MAIN MENU SELECTIONS														
Chik'n Bites	1 sm	310	19	8	55	17	16	0	1	200	790	—	—	6
Chik'n Bites Salad	1 serv	290	20	11	66	20	12	1	4	—	490	—	—	—
Fries	1 med	470	20	8	20	4	53	0	7	200	90	—	—	—
Fries Chili Cheese	1 serv	540	28	13	45	13	59	1	5	150	800	—	—	—
Krystal	1	160	7	3	20	7	17	1	1	60	260	—	—	—
Krystal Bacon Cheese	1	190	10	5	25	10	16	2	2	100	430	—	—	—
Krystal Cheese	1	180	9	4	25	9	17	1	2	100	430	—	—	—
Krystal Chik	1	240	11	4	25	11	24	1	2	—	640	—	—	—
Krystal Chili	1 serv	200	7	4	25	13	22	2	7	150	1130	—	—	—
Krystal Double	1	260	13	6	40	13	24	2	2	150	550	—	—	—
Krystal Double Cheese	1	310	16	7	65	16	26	2	tr	200	800	—	—	—
Pup	1	170	9	4	25	6	15	—	1	40	500	—	—	—
Pup Chili Cheese	1	210	12	5	40	9	17	2	2	100	510	—	—	—
Pup Corn	1	260	19	8	50	6	19	5	1	—	490	—	—	—

LITTLE CAESARS

FOOD	PORTION	CALS	FAT	SAT FAT	CHOL	PROT	CARB	SUGAR	FIBER	CALCI	SOD	POTAS	FOLIC	VIT C
MAIN MENU SELECTIONS														
Baby Pan! Pan!	1 piece	360	16	7	30	17	34	3	2	—	630	—	—	—
Crazy Bread	1 piece	90	3	tr	tr	3	15	tr	0	—	140	—	—	—
Crazy Bread Cinnamon	2 pieces	100	2	tr	tr	3	19	5	0	—	95	—	—	—
Crazy Sauce	1 serv (4 oz)	45	0	0	0	0	9	5	3	—	380	—	—	—
Deli Sandwich Italian	1	800	45	10	90	35	66	6	3	—	1950	—	—	—
Deli Sandwich Veggie	1	600	28	3	30	24	67	5	3	—	980	—	—	—
Deli Sandwich Ham & Cheese	1	640	29	3	50	32	66	5	3	—	1540	—	—	—
Italian Cheese Bread	1 piece	130	6	3	10	7	13	tr	0	—	310	—	—	—
PIZZA														
14 Inch Round Meatsa	1/10 pie	280	13	6	30	15	26	2	2	—	630	—	—	—
14 Inch Round Supreme	1/10 pie	270	10	5	25	13	31	4	3	—	510	—	—	—
14 Inch Round Veggie	1/10 pie	240	8	4	15	12	32	5	3	—	710	—	—	—

FOOD	PORTION	CALS	FAT	SAT FAT	CHOL	PROT	CARB	SUGAR	FIBER	CALCI	SOD	POTAS	FOLIC	VIT C
14 Inch Thin Crust Cheese	⅒ pie	160	7	4	15	8	14	1	0	—	210	—	—	—
16 Inch Round Cheese	1/12 pie	220	7	4	15	11	27	2	1	—	340	—	—	—
18 Inch Round Cheese	1/14 pie	230	7	4	15	12	30	2	1	—	350	—	—	—
Deep Dish Large	⅛ pie	320	12	5	20	15	37	3	2	—	460	—	—	—
Deep Dish Medium	⅛ pie	230	9	4	15	11	27	2	1	—	340	—	—	—
SALAD DRESSINGS														
Caesar	1 serv (1.5 oz)	230	25	4	55	1	1	0	0	—	360	—	—	—
Greek	1 serv (1.5 oz)	270	29	5	0	0	0	0	0	—	200	—	—	—
Italian	1 serv (1.5 oz)	220	23	4	0	0	2	2	0	—	370	—	—	—
Italian Fat Free	1 serv (1.5 oz)	25	0	0	0	0	5	3	0	—	390	—	—	—
Ranch	1 serv (1.5 oz)	230	24	4	10	1	2	1	0	—	380	—	—	—
SALADS														
Antipasto	1 serv	140	8	2	20	9	6	4	2	—	560	—	—	—
Caesar	1 serv	90	3	1	0	4	12	2	3	—	190	—	—	—
Greek	1 serv	128	7	5	25	6	11	8	3	—	590	—	—	—
Tossed Salad	1 serv	100	3	1	0	2	15	4	3	—	190	—	—	—
TOPPINGS PER SLICE														
Bacon	1 serv	41	4	1	7	2	tr	tr	tr	—	125	—	—	—
Beef	1 serv	20	2	1	2	1	tr	tr	tr	—	55	—	—	—
Black Olives	1 serv	12	2	tr	—	tr	tr	—	tr	—	47	—	—	—
Extra Cheese	1 serv	26	2	1	6	2	tr	tr	—	—	48	—	—	—
Green Peppers	1 serv	2	tr	—	—	tr	tr	tr	tr	—	tr	—	—	—
Ham	1 serv	5	tr	tr	2	1	tr	tr	tr	—	66	—	—	—
Italian Sausage	1 serv	22	2	1	5	1	tr	tr	tr	—	68	—	—	—
Mushrooms	1 serv	2	tr	tr	—	tr	tr	tr	tr	—	40	—	—	—
Onion	1 serv	3	tr	—	—	tr	1	tr	tr	—	tr	—	—	—
Pepperoni	1 serv	26	2	1	4	1	tr	—	—	—	110	—	—	—
Pineapple	1 serv	7	—	—	—	tr	2	2	tr	—	tr	—	—	—
Tomato	1 serv	2	tr	—	—	tr	tr	tr	tr	—	1	—	—	—

LONG JOHN SILVER'S

FOOD	PORTION	CALS	FAT	SAT FAT	CHOL	PROT	CARB	SUGAR	FIBER	CALCI	SOD	POTAS	FOLIC	VIT C
MAIN MENU SELECTIONS														
Batter-Dipped Fish	1 piece (3 oz)	170	11	3	30	11	12	—	5	—	470	—	—	—
Breaded Chicken Strips	1 piece (1.15 oz)	100	5	1	10	6	6	0	0	—	360	—	—	—
Breaded Clams	1 serv (3 oz)	300	17	4	40	11	31	—	5	—	670	—	—	—
Breaded Fish	1 piece (1.6 oz)	110	5	1	20	5	11	0	0	—	340	—	—	—
Cheese Sticks	1 serv (1.6 oz)	160	9	4	10	6	12	tr	tr	—	360	—	—	—
Chicken Salsa	1 reg (11 oz)	690	32	7	20	18	81	5	5	—	1690	—	—	—
Corn Cobbette w/ Butter	1 piece (3.3 oz)	140	8	2	0	3	19	2	0	—	0	—	—	—

FOOD	PORTION	CALS	FAT	SAT FAT	CHOL	PROT	CARB	SUGAR	FIBER	CALCI	SOD	POTAS	FOLIC	VIT C
Corn Cobbette w/o Butter	1 (3.1 oz)	80	1	0	0	3	19	2	0	—	0	—	—	—
Fish Cajun	1 lg (23 oz)	1450	70	15	60	18	85	10	10	—	3630	—	—	—
Flavorbaked Chicken	1 piece (2.6 oz)	110	3	1	55	19	tr	tr	tr	—	600	—	—	—
Flavorbaked Fish	1 piece (2.3 oz)	90	3	1	35	14	1	1	0	—	320	—	—	—
Fries	1 reg (3 oz)	250	15	3	0	3	28	0	3	—	500	—	—	—
Fries	1 lg (5 oz)	420	24	4	0	5	46	tr	4	—	830	—	—	—
Honey Mustard Sauce	1 serv (0.4 oz)	20	0	0	0	0	5	—	0	—	60	—	—	—
Hushpuppy	1 (0.8 oz)	60	3	0	0	1	9	—	0	—	25	—	—	—
Ketchup	1 serv (.32 oz)	10	0	0	0	0	2	1	0	—	110	—	—	—
Popcorn Chicken Munchers	1 serv (4 oz)	380	23	4	35	23	20	0	2	—	1030	—	—	—
Popcorn Fish Munchers	1 serv (4 oz)	300	14	3	50	14	29	tr	tr	—	1220	—	—	—
Popcorn Shrimp Munchers	1 serv (4 oz)	320	15	3	85	15	33	tr	1	—	1440	—	—	—
Rice	1 serv (3 oz)	140	3	1	0	3	26	0	tr	—	210	—	—	—
Sandwich Batter Dipped Fish No Sauce	1 (5.4 oz)	320	13	4	30	17	40	0	6	—	800	—	—	—
Sandwich Flavorbaked Chicken	1 (5.8 oz)	290	10	2	60	24	27	1	2	—	970	—	—	—
Sandwich Flavorbaked Fish	1 (6 oz)	320	14	7	55	23	28	2	2	—	930	—	—	—
Sandwich Ultimate Fish	1 (6.4 oz)	430	21	7	35	18	44	—	3	—	1340	—	—	—
Shrimp Sauce	1 serv (0.4 oz)	15	0	0	0	0	3	—	0	—	180	—	—	—
Side Salad	1 (4.3 oz)	25	0	0	0	1	4	3	tr	—	15	—	—	—
Slaw	1 serv (3.4 oz)	140	6	—	0	1	20	—	3	—	260	—	—	—
Sweet'N'Sour Sauce	1 serv (0.4 oz)	20	0	0	0	0	5	—	0	—	45	—	—	—
Tartar Sauce	1 serv (0.4 oz)	35	2	—	0	0	5	—	0	—	35	—	—	—
Wraps Chicken Cajun	1 lg (22 oz)	1440	71	14	50	37	165	10	11	—	3730	—	—	—
Wraps Chicken Cajun	1 reg (11 oz)	720	35	7	25	18	83	5	5	—	1860	—	—	—
Wraps Chicken Ranch	1 lg (22 oz)	1450	72	14	50	36	165	10	10	—	3620	—	—	—
Wraps Chicken Ranch	1 reg (11 oz)	730	36	7	25	18	82	5	5	—	1810	—	—	—
Wraps Chicken Salsa	1 lg (22 oz)	1370	64	13	35	36	162	10	10	—	3370	—	—	—

FOOD	PORTION	CALS	FAT	SAT FAT	CHOL	PROT	CARB	SUGAR	FIBER	CALCI	SOD	POTAS	FOLIC	VIT C
Wraps Chicken Tartar	1 reg (11 oz)	730	36	7	25	18	83	5	6	—	1780	—	—	—
Wraps Chicken Tartar	1 lg (22 oz)	1450	72	14	45	36	165	9	11	—	3560	—	—	—
Wraps Fish Cajun	1 reg (11.5 oz)	730	35	8	30	18	85	5	5	—	1820	—	—	—
Wraps Fish Ranch	1 reg (11.5 oz)	730	36	8	30	18	85	5	5	—	1760	—	—	—
Wraps Fish Ranch	1 lg (23 oz)	1460	72	15	60	35	170	10	10	—	3520	—	—	—
Wraps Fish Salsa	1 lg (23 oz)	1380	64	14	45	35	167	9	10	—	3280	—	—	—
Wraps Fish Salsa	1 reg (11.5 oz)	690	32	7	25	18	84	5	5	—	1640	—	—	—
Wraps Fish Tartar	1 reg (11.5 oz)	730	36	8	25	18	85	5	5	—	1730	—	—	—
Wraps Fish Tartar	1 lg (23 oz)	1470	72	15	55	35	170	11	10	—	3460	—	—	—
Wraps Popcorn Shrimp Cajun	1 reg (11 oz)	720	35	9	50	16	86	5	5	—	1830	—	—	—
Wraps Popcorn Shrimp Cajun	1 lg (22 oz)	1450	71	18	95	32	172	10	10	—	3660	—	—	—
Wraps Popcorn Shrimp Ranch	1 lg (22 oz)	1460	72	18	100	32	171	10	10	—	3560	—	—	—
Wraps Popcorn Shrimp Ranch	1 reg (11 oz)	720	35	9	50	16	86	5	5	—	1830	—	—	—
Wraps Popcorn Shrimp Salsa	1 reg (11 oz)	690	32	9	40	16	84	5	5	—	1660	—	—	—
Wraps Popcorn Shrimp Salsa	1 lg (22 oz)	1380	64	17	85	32	169	10	9	—	3310	—	—	—
Wraps Popcorn Shrimp Tartar	1 lg (22 oz)	1460	72	18	95	32	172	10	10	—	3500	—	—	—
Wraps Popcorn Shrimp Tartar	1 reg (11 oz)	730	36	9	45	16	86	5	5	—	1750	—	—	—
SALAD DRESSINGS														
Fat-Free French	1 serv (1.5 oz)	50	0	0	0	0	14	—	—	—	360	—	—	—
Fat-Free Ranch	1 serv (1.5 oz)	50	0	0	0	2	13	—	—	—	380	—	—	—
Italian	1 serv (1 oz)	130	14	2	0	0	2	—	—	—	280	—	—	—
Malt Vinegar	1 serv (0.3 oz)	0	0	0	0	0	0	—	0	—	15	—	—	—
Ranch Dressing	1 serv (1 oz)	170	18	3	5	0	1	—	—	—	260	—	—	—
Thousand Island	1 serv (1 oz)	110	10	2	15	0	5	—	—	—	280	—	—	—

MAGGIE MOO'S

FOOD	PORTION	CALS	FAT	SAT FAT	CHOL	PROT	CARB	SUGAR	FIBER	CALCI	SOD	POTAS	FOLIC	VIT C
Ice Cream Fat Free	½ cup	80	0	0	0	3	18	13	0	—	50	—	—	—
Ice Cream Low Carb Sugar Added	½ cup	100	6	4	30	2	11	4	0	—	60	—	—	—
Ice Cream Udderly Cream	½ cup	180	11	8	45	3	18	16	0	—	40	—	—	—
Sorbet	½ cup	90	0	0	0	0	22	20	0	—	5	—	—	—

MANHATTAN BAGEL

FOOD	PORTION	CALS	FAT	SAT FAT	CHOL	PROT	CARB	SUGAR	FIBER	CALCI	SOD	POTAS	FOLIC	VIT C
Blueberry	1	260	tr	0	0	9	54	4	2	20	560	—	—	0
Cheddar Cheese	1	270	4	2	10	11	48	3	2	80	560	—	—	0

FOOD	PORTION	CALS	FAT	SAT FAT	CHOL	PROT	CARB	SUGAR	FIBER	CALCI	SOD	POTAS	FOLIC	VIT C
Chocolate Chip	1	290	3	2	0	9	56	3	2	40	530	—	—	0
Cinnamon Raisin	1	280	tr	0	0	10	57	9	3	40	560	—	—	0
Cranberry Orange	1	270	1	0	0	10	55	5	2	20	520	—	—	0
Egg	1	270	2	0	0	10	53	3	2	40	710	—	—	0
Everything	1	290	3	0	0	11	54	3	3	60	2000	—	—	1
Garlic	1	270	tr	0	0	10	55	3	2	40	560	—	—	2
Jalapeño Cheddar	1	260	2	0	0	16	53	2	2	40	310	—	—	1
Marble	1	260	tr	0	0	10	52	3	3	40	540	—	—	0
Oat Bran	1	260	1	0	0	10	53	3	3	20	470	—	—	0
Oat Bran Raisin Walnut	1	270	3	0	0	10	54	5	3	20	450	—	—	0
Onion	1	270	tr	0	0	10	55	3	2	40	560	—	—	2
Plain	1	260	tr	0	0	10	52	3	2	20	560	—	—	0
Poppy	1	300	4	1	0	11	54	3	5	150	560	—	—	0
Pumpernickel	1	250	1	0	0	10	52	3	3	20	530	—	—	0
Rye	1	260	1	0	0	10	52	3	3	40	560	—	—	0
Salt	1	260	tr	tr	0	10	53	3	2	80	7100	—	—	0
Sesame	1	310	5	1	0	11	55	3	3	100	560	—	—	0
Spinach	1	270	tr	0	0	10	54	3	3	40	580	—	—	2
Sun-Dried Tomato	1	260	1	0	0	10	53	3	3	40	340	—	—	1
Whole Wheat	1	260	tr	0	0	10	52	3	3	20	470	—	—	0
MARBLE SLAB CREAMERY														
Cone Honey Wheat	1	130	3	0	15	3	24	12	tr	20	10	—	—	0
Cone Sugar	1	130	3	0	15	2	23	12	0	20	10	—	—	0
Cone Vanilla Cinnamon	1	130	3	0	15	2	24	12	tr	20	10	—	—	0
Frozen Yogurt Nonfat	½ cup	100	1	1	0	3	22	17	1	100	55	—	—	0
Frozen Yogurt Nonfat No Sugar Added	½ cup	90	1	1	0	4	17	6	1	150	85	—	—	0
Ice Cream Reduced Fat	1 serv (6.75 oz)	390	20	13	80	6	47	45	0	250	130	—	—	1
Ice Cream Superpremium	1 serv (6.75 oz)	450	28	18	115	8	44	43	0	300	135	—	—	1
Sorbet	½ cup	90	0	0	0	0	22	19	0	150	5	—	—	0
MAUI WOWI														
Smoothie Rip Sticks All Flavors	1	88	0	0	0	2	22	17	0	60	25	—	—	11
MAX & ERMA'S														
Black Bean Roll Up	1 serv	401	8	3	13	—	71	—	8	—	534	—	—	—
Black Bean Salsa	½ cup	215	15	2	0	—	17	—	5	—	338	—	—	—
Fruit Smoothie	1 serv	124	tr	tr	0	—	29	—	1	—	4	—	—	—

FOOD	PORTION	CALS	FAT	SAT FAT	CHOL	PROT	CARB	SUGAR	FIBER	CALCI	SOD	POTAS	FOLIC	VIT C
Garden Grill Sandwich w/ Tex Mex Dressing	1	569	7	tr	19	—	101	—	14	—	983	—	—	—
Garlic Breadstick	1	156	6	0	0	—	21	—	0	—	293	—	—	—
Hula Bowl w/ Fat Free Honey Mustard Dressing w/o Breadsticks	1 serv	583	10	1	111	—	73	—	5	—	1580	—	—	—
Salad Dressing Fat Free French	2 tbsp	126	tr	0	0	—	31	—	2	—	1034	—	—	—
Salad Dressing Fat Free Honey Mustard	2 tbsp	60	0	0	0	—	14	—	0	—	360	—	—	—
Salad Dressing Tex Mex	2 tbsp	33	tr	0	5	—	2	—	tr	—	262	—	—	—
Sugar Snap Peas w/ Lemon Pepper Butter	1 serv (4 oz)	106	6	4	15	—	8	—	3		100	—	—	—

MCDONALD'S

BAKED SELECTIONS

FOOD	PORTION	CALS	FAT	SAT FAT	CHOL	PROT	CARB	SUGAR	FIBER	CALCI	SOD	POTAS	FOLIC	VIT C
Apple Pie Baked	1 (2.7 oz)	260	13	4	0	3	34	13	tr	20	200	—	—	24
Cinnamon Roll	1 (3.5 oz)	340	15	5	35	5	52	28	3	250	250	—	—	—
Cookie Chocolate Chip	1 (1.4 oz)	170	9	3	5	2	23	14	tr	—	150	—	—	—
McDonaldland Cookies	1 pkg (2 oz)	230	8	2	0	3	38	12	1	—	250	—	—	—

BEVERAGES

FOOD	PORTION	CALS	FAT	SAT FAT	CHOL	PROT	CARB	SUGAR	FIBER	CALCI	SOD	POTAS	FOLIC	VIT C
Coca-Cola Classic	1 sm (16 oz)	150	0	0	0	0	40	40	0	—	15	—	—	—
Cocoa-Cola Classic	1 lg (32 oz)	310	0	0	0	0	86	86	0	—	30	—	—	—
Coffee	1 sm (8 oz)	0	0	0	0	0	tr	0	0	—	0	—	—	—
Coffee	1 lg (16 oz)	10	0	0	0	0	2	0	0	—	10	—	—	—
Diet Coke	1 lg (32 oz)	0	0	0	0	0	0	0	0	—	60	—	—	—
Diet Coke	1 sm (16 oz)	0	0	0	0	0	0	0	0	—	30	—	—	—
Half & Half Creamer	1 pkg	15	2	1	5	0	0	0	0	—	0	—	—	—
Hi-C Orange	1 sm (16 oz)	160	0	0	0	0	44	44	0	—	30	—	—	90
Hi-C Orange	1 lg (32 oz)	350	0	0	0	0	94	94	0	—	60	—	—	192
Iced Tea	1 lg (32 oz)	0	0	0	0	0	tr	0	0	—	20	—	—	—
Iced Tea	1 sm (16 oz)	0	0	0	0	0	0	0	0	—	0	—	—	—
Milk Lowfat 1%	1 serv (8 oz)	100	3	2	10	8	13	13	0	300	115	—	—	2
Orange Juice	1 (12 oz)	140	0	0	0	2	33	29	0	20	5	—	—	96
Shake Strawberry	1 (12 oz)	420	12	8	50	11	67	59	tr	350	140	—	—	6
Sprite	1 lg (32 oz)	310	0	0	0	0	83	83	—	—	115	—	—	—
Sprite	1 sm (16 oz)	150	0	0	0	0	39	39	0	—	55	—	—	—
Triple Shake Chocolate	1 (12 oz)	430	12	8	50	11	70	61	1	350	210	—	—	1

FOOD	PORTION	CALS	FAT	SAT FAT	CHOL	PROT	CARB	SUGAR	FIBER	CALCI	SOD	POTAS	FOLIC	VIT C
Triple Shake Vanilla	1 (12 oz)	430	12	8	50	11	67	57	0	350	300	—	—	1
BREAKFAST SELECTIONS														
Bagel Ham Egg Cheese	1 (7.7 oz)	550	23	8	255	26	58	10	2	200	1500	—	—	—
Bagel Spanish Omelet	1 (9.1 oz)	710	40	15	275	27	59	10	3	250	1520	—	—	15
Bagel Steak Egg Cheese	1 (8.5 oz)	640	31	12	265	31	57	9	2	200	1540	—	—	—
Big Breakfast	1 serv (9.4 oz)	710	48	13	455	24	45	3	3	100	1430	—	—	2
Biscuit	1 (2.4 oz)	240	11	3	0	4	30	1	1	40	640	—	—	—
Biscuit Bacon Egg Cheese	1 (5.4 oz)	480	31	10	250	21	31	3	1	150	1360	—	—	—
Biscuit Sausage	1 (4 oz)	410	28	8	35	10	30	2	1	40	930	—	—	—
Biscuit Sausage w/ Egg	1 (5.7 oz)	490	33	10	245	16	31	2	1	80	1010	—	—	—
Breakfast Burrito Sausage	1 (4 oz)	290	16	6	170	13	24	2	2	150	680	—	—	12
English Muffin	1 (2 oz)	150	2	1	0	5	27	2	2	200	270	—	—	—
Hash Browns	1 serv (1.9 oz)	130	8	2	0	1	14	0	1	—	330	—	—	2
Hotcakes Margarine & Syrup	1 serv (8 oz)	600	17	3	20	9	104	40	0	100	770	—	—	—
McGriddles Bacon Egg & Cheese	1 (5.9 oz)	450	23	8	240	19	43	16	1	200	1270	—	—	—
McGriddles Sausage Egg Cheese	1 (7 oz)	550	33	11	260	20	43	16	1	200	1290	—	—	—
McMuffin Sausage	1 (4 oz)	370	23	9	50	14	28	2	2	250	790	—	—	—
McMuffin Sausage w/ Egg	1 (5.8 oz)	450	28	10	260	20	29	3	2	300	930	—	—	—
McMuffin Egg	1 (4.9 oz)	300	12	5	235	18	29	3	2	300	840	—	—	1
Sausage	1 (1.5 oz)	170	16	5	35	6	0	0	0	—	290	—	—	—
Scrambled Eggs	2 (3.6 oz)	160	11	4	425	13	1	1	0	60	170	—	—	—
DESSERTS														
Fruit 'n Yogurt Parfait	1 serv (11.9 oz)	380	5	2	15	10	76	49	2	300	240	—	—	24
Fruit 'n Yogurt Parfait	1 snack size (5.3 oz)	160	2	1	5	4	30	21	tr	150	85	—	—	9
Fruit 'n Yogurt Parfait w/o Granola	1 serv (10.9 oz)	280	4	2	15	8	53	40	tr	250	115	—	—	24
Fruit 'n Yogurt Parfait w/o Granola	1 serv (5 oz)	130	2	1	5	4	25	19	0	100	55	—	—	9
Kiddo Cone	1 (1 oz)	45	2	1	5	1	7	6	0	40	20	—	—	—

FOOD	PORTION	CALS	FAT	SAT FAT	CHOL	PROT	CARB	SUGAR	FIBER	CALCI	SOD	POTAS	FOLIC	VIT C
McDonaldland Chocolate Chip Cookies	1 pkg (2 oz)	280	14	8	40	3	37	20	1	20	170	—	—	—
McFlurry Butterfinger	1 (12 oz)	620	22	14	70	16	90	76	tr	450	260	—	—	2
McFlurry M&M	1 (12 oz)	630	23	15	75	16	90	81	1	500	210	—	—	2
McFlurry Nestlé Crunch	1 (12 oz)	630	24	16	75	16	89	78	tr	500	230	—	—	2
McFlurry Oreo	1 (12 oz)	570	20	12	70	15	82	69	tr	450	280	—	—	2
Nuts For Sundaes	1 serv (7 g)	40	4	0	0	2	2	0	tr	—	55	—	—	—
Reduced Fat Ice Cream Cone Vanilla	1 (3.2 oz)	150	5	3	20	4	23	17	0	100	75	—	—	1
Sundae Hot Caramel	1 (6.4 oz)	360	10	6	35	7	61	47	0	250	180	—	—	1
Sundae Hot Fudge	1 (6.3 oz)	340	12	9	30	8	52	47	1	250	170	—	—	1
Sundae Strawberry	1 (6.3 oz)	290	7	5	30	7	50	46	tr	200	95	—	—	1
Triple Shake Chocolate	1 (32 oz)	1150	33	32	125	30	187	163	3	900	550	—	—	5
Triple Shake Raspberry	1 (32 oz)	1120	32	22	135	28	179	154	2	900	390	—	—	9
Triple Shake Raspberry	1 (12 oz)	420	12	8	50	11	67	58	tr	350	150	—	—	4
Triple Shake Strawberry	1 (32 oz)	1120	32	22	135	28	178	158	2	900	380	—	—	27
Triple Shake Vanilla	1 (32 oz)	1140	32	22	125	28	178	152	tr	900	810	—	—	5
MAIN MENU SELECTIONS														
Barbeque Sauce	1 pkg (1 oz)	45	0	0	0	0	10	10	0	—	250	—	—	4
Big Mac	1 (7.6 oz)	560	33	11	85	24	47	7	3	350	1050	—	—	2
Big N' Tasty	1 (8.2 oz)	530	32	10	80	24	37	8	2	200	790	—	—	9
Big N' Tasty w/ Cheese	1 (8.7 oz)	580	37	12	95	28	38	8	2	300	1030	—	—	6
Cheeseburger	1 (4.2 oz)	330	14	6	45	15	35	7	2	250	800	—	—	2
Cheeseburger Double	1 (6.1 oz)	480	27	12	85	25	37	7	2	350	1220	—	—	2
Chicken McNuggets	20 pieces (12.7 oz)	1030	65	13	170	49	61	0	5	50	2280	—	—	3
Chicken McNuggets	6 pieces (3.8 oz)	310	20	4	50	15	18	0	2	20	680	—	—	1
Chicken McNuggets	4 pieces (2.5 oz)	210	13	3	35	10	12	0	1	—	400	—	—	1
Chicken McNuggets	10 pieces (6.3 oz)	510	33	6	85	25	30	0	3	20	1140	—	—	2
Chicken McGrill	1 (7.5 oz)	400	17	3	60	25	37	6	2	200	890	—	—	6
Crispy Chicken	1 serv (7.7 oz)	500	26	5	50	22	46	6	2	20	1100	—	—	6
Filet-O-Fish	1 (5.5 oz)	470	26	5	50	15	45	5	1	200	730	—	—	—

FOOD	PORTION	CALS	FAT	SAT FAT	CHOL	PROT	CARB	SUGAR	FIBER	CALCI	SOD	POTAS	FOLIC	VIT C
French Fries	1 med (5.2 oz)	450	22	4	0	6	57	0	5	20	290	—	—	18
French Fries	1 lg (6.2 oz)	540	26	5	0	8	68	0	6	20	350	—	—	21
French Fries	1 sm (2.4 oz)	210	10	2	0	3	26	0	2	—	135	—	—	9
French Fries	1 McValue (3.7 oz)	320	16	3	0	5	40	0	4	10	210	—	—	12
Hamburger	1 (3.7 oz)	280	10	4	30	12	35	7	2	200	560	—	—	2
Honey	1 pkg (0.5 oz)	45	0	0	0	0	12	11	0	—	0	—	—	—
Honey Mustard	1 pkg (0.5 oz)	50	5	1	10	0	3	3	0	—	95	—	—	—
Hot Mustard	1 pkg (1 oz)	60	4	0	5	tr	7	6	tr	—	240	—	—	—
Light Mayonnaise	1 pkg (0.4 oz)	40	5	1	10	0	tr	0	0	—	100	—	—	—
McChicken	1 (5.2 oz)	430	23	5	45	14	41	6	3	200	840	—	—	—
McChicken Hot 'n Spicy	1 (5.1 oz)	450	26	5	45	15	39	5	1	350	830	—	—	—
Quarter Pounder	1 (6.1 oz)	420	21	8	70	23	36	8	2	200	780	—	—	2
Quarter Pounder Double w/ Cheese	1 (9.9 oz)	760	48	20	165	46	38	9	2	400	1450	—	—	2
Quarter Pounder w/ Cheese	1 (7 oz)	530	30	13	95	28	38	9	2	350	1250	—	—	2
Sweet 'N Sour Sauce	1 pkg (1 oz)	50	0	0	0	0	11	10	0	—	140	—	—	—
SALAD DRESSINGS														
Newman's Own Cobb	1 pkg (2 oz)	120	9	2	10	1	9	5	0	40	440	—	—	—
Newman's Own Creamy Caesar	1 pkg (2 oz)	190	18	4	20	2	4	2	0	60	500	—	—	—
Newman's Own Low Fat Balsamic Vinaigrette	1 pkg (1.5 oz)	40	0	0	0	0	4	3	0	—	730	—	—	2
Newman's Own Ranch	1 pkg (2 oz)	290	30	5	20	1	4	3	0	40	530	—	—	—
SALADS AND SALAD BARS														
Bacon Ranch w/o Chicken	1 serv (7.1 oz)	140	10	5	25	9	7	3	3	150	310	—	—	30
Caesar w/o Chicken	1 serv (6.7 oz)	90	4	3	10	7	7	3	3	200	170	—	—	30
California Cobb w/o Chicken	1 serv (7.6 oz)	160	11	5	85	11	7	4	3	150	450	—	—	30
Crispy Chicken Bacon Ranch	1 serv (10.4 oz)	370	21	7	65	28	20	4	3	150	1040	—	—	30
Crispy Chicken Caesar	1 serv (10 oz)	310	16	5	50	23	20	4	3	200	890	—	—	30
Crispy Chicken California Cobb	1 serv (10.9 oz)	380	23	7	125	27	20	4	3	150	1170	—	—	30
Croutons Butter Garlic	1 pkg (0.5 oz)	50	2	0	0	1	8	0	0	—	140	—	—	—

FOOD	PORTION	CALS	FAT	SAT FAT	CHOL	PROT	CARB	SUGAR	FIBER	CALCI	SOD	POTAS	FOLIC	VIT C
Grilled Chicken Bacon Ranch	1 serv (10.2 oz)	270	13	5	75	28	11	4	3	150	830	—	—	30
Grilled Chicken Caesar	1 serv (9.8 oz)	210	7	4	60	28	11	3	3	200	680	—	—	30
Grilled Chicken California Cobb	1 serv (10.7 oz)	280	14	6	130	30	11	4	3	150	960	—	—	30
Side Salad	1 (3.1 oz)	15	0	0	0	1	3	1	1	20	10	—	—	15

MIAMI SUBS

FOOD	PORTION	CALS	FAT	SAT FAT	CHOL	PROT	CARB	SUGAR	FIBER	CALCI	SOD	POTAS	FOLIC	VIT C
Burger Deluxe	1	784	59	17	30	28	31	3	1	89	532	—	—	13
Cheeseburger Deluxe	1	859	65	21	47	34	32	3	1	191	736	—	—	13
Cheeseburger Deluxe Bacon	1	919	70	23	61	34	32	3	1	191	963	—	—	13
Cheesesteak Classic	1 (6 inch)	420	11	7	77	32	48	5	2	113	993	—	—	22
Cheesesteak Original	1 (6 inch)	409	11	7	77	31	45	5	1	110	925	—	—	8
Cheesesteak Works	1 (6 inch)	532	23	8	87	34	51	7	2	122	1063	—	—	30
Chicken Philly Classic	1 (6 inch)	551	27	8	92	30	47	4	2	113	1033	—	—	22
Mozzarella Sticks	1 serv	757	57	16	60	25	34	9	1	609	1607	—	—	4
Onion Rings	1 serv	869	68	10	0	5	56	7	2	0	895	—	—	6
Pita Chicken	1	392	13	3	75	34	34	6	5	111	546	—	—	12
Pita Gyros	1	662	39	27	84	32	47	6	5	98	1998	—	—	12
Platter Chicken Breast	1 serv	743	41	11	80	34	57	3	5	119	186	—	—	22
Platter Gyros	1 serv	1420	93	9	186	61	81	3	5	94	4055	—	—	21
Salad Caesar w/ Dressing	1 serv	459	34	6	14	12	26	4	4	221	1089	—	—	48
Salad Chicken Caesar w/ Dressing	1 serv	609	39	7	74	35	28	4	4	241	1929	—	—	48
Salad Chicken Club	1 serv	490	25	10	210	42	23	6	5	321	1433	—	—	40
Salad Garden	1 serv	310	18	7	136	16	21	6	5	301	477	—	—	40
Salad Greek	1 serv	284	15	5	123	14	24	6	5	167	906	—	—	66
Salad Greek Side w/ Dressing	1 serv	78	5	2	8	3	4	2	1	45	349	—	—	13
Spicy Fries	1 reg	532	39	10	19	4	39	0	4	0	575	—	—	11
Subs 6 Inch Ham And Cheese	1	452	18	5	59	23	49	6	2	113	2051	—	—	30
Subs 6 Inch Italian Deli	1	516	25	8	69	24	49	6	2	107	2151	—	—	20
Subs 6 Inch Meatball	1	491	22	9	76	28	49	4	4	280	1319	—	—	8

FOOD	PORTION	CALS	FAT	SAT FAT	CHOL	PROT	CARB	SUGAR	FIBER	CALCI	SOD	POTAS	FOLIC	VIT C
Subs 6 Inch Tuna	1	468	18	2	67	34	44	3	2	29	1068	—	—	15
Subs 6 Inch Turkey	1	484	18	5	68	29	51	6	2	104	2009	—	—	15
Wings w/ Fries Celery & Blue Cheese	1 serv	1020	67	17	179	48	50	1	4	75	2840	—	—	18

MR. HERO

DESSERTS

FOOD	PORTION	CALS	FAT	SAT FAT	CHOL	PROT	CARB	SUGAR	FIBER	CALCI	SOD	POTAS	FOLIC	VIT C
Cheesecake	1 serv	350	27	15	—	6	26	—	—	—	—	—	—	—
Cheesecake w/ Cherries	1 serv	385	25	15	—	6	35	—	—	—	—	—	—	—

MAIN MENU SELECTIONS

FOOD	PORTION	CALS	FAT	SAT FAT	CHOL	PROT	CARB	SUGAR	FIBER	CALCI	SOD	POTAS	FOLIC	VIT C
Breadsticks w/ Sauce	1 serv	291	9	2	—	8	47	—	—	—	—	—	—	—
Cheddar Cheese Sauce	1 serv	60	5	1	—	2	5	—	—	—	—	—	—	—
Onion Rings	1 serv	564	32	14	—	8	64	—	—	—	—	—	—	—
Potato Waffers	1 serv	334	18	5	—	4	42	—	—	—	—	—	—	—
Spaghetti Dinner	1 serv	606	8	2	—	22	112	—	—	—	—	—	—	—
Spaghetti w/ Meatballs	1 serv	846	26	2	—	37	116	—	—	—	—	—	—	—

SALAD DRESSINGS

FOOD	PORTION	CALS	FAT	SAT FAT	CHOL	PROT	CARB	SUGAR	FIBER	CALCI	SOD	POTAS	FOLIC	VIT C
Buttermilk	1 serv (2 oz)	290	29	—	—	tr	6	—	—	—	—	—	—	—
Creamy Italian	1 serv (2 oz)	190	17	—	—	tr	11	—	—	—	—	—	—	—
Fat Free French	1 serv (2 oz)	70	0	0	—	tr	18	—	—	—	—	—	—	—
Fat Free Ranch	1 serv (2 oz)	70	0	—	—	tr	16	—	—	—	—	—	—	—

SALADS AND SALAD BARS

FOOD	PORTION	CALS	FAT	SAT FAT	CHOL	PROT	CARB	SUGAR	FIBER	CALCI	SOD	POTAS	FOLIC	VIT C
Croutons	1 serv	59	2	—	—	2	9	—	—	—	—	—	—	—
Garden Salad	1 serv	36	tr	0	—	2	7	—	—	—	—	—	—	—
Grilled Chicken	1 serv	225	10	3	—	27	7	—	—	—	—	—	—	—
Seafood Crab	1 serv	452	37	7	—	13	18	—	—	—	—	—	—	—
Side Salad	1 serv	27	tr	0	—	1	6	—	—	—	—	—	—	—
Tuna	1 serv	745	69	13	—	21	8	—	—	—	—	—	—	—

SANDWICHES

FOOD	PORTION	CALS	FAT	SAT FAT	CHOL	PROT	CARB	SUGAR	FIBER	CALCI	SOD	POTAS	FOLIC	VIT C
Cheesesteaks Grilled Steak Philly	7 inch	450	14	6	—	37	48	—	—	—	—	—	—	—
Cheesesteaks Hot Buttered Deluxe	7 inch	566	33	18	—	25	48	—	—	—	—	—	—	—
Cold Subs Classic Italian	7 inch	586	36	9	—	21	50	—	—	—	—	—	—	—
Cold Subs Tuna & Cheese	7 inch	666	47	9	—	19	47	—	—	—	—	—	—	—
Cold Subs Turkey & Cheese	7 inch	453	21	5	—	25	46	—	—	—	—	—	—	—

FOOD	PORTION	CALS	FAT	SAT FAT	CHOL	PROT	CARB	SUGAR	FIBER	CALCI	SOD	POTAS	FOLIC	VIT C
Cold Subs Ultimate Italian	7 inch	608	33	11	—	31	51	—	—	—	—	—	—	—
Hot Subs Grilled Chicken Philly	7 inch	438	14	5	—	34	48	—	—	—	—	—	—	—
Hot Subs Meatball	7 inch	620	32	3	—	35	53	—	—	—	—	—	—	—
Hot Subs Romanburger	7 inch	717	47	15	—	30	49	—	—	—	—	—	—	—
Round Bacon Cheeseburger	1	352	23	7	—	14	23	—	—	—	—	—	—	—
Round Chicken	1	420	23	5	—	31	23	—	—	—	—	—	—	—
Round Fish	1	412	23	4	—	21	31	—	—	—	—	—	—	—
Round Tuna	1	302	34	6	—	11	23	—	—	—	—	—	—	—

MR. PITA

FOOD	PORTION	CALS	FAT	SAT FAT	CHOL	PROT	CARB	SUGAR	FIBER	CALCI	SOD	POTAS	FOLIC	VIT C
Cranberry Turkey	1 reg	424	1	tr	45	25	77	17	3	—	1099	—	—	—
Grilled Raspberry Chicken	1 reg	342	3	1	34	22	56	5	1	—	1426	—	—	—
Grilled Chicken & Broccoli	1 reg	373	4	1	41	24	57	4	2	—	878	—	—	—
Grilled Chicken Caesar	1 reg	353	4	1	42	24	50	3	1	—	986	—	—	—
Grilled Hawaiian Chicken	1 reg	375	4	1	41	25	57	5	1	—	1784	—	—	—
Ultra Combo	1 reg	354	3	1	43	24	56	4	2	—	1058	—	—	—
Ultra Grilled Chicken	1 reg	367	4	1	41	23	56	5	2	—	1080	—	—	—
Ultra Supreme	1 reg	350	3	1	37	23	56	5	1	—	1314	—	—	—
Ultra Turkey	1 reg	343	1	tr	45	25	56	4	2	—	1099	—	—	—

MRS. FIELDS

FOOD	PORTION	CALS	FAT	SAT FAT	CHOL	PROT	CARB	SUGAR	FIBER	CALCI	SOD	POTAS	FOLIC	VIT C
Brownie Double Fudge	1 (2.7 oz)	360	19	11	80	4	59	49	2	20	240	—	—	0
Brownie Frosted Fudge	1 (3.7 oz)	440	21	12	80	4	62	41	2	20	265	—	—	0
Brownie Pecan Fudge	1 (2.7 oz)	340	21	9	70	4	40	30	2	20	220	—	—	0
Brownie Pecan Pie	1 (2.7 oz)	340	20	9	70	5	40	30	2	20	220	—	—	0
Brownie Walnut Fudge	1 (2.7 oz)	380	23	10	80	5	45	23	tr	20	240	—	—	0
Bundt Cake Banana Walnut	1 piece (2.9 oz)	350	21	5	40	6	35	18	3	40	300	—	—	2
Bundt Cake Banana Walnut w/ Chocolate Chips	1 piece (2.9 oz)	370	22	7	35	6	39	25	3	40	240	—	—	1
Bundt Cake Blueberry	1 piece (2.9 oz)	270	12	5	50	4	36	19	1	40	330	—	—	0

FOOD	PORTION	CALS	FAT	SAT FAT	CHOL	PROT	CARB	SUGAR	FIBER	CALCI	SOD	POTAS	FOLIC	VIT C
Bundt Cake Raspberry	1 piece (2.9 oz)	270	12	5	50	4	36	19	tr	40	330	—	—	2
Bundt Cake White w/ Chocolate Chips	1 piece (2.9 oz)	350	17	8	50	4	45	27	tr	40	330	—	—	0
Cookie Butter Toffee	1 (2.3 oz)	290	13	8	55	3	40	24	tr	40	190	—	—	0
Cookie Cinnamon Sugar	1 (2.3 oz)	300	12	8	50	3	41	23	tr	40	250	—	—	0
Cookie Coconut Macadamia	1 (2.3 oz)	280	13	5	20	3	39	23	tr	20	220	—	—	0
Cookie Debra's Special	1 (2.3 oz)	280	12	6	40	4	39	25	2	40	180	—	—	0
Cookie Milk Chocolate	1 (2.3 oz)	280	13	8	40	3	38	18	tr	20	180	—	—	0
Cookie Milk Chocolate & Walnuts	1 (2.3 oz)	320	17	9	40	4	37	26	1	60	180	—	—	0
Cookie Milk Chocolate Macadamia	1 (2.3 oz)	320	18	9	40	4	36	25	tr	60	180	—	—	0
Cookie Oatmeal Chocolate Chip	1 (2.3 oz)	280	13	8	35	3	40	17	1	40	140	—	—	0
Cookie Oatmeal Raisin & Walnuts	1 (2.3 oz)	280	12	6	40	4	39	25	2	40	180	—	—	0
Cookie Peanut Butter	1 (2.3 oz)	310	16	8	45	5	34	18	tr	40	260	—	—	0
Cookie Peanut Butter w/ Milk Chocolate Chips	1 (2.3 oz)	300	17	8	40	5	35	16	tr	40	160	—	—	0
Cookie Semi-Sweet Chocolate	1 (2.3 oz)	280	14	8	30	2	40	26	1	20	160	—	—	0
Cookie Semi-Sweet Chocolate & Walnuts	1 (2.3 oz)	310	16	8	35	3	38	25	2	40	170	—	—	0
Cookie White Chunk Macadamia	1 (2.3 oz)	310	17	9	35	4	37	25	tr	80	170	—	—	0
Jumbo Cookie Snickerdoodle	1 (5 oz)	640	29	17	110	7	90	49	2	20	540	—	—	0
Nibbler Cookies	2 (0.9 oz)	110	5	3	15	1	15	9	0	0	90	—	—	0
Nibbler Cookies Chewy Chocolate Fudge	2 (0.9 oz)	110	5	4	10	1	15	10	tr	0	130	—	—	0
Nibbler Cookies Cinnamon Sugar	2 (0.9 oz)	120	5	3	15	1	17	11	0	0	90	—	—	0
Nibbler Cookies Debra's Special	2 (0.9 oz)	100	5	2	10	1	13	8	0	0	80	—	—	0

FOOD	PORTION	CALS	FAT	SAT FAT	CHOL	PROT	CARB	SUGAR	FIBER	CALCI	SOD	POTAS	FOLIC	VIT C
Nibbler Cookies M&M	2 (0.9 oz)	110	5	4	15	1	16	10	0	0	55	—	—	0
Nibbler Cookies Milk Chocolate	2 (0.9 oz)	110	5	3	15	1	15	10	tr	0	70	—	—	0
Nibbler Cookies Milk Chocolate w/ Walnuts	2 (0.9 oz)	120	6	3	10	1	14	9	tr	20	65	—	—	0
Nibbler Cookies Peanut Butter	2 (0.9 oz)	110	6	3	15	2	13	7	0	0	95	—	—	0
Nibbler Cookies Semi-Sweet Chocolate	2 (0.9 oz)	110	5	3	10	1	15	10	tr	0	60	—	—	0
Nibbler Cookies Triple Chocolate	2 (0.9 oz)	110	6	3	15	1	15	11	tr	0	65	—	—	0
Nibbler Cookies White Chunk Macadamia	2 (0.9 oz)	120	7	4	10	1	13	5	tr	20	60	—	—	0
NATHAN'S														
¼ Pound Burger	1	537	30	12	90	25	42	11	2	77	813	—	—	8
¼ Pound Burger w/ Cheese	1	850	61	21	136	30	45	11	2	229	1239	—	—	8
Bacon Cheeseburger	1	707	44	20	128	32	43	11	2	229	1340	—	—	8
Cheesesteak Chicken	1 serv	565	19	10	81	38	62	11	5	253	1786	—	—	5
Cheesesteak Original	1	741	43	19	124	44	50	7	4	235	1239	—	—	4
Cheesesteak Supreme	1 serv	786	43	19	124	45	61	11	5	233	1525	—	—	4
Chicken Tender Pita	1	610	38	5	65	22	45	8	2	52	1009	—	—	11
Chicken Tenders	3 pieces	512	37	5	30	21	24	8	3	0	900	—	—	2
Cole Slaw	1 serv	213	9	1	7	1	34	30	3	57	326	—	—	30
Corn Muffin	1	163	6	1	0	2	25	10	1	13	244	—	—	tr
Famous Hot Dog	1	309	20	8	35	11	23	0	1	51	684	—	—	tr
Fish N Chips	1 serv	1538	101	17	111	31	132	39	9	180	2152	—	—	38
French Fries	1 reg	547	38	4	0	6	46	0	6	tr	200	—	—	10
Hot Dog Nuggets	6 pieces	351	28	4	20	5	20	5	0	0	400	—	—	0
Hush Puppy	2 pieces	277	10	2	5	5	42	7	2	107	967	—	—	1
Onion Rings	1 sm	559	44	6	0	3	36	5	2	0	576	—	—	4
Platter Chicken Breast	1 serv	943	54	7	84	28	89	32	9	102	978	—	—	41
Platter Chicken Tender	1 serv	1301	83	10	105	33	109	32	9	77	1059	—	—	39
Sandwich Chicken Tender	1	725	47	7	65	22	56	9	2	70	1008	—	—	15
Sandwich Fish	1	469	20	4	34	14	42	14	13	66	750	—	—	5

FOOD	PORTION	CALS	FAT	SAT FAT	CHOL	PROT	CARB	SUGAR	FIBER	CALCI	SOD	POTAS	FOLIC	VIT C
Sandwich Grilled Chicken	1	524	29	5	67	25	42	9	2	87	1179	—	—	13
Seafood Sampler	1 serv	3379	270	29	156	56	227	49	15	344	3553	—	—	41
Shrimp N Chips	1 serv	2051	124	13	222	51	225	51	12	326	3433	—	—	41
Super Burger	1	864	62	21	136	30	42	13	3	242	1245	—	—	21

NEWPORT CREAMERY

BEVERAGES

FOOD	PORTION	CALS	FAT	SAT FAT	CHOL	PROT	CARB	SUGAR	FIBER	CALCI	SOD	POTAS	FOLIC	VIT C
Skim Milk	1 serv (16 oz)	206	5	—	20	—	—	—	—	—	—	—	—	—

ICE CREAM

FOOD	PORTION	CALS	FAT	SAT FAT	CHOL	PROT	CARB	SUGAR	FIBER	CALCI	SOD	POTAS	FOLIC	VIT C
Reduced Fat No Sugar Added Chocolate	½ cup (2.6 oz)	110	3	2	0	4	22	5	1	100	80	—	—	0
Reduced Fat No Sugar Added Coffee	½ cup (2.6 oz)	100	4	2	15	4	18	6	0	150	70	—	—	0
Soft Serve Nonfat Frozen Yogurt Cone or Dish	1 reg (5 oz)	125	0	0	0	—	—	—	—	—	—	—	—	—

SALAD DRESSINGS

FOOD	PORTION	CALS	FAT	SAT FAT	CHOL	PROT	CARB	SUGAR	FIBER	CALCI	SOD	POTAS	FOLIC	VIT C
Corn Oil & Vinegar	1 tbsp	45	6	0	0	—	—	—	—	—	—	—	—	—
Fat Free Ranch	1½ oz	48	0	0	0	—	—	—	—	—	—	—	—	—
Low-Cal French	1½ oz	48	0	0	0	—	—	—	—	—	—	—	—	—

SALADS AND SALAD BARS

FOOD	PORTION	CALS	FAT	SAT FAT	CHOL	PROT	CARB	SUGAR	FIBER	CALCI	SOD	POTAS	FOLIC	VIT C
Chef's Salad	1 serv	215	8	—	50	—	—	—	—	—	—	—	—	—
Chicken Fajita	1 serv	295	20	—	44	—	—	—	—	—	—	—	—	—
Grilled Chicken	1 serv	247	13	—	48	—	—	—	—	—	—	—	—	—

SANDWICHES

FOOD	PORTION	CALS	FAT	SAT FAT	CHOL	PROT	CARB	SUGAR	FIBER	CALCI	SOD	POTAS	FOLIC	VIT C
Lite Chicken Salad	1	379	19	—	63	—	—	—	—	—	—	—	—	—
Lite Grilled Cheese	1	274	17	—	30	—	—	—	—	—	—	—	—	—
Lite Grilled Chicken Breast Pocket	1	327	12	—	74	—	—	—	—	—	—	—	—	—
Lite Sliced Turkey	1	288	12	—	32	—	—	—	—	—	—	—	—	—
Lite Tuna Salad	1	358	21	—	23	—	—	—	—	—	—	—	—	—
Lite Vegetarian Pocket Broccoli Mushrooms Onions Peppers Cheese	1	211	5	—	15	—	—	—	—	—	—	—	—	—
Lite Vegetarian Pocket Broccoli Cheese	1	214	5	—	15	—	—	—	—	—	—	—	—	—

FOOD	PORTION	CALS	FAT	SAT FAT	CHOL	PROT	CARB	SUGAR	FIBER	CALCI	SOD	POTAS	FOLIC	VIT C
Lite Vegetarian Pocket Peppers Onions Mushrooms Cheese	1	230	6	—	15	—	—	—	—	—	—	—	—	—
Low Fat Cheese	1 slice	73	4	—	15	—	—	—	—	—	—	—	—	—
Mayonnaise	2 tsp	71	8	—	5	—	—	—	—	—	—	—	—	—
Smart Sides Broccoli	1 serv	23	tr	—	0	—	—	—	—	—	—	—	—	—
Smart Sides Cottage Cheese	1 serv	90	4	—	13	—	—	—	—	—	—	—	—	—
Smart Sides Side Salad	1 serv	30	0	0	0	—	—	—	—	—	—	—	—	—

OLD SPAGHETTI FACTORY

MAIN MENU SELECTIONS

FOOD	PORTION	CALS	FAT	SAT FAT	CHOL	PROT	CARB	SUGAR	FIBER	CALCI	SOD	POTAS	FOLIC	VIT C
Caesar Salad	1 sm	330	30	6	30	9	8	—	2	—	610	—	—	—
Caesar Salad Dinner Chicken	1 serv	1280	85	23	250	87	42	—	4	—	2170	—	—	—
Pot Pourri	1 dinner serv	710	30	17	95	26	84	—	6	—	1240	—	—	—
Sandwich Meatball	1	860	41	15	140	49	74	—	4	—	2800	—	—	—
Sandwich Sausage	1	730	40	14	105	40	53	—	4	—	2450	—	—	—
Sandwich Tuscan Chicken	1	1060	60	12	175	76	53	—	4	—	1110	—	—	—
Seafood Cheddar Melt	1 serv	790	42	14	165	40	65	—	4	—	1850	—	—	—
Spaghetti w/ Clam Sauce	1 dinner serv	690	28	16	125	22	84	—	5	—	850	—	—	—
Spaghetti w/ Meat Sauce	1 dinner serv	470	5	1	15	21	83	—	6	—	1110	—	—	—
Spaghetti w/ Meat Sauce & Sausage	1 dinner serv	830	35	11	105	43	85	—	6	—	2150	—	—	—
Spaghetti w/ Meatballs	1 dinner serv	840	33	12	130	47	86	—	5	—	1430	—	—	—
Spaghetti w/ Mizithra	1 dinner serv	1010	64	40	180	37	74	—	4	—	1150	—	—	—
Spaghetti w/ Mushroom Sauce	1 dinner serv	460	7	1	0	14	83	—	6	—	810	—	—	—
Spaghetti w/ Tomato Sauce	1 dinner serv	440	5	1	0	14	84	—	7	—	1020	—	—	—
Spaghetti w/ Tomato Sauce & Clam Sauce	1 dinner serv	560	17	9	65	18	84	—	6	—	940	—	—	—

FOOD	PORTION	CALS	FAT	SAT FAT	CHOL	PROT	CARB	SUGAR	FIBER	CALCI	SOD	POTAS	FOLIC	VIT C
Starter Garlic Cheese Bread	1 serv	1220	85	21	0	17	105	—	5	—	2230	—	—	—
Starter Meatballs	1 serv	910	61	22	245	65	23	—	1	—	2450	—	—	—
Starter Sausage	1 serv	690	56	21	140	31	7	—	tr	—	1790	—	—	—
Starter Tortellini	1 serv	930	56	33	205	25	82	—	2	—	1420	—	—	—
SOUPS														
Chicken Mulligatawny	1 serv	250	14	8	60	10	20	—	2	—	990	—	—	—
Chicken Orzo	1 serv	90	3	1	20	8	9	—	tr	—	830	—	—	—
Clam Chowder	1 serv	380	29	18	95	6	25	2	—	—	850	—	—	—
Cream Of Broccoli	1 serv	220	12	7	40	9	19	—	2	—	1110	—	—	—
Mediterranean White Bean	1 serv	150	6	1	0	6	19	—	6	—	470	—	—	—
Minestrone	1 serv	120	5	1	5	5	15	—	3	—	890	—	—	—

OLIVE GARDEN

FOOD	PORTION	CALS	FAT	SAT FAT	CHOL	PROT	CARB	SUGAR	FIBER	CALCI	SOD	POTAS	FOLIC	VIT C
Garden Fare Apple Carmellina	1 serv (12.2 oz)	560	2	1	5	6	131	—	—	—	190	—	—	—
Garden Fare Dinner Capellini Pomodoro	1 serv (21.1 oz)	610	16	3	5	19	98	—	—	—	940	—	—	—
Garden Fare Dinner Capellini Primavera	1 serv (20.1 oz)	400	7	4	15	18	68	—	—	—	950	—	—	—
Garden Fare Dinner Capellini Primavera w/ Chicken	1 serv (23.8 oz)	560	10	5	95	47	71	—	—	—	1030	—	—	—
Garden Fare Dinner Chicken Giardino	1 serv (20.6 oz)	550	11	4	85	42	71	—	—	—	1000	—	—	—
Garden Fare Dinner Linguine Alla Marinara	1 serv (16.3 oz)	500	9	2	0	16	89	—	—	—	160	—	—	—
Garden Fare Dinner Penne Fra Diavolo	1 serv (14.3 oz)	420	7	3	10	13	77	—	—	—	940	—	—	—
Garden Fare Dinner Shrimp Primavera	1 serv (28.4 oz)	740	15	5	290	48	104	—	—	—	1630	—	—	—
Garden Fare Lunch Capellini Pomodoro	1 serv (11.7 oz)	360	9	2	5	12	57	—	—	—	540	—	—	—
Garden Fare Lunch Capellini Primavera	1 serv (11.2 oz)	260	5	3	15	12	42	—	—	—	560	—	—	—

FOOD	PORTION	CALS	FAT	SAT FAT	CHOL	PROT	CARB	SUGAR	FIBER	CALCI	SOD	POTAS	FOLIC	VIT C
Garden Fare Lunch Capellini Primavera w/ Chicken	1 serv (14.9 oz)	420	8	4	90	41	45	—	—	—	640	—	—	—
Garden Fare Lunch Chicken Giardino	1 serv (12.8 oz)	360	9	4	50	23	47	—	—	—	900	—	—	—
Garden Fare Lunch Linguine Alla Marinara	1 serv (10.2 oz)	310	6	1	0	10	54	—	—	—	105	—	—	—
Garden Fare Lunch Penne Fra Diavolo	1 serv (10.2 oz)	300	5	2	10	9	57	—	—	—	640	—	—	—
Garden Fare Lunch Shrimp Primavera	1 serv (15.2 oz)	410	8	3	145	25	60	—	—	—	840	—	—	—
Minestrone Soup	1 serv (6 oz)	80	1	0	0	4	15	—	—	—	450	—	—	—

P.J. CHANG'S CHINA BISTRO

FOOD	PORTION	CALS	FAT	SAT FAT	CHOL	PROT	CARB	SUGAR	FIBER	CALCI	SOD	POTAS	FOLIC	VIT C
Cantonese Scallops	1 serv	305	8	—	—	42	15	—	—	—	—	—	—	—
Chicken w/ Black Bean Sauce	1 serv	426	11	—	—	63	19	—	—	—	—	—	—	—
Pin Rice Noodles	1 serv	270	2	—	—	12	55	—	—	—	—	—	—	—
Vegetable Chow Fun	1 serv	677	18	—	—	16	112	—	—	—	—	—	—	—

PANDA EXPRESS

FOOD	PORTION	CALS	FAT	SAT FAT	CHOL	PROT	CARB	SUGAR	FIBER	CALCI	SOD	POTAS	FOLIC	VIT C
Beef & Broccoli	1 serv (5 oz)	180	9	2	—	—	—	—	—	—	910	—	—	—
Black Pepper Chicken	1 serv (5 oz)	210	9	2	—	—	—	—	—	—	570	—	—	—
Chicken w/ Mushrooms	1 serv (5 oz)	170	3	0	—	—	—	—	—	—	570	—	—	—
Chicken w/ String Beans	1 serv (5 oz)	180	9	2	—	—	—	—	—	—	620	—	—	—
Egg Flower Soup	1½ cups	80	0	0	—	—	—	—	—	—	640	—	—	—
Egg Rolls	2 (3 oz)	190	6	1	—	—	—	—	—	—	490	—	—	—
Hot & Sour Soup	1½ cups	110	4	1	—	—	—	—	—	—	890	—	—	—
Lo Mein	1 serv (8 oz)	300	10	2	—	—	—	—	—	—	1090	—	—	—
Mixed Vegetables	1 serv (5 oz)	80	3	—	0	—	—	—	—	—	450	—	—	—
Orange Chicken	1 serv (5 oz)	310	13	3	—	—	—	—	—	—	420	—	—	—
Spicy Chicken w/ Peanuts	1 serv (5 oz)	510	29	5	—	—	—	—	—	—	1250	—	—	—
Steamed Rice	1 serv (8 oz)	220	0	0	0	—	—	—	—	—	0	—	—	—
Sweet & Sour Pork	1 serv (4 oz)	310	20	7	—	—	—	—	—	—	250	—	—	—
Sweet & Sour Sauce	1 serv (2 oz)	60	0	0	0	—	—	—	—	—	150	—	—	—
Vegetable Chow Mein	1 serv (8 oz)	300	10	2	—	—	—	—	—	—	610	—	—	—

FOOD	PORTION	CALS	FAT	SAT FAT	CHOL	PROT	CARB	SUGAR	FIBER	CALCI	SOD	POTAS	FOLIC	VIT C
Vegetable Fried Rice	1 serv (8 oz)	410	19	3	—	—	—	—	—	—	440	—	—	—

PANERA BREAD

BAGELS AND SPREADS

FOOD	PORTION	CALS	FAT	SAT FAT	CHOL	PROT	CARB	SUGAR	FIBER	CALCI	SOD	POTAS	FOLIC	VIT C
Bagel Asiago Cheese	1	330	5	3	15	15	58	5	2	—	480	—	—	—
Bagel Blueberry	1	320	2	0	0	12	67	11	3	—	490	—	—	—
Bagel Cinnamon Crunch	1	490	9	5	0	12	91	35	3	—	500	—	—	—
Bagel Dutch Apple & Raisin	1	340	3	0	0	10	70	21	3	—	410	—	—	—
Bagel Everything	1	290	2	0	0	11	58	4	2	—	540	—	—	—
Bagel French Toast	1	340	5	1	0	10	65	16	2	—	610	—	—	—
Bagel Mochachip Swirl	1	340	4	2	0	12	68	13	3	—	460	—	—	—
Bagel Nine Grain	1	290	1	0	0	11	58	4	3	—	390	—	—	—
Bagel Peanut Butter Crunch	1	400	6	3	0	11	77	27	3	—	480	—	—	—
Bagel Plain	1	280	1	0	0	11	57	4	2	—	450	—	—	—
Bagel Sesame	1	310	3	0	0	12	60	4	3	—	460	—	—	—
Cream Cheese Hazelnut Reduced Fat	1 serv (2 oz)	150	11	7	35	5	6	6	tr	—	210	—	—	—
Cream Cheese Honey Walnut Reduced Fat	1 serv (2 oz)	150	11	7	30	4	9	6	tr	—	200	—	—	—
Cream Cheese Mocha Reduced Fat	1 serv (2 oz)	160	11	30	7	5	10	8	1	—	180	—	—	—
Cream Cheese Plain	1 serv (2 oz)	190	18	12	55	3	2	1	0	—	210	—	—	—
Cream Cheese Plain Reduced Fat	1 serv (2 oz)	130	12	8	35	5	2	1	tr	—	230	—	—	—
Cream Cheese Raspberry Reduced Fat	1 serv (2 oz)	120	10	7	30	4	3	2	0	—	200	—	—	—
Cream Cheese Smoked Salmon Reduced Fat	1 serv (2 oz)	120	10	6	35	7	2	1	0	—	180	—	—	—
Cream Cheese Sun Dried Tomato Reduced Fat	1 serv (2 oz)	140	11	7	35	5	4	2	tr	—	220	—	—	—
Cream Cheese Veggie Reduced Fat	1 serv (2 oz)	130	11	7	35	5	4	2	1	—	230	—	—	—

FOOD	PORTION	CALS	FAT	SAT FAT	CHOL	PROT	CARB	SUGAR	FIBER	CALCI	SOD	POTAS	FOLIC	VIT C
Hummus Roasted Garlic	1 serv (2 oz)	100	5	1	0	3	11	7	4	—	260	—	—	—
BEVERAGES														
Caffe Mocha	1 serv (11.5 oz)	360	16	55	10	11	47	39	2	—	190	—	—	—
Homestyle Lemonade	1 serv (16 oz)	80	0	0	0	0	19	—	0	—	10	—	—	—
Hot Chocolate	1 serv (11 oz)	350	15	10	50	11	45	38	2	—	190	—	—	—
IC Cappuccino Chip	1 serv (16 oz)	590	35	26	70	5	64	56	0	—	125	—	—	—
IC Caramel	1 serv (16 oz)	550	24	15	80	6	76	63	0	—	400	—	—	—
IC Honeydew Green Tea	1 serv (16 oz)	270	13	0	30	2	36	31	0	—	140	—	—	—
IC Mocha	1 serv (16 oz)	520	24	15	75	7	70	56	2	—	140	—	—	—
IC Spice	1 serv (16 oz)	470	22	13	70	4	66	56	0	—	80	—	—	—
Iced Green Tea	1 serv (16 oz)	60	0	0	0	0	15	14	0	—	5	—	—	—
Latte Caffe	1 serv (8.5 oz)	170	5	3	20	7	12	11	0	—	120	—	—	—
Latte Caramel	1 serv (11 oz)	400	16	9	55	9	54	46	0	—	450	—	—	—
Latte Chai Tea	1 serv (10 oz)	210	5	3	15	7	37	33	0	—	115	—	—	—
Latte House	1 serv (10.8 oz)	320	13	8	50	8	43	39	0	—	135	—	—	—
BREADS														
Artisan Country	1 slice	120	0	0	0	5	25	1	1	—	290	—	—	—
Artisan French	1 slice (2 oz)	110	0	0	0	4	23	1	tr	—	310	—	—	—
Artisan Kalamata Olive	1 slice (2 oz)	140	2	0	0	5	26	1	1	—	270	—	—	—
Artisan Multigrain	1 slice (2 oz)	120	1	0	0	4	24	1	1	—	230	—	—	—
Artisan Raisin Pecan	1 slice (2 oz)	140	3	0	0	4	25	5	1	—	280	—	—	—
Artisan Sesame Semolina	1 slice (2 oz)	120	0	0	0	4	24	1	4	—	300	—	—	—
Artisan Stone Milled Rye	1 slice (2 oz)	110	0	0	0	4	22	1	2	—	320	—	—	—
Artisan Three Cheese	1 slice (2 oz)	120	2	1	5	5	21	1	tr	—	270	—	—	—
Artisan Three Seed	1 slice	130	2	0	0	5	23	1	1	—	250	—	—	—
Ciabatta	1 (6 oz)	430	10	2	0	14	70	2	3	—	990	—	—	—
Cinnamon Raisin	1 slice (2 oz)	160	3	1	0	4	31	12	1	—	300	—	—	—
Focaccia Asiago Cheese	1 slice (2 oz)	150	6	2	5	5	19	1	1	—	300	—	—	—
Focaccia Basil Pesto	1 slice (2 oz)	150	6	2	5	4	19	1	1	—	300	—	—	—
Focaccia Rosemary & Onion	1 slice (2 oz)	140	5	1	5	4	19	1	1	—	280	—	—	—
French	1 slice (2 oz)	130	1	0	0	5	24	1	1	—	270	—	—	—
French Roll	1 (2.25 oz)	140	1	0	0	6	28	1	1	—	310	—	—	—

FOOD	PORTION	CALS	FAT	SAT FAT	CHOL	PROT	CARB	SUGAR	FIBER	CALCI	SOD	POTAS	FOLIC	VIT C
Holiday	1 slice (2 oz)	150	1	0	5	2	33	23	tr	—	135	—	—	—
Honey Wheat	1 slice (2 oz)	140	3	1	0	5	25	3	1	—	260	—	—	—
Nine Grain	1 slice (2 oz)	150	3	1	0	5	26	3	2	—	270	—	—	—
Rye	1 slice (2 oz)	140	3	1	0	5	25	3	1	—	290	—	—	—
Sourdough	1 slice (2 oz)	120	0	0	0	5	25	1	1	—	270	—	—	—
Sourdough Roll	1 (2.5 oz)	160	0	0	0	6	32	1	1	—	340	—	—	—
Sourdough Soup Bowl	1 serv (8 oz)	500	2	0	0	20	102	2	4	—	1090	—	—	—
Sunflower	1 slice (2 oz)	160	5	1	0	6	24	4	1	—	320	—	—	—
Tomato Basil	1 slice (2 oz)	130	1	0	0	5	27	1	1	—	350	—	—	—
DESSERTS														
Bear Claw	1	380	21	11	70	7	37	14	1	—	310	—	—	—
Brownie Caramel Pecan	1	470	24	5	80	5	60	47	2	—	150	—	—	—
Brownie Chocolate Raspberry	1	370	18	5	75	2	47	37	2	—	130	—	—	—
Brownie Very Chocolate	1	460	22	5	80	5	62	47	2	—	150	—	—	—
Cinnamon Roll	1	560	26	12	90	12	64	21	3	—	480	—	—	—
Cobblestone	1	560	9	2	0	8	100	42	4	—	620	—	—	—
Coffee Cake Cherry Cheese	1	190	10	5	30	3	21	11	1	—	130	—	—	—
Cookie Chocolate Chipper	1	420	22	13	60	5	51	21	2	—	320	—	—	—
Cookie Chocolate Duet w/ Walnuts	1	410	25	17	60	6	47	24	3	—	320	—	—	—
Cookie Nutty Chocolate Chipper	1	440	26	12	55	6	46	20	3	—	300	—	—	—
Cookie Nutty Oatmeal Raisin	1	350	14	7	45	5	51	22	5	—	260	—	—	—
Cookie Shortbread	1	340	21	13	60	3	36	11	1	—	160	—	—	—
Croissant Apple	1	260	11	7	30	4	34	17	1	—	230	—	—	—
Croissant Cheese	1	300	16	10	45	6	34	11	1	—	220	—	—	—
Croissant Chocolate	1	440	23	13	35	7	56	27	4	—	180	—	—	—
Croissant French	1	265	15	9	40	5	28	3	1	—	190	—	—	—
Croissant Raspberry Cheese	1	280	13	8	35	5	37	14	1	—	190	—	—	—
Danish Apple	1	510	30	15	85	9	50	17	2	—	350	—	—	—
Danish Cheese	1	590	35	19	110	10	55	25	1	—	430	—	—	—
Danish Cherry	1	520	26	14	85	8	60	31	1	—	340	—	—	—
Danish Georgia Peach	1	580	30	15	85	9	67	28	2	—	390	—	—	—

FOOD	PORTION	CALS	FAT	SAT FAT	CHOL	PROT	CARB	SUGAR	FIBER	CALCI	SOD	POTAS	FOLIC	VIT C
Danish German Chocolate	1	770	46	24	85	10	83	37	4	—	570	—	—	—
Macaroon Chocolate Hazelnut	1	270	15	10	0	3	30	18	3	—	90	—	—	—
Mini Bundt Cake Carrot Walnut	1	430	21	3	75	6	51	31	2	—	340	—	—	—
Mini Bundt Cake Lemon Poppyseed	1	460	20	4	90	6	62	33	1	—	430	—	—	—
Mini Bundt Cake Pineapple Upside Down	1	450	20	8	70	5	64	36	2	—	490	—	—	—
Muffie Banana Nut	1	260	12	2	15	5	34	15	3	—	250	—	—	—
Muffie Chocolate Chip	1	240	10	3	15	4	36	18	2	—	240	—	—	—
Muffie Pumpkin	1	270	6	2	30	3	43	26	1	—	270	—	—	—
Muffin Banana Nut	1	470	20	3	30	9	57	31	5	—	500	—	—	—
Muffin Blueberry	1	450	15	3	35	8	73	33	4	—	570	—	—	—
Muffin Chocolate Chip	1	540	22	8	30	8	83	42	5	—	550	—	—	—
Muffin Pumpkin	1	510	12	3	60	6	80	48	1	—	530	—	—	—
Muffin Low Fat Tripleberry	1	300	3	1	30	6	63	28	3	—	320	—	—	—
Pecan Roll	1	520	31	6	40	6	60	26	2	—	260	—	—	—
Scone Cinnamon Chip	1	560	27	16	150	10	70	23	2	—	440	—	—	—
Scone Orange	1	530	25	15	140	10	67	22	3	—	370	—	—	—
Strudel Apple Raisin	1	390	22	6	0	4	40	18	1	—	330	—	—	—
Strudel Cherry	1	400	24	6	0	5	38	20	1	—	290	—	—	—
SALADS														
Asian Sesame Chicken	1 serv	370	19	3	60	25	45	19	5	—	1280	—	—	—
Caesar	1 serv	350	26	7	110	11	15	1	3	—	1010	—	—	—
Caesar Grilled Chicken	1 serv	470	27	7	165	31	22	1	3	—	1550	—	—	—
Classic Cafe	1 serv	380	36	5	0	3	15	10	4	—	340	—	—	—
Fandango	1 serv	400	28	7	25	7	21	15	6	—	480	—	—	—
Greek	1 serv	520	48	10	20	9	17	4	5	—	1560	—	—	—
SANDWICHES														
Asiago Roast Beef	1	730	35	16	115	50	54	4	2	—	1620	—	—	—
Bacon Turkey Bravo	1	770	28	9	45	47	84	6	5	—	2850	—	—	—

FOOD	PORTION	CALS	FAT	SAT FAT	CHOL	PROT	CARB	SUGAR	FIBER	CALCI	SOD	POTAS	FOLIC	VIT C
Chicken Salad On Artisan Sesame Semolina	1	730	26	4	90	39	80	12	6	—	1750	—	—	—
Chicken Salad On Nine Grain	1	640	29	5	90	35	56	15	4	—	1340	—	—	—
Garden Veggie	1	570	23	7	15	15	74	6	5	—	1490	—	—	—
Italian Combo	1	1050	54	18	165	60	80	5	5	—	3570	—	—	—
Panini Coronado Carnitas	1	810	35	11	95	47	77	4	3	—	2210	—	—	—
Panini Portobello & Mozzarella	1	650	29	10	40	25	73	7	8	—	1100	—	—	—
Panini Turkey Artichoke	1	810	38	11	25	41	76	10	6	—	2470	—	—	—
Peanut Butter & Jelly On French	1	450	15	3	0	15	63	23	3	—	580	—	—	—
Panini Frontega Chicken	1	860	42	12	110	49	71	5	5	—	2260	—	—	—
Sierra Turkey	1	950	55	13	40	40	71	4	4	—	2380	—	—	—
Smoked Ham On Artisan Stone Milled Rye	1	930	31	10	110	52	106	6	6	—	3000	—	—	—
Smoked Ham On Rye	1	650	34	11	110	42	47	7	4	—	2350	—	—	—
Smoked Turkey Breast On Artisan Country	1	590	16	2	10	34	73	4	5	—	2320	—	—	—
Smoked Turkey On Sourdough	1	440	15	2	10	29	44	4	3	—	1950	—	—	—
Tuna Salad On Artisan Multigrain	1	830	41	5	65	32	78	7	5	—	1790	—	—	—
Tuna Salad On Honey Wheat	1	720	43	6	65	28	50	10	4	—	1570	—	—	—
Turkey Fresco	1	580	17	5	0	35	74	5	4	—	2430	—	—	—
Tuscan Chicken	1	950	56	10	80	35	76	8	6	—	2130	—	—	—
SOUPS														
Baked Potato	1 serv	260	16	8	35	6	23	2	1	—	750	—	—	—
Boston Clam Chowder	1 serv	210	11	6	40	6	19	2	tr	—	990	—	—	—
Broccoli Cheddar	1 serv	230	16	9	45	8	13	4	1	—	1000	—	—	—
Cream Of Chicken & Wild Rice	1 serv	200	12	6	35	5	19	2	tr	—	970	—	—	—
Forest Mushroom	1 serv	140	7	4	15	4	15	3	2	—	920	—	—	—
French Onion	1 serv	220	10	5	20	9	23	6	2	—	1810	—	—	—
Low Fat Chicken Noodle	1 serv	100	2	0	15	5	15	1	1	—	1080	—	—	—

FOOD	PORTION	CALS	FAT	SAT FAT	CHOL	PROT	CARB	SUGAR	FIBER	CALCI	SOD	POTAS	FOLIC	VIT C
Low Fat Vegetarian Garden Vegetable	1 serv	90	1	0	0	4	17	4	2	—	860	—	—	—
Low Fat Vegetarian Black Bean	1 serv	100	1	0	0	10	29	2	17	—	840	—	—	—
Vegetarian Santa Fe Roasted Corn	1 serv	130	4	1	0	4	22	4	3	—	940	—	—	—

PAPA JOHNS

OTHER MENU SELECTIONS

FOOD	PORTION	CALS	FAT	SAT FAT	CHOL	PROT	CARB	SUGAR	FIBER	CALCI	SOD	POTAS	FOLIC	VIT C
Bread Sticks	1 serv	140	2	0	0	4	26	3	1	8	260	—	—	—
Cheese Sticks	1 serv	180	8	3	13	8	20	2	1	120	380	—	—	—
Chickenstrips	1	83	4	1	13	6	5	tr	tr	4	178	—	—	—
Cinnapie	1 serv	114	6	1	0	1	14	6	0	0	145	—		—

PIZZA 14 INCH

FOOD	PORTION	CALS	FAT	SAT FAT	CHOL	PROT	CARB	SUGAR	FIBER	CALCI	SOD	POTAS	FOLIC	VIT C
Original All The Meats	⅛ pie	405	20	7	41	18	39	5	2	134	1114	—	—	—
Original BBQ Chicken & Bacon	⅛ pie	369	14	4	31	17	44	6	2	137	929	—	—	—
Original Cheese	⅛ pic	290	10	3	17	12	39	5	2	155	699	—	—	—
Original Chicken Alfredo	⅛ pie	310	12	4	31	15	37	4	2	142	743	—	—	—
Original Garden Fresh	⅛ pie	287	9	3	14	12	40	6	3	135	685	—	—	—
Original Hawaiian BBQ Chicken	⅛ pie	376	14	4	31	17	46	6	2	136	1029	—		—
Original Pepperoni	⅛ pie	343	15	5	27	14	39	5	2	155	913	—	—	—
Original Sausage	⅛ pie	336	14	4	28	14	38	5	2	135	894	·	—	—
Original Spinach Alfredo	⅛ pie	303	12	5	25	13	37	4	2	176	694	—	—	—
Original The Works	⅛ pie	370	16	5	34	17	40	6	3	165	1013	—	—	—
Thin Crust All The Meat	⅛ pie	371	24	7	44	17	24	3	2	178	945	—	—	—
Thin Crust BBQ Chicken & Bacon	⅛ pie	336	18	5	34	15	30	4	1	181	759	—	—	—
Thin Crust Cheese	⅛ pie	238	13	3	17	10	23	3	1	171	490	—	—	—
Thin Crust Chicken Alfredo	⅛ pie	276	15	5	35	14	22	1	1	186	573	—	—	—
Thin Crust Garden Fresh	⅛ pie	228	11	3	14	9	24	2	2	151	447	—	—	—
Thin Crust Hawaiian BBQ Chicken	⅛ pie	324	17	5	31	14	31	5	1	154	805	—	—	—

FOOD	PORTION	CALS	FAT	SAT FAT	CHOL	PROT	CARB	SUGAR	FIBER	CALCI	SOD	POTAS	FOLIC	VIT C
Thin Crust Pepperoni	⅛ pie	294	18	5	28	12	23	3	2	176	675	—	—	—
Thin Crust Sausage	⅛ pie	303	18	5	31	13	24	3	2	179	724	—	—	—
Thin Crust Spinach Alfredo	⅛ pie	251	15	5	26	10	22	1	1	192	470	—	—	—
Thin Crust The Works	⅛ pie	315	18	5	32	14	25	3	2	185	809	—	—	—
SALAD DRESSINGS AND SAUCES														
BBQ Sauce	1 serv	48	0	0	0	0	10	9	0	0	310	—	—	—
Buffalo Sauce	1 serv	25	1	0	0	0	3	1	0	0	1470	—	—	—
Cheese Sauce	1 serv	60	5	4	19	4	0	0	0	0	300	—	—	—
Garlic Sauce	1 serv	235	26	3	0	0	0	0	0	0	300	—	—	—
Honey Mustard Dressing	1 serv	170	19	3	10	0	6	6	0	0	150	—	—	—
Pizza Sauce	1 serv	25	2	0	0	0	3	1	2	102	125	—	—	—
Ranch Dressing	1 serv	140	14	3	15	1	2	1	0	24	280	—	—	—
PAPA MURPHY'S														
PIZZA														
Deeper Dish Traditional	⅛ pie	440	24	10	40	23	34	1	2	400	900	—	—	9
Delite Large Cheese	1/10 pie	130	6	4	15	8	11	0	0	—	240	—	—	1
Delite Large Hawaiian	1/10 pie	140	7	4	15	9	14	2	1	—	300	—	—	4
Delite Large Meat	1/10 pie	190	12	5	25	11	11	0	0	—	430	—	—	1
Delite Large Pepperoni	1/10 pie	160	9	5	20	9	11	0	0	—	350	—	—	1
Delite Large Veggie	1/10 pie	150	8	4	15	8	11	1	0	—	200	—	—	4
Family Size Cheese	1/12 pie	270	10	5	20	14	29	1	2	250	470	—	—	6
Gourmet Family Size Chicken Garlic	1/12 pie	320	15	6	35	18	30	1	1	300	600	—	—	9
Gourmet Family Size Classic Italian	1/12 pie	360	19	8	35	18	30	1	2	300	730	—	—	9
Gourmet Family Size Veggie	1/12 pie	300	14	6	25	15	31	1	2	300	570	—	—	12
Papa's Family Size All Meat	1/12 pie	370	19	8	40	20	31	1	2	300	860	—	—	9
Papa's Family Size Cheese	1/12 pie	270	10	5	20	14	29	1	2	250	470	—	—	6
Papa's Family Size Cowboy	1/12 pie	370	19	7	35	18	31	1	2	300	850	—	—	6

FOOD	PORTION	CALS	FAT	SAT FAT	CHOL	PROT	CARB	SUGAR	FIBER	CALCI	SOD	POTAS	FOLIC	VIT C
Papa's Family Size Favorite	¹⁄₁₂ pie	380	20	8	35	18	32	2	2	300	860	—	—	15
Papa's Family Size Hawaiian	¹⁄₁₂ pie	290	11	5	25	16	34	4	2	250	580	—	—	9
Papa's Family Size Murphy's Combo	¹⁄₁₂ pie	480	20	7	35	18	32	2	2	300	910	—	—	9
Papa's Family Size Pepperoni	¹⁄₁₂ pie	310	15	7	30	16	29	1	2	300	650	—	—	6
Papa's Family Size Perfect	¹⁄₁₂ pie	300	13	6	25	16	32	4	2	300	620	—	—	6
Papa's Family Size Rancher	¹⁄₁₂ pie	330	15	7	30	18	31	2	2	300	720	—	—	6
Papa's Family Size Specialty	¹⁄₁₂ pie	340	17	6	30	17	31	1	2	300	740	—	—	6
Papa's Family Size Veggie Combo	¹⁄₁₂ pie	300	13	5	20	14	32	2	2	300	570	—	—	18
Stuffed Big Murphy	⅛ pie	380	17	7	30	18	39	1	2	300	800	—	—	12
Stuffed Chicago Style	⅛ pie	370	16	7	30	17	39	2	2	250	770	—	—	9
SALADS														
Club	1 serv	190	21	8	50	21	11	2	4	250	930	—	—	42
Garden	1 serv	160	11	5	20	11	9	3	4	250	270	—	—	72
Italian	1 serv	220	17	6	30	13	7	2	3	250	510	—	—	42

PERKINS

FOOD	PORTION	CALS	FAT	SAT FAT	CHOL	PROT	CARB	SUGAR	FIBER	CALCI	SOD	POTAS	FOLIC	VIT C
Low Fat Brownie	1 (5.4 oz)	260	1	—	—	—	—	—	—	—	—	—	—	—
Low Fat Muffin Banana	1 (5.8 oz)	330	3	—	—	—	—	—	—	—	—	—	—	—
Low Fat Muffin Blueberry	1 (5.8 oz)	270	3	—	—	—	—	—	—	—	—	—	—	—
Low Fat Muffin Honey Bran	1 (5.8 oz)	270	3	—	—	—	—	—	—	—	—	—	—	—
Low Fat Muffin Plain	1 (5.8 oz)	300	3	—	—	—	—	—	—	—	—	—	—	—

PICCADILLY CAFETERIA

FOOD	PORTION	CALS	FAT	SAT FAT	CHOL	PROT	CARB	SUGAR	FIBER	CALCI	SOD	POTAS	FOLIC	VIT C
DESSERTS														
Gelatin Sugar Free	1 serv	0	0	0	0	0	0	0	0	—	5	—	—	—
Sugar Free Blueberry Pie	1 serv	314	17	5	0	5	42	—	3	—	253	—	—	—
Sugar Free Cherry Pie	1 serv	334	17	5	0	5	45	—	1	—	253	—	—	—
Sugar Free Chocolate Almond Pie	1 serv	611	44	34	1	5	49	—	2	—	564	—	—	—

FOOD	PORTION	CALS	FAT	SAT FAT	CHOL	PROT	CARB	SUGAR	FIBER	CALCI	SOD	POTAS	FOLIC	VIT C
MAIN MENU SELECTIONS														
Bass Blackened	1 serv	408	32	7	28	26	2	—	1	—	616	—	—	—
Bass Cajun Baked	1 serv	260	15	4	28	27	4	—	1	—	600	—	—	—
Bass Stuffed	1 serv	447	30	7	64	34	8	—	1	—	1007	—	—	—
Beef Chopped Steak	1 serv	382	31	11	74	21	4	—	0	—	160	—	—	—
Beef Chopped Steak Fried	1 serv	225	12	4	59	26	2	—	0	—	1604	—	—	—
Beef Roast Leg	1 sm serv	353	22	9	103	35	2	—	1	—	213	—	—	—
Broccoli Florets	1 serv	90	7	1	0	3	5	—	3	—	174	—	—	—
Broccoli w/ Cheese Sauce	1 serv	55	1	0	4	3	9	—	3	—	284	—	—	—
Brussels Sprouts	1 serv	92	6	1	0	3	8	—	4	—	119	—	—	—
Cabbage Steamed Bacon Seasoned	1 serv	108	8	3	9	2	6	—	2	—	191	—	—	—
Cabbage Steamed Buttered	1 serv	68	5	1	0	1	6	—	2	—	132	—	—	—
Catfish Filet Blackened	1 serv	523	43	8	87	29	2	—	1	—	647	—	—	—
Catfish Filet Cajun Baked	1 serv	401	28	6	87	30	5	—	1	—	927	—	—	—
Catfish Filet Stuffed	1 serv	561	41	8	123	37	8	—	1	—	1036	—	—	—
Cauliflower Buttered	1 serv	73	4	1	0	1	5	—	1	—	153	—	—	—
Chicken Barbecued Quarters	1 serv	472	52	15	255	65	9	—	1	—	871	—	—	—
Chicken Grilled Breast	1 serv	345	21	5	136	34	2	—	1	—	512	—	—	—
Chicken Rotisserie Herb Dark Meat	1 serv	823	63	16	276	57	3	—	1	—	877	—	—	—
Chicken Rotisserie Herb White Meat	1 serv	602	32	9	218	71	3	—	1	—	843	—	—	—
Chicken Baked Cajun Boneless Breast	1 serv	428	27	6	136	35	9	—	1	—	1597	—	—	—
Chicken Baked Quarters	1 serv	828	59	16	255	64	5	—	1	—	972	—	—	—
Chicken Breast Italian Boneless Breast	1 serv	371	41	7	139	34	7	—	1	—	1773	—	—	—
Chicken Breast Mesquite Smoke	1 serv	212	8	2	86	34	1	—	1	—	1215	—	—	—
Chicken Breast Mesquite w/ BBQ Sauce	1 serv	240	9	3	86	35	6	—	0	—	1462	—	—	—

FOOD	PORTION	CALS	FAT	SAT FAT	CHOL	PROT	CARB	SUGAR	FIBER	CALCI	SOD	POTAS	FOLIC	VIT C
Chicken Breast Southwestern	1 serv	315	35	14	133	44	8	—	1	—	1837	—	—	—
Chicken Half Rotisserie Herb	1 serv	833	21	5	478	146	4	—	2	—	1781	—	—	—
Corn	1 serv	125	6	1	0	3	18	—	1	—	128	—	—	—
Cottage Cheese	1 serv	117	5	3	17	14	3	—	0	—	813	—	—	—
Filet Mignon	1 (6 oz)	184	20	8	105	36	1	—	0	—	286	—	—	—
Green Beans	1 serv	136	11	4	12	3	8	—	4	—	291	—	—	—
Green Collard Mustard Turnip	1 serv	135	10	4	12	4	3	—	2	—	224	—	—	—
Greens Turnip w/ Diced Turnips	1 serv	150	12	4	14	4	4	—	2	—	242	—	—	—
Grouper Filet Baked	1 piece (6 oz)	305	9	2	84	46	8	—	1	—	424	—	—	—
New York Strip	1 (10 oz)	871	71	26	190	55	1	—	0	—	360	—		—
Okra Creole	1 serv	77	4	2	5	2	8	—	3	—	205	—	—	—
Okra Fried	1 serv	240	13	4	0	4	26	—	4	—	473	—	—	—
Peas & Sugar Snapped Mixed	1 serv	102	5	1	0	3	10	—	3	—	115	—	—	—
Pork Loin Marinated Boneless	1 serv	365	24	8	102	34	1	—	0	—	529	—	—	—
Pork Loin Roast Bone In	1 serv	373	13	5	120	49	10	—	1	—	335	—	—	—
Ribeye	1 (10 oz)	1038	91	34	193	50	2	—	1	—	542	—	—	—
Roast Beef	1 serv	481	30	13	141	46	3	—	1	—	292	—	—	—
Roll Parker House	1	147	5	1	0	3	22	—	1	—	198	—	—	—
Roll Whole Wheat	1	231	8	2	0	6	37	—	5	—	376	—	—	—
Shrimp Fried	1 serv	499	22	12	277	26	45	—	0	—	907	—	—	—
Tilapia Baked	1 serv	210	11	2	0	17	10	—	1	—	560	—	—	—
Tilapia Cajun Baked	1 serv	263	19	4	0	17	6	—	1	—	1039	—	—	—
Trout Almondine Baked	1 lg serv	457	18	3	167	60	10	—	1	—	398	—	—	—
Trout Cajun Baked	1 lg serv	517	27	5	167	59	6	—	1	—	1082	—	—	—
Trout Filet Baked	1 lg serv	464	19	4	167	59	10	—	1	—	594	—	—	—
Turkey Breast Carved	1 serv	302	11	3	123	45	2	—	0	—	2605	—	—	—
Vegetables Mixed	1 serv	95	6	1	0	1	8	—	3	—	137	—	—	—
SALAD DRESSINGS AND TOPPINGS														
Au Jus	1 serv	6	0	0	0	0	1	—	0	—	457	—	—	—
Blue Cheese	2 tbsp	160	18	3	20	1	1	—	0	—	210	—	—	—
Cheese Sauce	2 oz	35	1	0	4	1	5	—	0	—	274	—	—	—
French	2 tbsp	130	13	2	0	0	5	—	0	—	240	—	—	—
Italian	2 tbsp	140	14	2	0	0	3	—	0	—	421	—	—	—

FOOD	PORTION	CALS	FAT	SAT FAT	CHOL	PROT	CARB	SUGAR	FIBER	CALCI	SOD	POTAS	FOLIC	VIT C
Ranch	2 tbsp	150	17	2	15	1	1	—	0	—	210	—	—	—
Ranch Fat Free	2 tbsp	36	0	0	0	1	7	—	1	—	352	—	—	—
SALADS														
Asparagus & Tomato	1 serv	86	5	1	4	2	10	—	2	—	118	—	—	—
Caesar	1 serv	141	11	3	12	4	7	—	1	—	317	—	—	—
Cauilflower	1 serv	118	8	2	33	4	9	—	2	—	361	—	—	—
Chef	1 sm serv	146	9	4	150	13	4	—	1	—	475	—	—	—
Cole Slaw Kosher Style	1 serv	140	13	2	0	1	7	—	2	—	76	—	—	—
Coleslaw Italian	1 serv	163	16	2	0	1	5	—	2	—	645	—	—	—
Combination	1 serv	63	3	1	125	5	4	—	2	—	48	—	—	—
Cucumber & Celery	1 serv	74	4	1	0	1	9	—	1	—	141	—	—	—
Cucumber & Tomato	1 serv	41	0	0	0	1	10	—	1	—	109	—	—	—
Cucumber Mix	1 serv	61	4	1	0	1	7	—	2	—	107	—	—	—
Cucumbers & Sour Cream	1 serv	90	7	4	22	2	6	—	1	—	122	—	—	—
Louisianne Bowl	1 serv	42	2	1	9	4	2	—	1	—	112	—	—	—
Mexican	1 serv	58	3	0	0	1	8	—	1	—	54	—	—	—
Piccadilly Bowl	1 serv	27	0	0	0	1	6	—	2	—	30	—	—	—
Piccadilly Fruit	1 serv	76	0	0	0	1	20	—	3	—	3	—	—	—
Shrimp Remoulade	1 serv	521	29	4	410	31	33	—	5	—	871	—	—	—
Spring Bowl	1 reg serv	24	0	0	0	2	5	—	2	—	16	—	—	—
Tomato Cucumber & Onion	1 serv	44	0	0	0	1	10	—	1	—	106	—	—	—
Vegetable Combo w/ Cherry Tomatoes	1 serv	66	4	0	0	1	9	—	2	—	114	—	—	—
SOUPS														
Gumbo Chicken & Sausage No Rice	1 serv	224	15	3	39	12	10	—	1	—	649	—	—	—
Gumbo Chicken No Rice	1 serv	89	2	1	23	8	9	—	1	—	8463	—	—	—

PIZZA HUT

FOOD	PORTION	CALS	FAT	SAT FAT	CHOL	PROT	CARB	SUGAR	FIBER	CALCI	SOD	POTAS	FOLIC	VIT C
APPETIZERS														
Breadstick	1	150	6	1	0	4	20	4	tr	0	220	—	—	0
Breadstick Cheese	1	200	10	4	15	7	21	4	tr	100	340	—	—	0
Breadstick Dipping Sauce	1 serv (3 oz)	50	0	0	0	1	11	6	2	20	270	—	—	9
Hot Wings	2 pieces	110	6	2	70	11	1	0	0	0	450	—	—	0
Mild Wings	2 pieces	110	7	2	70	11	tr	0	0	0	320	—	—	0

FOOD	PORTION	CALS	FAT	SAT FAT	CHOL	PROT	CARB	SUGAR	FIBER	CALCI	SOD	POTAS	FOLIC	VIT C
Wing Blue Cheese Dipping Sauce	1 serv (1.5 oz)	230	24	5	25	2	2	2	0	20	550	—	—	0
Wing Ranch Dipping Sauce	1 serv (1.5 oz)	210	22	4	10	tr	4	2	0	0	340	—	—	0
BEVERAGES														
Diet Pepsi	1 med (14 oz)	0	0	0	0	0	0	0	0	0	45	—	—	0
Mt. Dew	1 med (14 oz)	190	0	0	0	0	54	54	0	0	60	—	—	0
Pepsi	1 med (14 oz)	180	0	0	0	0	47	47	0	0	45	—	—	0
DESSERTS														
Apple Pizza	1 slice	260	4	1	0	4	53	14	1	20	250	—	—	0
Cherry Pizza	1 slice	240	4	1	0	4	47	24	1	20	250	—	—	6
Cinnamon Sticks	2	170	5	1	0	4	27	10	tr	0	170	—	—	0
White Icing Dipping Cup	1 serv (2 oz)	170	0	0	0	0	46	39	0	0	0	—	—	0
PIZZA														
Fit 'N Delicious Diced Chicken Mushroom Jalapeño	1 med slice	170	5	2	15	10	22	5	2	80	630	—	—	5
Fit 'N Delicious Diced Chicken Red Onion Green Pepper	1 med slice	170	5	2	15	10	23	6	2	80	460	—	—	18
Fit 'N Delicious Green Pepper Red Onion Diced Red Tomato	1 med slice	150	4	2	10	6	24	6	2	80	360	—	—	21
Fit 'N Delicious Ham Pineapple Diced Red Tomato	1 med slice	160	4	2	15	8	24	7	2	80	470	—	—	12
Fit 'N Delicious Ham Red Onion Mushroom	1 med slice	160	5	2	15	8	22	6	2	80	470	—	—	6
Fit 'N Delicious Tomato Mushroom Jalapeño	1 med slice	150	4	2	10	6	22	5	2	80	590	—	—	6
Hand Tossed Cheese	1 med slice	240	8	5	25	12	30	5	2	200	520	—	—	1
Hand Tossed Chicken Supreme	1 med slice	230	6	3	25	14	30	6	2	150	550	—	—	6
Hand Tossed Ham	1 med slice	220	6	3	20	12	29	5	2	150	550	—	—	6
Hand Tossed Meat Lover's	1 med slice	300	13	6	35	15	29	6	2	150	760	—	—	6
Hand Tossed Pepperoni	1 med slice	250	9	5	25	12	29	6	2	150	570	—	—	2

FOOD	PORTION	CALS	FAT	SAT FAT	CHOL	PROT	CARB	SUGAR	FIBER	CALCI	SOD	POTAS	FOLIC	VIT C
Hand Tossed Pepperoni Lover's	1 med slice	300	13	7	40	15	30	6	2	200	710	—	—	2
Hand Tossed Sausage Lover's	1 med slice	280	12	5	30	13	30	8	2	150	650	—	—	4
Hand Tossed Super Supreme	1 med slice	300	13	6	35	13	30	6	2	150	780	—	—	9
Hand Tossed Supreme	1 med slice	270	11	5	25	13	30	6	2	150	660	—	—	9
Hand Tossed Veggie Lover's	1 med slice	220	6	3	15	10	31	6	2	150	490	—	—	9
Marinara Dipping Sauce	1 serv (3 oz)	45	0	0	0	2	9	6	2	0	380	—	—	5
Pan Cheese	1 med slice	280	13	5	25	11	29	6	1	200	500	—	—	1
Pan Chicken Supreme	1 med slice	280	12	4	25	13	30	7	2	150	530	—	—	6
Pan Ham	1 med slice	260	11	4	20	11	29	6	1	150	540	—	—	6
Pan Meat Lover's	1 med slice	340	19	2	35	15	29	6	2	150	750	—	—	6
Pan Pepperoni	1 med slice	290	15	5	25	11	29	6	2	150	560	—	—	2
Pan Pepperoni Lover's	1 med slice	340	19	7	40	15	29	6	2	200	690	—	—	2
Pan Sausage Lover's	1 med slice	330	17	6	30	13	29	6	2	150	640	—	—	4
Pan Super Supreme	1 med slice	340	18	6	35	14	30	7	2	150	760	—	—	9
Pan Supreme	1 med slice	320	16	6	25	13	30	7	2	150	650	—	—	6
Pizone Classic	1	1220	42	22	100	66	142	18	6	800	2420	—	—	24
Pizone Pepperoni	1	1220	44	22	110	68	138	16	6	800	2560	—	—	2
Thin'N Crispy Cheese	1 med slice	200	8	5	25	10	27	4	1	200	490	—	—	1
Thin'N Crispy Chicken Supreme	1 med slice	200	7	4	25	13	23	6	2	150	520	—	—	12
Thin'N Crispy Ham	1 med slice	180	6	3	20	9	21	5	1	150	530	—	—	6
Thin'N Crispy Meat Lover's	1 med slice	270	14	6	35	13	21	5	2	150	740	—	—	6
Thin'N Crispy Pepperoni	1 med slice	170	10	5	25	10	21	5	1	150	550	—	—	2
Thin'N Crispy Pepperoni Lover's	1 med slice	260	14	7	40	13	21	5	2	200	690	—	—	2
Thin'N Crispy Super Supreme	1 med slice	260	13	6	35	13	23	6	2	150	760	—	—	12
Thin'N Crispy Supreme	1 med slice	240	11	5	25	11	22	5	2	150	640	—	—	9
Thin'N Crispy Veggie Lover's	1 med slice	180	7	3	15	8	23	5	2	150	480	—	—	9

FOOD	PORTION	CALS	FAT	SAT FAT	CHOL	PROT	CARB	SUGAR	FIBER	CALCI	SOD	POTAS	FOLIC	VIT C
QUINCY'S														
BAKED SELECTIONS														
Banana Nut Bread	1 serv (2 oz)	165	7	1	5	2	22	—	—	—	195	—	—	—
Biscuit	1 (2.5 oz)	270	15	4	11	5	29	—	—	—	610	—	—	—
Cornbread	1 serv (2 oz)	140	5	1	0	3	19	—	—	—	340	—	—	—
Yeast Roll	1 (2 oz)	160	4	tr	0	1	29	—	—	—	285	—	—	—
BREAKFAST SELECTIONS														
Bacon	1 serv (0.25 oz)	35	3	1	5	2	0	—	—	—	100	—	—	—
Corned Beef Hash	1 serv (4.5 oz)	210	15	8	45	10	11	—	—	—	795	—	—	—
Country Ham	1 serv (1.5 oz)	90	6	2	35	9	1	—	—	—	1100	—	—	—
Escalloped Apples	1 serv (3.5 oz)	120	2	0	0	0	26	—	—	—	20	—	—	—
Oatmeal	1 serv (1 oz)	175	2	0	0	4	18	—	—	—	285	—	—	—
Pancakes	1 (1.5 oz)	95	3	1	30	3	12	—	—	—	250	—	—	—
Sausage Gravy	1 serv (4 oz)	70	6	2	10	2	3	—	—	—	150	—	—	—
Sausage Links	1 (2 oz)	225	22	8	20	7	0	–	—	—	390	—	—	—
Sausage Patties	1 (2 oz)	230	23	9	45	7	0	—	—	—	350	—	—	—
Scrambled Eggs	1 serv (2 oz)	95	7	2	215	7	1	—	—	—	270	—	—	—
Steak Fingers	1 serv (3.5 oz)	360	25	11	50	16	18	—	—	—	690	—	—	—
Syrup	1 oz	75	0	0	0	0	20	—	—	—	15	—	—	—
DESSERTS														
Banana Pudding	1 serv (5 oz)	240	12	9	10	3	30	–	—	—	240	—	—	—
Brownie Pudding Cake	1 serv (4 oz)	310	5	tr	0	4	66	—	—	—	395	—	—	—
Caramel Topping	1 serv (1 oz)	105	1	tr	0	0	24	—	—	—	120	—	—	—
Chocolate Chip Cookies	1 (0.5 oz)	60	8	1	5	1	8	—	—	–	35	—	—	—
Cobbler Apple	1 serv (6 oz)	255	8	2	5	1	49	—	—	—	285	—	—	—
Cobbler Cherry	1 serv (6 oz)	410	8	2	5	1	55	—	—	—	185	—	—	—
Cobbler Peach	1 serv (6 oz)	305	8	2	5	1	50	—	—	—	190	—	—	—
Frozen Yogurt	1 serv (4 oz)	135	2	1	5	5	25	–	—	—	85	—	—	—
Fudge Topping	1 serv (1 oz)	105	4	1	0	1	15	–	—	—	75	—	—	—
Sugar Cookie	1 (0.5 oz)	60	3	1	5	tr	8	–	—	—	30	—	—	—
MAIN MENU SELECTIONS														
⅓ Pound Hamburger	1 serv (8 oz)	565	33	16	66	32	32	—	—	—	603	—	—	—
Bacon Cheese Burger	1 (9 oz)	663	41	17	87	37	33	—	—	—	997	—	—	—
Baked Potato	1 (6 oz)	115	0	0	0	5	30	—	—	—	0	—	—	—
BBQ Beans	1 serv (4 oz)	114	1	1	0	4	21	—	—	—	604	—	—	—
Broccoli	1 serv (4 oz)	34	0	0	0	3	5	—	—	—	50	—	—	—
Cheese Sauce	1 serv (1 oz)	58	5	2	11	2	1	—	—	—	212	—	—	—
Chopped Steak	1 serv (8 oz)	499	42	20	89	31	0	—	—	—	348	—	—	—
Cinnamon Apples	1 serv (4 oz)	172	5	1	0	0	34	—	—	—	149	—	—	—
Corn	1 serv (4 oz)	96	1	0	0	3	24	—	—	—	271	—	—	—

FOOD	PORTION	CALS	FAT	SAT FAT	CHOL	PROT	CARB	SUGAR	FIBER	CALCI	SOD	POTAS	FOLIC	VIT C
Country Steak w/ Gravy	1 serv (8 oz)	530	25	7	54	32	44	—	—	—	1161	—	—	—
Cowboy Steak	1 serv (14 oz)	580	33	15	176	61	9	—	—	—	1308	—	—	—
Filet w/ Bacon	1 serv (8 oz)	340	17	7	124	48	2	—	—	—	311	—	—	—
Green Beans	1 serv (4 oz)	61	4	1	0	1	6	—	—	—	796	—	—	—
Grilled Chicken	1 reg serv (5 oz)	120	2	0	55	25	1	—	—	—	540	—	—	—
Grilled Chicken Sandwich	1 (9 oz)	324	4	1	55	33	39	—	—	—	1183	—	—	—
Grilled Salmon	1 serv (7 oz)	228	4	1	109	46	1	—	—	—	112	—	—	—
Homestyle Chicken Fillet	1 serv (3 oz)	217	9	2	25	13	21	—	—	—	682	—	—	—
Junior Sirloin Steak	1 serv (5.5 oz)	194	10	5	69	25	0	—	—	—	199	—	—	—
Large Sirloin Steak	1 serv (10 oz)	368	20	9	119	46	2	—	—	—	390	—	—	—
Mashed Potatoes	1 serv (4 oz)	54	6	1	0	1	11	—	—	—	195	—	—	—
NY Strip Steak	1 serv (10 oz)	450	26	13	148	53	1	—	—	—	156	—	—	—
Philly Cheese Steak	1 serv (11 oz)	588	30	11	87	37	38	—	—	—	1684	—	—	—
Porterhouse Steak	1 serv (17 oz)	683	46	23	154	67	0	—	—	—	346	—	—	—
Regular Sirloin Steak	1 serv (8 oz)	285	16	7	71	34	0	—	—	—	317	—	—	—
Ribeye Steak	1 serv (10 oz)	452	29	13	116	48	0	—	—	—	156	—	—	—
Rice Pilaf	1 serv (4 oz)	119	2	0	0	2	23	—	1	—	1283	—	—	—
Roasted BBQ Chicken	1 serv (14 oz)	941	65	17	340	70	21	—	—	—	1548	—	—	—
Roasted Herb Chicken	1 serv (14 oz)	875	65	17	340	70	4	—	—	—	1238	—	—	—
Sirloin Tips w/ Mushroom Gravy	1 serv (6 oz)	196	7	3	64	28	5	—	—	—	578	—	—	—
Sirloin Tips w/ Peppers & Onions	1 serv (5 oz)	203	8	3	63	27	4	—	—	—	793	—	—	—
Smothered Steak Sandwich	1 (9 oz)	429	15	6	69	34	36	—	—	—	846	—	—	—
Smothered Strip Steak	1 serv (10 oz)	622	41	16	148	55	12	—	—	—	239	—	—	—
Southern Breaded Shrimp	1 serv (7 oz)	546	31	6	135	19	47	—	—	—	821	—	—	—
Spicy BBQ Chicken Sandwich	1 (10 oz)	368	1	1	55	34	45	—	—	—	1608	—	—	—
Steak & Shrimp	1 serv (9 oz)	677	39	12	170	48	33	—	—	—	816	—	—	—
Steak Fries	1 serv (4 oz)	358	19	6	0	5	45	—	—	—	245	—	—	—
T-Bone Steak	1 serv (13 oz)	521	35	18	118	51	0	—	—	—	265	—	—	—

FOOD	PORTION	CALS	FAT	SAT FAT	CHOL	PROT	CARB	SUGAR	FIBER	CALCI	SOD	POTAS	FOLIC	VIT C
SALAD DRESSINGS														
Blue Cheese	1 serv (1 oz)	155	16	3	10	2	2	—	—	—	165	—	—	—
French	1 serv (1 oz)	125	12	1	0	0	4	—	—	—	500	—	—	—
Honey Mustard	1 serv (1 oz)	100	6	tr	0	2	10	—	—	—	220	—	—	—
Italian	1 serv (1 oz)	135	14	2	0	0	3	—	—	—	230	—	—	—
Light Creamy Italian	1 serv (1 oz)	65	4	0	0	2	8	—	—	—	485	—	—	—
Light French	1 serv (1 oz)	85	4	0	0	2	13	—	—	—	285	—	—	—
Light Italian	1 serv (1 oz)	20	2	0	0	2	2	—	—	—	485	—	—	—
Light Thousand Island	1 serv (1 oz)	65	4	0	20	2	8	—	—	—	340	—	—	—
Parmesan Peppercorn	1 serv (1 oz)	150	14	0	0	1	4	—	—	—	280	—	—	—
Ranch	1 serv (1 oz)	110	11	2	10	1	1	—	—	—	195	—	—	—
SOUPS														
Chili With Beans	1 serv (6 oz)	235	11	2	15	13	21	—	—	—	920	—	—	—
Clam Chowder	1 serv (6 oz)	180	9	1	0	3	21	—	—	—	835	—	—	—
Cream Of Broccoli	1 serv (6 oz)	170	10	1	0	2	18	—	—	—	770	—	—	—
Vegetable Beef	1 serv (6 oz)	90	2	1	0	5	14	—	—	—	325	—	—	—
QUIZNO'S														
Cookie Oatmeal Chocolate Chip	1	360	17	5	25	5	48	23	1	40	120	—	—	0
Cookie w/ Reese's Pieces	1	360	17	3	20	6	48	22	1	40	130	—	—	0
Sub Honey Bourbon Chicken	1 sm	329	6	1	38	24	45	—	3	110	1494	—	—	—
Sub Sierra Turkey w/ Raspberry Chipotle Sauce	1 sm	350	6	0	25	23	53	—	3	—	1140	—	—	—
Sub Turkey Lite	1 sm	334	6	1	19	24	52	—	3	96	1909	—	—	—
Sub Tuscan Chicken Salad	1 sm	326	6	1	35	21	45	—	4	96	1271	—	—	—
RALLY'S														
BEVERAGES														
Coke	1 serv (32 oz)	264	0	—	0	0	70	—	—	—	26	—	—	—
Coke	1 serv (16 oz)	132	0	—	0	0	35	—	—	—	13	—	—	—
Coke	1 serv (20 oz)	177	0	—	0	0	47	—	—	—	17	—	—	—
Coke	1 serv (42 oz)	372	0	—	0	0	99	—	—	—	36	—	—	—
Diet Coke	1 serv (20 oz)	1	0	—	0	0	0	—	—	—	18	—	—	—
Diet Coke	1 serv (32 oz)	1	0	—	0	0	1	—	—	—	27	—	—	—
Diet Coke	1 serv (42 oz)	2	0	—	0	0	0	—	—	—	38	—	—	—
Fanta Orange	1 serv (16 oz)	150	0	—	0	0	38	—	—	—	11	—	—	—
Fanta Orange	1 serv (20 oz)	202	0	—	0	0	52	—	—	—	15	—	—	—
Fanta Orange	1 serv (42 oz)	424	0	—	0	0	109	—	—	—	32	—	—	—
Fanta Orange	1 serv (32 oz)	301	0	—	0	0	77	—	—	—	22	—	—	—

FOOD	PORTION	CALS	FAT	SAT FAT	CHOL	PROT	CARB	SUGAR	FIBER	CALCI	SOD	POTAS	FOLIC	VIT C
Mr. Pibb	1 serv (16 oz)	113	0	—	0	0	29	—	—	—	16	—	—	—
Mr. Pibb	1 serv (32 oz)	237	0	—	0	0	60	—	—	—	33	—	—	—
Mr. Pibb	1 serv (20 oz)	159	0	—	0	0	40	—	—	—	22	—	—	—
Mr. Pibb	1 serv (42 oz)	334	0	—	0	0	84	—	—	—	46	—	—	—
Root Beer	1 serv (32 oz)	294	0	—	0	0	77	—	—	—	33	—	—	—
Root Beer	1 serv (20 oz)	197	0	—	0	0	52	—	—	—	22	—	—	—
Root Beer	1 serv (16 oz)	146	0	—	0	0	38	—	—	—	16	—	—	—
Root Beer	1 serv (42 oz)	414	0	—	0	0	109	—	—	—	46	—	—	—
Shake Banana	1 serv	399	11	—	38	9	70	—	—	—	223	—	—	—
Shake Chocolate	1 serv	411	12	—	38	10	73	—	—	—	262	—	—	—
Shake Strawberry	1 serv	399	11	—	38	9	70	—	—	—	223	—	—	—
Shake Vanilla	1 serv	320	11	—	38	9	49	—	—	—	197	—	—	—
Sprite	1 serv (42 oz)	338	0	—	0	0	84	—	—	—	76	—	—	—
Sprite	1 serv (32 oz)	264	0	—	0	0	66	—	—	—	59	—	—	—
Sprite	1 serv (20 oz)	161	0	—	0	0	40	—	—	—	36	—	—	—
Sprite	1 serv (16 oz)	132	0	—	0	0	33	—	—	—	29	—	—	—
MAIN MENU SELECTIONS														
Big Buford	1	743	46	—	151	41	35	—	—	—	1860	—	—	—
Chicken Fillet Sandwich	1	399	15	—	42	21	43	—	—	—	790	—	—	—
Chili w/ Cheese & Onion	1 serv (7 oz)	360	22	—	74	23	20	—	—	—	1144	—	—	—
Chili w/ Cheese & Onion	1 serv (13 oz)	669	41	—	137	43	37	—	—	—	2125	—	—	—
French Fries	1 lg (6 oz)	317	16	—	10	5	39	—	—	—	439	—	—	—
French Fries	1 extra lg (8 oz)	423	21	—	13	7	52	—	—	—	585	—	—	—
French Fries	1 reg (4 oz)	211	11	—	7	3	26	—	—	—	293	—	—	—
Onion Rings	1 serv	210	2	—	0	6	45	—	—	—	855	—	—	—
Rallyburger	1	433	22	—	63	20	35	—	—	—	1176	—	—	—
Rallyburger w/ Cheese	1	488	35	—	27	23	35	—	—	—	1376	—	—	—
Spicy Chicken Sandwich	1	437	18	—	40	18	50	—	—	—	887	—	—	—
Super Barbecue Bacon	1	593	31	—	88	29	49	—	—	—	1709	—	—	—
Super Double Cheeseburger	1	762	48	—	154	41	37	—	—	—	1734	—	—	—

RANCH 1

FOOD	PORTION	CALS	FAT	SAT FAT	CHOL	PROT	CARB	SUGAR	FIBER	CALCI	SOD	POTAS	FOLIC	VIT C
MAIN MENU SELECTIONS														
Baked Potato w/ Broccoli	1 serv	510	1	0	0	12	117	8	12	80	50	—	—	102
Baked Potato w/ Cheese	1 serv	790	25	12	50	23	118	9	11	400	850	—	—	60
Baked Potato w/ Chicken	1 serv	610	4	1	55	30	114	7	11	60	135	—	—	60
Chicken Tenders	1 serv	370	15	3	140	52	7	0	0	40	620	—	—	—

FOOD	PORTION	CALS	FAT	SAT FAT	CHOL	PROT	CARB	SUGAR	FIBER	CALCI	SOD	POTAS	FOLIC	VIT C
Fajita Grilled Chicken	1	330	16	7	50	22	25	4	4	350	560	—	—	12
Fruit Cup	1 serv	90	1	0	0	3	21	18	2	20	20	—	—	48
Hot Pasta Grilled Chicken	1 serv	590	10	2	60	37	86	7	6	80	840	—	—	18
Platter Grilled Chicken & Vegetables	1 serv	790	7	2	105	54	129	12	16	100	270	—	—	60
Ranch Fries	1 lg	420	17	5	0	6	62	2	7	—	340	—	—	18
Ranch Fries	1 reg	350	14	5	0	5	51	1	5	—	280	—	—	15
Sandwich American Rancher	1	390	10	4	50	25	51	4	3	150	780	—	—	12
Sandwich Grilled Chicken Philly	1	450	14	5	50	28	53	4	3	200	500	—	—	27
Sandwich Ranch Classic	1	370	5	1	50	26	53	4	3	60	550	—	—	9
Sandwich Spicy Grilled Chicken	1	420	11	2	35	23	58	7	3	60	620	—	—	6
Sandwich Club	1	470	16	6	60	29	53	4	3	150	750	—	—	12
SALADS														
Gourmet Greens	1 serv	220	7	3	10	10	31	7	5	150	370	—	—	27
Gourmet Greens w/ Chicken	1 serv	350	11	4	70	32	31	7	5	200	470	—	—	27
Zesty Caesar	1 serv	180	3	2	5	8	31	4	4	150	350	—	—	36
Zesty Chicken Caesar	1 serv	290	6	2	50	26	31	4	4	150	440	—	—	36

RAX

MAIN MENU SELECTIONS

FOOD	PORTION	CALS	FAT	SAT FAT	CHOL	PROT	CARB	SUGAR	FIBER	CALCI	SOD	POTAS	FOLIC	VIT C
Baked Potato	1	207	0	0	0	—	60	—	—	—	9	—	—	—
Baked Potato w/ Butter	1	306	11	—	0	—	60	—	—	—	94	—	—	—
Baked Potato w/ Cheese	1 serv	270	tr	—	4	—	70	—	—	—	620	—	—	—
Baked Potato w/ Cheese Bacon	1 serv	336	19	—	82	—	70	—	—	—	876	—	—	—
Baked Potato w/ Cheese Broccoli	1 serv	281	tr	—	4	—	71	—	—	—	621	—	—	—
Baked Potato w/ Sour Topping	1 serv	257	4	—	0	—	62	—	—	—	29	—	—	—
BBQ Beef Sandwich	1	399	20	—	40	—	43	—	—	—	1030	—	—	—
BBQ Sandwich	1	716	51	—	102	—	37	—	—	—	1453	—	—	—
Cheddar Melt	1	346	23	—	41	—	26	—	—	—	539	—	—	—
Deluxe Sandwich	1	521	34	—	68	—	34	—	—	—	785	—	—	—

FOOD	PORTION	CALS	FAT	SAT FAT	CHOL	PROT	CARB	SUGAR	FIBER	CALCI	SOD	POTAS	FOLIC	VIT C
Grilled Chicken Sandwich	1	526	33	—	69	—	32	—	—	—	994	—	—	—
Jr. Deluxe Sandwich	1	367	25	—	42	—	25	—	—	—	509	—	—	—
Mushroom Melt	1	599	37	—	104	—	35	—	—	—	1688	—	—	—
Philly Melt	1	537	32	—	79	—	35	—	—	—	1296	—	—	—
Regular Rax	1	388	22	—	54	—	31	—	—	—	708	—	—	—
Turkey Bacon Club	1	680	47	—	76	—	37	—	—	—	1898	—	—	—
Turkey Sandwich	1	484	32	—	50	—	32	—	—	—	1286	—	—	—
SALAD DRESSINGS														
1000 Island	1 serv	130	13	—	10	—	5	—	—	—	230	—	—	—
Blue Cheese	1 serv	145	16	—	25	—	1	—	—	—	300	—	—	—
Buttermilk Ranch	1 serv	175	20	—	0	—	1	—	—	—	240	—	—	—
Catalina Fat Free	1 serv	32	0	0	0	—	6	—	—	—	240	—	—	—
Creamy Caesar	1 serv	140	15	—	5	—	1	—	—	—	290	—	—	—
Honey French	1 serv	140	5	—	0	—	9	—	—	—	210	—	—	—
Italian Fat Free	1 serv	12	0	0	0	—	2	—	—	—	420	—	—	—
Ranch Fat Free	1 serv	30	0	0	0	—	6	—	—	—	300	—	—	—
Vinaigrette	1 serv	30	2	—	0	—	4	—	—	—	150	—	—	—
SALADS														
Garden	1 serv	220	9	—	5	—	12	—	—	—	840	—	—	—
Grilled Chicken	1 serv	160	5	—	50	—	6	—	—	—	1150	—	—	—
Side Salad	1 serv (19 oz)	40	4	—	0	—	2	—	—	—	90	—	—	—
SOUPS														
Chicken Noodle	1 serv	113	1	—	45	—	20	—	—	—	304	—	—	—
Chili	1 serv	158	9	—	31	—	11	—	—	—	421	—	—	—
Cream Of Broccoli	1 serv	95	4	—	1	—	14	—	—	—	512	—	—	—

RED LOBSTER

FOOD	PORTION	CALS	FAT	SAT FAT	CHOL	PROT	CARB	SUGAR	FIBER	CALCI	SOD	POTAS	FOLIC	VIT C
BEVERAGES														
Dannon Spring Water	1 glass	0	0	0	—	0	0	0	0	—	—	—	—	—
Diet Coke	1 serv	0	0	0	0	0	0	0	0	—	—	—	—	—
Hot Tea	1 cup	0	0	0	0	0	0	0	0	—	—	—	—	—
Iced Tea Unsweetened	1 glass	0	0	0	—	0	0	0	0	—	—	—	—	—
Michelob Ultra	1 glass	95	0	—	—	—	2	—	0	—	—	—	—	—
Perrier Water	1 glass	0	2	0	—	0	0	0	0	—	—	—	—	—
Sutter Home Cabernet Sauvignon	1 glass	138	0	0	—	—	5	—	0	—	—	—	—	—
Sutter Home Chardonnay	1 glass	147	0	0	—	—	5	—	0	—	—	—	—	—
MAIN MENU SELECTIONS														
Baked Potato Plain	1	170	2	—	—	—	36	—	4	—	—	—	—	—

FOOD	PORTION	CALS	FAT	SAT FAT	CHOL	PROT	CARB	SUGAR	FIBER	CALCI	SOD	POTAS	FOLIC	VIT C
Baked Potato w/ Pico De Gallo Topping	1 serv	185	2	—	—	—	37	—	5	—	—	—	—	—
Cheddar Bay Biscuit	1	160	9	—	—	—	17	—	0	—	—	—	—	—
Fresh Buttered Vegetables	1 serv	143	12	—	—	—	9	—	3	—	—	—	—	—
Garden Salad	1 serv	52	2	—	—	—	9	—	0	—	—	—	—	—
Light House Broiled Flounder	1 serv	240	5	—	—	—	0	—	0	—	—	—	—	—
Light House Grilled Chicken	1 serv	527	14	—	—	—	38	—	2	—	—	—	—	—
Light House Jumbo Shrimp Cocktail Dinner	1 serv	243	3	—	—	—	2	—	0	—	—	—	—	—
Light House King Crab Legs	1 serv	490	9	—	—	—	0	—	0	—	—	—	—	—
Light House Live Maine Lobster	1 serv	145	1	—	—	—	2	—	0	—	—	—	—	—
Light House Maine Lobster Tail	1 serv	104	5	—	—	—	2	—	0	—	—	—	—	—
Light House Rainbow Trout	1 lunch serv	273	14	—	—	—	2	—	0	—	—	—	—	—
Light House Rock Lobster Tail	1 serv	256	3	—	—	—	2	—	0	—	—	—	—	—
Light House Salmon	1 serv	578	31	—	—	—	0	—	0	—	—	—	—	—
Light House Salmon	1 lunch serv	258	12	—	—	—	0	—	0	—	—	—	—	—
Light House Snow Crab Legs	1 serv	262	5	—	—	—	0	—	0	—	—	—	—	—
Light House Tilapia	1 lunch serv	186	6	—	—	—	0	—	0	—	—	—	—	—
Light House Tilapia	1 serv	346	10	—	—	—	0	—	0	—	—	—	—	—
Seasoned Fresh Broccoli	1 serv	60	0	0	—	—	12	—	5	—	—	—	—	—
Shrimp Cocktail	1 jumbo	146	2	—	—	—	2	—	0	—	—	—	—	—
Wild Rice Pilaf	1 serv	2080	5	—	—	—	36	—	2	—	—	—	—	—
SALAD DRESSINGS AND TOPPINGS														
Large Cocktail Sauce	1 serv	68	0	0	—	—	17	—	0	—	—	—	—	—
Lemon Wedge	1 serv	8	0	0	—	—	2	—	0	—	—	—	—	—
Melted Butter	1 serv	183	21	—	—	—	0	—	0	—	—	—	—	—
Red Wine Vinaigrette	1 serv	49	3	—	—	—	5	—	0	—	—	—	—	—
Topping Petite Shrimp	1 serv	30	1	—	—	—	1	—	0	—	—	—	—	—

FOOD	PORTION	CALS	FAT	SAT FAT	CHOL	PROT	CARB	SUGAR	FIBER	CALCI	SOD	POTAS	FOLIC	VIT C
RUBIO'S														
MAIN MENU SELECTIONS														
Black Beans	1 serv	220	3	1	5	12	37	0	12	150	840	—	—	0
Burritos Baja Carne Asada	1	710	33	13	100	38	63	6	5	400	2270	—	—	18
Burritos Baja Carnitas	1	660	30	12	85	36	64	8	5	400	1950	—	—	24
Burritos Baja Chicken	1	640	28	9	85	42	61	5	5	400	1740	—	—	18
Burritos Carne Asada Especial w/ Black Beans	1	970	37	10	65	40	117	6	13	250	2740	—	—	12
Burritos Carne Asada Especial w/ Pinto	1	950	38	10	65	35	118	6	14	300	2530	—	—	12
Burritos Chicken Especial w/ Black Beans	1	920	32	7	50	42	116	5	13	250	2320	—	—	12
Burritos Chicken Especial w/ Pinto	1	900	32	7	50	37	116	5	14	250	2200	—	—	12
Burritos Fish	1	780	41	8	50	25	76	4	7	200	1220	—	—	15
Burritos HealthMex Chicken	1	520	11	2	40	33	75	6	9	250	1570	—	—	15
Burritos HealthMex Veggie	1	470	8	1	0	15	81	12	13	250	1100	—	—	15
Burritos Lobster	1	660	26	5	190	24	82	5	9	200	1630	—	—	15
Burritos Mahi	1	630	30	9	65	40	58	4	5	200	1070	—	—	12
Burritos Shrimp	1	650	25	7	170	26	77	4	6	350	1680	—	—	6
Carne Asada	1 serv	1430	87	31	170	54	114	3	19	1000	2680	—	—	12
Chips	1 serv	430	22	2	0	5	56	0	7	100	480	—	—	0
Grilled Grande Bowl Asada Black Beans	1 serv	770	37	12	85	41	70	3	11	300	2350	—	—	36
Grilled Grande Bowl Asada Pinto	1 serv	760	37	12	85	38	70	4	12	300	2230	—	—	36
Grilled Grande Bowl Chicken Black Beans	1 serv	710	31	9	75	44	69	3	11	250	1930	—	—	36
Grilled Grande Bowl Chicken Pinto	1 serv	700	32	9	75	38	69	3	12	250	1810	—	—	36
Guacamole	1 sm	170	16	3	0	2	8	1	5	20	75	—	—	9
Nachos Grande	1 serv	1270	79	27	120	37	112	3	19	1000	1790	—	—	12
Nachos Grande w/ Chicken	1 serv	1380	82	28	160	56	112	2	19	1000	2280	—	—	12
Pinto Beans	1 serv	190	3	2	5	4	44	1	16	100	600	—	—	0

FOOD	PORTION	CALS	FAT	SAT FAT	CHOL	PROT	CARB	SUGAR	FIBER	CALCI	SOD	POTAS	FOLIC	VIT C
Quesadillas Carne Asada	1	1010	61	30	175	53	62	4	4	1000	2340	—	—	9
Quesadillas Cheese	1	860	53	27	125	36	60	3	4	1000	1450	—	—	6
Quesadillas Grilled Chicken	1	860	56	28	165	56	61	3	4	1000	1820	—	—	6
Quesadillas Lobster	1	820	54	27	280	48	62	3	5	1000	1820	—	—	6
Quesadillas Shrimp	1	810	54	27	285	48	61	3	4	1000	1850	—	—	6
Salsa Picante	1 serv (1.5 oz)	30	2	0	0	1	3	0	2	0	290	—	—	0
Salsa Regular	1 serv (1.5 oz)	15	0	0	0	1	2	2	1	0	330	—	—	9
Salsa Verde	1 serv (1.5 oz)	5	0	0	0	0	1	0	1	0	230	—	—	0
Tacos Carne Asada	1	220	8	3	25	13	23	1	2	250	420	—	—	6
Tacos Fish	1	310	18	3	20	11	28	1	2	150	280	—	—	9
Tacos Fish Especial	1	370	21	6	35	14	38	2	3	250	360	—	—	12
Tacos Grilled Chicken	1	300	16	4	30	15	23	1	2	250	400	—	—	6
Tacos Grilled Fish	1	310	16	5	30	18	24	2	2	250	230	—	—	12
Tacos HealthMex w/ Chicken	1	170	3	1	15	12	23	2	2	150	270	—	—	12
Taquitos	3	310	11	2	45	16	37	1	5	40	310	—	—	9
SALADS AND SALAD DRESSINGS														
Grilled Chicken Chopped Salad	1 serv	540	33	9	75	33	33	4	5	350	1480	—	—	54
HealthMex Chicken	1 serv	220	4	1	40	22	27	16	2	80	890	—	—	54
Low Carb Chicken	1 serv	480	34	10	95	37	11	3	5	300	980	—	—	24
Serrano Grape Dressing	1 serv (1.3 oz)	10	0	0	0	0	2	1	0	0	160	—	—	2

RUBY TUESDAY'S

FOOD	PORTION	CALS	FAT	SAT FAT	CHOL	PROT	CARB	SUGAR	FIBER	CALCI	SOD	POTAS	FOLIC	VIT C
Cajun Chicken Salad w/ Ranch Dressing	1 serv	636	46	—	—	—	16	—	—	—	—	—	—	—
Peppercorn Mushroom Sirloin	1 serv	947	57	—	—	—	19	—	—	—	—	—	—	—

SBARRO

FOOD	PORTION	CALS	FAT	SAT FAT	CHOL	PROT	CARB	SUGAR	FIBER	CALCI	SOD	POTAS	FOLIC	VIT C
Baked Ziti	1 serv (14 oz)	830	42	21	—	—	—	—	—	—	950	—	—	—
Meat Lasagna	1 serv (17 oz)	730	38	17	—	—	—	—	—	—	1660	—	—	—
Pizza Cheese	1 serv (6 oz)	450	14	7	—	—	—	—	—	—	990	—	—	—
Pizza Pepperoni	1 serv (6 oz)	510	21	10	—	—	—	—	—	—	1240	—	—	—
Pizza Sausage	1 serv (10 oz)	640	29	14	—	—	—	—	—	—	1560	—	—	—
Pizza Sausage & Pepperoni Stuffed	1 serv (11 oz)	880	44	19	—	—	—	—	—	—	2230	—	—	—

FOOD	PORTION	CALS	FAT	SAT FAT	CHOL	PROT	CARB	SUGAR	FIBER	CALCI	SOD	POTAS	FOLIC	VIT C
Pizza Spinach & Broccoli Stuffed	1 serv (11 oz)	710	26	10	—	—	—	—	—	—	1490	—	—	—
Pizza Supreme	1 serv (10 oz)	600	25	12	—	—	—	—	—	—	1580	—	—	—
Pizza Veggie Slice	1 serv (10 oz)	490	12	5	15	20	75	3	1	150	1350	—	—	tr
Spaghetti w/ Sauce	1 serv (18 oz)	630	18	3	—	—	—	—	—	—	1260	—	—	—

SCHLOTZSKY'S DELI

SALADS AND SALAD BARS

FOOD	PORTION	CALS	FAT	SAT FAT	CHOL	PROT	CARB	SUGAR	FIBER	CALCI	SOD	POTAS	FOLIC	VIT C
Caesar	1 serv (7 oz)	150	8	4	—	—	—	—	—	—	510	—	—	—
Chicken Caesar	1 serv (9 oz)	250	10	5	—	—	—	—	—	—	940	—	—	—
Chinese Chicken	1 serv (9 oz)	150	3	1	—	—	—	—	—	—	450	—	—	—
Choice Potato Salad	1 serv (5 oz)	250	18	3	—	—	—	—	—	—	530	—	—	—
Country Style Cole Slaw	1 serv (4 oz)	230	16	3	—	—	—	—	—	—	290	—	—	—
Garden	1 serv (9 oz)	60	1	0	—	—	—	—	—	—	120	—	—	—
Greek	1 serv (12 oz)	220	12	8	—	—	—	—	—	—	560	—	—	—
Smoked Turkey Chef	1 serv (13 oz)	240	10	5	—	—	—	—	—	—	1280	—	—	—

SANDWICHES

FOOD	PORTION	CALS	FAT	SAT FAT	CHOL	PROT	CARB	SUGAR	FIBER	CALCI	SOD	POTAS	FOLIC	VIT C
Light & Flavorful Albacore Tuna	1 (13 oz)	530	16	4	—	—	—	—	—	—	1660	—	—	—
Light & Flavorful Chicken Breast	1 (15 oz)	540	10	3	—	—	—	—	—	—	2370	—	—	—
Light & Flavorful Dijon Chicken	1 (15 oz)	500	6	1	—	—	—	—	—	—	2090	—	—	—
Light & Flavorful Dijon Chicken	1 sm (10 oz)	330	4	1	—	—	—	—	—	—	1370	—	—	—
Light & Flavorful Pesto Chicken	1 (14 oz)	510	9	2	—	—	—	—	—	—	1930	—	—	—
Light & Flavorful Santa Fe Chicken	1 (17 oz)	640	19	9	—	—	—	—	—	—	2300	—	—	—
Light & Flavorful Smoked Turkey Breast	1 (13 oz)	500	7	1	—	—	—	—	—	—	2120	—	—	—
Light & Flavorful The Vegetarian	1 (12 oz)	520	17	7	—	—	—	—	—	—	1330	—	—	—
Original Cheese	1 (14 oz)	850	44	23	—	—	—	—	—	—	2110	—	—	—
Original Ham & Cheese	1 (17 oz)	790	32	12	—	—	—	—	—	—	3430	—	—	—
Original Turkey	1 (17 oz)	1020	51	20	—	—	—	—	—	—	3740	—	—	—
Specialty Deli Albacore Tuna Melt	1 (16 oz)	820	40	16	—	—	—	—	—	—	2290	—	—	—
Specialty Deli BLT	1 (10 oz)	580	24	7	—	—	—	—	—	—	1550	—	—	—

FOOD	PORTION	CALS	FAT	SAT FAT	CHOL	PROT	CARB	SUGAR	FIBER	CALCI	SOD	POTAS	FOLIC	VIT C
Specialty Deli Chicken Club	1 (16 oz)	690	23	9	—	—	—	—	—	—	2400	—	—	—
Specialty Deli Corned Beef	1 (12 oz)	590	15	3	—	—	—	—	—	—	2490	—	—	—
Specialty Deli Corned Beef Reuben	1 (15 oz)	830	35	13	—	—	—	—	—	—	3510	—	—	—
Specialty Deli Pastrami & Swiss	1 (15 oz)	860	37	17	—	—	—	—	—	—	3720	—	—	—
Specialty Deli Pastrami Reuben	1 (16 oz)	920	43	18	—	—	—	—	—	—	3920	—	—	—
Specialty Deli Roast Beef	1 (14 oz)	620	17	3	—	—	—	—	—	—	1730	—	—	—
Specialty Deli Roast Beef & Cheese	1 (17 oz)	850	34	14	—	—	—	—	—	—	2450	—	—	—
Specialty Deli Texas Schlotzsky	1 (16 oz)	820	37	16	—	—	—	—	—	—	3360	—	—	—
Specialty Deli The Philly	1 (16 oz)	820	32	14	—	—	—	—	—	—	2190	—	—	—
Specialty Deli Turkey & Bacon Club	1 (17 oz)	870	40	15	—	—	—	—	—	—	3010	—	—	—
Specialty Deli Turkey Guacamole	1 (16 oz)	680	24	3	—	—	—	—	—	—	2680	—	—	—
Specialty Deli Turkey Reuben	1 (16 oz)	860	39	16	—	—	—	—	—	—	3890	—	—	—
Specialty Deli Vegetable Club	1 (13 oz)	580	24	7	—	—	—	—	—	—	1440	—	—	—
Specialty Deli Western Vegetarian	1 (12 oz)	650	33	14	—	—	—	—	—	—	1160	—	—	—
The Original	1 (14 oz)	940	50	22	—	—	—	—	—	—	3170	—	—	—
SEE'S CANDIES														
Bridge Mix	14 pieces (1.4 oz)	200	12	6	10	2	24	19	1	40	45	—	—	0
Dark Chocolate Bordeaux	2 (1.4 oz)	170	27	1	25	tr	27	25	1	0	40	—	—	0
Dark Chocolates	2 (1.2 oz)	160	10	5	10	2	19	15	2	0	35	—	—	0
Lollypop Butterscotch	1	90	3	2	10	0	17	12	0	—	75	—	—	—
Lollypop Cafe Latte	1	90	3	2	10	0	16	8	0	—	40	—	—	—
Lollypop Chocolate	1	90	5	3	5	tr	14	9	tr	—	40	—	—	—
Lollypop Peanut Butter	1	90	4	1	0	2	14	8	0	—	95	—	—	—

FOOD	PORTION	CALS	FAT	SAT FAT	CHOL	PROT	CARB	SUGAR	FIBER	CALCI	SOD	POTAS	FOLIC	VIT C
Marshmints	3 (1.4 oz)	140	4	3	0	tr	27	21	tr	0	10	—	—	0
Milk Chocolate Bordeaux	2 (1.4 oz)	170	8	5	15	1	27	25	tr	40	45	—	—	0
Milk Chocolate Butter	2 (1.4 oz)	190	9	6	15	1	27	24	tr	20	50	—	—	0
Milk Chocolate Buttercreams	2 (1.4 oz)	180	8	5	15	1	27	25	0	20	50	—	—	0
Milk Chocolate California Brittle	2 (1.3 oz)	220	16	8	25	3	19	17	0	40	115	—	—	0
Milk Chocolate Nuts & Chews	3 (1.7 oz)	250	16	7	15	4	26	19	2	60	60	—	—	0
Milk Chocolate Peanuts	3 (1.5 oz)	230	17	6	5	6	18	14	2	60	90	—	—	0
Milk Chocolate Soft Centers	2 (1.4 oz)	170	9	5	15	1	25	21	tr	20	40	—	—	0
Milk Chocolates	2 (1.2 oz)	160	9	5	10	2	20	17	tr	40	40	—	—	0
Nuts & Chews	3 (1.6 oz)	240	16	6	10	4	25	18	2	60	50	—	—	0
Peanut Brittle	1.5 oz	230	16	6	25	4	21	15	0	0	280	—	—	0
Pecan Buds	3 (1.7 oz)	270	21	6	10	3	22	16	tr	40	30	—	—	0
P-Nut Crunch	2 (1.4 oz)	220	15	6	10	4	21	17	1	40	80	—	—	0
Red Hot Swamp Goo	3 pieces (1.4 oz)	140	4	3	0	tr	27	21	tr	0	10	—	—	0
Soft Centers	2 (1.4 oz)	170	9	5	10	1	25	21	tr	20	40	—	—	0
Truffles Black or Gold	2 (1.4 oz)	180	11	6	10	2	22	13	1	20	25	—	—	0
Truffles Mint	3 (1.6 oz)	200	11	7	15	2	26	22	tr	40	30	—	—	0
Victoria Toffee	1.5 oz	250	19	7	20	4	19	15	1	60	115	—	—	0

SKIPPERS

CHILDREN'S MENU SELECTIONS

FOOD	PORTION	CALS	FAT	SAT FAT	CHOL	PROT	CARB	SUGAR	FIBER	CALCI	SOD	POTAS	FOLIC	VIT C
Kids Catch Chicken Tenderloin + Chips & Kids Side	1 serv	560	11	4	30	20	79	24	1	—	1040	—	—	—
Kids Catch Fish Bites + Chips & Kids Side	1 serv	490	15	8	0	15	84	26	3	—	1270	—	—	—
Kids Catch Sandwich Grilled Cheese + Chips & Kids Side	1 serv	620	19	7	20	14	97	27	3	—	1150	—	—	—
Kids Catch Shrimp + Chips & Kids Side	1 serv	520	11	3	50	14	91	25	2	—	1150	—	—	—

MAIN MENU SELECTIONS

FOOD	PORTION	CALS	FAT	SAT FAT	CHOL	PROT	CARB	SUGAR	FIBER	CALCI	SOD	POTAS	FOLIC	VIT C
Baked Potato Plain	1	210	0	0	0	6	48	3	4	—	25	—	—	—

FOOD	PORTION	CALS	FAT	SAT FAT	CHOL	PROT	CARB	SUGAR	FIBER	CALCI	SOD	POTAS	FOLIC	VIT C
Basket Chicken & Fish + Chips & Slaw	1 serv	620	27	9	45	26	59	5	1	—	1650	—	—	—
Basket Chicken & Shrimp + Chips & Slaw	1 serv	760	25	5	120	33	84	5	1	—	2060	—	—	—
Basket Chicken + Chips & Slaw	1 piece	730	25	7	70	33	60	4	0	—	1650	—	—	—
Basket Clam Strips + Chips & Slaw	1 serv	890	34	6	75	38	113	4	12	—	1670	—	—	—
Basket Clams & Fish + Chips & Slaw	1 serv	740	32	9	50	30	91	5	8	—	1720	—	—	—
Basket Original Recipe Shrimp + Chips & Slaw	1 serv	800	25	4	165	32	107	6	3	—	2470	—	—	—
Basket Popcorn Shrimp + Chips & Slaw	1 serv	750	25	5	180	33	96	5	2	—	2090	—	—	—
Basket Prawn & Fish + Chips & Slaw	1 serv	730	41	10	235	38	61	5	2	—	1600	—	—	—
Basket Prawn Seafood + Chips & Slaw	1 serv	720	40	7	280	36	52	4	tr	—	1200	—	—	—
Basket Shrimp & Fish + Chips & Slaw	1 serv	650	27	8	90	25	83	6	2	—	2060	—	—	—
Basket Shrimp Trio + Chips & Slaw	1 serv	1040	38	9	305	56	123	7	4	—	3020	—	—	—
Clam Chowder	1 cup	120	8	0	5	3	14	1	tr	—	600	—	—	—
Clam Strips	1 serv	270	6	1	30	17	39	0	6	—	490	—	—	—
Fish Bites + Chips & Slaw	6 pieces	490	17	4	0	7	94	0	7	—	1630	—	—	—
French Fries	1 reg	180	6	2	0	3	27	0	0	—	500	—	—	—
Grilled Veggies	1 serv	35	0	0	0	2	8	3	3	—	50	—	—	—
Halibut + Chips & Slaw	1 serv	580	30	5	45	23	51	4	0	—	1280	—	—	—
Homestyle Chicken Tenderloin	1 piece	190	2	2	30	15	13	0	0	—	480	—	—	—
Hush Puppies	3 pieces	240	9	2	0	3	47	0	3	—	820	—	—	—
Original Fish Fillet	1 piece	80	4	4	0	7	12	1	1	—	480	—	—	—
Original Fish + Chips & Slaw	2 pieces	510	29	11	15	18	59	6	2	—	1650	—	—	—
Original Shrimp	9 pieces	220	2	0	75	14	36	1	1	—	890	—	—	—

FOOD	PORTION	CALS	FAT	SAT FAT	CHOL	PROT	CARB	SUGAR	FIBER	CALCI	SOD	POTAS	FOLIC	VIT C
Sandwich Fish + Chips & Slaw	1 serv	800	34	9	20	22	105	14	4	—	1780	—	—	—
Sandwich Fried Chicken + Chips & Slaw	1	1260	49	15	105	52	117	12	3	—	2390	—	—	—
Sandwich Grilled Chicken + Chips & Slaw	1	1070	50	13	145	57	92	12	3	—	1510	—	—	—
Skipper's Platter + Chips & Slaw	1 serv	930	33	9	12	42	122	6	8	—	2550	—	—	—
SALADS														
Caesar	1 sm	150	13	3	5	2	8	4	2	—	300	—	—	—
Caesar w/ Chicken	1 sm	340	17	4	100	27	8	4	2	—	380	—	—	—
Caesar w/ Salmon	1 sm	350	19	4	80	35	8	4	2	—	380	—	—	—
Green Salad w/o Dressing	1 sm	25	0	0	0	1	5	3	2	—	20	—	—	—

SMOOTHIE KING

FOOD	PORTION	CALS	FAT	SAT FAT	CHOL	PROT	CARB	SUGAR	FIBER	CALCI	SOD	POTAS	FOLIC	VIT C
Activator Chocolate	1 (20 oz)	429	1	tr	2	19	90	—	4	230	260	—	—	31
Activator Strawberry	1 (20 oz)	559	1	tr	2	20	123	—	5	250	260	—	—	73
Activator Vanilla	1 (20 oz)	429	1	tr	2	19	90	—	4	230	260	—	—	31
Banana Boat	1 (20 oz)	520	14	8	80	11	93	—	5	—	230	—	—	—
Coconut Surprise	1 (20 oz)	457	6	2	3	8	99	—	5	300	126	—	—	18
Coffee Smoothies Hazelnut	1 (20 oz)	118	tr	tr	1	6	23	—	tr	—	124	—	—	—
Coffee Smoothies Amaretto	1 (20 oz)	118	tr	tr	1	6	23	—	tr	—	124	—	—	—
Coffee Smoothies French Roast	1 (20 oz)	164	tr	tr	1	6	35	—	tr	—	124	—	—	—
Coffee Smoothies French Vanilla	1 (20 oz)	118	tr	tr	1	6	23	—	tr	—	124	—	—	—
Coffee Smoothies Irish Creme	1 (20 oz)	118	tr	tr	1	6	23	—	tr	—	124	—	—	—
Coffee Smoothies Mocha	1 (20 oz)	206	1	tr	1	8	42	—	1	—	215	—	—	—
HeaterZ Banana Nut	1	400	22	—	5	14	67	—	3	—	—	—	—	—
HeaterZ Blueberry Muffin	1	370	26	—	<5	19	15	—	9	—	—	—	—	—
HeaterZ Chocolate Peanut Butter Cup	1	380	13	—	5	23	48	—	6	—	—	—	—	—
HeaterZ Cinnamon Oatmeal Raisin	1	420	3	—	0	19	36	—	9	—	—	—	—	—
HeaterZ Coconut	1	440	13	—	5	17	3	—	3	—	—	—	—	—

FOOD	PORTION	CALS	FAT	SAT FAT	CHOL	PROT	CARB	SUGAR	FIBER	CALCI	SOD	POTAS	FOLIC	VIT C
HeaterZ Coffee Amaretto	1 (12 oz)	177	2	1	1	9	34	—	4	—	126	—	—	—
HeaterZ Coffee French Roast	1 (12 oz)	172	2	1	1	9	33	—	4	—	125	—	—	—
HeaterZ Coffee French Vanilla	1 (12 oz)	177	2	1	1	9	34	—	4	—	126	—	—	—
HeaterZ Coffee Hazelnut	1 (12 oz)	177	2	1	1	9	34	—	4	—	126	—	—	—
HeaterZ Coffee Irish Creme	1 (12 oz)	177	2	1	1	9	34	—	4	—	126	—	—	—
HeaterZ Coffee Mocha	1 (12 oz)	266	2	1	1	10	55	—	5	—	171	—	—	—
High Protein Almond Mocha	1 (20 oz)	402	13	2	17	31	45	—	4	450	245	—	—	10
High Protein Banana	1 (20 oz)	412	14	2	14	34	44	—	6	470	315	—	—	26
High Protein Chocolate	1 (20 oz)	401	13	2	17	31	45	—	4	450	244	—	—	10
High Protein Lemon	1 (20 oz)	390	13	2	12	29	41	—	3	310	177	—	—	21
High Protein Pineapple	1 (20 oz)	380	13	2	12	31	41	—	7	340	206	—	—	27
Hot Coffee Amaretto	1 (12 oz)	168	tr	tr	1	6	35	—	tr	—	125	—	—	—
Hot Coffee French Roast	1 (12 oz)	164	tr	tr	1	6	35	—	tr	—	124	—	—	—
Hot Coffee French Vanilla	1 (12 oz)	168	tr	tr	1	6	35	—	tr	—	125	—	—	—
Hot Coffee Hazelnut	1 (12 oz)	168	tr	tr	1	6	35	—	tr	—	125	—	—	—
Hot Coffee Irish Creme	1 (12 oz)	168	tr	tr	1	6	35	—	tr	—	125	—	—	—
Hot Coffee Mocha	1 (12 oz)	209	1	tr	1	7	44	—	1	—	169	—	—	—
Iced Coffee Amaretto	1 (20 oz)	168	tr	tr	1	6	35	—	tr	—	125	—	—	—
Iced Coffee French Roast	1 (20 oz)	164	tr	tr	1	6	35	—	tr	—	125	—	—	—
Iced Coffee French Vanilla	1 (20 oz)	168	tr	tr	1	6	35	—	tr	—	125	—	—	—
Iced Coffee Hazelnut	1 (20 oz)	168	tr	tr	1	6	35	—	tr	—	125	—	—	—
Iced Coffee Irish Creme	1 (20 oz)	168	tr	tr	1	6	35	—	tr	—	125	—	—	—
Iced Coffee Mocha	1 (20 oz)	209	1	tr	1	7	44	—	1	—	169	—	—	—
Kid Cup Berry Interesting	1	150	0	0	0	1	37	—	2	—	5	—	—	—

FOOD	PORTION	CALS	FAT	SAT FAT	CHOL	PROT	CARB	SUGAR	FIBER	CALCI	SOD	POTAS	FOLIC	VIT C
Kid Cup Choc-A-Laka	1	210	2	0	0	4	44	—	2	—	200	—	—	—
Kid Cup Gimmi-Grape	1	170	0	0	0	1	42	—	1	—	5	—	—	—
Kid Cup Smarti Tarti	1	150	0	0	0	1	36	—	0	—	5	—	—	—
Low Carb All Flavors	1 (20 oz)	225	6	3	6	35	4	—	2	—	207	—	—	—
Low Fat Angel Food	1 (20 oz)	330	1	tr	2	6	79	—	4	170	71	—	—	49
Low Fat Blackberry Dream	1 (20 oz)	343	tr	tr	0	2	86	—	3	100	39	—	—	18
Low Fat Carribean Way	1 (20 oz)	392	tr	tr	0	2	96	—	5	50	18	—	—	109
Low Fat Celestial Cherry High	1 (20 oz)	285	tr	tr	0	1	69	—	4	40	22	—	—	107
Low Fat Cherry Picker	1 (20 oz)	360	1	tr	0	6	98	—	2	—	231	—	—	—
Low Fat Cranberry Supreme	1 (20 oz)	577	1	tr	24	3	139	—	3	190	120	—	—	563
Low Fat Cranberry Cooler	1 (20 oz)	538	tr	tr	0	1	132	—	3	50	95	—	—	4
Low Fat Grape Expectations	1 (20 oz)	399	tr	tr	0	3	96	—	2	30	24	—	—	27
Low Fat Grape Expectations II	1 (20 oz)	529	tr	tr	0	4	129	—	4	50	24	—	—	68
Low Fat Healthy Apple	1 (20 oz)	380	2	1	25	12	81	—	2	—	276	—	—	—
Low Fat Immune Builder	1 (20 oz)	333	1	tr	24	5	80	—	4	190	47	—	—	607
Low Fat Instant Vigor	1 (20 oz)	359	1	tr	0	2	87	—	2	60	38	—	—	70
Low Fat Island Treat	1 (20 oz)	334	1	tr	0	2	81	—	5	40	29	—	—	74
Low Fat Lemon Twist Banana	1 (20 oz)	339	tr	tr	0	3	82	—	2	30	24	—	—	43
Low Fat Lemon Twist Strawberry	1 (20 oz)	399	tr	tr	0	3	97	—	2	50	23	—	—	77
Low Fat Light & Fluffy	1 (20 oz)	389	tr	tr	0	2	98	—	4	60	12	—	—	112
Low Fat Mangofest	1 (20 oz)	320	0	0	0	1	78	—	2	40	50	—	—	42
Low Fat Muscle Punch	1 (20 oz)	339	1	tr	2	6	80	—	4	180	75	—	—	49
Low Fat Muscle Punch Plus	1 (20 oz)	340	1	tr	2	6	80	—	5	180	65	—	—	50

FOOD	PORTION	CALS	FAT	SAT FAT	CHOL	PROT	CARB	SUGAR	FIBER	CALCI	SOD	POTAS	FOLIC	VIT C
Low Fat Orange Ka-BAM	1 (20 oz)	320	0	0	0	2	104	—	3	—	200	—	—	—
Low Fat Peach Slice	1 (20 oz)	341	tr	tr	2	5	80	—	3	160	93	—	—	49
Low Fat Pep Upper	1 (20 oz)	334	1	tr	0	3	80	—	5	60	39	—	—	107
Low Fat Pineapple Pleasure	1 (20 oz)	331	tr	tr	0	2	76	—	4	50	29	—	—	76
Low Fat Pineapple Surf	1 (20 oz)	440	1	0	3	8	104	—	4	—	190	—	—	—
Low Fat Raspberry Sunrise	1 (20 oz)	335	1	tr	0	3	85	—	4	100	39	—	—	62
Low Fat Strawberry X-Treme	1 (20 oz)	370	0	0	0	3	91	—	4	—	40	—	—	—
Low Fat Strawberry Kiwi Breeze	1 (20 oz)	300	0	0	0	4	70	—	2	—	120	—	—	—
Low Fat Youth Fountain	1 (20 oz)	267	tr	tr	0	3	65	—	5	50	40	—	—	73
Malts	1 (20 oz)	887	41	26	166	17	119	—	tr	630	370	—	—	3
Mo'cuccino	1 (20 oz)	420	12	7	75	9	71	—	1	—	190	—	—	—
Peanut Power	1 (20 oz)	502	21	4	2	15	72	—	4	190	88	—	—	5
Peanut Power Plus Grape	1 (20 oz)	703	21	4	2	16	119	—	4	180	87	—	—	5
Peanut Power Plus Strawberry	1 (20 oz)	632	21	4	2	15	104	—	5	200	87	—	—	47
Piña Colada Island	1 (20 oz)	550	11	9	5	16	102	—	6	—	300	—	—	—
Power Punch	1 (20 oz)	430	1	tr	2	6	102		4	190	91	—	—	49
Power Punch Plus	1 (20 oz)	499	2	tr	2	10	113	—	4	330	91	—	—	188
Shakes	1 (20 oz)	875	41	25	166	16	117	—	0	620	359	—	—	3
Slim-N-Trim Chocolate	1 (20 oz)	270	2	1	4	12	55	—	3	340	261	—	—	23
Slim-N-Trim Orange Vanilla	1 (20 oz)	199	1	0	0	5	43	—	1	—	150	—	—	—
Slim-N-Trim Strawberry	1 (20 oz)	357	1	tr	2	7	79	—	3	200	149	—	—	55
Slim-N-Trim Vanilla	1 (20 oz)	227	1	tr	2	6	51	—	2	190	150	—	—	16
Super Punch	1 (20 oz)	425	tr	tr	0	2	95	—	6	70	179	—	—	109
Super Punch Plus	1 (20 oz)	516	tr	tr	0	2	118	—	6	80	195	—	—	109
The Hulk Chocolate	1 (20 oz)	846	29	17	102	23	129	—	6	550	626	—	—	21
The Hulk Strawberry	1 (20 oz)	953	29	16	102	24	156	—	6	400	645	—	—	61

FOOD	PORTION	CALS	FAT	SAT FAT	CHOL	PROT	CARB	SUGAR	FIBER	CALCI	SOD	POTAS	FOLIC	VIT C
The Hulk Vanilla	1 (20 oz)	846	29	16	102	23	129	—	5	390	646	—	—	21
Yogurt D-Lite	1 (20 oz)	335	4	2	43	17	58	—	0	—	271	—	—	—

SONIC DRIVE-IN

ADD-ONS

FOOD	PORTION	CALS	FAT	SAT FAT	CHOL	PROT	CARB	SUGAR	FIBER	CALCI	SOD	POTAS	FOLIC	VIT C
Bacon	1 serv (0.5 oz)	80	7	3	15	5	0	0	0	—	330	—	—	—
Cheddar Cheese Shredded	1 serv (1 oz)	104	9	6	28	6	1	0	0	—	491	—	—	—
Cheese	1 serv (0.7 oz)	70	6	4	15	4	1	0	0	—	350	—	—	—
Chili	1 serv (1 oz)	52	4	2	8	2	1	0	0	—	59	—	—	—
Cone Coat Chocolate	1 serv (1 oz)	143	8	7	0	1	16	15	1	—	40	—	—	—
Green Chilies	1 serv (1 oz)	10	0	0	0	0	3	0	0	—	24	—	—	—
Hickory Barbecue Sauce	1 serv (1 oz)	41	0	0	—	—	10	1	—	—	429	—	—	—
Honey Mustard Dressing	1 serv (1.1 oz)	110	9	1	10	0	9	7	0	—	300	—	—	—
Jalapeños Nachos Sliced	1 serv (1 oz)	5	0	0	0	0	1	0	1	—	302	—	—	—
Malt	1 serv (1 oz)	104	1	0	0	4	22	—	—	—	23	—	—	—
Maraschino Cherry	1 serv (8 g)	10	0	0	0	0	3	3	0	—	0	—	—	—
Marinara Sauce	1 serv (1 oz)	15	0	0	0	0	3	2	1	—	260	—	—	—
Ranch Dressing	1 serv (1 oz)	147	16	2	5	0	2	1	0	—	215	—	—	—
Slaw	1 serv (0.9 oz)	45	3	0	0	0	4	3	1	—	45	—	—	—
Sweet Pickle Relish	1 serv (1.1 oz)	40	0	0	0	0	11	10	0	—	248	—	—	—
Syrup Blue Coconut	1 serv (1 oz)	65	0	0	0	0	16	15	0	—	23	—	—	—
Syrup Cherry	1 serv (1 oz)	64	0	0	0	0	16	16	0	—	0	—	—	—
Syrup Chocolate	1 serv (1 oz)	74	0	0	0	0	16	16	0	—	52	—	—	—
Syrup Grape	1 serv (1 oz)	63	0	0	0	0	16	15	0	—	19	—	—	—
Syrup Vanilla	1 serv (1 oz)	61	0	0	0	0	15	—	0	—	0	—	—	—
Syrup Watermelon	1 serv (1 oz)	71	0	0	0	0	18	12	0	—	28	—	—	—
Thousand Island Dressing	1 serv (1 oz)	150	15	2	10	0	3	3	0	—	170	—	—	—
Topping Pineapple	1 serv (1.5 oz)	108	0	0	0	0	28	28	0	—	27	—	—	—
Topping Strawberry	1 serv (1.2 oz)	38	0	0	0	0	10	9	1	—	0	—	—	—
Topping Strawberry	1 serv (1 oz)	101	4	3	0	1	16	15	0	—	39	—	—	—

BEVERAGES

FOOD	PORTION	CALS	FAT	SAT FAT	CHOL	PROT	CARB	SUGAR	FIBER	CALCI	SOD	POTAS	FOLIC	VIT C
Barqs Root Beer	1 sm	160	0	0	0	0	43	43	0	—	35	—	—	—
Barqs Root Beer	1 lg	333	0	0	0	0	90	90	0	—	72	—	—	—
Coca-Cola	1 sm	139	0	0	0	0	39	39	0	—	13	—	—	—
Coca-Cola	1 lg	291	0	0	0	0	81	81	0	—	27	—	—	—

FOOD	PORTION	CALS	FAT	SAT FAT	CHOL	PROT	CARB	SUGAR	FIBER	CALCI	SOD	POTAS	FOLIC	VIT C
Diet Coca-Cola	1 lg	3	0	0	0	0	0	0	0	—	12	—	—	—
Diet Coca-Cola	1 sm	1	0	0	0	0	0	0	0	—	6	—	—	—
Diet Sprite	1 lg	8	0	0	0	0	0	0	0	—	0	—	—	—
Diet Sprite	1 sm	4	0	0	0	0	0	0	0	—	0	—	—	—
Dr Pepper	1 sm	144	0	0	0	0	39	39	0	—	50	—	—	—
Dr Pepper	1 lg	300	0	0	0	0	81	81	0	—	105	—	—	—
Float Or Flurry Blue Coconut Slush	1 reg	424	12	12	30	61	57	52	0	—	255	—	—	—
Limeade	1 sm	143	0	0	0	0	39	37	1	—	33	—	—	—
Limeade	1 lg	303	0	0	0	0	83	78	2	—	69	—	—	—
Limeade Cherry	1 sm	169	0	0	0	0	46	44	1	—	33	—	—	—
Limeade Cherry	1 lg	361	0	0	0	0	98	93	2	—	69	—	—	—
Limeade Strawberry	1 sm	172	0	0	0	0	47	45	1	—	33	—	—	—
Limeade Strawberry	1 lg	341	0	0	0	0	93	88	2	—	69	—	—	—
Slush Blue Coconut	1 lg	521	0	0	0	0	134	132	0	—	27	—	—	—
Slush Watermelon	1 lg	526	0	0	0	0	136	130	0	—	31	—	—	—
Sprite	1 lg	288	0	0	0	0	78	78	0	—	69	—	—	—
Sprite	1 sm	138	0	0	0	0	37	37	0	—	33	—	—	—
BREAKFAST SELECTIONS														
Breakfast Burrito	1	731	47	22	167	29	47	2	3	—	1535	—	—	—
Fruit Taquitos	1 serv	302	7	1	0	6	51	12	3	—	300	—	—	—
Sunrise	1 lg	368	0	0	0	0	100	94	2	—	72	—	—	—
Sunrise	1 reg	224	0	0	0	0	60	56	1	—	41	—	—	—
Toaster Bacon Egg & Cheese	1	500	20	11	156	28	40	3	2	—	1698	—	—	—
Toaster Ham Egg & Cheese	1	436	19	7	174	33	41	4	2	—	2079	—	—	—
Toaster Sausage Egg & Cheese	1	570	36	14	126	24	44	3	2	—	100	—	—	—
DESSERTS														
Banana Split	1 serv	467	11	10	23	6	75	72	3	—	224	—	—	—
Chocolate Covered Shake Banana	1 reg	625	25	23	46	10	66	60	2	—	383	—	—	—
Chocolate Covered Shake Cherry	1 reg	587	24	23	46	10	59	51	1	—	383	—	—	—
Chocolate Covered Shake Peanut Butter	1 reg	678	34	25	46	12	57	50	1	—	469	—	—	—
Chocolate Covered Shake Strawberry	1 reg	608	24	23	46	10	64	56	1	—	383	—	—	—

FOOD	PORTION	CALS	FAT	SAT FAT	CHOL	PROT	CARB	SUGAR	FIBER	CALCI	SOD	POTAS	FOLIC	VIT C
Cream Pie Shake Banana	1 reg	775	27	21	47	12	92	82	2	—	474	—	—	—
Cream Pie Shake Chocolate	1 reg	795	27	21	47	12	96	86	1	—	525	—	—	—
Cream Pie Shake Coconut	1 reg	721	26	21	47	11	79	71	1	—	474	—	—	—
Dish Of Vanilla	1 serv	265	11	11	26	5	24	19	0	—	212	—	—	—
Float Or Flurry Cherry Slush	1 reg	421	12	12	30	6	57	52	0	—	249	—	—	—
Float Or Flurry Coca-Cola	1 reg	379	12	12	30	6	47	41	0	—	246	—	—	—
Float Or Flurry Dr Pepper	1 reg	377	12	12	30	6	47	41	0	—	268	—	—	—
Float Or Flurry Grape Slush	1 reg	423	12	12	30	6	57	52	0	—	253	—	—	—
Float Or Flurry Orange Slush	1 reg	422	12	12	30	6	56	52	0	—	244	—	—	—
Float Or Flurry Rootbeer	1 reg	386	12	12	30	6	50	44	0	—	260	—	—	—
Float Or Flurry Watermelon Slush	1 reg	427	12	12	30	6	56	53	0	—	258	—	—	—
Ice Cream Cone	1	285	11	11	26	6	24	23	0	—	223	—	—	—
Shake Banana	1 reg	508	18	18	45	10	52	46	1	—	363	—	—	—
Shake Chocolate	1 reg	564	18	18	45	10	64	58	0	—	440	—	—	—
Shake Pineapple	1 reg	615	18	18	45	9	83	74	1	—	403	—	—	—
Shake Strawberry	1 reg	510	18	18	45	9	54	46	1	—	363	—	—	—
Shake Vanilla	1 reg	454	18	18	45	9	41	32	0	—	363	—	—	—
Sonic Blast Butterfinger	1 reg	636	26	23	46	13	59	56	1	—	436	—	—	—
Sonic Blast M&M	1 reg	641	27	24	50	11	64	58	1	—	387	—	—	—
Sonic Blast Oreo	1 reg	638	27	21	45	11	57	56	1	—	602	—	—	—
Sonic Blast Reese's	1 reg	658	30	23	47	13	56	52	1	—	478	—	—	—
Sundae Chocolate	1 serv	362	11	11	26	6	45	41	0	—	270	—	—	—
Sundae Hot Fudge	1 serv	392	15	15	27	6	44	40	0	—	255	—	—	—
Sundae Pineapple	1 serv	399	11	11	26	5	58	53	0	—	242	—	—	—
Sundae Strawberry	1 serv	322	11	11	26	6	37	32	1	—	213	—	—	—
MAIN MENU SELECTIONS														
Ched'R'Peppers	1 serv	256	12	5	28	8	29	5	4	—	1056	—	—	—
Cheese Fries	1 reg	265	17	6	15	6	23	1	4	—	998	—	—	—
Cheese Fries	1 lg	322	19	6	15	7	31	2	5	—	1108	—	—	—
Cheese Tater Tots	1 reg	329	22	7	15	4	28	1	3	—	1396	—	—	—
Cheese Tots	1 lg	435	27	8	15	4	41	2	4	—	1708	—	—	—
Chicken Strip Dinner	1 serv	749	32	5	47	32	86	5	5	—	1973	—	—	—
Chicken Strip Snack	1 serv	272	13	2	35	19	22	—	0	—	760	—	—	—

FOOD	PORTION	CALS	FAT	SAT FAT	CHOL	PROT	CARB	SUGAR	FIBER	CALCI	SOD	POTAS	FOLIC	VIT C
Chicken Strips	2	184	9	1	23	13	15	—	0	—	507	—	—	—
Chili Cheese Fries	1 reg	299	19	6	22	8	24	2	4	—	952	—	—	—
Chili Cheese Fries	1 lg	357	22	7	22	8	32	2	5	—	1062	—	—	—
Chili Cheese Tater Tots	1 reg	363	25	7	22	5	28	2	3	—	1350	—	—	—
Chili Cheese Tots	1 lg	547	36	11	37	9	43	3	5	—	1844	—	—	—
Corn Dog	1	262	17	5	15	6	23	5	1	—	480	—	—	—
Extra Long Coney Cheese	1	666	42	17	87	23	47	9	2	—	1648	—	—	—
Extra Long Coney Plain	1	483	27	10	50	14	44	9	1	—	1182	—	—	—
French Fries	1 reg	195	11	2	0	2	22	1	4	—	648	—	—	—
French Fries	1 lg	252	13	2	0	3	30	2	5	—	758	—	—	—
Fritos Chili Pie	1 serv	611	44	13	53	18	36	3	36	—	816	—	—	—
Hot Dog Plain	1	262	16	5	30	8	22	5	1	—	657	—	—	—
Jr. Burger	1	353	21	6	45	14	27	7	1	—	1294	—	—	—
Mozzarella Sticks	1 serv	382	19	11	50	20	35	5	0	—	1300	—	—	—
No.1 Hamburger	1	577	36	7	37	14	43	7	2	—	753	—	—	—
No.1 Sonic Cheeseburger	1	647	42	11	52	18	44	7	2	—	1103	—	—	—
No.2 Hamburger	1	481	25	5	29	14	43	7	2	—	761	—	—	—
No.2 Sonic Cheeseburger	1	551	31	9	44	18	44	7	2	—	1111	—	—	—
Onion Rings	1 lg	507	35	7	0	12	102	35	10	—	486	—	—	—
Onion Rings	1 reg	331	23	5	0	8	66	23	7	—	311	—	—	—
Regular Coney Cheese	1	366	24	10	52	13	24	5	1	—	962	—	—	—
Regular Coney Plain	1	262	16	5	30	8	22	5	1	—	657	—	—	—
Sandwich Breaded Chicken	1	582	23	4	53	28	66	6	2	—	427	—	—	—
Sandwich Country Fried Steak	1	748	47	12	60	24	56	7	2	—	804	—	—	—
Sandwich Grilled Chicken	1	343	13	2	70	27	31	6	2	—	829	—	—	—
Super Sonic No.1	1	929	66	19	964	28	45	7	2	—	1476	—	—	—
Super Sonic No.2	1	839	56	17	88	28	46	7	3	—	1571	—	—	—
SuperSonic Onion Rings	1 serv	706	10	1	1	16	141	39	11	—	788	—	—	—
SuperSonic Tots	1 serv	485	28	5	0	0	53	3	5	—	1570	—	—	—
SuperSonic Fries	1 serv	358	18	3	0	5	44	2	7	—	963	—	—	—
Tater Tots	1 lg	365	21	4	0	0	40	2	4	—	1358	—	—	—
Tater Tots	1 reg	259	16	3	0	0	27	1	3	—	1046	—	—	—
Toaster Sandwich Bacon Cheddar Burger	1	675	38	11	59	26	60	6	4	—	1786	—	—	—

FOOD	PORTION	CALS	FAT	SAT FAT	CHOL	PROT	CARB	SUGAR	FIBER	CALCI	SOD	POTAS	FOLIC	VIT C
Toaster Sandwich BLT	1	581	41	9	47	19	42	4	3	—	1307	—	—	—
Toaster Sandwich Chicken Club	1	675	29	8	85	39	75	10	3	—	1458	—	—	—
Toaster Sandwich Country Fried Steak	1	708	45	11	60	26	55	4	3	—	944	—	—	—
Toaster Sandwich Grilled Cheese	1	282	12	5	15	12	39	2	2	—	830	—	—	—
Wrap Chicken Strip	1	574	29	5	28	20	55	2	2	—	1071	—	—	—
Wrap Grilled Chicken	1	539	27	5	70	29	40	2	2	—	1035	—	—	—
Wrap w/o Ranch Chicken Strip	1	428	13	2	23	20	53	1	2	—	856	—	—	—
Wrap w/o Ranch Grilled Chicken	1	393	12	3	65	29	38	1	2	—	820	—	—	—

SOUPLANTATION

BREADS AND MUFFINS

FOOD	PORTION	CALS	FAT	SAT FAT	CHOL	PROT	CARB	SUGAR	FIBER	CALCI	SOD	POTAS	FOLIC	VIT C
Bread Low Fat Sourdough	1 slice	150	1	0	0	9	27	0	0	—	240	—	—	—
Breads Indian Grain Low Fat	1 slice	200	2	0	15	11	35	5	0	—	260	—	—	—
Cornbread Buttermilk Low Fat	1 piece	140	2	0	10	3	27	4	2	—	270	—	—	—
Focaccia Big Hearth Pizza	1	140	6	2	10	5	16	2	1	—	220	—	—	—
Focaccia Bruschetta	1 piece	130	6	2	5	4	15	1	1	—	260	—	—	—
Focaccia Pepperoni	1 piece	160	7	3	15	5	19	1	1	—	340	—	—	—
Focaccia Roasted Potato	1 piece	150	6	2	10	6	17	1	2	—	220	—	—	—
Focaccia Sauteed Vegetables	1 piece	150	7	2	10	3	18	3	1	—	230	—	—	—
Focaccia Tomatillo	1 piece	140	6	2	10	5	16	2	1	—	270	—	—	—
Focaccia Low Fat Garlic Parmesan	1 piece	100	3	0	0	2	15	1	1	—	170	—	—	—
Muffin Apple Cinnamon Bran 96% Fat Free	1	80	1	0	0	2	17	13	1	—	110	—	—	—
Muffin Apple Raisin	1	150	7	1	10	2	22	9	1	—	190	—	—	—
Muffin Banana Nut	1	150	7	1	10	2	22	9	1	—	190	—	—	—

FOOD	PORTION	CALS	FAT	SAT FAT	CHOL	PROT	CARB	SUGAR	FIBER	CALCI	SOD	POTAS	FOLIC	VIT C
Muffin Big Blue Blueberry	1	310	12	2	20	5	46	20	2	—	380	—	—	—
Muffin Black Forest	1	230	9	2	10	2	36	19	1	—	190	—	—	—
Muffin Cappuccino Chip	1	160	4	2	25	3	28	15	1	—	160	—	—	—
Muffin Caribbean Key Lime	1	170	6	1	10	2	28	15	1	—	210	—	—	—
Muffin Cherry Nut	1	150	7	1	10	2	22	9	1	—	190	—	—	—
Muffin Chocolate Brownie	1	170	8	2	10	3	22	10	1	—	190	—	—	—
Muffin Chocolate Chip	1	170	8	2	10	3	22	10	1	—	190	—	—	—
Muffin Country Blackberry	1	170	6	2	15	2	27	13	1	—	190	—	—	—
Muffin French Quarter Praline	1	290	15	2	20	4	38	21	2	—	100	—	—	—
Muffin Georgia Peach Poppyseed	1	150	6	1	10	2	20	10	1	—	210	—	—	—
Muffin Lemon	1	140	4	1	10	2	24	13	1	—	190	—	—	—
Muffin Macadamia Nut Spice	1	220	9	2	20	3	33	18	1	—	260	—	—	—
Muffin Maple Walnut	1	230	10	2	5	3	33	21	1	—	230	—	—	—
Muffin Nutty Peanut Butter	1	170	8	1	10	4	21	9	1	—	210	—	—	—
Muffin Pumpkin Raisin	1	150	6	1	10	2	25	14	1	—	210	—	—	—
Muffin Strawberry Buttermilk	1	140	6	1	10	2	21	8	1	—	210	—	—	—
Muffin Sweet Orange & Cranberry	1	200	7	1	5	2	33	20	1	—	220	—	—	—
Muffin Taffy Apple	1	160	6	1	10	2	25	18	1	—	190	—	—	—
Muffin Tropical Papaya Coconut	1	180	7	2	10	2	28	18	1	—	210	—	—	—
Muffin Zucchini Nut	1	150	7	1	10	2	22	9	1	—	190	—	—	—
Muffin 96% Fat Free Cranberry Orange Bran	1	80	1	0	0	2	17	15	1	—	110	—	—	—
Muffin 96% Fat Free Fruit Medley Bran	1	80	1	0	0	2	17	15	1	—	110	—	—	—

FOOD	PORTION	CALS	FAT	SAT FAT	CHOL	PROT	CARB	SUGAR	FIBER	CALCI	SOD	POTAS	FOLIC	VIT C
Muffin Low Fat Chile Corn	1	140	3	1	10	3	27	5	2	—	320	—	—	—
DESSERTS														
Cobbler Apple	½ cup	350	10	2	0	2	64	10	1	—	160	—	—	—
Cobbler Blissful Blueberry	½ cup	380	10	2	0	3	70	45	3	—	230	—	—	—
Cobbler Cherry	½ cup	340	10	2	0	2	61	10	2	—	180	—	—	—
Cobbler Cranberry Apple	½ cup	370	10	2	0	3	58	42	3	—	210	—	—	—
Cobbler Peach	½ cup	360	10	2	0	2	65	40	2	—	220	—	—	—
Cookie Chocolate Chip	1 sm	70	3	1	5	1	10	6	0	—	90	—	—	—
Fat Free Apple Medley	½ cup	70	0	0	0	1	18	12	1	—	5	—	—	—
Fat Free Banana Royale	½ cup	80	0	0	0	1	20	12	1	—	5	—	—	—
Fat Free Frozen Yogurt Chocolate	½ cup	95	0	0	0	3	21	15	0	—	80	—	—	—
Jello Fat Free All Flavors	½ cup	80	0	0	0	1	20	19	0	—	40	—	—	—
Jello Fat Free Sugar Free All Flavors	½ cup	10	0	0	0	1	0	0	0	—	10	—	—	—
Pudding Banana	½ cup	160	4	0	10	4	27	26	1	—	220	—	—	—
Pudding Vanilla	½ cup	140	4	0	10	4	24	24	0	—	160	—	—	—
Pudding Low Fat Butterscotch	½ cup	140	3	0	10	4	24	24	0	—	160	—	—	—
Pudding Low Fat Chocolate	½ cup	140	3	0	10	4	23	23	0	—	220	—	—	—
Pudding Low Fat Rice	½ cup	110	2	1	10	3	20	12	1	—	50	—	—	—
Soft Serve Reduced Fat Vanilla	½ cup	140	4	3	20	3	22	19	0	—	70	—	—	—
Tapioca Low Fat	½ cup	140	3	0	10	4	24	24	0	—	160	—	—	—
MAIN MENU SELECTIONS														
Alfredo Broccoli w/ Basil	1 cup	380	17	8	40	12	45	5	1	—	790	—	—	—
Alfredo Fettuccine	1 cup	390	18	10	50	15	41	4	2	—	580	—	—	—
Alfredo Four Cheese	1 cup	390	13	7	30	19	50	3	3	—	690	—	—	—
Alfredo Roasted Garlic & Asiago	1 cup	330	11	6	25	13	45	5	2	—	650	—	—	—
Alfredo Roasted w/ Rosemary	1 cup	380	14	8	35	19	44	4	2	—	850	—	—	—
Alfredo Southwestern	1 cup	350	16	9	50	10	42	3	1	—	420	—	—	—
Beef Stroganoff	1 cup	340	21	11	75	9	28	4	2	—	590	—	—	—

FOOD	PORTION	CALS	FAT	SAT FAT	CHOL	PROT	CARB	SUGAR	FIBER	CALCI	SOD	POTAS	FOLIC	VIT C
Carbonara Pasta	1 cup	280	8	4	20	10	43	3	2	—	250	—	—	—
Chili Arizona	1 cup	220	8	4	20	14	25	3	7	—	690	—	—	—
Chili Longhorn Beef	1 cup	190	6	3	20	10	25	5	4	—	790	—	—	—
Chili Rock N' Mole	1 cup	240	13	5	25	7	22	6	5	—	690	—	—	—
Chili Santa Fe Black Bean Low Fat	1 cup	190	3	0	0	9	26	2	8	—	580	—	—	—
Chili Texas Red	1 cup	240	8	4	20	14	30	4	7	—	680	—	—	—
Chili Three Bean Turkey Low Fat	1 cup	140	3	1	20	9	19	4	5	—	560	—	—	—
Chili Vegetarian	1 cup	150	3	0	0	5	25	6	6	—	770	—	—	—
Chili Cheatin' Heart	1 cup	300	19	5	60	18	23	6	6	—	800	—	—	—
Chili Deep Kettle House Low Fat	1 cup	230	3	2	15	15	26	4	7	—	560	—	—	—
Creamy Herb Chicken	1 cup	310	17	8	80	8	32	7	2	—	360	—	—	—
Creamy Pepper Jack	1 cup	290	15	6	50	6	35	6	2	—	360	—	—	—
Garden Vegetable w/ Italian Sausage	1 cup	300	10	3	20	12	42	2	3	—	540	—	—	—
Garden Vegetable w/ Meatballs	1 cup	270	7	3	10	11	42	2	3	—	460	—	—	—
Greek Mediterranean	1 cup	290	8	3	15	10	45	4	2	—	520	—	—	—
Italian Vegetable Beef	1 cup	270	6	2	10	10	43	3	4	—	470	—	—	—
Italian Sausage w/ Red Pepper Puree	1 cup	250	10	4	45	6	35	7	2	—	380	—	—	—
Lemon Cream & Asparagus	1 cup	230	9	2	0	6	34	4	1	—	470			—
Linguini w/ Clam Sauce	1 cup	380	10	5	40	16	56	3	1	—	890	—	—	—
Low Fat Oriental Green Bean & Noodle	1 cup	240	3	0	0	7	45	4	2	—	780	—	—	—
Macaroni & Cheese	1 cup	260	6	3	15	10	40	2	2	—	480	—	—	—
Nutty Mushroom	1 cup	390	20	9	45	12	42	4	2	—	410	—	—	—
Pasta Florentine	1 cup	360	10	4	15	18	54	4	7	—	920	—	—	—
Penne Arrabbiatta	1 cup	340	10	6	20	18	43	3	3	—	710	—	—	—
Pesto Cilantro Lime	1 cup	370	21	3	20	9	36	3	2	—	760	—	—	—
Roasted Eggplant Marinara	1 cup	340	10	6	20	18	43	3	3	—	700	—	—	—

FOOD	PORTION	CALS	FAT	SAT FAT	CHOL	PROT	CARB	SUGAR	FIBER	CALCI	SOD	POTAS	FOLIC	VIT C
Smoked Salmon & Dill	1 cup	360	16	8	45	13	41	2	2	—	390	—	—	—
Tuscany Sausage w/ Capers & Olives	1 cup	240	10	4	15	10	29	3	2	—	920	—	—	—
Vegetable Ragu	1 cup	250	5	2	10	9	41	4	3	—	480	—	—	—
Vegetarian Marinara w/ Basil	1 cup	260	4	2	10	10	44	3	3	—	750	—	—	—
Walnut Pesto	1 cup	310	9	3	10	10	42	4	2	—	610	—	—	—
SALAD DRESSINGS														
Bacon	2 tbsp	120	11	2	0	1	5	5	0	—	320	—	—	—
Balsamic Vinaigrette	1 tbsp	180	19	2	0	0	1	1	0	—	190	—	—	—
Basil Vinaigrette	2 tbsp	160	17	1	0	0	1	0	0	—	160	—	—	—
Blue Cheese	1 tbsp	140	14	3	10	1	3	2	0	—	230	—	—	—
Creamy Italian	2 tbsp	120	13	2	10	0	1	1	0	—	300	—	—	—
Fat Free Honey Mustard	2 tbsp	45	0	0	10	0	10	9	0	—	160	—	—	—
Honey Mustard	2 tbsp	150	13	2	10	0	8	6	0	—	230	—	—	—
Italian Fat Free	2 tbsp	20	0	0	0	0	5	4	0	—	340	—	—	—
Kahlena French	2 tbsp	120	9	2	0	0	10	9	0	—	520	—	—	—
Parmesan Pepper Cream	2 tbsp	160	17	3	5	1	2	1	0	—	330	—	—	—
Ranch	2 tbsp	130	13	2	10	1	1	1	0	—	180	—	—	—
Ranch Fat Free	2 tbsp	50	0	0	0	1	2	1	0	—	180	—	—	—
Reduced Calorie Cucumber	2 tbsp	80	7	1	0	0	4	3	0	—	290	—	—	—
Roasted Garlic	2 tbsp	140	14	2	5	1	2	1	0	—	300	—	—	—
Thousand Island	2 tbsp	110	11	2	5	0	3	2	0	—	250	—	—	—
SALADS														
Ambrosia w/ Coconut	½ cup	170	6	3	5	1	30	20	2	—	80	—	—	—
Antipasto w/ Peppered Salami	1 cup	140	10	3	10	5	6	2	2	—	370	—	—	—
Artichoke Rice	½ cup	160	8	1	3	3	21	2	2	—	780	—	—	—
Aunt Doris' Red Pepper Slaw Fat Free	½ cup	70	0	0	0	1	18	13	3	—	480	—	—	—
Baja Bean & Cilantro Low Fat	½ cup	180	3	0	0	9	29	2	5	—	190	—	—	—
Bartlett Pear & Walnut	1 cup	180	12	2	5	4	13	10	2	—	220	—	—	—
BBQ Julienne Chopped	1 cup	190	10	2	20	5	20	5	3	—	430	—	—	—

FOOD	PORTION	CALS	FAT	SAT FAT	CHOL	PROT	CARB	SUGAR	FIBER	CALCI	SOD	POTAS	FOLIC	VIT C
BBQ Smokehouse w/ Bacon & Peanuts	1 cup	190	10	3	10	6	19	4	3	—	530	—	—	—
Caesar Asiago	1 cup	190	14	2	10	5	10	4	1	—	280	—	—	—
California Cobb	1 cup	180	8	2	25	3	4	1	2	—	190	—	—	—
Carrot Ginger w/ Herb Vinaigrette	½ cup	150	12	1	0	1	9	6	3	—	40	—	—	—
Carrot Raisin Low Fat	½ cup	90	3	0	5	1	17	15	2	—	80	—	—	—
Chinese Krab	½ cup	160	8	1	3	5	19	4	3	—	260	—	—	—
Citrus Noodle w/ Snow Peas	½ cup	140	6	1	0	3	19	5	2	—	240	—	—	—
Country French w/ Bacon	1 cup	210	18	6	20	10	7	1	2	—	420	—	—	—
Ensalada Azteca	1 cup	130	9	3	15	6	7	3	4	—	230	—	—	◢
Field Corn & Very Wild Rice	½ cup	170	9	1	0	4	19	3	3	—	420	—	—	—
Greek	1 cup	120	9	3	10	3	4	2	2	—	230	—	—	—
Greek Couscous w/ Feta	½ cup	170	9	1	4	6	19	3	3	—	480	—	—	—
Indian Summer Spinach	1 cup	200	15	4	15	6	11	5	6	—	220	—	—	—
Italian Garden Vegetable	½ cup	110	8	1	0	1	9	2	2	—	240	—	—	—
Italian Sub Salad w/ Turkey & Salami	1 cup	260	17	6	20	9	18	5	2	—	470	—	—	—
Italian White Bean	½ cup	140	5	0	0	6	19	2	4	—	480	—	—	—
Joan's Blue BLT	1 cup	250	16	5	25	6	20	4	3	—	600	—	—	—
Joan's Broccoli Madness	½ cup	180	14	3	10	2	11	9	3	—	250	—	—	—
Lemon Rice w/ Cashews	½ cup	160	7	2	0	2	23	3	1	—	290	—	—	—
Mandarin Noodles w/ Broccoli Low Fat	½ cup	120	3	0	0	3	19	5	2	—	380	—	—	—
Mandarin Shells w/ Almonds	½ cup	120	3	0	0	3	19	4	2	—	360	—	—	—
Mandarin Spinach w/ Carmelized Walnuts	1 cup	170	11	1	0	3	14	11	3	—	150	—	—	—
Marinated Summer Vegetables Fat Free	½ cup	80	0	0	0	1	19	14	4	—	210	—	—	—
Mediterranean	1 cup	150	11	2	5	4	9	2	4	—	430	—	—	—

FOOD	PORTION	CALS	FAT	SAT FAT	CHOL	PROT	CARB	SUGAR	FIBER	CALCI	SOD	POTAS	FOLIC	VIT C
Monterey Blue w/ Peanuts	1 cup	200	12	4	5	3	20	5	2	—	330	—	—	—
Moroccan Marinated Vegetables Low Fat	½ cup	90	3	0	0	2	9	2	2	—	230	—	—	—
Old Fashioned Macaroni Salad w/ Ham	½ cup	180	11	2	10	4	15	3	3	—	360	—	—	—
Oriental Ginger Slaw w/ Krab Low Fat	½ cup	70	3	0	2	2	8	3	4	—	80	—	—	—
Penne w/ Chicken In Citrus Vinaigrette Low Fat	½ cup	130	3	0	5	5	20	5	2	—	380	—	—	—
Pesto Orzo w/ Pinenuts	1 cup	220	17	3	10	4	14	5	2	—	320	—	—	—
Pesto Pasta	½ cup	160	7	1	2	4	18	2	2	—	320	—	—	—
Pineapple Coconut Slaw	½ cup	150	10	3	15	1	14	10	2	—	190	—	—	—
Poppyseed Coleslaw	½ cup	120	9	1	10	1	9	5	3	—	130	—	—	—
Potato BBQ	½ cup	160	8	1	5	2	20	3	2	—	270	—	—	—
Potato Dijon w/ Garlic Dill Vinaigrette	½ cup	150	12	1	0	1	9	6	3	—	40	—	—	—
Potato German	½ cup	120	3	1	0	2	18	3	2	—	260	—	—	—
Potato Jalapeño	½ cup	140	5	1	0	2	20	3	2	—	490	—	—	—
Potato Picnic	½ cup	150	7	1	80	3	19	3	2	—	320	—	—	—
Potato Southern Dill Low Fat	½ cup	120	3	2	5	4	20	2	2	—	300	—	—	—
Ragin' Cajun	1 cup	200	14	2	15	7	12	7	2	—	450	—	—	—
Ranch House BLT Salad w/ Turkey	1 cup	180	11	4	15	6	10	2	6	—	390	—	—	—
Red Potato & Tomato	½ cup	120	10	2	5	2	8	1	3	—	540	—	—	—
Roasted Vegetables w/ Feta & Olives	1 cup	140	11	2	10	2	5	2	4	—	340	—	—	—
Roasted Potato Salad w/ Chipotle Chili Vinaigrette	½ cup	140	6	1	0	3	18	3	4	—	250	—	—	—
Roma Tomatoes Mozzarella & Basil	1 cup	120	9	2	10	4	7	2	1	—	180	—	—	—
San Francisco Herb Rice	½ cup	170	5	2	5	4	25	1	1	—	380	—	—	—
Shrimp & Seafood	½ cup	200	11	2	20	5	20	3	2	—	380	—	—	—

FOOD	PORTION	CALS	FAT	SAT FAT	CHOL	PROT	CARB	SUGAR	FIBER	CALCI	SOD	POTAS	FOLIC	VIT C
Smoked Turkey & Spinach w/ Almonds	1 cup	190	10	2	15	6	20	15	2	—	480	—	—	—
Sonoma Spinach w/ Honey Dijon Vinaigrette	1 cup	210	14	3	10	5	16	8	2	—	270	—	—	—
Southern Black Eyed Pea	½ cup	130	6	0	0	2	18	4	3	—	220	—	—	—
Southwestern Rice & Beans	½ cup	90	3	0	0	1	15	2	3	—	480	—	—	—
Spiced Pecans & Roasted Vegetables	1 cup	180	11	3	15	5	15	7	2	—	390	—	—	—
Spicy Southwestern Pasta Low Fat	½ cup	130	3	0	0	5	21	3	4	—	350	—	—	—
Spinach Gorgonzola w/ Spiced Pecans	1 cup	210	19	4	10	5	5	3	4	—	430	—	—	—
Strawberry Fields w/ Carmelized Walnuts	1 cup	130	8	1	0	3	15	12	3	—	75	—	—	—
Summer Barley w/ Black Beans Low Fat	½ cup	110	3	0	0	4	19	1	4	—	280	—	—	—
Summer Lemon w/ Spiced Pecans	1 cup	220	15	3	10	2	18	13	2	—	250	—	—	—
Thai Noodle w/ Peanut Sauce	½ cup	170	8	1	0	5	17	4	3	—	310	—	—	—
Three Bean Marinade	½ cup	170	6	1	0	4	27	11	3	—	320	—	—	—
Tomato Cucumber Marinade	½ cup	80	5	0	0	0	8	2	1	—	220	—	—	—
Traditional Spinach w/ Bacon	1 cup	160	11	4	40	5	7	3	3	—	310	—	—	—
Tuna Tarragon	½ cup	240	14	2	10	6	21	3	3	—	480	—	—	—
Turkey Chutney Pasta	½ cup	230	9	2	30	14	21	6	2	—	310	—	—	—
Watercress & Orange	1 cup	90	4	1	0	1	12	6	2	—	90	—	—	—
Wild Rice & Chicken	½ cup	300	22	5	20	5	20	4	1	—	490	—	—	—
Won Ton Chicken Happiness	1 cup	150	8	1	10	6	12	4	2	—	220	—	—	—
Zesty Tortellini	½ cup	190	15	2	10	4	18	3	2	—	460	—	—	—

FOOD	PORTION	CALS	FAT	SAT FAT	CHOL	PROT	CARB	SUGAR	FIBER	CALCI	SOD	POTAS	FOLIC	VIT C
SOUPS														
Albino Bean Chicken	1 cup	190	6	3	40	14	18	3	4	—	990	—	—	—
Albondigas Locas	1 cup	210	10	4	30	10	19	4	2	—	860	—	—	—
Autumn Root Vegetable w/ Wild Rice	1 cup	80	0	0	0	1	18	3	2	—	970	—	—	—
Baked Potato & Cheese w/ Bacon	1 cup	290	18	10	50	11	22	6	2	—	670	—	—	—
Be Wild With Mushroom	1 cup	220	16	9	50	4	14	5	2	—	830	—	—	—
Big Chunk Chicken Noodle Low Fat	1 cup	160	3	2	20	15	17	3	2	—	480	—	—	—
Black Bean Sausage Fling	1 cup	350	23	11	60	14	21	3	5	—	1900	—	—	—
Black Bean & Chorizo	1 cup	230	9	3	15	11	27	6	6	—	830	—	—	—
Bombay Lentil Low Fat	1 cup	160	3	2	0	8	25	5	9	—	880	—	—	—
Broc On	1 cup	220	18	11	60	3	13	4	2	—	930	—	—	—
Broccoli Cheese	1 cup	280	20	11	50	11	15	7	2	—	810	—	—	—
Butternut Squash	1 cup	140	6	4	17	3	15	4	4	—	670	—	—	—
Cheese Stuffed Cappelletti	1 cup	130	4	2	10	5	20	8	1	—	1580	—	—	—
Chesapeake Corn Chowder	1 cup	280	16	8	35	7	30	8	2	—	750	—	—	—
Chicken Got Smoked	1 cup	350	21	14	85	11	28	6	2	—	750	—	—	—
Chicken Tortilla w/ Jalapeño Chiles & Tomatoes Low Fat	1 cup	100	3	1	20	12	5	2	1	—	990	—	—	—
Chunky Potato Cheese w/ Thyme	1 cup	210	10	6	30	10	19	3	2	—	480	—	—	—
Classical French Onion	1 cup	130	5	2	5	2	16	12	2	—	1280	—	—	—
Classical Minestrone Low Fat	1 cup	120	2	0	0	4	20	4	3	—	510	—	—	—
Classical Shrimp Bisque	1 cup	240	16	7	70	9	15	5	1	—	230	—	—	—
Country Corn & Red Potato Chowder	1 cup	160	6	3	15	3	24	6	4	—	330	—	—	—
Cream Of Broccoli	1 cup	210	15	6	25	4	14	3	7	—	960	—	—	—

FOOD	PORTION	CALS	FAT	SAT FAT	CHOL	PROT	CARB	SUGAR	FIBER	CALCI	SOD	POTAS	FOLIC	VIT C
Cream Of Mushroom	1 cup	290	21	8	30	10	15	3	2	—	820	—	—	—
Cream Of Rosemary Potato	1 cup	270	19	10	50	3	22	4	2	—	790	—	—	—
Cream Of Chicken	1 cup	260	18	9	55	8	17	7	1	—	770	—	—	—
Creamy Vegetable Chowder	1 cup	200	10	4	20	6	23	6	3	—	610	—	—	—
Devotion To The Ocean	1 cup	220	12	7	100	13	14	7	2	—	800	—	—	—
El Paso Lime & Chicken	1 cup	160	4	1	15	7	24	5	2	—	1250	—	—	—
Field Of Creams Cauliflower w/ Cheese	1 cup	260	20	9	40	5	15	3	1	—	990	—	—	—
Field Of Creams Celery	1 cup	210	15	7	30	2	15	2	2	—	800	—	—	—
Field Of Creams Spinach	1 cup	280	22	10	45	4	18	3	2	—	950	—	—	—
Field Of Creams Tomato Basil	1 cup	220	15	7	30	3	20	4	2	—	990	—	—	—
Fire Roasted Green Chili & Corn Chowder	1 cup	230	14	6	25	5	21	7	1	—	670	—	—	—
Garden Fresh Vegetable Low Fat	1 cup	110	1	0	0	4	22	4	4	—	890	—	—	—
Garlic Kickin Roasted Chicken	1 cup	140	6	3	30	10	10	4	3	—	310	—	—	—
Hungarian Vegetable Low Fat	1 cup	120	2	0	0	2	20	5	2	—	520	—	—	—
Irish Potato Leek	1 cup	250	15	7	35	5	23	7	1	—	940	—	—	—
Living On The Veg	1 cup	90	1	0	0	2	15	3	3	—	380	—	—	—
Manhattan Clam Chowder	1 cup	130	4	1	20	7	16	4	2	—	990	—	—	—
Mulligatawny	1 cup	210	12	5	40	8	18	5	2	—	690	—	—	—
Navy Bean w/ Ham	1 cup	340	10	4	40	35	30	3	6	—	980	—	—	—
Neighbor Joe's Gumbo	1 cup	280	8	3	50	14	36	5	3	—	850	—	—	—
Posole	1 cup	150	6	2	35	12	8	1	2	—	980	—	—	—
Ratatouille Provençale Fat Free	1 cup	110	0	0	0	2	25	3	2	—	600	—	—	—
Roasted Mushroom w/ Sage	1 cup	320	25	11	50	5	20	7	1	—	910	—	—	—
Spicy Sausage & Pasta	1 cup	310	12	5	30	15	36	8	5	—	1270	—	—	—

FOOD	PORTION	CALS	FAT	SAT FAT	CHOL	PROT	CARB	SUGAR	FIBER	CALCI	SOD	POTAS	FOLIC	VIT C
Split Pea w/ Ham	1 cup	350	10	4	40	36	32	3	6	—	980	—	—	—
Tomato Chipotle Bisque	1 cup	240	16	8	40	5	21	7	2	—	1140	—	—	—
Tomato Parmesan & Vegetables Low Fat	1 cup	120	3	1	5	4	18	3	3	—	460	—	—	—
Toot Your Horn For Crab & Corn	1 cup	290	20	12	90	10	18	8	2	—	750	—	—	—
Vegetarian Lentils & Brown Rice Low Fat	1 cup	130	1	0	0	6	25	2	6	—	740	—	—	—
Yankee Clipper Clam Chowder w/ Bacon	1 cup	330	20	10	80	18	21	3	2	—	630	—	—	—

STARBUCKS

BAKED SELECTIONS

FOOD	PORTION	CALS	FAT	SAT FAT	CHOL	PROT	CARB	SUGAR	FIBER	CALCI	SOD	POTAS	FOLIC	VIT C
Baby Bundt Cake Chocolate	1	330	15	7	25	5	45	29	4	—	380	—	—	—
Bagel	1	430	1	0	0	15	92	5	3	20	660	—	—	0
Bagel Cinnamon Raisin	1	440	1	0	0	13	96	14	3	40	570	—	—	0
Bagel Sesame	1	440	3	0	0	16	92	5	6	40	630	—	—	0
Bar Caramel Apple	1	310	16	8	40	3	38	21	2	20	150	—	—	0
Bar Carrot Cake	1	420	25	9	85	4	46	35	tr	—	440	—	—	—
Bar Lemon	1	310	14	8	140	4	44	32	0	—	130	—	—	—
Bar Oreo Dream	1	420	30	15	65	5	33	22	2	—	200	—	—	—
Bar Toffee Crunch	1	430	21	8	50	4	56	37	1	—	420	—	—	—
Biscotti Chocolate Hazelnut	1	110	5	2	25	2	15	8	1	20	80	—	—	0
Biscotti Vanilla Almond	1	110	5	2	25	2	15	8	1	—	75	—	—	—
Brownie Caramel	1	580	36	12	100	5	60	44	2	—	230	—	—	—
Brownie Enrobed Espresso	1	430	25	16	75	5	48	32	3	—	140	—	—	—
Brownie Espresso	1	370	21	13	85	4	43	30	2	—	115	—	—	—
Brownie Milk Chocolate Peanut Butter	1	460	29	9	50	6	45	34	2	—	170	—	—	—
Bundt Cake Lemon Yogurt	1 serv	350	13	5	55	4	56	34	tr	—	250	—	—	—
Caramel Pecan Sticky Roll	1	730	40	7	40	10	75	39	7	150	860	—	—	1
Cinnamon Roll	1	620	29	7	45	9	80	41	3	100	740	—	—	0
Cinnamon Twist	1	320	17	2	25	5	37	13	1	40	280	—	—	0
Coffee Cake	1 serv	570	28	10	75	7	75	45	2	—	310	—	—	—

FOOD	PORTION	CALS	FAT	SAT FAT	CHOL	PROT	CARB	SUGAR	FIBER	CALCI	SOD	POTAS	FOLIC	VIT C
Coffee Cake Apple Walnut	1 serv	320	17	5	55	4	41	28	1	—	330	—	—	—
Coffee Cake Blueberry Walnut	1 serv	340	18	5	60	4	43	30	1	—	360	—	—	—
Coffee Cake Cinnamon Walnut	1 serv	360	18	5	65	4	46	31	1	—	390	—	—	—
Coffee Cake Crumble Berry	1 serv	520	26	10	75	6	69	40	2	—	350	—	—	—
Coffee Cake Hazelnut	1 serv	630	35	14	125	9	74	43	2	—	460	—	—	—
Coffee Cake Sour Cream	1 serv	420	25	12	95	5	43	29	1	—	260	—	—	—
Cookie Black And White	1	430	17	3	50	4	68	53	2	—	210	—	—	—
Cookie Double Chocolate Chunk	1 serv	430	21	7	15	5	58	37	3	—	350	—	—	—
Cookie Oatmean Raisin	1	390	15	2	15	6	65	34	3	—	340	—	—	—
Cookie White Chocolate Macadamia Nut	1	470	27	8	15	6	54	34	2	—	350	—	—	—
Crisp Cinnamon Twist	1	60	2	1	0	0	9	4	0	100	25	—	—	0
Croissant Almond	1	330	18	7	30	6	39	16	2	—	230	—	—	—
Croissant Butter w/ Apricot Glaze	1	320	17	2	25	5	37	13	1	—	280	—	—	—
Croissant Raspberry & Cream Cheese	1	260	12	7	30	4	34	11	1	—	270	—	—	—
Crumb Cake	1 serv	670	32	15	115	8	89	44	1	—	360	—	—	—
Crumb Cake Key Lime	1 serv	550	27	10	190	8	71	44	1	—	370	—	—	—
Danish Apple w/ Mocha Swirls	1	370	19	2	25	5	44	18	2	—	330	—	—	—
Danish Cheese w/ Mocha Swirls	1	460	28	7	50	7	44	18	1	—	400	—	—	—
Danish Raspberry w/ Mocha Swirls	1	370	19	2	25	5	45	17	1	—	380	—	—	—
Graham Dark Chocolate	1	140	8	5	<5	2	17	12	tr	—	60	—	—	—
Graham Milk Chocolate	1	140	8	5	<5	2	17	12	tr	20	60	—	—	0
Madeleine	1	80	4	2	25	1	11	6	0	—	30	—	—	—
Muffin Blueberry	1	380	19	4	70	5	49	28	1	20	380	—	—	0

FOOD	PORTION	CALS	FAT	SAT FAT	CHOL	PROT	CARB	SUGAR	FIBER	CALCI	SOD	POTAS	FOLIC	VIT C
Muffin Chocolate Cream Cheese	1	450	24	6	80	5	53	31	1	60	420	—	—	0
Muffin Cranberry Orange	1	410	20	4	70	5	53	31	2	—	400	—	—	—
Muffin Morning Sunrise	1	330	12	5	35	5	54	32	2	—	550	—	—	—
Pound Cake Banana	1 serv	360	18	11	100	4	47	24	1	—	380	—	—	—
Pound Cake Cranberry Walnut	1 serv	390	21	9	110	6	45	26	1	—	310	—	—	—
Pound Cake Iced Carrot	1 serv	540	13	3	35	5	101	64	3	—	320	—	—	—
Pound Cake Iced Lemon	1 serv	500	23	12	145	6	69	46	tr	—	390	—	—	—
Pound Cake Marble	1 serv	400	21	11	130	6	49	29	tr	—	370	—	—	—
Pound Cake Orange Poppy	1 serv	490	27	12	140	8	55	32	2	—	380	—	—	—
Pound Cake Pumpkin	1 serv	310	12	2	65	5	47	27	2	—	360	—	—	—
Pound Cake Zucchini	1 serv	370	19	2	55	5	47	27	2	—	250	—	—	—
Pullman Banana	1 serv	400	17	5	65	5	57	31	2	—	320	—	—	—
Pullman Chocolate	1	380	17	7	55	5	54	33	2	—	270	—	—	—
Pullman Cranberry Walnut	1	360	15	4	25	5	53	28	2	—	240	—	—	—
Pullman Lemon Glazed	1	370	15	9	90	5	55	31	tr	—	180	—	—	—
Pullman Marble Chocolate Chip	1	440	20	12	95	6	61	37	1	—	250	—	—	—
Pullman Orange Poppy Cheese	1	450	22	13	110	7	55	34	1	—	290	—	—	—
Pullman Pumpkin	1	370	17	3	60	4	51	22	2	—	340	—	—	—
Scone Blueberry	1	460	18	4	50	5	68	24	3	—	400	—	—	—
Scone Butterscotch Pecan	1	520	27	11	50	7	64	22	2	—	390	—	—	—
Scone Cinnamon Chip w/ Icing	1	510	23	10	50	6	71	29	2	—	480	—	—	—
Scone Maple Oat w/ Icing	1	490	22	9	45	7	69	28	2	—	430	—	—	—
Scone Apricot Currant	1	450	17	8	60	7	67	17	3	40	360	—	—	0

FOOD	PORTION	CALS	FAT	SAT FAT	CHOL	PROT	CARB	SUGAR	FIBER	CALCI	SOD	POTAS	FOLIC	VIT C
Scone Raspberry	1	440	18	8	50	7	65	20	2	20	360	—	—	4
Shortbread	1	100	6	3	15	1	12	4	0	—	65	—	—	—
BEVERAGES														
Apple Juice	1 grande	230	0	0	0	0	57	52	0	—	20	—	—	—
Blended Coffee Of The Week	1 grande	10	0	0	0	0	2	0	0	—	0	—	—	—
Cafe Americano	1 grande	150	0	0	0	1	3	0	0	—	15	—	—	—
Cafe Au Lait Nonfat Milk	1 grande	90	0	0	<5	9	13	11	0	—	120	—	—	—
Cafe Au Lait Soy Milk	1 grande	110	3	0	0	6	15	12	tr	—	90	—	—	—
Cafe Latte Whole Milk	1 grande	260	14	9	55	14	21	19	0	—	200	—	—	—
Cafe Misto Cafe Au Lait Whole Milk	1 grande	140	8	5	30	8	11	11	0	—	115	—	—	—
Cafe Mocha Whip Whole Milk	1 grande	400	22	13	80	13	42	33	2	—	160	—	—	—
Caffe Latte Soy Milk	1 grande	210	6	1	0	11	28	21	2	—	160	—	—	—
Caffe Mocha No Whip Whole Milk	1 grande	300	12	7	40	13	41	31	2	—	150	—	—	—
Caffe Mocha No Whip Nonfat Milk	1 grande	230	2	0	5	14	43	32	2	—	160	—	—	—
Caffe Mocha No Whip Soy Milk	1 grande	260	6	1	0	10	46	33	3	—	120	—	—	—
Caffe Mocha Whip Nonfat Milk	1 grande	330	12	7	45	14	44	34	2	—	170	—	—	—
Caffe Mocha Whip Soy Milk	1 grande	360	16	7	40	10	48	35	3	—	125	—	—	—
Caffe Latte Nonfat Milk	1 grande	160	0	0	10	16	24	20	0	—	220			
Cappuccino Nonfat Milk	1 grande	100	0	0	<5	9	14	11	0	—	125	—		—
Cappuccino Soy Milk	1 grande	120	3	0	0	6	17	12	tr	—	90	—	—	—
Caramel Mocha No Whip Soy Milk	1 grande	340	6	1	0	10	66	52	3	—	120	—	—	—
Caramel Macchiato Nonfat Milk	1 grande	230	2	2	15	14	40	35	0	—	200	—	—	—
Caramel Macchiato Soy Milk	1 grande	300	8	2	5	9	49	36	1	—	160	—	—	—

FOOD	PORTION	CALS	FAT	SAT FAT	CHOL	PROT	CARB	SUGAR	FIBER	CALCI	SOD	POTAS	FOLIC	VIT C
Caramel Macchiato Whole Milk	1 grande	320	14	8	55	12	37	34	0	—	190	—	—	—
Caramel Mocha Whip Soy Milk	1 grande	440	16	7	40	10	68	54	3	—	125	—	—	—
Caramel Apple Cider No Whip	1 grande	300	0	0	0	0	72	64	0	—	15	—	—	—
Caramel Apple Cider Whip	1 grande	410	10	7	40	0	76	68	0	—	30	—	—	—
Caramel Mocha No Whip Whole Milk	1 grande	370	11	6	35	13	61	50	2	—	140	—	—	—
Caramel Mocha Whip Nonfat Milk	1 grande	410	12	7	45	14	65	52	2	—	160	—	—	—
Caramel Mocha Whip Whole Milk	1 grande	470	21	12	75	13	63	52	2	—	150	—	—	—
Caramel Mocha Whip Nonfat Milk	1 grande	300	3	0	5	14	63	51	2	—	150	—	—	—
Chocolate Nonfat Milk	1 grande	240	2	0	10	16	45	36	2	—	200	—	—	—
Chocolate Whole Milk	1 grande	340	15	8	50	15	42	35	2	—	—	—	—	—
Cinnamon Spice Mocha No Whip Nonfat Milk	1 grande	250	1	0	5	14	47	40	tr	—	180	—	—	—
Cinnamon Spice Mocha No Whip Whole Milk	1 grande	330	12	7	45	13	45	45	tr	—	170	—	—	—
Cinnamon Spice Mocha Whip Nonfat Milk	1 grande	350	11	6	45	14	49	41	tr	—	190	—	—	—
Cinnamon Spice Mocha Whip Whole Milk	1 grande	430	22	14	85	13	47	41	tr	—	180	—	—	—
Cinnamon Spice No Whip Soy Milk	1 grande	290	6	1	0	10	51	41	2	—	130	—	—	—
Cinnamon Spice Whip Soy Milk	1 grande	390	15	7	40	10	53	42	2	—	140	—	—	—
Espresso Decaf Coffee Of The Week	1 grande	10	0	0	0	0	2	0	0	—	0	—	—	—
Frappuccino Blended Coffee	1 grande	230	3	2	10	5	46	38	0	—	220	—	—	—

FOOD	PORTION	CALS	FAT	SAT FAT	CHOL	PROT	CARB	SUGAR	FIBER	CALCI	SOD	POTAS	FOLIC	VIT C
Frappuccino Blended Coffee Mocha Coconut No Whip Whole Milk	1 grande	400	10	7	15	7	75	60	2	—	310	—	—	—
Frappuccino Caramel Blended Coffee No Whip	1 grande	280	4	2	15	5	57	48	0	—	250	—	—	—
Frappuccino Caramel Blended Coffee Whip	1 grande	430	16	10	65	6	61	52	0	—	270	—	—	—
Frappuccino Chocolate Blended Creme Whip	1 grande	530	19	10	55	18	75	65	1	—	420	—	—	—
Frappuccino Chocolate Blended Creme No Whip	1 grande	400	7	2	<5	18	73	63	1	—	410	—	—	—
Frappuccino Chocolate Brownie Blended Coffee No Whip	1 grande	370	9	6	15	7	69	56	2	—	310	—	—	—
Frappuccino Chocolate Brownie Blended Coffee Whip	1 grande	510	22	15	65	7	72	59	2		320	—	—	—
Frappuccino Chocolate Malt Blended Creme No Whip	1 grande	470	10	4	15	15	87	69	2	—	420	—	—	—
Frappuccino Chocolate Malt Blended Creme Whip	1 grande	610	22	11	65	15	90	72	2	—	430	—	—	—
Frappuccino Mocha Blended Coffee No Whip	1 grande	290	4	2	15	6	58	48	0	—	250	—	—	—
Frappuccino Mocha Blended Coffee Whip	1 grande	420	16	10	65	6	61	51	0	—	260	—	—	—
Frappuccino Mocha Coconut Blended Coffee Whip	1 grande	550	22	16	65	7	80	64	2	—	320	—	—	—
Frappuccino Mocha Malt Blended Coffee No Whip	1 grande	430	7	4	20	14	91	65	1	—	390	—	—	—

FOOD	PORTION	CALS	FAT	SAT FAT	CHOL	PROT	CARB	SUGAR	FIBER	CALCI	SOD	POTAS	FOLIC	VIT C
Frappuccino Mocha Malt Blended Coffee Whip	1 grande	570	20	12	75	14	95	68	1	—	400	—	—	—
Frappuccino Tazo Chai Creme Blended Tea No Whip	1 grande	370	5	1	<5	15	69	64	0	—	370	—	—	—
Frappuccino Tazo Chai Creme Blended Tea Whip	1 grande	500	17	9	55	15	72	66	0	—	380	—	—	—
Frappuccino Tazoberry Blended Tea	1 grande	190	0	0	0	tr	49	46	tr	—	40	—	—	—
Frappuccino Tazoberry Creme Blended Tea No Whip	1 grande	330	2	0	0	6	74	60	tr	—	180	—	—	—
Frappuccino Tazoberry Creme Blended Tea Whip	1 grande	460	14	9	50	6	76	71	tr	—	190	—	—	—
Frappuccino Vanilla Blended Creme No Whip	1 grande	350	5	1	<5	15	64	60	0	—	370	—	—	—
Frappuccino Vanilla Blended Creme Whip	1 grande	480	17	9	55	15	66	62	0	—	380	—	—	—
Frappuccino White Chocolate Mocha Blended Coffee No Whip	1 grande	320	5	3	15	6	62	54	0	—	280	—	—	—
Frappuccino White Chocolate Mocha Blended Coffee Whip	1 grande	450	17	11	65	6	65	56	0	—	290	—	—	—
Hot Chocolate No Whip Whole Milk	1 grande	340	15	8	50	15	42	35	2	—	190	—	—	—
Hot Chocolate No Whip Nonfat Milk	1 grande	240	2	0	10	16	45	36	2	—	200	—	—	—
Hot Chocolate Whip Nonfat Milk	1 grande	340	12	7	45	16	47	37	2	—	210	—	—	—
Hot Chocolate Whip Whole Milk	1 grande	440	24	15	90	15	44	37	2	—	200	—	—	—

FOOD	PORTION	CALS	FAT	SAT FAT	CHOL	PROT	CARB	SUGAR	FIBER	CALCI	SOD	POTAS	FOLIC	VIT C
Iced Caffe Mocha Whip Milk	1 grande	350	20	12	75	9	37	27	2	—	105	—	—	—
Iced Caffe Latte Whole Milk	1 grande	160	8	5	30	8	13	11	0	—	120	—	—	—
Iced Caffe Mocha Whip Nonfat Milk	1 grande	310	14	9	55	9	38	28	2	—	110	—	—	—
Iced Caffe Mocha Whip Soy Milk	1 grande	330	17	9	50	7	40	28	3	—	85	—	—	—
Iced Caffe Americano	1 grande	20	0	0	0	1	3	0	0	—	15	—	—	—
Iced Caffe Mocha No Whip Whole Milk	1 grande	220	8	4	25	9	35	25	2	—	95	—	—	—
Iced Caffe Latte Nonfat Milk	1 grande	100	0	0	<5	9	14	11	0	—	130	—	—	—
Iced Caffe Latte Soy Milk	1 grande	120	5	0	0	6	17	12	tr	—	95	—	—	—
Iced Caffe Mocha No Whip Nonfat Milk	1 grande	180	2	0	<5	9	36	26	2	—	100	—	—	—
Iced Caffe Mocha No Whip Soy Milk	1 grande	200	5	1	0	7	38	26	3	—	75	—	—	—
Iced Caramel Macchiato Nonfat Milk	1 grande	100	1	1	10	11	36	32	0	—	160	—	—	—
Iced Caramel Macchiato Soy Milk	1 grande	230	5	1	<5	7	39	33	1	—	120	—	—	—
Iced Caramel Macchiato Whole Milk	1 grande	270	10	6	40	10	34	31	0	—	150	—	—	—
Iced Shaken Coffee	1 grande	80	0	0	0	0	20	19	0	—	5	—	—	—
Iced Tazo Chai Nonfat Milk	1 grande	230	0	0	0	8	50	45	0	—	120	—	—	—
Iced Tazo Chai Whole Milk	1 grande	270	7	4	25	7	48	45	0	—	110	—	—	—
Iced White Chocolate Mocha No Whip Soy Milk	1 grande	340	8	5	<5	9	59	53	tr	—	190	—	—	—
Iced White Chocolate Mocha No Whip Whole Milk	1 grande	360	11	8	25	11	56	52	0	—	210	—	—	—

FOOD	PORTION	CALS	FAT	SAT FAT	CHOL	PROT	CARB	SUGAR	FIBER	CALCI	SOD	POTAS	FOLIC	VIT C
Iced White Chocolate Mocha Whip Nonfat Milk	1 grande	450	18	12	55	11	59	55	0	—	220	—	—	—
Iced White Chocolate Mocha Whip Soy Milk	1 grande	470	20	13	55	9	61	55	tr	—	200	—	—	—
Iced White Chocolate Mocha Whip Whole Milk	1 grande	490	24	16	75	11	58	54	0	—	220	—	—	—
Iced White Chocolate No Whip Nonfat Milk	1 grande	320	6	5	5	11	57	53	0	—	210	—	—	—
Milk Nonfat	1 grande	160	0	0	10	16	23	22	0	—	230	—	—	—
Steamed Apple Cider	1 grande	230	0	0	0	0	57	52	0	—	20	—	—	—
Steamed Nonfat Milk	1 grande	160	0	0	0	16	23	22	0	—	230	—	—	—
Steamed Whole Milk	1 grande	270	15	9	60	15	21	21	0	—	220	—	—	—
Tazo Chai Whole Milk	1 grande	290	7	5	30	8	50	46	0	—	120	—	—	—
Tazo Chai Nonfat Milk	1 grande	230	0	0	5	8	51	47	0	—	125	—	—	—
Tazo Iced Tea	1 grande	80	0	0	0	0	20	19	0	—	0	—	—	—
Tazo Tea Lemonade	1 grande	120	0	0	0	0	31	29	0	—	15	—	—	—
Vanilla Creme Whip Nonfat Milk	1 grande	340	9	6	50	16	44	42	0	—	230	—	—	—
Vanilla Creme Whip Whole Milk	1 grande	440	24	15	95	14	42	41	0	—	220	—	—	—
Vanilla Creme No Whip Nonfat Milk	1 grande	240	0	0	10	16	43	40	0	—	230	—	—	—
Vanille Creme No Whip Whole Milk	1 grande	340	14	9	60	14	40	39	0	—	210	—	—	—
White Chocolate Mocha No Whip Nonfat Milk	1 grande	340	5	4	10	16	58	54	0	—	260	—	—	—
White Chocolate Mocha No Whip Whole Milk	1 grande	410	15	10	45	14	56	53	0	—	250	—	—	—

FOOD	PORTION	CALS	FAT	SAT FAT	CHOL	PROT	CARB	SUGAR	FIBER	CALCI	SOD	POTAS	FOLIC	VIT C
White Chocolate Mocha Whip Nonfat Milk	1 grande	440	14	10	45	16	60	56	0	—	270	—	—	—
White Chocolate Mocha Whip Milk	1 grande	510	24	16	80	14	58	55	0	—	260	—	—	—
White Chocolate No Whip Soy Milk	1 grande	370	14	22	0	12	62	55	1	—	220	—	—	—
White Chocolate Whip Soy Milk	1 grande	440	15	8	20	13	65	58	1	—	250	—	—	—
White Hot Chocolate No Whip Nonfat Milk	1 grande	390	6	5	10	18	66	63	0	—	320	—	—	—
White Hot Chocolate No Whip Whole Milk	1 grande	480	18	12	55	17	63	62	0	—	300	—	—	—
White Hot Chocolate Whip Nonfat Milk	1 grande	490	15	11	50	18	68	65	0	—	330	—	—	—
White Hot Chocolate Whip Whole Milk	1 grande	580	28	19	95	17	65	64	0	—	310	—	—	—
Whole Milk	1 grande	270	15	9	60	15	21	21	0	—	220	—	—	—
TOPPINGS														
Caramel	1 tbsp	15	1	0	0	0	2	2	0	0	5	—	—	0
Chocolate	1 tsp	5	0	0	0	0	1	1	0	0	0	—	—	0
Flavored Sugar Free Syrup	1 pump	0	0	0	0	0	0	0	0	0	0	—	—	0
Flavored Syrup	1 pump	20	0	0	0	0	5	5	0	0	0	—	—	0
Mocha Syrup	1 pump	25	1	0	0	1	6	4	0	0	0	—	—	0
Sprinkles	1 serv	0	0	0	0	0	tr	tr	0	0	0	—	—	0

STEAK ESCAPE

FOOD	PORTION	CALS	FAT	SAT FAT	CHOL	PROT	CARB	SUGAR	FIBER	CALCI	SOD	POTAS	FOLIC	VIT C
BEVERAGES														
Coca Cola	12 oz	110	0	0	0	0	29	—	—	—	10	—	—	—
Coca Cola	44 oz	430	0	0	0	0	118	—	—	—	40	—	—	—
Diet Coke	44 oz	0	0	0	0	0	0	0	0	—	75	—	—	—
Diet Coke	12 oz	0	0	0	0	0	0	0	0	—	20	—	—	—
Hi-C Fruit Punch	44 oz	452	0	0	0	0	123	—	—	—	60	—	—	—
Hi-C Fruit Punch	12 oz	116	0	0	0	0	30	—	—	—	15	—	—	—
Lemonade	12 oz	126	0	0	0	0	34	—	—	—	0	—	—	—
Lemonade	44 oz	488	0	0	0	0	130	—	—	—	2	—	—	—
Sprite	44 oz	430	0	0	0	0	114	—	—	—	157	—	—	—
Sprite	12 oz	110	0	0	0	0	28	—	—	—	40	—	—	—
CHILDREN'S MENU SELECTIONS														
Kids Fries	1 serv	249	13	—	0	4	34	—	—	—	205	—	—	—

FOOD	PORTION	CALS	FAT	SAT FAT	CHOL	PROT	CARB	SUGAR	FIBER	CALCI	SOD	POTAS	FOLIC	VIT C
Kids Tenders	2 pieces	240	11	—	35	15	21	—	—	—	1050	—	—	—
Sandwich Chicken	1	205	7	—	32	12	32	—	—	—	470	—	—	—
Sandwich Ham	1	183	1	—	13	6	32	—	—	—	765	—	—	—
Sandwich Steak	1	210	3	—	13	9	31	—	—	—	445	—	—	—
Sandwich Turkey	1	183	1	—	13	6	32	—	—	—	765	—	—	—
MAIN MENU SELECTIONS														
12 Inch Sandwich Grand Cobbler	1	680	4	—	60	49	116	—	—	—	3094	—	—	—
12 Inch Sandwich Grand Escape	1	776	12	—	100	55	108	—	—	—	1590	—	—	—
12 Inch Sandwich Grandest Chicken	1	770	10	—	110	61	110	—	—.	—	1914	—	—	—
12 Inch Sandwich Great Escape	1	776	12	—	100	55	108	—	—	—	1590	—	—	—
12 Inch Sandwich Hambrosia	1	684	4	—	60	47	119	—	—	—	3090	—	—	—
12 Inch Sandwich Ragin' Cajun	1	756	10	—	110	59	108	—	—	—	1965	—	—	—
12 Inch Sandwich Turkey Club	1	675	4	—	70	52	111	—	—	—	3430	—	—	—
12 Inch Sandwich Vegetarian	1	524	2	—	0	18	109	—	—	—	1053	—	—	—
12 Inch Sandwich Wild West BBQ	1	841	12	—	100	55	126	—	—	—	2092	—	—	—
7 Inch Sandwich Grand Cobbler	1	380	2	—	30	26	67	—	—	—	1842	—	—	—
7 Inch Sandwich Grand Escape	1	435	6	—	50	30	64	—	—	—	892	—	—	—
7 Inch Sandwich Grandest Chicken	1	425	5	—	55	32	64	—	—	—	1052	—	—	—
7 Inch Sandwich Great Escape	1	428	6	—	50	29	63	—	—	—	890	—	—	—
7 Inch Sandwich Hambrosia	1	382	2	—	30	25	69	—	—	—	1640	—	—	—
7 Inch Sandwich Ragin' Cajun	1	418	5	—	55	31	63	—	—	—	1107	—	—	—
7 Inch Sandwich Turkey Club	1	390	2	—	40	30	65	—	—	—	1980	—	—	—
7 Inch Sandwich Vegetarian	1	302	1	—	0	10	64	—	—	—	622	—	—	—
7 Inch Sandwich Wild West BBQ	1	469	6	—	50	29	72	—	—	—	1141	—	—	—
Fries	1 serv (12 oz)	498	26	—	0	8	67	—	—	—	409	—	—	—
Fries	1 serv (32 oz)	996	52	—	0	16	134	—	—	—	818	—	—	—

FOOD	PORTION	CALS	FAT	SAT FAT	CHOL	PROT	CARB	SUGAR	FIBER	CALCI	SOD	POTAS	FOLIC	VIT C
Fries Loaded Bacon & Cheddar	1 serv	905	44	—	29	18	88	—	—	—	1587	—	—	—
Fries Loaded Ranch & Bacon	1 serv	1044	71	—	39	18	84	—	—	—	1398	—	—	—
Smashed Potatoes Loaded Bacon & Cheddar	1 serv	636	26	—	24	13	91	—	—	—	827	—	—	—
Smashed Potatoes Loaded Ranch & Bacon	1 serv	692	34	—	29	14	87	—	—	—	501	—	—	—
Smashed Potatoes Plain	1 serv	246	0	—	0	11	53	—	—	—	43	—	—	—
Smashed Potatoes w/ Chicken	1 serv	318	4	—	55	33	56	—	—	—	475	—	—	—
Smashed Potatoes w/ Ham	1 serv	336	2	—	30	27	59	—	—	—	1065	—	—	—
Smashed Potatoes w/ Steak	1 serv	391	5	—	50	31	56	—	—	—	313	—	—	—
Smashed Potatoes w/ Turkey	1 serv	336	2	—	30	27	59	—	—	—	1065	—	—	—
SALAD DRESSINGS AND TOPPINGS														
American Cheese	1 slice	101	9	—	26	6	3	—	—	—	437	—	—	—
Bacon	1 serv (1 oz)	80	7	—	10	5	0	0	0	—	374	—	—	—
BBQ Sauce	1 serv (1 oz)	40	0	0	0	0	9	—	—	—	252	—	—	—
Black Olives	1 serv (1 oz)	32	3	—	0	0	2	—	—	—	248	—	—	—
Brown Mustard	1 serv (1 oz)	0	0	0	0	0	0	0	0	—	340	—	—	—
Cheddar Cheese	1 slice	116	9	—	30	8	1	—	—	—	179	—	—	—
Dressing Italian	1 serv (0.5 oz)	51	5		0	0	1	—	—	—	248	—	—	—
Dressing Ranch	1 serv (0.5 oz)	83	9	—	5	0	0	0	0	—	137	—	—	—
Lettuce	1 serv (1 oz)	2	0	0	0	1	0	—	—	—	2	—	—	—
Margarine	1 serv (1 oz)	203	23	—	0	0	0	0	0	—	306	—	—	—
Mayonnaise	1 serv (1 oz)	101	11	—	5	0	0	—	—	—	76	—	—	—
Peppers Jalapeño	1 serv (1.5 oz)	11	0	—	0	0	2	—	—	—	415	—	—	—
Peppers Mild	1 serv (1.5 oz)	11	0	0	0	0	4	—	—	—	500	—	—	—
Provolone Cheese	1 slice	80	6	—	15	5	0	—	—	—	190	—	—	—
Sour Cream	1 serv (1 oz)	61	6	—	13	1	1	—	—	—	15	—	—	—
Swiss Cheese	1 slice	100	8	—	26	8	1	—	—	—	60	—	—	—
Tomatoes	1 serv (2 oz)	24	0	0	0	2	2	—	—	—	5	—	—	—
SALADS														
Grilled Salad w/ Chicken	1 serv	175	5	—	55	25	11	—	—	—	652	—	—	—
Grilled Salad w/ Ham	1 serv	130	2	—	30	19	8	—	—	—	1042	—	—	—
Grilled Salad w/ Steak	1 serv	185	6	—	50	23	11	—	—	—	292	—	—	—

FOOD	PORTION	CALS	FAT	SAT FAT	CHOL	PROT	CARB	SUGAR	FIBER	CALCI	SOD	POTAS	FOLIC	VIT C
Grilled Salad w/ Turkey	1 serv	130	2	—	30	19	8	—	—	—	1042	—	—	—
Side	1 serv	40	5	—	0	3	8	—	—	—	20	—	—	—

SUBWAY

BEVERAGES

FOOD	PORTION	CALS	FAT	SAT FAT	CHOL	PROT	CARB	SUGAR	FIBER	CALCI	SOD	POTAS	FOLIC	VIT C
Fruizle Smoothie Berry Lishus	1 sm (13 oz)	113	0	0	15	1	28	27	1	5	30	—	—	66
Fruizle Smoothie Berry Lishus w/ Banana	1 sm (17 oz)	221	1	0	15	1	56	27	4	20	30	—	—	78
Fruizle Smoothie Peach Pizazz	1 sm (12 oz)	103	0	0	0	1	26	26	0	0	25	—	—	66
Fruizle Smoothie Pineapple Delight w/ Banana	1 sm (17 oz)	241	1	0	0	1	61	33	4	20	25	—	—	96
Fruizle Smoothie Pineapple Delite	1 sm (13 oz)	133	0	0	0	1	33	33	1	0	25	—	—	90
Fruizle Smoothie Sunrise Refresher	1 sm (12 oz)	119	0	0	0	1	29	28	1	23	20	—	—	126

COOKIES

FOOD	PORTION	CALS	FAT	SAT FAT	CHOL	PROT	CARB	SUGAR	FIBER	CALCI	SOD	POTAS	FOLIC	VIT C
Chocolate Chip	1	215	10	4	13	2	30	18	1	0	160	—	—	0
Chocolate Chunk	1	217	10	4	12	2	30	17	1	0	105	—	—	0
Double Chocolate	1	209	10	4	15	2	30	20	1	0	170	—	—	0
M&M	1	215	10	4	13	2	30	17	1	0	105	—	—	0
Oatmeal Raisin	1	210	8	3	14	3	30	16	2	0	180	—	—	0
Peanut Butter	1	221	12	4	12	4	26	16	1	0	200	—	—	0
Sugar	1	227	12	4	17	2	28	14	0	0	135	—	—	0
White Macadamia Nut	1	221	11	4	15	2	28	17	1	0	160	—	—	0

SALAD DRESSINGS

FOOD	PORTION	CALS	FAT	SAT FAT	CHOL	PROT	CARB	SUGAR	FIBER	CALCI	SOD	POTAS	FOLIC	VIT C
Fat Free French	1 serv (2 oz)	70	0	0	0	0	17	12	0	0	390	—	—	0
Fat Free Italian	1 serv (2 oz)	20	0	0	0	0	4	3	0	0	610	—	—	0
Fat Free Ranch	1 serv (2 oz)	60	0	0	0	0	14	6	0	0	530	—	—	0

SALADS AND SALAD BARS

FOOD	PORTION	CALS	FAT	SAT FAT	CHOL	PROT	CARB	SUGAR	FIBER	CALCI	SOD	POTAS	FOLIC	VIT C
BMT	1 serv	275	19	8	55	16	11	1	3	100	1590	—	—	30
Cold Cut Trio	1 serv	234	15	6	57	14	11	1	3	150	1370	—	—	30
Ham	1 serv	112	3	1	25	11	11	1	3	40	1070	—	—	30
Meatball	1 serv	320	20	9	56	17	17	2	4	100	1050	—	—	36
Roast Beef	1 serv	117	3	1	25	12	10	1	3	40	720	—	—	30
Roasted Chicken Breast	1 serv	130	3	1	50	18	9	0	3	40	630	—	—	36
Seafood & Crab	1 serv	197	11	4	24	9	17	1	4	100	970	—	—	30
Steak & Cheese	1 serv	181	8	4	37	17	12	2	4	100	890	—	—	30
Subway Club	1 serv	146	4	2	33	17	12	2	3	40	1110	—	—	30

FOOD	PORTION	CALS	FAT	SAT FAT	CHOL	PROT	CARB	SUGAR	FIBER	CALCI	SOD	POTAS	FOLIC	VIT C
Subway Melt	1 serv	203	10	5	44	17	11	1	3	100	1410	—	—	30
Tuna	1 serv	238	16	2	42	13	10	0	3	100	880	—	—	30
Turkey Breast	1 serv	105	2	0	20	11	11	1	3	40	820	—	—	30
Turkey Breast & Ham	1 serv	117	3	1	26	13	11	1	3	40	1030	—	—	30
Veggie Delight	1 serv	50	1	0	0	2	9	0	3	40	310	—	—	30
SANDWICHES														
6 Inch Steak & Cheese	1	362	13	5	37	23	41	7	4	100	1200	—	—	24
6 Inch Subway Melt	1	384	15	5	44	23	40	6	3	100	1720	—	—	24
6 Inch Sub BMT	1	456	24	9	55	21	40	6	3	100	1890	—	—	24
6 Inch Sub Cold Cut Trio	1	415	20	7	57	19	40	5	3	150	1670	—	—	24
6 Inch Sub Ham	1	261	5	2	25	17	39	6	3	40	1260	—	—	21
6 Inch Sub Meatball	1	501	25	10	56	23	46	7	4	100	1350	—	—	30
6 Inch Sub Roast Beef	1	267	5	2	20	17	39	6	3	40	900	—	—	21
6 Inch Sub Roasted Chicken Breast	1	291	5	2	46	21	40	6	3	40	990	—	—	21
6 Inch Sub Seafood & Crab	1	378	16	5	24	14	46	6	3	100	1270	—	—	24
6 Inch Sub Subway Club	1	296	5	2	33	22	40	6	3	40	1290	—	—	21
6 Inch Sub Tuna	1	419	21	5	42	18	39	5	3	100	1180	—	—	24
6 Inch Sub Turkey Breast	1	254	4	1	20	17	39	5	3	40	1000	—	—	21
6 Inch Sub Turkey Breast & Ham	1	267	5	1	26	18	40	5	3	40	1210	—	—	21
6 Inch Sub Veggie Delight	1	200	3	1	0	7	37	4	3	40	500	—	—	21
American Cheese Triangles	2	41	4	2	10	2	0	0	0	80	200	—	—	0
Asiago Caesar Sauce	1.5 tbsp	110	11	2	10	1	2	1	0	0	230	—	—	0
Bacon Strips	2	45	4	2	8	3	0	0	0	0	180	—	—	0
Breakfast Bacon & Egg	1	321	16	5	184	14	34	3	3	80	520	—	—	4
Breakfast Cheese & Egg	1	317	15	5	187	14	34	3	3	150	550	—	—	4
Breakfast Ham & Egg	1	338	14	4	201	21	34	4	3	80	1100	—	—	4
Breakfast Western Egg	1	300	12	4	182	14	36	3	3	80	540	—	—	12
Cheddar Triangles	2	59	5	3	15	4	0	0	0	100	95	—	—	0

FOOD	PORTION	CALS	FAT	SAT FAT	CHOL	PROT	CARB	SUGAR	FIBER	CALCI	SOD	POTAS	FOLIC	VIT C
Cucumber Slices	3	2	0	0	0	0	0	0	0	0	0	—	—	0
Deli Ham	1	210	4	2	12	11	35	3	3	60	770	—	—	12
Deli Roast Beef	1	223	5	2	13	13	35	3	3	60	660	—	—	12
Deli Tuna	1	325	16	5	26	13	36	2	3	150	830	—	—	12
Deli Turkey Breast	1	215	4	2	13	13	36	3	3	60	730	—	—	12
Deli Style Roll	1	165	3	1	0	6	32	2	3	40	280	—	—	4
Dijon Horseradish	1.5 tbsp	91	10	2	8	0	1	0	0	0	160	—	—	0
Dijon Horseradish Melt	6 inch	465	22	7	52	25	47	67	4	150	1620	—	—	24
Fat Free Red Wine Vinaigrette	1.5 tbsp	29	0	0	1	0	6	3	0	0	340	—	—	0
Fat Free Sweet Onion	1.5 tbsp	38	0	0	0	0	9	8	0	0	85	—	—	0
Green Pepper Strips	3 (0.2 oz)	2	0	0	0	0	0	0	0	0	0	—	—	6
Hearty Italian Bread	6 inch	207	3	2	0	8	41	5	3	40	340	—	—	5
Honey Mustard	1.5 tbsp	28	0	0	0	0	7	6	0	0	140	—	—	0
Honey Mustard Ham	6 inch	311	5	2	25	18	52	12	4	60	1260	—	—	24
Honey Oat Bread	6 inch	249	4	1	0	10	48	9	4	60	380	—	—	9
Italian Bread	6 inch	178	2	1	0	7	33	4	2	20	350	—	—	9
Lettuce	1 serv (0.7 oz)	3	0	0	0	0	0	0	0	0	0	—	—	0
Mayonnaise	1 tbsp	111	12	3	9	0	0	0	0	0	80	—	—	0
Mayonnaise Light	1 tbsp	46	5	1	6	0	1	0	0	0	100	—	—	0
Monterey Cheddar Bread	6 inch	235	6	4	10	10	39	5	3	100	400	—	—	5
Mustard	2 tsp	7	0	0	0	0	1	0	0	0	115	—	—	0
Olive Oil Blend	1 tsp	45	5	1	0	0	0	0	0	0	0	—	—	0
Olive Rings	3 (3 g)	3	tr	0	0	0	0	0	0	0	25	—	—	0
Onions	1 serv (0.5 oz)	5	0	0	0	0	1	0	0	0	0	—	—	0
Parmesan Oregano Bread	6 inch	211	4	2	0	8	40	5	3	40	530	—	—	5
Pepperjack Cheese Triangles	2	40	4	2	11	2	0	0	0	100	210	—	—	0
Pickle Chips	3 pieces (0.3 oz)	1	0	0	0	0	0	0	0	0	125	—	—	0
Provolone Circles	2 halves	51	4	2	11	4	0	0	0	100	125	—	—	0
Red Wine Vinaigrette Club	6 inch	350	6	3	33	24	53	9	4	60	1520	—	—	24
Roasted Garlic Bread	6 inch	225	3	2	0	8	45	7	4	40	1210	—	—	5
Sourdough Bread	6 inch	208	3	1	0	8	41	2	3	40	210	—	—	4
Southwest Sauce	1.5 tbsp	86	9	2	7	0	2	1	0	0	190	—	—	0
Southwest Turkey Bacon	6 inch	407	17	5	35	21	48	7	4	60	1230	—	—	24

FOOD	PORTION	CALS	FAT	SAT FAT	CHOL	PROT	CARB	SUGAR	FIBER	CALCI	SOD	POTAS	FOLIC	VIT C
Sweet Onion Chicken Teriyaki	6 inch	374	5	2	50	26	59	17	4	80	1090	—	—	27
Swiss Triangles	2	53	4	3	13	4	0	0	0	150	30	—	—	0
Tomato Slices	3 (1.2 oz)	7	0	0	0	0	2	0	0	0	0	—	—	6
Vinegar	1 tsp	1	0	0	0	0	0	0	0	0	0	—	—	0
Wheat Sub	6 inch	186	2	0	0	7	36	5	3	20	360	—	—	9
Wrap Chicken Bacon Ranch w/ Swiss	1	480	27	—	—	—	19	—	—	—	—	—	—	—
Wrap Turkey Bacon Melt	1	430	25	—	—	—	22	—	—	—	—	—	—	—
SOUPS														
Black Bean	1 cup	180	5	2	5	9	27	4	15	60	1160	—	—	5
Brown & Wild Rice w/ Chicken	1 cup	190	11	5	20	6	17	3	2	300	990	—	—	24
Cheese w/ Ham & Bacon	1 cup	230	16	6	20	8	13	4	2	200	1270	—	—	0
Chicken & Dumplings	1 cup	130	5	3	30	7	16	2	1	20	1030	—	—	0
Cream Of Broccoli	1 cup	130	7	2	15	4	12	5	1	100	890	—	—	12
Cream Of Potato w/ Bacon	1 cup	210	12	4	20	5	20	3	4	100	970	—	—	6
Golden Broccoli Cheese	1 cup	180	12	4	10	6	12	4	9	150	910	—	—	9
Hearty Chili Beef	1 cup	250	7	3	20	15	31	9	9	100	1450	—	—	12
Minestrone	1 cup	70	1	0	5	3	11	2	0	40	1030	—	—	6
New England Clam Chowder	1 cup	140	5	1	15	5	19	2	1	40	900	—	—	0
Potato Cheese Chowder	1 cup	210	10	7	25	7	22	3	2	200	1010	—	—	0
Roasted Chicken Noodle	1 cup	90	4	1	20	7	7	1	1	20	1180	—	—	4
Tomato Bisque	1 cup	90	3	1	0	1	15	7	3	20	750	—	—	5
Vegetable Beef	1 cup	90	2	1	5	5	14	4	2	20	1340	—	—	4

TACO BELL

FOOD	PORTION	CALS	FAT	SAT FAT	CHOL	PROT	CARB	SUGAR	FIBER	CALCI	SOD	POTAS	FOLIC	VIT C
BEVERAGES														
2% Lowfat Milk	1 serv (8 oz)	110	5	3	15	8	11	10	0	300	115	—	—	2
Coffee Black	1 serv (12 oz)	5	0	0	0	0	1	0	0	0	5	—	—	0
Diet Pepsi	1 serv (16 oz)	0	0	0	0	0	0	0	0	0	47	—	—	0
Lipton Iced Tea Sweetened	1 serv (16 oz)	140	0	0	0	0	40	40	0	0	60	—	—	0
Lipton Iced Tea Unsweetened	1 serv (16 oz)	0	0	0	0	0	0	0	0	0	60	—	—	0
Mountain Dew	1 serv (16 oz)	227	0	0	0	0	61	61	0	0	93	—	—	0
Orange Juice	1 serv (6 oz)	80	0	0	0	1	18	18	0	20	0	—	—	66

FOOD	PORTION	CALS	FAT	SAT FAT	CHOL	PROT	CARB	SUGAR	FIBER	CALCI	SOD	POTAS	FOLIC	VIT C
Pepsi Cola	1 serv (16 oz)	200	0	0	0	0	51	55	0	0	47	—	—	0
Slice	1 serv (16 oz)	200	0	0	0	0	53	52	0	0	73	—	—	0
BREAKFAST SELECTIONS														
Breakfast Quesadilla Cheese	1 (5.5 oz)	380	21	9	280	15	33	1	1	300	1010	—	—	0
Breakfast Quesadilla w/ Bacon	1 (6 oz)	450	27	11	290	19	33	1	2	300	1200	—	—	0
Breakfast Quesadilla w/ Sausage	1 (6 oz)	430	25	10	285	17	33	1	1	300	1090	—	—	0
Country Breakfast Burrito	1 (4 oz)	270	14	5	195	8	26	1	2	100	690	—	—	0
Double Bacon & Egg Burrito	1 (6.25 oz)	480	27	9	405	18	39	2	2	150	1240	—	—	0
Fiesta Breakfast Burrito	1 (3.5 oz)	280	16	6	25	9	25	1	2	80	580	—	—	0
Grande Breakfast Burrito	1 (6.25 oz)	420	22	7	205	13	43	2	3	100	1050	—	—	0
Hash Brown Nuggets	1 serv (3.5 oz)	280	18	5	0	2	29	0	1	0	570	—	—	0
MAIN MENU SELECTIONS														
7-Layer Burrito	1 (10 oz)	530	23	7	25	16	66	4	13	200	1280	—	—	6
Bacon Cheeseburger Burrito	1 (8.5 oz)	570	31	12	70	27	46	5	6	200	1460	—	—	5
Bean Burrito	1 (7 oz)	380	12	4	10	13	55	3	13	150	1100	—	—	0
Big Beef Burrito Supreme	1 (10.5 oz)	520	23	10	55	24	54	4	11	150	1520	—	—	5
Big Beef MexiMelt	1 (4.75 oz)	290	15	7	45	16	23	2	4	200	850	—	—	4
Big Chicken Burrito Supreme	1 (9 oz)	510	24	7	95	23	52	3	4	150	1900	—	—	0
BLT Soft Taco	1 (4.5 oz)	340	23	8	40	11	22	8	7	100	610	—	—	4
Border Sauce Fire	1 serv (0.3 oz)	0	0	0	0	0	0	0	0	0	110	—	—	0
Border Sauce Hot	1 serv (0.3 oz)	0	0	0	0	0	0	0	0	0	85	—	—	0
Border Sauce Mild	1 serv (0.3 oz)	0	0	0	0	0	0	0	0	0	75	—	—	0
Burger Sauce	1 serv (0.5 oz)	60	5	1	5	0	2	2	0	0	110	—	—	0
Burrito Supreme	1 (9 oz)	440	19	8	35	17	51	4	10	150	1230	—	—	5
Cheddar Cheese	1 serv (0.25 oz)	30	2	2	5	2	0	0	0	60	45	—	—	0
Cheese Quesadilla	1 (4.25 oz)	350	18	9	50	16	32	1	2	450	860	—	—	0
Chicken Fajita Wrap	1 (8 oz)	470	22	6	60	17	51	3	4	150	1290	—	—	4
Chicken Fajita Wrap Supreme	1 (9 oz)	520	25	8	70	18	53	4	4	150	1300	—	—	6

FOOD	PORTION	CALS	FAT	SAT FAT	CHOL	PROT	CARB	SUGAR	FIBER	CALCI	SOD	POTAS	FOLIC	VIT C
Chicken Quesadilla	1 (6 oz)	410	21	10	90	23	34	2	3	450	1170	—	—	0
Chicken Club Burrito	1 (8 oz)	540	32	10	80	20	43	5	4	100	1250	—	—	5
Chili Cheese Burrito	1 (5 oz)	330	13	6	35	14	37	2	5	200	870	—	—	0
Choco Taco Ice Cream Dessert	1 serv (4 oz)	310	17	10	20	3	37	27	1	60	100	—	—	0
Cinnamon Twists	1 serv (1 oz)	140	6	0	0	1	19	0	0	0	190	—	—	0
Club Sauce	1 serv (0.5 oz)	80	8	1	10	0	1	0	0	0	105	—	—	0
Double Decker Taco	1 (5.75 oz)	340	15	5	25	14	38	2	9	100	750	—	—	0
Double Decker Taco Supreme	1 (7 oz)	390	19	8	35	15	40	3	9	150	760	—	—	4
Fajita Sauce	1 serv (0.5 oz)	70	7	1	5	0	1	0	0	0	130	—	—	0
Green Sauce	1 serv (1 oz)	5	0	0	0	0	1	0	0	0	150	—	—	2
Grilled Chicken Burrito	1 (7 oz)	410	15	5	55	17	50	3	4	150	1380	—	—	1
Grilled Chicken Soft Taco	1 (4.5 oz)	240	12	4	45	12	21	2	3	80	1110	—	—	0
Grilled Steak Soft Taco	1 (4.5 oz)	230	10	3	25	15	20	1	2	80	1020	—	—	0
Grilled Steak Soft Taco Supreme	1 (5.75 oz)	290	14	5	35	16	24	4	3	100	1040	—	—	12
Guacamole	1 serv (0.75 oz)	35	3	0	0	0	1	1	1	0	80	—	—	1
Mexican Pizza	1 serv (7.75 oz)	570	35	10	45	21	42	1	8	250	1040	—	—	5
Mexican Rice	1 serv (4.75 oz)	190	9	4	15	5	23	1	1	150	760	—	—	1
Nacho Cheese Sauce	2 serv (2 oz)	120	10	3	5	2	5	2	0	40	470	—	—	0
Nachos	1 serv (3.5 oz)	320	18	4	5	5	34	2	3	100	570	—	—	0
Nachos Beef Supreme	1 serv (7 oz)	450	24	8	30	14	45	3	9	150	810	—	—	4
Nachos Bellgrande	1 serv (11 oz)	770	39	11	35	21	84	4	17	200	1310	—	—	4
Picante Sauce	1 serv (0.3 oz)	0	0	0	0	0	0	0	0	0	110	—	—	1
Pico De Gallo	1 serv (0.75 oz)	5	0	0	0	0	1	1	0	0	65	—	—	4
Pintos 'n Cheese	1 serv (4.5 oz)	190	9	4	15	9	18	1	10	150	650	—	—	0
Red Sauce	1 serv (1 oz)	10	0	0	0	0	2	0	0	0	320	—	—	0
Soft Taco	1 (3.5 oz)	220	10	5	25	11	21	1	3	80	580	—	—	0
Soft Taco Supreme	1 (5 oz)	260	14	7	35	12	23	3	3	100	590	—	—	4
Sour Cream	1 serv (0.75 oz)	40	4	3	10	1	1	0	0	0	10	—	—	0
Steak Fajita Wrap	1 (8 oz)	470	21	6	40	20	50	3	3	150	1190	—	—	4
Steak Fajita Wrap Supreme	1 (9 oz)	510	25	8	50	21	52	4	3	150	1200	—	—	6
Taco	1 (2.75 oz)	180	10	4	25	9	12	1	3	80	330	—	—	0
Taco Supreme	1 (4 oz)	220	14	7	35	10	14	2	3	100	350	—	—	4

FOOD	PORTION	CALS	FAT	SAT FAT	CHOL	PROT	CARB	SUGAR	FIBER	CALCI	SOD	POTAS	FOLIC	VIT C
Taco Salad w/ Salsa	1 (19 oz)	850	52	15	60	30	65	9	16	300	1780	—	—	24
Taco Salad w/ Salsa w/o Shell	1 (16.5 oz)	420	22	11	60	24	32	9	15	250	1520	—	—	21
Three Cheese Blend	1 serv (0.25 oz)	25	2	1	5	2	0	0	0	40	50	—	—	0
Tostada	1 (6.25 oz)	300	15	5	15	10	31	2	12	150	650	—	—	1
Veggie Fajita Wrap	1 (8 oz)	420	19	5	20	10	53	3	3	150	980	—	—	4
Veggie Fajita Wrap Supreme	1 (9 oz)	470	22	7	30	11	55	4	3	150	990	—	—	6

TACO CABANA

FOOD	PORTION	CALS	FAT	SAT FAT	CHOL	PROT	CARB	SUGAR	FIBER	CALCI	SOD	POTAS	FOLIC	VIT C
Black Beans	1 serv (4 oz)	111	tr	—	—	6	21	—	—	—	—	—	—	—
Borracho Beans	1 serv (4 oz)	108	3	—	—	4	17	—	—	—	—	—	—	—
Breakfast Taco Bacon & Egg	1	246	12	—	—	13	22	—	—	—	—	—	—	—
Breakfast Taco Barbacoa	1	307	15	—	—	22	2	—	—	—	—	—	—	—
Breakfast Taco Chorizo & Egg	1	248	12	—	—	12	22	—	—	—	—	—	—	—
Breakfast Taco Potato & Egg	1	234	10	—	—	10	27	—	—	—	—	—	—	—
Burrito Bean & Cheese	1	710	27	—	—	28	85	—	—	—	—	—	—	—
Burrito Beef	1	653	24	—	—	30	76	—	—	—	—	—	—	—
Burrito Black Bean	1	559	11	—	—	16	95	—	—	—	—	—	—	—
Burrito Chicken	1	665	26	—	—	31	74	—	—	—	—	—	—	—
Calabacita	1 serv (4 oz)	78	5	—	—	2	6	—	—	—	—	—	—	—
Chips	1 serv (2 oz)	285	14	—	—	5	36	—	—	—	—	—	—	—
Elotes	1	220	11	—	—	7	26	—	—	—	—	—	—	—
Fajitas Beef	1 serv (4 oz)	245	12	—	—	31	3	—	—	—	—	—	—	—
Fajitas Chicken Dark	1 serv (4 oz)	236	11	—	—	33	2	—	—	—	—	—	—	—
Fajitas Chicken White	1 serv (4 oz)	191	6	—	—	30	3	—	—	—	—	—	—	—
Grilled Chicken Dark	1 serv (4.5 oz)	298	18	—	—	33	1	—	—	—	—	—	—	—
Grilled Chicken Dark No Skin	1 serv (3.4 oz)	170	7	—	—	26	1	—	—	—	—	—	—	—
Grilled Chicken White	1 serv (5 oz)	295	14	—	—	42	1	—	—	—	—	—	—	—
Grilled Chicken White No Skin	1 serv (3.8 oz)	167	3	—	—	35	tr	—	—	—	—	—	—	—
Guacamole	1 serv (1 oz)	48	4	—	—	tr	2	—	—	—	—	—	—	—
Queso	1 serv (3 oz)	184	12	—	—	9	7	—	—	—	—	—	—	—
Refried Beans	1 serv (4 oz)	171	6	—	—	7	21	—	—	—	—	—	—	—
Sour Cream	1 serv (1 oz)	57	5	—	—	1	1	—	—	—	—	—	—	—
Spanish Rice	1 serv (4 oz)	181	5	—	—	3	30	—	—	—	—	—	—	—

FOOD	PORTION	CALS	FAT	SAT FAT	CHOL	PROT	CARB	SUGAR	FIBER	CALCI	SOD	POTAS	FOLIC	VIT C
Taco Bean & Cheese	1	292	12	—	—	12	35	—	—	—	—	—	—	—
Taco Black Bean	1	216	5	—	—	8	37	—	—	—	—	—	—	—
Taco Carne Guisada	1	202	8	—	—	14	20	—	—	—	—	—	—	—
Taco Crispy Beef	1	148	7	—	—	9	13	—	—	—	—	—	—	—
Taco Soft Chicken	1	217	9	—	—	13	21	—	—	—	—	—	—	—
Tortilla Corn	1 6-inch	70	1	—	—	2	11	—	—	—	—	—	—	—
Tortilla Flour	1 6-inch	129	3	—	—	3	22	—	—	—	—	—	—	—
Tortilla Soup	1 sm	249	8	—	—	18	26	—	—	—	—	—	—	—
Tortilla Soup	1 lg	371	13	—	—	33	32	—	—	—	—	—	—	—

TACO JOHN'S

DESSERTS

FOOD	PORTION	CALS	FAT	SAT FAT	CHOL	PROT	CARB	SUGAR	FIBER	CALCI	SOD	POTAS	FOLIC	VIT C
Apple Grande	1 scrv	240	9	3	5	5	36	15	0	—	220	—	—	—
Choco Taco	1 serv	300	15	7	15	4	38	24	1	—	110	—	—	—
Churro	1 serv	230	11	2	10	2	31	19	1	—	120	—	—	—
Cinnamon Mini Swirl	1 piece	10	0	0	0	0	3	3	0	—	0	—	—	—

MAIN MENU SELECTIONS

FOOD	PORTION	CALS	FAT	SAT FAT	CHOL	PROT	CARB	SUGAR	FIBER	CALCI	SOD	POTAS	FOLIC	VIT C
Burrito Bean	1	380	12	5	15	15	53	1	10	—	830	—	—	—
Burrito Beefy	1	430	20	9	55	22	41	1	8	—	870	—	—	—
Burrito Chicken & Potato	1	460	19	7	35	18	54	1	8	—	1470	—	—	—
Burrito Combination	1	400	16	7	35	18	47	1	9	—	850	—	—	—
Burrito Meat & Potato	1	490	23	8	30	15	55	1	9	—	1190	—	—	—
Burrito Super	1	450	20	9	40	19	49	2	10	—	920	—	—	—
Crispy Taco	1 serv	180	10	4	25	9	13	0	3	—	270	—	—	—
Mexican Rice	1 serv	250	5	1	0	5	45	2	2	—	860	—	—	—
Nachos	1 serv	380	23	6	10	6	38	0	tr	—	970	—	—	—
Potato Oles	1 sm	440	26	6	0	4	48	0	5	—	1270	—	—	—
Potato Oles	1 lg	790	47	11	0	7	86	0	8	—	2290	—	—	—
Potato Oles Bravo	1 serv	580	36	11	20	9	55	1	6	—	1760	—	—	—
Potato Oles Super	1 serv	980	62	22	60	22	82	2	10	—	2950	—	—	—
Potato Oles w/ Nacho Cheese	1 serv	550	35	10	10	7	52	0	5	—	2000	—	—	—
Quesadilla Cheese	1	480	28	15	50	20	39	1	6	—	960	—	—	—
Quesadilla Chicken	1	540	29	15	75	29	41	1	7	—	1430	—	—	—
Refried Beans	1 serv	400	14	5	15	18	50	2	11	—	1110	—	—	—
Sierra Taco Beef	1	430	23	8	45	17	38	3	1	—	980	—	—	—
Sierra Taco Chicken	1	390	17	5	50	21	37	3	3	—	1350	—	—	—
Softshell Taco	1	220	10	5	25	11	21	1	4	—	470	—	—	—

FOOD	PORTION	CALS	FAT	SAT FAT	CHOL	PROT	CARB	SUGAR	FIBER	CALCI	SOD	POTAS	FOLIC	VIT C
Softshell Taco Chicken	1	190	6	3	30	14	19	0	4	—	760	—	—	—
Super Nachos	1 serv	830	51	17	60	22	73	2	5	—	1730	—	—	—
Super Nachos Chicken	1 serv	780	45	15	90	31	62	2	3	—	2250	—	—	—
Taco Bravo	1 serv	340	14	5	25	15	30	1	8	—	650	—	—	—
Taco Burger	1	280	12	5	35	14	28	3	3	—	600	—	—	—
Texas Chili	1 serv	270	12	6	35	15	26	3	4	—	1400	—	—	—
SALAD DRESSINGS AND TOPPINGS														
Bacon Ranch Dressing	1 serv (3 oz)	250	19	3	20	2	21	14	0	—	740	—	—	—
Barbecue Sauce	1 serv (2 oz)	70	0	0	0	0	15	9	0	—	490	—	—	—
Chipotle Cream Sauce	1 serv (3 oz)	450	45	9	30	—	6	3	0	—	1020	—	—	—
Creamy Italian Dressing	1 serv (3 oz)	260	29	5	0	0	6	3	0	—	600	—	—	—
Guacamole	1 serv (2 oz)	90	9	3	0	0	6	2	—	—	360	—	—	—
Hot Sauce	1 serv (1 oz)	5	0	0	0	0	1	0	0	—	135	—	—	—
House Dressing	1 serv (3 oz)	140	15	2	0	0	5	2	tr	—	540	—	—	—
Jalapeños	1 serv (2 oz)	15	1	0	0	1	3	1	1	—	950	—	—	—
Mild Sauce	1 serv (1 oz)	5	0	0	0	0	1	0	0	—	140	—	—	—
Nacho Cheese	1 serv (3 oz)	120	9	4	10	4	5	0	0	—	740	—	—	—
Pico De Gallo	1 serv (2 oz)	15	0	0	0	1	4	2	tr	—	160	—	—	—
Ranch Dressing	1 serv (3 oz)	280	31	5	45	3	6	3	0	—	710	—	—	—
Salsa	1 serv (2 oz)	20	0	0	0	0	5	4	0	—	390	—	—	—
Sour Cream	1 serv (2 oz)	120	12	7	25	2	2	0	0	—	30	—	—	—
Super Hot Sauce	1 serv (1 oz)	10	0	0	0	1	2	1	tr	—	25	—	—	—
SALADS														
Chicken Festiva w/o Dressing	1 serv	400	23	10	70	24	24	2	4	—	830	—	—	—
Chicken Taco w/o Dressin	1	530	27	11	70	27	45	5	3	—	1330	—	—	—
Side w/o Dressing	1 serv	80	5	2	5	3	6	1	1	—	50	—	—	—
Taco w/o Dressing	1 serv	580	32	13	60	23	46	5	4	—	960	—	—	—

TACOTIME

FOOD	PORTION	CALS	FAT	SAT FAT	CHOL	PROT	CARB	SUGAR	FIBER	CALCI	SOD	POTAS	FOLIC	VIT C
DESSERTS														
Cinnamon Crustos	1 serv	373	15	—	0	9	47	—	—	—	86	—	—	—
Fruit Filled Empanada	1 serv	250	9	—	0	5	37	—	—	—	46	—	—	—
MAIN MENU SELECTIONS														
Burrito Beef Bean & Cheese	1 serv	617	23	10	63	39	66	—	18	—	1343	—	—	—
Burrito Casita	1 serv	647	31	15	89	40	54	—	16	—	1233	—	—	—
Burrito Chicken & Black Bean	1 serv	400	18	7	36	19	45	—	5	—	580	—	—	—

FOOD	PORTION	CALS	FAT	SAT FAT	CHOL	PROT	CARB	SUGAR	FIBER	CALCI	SOD	POTAS	FOLIC	VIT C
Burrito Chicken BLT	1 serv	580	39	12	50	23	36	—	5	—	1020	—	—	—
Burrito Crisp Bean	1 serv	427	18	5	12	15	53	—	9	—	453	—	—	—
Burrito Crisp Chicken	1	422	25	8	54	17	32	—	2	—	795	—	—	—
Burrito Crisp Meat	1 serv	552	30	10	58	34	39	—	7	—	1000	—	—	—
Burrito Soft Bean	1	380	10	4	15	16	58	—	13	—	715	—	—	—
Burrito Soft Meat	1 serv	491	21	8	56	31	48	—	12	—	1197	—	—	—
Burrito Veggie	1 serv	491	16	6	24	21	70	—	10	—	643	—	—	—
Burrito Big Juan Beef	1 serv	640	25	12	60	34	71	—	15	—	1120	—	—	—
Burrito Big Juan Chicken	1 serv	620	24	11	65	34	69	—	12	—	1230	—	—	—
Cheddar Cheese	1 serv (0.75 oz)	86	7	4	22	5	0	—	0	—	132	—	—	—
Cheddar Fries	1 sm	352	24	—	—	6	27	—	—	—	931	—	—	—
Cheddar Fries	1 lg	704	48	—	—	16	54	—	—	—	1862	—	—	—
Cheddar Melt	1 serv	205	11	6	30	11	17	—	1	—	255	—	—	—
Mexi-Fries	1 lg	532	34	—	—	6	54	—	—	—	1598	—	—	—
Mexi-Fries	1 sm	266	17	—	—	3	27	—	—	—	799	—	—	—
Mexi-Rice	1 serv	159	2	1	0	3	30	—	1	—	530	—	—	—
Nachos	1 serv	680	38	19	78	26	61	—	11	—	1250	—	—	—
Nachos Deluxe	1 serv	1048	57	23	109	46	91	—	17	—	2252	—	—	—
Refritos Cheese Sauce Chips	1 serv	326	10	5	22	18	44	—	13	—	525	—	—	—
Stuffed Fries	1 sm	490	37	10	20	6	34	—	3	—	1400	—	—	—
Stuffed Fries	1 lg	990	73	19	35	16	88	—	6	—	2580	—	—	—
Taco Cheeseburger	1	633	36	10	66	31	48	—	7	—	1291	—	—	—
Taco Crisp	1	295	17	7	48	22	16	—	5	—	609	—	—	—
Taco Soft	1 serv	316	15	7	48	24	23	—	5	—	599	—	—	—
Taco Soft ½ lb	1 serv	512	23	10	63	33	46	—	12	—	1111	—	—	—
Taco Soft ½ lb Chicken	1 serv	387	16	6	48	21	41	—	7	—	933	—	—	—
Taco Super Soft	1 serv	510	23	12	60	29	50	—	11	—	590	—	—	—
SALAD DRESSINGS AND TOPPINGS														
1000 Island Dressing	1 serv (1 oz)	120	12	2	5	0	3	—	0	—	120	—	—	—
Green Sauce	1 serv (1 oz)	5	0	0	0	0	2	—	tr	—	115	—	—	—
Original Hot Sauce	1 serv (1 oz)	10	0	0	0	0	2	—	0	—	120	—	—	—
Salsa Fresca	1 serv (1 oz)	65	0	0	0	0	16	—	0	—	3508	—	—	—
SALADS														
Chicken Fiesta	1 serv	390	19	6	45	20	35	—	4	—	840	—	—	—
Taco	1 reg	479	28	11	63	30	30	—	7	—	895	—	—	—

FOOD	PORTION	CALS	FAT	SAT FAT	CHOL	PROT	CARB	SUGAR	FIBER	CALCI	SOD	POTAS	FOLIC	VIT C
Taco Salad Chicken	1 serv	370	21	7	48	19	27	—	3	—	861	—	—	—
Tostada	1 serv	628	33	14	82	36	48	—	13	—	1004	—	—	—

TCBY

FOOD	PORTION	CALS	FAT	SAT FAT	CHOL	PROT	CARB	SUGAR	FIBER	CALCI	SOD	POTAS	FOLIC	VIT C
Hand Dipped All Flavors 96% Fat Free	½ cup (3 oz)	140	3	2	5	3	26	22	0	100	26	—	—	0
Hand Dipped All Flavors Nonfat	½ cup (2.9 oz)	120	0	0	0	4	25	18	1	100	60	—	—	0
Lowfat Ice Cream All Flavors No Sugar Added	½ cup (2.6 oz)	110	3	2	10	3	19	6	0	100	60	—	—	0
Nonfat Ice Cream All Flavors	½ cup (2.9 oz)	120	0	0	0	3	26	19	1	100	55	—	—	1
Soft Serve All Flavors 96% Fat Free	½ cup (3.4 fl oz)	140	3	2	15	4	23	20	0	80	60	—	—	0
Soft Serve All Flavors No Sugar Added Nonfat	½ cup (2.8 oz)	80	0	0	<5	4	20	7	0	100	35	—	—	0
Soft Serve All Flavors Nonfat	½ cup (3.4 oz)	110	0	0	<5	4	23	20	0	100	60	—	—	0
Sorbet All Flavors Nonfat & Nondairy	½ cup (3.4 oz)	100	0	0	0	0	24	19	0	0	30	—	—	0

TGI FRIDAY'S

FOOD	PORTION	CALS	FAT	SAT FAT	CHOL	PROT	CARB	SUGAR	FIBER	CALCI	SOD	POTAS	FOLIC	VIT C
Sizzling Chicken & Broccoli	1 serv	700	40	—	—	—	15	—	—	—	—	—	—	—
Sizzling NY Strip Steak w/ Blue Cheese & Broccoli	1 serv	684	36	—	—	—	15	—	—	—	—	—	—	—

TIM HORTONS

BAGELS AND CREAM CHEESE

FOOD	PORTION	CALS	FAT	SAT FAT	CHOL	PROT	CARB	SUGAR	FIBER	CALCI	SOD	POTAS	FOLIC	VIT C
Blueberry	1	200	2	0	0	11	59	10	3	0	520	—	—	0
Cinnamon Raisin	1	300	2	0	0	11	58	12	4	20	390	—	—	0
Cream Cheese Light	1.5 oz	90	7	5	20	4	3	3	0	50	200	—	—	0
Cream Cheese Plain	1.5 oz	140	14	10	45	3	1	1	0	30	140	—	—	0
Everything	1	300	2	0	0	12	57	8	3	20	560	—	—	0
Multigrain	1	300	3	0	0	12	58	8	6	20	655	—	—	0
Onion	1	295	2	0	0	11	58	8	3	20	530	—	—	0
Plain	1	290	2	0	0	11	57	8	3	0	800	—	—	0
Poppy Seed	1	300	3	0	0	11	58	8	4	20	500	—	—	0

FOOD	PORTION	CALS	FAT	SAT FAT	CHOL	PROT	CARB	SUGAR	FIBER	CALCI	SOD	POTAS	FOLIC	VIT C
Sesame Seed	1	300	3	0	0	11	57	7	4	0	570	—	—	0
Whole Wheat & Honey	1	300	2	0	0	11	59	11	6	20	590	—	—	0
BAKED SELECTIONS														
Biscuit Southern Country Cranberry	1	470	19	5	0	7	68	21	2	150	1050	—	—	2
Biscuit Southern Country Raspberry	1	470	19	5	0	7	68	19	2	150	1050	—	—	5
Cake Black Forest	1 serv	500	21	14	0	4	75	44	3	60	790	—	—	2
Cake Celebration	1 serv	500	16	8	5	4	85	56	1	60	530	—	—	0
Cake Chocolot Fantasy	1 serv	420	15	7	35	5	72	51	3	40	630	—	—	0
Cake Shadow	1 serv	430	19	10	35	4	63	43	2	40	470	—	—	0
Cookie Chocolate Chip	1	150	7	3	20	2	21	12	1	20	140	—	—	0
Cookie Macaroon	1	140	8	7	0	1	14	11	3	0	60	—	—	0
Cookie Oatcakes	1	190	10	4	0	2	22	10	1	20	150	—	—	0
Cookie Oatmeal Raisin	1	150	6	2	15	2	22	13	1	20	140	—	—	0
Cookie Peanut Butter	1	170	10	3	20	3	17	8	1	20	190	—	—	0
Cookie Peanut Butter Chocolate Chunk	1	170	10	4	15	3	18	11	1	20	190	—	—	0
Croissant Butter	1	210	11	6	30	5	25	3	1	0	370	—	—	0
Croissant Cheese	1	240	12	5	20	6	27	3	1	40	370	—	—	0
Danish Cherry Cheese	1	380	23	9	45	7	33	11	1	40	410	—	—	6
Donut Apple Fritter	1	300	14	5	0	5	40	14	2	20	280	—	—	1
Donut Chocolate Dip	1	230	10	3	0	4	33	11	0	20	270	—	—	0
Donut Chocolate Glazed	1	360	22	7	10	3	36	19	1	20	340	—	—	0
Donut Dutchie	1	280	13	4	0	4	39	18	1	20	240	—	—	0
Donut Honey Dip	1	230	10	3	0	4	32	10	0	20	250	—	—	0
Donut Maple Dip	1	250	10	3	0	4	36	15	0	20	280	—	—	0
Donut Old Fashion Glazed	1	270	12	4	15	3	39	22	0	20	280	—	—	0
Donut Old Fashion Plain	1	220	12	4	15	3	24	8	0	20	260	—	—	0
Donut Sour Cream Plain	1	280	18	6	20	3	25	11	0	20	230	—	—	0
Donut Sugar Twist	1	230	10	3	0	5	32	9	0	20	280	—	—	0

FOOD	PORTION	CALS	FAT	SAT FAT	CHOL	PROT	CARB	SUGAR	FIBER	CALCI	SOD	POTAS	FOLIC	VIT C
Donut Walnut Crunch	1	320	18	5	10	5	36	17	2	20	410	—	—	0
Donut Filled Angel Cream	1	280	13	4	0	4	36	15	0	20	280	—	—	0
Donut Filled Blueberry	1	220	8	3	0	4	33	11	0	20	280	—	—	1
Donut Filled Boston Cream	1	230	8	3	0	4	36	13	0	20	320	—	—	0
Donut Filled Canadian Maple	1	230	8	3	0	4	36	13	0	20	320	—	—	0
Donut Filled Strawberry	1	220	8	3	0	4	33	10	0	20	310	—	—	2
Donuts Honey Stick	1	280	15	5	30	4	34	13	0	20	350	—	—	0
Muffin Blueberry Bran	1	300	9	2	10	5	51	21	5	60	690	—	—	4
Muffin Carrot Whole Wheat	1	410	22	2	10	5	52	24	4	40	580	—	—	5
Muffin Chocolate Chip	1	390	15	4	20	5	62	32	2	60	580	—	—	0
Muffin Oatbran Carrot 'n Raisin	1	340	11	2	0	5	57	26	4	40	390	—	—	1
Muffin Oatbran 'n Apple	1	350	12	3	0	5	58	24	4	40	430	—	—	1
Muffin Oatmeal Raisin	1	430	11	2	20	6	80	48	3	40	520	—	—	2
Muffin Raisin Bran	1	380	10	2	10	6	66	36	6	100	750	—	—	1
Muffin Wild Blueberry	1	330	11	2	15	4	54	27	2	60	520	—	—	2
Muffin Low Fat Carrot	1	260	2	0	0	5	60	30	6	100	620	—	—	4
Muffin Low Fat Cranberry	1	260	2	0	0	5	60	30	6	100	610	—	—	4
Muffin Low Fat Honey	1	290	2	0	0	6	66	33	6	100	700	—	—	2
Pie Apple	1 serv	540	31	6	0	4	62	26	3	20	230	—	—	9
Pie Banana Cream	1 serv	440	26	13	0	2	50	21	1	0	135	—	—	2
Pie Cherry	1 serv	570	31	6	0	4	70	35	2	20	320	—	—	12
Pie Chocolate Cream	1 serv	490	31	16	10	2	52	23	1	0	170	—	—	0
Tart Fresh Strawberry	1 serv	220	9	2	0	1	36	10	2	20	140	—	—	30
Tart Raisin Butter	1 serv	330	11	3	15	3	54	25	1	20	200	—	—	0
Tea Biscuit Plain	1	220	6	2	0	5	36	3	1	20	590	—	—	0
Tea Biscuit	1	250	6	2	0	5	47	15	2	20	570	—	—	0

FOOD	PORTION	CALS	FAT	SAT FAT	CHOL	PROT	CARB	SUGAR	FIBER	CALCI	SOD	POTAS	FOLIC	VIT C
Raisin														
Timbits Chocolate Glazed	1	70	3	1	5	1	9	5	0	0	95	—	—	0
Timbits Dutchie	1	60	2	0	0	1	10	5	0	0	90	—	—	0
Timbits Honey Dip	1	50	1	0	0	1	10	3	0	0	70	—	—	0
Timbits Old Fashion Plain	1	45	2	0	5	1	7	2	0	0	70	—	—	0
Timbits Filled Banana Cream	1	45	1	0	0	1	8	2	0	0	70	—	—	0
Timbits Filled Lemon	1	50	2	0	0	1	9	3	0	0	75	—	—	1
Timbits Filled Spiced Apple	1	80	1	0	0	1	9	3	0	0	75	—	—	0
Timbits Filled Strawberry	1	50	1	0	0	1	9	3	0	0	80	—	—	0
BEVERAGES														
Apple Juice	1 (9 oz)	140	0	0	0	0	36	34	0	20	16	—	—	60
Cafe Mocha	1 (10 oz)	250	10	4	0	3	34	3	0	0	330	—	—	0
Cappuccino English Toffee	1 (10 oz)	130	5	4	0	3	20	16	0	80	120	—	—	0
Cappuccino French Vanilla	1 (10 oz)	130	5	4	0	3	20	16	0	80	120	—	—	0
Cappuccino Iced	1 (16 oz)	430	23	14	80	3	54	52	0	100	50	—	—	1
Chocolate Milk	1 (14 oz)	280	5	3	15	15	46	39	0	500	270	—	—	4
Coffee Decaffeinated + Sugar & Cream	1 (10 oz)	80	4	2	12	1	10	10	0	20	20	—	—	0
Coffee + Sugar & Cream	1 (10 oz)	80	4	2	12	1	10	10	0	20	20	—	—	0
Coke	1 (14 oz)	170	0	0	0	0	44	44	0	0	12	—	—	0
Diet Coke	1 (14 oz)	1	0	0	0	0	0	0	0	0	20	—	—	0
Fruit Punch	1 (10 oz)	150	0	0	0	0	38	36	0	20	10	—	—	60
Hot Chocolate	1 (10 oz)	200	6	2	0	2	44	43	0	0	370	—	—	0
Iced Tea	1 (14 oz)	130	0	0	0	0	34	34	0	0	0	—	—	0
Milk 2%	1 (14 oz)	210	6	5	30	14	20	20	0	500	210	—	—	4
Orange Juice	1 (10 oz)	140	0	0	0	2	36	33	0	20	14	—	—	60
Sprite	1 (14 oz)	160	0	0	0	0	41	41	0	0	40	—	—	0
Tea + Sugar & Milk	1 (10 oz)	45	0	0	0	1	9	9	0	20	20	—	—	0

FOOD	PORTION	CALS	FAT	SAT FAT	CHOL	PROT	CARB	SUGAR	FIBER	CALCI	SOD	POTAS	FOLIC	VIT C
SANDWICHES														
Albacore Tuna Salad	1 serv	350	8	1	15	21	49	50	3	20	1100	—	—	9
Black Forest Ham & Swiss	1 serv	640	27	9	75	33	53	4	2	450	1540	—	—	12
Chunky Chicken Salad	1 serv	380	10	1	45	23	50	6	3	20	770	—	—	12
Fireside Roast Beef	1 serv	470	19	3	36	22	48	4	2	20	1470	—	—	9
Garden Vegetable	1 serv	460	24	11	45	12	50	6	3	20	730	—	—	9
Harvest Turkey Breast	1 serv	470	18	2	30	22	53	4	2	20	1460	—	—	9
SOUPS														
Barley & Wild Rice	1 serv	120	2	0	6	22	22	1	1	20	330	—	—	15
Chicken Noodle	1 serv	100	3	1	14	8	15	4	1	20	710	—	—	12
Chili	1 serv	320	9	3	65	29	32	10	8	150	960	—	—	36
Cream Of Broccoli	1 serv	190	7	2	6	7	27	9	1	200	1120	—	—	27
Cream of Mushroom	1 serv	195	10	3	8	4	21	4	1	60	900	—	—	2
Hearty Vegetable	1 serv	130	2	0	0	3	27	4	2	60	830	—	—	42
Minestrone	1 serv	125	2	0	1	4	25	4	2	80	910	—	—	27
Potato Bacon	1 serv	195	7	2	5	4	29	3	1	200	1100	—	—	27
Vegetable Beef Barley	1 serv	110	2	0	9	5	14	5	2	60	840	—	—	18
TJ CINNAMONS														
Cinnachips	1 bag (10 oz)	1130	50	6	42	—	157	—	3	—	700	—	—	—
Cinnamon Twist	1	260	13	3	5	—	33	—	10	—	190	—	—	—
Coffee Black	1 (12 oz)	0	0	0	0	0	0	0	0	—	0	—	—	—
Mocha Chill w/ Whipped Cream	1 (12.5 oz)	310	6	3	25	—	49	—	10	—	190	—	—	—
Mocha Chill w/o Whipped Cream	1 (12.5 oz)	260	4	1	15	—	48	—	10	—	190	—	—	—
Original Roll w/o Icing	1	500	17	4	30	—	81	—	0	—	370	—	—	—
Original Roll w/ Cream Cheese Icing	1	651	37	7	40	—	103	—	0	—	420	—	—	—
Pecan Sticky Roll	1	690	28	5	32	—	97	—	0	—	400	—	—	—
TOGO'S														
SALAD DRESSINGS														
1000 Island	1 serv (2.3 oz)	231	22	—	30	1	9	—	0	—	532	—	—	—
Caesar	1 serv (2.3 oz)	241	23	—	20	2	8	—	0	—	633	—	—	—
Oriental	1 serv (2.3 oz)	221	14	—	5	0	24	—	0	—	512	—	—	—

FOOD	PORTION	CALS	FAT	SAT FAT	CHOL	PROT	CARB	SUGAR	FIBER	CALCI	SOD	POTAS	FOLIC	VIT C
Ranch	1 serv (2.3 oz)	321	33	—	15	2	5	—	0	—	643	—	—	—
Reduced Calorie Italian	1 serv (2.3 oz)	60	5	—	0	0	4	—	0	—	693	—	—	—
Reduced Calorie Ranch	1 serv (2.3 oz)	191	16	—	25	1	10	—	0	—	603	—	—	—
SALADS AND SALAD BARS														
Caesar Salad	1 serv	471	31	—	72	30	23	—	2	—	1189	—	—	—
Garden Salad	1 serv	256	10	—	214	12	31	—	2	—	579	—	—	—
Oriental Salad	1 serv	499	21	—	41	25	49	—	3	—	1062	—	—	—
Taco Salad	1 serv	943	59	—	71	29	76	—	11	—	1623	—	—	—
SANDWICHES														
Albacore Tuna	1 sm	701	30	—	67	32	78	—	3	—	1653	—	—	—
Avocado & Turkey	1 sm	675	28	—	80	27	80	—	6	—	1606	—	—	—
Avocado Cucumber & Alfalfa Sprouts	1 sm	637	28	—	85	16	85	—	7		1150		—	—
Bar-B-Q Beef	1 sm	724	22	—	88	39	94	—	3	—	2120	—	—	—
California Roasted Chicken	1 sm	510	15	—	65	36	73	—	3	—	1768	—	—	—
Cheese Swiss American Provolone	1 sm	859	46	—	107	42	77	—	3	—	2196	—	—	—
Chunky Chicken Salad	1 sm	636	26	—	42	40	72	—	3	—	1562	—	—	—
Egg Salad w/ Cheese	1 sm	728	35	—	456	29	76	—	3	—	1765	—	—	—
Ham & Cheese	1 sm	661	26	—	68	33	76	—	3	—	2900	—	—	—
Hot Pastrami	1 sm	705	26	—	72	34	85	—	3	—	2260	—	—	—
Hummus	1 sm	668	21	—	9	20	102	—	4	—	1510	—	—	—
Italian Salami & Cheese	1 sm	770	33	—	118	42	78	—	3	—	3288	—	—	—
Italian Salami Capicolla Mortadella Cotto & Provolone	1 sm	736	32	—	85	31	74	—	3	—	2191	—	—	—
Meatballs w/ Pizza Sauce & Parmesan	1 sm	707	28	—	97	36	78	—	4	—	1602	—	—	—
Pastrami Reuben	1 sm	875	45	—	111	44	85	—	2	—	2460	—	—	—
Roast Beef Hot & Cold	1 sm	552	11	—	84	42	73	—	3	—	1537	—	—	—
Turkey & Cranberry	1 sm	623	13	—	49	30	96	—	4	—	1904	—	—	—
Turkey & Bacon Club	1 sm	667	26	—	81	37	73	—	3	—	2108	—	—	—
Turkey & Cheese	1 sm	638	23	—	71	34	75	—	3	—	2277	—	—	—
Turkey & Ham w/ Cheese	1 sm	670	25	—	76	37	76	—	3	—	2772	—	—	—

WENDY'S

FOOD	PORTION	CALS	FAT	SAT FAT	CHOL	PROT	CARB	SUGAR	FIBER	CALCI	SOD	POTAS	FOLIC	VIT C
BEVERAGES														
Cola	11 oz	130	0	0	0	0	36	36	0	0	10	—	—	0
Diet Cola	11 oz	0	0	0	0	0	0	0	0	0	15	—	—	0
Frosty Junior	6 oz	170	4	3	20	4	26	21	0	160	100	—	—	0
Frosty Medium	16 oz	440	11	7	50	11	73	56	0	410	260	—	—	0
Frosty Small	12 oz	330	8	5	35	8	56	43	0	310	200	—	—	0
Lemon-Lime Soda	11 oz	130	0	0	0	0	34	34	0	0	30	—	—	0
CHILDREN'S MENU SELECTIONS														
French Fries Kid's Meal	1 serv (3.2 oz)	270	13	2	0	4	35	0	3	10	85	—	—	5
Kid's Meal Cheeseburger	1 (4.2 oz)	310	12	6	45	17	33	6	2	150	800	—	—	4
Kid's Meal Hamburger	1 (3.9 oz)	270	9	3	30	14	33	6	1	100	620	—	—	4
Kids' Meal Chicken Nuggets	4 pieces (2.1 oz)	190	13	3	25	9	9	0	0	20	380	—	—	1
MAIN MENU SELECTIONS														
¼ lb Hamburger Patty	1 (2.6 oz)	200	14	6	65	19	0	0	0	20	290	—	—	0
2 Oz Hamburger Patty	1 (1.3 oz)	100	7	3	30	9	0	0	0	10	150	—	—	0
American Cheese	1 slice (0.6 oz)	70	6	4	15	4	0	0	0	100	260	—	—	0
American Cheese Jr.	1 slice (0.4 oz)	45	4	3	10	3	0	0	0	80	170	—	—	0
Bacon	1 strip (4 g)	20	2	1	5	1	0	0	0	0	90	—	—	0
Big Bacon Classic	1 (9.9 oz)	580	30	12	100	34	46	10	3	250	1460	—	—	15
Breaded Chicken Fillet	1 (3.5 oz)	230	11	2	50	22	13	0	0	0	390	—	—	5
Cheddar Shredded	2 tbsp (0.6 oz)	70	6	4	15	4	1	0	0	100	110	—	—	0
Chicken Breast Filet Sandwich	1 (7.3 oz)	430	16	3	56	27	46	6	2	100	750	—	—	12
Chicken Club Sandwich	1 (7.6 oz)	470	20	5	65	30	47	6	2	100	940	—	—	12
Chicken Nuggets	5 pieces (2.6 oz)	230	16	3	30	11	11	0	0	20	470	—	—	1
Chili	1 lg (12 oz)	310	10	4	45	23	32	8	7	120	1190	—	—	6
Chili	1 sm (8 oz)	210	7	3	30	15	21	5	5	80	800	—	—	4
Classic Single w/ Everything	1 (7.6 oz)	410	19	7	70	25	37	6	2	100	920	—	—	9
French Fries	1 Great Biggie (6.7 oz)	570	27	4	0	8	73	1	7	30	180	—	—	9
French Fries	1 Biggie (5.6 oz)	470	23	4	0	7	61	0	6	30	150	—	—	9
French Fries	1 med (5 oz)	420	20	3	0	6	50	0	5	20	130	—	—	6

FOOD	PORTION	CALS	FAT	SAT FAT	CHOL	PROT	CARB	SUGAR	FIBER	CALCI	SOD	POTAS	FOLIC	VIT C
Grilled Chicken Fillet	1 (2.9 oz)	110	3	1	55	19	1	0	0	0	400	—	—	1
Grilled Chicken Sandwich	1 (6.6 oz)	300	7	2	56	24	36	8	2	60	740	—	—	9
Honey Mustard Reduced Calorie	1 tsp (7 g)	25	2	0	0	0	2	2	0	0	40	—	—	0
Hot Stuffed Bake Potato Plain	1 (10 oz)	310	0	0	0	7	72	5	6	20	25	—	—	36
Hot Stuffed Baked Potato Bacon & Cheese	1 (12.6 oz)	530	18	4	25	16	78	5	7	100	820	—	—	36
Hot Stuffed Baked Potato Broccoli & Cheese	1 (14.4 oz)	470	14	3	5	9	80	6	9	150	470	—	—	72
Jr. Bacon Cheeseburger	1 (5.8 oz)	380	19	7	55	20	34	5	2	150	870	—	—	9
Jr. Cheeseburger	1 (4.5 oz)	310	12	6	45	17	34	6	2	150	800	—	—	4
Jr. Cheeseburger Deluxe	1 (6.3 oz)	360	16	6	50	18	36	7	2	150	860	—	—	9
Kaiser Bun	1 (2.5 oz)	200	3	1	0	6	38	6	2	80	340	—	—	2
Ketchup	1 tsp (7 g)	10	0	0	0	0	2	1	0	0	80	—	—	0
Lettuce	1 leaf (0.5 oz)	0	0	0	0	0	0	0	0	0	0	—	—	0
Mayonnaise	1½ tsp (9 g)	30	3	0	5	0	1	0	0	0	60	—	—	0
Mustard	½ tsp (5 g)	5	0	0	0	0	0	0	0	0	50	—	—	0
Nuggets Sauce Barbeque	1 pkg (1 oz)	45	0	0	0	1	10	7	0	0	160	—	—	0
Nuggets Sauce Honey Mustard	1 pkg (1 oz)	130	12	2	10	0	6	5	0	0	220	—	—	0
Nuggets Sauce Sweet & Sour	1 pkg (1 oz)	50	0	0	0	0	12	10	0	0	120	—	—	1
Onion	4 rings (0.5 oz)	5	0	0	0	0	1	1	0	0	0	—	—	1
Pickles	4 slices (0.4 oz)	0	0	0	0	0	0	0	0	0	140	—	—	0
Saltines	2 (0.2 oz)	25	1	0	0	1	4	0	0	10	80	—	—	0
Sandwich Bun	1 (2 oz)	160	2	0	0	5	31	4	1	80	300	—	—	2
Spicy Chicken Fillet	1 (3.6 oz)	210	9	2	60	22	10	0	0	10	920	—	—	1
Spicy Chicken Sandwich	1 (7.5 oz)	410	14	3	65	28	43	5	2	100	1280	—	—	9
Tomatoes	1 slice (0.9 oz)	5	0	0	0	0	1	1	1	0	0	—	—	5
Whipped Margarine	1 pkg (0.5 oz)	70	7	2	0	0	0	0	0	0	115	—	—	0
SALAD DRESSINGS														
Blue Cheese	1 pkg (2 oz)	360	36	7	30	2	1	0	0	40	350	—	—	0
French	1 pkg (2 oz)	250	21	3	0	0	13	11	0	0	670	—	—	1
Hidden Valley Ranch	1 pkg (2 oz)	200	20	3	25	1	3	1	0	20	410	—	—	0

FOOD	PORTION	CALS	FAT	SAT FAT	CHOL	PROT	CARB	SUGAR	FIBER	CALCI	SOD	POTAS	FOLIC	VIT C
Hidden Valley Ranch Reduced Fat Reduced Calorie	1 pkg (2 oz)	120	11	2	20	1	4	1	0	20	470	—	—	0
Italian Reduced Fat Reduced Calorie	1 pkg (2 oz)	80	7	1	0	0	6	4	0	0	690	—	—	2
Italian Caesar	1 pkg (1.5 oz)	230	24	4	25	1	1	0	0	20	350	—	—	1
Thousand Island	1 pkg (2 oz)	260	25	4	20	1	7	6	0	0	380	—	—	1
SALADS AND SALAD BARS														
Ceasar Side Salad w/o Dressing	1 (3.2 oz)	110	5	3	15	9	6	1	1	150	360	—	—	9
Deluxe Garden Salad w/o Dressing	1 (9.5 oz)	110	6	1	0	7	10	5	4	200	320	—	—	36
Grilled Chicken Salad w/o Dressing	1 (11.9 oz)	200	7	2	55	27	10	5	4	200	780	—	—	36
Side Salad w/o Dressing	1 (5.4 oz)	60	3	1	0	4	5	2	2	100	160	—	—	18
Soft Breadstick	1 (1.5 oz)	130	3	1	5	4	23	—	1	40	250	—	—	0
Taco Chips	15 (1.5 oz)	210	9	2	0	3	28	0	2	40	160	—	—	0
Taco Salad w/o Dressing	1 (16.4 oz)	380	19	10	65	26	28	8	8	350	1040	—	—	27

WHATABURGER

FOOD	PORTION	CALS	FAT	SAT FAT	CHOL	PROT	CARB	SUGAR	FIBER	CALCI	SOD	POTAS	FOLIC	VIT C
BAKED SELECTIONS														
Cinnamon Roll	1	860	34	—	50	12	126	—	4	—	320	—	—	—
BEVERAGES														
Cherry Coke	1 lg (44 oz)	343	0	0	0	0	92	—	0	—	13	—	—	—
Cherry Coke	1 sm (20 oz)	169	0	0	0	0	46	—	0	—	7	—	—	—
Coca Cola Classic	1 lg (44 oz)	327	0	0	0	0	89	—	0	—	20	—	—	—
Coca Cola Classic	1 sm (20 oz)	161	0	0	0	0	44	—	0	—	10	—	—	—
Coffee	1 sm (8 oz)	30	1	—	0	0	4	—	0	—	5	—	—	—
Creamer Nondairy	1 pkg	15	1	—	0	0	1	—	0	—	0	—	—	—
Diet Coke	1 lg (44 oz)	0	0	0	0	0	0	0	0	—	34	—	—	—
Diet Coke	1 sm (20 oz)	0	0	0	0	0	0	0	0	—	16	—	—	—
Diet Dr Pepper	1 sm (20 oz)	0	0	0	0	0	0	0	0	—	73	—	—	—
Dr. Pepper	1 sm (20 oz)	147	0	0	0	0	42	—	0	—	49	—	—	—
Fanta Strawberry	1 lg (44 oz)	360	0	0	0	0	96	—	0	—	26	—	—	—
Fanta Strawberry	1 sm (20 oz)	177	0	0	0	0	47	—	0	—	13	—	—	—
Fruit Drink	1 sm (20 oz)	121	0	0	0	0	31	—	0	—	46	—	—	—
Fruit Drink	1 lg (44 oz)	244	0	0	0	0	63	—	0	—	92	—	—	—
Lemonade	1 sm (20 oz)	158	0	0	0	0	42	—	0	—	67	—	—	—
Lemonade	1 lg (44 oz)	320	0	0	0	0	86	—	0	—	135	—	—	—

FOOD	PORTION	CALS	FAT	SAT FAT	CHOL	PROT	CARB	SUGAR	FIBER	CALCI	SOD	POTAS	FOLIC	VIT C
Lipton Iced Tea	1 med	0	0	0	0	0	0	0	0	—	0	—	—	—
Milk 2%	8 oz	120	5	—	20	8	11	—	0	—	115	—	—	—
Orange Juice	1 serv	140	0	0	0	2	33	—	0	—	0	—	—	—
Orange Soda	1 lg (44 oz)	350	0	0	0	0	96	—	0	—	0	—	—	—
Orange Soda	1 sm (20 oz)	173	0	0	0	0	47	—	0	—	0	—	—	—
Shake Chocolate	1 sm (20 oz)	616	17	—	61	13	100	—	0	—	325	—	—	—
Shake Strawberry	1 sm (20 oz)	620	16	—	61	12	101	—	0	—	296	—	—	—
Shake Vanilla	1 sm (20 oz)	559	17	—	65	13	82	—	0	—	301	—	—	—
Sprite	1 sm	158	0	0	0	0	42	—	0	—	36	—	—	—
Sprite	1 lg (44 oz)	320	0	0	0	0	86	—	0	—	73	—	—	—
CHILDREN'S MENU SELECTIONS														
Kid's Justaburger	1	306	15	—	40	16	27	—	1	—	682	—	—	—
Kid's Chicken Strips	1 serv	382	24	—	33	19	22	—	4	—	705	—	—	—
MAIN MENU SELECTIONS														
Biscuit Buttermilk	1	300	16	—	0	5	34	—	0	—	470	—	—	—
Biscuit w/ Bacon	1	375	22	—	12	10	34	—	0	—	788	—	—	—
Biscuit w/ Bacon Egg & Cheese	1	476	29	—	252	17	35	—	0	—	875	—	—	—
Biscuit w/ Egg & Cheese	1	446	27	—	250	15	35	—	0	—	777	—	—	—
Biscuit w/ Sausage	1	517	35	—	35	16	34	—	1	—	947	—	—	—
Biscuit w/ Sausage Egg & Cheese	1	663	46	—	285	26	35	—	1	—	1254	—	—	—
Biscuit w/ Sausage Gravy	1	491	33	—	19	8	47	—	tr	—	1249	—	—	—
Breakfast Platter w/ Bacon	1 serv	698	43	—	466	23	52	—	3	—	1362	—	—	—
Breakfast Platter w/ Sausage	1 serv	840	56	—	489	29	52	—	4	—	1521	—	—	—
Breakfast On A Bun Ranchero w/ Bacon	1	404	23	—	262	20	29	—	3	—	1183	—	—	—
Breakfast On A Bun Ranchero w/ Sausage	1	546	36	—	285	27	29	—	3	—	1342	—	—	—
Breakfast On A Bun w/ Bacon	1	398	23	—	262	20	28	—	2	—	965	—	—	—
Breakfast On A Bun w/ Sausage	1	540	36	—	285	27	28	—	2	—	1124	—	—	—
Chicken Strips	2	382	24	—	33	19	22	—	4	—	705	—	—	—
Croutons Njoy Seasoned	1 pkg	35	2	—	0	0	4	—	0	—	90	—	—	—
French Fries	1 lg	514	26	—	0	9	66	—	5	—	413	—	—	—
French Fries	1 sm	257	13	—	0	4	33	—	3	—	207	—	—	—
Grape Jelly	1 pkg	35	0	0	0	0	9	—	0	—	5	—	—	—

FOOD	PORTION	CALS	FAT	SAT FAT	CHOL	PROT	CARB	SUGAR	FIBER	CALCI	SOD	POTAS	FOLIC	VIT C
Gravy White Peppered	1 serv	53	5	—	0	0	8	—	0	—	345	—	—	—
Hashbrown Sticks	1 serv	140	8	—	0	0	16	—	3	—	440	—	—	—
Honey	1 pkg	25	0	0	0	0	7	—	0	—	0	—	—	—
Hot Apple Pie	1	240	12	—	5	2	31	—	1	—	290	—	—	—
Justaburger	1	309	15	—	40	17	28	—	1	—	682	—	—	—
Ketchup	1 pkg	40	0	0	0	1	8	—	0	—	350	—	—	—
Margarine	1 pkg	23	3	—	0	0	0	—	0	—	39	—	—	—
Onion Rings	1 med	201	11	—	0	3	23	—	1	—	477	—	—	—
Pancake Syrup	1 pkg	120	0	0	0	0	31	—	0	—	25	—	—	—
Pancakes	1 serv	614	8	—	0	19	118	—	3	—	2250	—	—	—
Pancakes w/ Bacon	1 serv	689	13	—	12	24	118	—	3	—	2568	—	—	—
Pancakes w/ Sausage	1 serv	831	27	—	35	30	118	—	5	—	2727	—	—	—
Picante Sauce	1 serv	5	0	0	0	0	1	—	0	—	110	—	—	—
Sandwich Egg	1	323	17	—	250	16	28	—	1	—	647	—	—	—
Sandwich Grilled Chicken	1	473	20	—	82	30	49	—	4	—	1167	—	—	—
Sandwich Grilled Chicken No Bun	1	190	7	—	73	22	10	—	1	—	609	—	—	—
Sandwich Whatacatch	1	473	26	—	59	20	45	—	2	—	936	—	—	—
Sandwich Whatachick'n	1	523	21	—	49	28	63	—	5	—	1524	—	—	—
Strawberry Jam	1 pkg	40	0	0	0	0	10	—	0	—	5	—	—	—
Taquito Bacon & Egg	1	387	22	—	352	19	25	—	1	—	839	—	—	—
Taquito Potato & Egg	1	382	20	—	340	14	33	—	4	—	741	—	—	—
Taquito Sausage & Egg	1	389	26	—	354	17	26	—	1	—	675	—	—	—
Taquito w/ Bacon Egg & Cheese	1	432	25	—	362	21	25	—	1	—	1059	—	—	—
Taquito w/ Potato Egg & Cheese	1	427	24	—	350	17	33	—	4	—	961	—	—	—
Taquito w/ Sausage Egg & Cheese	1	434	27	—	364	19	26	—	1	—	895	—	—	—
Texas Toast	1 serv	328	15	—	0	8	42	—	2	—	540	—	—	—
Whataburger	1	607	30	—	75	31	53	—	3	—	1158	—	—	—
Whataburger Double Meat	1	857	48	—	150	51	53	—	3	—	1297	—	—	—
Whataburger Double Meat No Bun	1	520	36	—	150	41	4	—	1	—	487	—	—	—

FOOD	PORTION	CALS	FAT	SAT FAT	CHOL	PROT	CARB	SUGAR	FIBER	CALCI	SOD	POTAS	FOLIC	VIT C
Whataburger Jr.	1	315	16	—	40	16	29	—	2	—	685	—	—	—
Whataburger No Bun	1	270	18	—	75	21	4	—	1	—	348	—	—	—
Whataburger Triple Meat	1	1107	66	—	225	71	53	—	4	—	1435	—	—	—
Whataburger w/ Bacon & Cheese	1	810	45	—	113	42	54	—	3	—	2065	—	—	—
Whatacatch	2 pieces	814	65	—	147	28	38	—	2	—	1360	—	—	—
SALAD DRESSINGS														
Low Fat Ranch	1 pkg	66	4	—	19	2	9	—	2	—	605	—	—	—
Low Fat Vinaigrette	1 pkg	35	2	—	0	0	6	—	0	—	890	—	—	—
Ranch	1 pkg	310	33	—	20	1	3	—	0	—	470	—	—	—
Thousand Island	1 pkg	150	13	—	20	0	11	—	0	—	490	—	—	—
SALADS														
Chicken Strips	1 serv	419	25	—	33	21	29	—	7	—	744	—	—	—
Chicken Strips w/ Cheddar Cheese	1 serv	600	39	—	76	31	32	—	8	—	957	—	—	—
Chicken Strips w/ Cheddar Cheese & Bacon	1 serv	675	45	—	88	36	33	—	8	—	1275	—	—	—
Garden Salad	1	49	1	—	0	3	10	—	4	—	49	—	—	—
Garden w/ Cheddar Cheese	1 serv	218	15	—	43	13	10	—	4	—	252	—	—	—
Garden w/ Cheddar Cheese & Bacon	1 serv	293	20	—	55	18	11	—	4	—	570	—	—	—
Grilled Chicken	1 serv	229	7	—	73	25	19	—	5	—	653	—	—	—
Grilled Chicken w/ Cheddar Cheese	1 serv	398	21	—	115	34	19	—	4	—	855	—	—	—
Grilled Chicken w/ Cheddar Cheese & Bacon	1 serv	473	27	—	127	39	19	—	5	—	1173	—	—	—

WHITE CASTLE

FOOD	PORTION	CALS	FAT	SAT FAT	CHOL	PROT	CARB	SUGAR	FIBER	CALCI	SOD	POTAS	FOLIC	VIT C
BEVERAGES														
Coca Cola	16 oz	200	0	0	0	0	54	—	—	—	15	—	—	—
Coffee Black	1 sm	6	0	0	0	0	1	—	—	—	5	—	—	—
Diet Coke	16 oz	0	0	0	0	0	0	0	0	—	20	—	—	—
Iced Tea	16 oz	90	0	0	0	0	24	—	—	—	35	—	—	—
Shake Chocolate	16 oz	250	15	8	30	9	37	27	—	—	160	—	—	—
Shake Vanilla	16 oz	260	15	8	30	9	40	28	—	—	170	—	—	—
MAIN MENU SELECTIONS														
Bacon Cheeseburger	1	200	13	6	25	10	12	0	3	—	430	—	—	—

FOOD	PORTION	CALS	FAT	SAT FAT	CHOL	PROT	CARB	SUGAR	FIBER	CALCI	SOD	POTAS	FOLIC	VIT C
Cheese Sticks	3	250	14	6	25	10	22	2	2	—	750	—	—	—
Cheeseburger	1	160	9	4	15	7	11	0	2	—	250	—	—	—
Chicken Rings	6	210	14	3	50	11	10	0	0	160	420	—	—	0
Double Cheeseburger	1	290	18	8	30	14	16	0	5	—	430	—	—	—
Double Hamburger	1	240	14	6	20	11	16	0	4	—	200	—	—	—
French Fries	1 sm	115	6	1	—	—	15	2	2	—	15	—	—	—
Hamburger	1	140	7	3	10	6	11	0	2	—	135	—	—	—
Onion Rings	6	260	13	2	0	4	31	4	3	160	520	—	—	0
Sandwich Breakfast	1	340	25	10	130	14	17	2	0	—	900	—	—	—
Sandwich Chicken	1	190	8	2	20	6	21	1	—	—	360	—	—	—
Sandwich Chicken Ring	1	180	8	2	25	8	20	2	0	—	370	—	—	—
Sandwich Fish	1	180	7	2	10	7	27	2	1	—	390	—	—	—

WINCHELL'S DONUTS

FOOD	PORTION	CALS	FAT	SAT FAT	CHOL	PROT	CARB	SUGAR	FIBER	CALCI	SOD	POTAS	FOLIC	VIT C
Chocolate Bar	1	240	16	—	—	4	29	—	—	—	125	—	—	—
Chocolate Round	1	240	16	—	—	4	29	—	—	—	125	—	—	—
Chocolate Twist	1	240	16	—	—	4	29	—	—	—	125	—	—	—
Croissant	1	260	17	—	—	5	28	—	—	—	280	—	—	—
Glazed Round	1	230	15	—	—	2	27	—	—	—	120	—	—	—
Glazed Twist	1	230	15	—	—	2	27	—	—	—	120	—	—	—
Iced Chocolate	1	230	15	—	—	2	28	—	—	—	220	—	—	—
Traditional	1	215	14	—	—	2	26	—	—	—	215	—	—	—